Konstantinos N. Syrigos · Christopher M. Nutting · Charis Roussos (Eds.)

Tumors of the Chest
Biology, Diagnosis and Management

Konstantinos N. Syrigos · Christopher M. Nutting
Charis Roussos (Eds.)

Tumors of the Chest

Biology, Diagnosis and Management

With 115 Figures, 55 in Color and 138 Tables

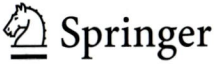 Springer

Konstantinos N. Syrigos, MD, PhD
Sotiria General Hospital
Athens Medical School
Athens, Greece

Christopher M. Nutting, MB BA, MD, FRCR
Royal Marsden NHS Trust Hospitals
London, UK

Charis Roussos, MD, MSc, PhD, MRS, FRCP(C)
Athens Medical School,
Evangelismos General Hospital
Athens, Greece
and Faculty of Medicine
McGill University, Montreal, Canada

Cover Illustration: My Inferno of Hell is a painting by Panos Tzortzinis, one of the most renowned of contemporary Greek painters. An artist who has participated in several domestic and international exhibitions, he was born in Kalamata, Peloponnesus in 1950 and is currently Professor of Art at the Egaleon School of Art. This painting, deriving from Tzortzini's own lung cancer diagnosis, attempts to visually convey his personal thoughts and feelings while undergoing chemotherapy.

Library of Congress Control Number 2005937528

ISBN-10   3-540-31039-8 Springer Berlin Heidelberg New York
ISBN-13   978-3-540-31039-6 Springer Berlin Heidelberg New York

Cataloging-in-Publication Data applied for
A catalog record for this book is available from the Library of Congress.

Springer is a part of Springer Science+Business Media
springeronline.com
© Springer Berlin Heidelberg 2006
Printed in Germany

Editor: Dr. Ute Heilmann
Desk Editor: Meike Stoeck
Production: LE-TeX Jelonek, Schmidt & Vöckler GbR, Leipzig
Typesetting: K + V Fotosatz, Beerfelden
Cover: Frido Steinen-Broo, EStudio Calamar, Spain

Printed on acid-free paper   21/3150/YL   5 4 3 2 1 0

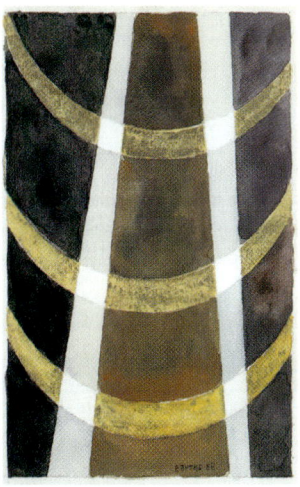

Production of this volume was partially supported by the THORAX FOUNDATION

Preface

Despite medical advances, lung cancer remains a formidable foe, claiming many lives every year and bringing physical and emotional agony – unimaginable to those that have not been touched by it – to both patients and their families. Apart from the physical pain and suffering caused by the disease, the traditional treatment options of surgery, radiotherapy, and chemotherapy often constitute complicated procedures or induce agonizing side effects without any guarantees that such measures will result in a cure or even the significant prolongation of life. This makes lung cancer not only a physically challenging disease, but also one that is psychologically devastating for patients – first and foremost – and subsequently for their families who are subjected to watching their loved ones suffer and are incapable of offering more than a token presence as they try desperately to comfort and support, while simultaneously being in need of the same.

Overall, chest malignancies represent an outstanding example of the new era we are witnessing in oncology – an era in which doctors and researchers are not focusing exclusively on discovering a cure, but on investigating the causes of the disease in an attempt to better understand and possibly prevent it, as well as make it possible for patients to live longer, more productive, and qualitative lives by rendering lung cancer a chronic, controllable affliction that can be treated comfortably and conveniently. In fact, over the last decade lung cancer has increasingly become the province of many scientific specialties including the medical oncologist, radiotherapist, chest physician, radiologist, palliative care physician, epidemiologist, and biologist. In an age of ever-increasing specialization, where web sites, journals, articles, and books addressed to specialists comprise the main source of information, we feel strongly that a comprehensive textbook on chest malignancies is still needed. As a result, the purpose of the volume at hand is to present a picture of lung cancer in its totality and to update the subject in one tome, based on the experience of well-established scientists. Authorship is derived from an international forum and consists primarily of those who have made major contributions in the area they have been asked to discuss. Through their chapters, the authors have attempted to combine clinical experience with the newest advances in the relevant sciences as well as to highlight the therapeutic aspects of each topic. Emphasis has been given to the multidisciplinary approach, providing overviews from various expert branches. It is expected that with this methodology, specialists associated with chest malignancies will not only get a feeling for the current practice in their own area of interest, but will also be able to obtain sufficient information about problems presenting in their patients and potential solutions offered by different areas of expertise. The rationale behind this policy is the perception that physicians acquainted with "adjacent" specialist branches, familiar with basic sciences and able to use this knowledge in the evaluation and treatment of their patients, are in a better position to analyze clinical problems and help their patients accordingly. Hence, a portion of this volume is dedicated to the biology and pathogenesis of chest malignancies, presented in an easy-to-understand format. In addition, a few chapters of this book deal with the quality of life issues associated with these malignancies, which were included in order to offer the reader a more complete and comprehensive framework of the clinical problems that arise in these patients. Finally, decision-making in lung cancer patients is surrounded by several controversies, such as the multimodality approach of locally advanced disease, the use of platinum-based regimens in the treatment of extensive disease, and the management of elderly and poor performance status patients. In this volume, an effort has been made to clearly and equably present all arguments for each approach in sequential chapters.

A comprehensive textbook is inevitably not fully up-to-date at the time of publication, and this applies particularly to areas where advances have been more rapid. It is therefore a tribute to our distinguished contributors and to the publisher Springer-Verlag that this edition has appeared within 2 years of its initiation. Gratitude should also be extended to our patients and relatives, students, and colleagues for providing the authors with ongoing education, stimulus, and purpose.

Finally, we wish to dedicate this volume to all of the generous donors who, being touched by the pain and suffering caused by this disease, have contributed benevolently to facilities and research projects around the world in the fight against lung cancer. In doing so, we would like to make a special mention of Mr. Aristidis I. Alafouzos, whose continued, generous support enables hundreds of patients with chest malignancies to be treated every day, while also funding several facilities and research projects currently in progress, thus furthering efforts to continue making the lung cancer patient more comfortable and providing much needed assistance to the family for the difficult road ahead.

Konstantinos Syrigos, Christopher M. Nutting,
and Charis Roussos

Foreword

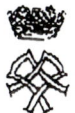

As someone who has been touched personally by this dreadful disease, I think it is reassuring that all of you – experts in your own field – have gathered together to produce this comprehensive book.

The 'elusive enemy' cancer does of course have a devastating effect – not only on the patient but the families who have to cope. I urge the men and women involved in the administration of existing therapies, as well as those working on the development of new treatments, to join forces on a global level by sharing information conducting more joint multi-centres and multi-national clinical trials and combining resources.

I wish you well in your endeavours.

Alexandra

Introduction

Tumors of the Chest: Biology, Diagnosis, and Management – A Shifting Paradigm

I'm pleased to have the opportunity to write the introduction for this new book on chest oncology. There are several ways to approach writing an introduction. One can assume the quality of the book from the reputations of the editors as a starting point or peruse the table of contents and/or read selected chapters, and then try to put the book into perspective, or one can actually read it. I have a special interest in textbooks and so I decided to do all of the above. I have confidence in the distinguished editors, who have selected a large number of highly qualified authors, and I read all or part of every chapter in the text, kindly provided to me in advance by the editors. Having done that, I feel secure in providing the proper context for this textbook.

And, the context is this. This is the right book, in the right place, at the right time. It's the right book because of the way it has been put together. It has an unusually strong international flavor for a textbook, with leaders in lung cancer research and management from all over the world providing varied and valuable contributions on virtually every aspect of chest tumors, including mesotheliomas. It is probably the most comprehensive textbook on lung cancer currently available. Its international flavor also positions the book in the right place. One can learn a great deal from variations in the incidence and management of lung cancer throughout the world, as well as from the nature of clinical trials in various countries, and these clinical trials are discussed in several chapters. This includes those international differences related to the regulations surrounding the development of new agents, always a major impediment to progress. It is the right time because in the past 2 years lung cancer has undergone a paradigm shift and physicians have some significant new tools on hand to help manage the disease. These tools should, if applied worldwide, have an impact on mortality and survival rates.

Lung cancer is caused largely by exposure to tobacco smoke, and we shouldn't forget that tobacco-related cancers are the most preventable cancers we know of. If smoking were eliminated, mortality rates from cancer would be 40% lower in 15 years, and we wouldn't need this book at all. In 2004, for example, tobacco use was responsible for 5 million deaths worldwide, and it is estimated that unless we do more to prevent its use, the yearly total of deaths from tobacco will have risen to 10 million by 2020. In the USA alone, about 450,000 people die each year from the effects of smoking. Therefore, despite concerns over exposure to chemicals, increased obesity, and other carcinogenic risks, the big concern in cancer causation is, and always has been, tobacco.

And here too, there has been a dramatic development in the past 2 years: the negotiation and signing of the Framework Convention on Tobacco Control. On November 30, 2004 an event occurred that, given its importance to the antitobacco movement, received surprisingly little attention. On that day, Peru became the 40th country to ratify the Framework Convention on Tobacco Control. The Framework Convention was adopted after 4 years of negotiation, by a voice vote of the 192 members of the World Health Assembly. The World Health Organization sponsored it in 2003, and it is the world's first public health treaty committed to stemming the globalization of the tobacco epidemic. To become legally binding, the Framework Convention had to be ratified by the legislative bodies of 40 nations, hence the importance of the ratification by the Peruvian government. The Framework Convention became legally binding for all ratifying parties on February 28, 2005. Its mandatory provisions include a comprehensive ban on advertising, sponsorship, and promotion, with narrow exceptions for countries such as the USA, which face constitutional conflicts. It also stipulates that warning labels on tobacco products cover at least 30% of the package, and the elimination of deceptive and misleading labels such as "light" and "low tar". In addition, it provides for protection of nonsmokers in public places and places of work, and contains specific measures to reduce tobacco smuggling. The treaty encourages parties to enact other tobacco-control policies, such as increasing tobacco taxes, eliminating duty-free sales of tobacco products, prohibiting the sale of tobacco to minors, and including tobacco cessation services in national health plans. In 2005, the ratifying member nations will begin negotiations to develop more detailed provisions of the treaty. Unlike most of the world, many of the provisions of the treaty are already in effect throughout the USA, but a worldwide treaty offers the chance to globalize the antitobacco effort in a way that has hitherto been considered impossible.

The American experience here is really quite important when one looks at the smoking rates around the world, which are covered nicely in several chapters in this book. In most of the developed countries, over 40% of adults still smoke. In the USA, due to the earlier application of effective methods of tobacco control, many now included in the Framework Convention on Tobacco Control protocols, smoking incidence has fallen from over 50% in the 1960s to about 23%, about half of that in developed countries. In developing countries, smoking rates are even higher than in Europe, although accurate data are less available. By emphasizing differential rates, and using methods proven to work to reduce tobacco usage, in the context of the new Framework Convention, public health officials can be more effective in reducing tobacco usage worldwide. As a result of reduced smoking rates in the USA, for example, incidence rates of lung cancer began to fall in the early nineties. Naturally, since you don't die of diseases you don't get, declines in mortality rates soon followed, something application of Framework Convention protocols will hopefully replicate in other countries. A text with a heavy international influence is certainly the right book at the right time to emphasize the importance of the Framework Convention protocols.

The medical costs of managing lung cancer worldwide are astronomical. However, the ancillary costs associated with smoking and lung cancer are often overlooked. There are two valuable chapters on this subject in the text that should also prove useful for public health officials. Ancillary costs, combined with medical costs, put the relatively small amounts of money spent trying to prevent smoking worldwide into stark perspective, and highlight not only the need for, but the financial benefits of smoking cessation programs.

The advances in management have also been dramatic and their implications are significant in several areas. These advances have been achieved by clinical investigators who have been working tirelessly in the trenches for years developing and testing one new drug after another in advanced lung cancer patients, combining them in doublets and triplets in large-scale clinical trials. Much of this work has been discouraging and has been disparaged by many people as not terribly useful. But in the end, standard therapies have been developed that have been shown to prolong survival in patients with all types of advanced lung cancer, when compared to supportive care, and to improve the quality of life of treated patients, compared to untreated con-

trols. The latter finding came as quite a surprise. After all, chemotherapy and radiotherapy are quite toxic. It turns out, however, that treatment, even when it cannot prolong survival, reduces the rate of complications and prevents hospitalizations, thereby improving, not disturbing quality of life, and reducing the cost of care.

The major impact of these trials in patients with advanced disease has been realized only recently with the important observation that adjuvant chemotherapy, given after surgery, has a substantial impact on median survival and 5-year survival rates in patients with stages IB and II non-small-cell lung cancer. The most recent study, published in the New England Journal of Medicine, was impressive enough to warrant an editorial in the New York Times. Not emphasized in the editorial or elsewhere in the excitement about the recent adjuvant trial was the fact that there were four studies in the previous 2 years that showed the same result, with less dramatic, but significant, improvements in survival. Pessimism is so prevalent in the chemotherapy of solid tumors like lung cancer, that people discounted the value of past positive studies with statistically significant improvements, because of their marginal clinical utility.

This has always been a dilemma for clinical investigators in the solid tumor area. There are three general end results when studying the effects of treatment in patients with advanced solid tumors. Those trials that show no effect, those that show a treatment having a dramatic clinical impact on the disease studied (rare), and those trials that have a statistically significant, but what might be considered a clinically insignificant impact in the study population; for example, a significant improvement in median survival, but of only 2 or 3 months. Treatments developed in the latter trials, however, if applied in a different set of clinical circumstances, can yield important clinical advantages, and this is the story of the development of effective adjuvant treatments in most solid tumors.

So now there are five adjuvant studies in localized non-small-cell lung cancer, all showing the effectiveness of chemotherapy in the postoperative period, and it is reasonable to conclude that, at the time of publication of this text, adjuvant therapy is indicated for all patients with these early stages of lung cancer – quite a shift in management. These studies were made possible by the arduous clinical trials in patients with advanced disease mentioned above and detailed in the text.

In the common solid tumors, patients with advanced disease have always been the proving ground for treatments useful in the adjuvant situation. This has been particularly advantageous for breast cancer patients who, 90% of the time, present with local or locoregional disease, and in colorectal cancers. As a result, in the last 10 years we have seen dramatic results with the application of chemotherapy in the adjuvant situation in both breast in colorectal cancer, with national mortality rates in the USA falling as a consequence. The effect of chemotherapy in both tumor types has also led to less morbid primary treatment methods. Lung cancer treatments are following the same path, and lung cancer patients can look forward to less morbid treatments. Again, the road to successful adjuvant applications and less morbid primary treatment in breast and colorectal cancer was the same long trek through the testing of new regimens in large numbers of patients with advanced disease, where results showed marginal improvements in those patients, but dramatic results, and cures, when used in the adjuvant situation. This fact is often lost on those more pessimistic among us who gauge the usefulness of chemotherapy only by its ability, or, in most cases, inability to cure patients with advanced disease.

Why some solid tumors are so drug resistant at the outset is a challenge for future investigators. Tumors like lung cancer, colorectal cancer, and to a lesser degree breast cancer, arise in an external environment with exposure to sometimes thousands of chemicals. The cells that become cancerous are not necessarily those that are damaged by toxins; those cells probably die. Rather, there is evidence that tumors may well arise from cells capable of surviving the toxic insult in that environment, which, when they emerge, are already quite efficient at dealing with and resisting external toxins, which in many ways resemble the agents they will see in treatment. We have a poor appreciation of this kind of drug resistance and yet it is a major roadblock to successful therapy. In other words, drug resistance is not the unified concept we have come to believe. It comes in different varieties and needs to be dealt with in different ways for different tumor types, and lung cancers, with their extraordinary history of exposure to a toxic chemical environment are the model systems to study.

We are also embarking on an era of targeted treatment that has already had an impact on non-small-cell lung cancer, again in the past 2 years. A feature of the new agents targeted at various signaling systems is that they appear to sensitize tumors that are resistant to the effects of both chemotherapy and radiotherapy. Since this is the major issue in lung tumors, they have the potential to produce another paradigm change in the management of patients with lung cancer in the next several years. The trials of these agents, which are in their early stages, are all collected in this volume, often by country of origin. Indeed, another source of optimism is that there are over 90 agents targeted at lung cancer that are either approved or under development in clinical trials around the world. Japan alone has approved 23 new agents, 9 of which were actually developed in Japan. The international flavor and influence of this text is never more apparent than here.

The dilemma of small-cell lung cancer is also well developed in this text. A responsive tumor with a veritable garden of molecular abnormalities, its high com-

plete response rates, even in patients with advanced disease, recognized years ago, caused much excitement and speculation that it would be a curable form of lung cancer. Results have reached a plateau, however, as it has resisted all aggressive attempts at improving the cure rate with high-dose chemotherapy. While patients with limited disease are sometimes cured by chemotherapy and radiotherapy, patients with advanced disease almost invariably die of their disease, despite high complete remission rates using doublet combination chemotherapy. The application of more than two drugs has not added much to the outcome, although the results of a recent trial from Japan in which a third drug was added to the therapy, have suggested that this impasse may also yield. The very high complete response rate coupled with an almost invariable high relapse rate is almost unique in oncology, and is just the opposite of what we see in non-small-cell lung cancer, and in stark contrast to the consequence of achieving complete remissions in patients with lymphomas and leukemias. The opportunity to target agents to the myriad molecular abnormalities in small-cell lung cancer is exciting, and emphasizes the need for the clinicians, like those who wrote the clinical chapters, to collaborate with basic scientists, like those who wrote the chapters about the biology of this fascinating tumor. That's where the future lies. One gets the feeling that, in the management of small-cell lung cancer, we are one effective targeted treatment away from converting many complete responders into cures.

Three more areas are worthy of comment and are well covered in this text: screening, chemoprevention, and the worldwide regulatory environment. The news in all three areas is not positive.

Even though we now have extraordinarily sensitive ways of screening patients for lung cancer, screening smokers for early cancers has not been shown to have any consistent affect on mortality rates. In fact, the expensive hypersensitive techniques have too many false positives and are a costly way to try to deal with the lung cancers that are detected. In addition, when early tumors are found, although a good number are curable with surgery alone, many have micrometastases because of their aggressive biology. Heretofore, we have had no effective way to deal with them. That situation could now change as the newer adjuvant programs are advanced to use in increasingly earlier cases. It may also be possible to make better use of older, less sensitive, and less expensive screening tests. Designing and executing trials to test these hypotheses is very complex and the studies themselves expensive. Newer ways of evaluating screening are necessary.

As the author of the chapter on the subject of chemoprevention points out, not only have the chemopreventive agents tested turned out not to prevent cancer, in some cases exposure to a putative chemopreventative agent increases the incidence of lung cancer. There is a bright side here as well, however. The apparent harm created by some agents appears to occur only in active smokers. There is some evidence that these agents can prevent cancers when used under the proper circumstances. This leaves the area of testing chemoprevention in those increasingly large numbers of people who have given up smoking, to attempt to accelerate the decline in the incidence of lung cancers, which are the slowest of the smoking-related cancers to decline after smoking is stopped. If such studies proved that chemoprevention could work under those conditions, it would provide one of the best motivations to stop smoking. Like screening studies, such trials are large, expensive, and time consuming, but they are important to consider nonetheless.

Finally, it seems appropriate to make a comment or two about the impact of the regulatory environment on the ability to find new drugs for cancer. We are simply overregulated. Cancer is not the common cold, nor is it rheumatoid arthritis or hypertension, where the interaction of drugs and disease takes place over years and decades. While cancer is the most curable of the chronic diseases, it is also the most fatal, and new drugs are tested under extreme circumstances in near-terminal patients. The outcome is noted in months, rarely more than 6 months. Yet the regulations surrounding the testing and development of new agents remains as rigid as for other, more chronic and infrequently fatal illnesses, and they not only increase the cost of development and discourage companies from getting involved with anti-cancer agents, but the slowness, in an era of a plethora of new opportunities, prevents innovation. Particularly onerous, in this author's opinion, is the requirement by the United States Food and Drug Administration to approve the use of drugs already approved for marketing for each new indication on a trial-by-trial basis. Post-

marketing innovation has always been the most effective way of finding out how to improve therapeutic outcomes. Most of the regimens we have that cure advanced cancers were developed this way. The requirement for approval of each new use has had a stifling effect on the development of novel approaches to treatment. I mention this because this is another positive feature of a text like this. There are several chapters on the development of drugs in different countries and under different regulatory environments, and as such, the text gives the reader some opportunity to compare and develop a consensus about the most effective way to regulate the development of drugs for cancer patients.

The stated goal of the editors of this text was to collect the most important advances in chest oncology together in a single volume, and they have done that. And there have been many advances in the past few years to chronicle. Textbooks, when they are carefully prepared and edited, serve both as a foundation stone and a launching pad. They serve as a foundation stone by allowing the reader to acquire all the important information in one volume and gain an important perspective on the state of the art and what's best for their patients. They are a launching pad because with this kind of overview in hand, investigators can see more clearly which areas need to be investigated. As I said at the beginning of this introduction, this is the right text in the right place at the right time. The challenge to the editors will be to plan for the second edition in a timely way. This first edition is arriving at the time of a shifting paradigm and should help with the transition. A timely second edition may well find itself right on the new paradigm it helped to create. Good textbooks do that.

Vincent T. DeVita Jr., M.D.

Contents

Section VIII:
Mesothelioma

Section IX:
Palliation of Lung Cancer Patients

Section X:
Social Issues in the Management
of Lung Cancer

List of Contributors

Alex A. Adjei
Department of Oncology
Mayo Clinic
Rochester, NY, USA

Fabrice Andre
Department of Medicine
Gustave Roussy Institute
Villejuif, France

Tim Benepal
Department of Clinical Oncology
Royal Marsden Hospital
London, UK

Gerold Bepler
H. Lee Moffitt Cancer Center and Research Institute
Thoracic Oncology Program
Tampa, FL, USA

Sebastian Belle
Department of Surgery
Heidelberg University Medical Center
Mannheim, Germany

Ricardo Bello
Department of Cardiothoracic Surgery
Montefiore Medical Center
New York, NY, USA

Benjamin Besse
Department of Medicine
Gustave Roussy Institute
Villejuif, France

Francesc Casas
Radiation Oncology Department
Hospital Clínic i Universitari
Barcelona, Spain

Adrianni Charpidou
Oncology Unit
3rd Department of Medicine
Sotiria General Hospital
Athens Medical School
Athens, Greece

Yuhchyau Chen
Department of Radiation Oncology
University of Rochester Medical Center
Rochester, NY, USA

Victor Cohen
Sir Mortimer B. Davis Jewish General Hospital
McGill University School of Medicine
Department of Oncology
Montreal, QC, Canada

Catherine M. Corbishley
Department of Cellular Pathology
St. George's Healthcare NHS Trust
London, UK

Daphne M. Coutroubis
Lung Cancer and Mesothelioma Unit
St Bartholomew's Hospital and Medical College
London, UK

Melanie Deberne
Department of Medicine
Gustave Roussy Institute
Villejuif, France

Geoff P. Delaney
Liverpool and Campbelltown Hospitals
Cancer Therapy Centre
Liverpool Hospital
Liverpool, BC, Australia

Vincent T. DeVita Jr.
Yale Cancer Center
Yale School of Medicine
New Haven, CT, USA

Chad M. DeYoung
Department of Radiation Oncology
University of Maryland School of Medicine
Baltimore, MD, USA

Martin J. Edelman
Medical Thoracic Oncology
University of Maryland Greenebaum Cancer Center
Baltimore, MD, USA

Tim Eisen
Department of Clinical Oncology
Royal Marsden Hospital
London, UK

Hugo Esteva
Thoracic Surgery Division
Hospital de Clínicas José de San Martín
Buenos Aires University
Buenos Aires, Argentina

Rosangela Filiberti
Epidemiology and Biostatistics
National Cancer Research Institute
Genoa, Italy

Bruce G. French
Cardiothoracic Surgery Department
Liverpool Hospital
Liverpool, BC, Australia

David Gandara
Department of Internal Medicine
UC Davis Cancer Center
University of California
Sacramento, CA, USA

Adi F. Gazdar
The Hamon Center for Therapeutic Oncology Research
Department of Pathology
The University of Texas Southwestern Medical Center
Dallas, TX, USA

Sebastien Gilbert
Division of Thoracic and Foregut Surgery
University of Pittsburgh Medical Center
Pittsburgh, PA, USA

Christine Godfrey
Department of Health Sciences and Centre
for Health Economics
University of York
York, UK

Ramaswamy Govindan
Alvin J. Siteman Cancer Center
Division of Medical Oncology
Washington University School of Medicine
St. Louis, MO, USA

Christina Gratziou
Pulmonary and Critical Care Department
Medical School, University of Athens
Evangelismos Hospital
Athens, Greece

Cesare Gridelli
Division of Medical Oncology
S. G. Moscati Hospital
Avellino, Italy

Nora Taubenslag Grigera
Department of Mental Health
Hospital de Clínicas José de San Martín
Buenos Aires University
Buenos Aires, Argentina

Heine H. Hansen
Department of Medicine
Oncology/Hematology Unit
Roskilde Hospital
Roskilde, Denmark

Kevin J. Harrington
Cancer Research UK Centre
for Cell and Molecular Biology
Institute of Cancer Research
London, UK

Kristin L. Hennenfent
St. Louis College of Pharmacy
St. Louis, MO, USA

Richard Houlston
Institute of Cancer Research
Sutton
Surrey, UK

J. Russell Hoverman
Clinical Resource Management Department
Texas Oncology PA
Dallas, TX, USA

Janssen-Heijnen Maryska LG
Eindhoven Cancer Registry
Comprehensive Cancer Centre South
Eindhoven, The Netherlands

Branislav Jeremic
Applied Radiation Biology and Radiotherapy Section
Division of Human Health, IAEA
Vienna, Austria

Michael R. Johnston
Division of Thoracic Surgery
Toronto General Hospital
Division of Surgical Oncology
Princess Margaret Hospital
University of Toronto
Toronto, ON, Canada

Eleni Karapanagiotou
3rd Department of Medicine
Athens Medical School
Sotiria General Hospital
Athens, Greece

Steven M. Keller
Albert Einstein College of Medicine
Division of Thoracic Surgery
Montefiore Medical Center
New York, NY, USA

Michael S. Kent
Division of Thoracic and Foregut Surgery
University of Pittsburgh Medical Center
Pittsburgh, PA, USA

Fadlo R. Khuri
Winship Cancer Institute
Emory University
Atlanta, GA, USA

George Ladas
Royal Brompton Hospital
Imperial College School of Medicine
London, UK

Thierry Le Chevalier
Department of Medicine
Gustave Roussy Institute
Villejuif, France

Zhongxing Liao
Department of Radiation Oncology
The University of Texas
M.D. Anderson Cancer Center
Houston, TX, USA

Rogerio Lilenbaum
University of Miami School of Medicine
Thoracic Oncology Program
The Mount Sinai Comprehensive Cancer Center
Miami Beach, FL, USA

Jiang Liu
Division of Thoracic Surgery
Toronto General Hospital
Division of Surgical Oncology
Princess Margaret Hospital
University of Toronto
Toronto, ON, Canada

James D. Luketich
Division of Thoracic and Foregut Surgery
University of Pittsburgh Medical Center
Pittsburgh, PA, USA

Paolo Maione
Division of Medical Oncology
S.G. Moscati Hospital
Avellino, Italy

Effrosyni D. Manali
4th Department of Internal Medicine
National and Kapodistrian University of Athens
Medical School of Athens
Attikon University Hospital
Athens, Greece

Christian Manegold
Heidelberg University Medical Center
Department of Surgery
Mannheim, Germany

Athena Matakidou
Institute of Cancer Research
Sutton
Surrey, UK

Christine C. Maurer
Oncology Unit
Third Department of Medicine
Sotiria General Hospital
Athens, Greece

Luka Milas
Department of Experimental Radiation Oncology
The University of Texas
M.D. Anderson Cancer Center
Houston, TX, USA

Julian R. Molina
Department of Oncology
Mayo Clinic
Rochester, NY, USA

Annette Mueller
Heidelberg University Medical Center
Department of Surgery
Mannheim, Germany

Katie Newbold
Academic Unit of Radiotherapy and Oncology
Institute of Cancer Research
Royal Marsden NHS Trust
Sutton, UK

Alejandro T. Newton
Thoracic Surgery Division
Hospital de Clínicas José de San Martín
Buenos Aires University
Buenos Aires, Argentina

Christopher M. Nutting
Royal Marsden NHS Trust Hospitals
London, UK

Yuichiro Ohe
Divisions of Thoracic Oncology and Internal Medicine
National Cancer Center Hospital
Tokyo, Japan

Simon Padley
Chelsea and Westminster Hospital
London, UK

Spyros A. Papiris
Second Pulmonary Department
National and Kapodistrian University of Athens
Attikon University Hospital
Athens, Greece

Steve Parrott
Centre for Health Economics
Alcuin College University of York
York, UK

Cristina Pecci
Department of Mental Health
Hospital de Clínicas José de San Martín
Buenos Aires University
Buenos Aires, Argentina

Branislav Perin
Institute of Lung Diseases
School of Medicine
University of Novi Sad
Novi Sad, Yugoslavia

Eleni Plaisia
Department of Anaesthesiology, Pain Clinic
Evangelismos General Hospital
Athens, Greece

Ekaterini N. Politi
Areteion University Hospital
Athens Medical School
Athens, Greece

Tamara Portas
Thoracic Surgery Division
Hospital de Clínicas José de San Martín
Buenos Aires University
Buenos Aires, Argentina

Riccardo Puntoni
Epidemiology and Biostatistics
National Cancer Research Institute
Genoa, Italy

Ritesh Rathore
Department of Internal Medicine
Roger Williams Medical Center
Providence, RI, USA

Jack A. Roth
Department of Thoracic and Cardiovascular Surgery
University of Texas
M.D. Anderson Cancer Center
Houston, TX, USA

Charis Roussos
Athens Medical School,
Evangelismos General Hospital
Athens, Greece
and Faculty of Medicine
McGill University, Montreal, Canada

Nagahiro Saijo
Divisions of Thoracic Oncology and Internal Medicine
National Cancer Center Hospital
Tokyo, Japan

Giorgio V. Scagliotti
Thoracic Oncology Unit
Department of Clinical and Biological Sciences
University of Turin
S. Luigi Hospital
Turin, Italy

Lidia Schapira
Harvard Medical School
Division of Hematology-Oncology
Boston, MA, USA

Joan H. Schiller
Section of Medical Oncology
University of Wisconsin Comprehensive Cancer Center
Madison, WI, USA

Ikuo Sekine
Divisions of Thoracic Oncology and Internal Medicine
National Cancer Center Hospital
Tokyo, Japan

Giovanni Selvaggi
Thoracic Oncology Unit
Department of Clinical and Biological Sciences
University of Turin
S. Luigi Hospital
Turin, Italy

Pallav L. Shah
Royal Brompton Hospital
London, UK

Jill M. Siegfried
Department of Pharmacology
University of Pittsburgh
Hillman Cancer Center
Pittsburgh, PA, USA

Michael J. Simoff
Pulmonary and Critical Care Medicine
Henry Ford Medical Center
Detroit, MI, USA

Mark A. Socinski
Multidisciplinary Thoracic Oncology Program
Department of Hematology/Oncology
University of North Carolina
Chapel Hill, NC, USA

Merrill Solan
Department of Radiation Oncology
Thomas Jefferson University Hospital
Philadelphia, PA, USA

Morten Sorensen
Department of Medicine
Oncology/Hematology Unit
Roskilde Hospital
Roskilde, Denmark

Jean-Charles Soria
Department of Medicine
Gustave Roussy Institute
Villejuif, France

Laura P. Stabile
Lung and Thoracic Malignancies Program
University of Pittsburgh Cancer Institute
Pittsburgh, PA, USA

Jeremy P. C. Steele
Lung Cancer and Mesothelioma Unit
St Bartholomew's Hospital and Medical College
London, UK

Thomas E. Stinchcombe
Multidisciplinary Thoracic Oncology Program
Department of Hematology/Oncology
University of North Carolina
Chapel Hill, NC, USA

Konstantinos N. Syrigos
Oncology Unit
Sotiria General Hospital
Athens Medical School
Athens, Greece

Tomohide Tamura
Divisions of Thoracic Oncology and Internal Medicine
National Cancer Center Hospital
Tokyo, Japan

Evagellos Terpos
Haematology Unit
251 Air Force and VA Hospital
Athens, Greece

Melvyn Tockman
Lee Moffitt Cancer Center and Research Institute
Thoracic Oncology Program
Tampa, FL, USA

Anne M. Traynor
Section of Medical Oncology
University of Wisconsin Comprehensive Cancer Center
Madison, WI, USA

Ifigenia Tzannou
Oncology Unit
3rd Department of Medicine
Sotiria General Hospital
Athens Medical School
Athens, Greece

Heather Wakelee
Department of Medicine
Division of Oncology
Stanford Cancer Center
Stanford, CA, USA

Alan B. Weitberg
Department of Internal Medicine
Roger Williams Medical Center
Providence, RI, USA

Maria Werner-Wasik
Department of Radiation Oncology
Thomas Jefferson University Hospital
Philadelphia, PA, USA

Ignacio I. Wistuba
Department of Pathology and Department of Thoracic/
Head and Neck Medical Oncology
The University of Texas
M.D. Anderson Cancer Center
Houston, TX, USA

Ying Zee
Department of Clinical Oncology
Royal Marsden Hospital
London, UK

Frank B. Zimmerman
Department of Radiation Oncology
Klinikum rechts der Isar
Technical University Munich
Munich, Germany

Section I:
Epidemiologie and Etiology of Lung Cancer

Epidemiology of Lung Cancer

1

Maryska L. G. Janssen-Heijnen

1.1   Introduction

At the beginning of the 20th century lung cancer was a very rare disease, but rates have increased so dramatically that lung cancer can be considered one of the major epidemics of the 20th century. Currently, lung cancer is still death cause number one among cancer [1]. Mortality is influenced by incidence and survival. In this chapter, the geographic variation in incidence, mortality, and survival of lung cancer and the time trends are described, as well as the factors underlying these trends.

1.2   Classification of Lung Cancer

Lung cancer is commonly classified as small-cell carcinoma and non-small-cell carcinoma [2]. The latter includes squamous cell carcinoma, adenocarcinoma, large-cell undifferentiated carcinoma, and some rare subtypes such as adenosquamous cell carcinoma, mu-

coepidermoid carcinoma, and adenoid cystic carcinoma. Large-cell undifferentiated carcinoma has frequently been called a "wastebasket" or nonentity, because the carcinomas are so poorly differentiated that squamous or glandular differentiation is no longer evident at the light-microscopic level. Thus, the incidence of this histological subtype varies with the criteria used to classify the other forms of non-small-cell lung cancer.

1.3   Incidence and Mortality

Since the prognosis for lung cancer is still very poor, mortality rates closely follow incidence rates.

1.3.1   Geographic Variation

The international variations in the incidence and mortality of lung cancer are striking. Worldwide male lung cancer incidence rates in the late 1990s were highest (>46 per 100,000 person-years) in Canada, the USA, Uruguay, the Philippines, most European countries, Russia, and Korea, moderate (25–46 per 100,000 person-years) in Argentina, Cuba, Iceland, Norway, Finland, Portugal, China, Ireland, Malta, Spain, Australia, and New Zealand, and low (<25 per 100,000 person-years) in Utah (USA), other Latin-American countries, Sweden, Africa, and most Asian countries. For women, lung cancer incidence rates were relatively high (>11.5 per 100,000 person-years) in Canada, the United States, Cuba, north-western Europe and central Europe, southeast Asia, Australia and New Zealand, moderate (6.5–11.5 per 100,000 person-years) in Mexico, Latin America, southern and eastern Europe, South Africa, and Russia, and low (<6.5 per 100,000 person-years) in Bolivia, Paraguay, Spain, India, and Africa.

1.3.2   Time Trends

Incidence and mortality rates for lung cancer have changed markedly over the past 5 decades [3, 4]. In North America, Australia, New Zealand, and most countries of northwestern Europe, the age-standardized rate for men has increased markedly up to the 1970s or 1980s and then started to decline, first among middle-aged men and later in the older age groups [5–18]. In southern and eastern Europe, the incidence of lung cancer among men has increased up to the late 1980s or even up to the late 1990s [4, 19–22]. In Latin America, Africa, and Asia, lung cancer mortality has been increasing, except for Cuba, Argentina, Paraguay, and Peru [23–25]. Among women, the incidence of lung cancer (being much lower than for men) started to increase later and is still on the rise in most countries. Dramatic increases have been seen in North America, Iceland, Ireland, the UK, and Denmark, but also in The Netherlands and Hungary [5, 13, 17, 26]. Female lung cancer rates were also relatively high in Norway and Sweden, both countries with relatively low rates among males, and have been increasing over time [4, 5]. In some countries (USA, Cuba, Argentina, Paraguay, Peru, Ireland, the UK, Hong Kong, Singapore, and Japan) the increase in incidence rates among women has already leveled off [4, 5, 23, 27, 28].

1.3.3   Variation Between Histological Types

Squamous cell carcinoma used to be the most common histological subtype of lung cancer among men. However, the incidence of squamous cell carcinoma among men has been decreasing since the early 1980s, in contrast to that of adenocarcinoma [4, 9, 10, 14–16, 18, 29–33]. The incidence of the latter type has been increasing up to the 1990s. In the mid-1990s adenocarcinoma had become the most common histological subtype of lung cancer among men in the USA. In other Western countries, squamous cell carcinoma was still the most common subtype among men [4]. Among women, adenocarcinoma used to be the most common histological subtype (about one-third), and the incidence rates of all histological subtypes have been increasing [10, 15, 18]. These trends have led to an overall increase in the incidence of adenocarcinoma.

1.3.4   Risk Factors

A lot of studies have indicated that smoking tobacco is the main cause of lung cancer, with a latency time between the start of smoking and lung cancer of 15–50 years [34–36]. In addition, the number of pack-years, the tar level of the cigarettes smoked, and the age at initiation of smoking are closely related to lung cancer risk [37, 38]. The relative risk (RR) of smoking is higher for squamous cell carcinoma and small-cell carcinoma (RR between 10 and 200) than for adenocarcinoma (RR between 2 and 40) [36, 39–46]. The decline in risk after quitting smoking is also more consistent for squamous cell and small-cell carcinoma than for adenocarcinoma [47]. However, the lower risk for adenocarcinoma could be spurious, because the risk of adenocarcinoma in nonsmokers (i.e., the reference group) is also higher [36, 43, 44, 47, 48]. The association between smoking and lung cancer cell types seems to be related to inhalation pattern [15, 49] and tumor location: adenocarcinoma is known to occur primarily in the peripheral lung zones, whereas squamous cell carcinoma and small-cell carcinoma occur mainly in central or hilar locations [36, 40, 47, 50].

The geographic variation and time trends in lung cancer incidence for both sexes are strongly related to smoking behavior [5, 43, 46, 51]. The percentage smokers among men in North America, Australia, New Zealand, and north-western Europe was much higher than among women, but has dropped since the 1950s/1960s, first among younger men [47, 52–55]. The percentage of low-tar filter cigarette smokers among male smokers has increased markedly [56–58]. The percentage of female smokers started to increase later and has only been decreasing since the end of the 1970s. In southwestern Europe, the percentage of smokers did not start to decrease until the 1980s, and in many eastern European countries the prevalence of smoking has increased until the 1990s [55]. The proportion of female smokers is still increasing in Austria and Spain [5, 59]. The low incidence in Utah is probably due to the high proportion (about 70%) of Mormons, who are discouraged from smoking. In Latin America the proportion of smokers among men and women has been increasing [60]. In Asia there has been a typically high, but decreasing smoking rate among men. The smoking rate among Asian women was low, but has been increasing among younger women [25]. In Africa the proportion of smokers has been increasing since the 1960s [61]. Traditionally only men smoked, but the proportion of female, children, and adolescents smokers has also been rising.

The decrease in incidence rates for squamous cell carcinoma and small-cell carcinoma among men was probably due to the decrease in the percentage of smokers since the 1950s and the change to low-tar filter cigarettes. The increase in adenocarcinoma is more difficult to explain. The extent to which changes in diagnostic techniques or classification were responsible for the increase is likely to be small [15, 30, 62, 63]. Furthermore, the interobserver reproducibility for adenocarcinoma was good [64–66]. The introduction of filter cigarettes since the mid-1950s may have led to an increase in the incidence of adenocarcinoma, because filters are less effective at eliminating smaller particles and filter use could also result in taking larger puffs and retaining smoke longer to compensate for the lower nicotine yield [15, 36, 47, 49, 67]. This leads to a higher deposition of small carcinogens in the peripheral lung zones. This is the area were adenocarcinoma generally occurs. A second, complementary hypothesis suggests that smoking low-tar filter cigarettes may increase the risk of adenocarcinoma because these cigarettes have a higher nitrate content [68]. The higher proportion of women and Americans who smoke low-tar filter cigarettes has resulted in a higher incidence rate of adenocarcinoma in these groups [58].

Un updated metaanalysis in the International Agency for Research on Cancer monograph showed that the risk of lung cancer for passive smoking was 20–35% higher than expected [38, 69]. A recent European study showed that frequent exposure to environmental tobacco smoke during childhood (daily exposure for many hours) was associated with lung cancer in adulthood [70].

Other causes of lung cancer have been identified, such as air pollution [71], occupational exposure to arsenic, asbestos, radon, chloromethyl ethers, chromium, mustard gas, nickel refining, and polycyclic hydrocarbons (however, only a small proportion of the population was exposed) [72–78]. Vitamin A deficiency [79–83], indoor radon [84, 85], possibly bird keeping [43, 86–90], and previous chronic lung diseases [91] have also been identified as possible risk factors, but the effects of smoking are so predominant that trends in other exposures seem unlikely to be largely responsible for the changes in incidence. However, despite the traditionally low prevalence of female smoking, the incidence rates of lung cancer among women in Hong Kong have been among the highest in the world [27, 92, 93]. Exposure to cooking oil vapors during high-temperature cooking might have played a role [93–95]. Genetic predisposition may also play a role in the etiology of lung cancer [96, 97].

1.4 Prognosis

1.4.1 Geographic Variation

Worldwide, the prognosis for patients with lung cancer is very poor, because metastases are often present at the time of diagnosis. In North America the 5-year survival rates in the late 1990s were about 15% [98]. Between 1990 and 1994, fairly large variations in lung cancer survival rates existed between European countries: 1-year rates varied between 23% and 43%, and 5-year rates between 6% and 16% (Fig. 1.1). Survival was highest in France, Germany, The Netherlands and Switzer-

land, and lowest in Denmark, England, Poland, and Scotland [99, 100].

Variation in survival may be explained by differences in access to specialized care (medically, financially, and geographically) [101]. This may explain the poor survival rates in the UK, where the number of consultants and the proportion of patients receiving curative treatment are lower than in most other European countries. Delays in diagnosing and treating patients might partly explain the lower patient survival in Denmark, because the lower survival rate was due to an unfavorable stage distribution [102].

1.4.2 Time Trends

The prognosis for lung cancer patients, regardless of histological type, has improved slightly over time [98, 103, 104].

1.4.2.1 Non-Small-Cell Lung Cancer

There has been only a slight improvement in the prognosis of non-small-cell lung cancer during the last decades. Nowadays, the 5-year survival rate is 13–19% [98, 101, 105–107]. Although non-small-cell lung cancer is often considered to be one clinically uniform category, several studies indicate that survival differs according to histological subtype, being better for squamous cell carcinoma and adenocarcinoma (1-year survival rates of 40–50%) than for large-cell undifferentiated carcinoma (1-year survival rates of 25–30%) [107–111].

1.4.2.2 Small-Cell Lung Cancer

Small-cell lung cancer can be distinguished from other forms of lung cancer. Its features are: rapid progression, short doubling time, high growth fraction, and sensitivity to multiple chemotherapeutic agents and radiation therapy. Short-term survival has improved since the introduction of chemotherapy in the 1970s, but 5-year survival still does not exceed 5% [98, 112–118]. Death from recurrent disease occurs within 2 years of diagnosis in 80–98% of the cases [119–123].

1.4.3 Prognostic Factors

As we have seen here, histological subtype is a strong prognostic factor. Survival of lung cancer is also closely associated with tumor stage and treatment [109]. Until now, the only chance for cure is tumor resection. Patients with stage I or II non-small-cell lung cancer are candidates for surgical resection [124]. Positron emission tomography (PET) scanning is useful for patients who are possible candidates for surgical resection. PET

A) Males

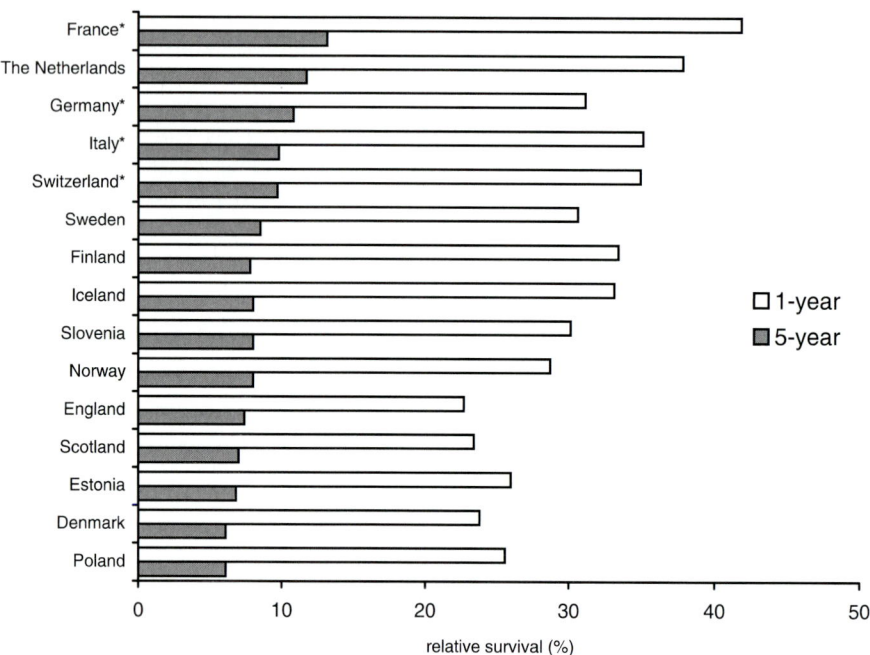

B) Females

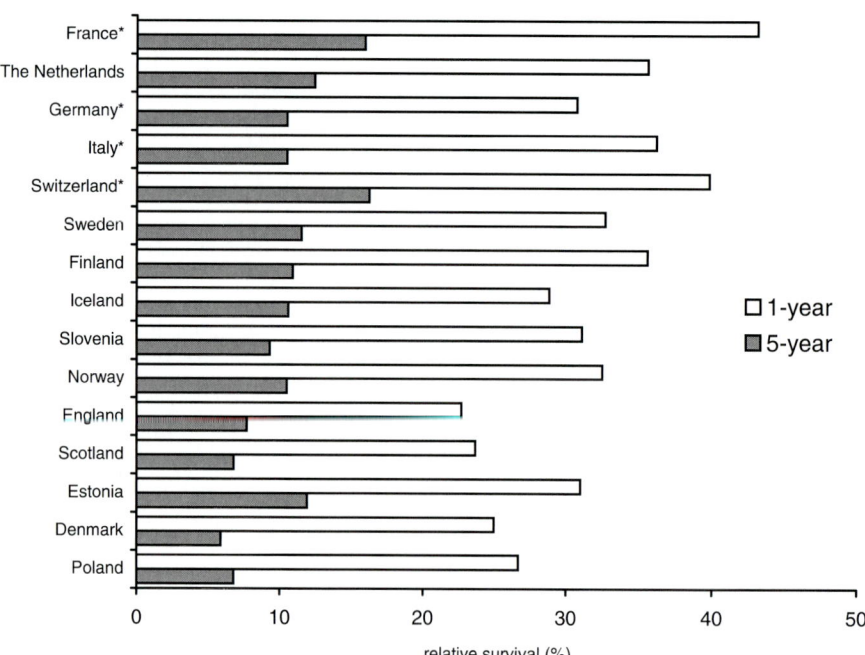

Fig. 1.1. Geographic variations in age-adjusted relative survival in Europe (1990–1994) in males (**A**) and females (**B**). Source: EURO-CARE III [101]. * <15% of the national population covered

is a new technology that can be used to investigate nodal as well as distant dissemination, and can be used for staging and follow-up. In this way, mediastinoscopy and unnecessary surgery can be avoided [125, 126].

For most patients with stage III disease, the preferred therapeutic modality is thoracic radiotherapy in combination with chemotherapy [124, 127–132]. For patients with stage IV lung cancer, no curative treatment or "standard therapy" is available [124, 133]. Currently, small-cell lung cancer patients with limited disease generally receive combination chemotherapy and radiotherapy [134], and approximately 50% experience complete clinical remission. Patients with extensive disease also exhibit an initial response to chemotherapy, but only 20–40% go into complete remission.

Although therapy for lung cancer has made progress in recent years, most patients will die of disease progression, and some current treatments are very toxic, in particular concomitant chemoradiotherapy for stage III disease. Therefore, the introduction of novel agents remains a high priority. Current interest is focused on molecular markers [135] and biological therapies, such as targeting growth factors and growth factor receptors, suppressing angiogenesis, and immunotherapy.

Prognosis for elderly lung cancer patients is worse compared to younger patients, even after adjustment for higher mortality in the general population [109, 136]. Elderly patients with localized non-small-cell lung cancer underwent less surgery than younger patients, and older patients with nonlocalized non-small-cell lung cancer received less chemotherapy [136, 137]. Since the proportion of elderly patients in most Western countries is growing, comorbidity or the coexistence of various chronic illnesses in addition to the index disease is of growing importance for the clinical management (especially surgical management) of lung cancer patients. Comorbidity may increase the risk of preoperative and postoperative complications [138–141], especially those of the cardiorespiratory system [142–145]. Comorbidity may also be an independent prognostic factor [146–151]. However, comorbidity is probably of less importance in case of a lethal disease as lung cancer [136, 149, 152]. Most patients die of lung cancer before they are at risk of dying from the comorbid condition. Pulmonary resection is justified even for elderly lung cancer patients. However, a careful preoperative assessment ought to be performed and standard resections should be preferred [144, 145]. In a recent study smoking was also found to be a prognostic factor, even after adjustment for age, gender, illicit drug use, adverse symptoms, histology, stage, comorbidity, and treatment [153].

Some studies found higher survival rates for females than for males [98, 154, 155]. Since survival rates are higher for younger persons than for older, some of the female–male survival differential may be due to a higher preponderance of younger-aged patients in the female group. The prognostic difference might also be due to a different histological distribution of the tumors or to the lower prevalence of comorbid conditions among women, such as chronic obstructive pulmonary diseases or cardiovascular diseases.

1.5 Prevention and Early Detection

Lung cancer is still death cause number one, and smoking is the most important risk factor. Since survival is very poor, prevention of lung cancer is important through quitting smoking and discouraging young people from starting smoking. Despite a decrease since the 1950s, the percentage of adult smokers is still 20–50%, and more teenagers have even been smoking since 1990 [55, 156]. Furthermore, the average number of cigarettes smoked per day has increased, because the smokers who continued smoking were the heavily addicted ones. Thus, the decrease in lung cancer incidence in Western countries will probably have reached a plateau at the beginning of the 21st century, and for those born after 1970, lung cancer incidence will probably even increase again after 2010.

Most cases of lung cancer are diagnosed at advanced stages, when the chance of cure is poor. The prognosis for patients with early-stage disease who can undergo surgical resection is much better than for those with advanced-stage disease. Therefore, screening might reduce mortality. Current screening methods include X-ray, sputum analysis, low-dose computed tomography (CT) or spiral CT, and fluorescence bronchoscopy [157–163]. Data from nonrandomized trials, however, are influenced by biases, such as lead-time, length, and overdiagnosis bias. All methods have to be validated in randomized controlled trials with the endpoint "mortality reduction". At the present time, screening for lung cancer is not recommended [164–166].

1.6 Conclusions

Although the peak of lung cancer incidence among men in North America, Australia, New Zealand, and northwestern Europe was reached in the 1980s, the rate for men in southern and eastern Europe and for women continued to increase, at least until the 1990s. In other parts of the world, where smoking is still increasing, mortality due to lung cancer will increase dramatically in the next decades.

The geographic variation and trends in incidence were closely associated with past smoking behavior. The trend toward smoking more low-tar filter cigarettes probably caused the increase in the incidence of adenocarcinoma. This tumor type is already the major histological subtype in North America and may also become the major type in other countries in the near future. Lymphatic and hematogenous metastases are often present at the time that lung cancer is diagnosed, and prognosis is still very poor. The prognosis for non-small-cell lung cancer has only slightly improved, while considerable progress has been made in the short-term survival of small-cell lung cancer since the introduction of chemotherapy in the 1970s. Due to a growing proportion of elderly lung cancer patients, more patients present with serious comorbidity at diagnosis of cancer. This may complicate treatment and indicates the need for adapted guidelines for these patients, who usually are not entered in clinical trials.

Key Points

- Although the peak of lung cancer incidence among men in North America, Australia, New Zealand, and north-western Europe was reached in the 1980s, the rate for men in southern and eastern Europe and for women continued to increase, at least until the 1990s. In other parts of the world, where smoking is still increasing, mortality due to lung cancer will increase dramatically in the next decades.

- Mortality associated with adenocarcinoma will probably increase worldwide, due to the increased use of low-tar filter cigarettes.

- Except for short-term survival of small-cell tumors, the prognosis for patients with lung cancer has not improved significantly and is still very poor. Screening is not yet recommended. Prevention, therefore, remains important.

- Due to a growing proportion of elderly lung cancer patients, more patients present with serious comorbidity at diagnosis of cancer. This may complicate treatment.

References

1. Levi F, Lucchini F, Negri E, Boyle P, La Vecchia C (2004) Cancer mortality in Europe, 1995–1999, and an overview of trends since 1960. Int J Cancer 2004; 110:155.
2. WHO. The World Health Organization histological typing of lung tumours. Second edition. Am J Clin Pathol 1982; 77:123.
3. Parkin DM, Whelan SL, Ferlay J, Raymond L, Young J. Cancer Incidence in Five Continents, vol. VII. IARC Scientific Publications, Lyon, 1997.
4. Parkin DM, Whelan SL, Ferlay J, Teppo L, Thomas DB. Cancer incidence in five continents, vol. VIII. IARC Scientific Publications, Lyon, 2002.
5. Bray F, Tyczynski JE, Parkin DM. Going up or coming down? The changing phases of the lung cancer epidemic from 1967 to 1999 in the 15 European Union countries. Eur J Cancer 2004; 40:96.
6. Devesa SS, Silverman DT, Young JL, et al. Cancer incidence and mortality trends among whites in the United States, 1947–84. J Natl Cancer Inst 1987; 79:701.
7. Dinse GE, Hoel DG. Exploring time trends in cancer incidence. Cancer Causes Control 1992; 3:409.
8. Horm JW, Kessler LG. Falling rates of lung cancer in men in the United States. Lancet 1986; 1:425.
9. Janssen-Heijnen ML, Nab HW, van Reek J, van der Heijden LH, Schipper R, Coebergh JW. Striking changes in smoking behaviour and lung cancer incidence by histological type in south-east Netherlands, 1960-1991. Eur J Cancer 1995; 31A:949.
10. Levi F, Franceschi S, La Vecchia C, Randimbison L, Te VC. Lung carcinoma trends by histologic type in Vaud and Neuchatel, Switzerland, 1974–1994. Cancer 1997; 79:906.
11. McCredie M, Coates MS, Ford JM. The changing incidence of cancer in adults in New South Wales. Int J Cancer 1988; 42:667.
12. McLaughlin JR, Kreiger N, Marrett LD, Holowaty EJ. Cancer incidence registration and trends in Ontario. Eur J Cancer 1991; 27:1520.
13. O'Lorcain P, Comber H. Lung cancer mortality predictions for Ireland 2001–2015 and current trends in North Western Europe. Lung Cancer 2004; 46:157.
14. Skuladottir H, Olsen JH, Hirsch FR. Incidence of lung cancer in Denmark: historical and actual status. Lung Cancer 2000; 27:107.
15. Thun MJ, Lally CA, Flannery JT, Calle EE, Flanders WD, Heath CW Jr. Cigarette smoking and changes in the histopathology of lung cancer. J Natl Cancer Inst 1997; 89:1580.
16. Travis WD, Lubin J, Ries L, Devesa S. United States lung carcinoma incidence trends: declining for most histologic types among males, increasing among females. Cancer 1996; 77:2464.
17. Tyczynski JE, Bray F, Aareleid T, et al. Lung cancer mortality patterns in selected Central, Eastern and Southern European countries. Int J Cancer 2004; 109:598.
18. Zheng T, Holford TR, Boyle P, Chen Y, Ward BA, Flannery J, Mayne ST. Time trend and the age-period-cohort effect on the incidence of histologic types of lung cancer in Connecticut, 1960–1989. Cancer 1994; 74:1556.
19. Muir CS, Waterhouse j, Mack T, Powell J, Whelan S. Cancer Incidence in Five Continents, vol V. IARC Scientific Publications, Lyon, 1987.
20. Parkin DM, Muir CS, Whelan S, Gao YT, Ferlay J, Powell J. Cancer Incidence in Five Continents, vol VI. IARC Scientific Publications, Lyon, 1992.
21. Russo A, Crosignani P, Franceschi S, Berrino F. Changes in lung cancer histological types in Varese Cancer Registry, Italy 1976–1992. Eur J Cancer 1997; 33:1643.
22. Waterhouse J, Muir CS, Powell J, Shanmugaratnam K. Cancer Incidence in Five Continents, vol IV. IARC Scientific Publications, Lyon, 1982.
23. Boffetta P, La Vecchia C, Levi F, Lucchini F. Mortality patterns and trends for lung cancer and other tobacco-related cancers in the Americas, 1955–1989. Int J Epidemiol 1993; 22:377.
24. La Vecchia C, Lucchini F, Negri E, Boyle P, Levi F. Trends in cancer mortality, 1955–1989: Asia, Africa and Oceania. Eur J Cancer 1993; 29A:2168.
25. Morita T. A statistical study of lung cancer in the annual of pathological autopsy cases in Japan, from 1958 to 1997, with reference to time trends of lung cancer in the world. Jpn J Cancer Res 2002; 93:15.
26. Siesling S, van Dijck JA, Visser O, Coebergh JW. Trends in incidence of and mortality from cancer in The Netherlands in the period 1989–1998. Eur J Cancer 2003; 39:2521.

27. Chiu YL, Yu IT, Wong TW. Time trends of female lung cancer in Hong Kong: age, period and birth cohort analysis. Int J Cancer 2004; 111:424.

28. Coleman MP, Estève J, Damiecki P, Arslan A, Renard H. Trends in Cancer Incidence and Mortality. IARC Scientific Publications, Lyon, 1993.

29. Dodds L, Davis S, Polissar L. A population-based study of lung cancer incidence trends by histologic type, 1974–81. J Natl Cancer Inst 1986; 76:21.

30. El-Torky M, el-Zeky F, Hall JC. Significant changes in the distribution of histologic types of lung cancer. A review of 4928 cases. Cancer 1990; 65:2361.

31. Perng DW, Perng RP, Kuo BI, Chiang SC. The variation of cell type distribution in lung cancer: a study of 10,910 cases at a medical center in Taiwan between 1970 and 1993. Jpn J Clin Oncol 1996; 26:229.

32. Vincent RG, Pickren JW, Lane WW, et al. The changing histopathology of lung cancer: a review of 1682 cases. Cancer 1977; 39:1647.

33. Wu AH, Henderson BE, Thomas DC, Mack TM. Secular trends in histologic types of lung cancer. J Natl Cancer Inst 1986; 77:53.

34. Doll R, Peto R, Wheatley K, Gray R, Sutherland I. Mortality in relation to smoking: 40 years' observations on male British doctors. BMJ 1994; 309:901.

35. Haldorsen T, Grimsrud TK. Cohort analysis of cigarette smoking and lung cancer incidence among Norwegian women. Int J Epidemiol 1999; 28:1032.

36. Lubin JH, Blot WJ. Assessment of lung cancer risk factors by histologic category. J Natl Cancer Inst 1984; 73:383.

37. Harris JE, Thun MJ, Mondul AM, Calle EE. Cigarette tar yields in relation to mortality from lung cancer in the cancer prevention study II prospective cohort, 1982–8. BMJ 2004; 328:72.

38. Sasco AJ, Secretan MB, Straif K. Tobacco smoking and cancer: a brief review of recent epidemiological evidence. Lung Cancer 2004; 45 Suppl 2:S3.

39. de Waard F, Kemmeren JM, van Ginkel LA, Stolker AA. Urinary cotinine and lung cancer risk in a female cohort. Br J Cancer 1995; 72:784.

40. Denissenko MF, Pao A, Tang M, Pfeifer GP. Preferential formation of benzo[a]pyrene adducts at lung cancer mutational hotspots in P53. Science 1996; 274:430.

41. Ellard GA, de Waard F, Kemmeren JM. Urinary nicotine metabolite excretion and lung cancer risk in a female cohort. Br J Cancer 1995; 72:788.

42. Engeland A, Haldorsen T, Andersen A, Tretli S. The impact of smoking habits on lung cancer risk: 28 years' observation of 26,000 Norwegian men and women. Cancer Causes Control 1996; 7:366.

43. Morabia A, Wynder EL. Cigarette smoking and lung cancer cell types. Cancer 1991; 68:2074.

44. Pezzotto SM, Mahuad R, Bay ML, Morini JC, Poletto L. Variation in smoking-related lung cancer risk factors by cell type among men in Argentina: a case-control study. Cancer Causes Control 1993; 4:231.

45. Siemiatycki J, Krewski D, Franco E, Kaiserman M. Associations between cigarette smoking and each of 21 types of cancer: a multi-site case-control study. Int J Epidemiol 1995; 24:504.

46. Simonato L, Agudo A, Ahrens W, et al. Lung cancer and cigarette smoking in Europe: an update of risk estimates and an assessment of inter-country heterogeneity. Int J Cancer 2001; 91:876.

47. Higgins IT, Wynder EL. Reduction in risk of lung cancer among ex-smokers with particular reference to histologic type. Cancer 1988; 62:2397.

48. Makitaro R, Paakko P, Huhti E, Bloigu R, Kinnula VL. An epidemiological study of lung cancer: history and histo-

49. logical types in a general population in northern Finland. Eur Respir J 1999; 13:436.

49. Stellman SD, Garfinkel L. Lung cancer risk is proportional to cigarette tar yield: evidence from a prospective study. Prev Med 1989; 18:518.

50. Wynder EL, Hoffmann D. Smoking and lung cancer: scientific challenges and opportunities. Cancer Res 1994; 54:5284.

51. Tyczynski JE, Bray F, Parkin DM. Lung cancer in Europe in 2000: epidemiology, prevention, and early detection. Lancet Oncol 2003; 4:45.

52. Brown CC, Kessler LG. Projections of lung cancer mortality in the United States: 1985–2025. J Natl Cancer Inst 1988; 80:43.

53. Devesa SS, Grauman DJ, Blot WJ, Fraumeni JF Jr. Cancer surveillance series: changing geographic patterns of lung cancer mortality in the United States, 1950 through 1994. J Natl Cancer Inst 1999; 91:1040.

54. Fiore MC, Novotny TE, Pierce JP, Hatziandreu EJ, Patel KM, Davis RM. Trends in cigarette smoking in the United States. The changing influence of gender and race. JAMA 1989; 261:49.

55. Franceschi S, Naett C. Trends in smoking in Europe. Eur J Cancer Prev 1995; 4:271.

56. Giovino GA, Henningfield JE, Tomar SL, Escobedo LG, Slade J. Epidemiology of tobacco use and dependence. Epidemiol Rev 1995; 17:48.

57. Stellman SD, Muscat JE, Thompson S, Hoffmann D, Wynder EL. Risk of squamous cell carcinoma and adenocarcinoma of the lung in relation to lifetime filter cigarette smoking. Cancer 1997; 80:382.

58. Wynder EL, Muscat JE. The changing epidemiology of smoking and lung cancer histology. Environ Health Perspect 1995; 103 Suppl 8:143.

59. Franco J, Perez-Hoyos S, Plaza P. Changes in lung-cancer mortality trends in Spain. Int J Cancer 2002; 97:102.

60. Da Costa e Silva VL, Koifman S. Smoking in Latin America: a major public health problem. Cad Saude Publica 1998; 14 Suppl 3:99.

61. Taha A, Ball K. Smoking in Africa: the coming epidemic. World Smoking Health 1982; 7:25.

62. Beard CM, Jedd MB, Woolner LB, Richardson RL, Bergstralh EJ, Melton LJ 3rd. Fifty-year trend in incidence rates of bronchogenic carcinoma by cell type in Olmsted County, Minnesota. J Natl Cancer Inst 1988; 80:1404.

63. Caldwell CJ, Berry CL. Is the incidence of primary adenocarcinoma of the lung increasing? Virchows Arch 1996; 429:359.

64. Brownson RC, Loy TS, Ingram E, Myers JL, Alavanja MC, Sharp DJ, Chang JC. Lung cancer in nonsmoking women. Histology and survival patterns. Cancer 1995; 75:29.

65. Campobasso O, Andrion A, Ribotta M, Ronco G. The value of the 1981 WHO histological classification in interobserver reproducibility and changing pattern of lung cancer. Int J Cancer 1993; 53:205.

66. Greenberg ER, Korson R, Baker J, Barrett J, Baron JA, Yates J. Incidence of lung cancer by cell type: a population-based study in New Hampshire and Vermont. J Natl Cancer Inst 1984; 72:599.

67. Wynder EL, Covey LS. Epidemiologic patterns in lung cancer by histologic type. Eur J Cancer Clin Oncol 1987; 23:1491.

68. Hecht SS, Hoffmann D. Tobacco-specific nitrosamines, an important group of carcinogens in tobacco and tobacco smoke. Carcinogenesis 1988; 9:875.

69. International Agency for Research on Cancer. Tobacco smoking and involuntary smoking. In: IARC Monographs on the Evaluation of Carcinogenic Risks to Humans, vol 83. IARC Scientific Publications, Lyon, 2004.

70. Vineis P, Airoldi L, Veglia P, et al. Environmental tobacco smoke and risk of respiratory cancer and chronic obstructive pulmonary disease in former smokers and never smokers in the EPIC prospective study. BMJ 2005; 330:277.

71. Vena JE. Air pollution as a risk factor in lung cancer. Am J Epidemiol 1982; 116:42.

72. Blot WJ, Fraumeni JF. Arsenic and lung cancer. In: Samet J (ed) The Epidemiology of Lung Cancer. Marcel Dekker, New York, 1994, p 207.

73. Coultas DB. Other occupational carcinogens. In: Samet J (ed) The Epidemiology of Lung Cancer. Marcel Dekker, New York, 1994, p 299.

74. Doll R. Report of the International Committee on Nickel Carcinogenesis in man. Scand J Work Environ Health 1990; 16:1.

75. Doll R, Vessey MP, Beasley RW, et al. Mortality of gasworkers – final report of a prospective study. Br J Ind Med 1972; 29:394.

76. Easton DF, Peto J, Doll R. Cancers of the respiratory tract in mustard gas workers. Br J Ind Med 1988; 45:652.

77. Gowers DS, DeFonso LR, Schaffer P, Karli A, Monroe CB, Bernabeu L, Renshaw FM. Incidence of respiratory cancer among workers exposed to chloromethyl-ethers. Am J Epidemiol 1993; 137:31.

78. Wada S, Miyanishi M, Nishimoto Y, Kambe S, Miller RW. Mustard gas as a cause of respiratory neoplasia in man. Lancet 1968; 1:1161.

79. Dorant E, van den Brandt PA, Goldbohm RA. A prospective cohort study on allium vegetable consumption, garlic supplement use, and the risk of lung carcinoma in The Netherlands. Cancer Res 1994; 54:6148.

80. Margetts BM, Jackson AA. Interactions between people's diet and their smoking habits: the dietary and nutritional survey of British adults. BMJ 1993; 307:1381.

81. Scali J, Astre C, Segala C, Gerber M. Relationship of serum cholesterol, dietary and plasma beta-carotene with lung cancer in male smokers. Eur J Cancer Prev 1995; 4:169.

82. Serdula MK, Byers T, Mokdad AH, Simoes E, Mendlein JM, Coates RJ. The association between fruit and vegetable intake and chronic disease risk factors. Epidemiology 1996; 7:161.

83. Ziegler RG, Colavito EA, Hartge P, McAdams MJ, Schoenberg JB, Mason TJ, Fraumeni JF Jr. Importance of alpha-carotene, beta-carotene, and other phytochemicals in the etiology of lung cancer. J Natl Cancer Inst 1996; 88:612.

84. Darby S, Hill D, Auvinen A, et al. Radon in homes and risk of lung cancer: collaborative analysis of individual data from 13 European case-control studies. BMJ 2004; 330:223.

85. Lubin JH, Boice JD Jr. Lung cancer risk from residential radon: meta-analysis of eight epidemiologic studies. J Natl Cancer Inst 1997; 89:49.

86. Alavanja MC, Brownson RC, Berger E, Lubin J, Modigh C. Avian exposure and risk of lung cancer in women in Missouri: population based case-control study. BMJ 1996; 313:1233.

87. Gardiner AJ, Forey BA, Lee PN. Avian exposure and bronchogenic carcinoma. BMJ 1992; 305:989.

88. Holst PA, Kromhout D, Brand R. For debate: pet birds as an independent risk factor for lung cancer. BMJ 1988; 297:1319.

89. Kohlmeier L, Arminger G, Bartolomeycik S, Bellach B, Rehm J, Thamm M. Pet birds as an independent risk factor for lung cancer: case-control study. BMJ 1992; 305:986.

90. Modigh C, Axelsson G, Alavanja M, Andersson L, Rylander R. Pet birds and risk of lung cancer in Sweden: a case-control study. BMJ 1996; 313:1236.

91. Littman AJ, Thornquist MD, White E, Jackson LA, Goodman GE, Vaughan TL. Prior lung disease and risk of lung cancer in a large prospective study. Cancer Causes Control 2004; 15:819.

92. Au JS, Mang OW, Foo W, Law SC. Time trends of lung cancer incidence by histologic types and smoking prevalence in Hong Kong 1983–2000. Lung Cancer 2004; 45:143.

93. Seow A, Duffy SW, Ng TP, McGee MA, Lee HP. Lung cancer among Chinese females in Singapore 1968–1992: time trends, dialect group differences and implications for aetiology. Int J Epidemiol 1998; 27:167.

94. Ko YC, Lee CH, Chen MJ, et al. Risk factors for primary lung cancer among non-smoking women in Taiwan. Int J Epidemiol 1997; 26:24.

95. Wu-Williams AH, Dai XD, Blot W, et al. Lung cancer among women in north-east China. Br J Cancer 1990; 62:982.

96. Khan S, Coulson JM, Woll PJ. Genetic abnormalities in plasma DNA of patients with lung cancer and other respiratory diseases. Int J Cancer 2004; 110:891.

97. Sy SM, Wong N, Lee TW, et al. Distinct patterns of genetic alterations in adenocarcinoma and squamous cell carcinoma of the lung. Eur J Cancer 2004; 40:1082.

98. Ries LA, Eisner MP, Kosary CL, et al. SEER Cancer Statistics Review, 1975–2001. National Cancer Institute. Bethesda, MD. http://seer.cancer.gov/csr/1975_2001/, 2004.

99. Janssen-Heijnen MLG, Coebergh JWW. The changing epidemiology of lung cancer in Europe. Lung Cancer 2003; 41:245.

100. Sant M, Aareleid T, Berrino F, et al. EUROCARE-3: survival of cancer patients diagnosed 1990–94 – results and commentary. Ann Oncol 2003; 14 Suppl 5:V61.

101. Janssen-Heijnen ML, Gatta G, Forman D, Capocaccia R, Coebergh JW. Variation in survival of patients with lung cancer in Europe, 1985–1989. EUROCARE Working Group. Eur J Cancer 1998; 34:2191.

102. Storm HH, Dickman PW, Engeland A, Haldorsen T, Hakulinen T. Do morphology and stage explain the inferior lung cancer survival in Denmark? Eur Respir J 1999; 13:430.

103. Capocaccia R, Micheli A, Berrino F, et al. Time trends of lung and larynx cancers in Italy. Int J Cancer 1994; 57:154.

104. Levi F, Randimbison L, Te VC, Franceschi S, La Vecchia C. Trends in cancer survival in Vaud, Switzerland. Eur J Cancer 1992; 28A:1490.

105. Foucher P, Coudert B, Arveux P, et al. Age and prognosis of non-small cell lung cancer. Usefulness of a relative survival model. Eur J Cancer 1993; 29A:1809.

106. Grosclaude P, Galat JP, Mace-Lesech J, Roumagnac-Machelard M, Mercier M, Robillard J. Differences in treatment and survival rates of non-small-cell lung cancer in three regions of France. Br J Cancer 1995; 72:1278.

107. Pastorino U, Berrino F, Valente M, et al. Incident lung cancer survival. Long-term follow-up of a population-based study in Italy. Tumori 1990; 76:199.

108. Janssen-Heijnen ML, Schipper RM, Klinkhamer PJ, Crommelin MA, Mooi WJ, Coebergh JW. Divergent changes in survival for histological types of non-small-cell lung cancer in the southeastern area of The Netherlands since 1975. Br J Cancer 1998; 77:2053.

109. Ries LA. Influence of extent of disease, histology, and demographic factors on lung cancer survival in the SEER population-based data. Semin Surg Oncol 1994; 10:21.

110. Sant M, Gatta G, Capocaccia R, et al. Survival for lung cancer in northern Italy. Cancer Causes Control 1992; 3:223.

111. Travis WD, Travis LB, Devesa SS. Lung cancer. Cancer 1995; 75:191.

112. Choi NC, Carey RW, Kaufman SD, Grillo HC, Younger J, Wilkins EW Jr. Small cell carcinoma of the lung. A progress report of 15 years' experience. Cancer 1987; 59:6.

113. Connolly CK, Jones WG, Thorogood J, Head C, Muers MF. Investigation, treatment and prognosis of bronchial carcinoma in the Yorkshire region of England 1976–1983. Br J Cancer 1990; 61:579.

114. Janssen-Heijnen ML, Schipper RM, Klinkhamer PJ, Crommelin MA, Coebergh JW. Improvement and plateau in survival of small-cell lung cancer since 1975: a population-based study. Ann Oncol 1998; 9:543.

115. Lassen U, Osterlind K, Hansen M, Dombernowsky P, Bergman B, Hansen HH. Long-term survival in small-cell lung cancer: posttreatment characteristics in patients surviving 5 to 18+ years–an analysis of 1,714 consecutive patients. J Clin Oncol 1995; 13:1215.

116. Skarin AT. Analysis of long-term survivors with small-cell lung cancer. Chest 1993; 103:440S.

117. Souhami RL, Law K. Longevity in small cell lung cancer. A report to the Lung Cancer Subcommittee of the United Kingdom Coordinating Committee for Cancer Research. Br J Cancer 1990; 61:584.

118. Watkin SW, Hayhurst GK, Green JA. Time trends in the outcome of lung cancer management: a study of 9,090 cases diagnosed in the Mersey Region, 1974–86. Br J Cancer 1990; 61:590.

119. Davis S, Wright PW, Schulman SF, Scholes D, Thorning D, Hammar S. Long-term survival in small-cell carcinoma of the lung: a population experience. J Clin Oncol 1985; 3:80.

120. Findlay MP, Griffin AM, Raghavan D, McDonald KE, Coates AS, Duval PJ, Gianoutsos P. Retrospective review of chemotherapy for small cell lung cancer in the elderly: does the end justify the means? Eur J Cancer 1991; 27:1597.

121. Osterlind K, Hansen HH, Hansen M, Dombernowsky P. Mortality and morbidity in long-term surviving patients treated with chemotherapy with or without irradiation for small-cell lung cancer. J Clin Oncol 1986; 4:1044.

122. Schiller JH, Ettinger DS, Larson MM, Gradishar W, Merkel D, Johnson DH. Phase II trial of oral etoposide plus cisplatin in extensive stage small cell carcinoma of the lung: an Eastern Cooperative Oncology Group study. Eur J Cancer 1994; 30A:158.

123. van der Gaast A, Postmus PE, Burghouts J, van Bolhuis C, Stam J, Splinter TA. Long term survival of small cell lung cancer patients after chemotherapy. Br J Cancer 1993; 67:822.

124. Bunn PA, Jr., Van Zandwijk N, Pastorino U, et al. European School of Oncology. First Euro-American forum on lung cancer treatment. Eur J Cancer 1994; 30A:710.

125. van Tinteren H, Hoekstra OS, Smit EF, et al. Effectiveness of positron emission tomography in the preoperative assessment of patients with suspected non-small-cell lung cancer: the PLUS multicentre randomised trial. Lancet 2002; 359:1388.

126. Vansteenkiste JF. FDG-PET for lymph node staging in NSCLC: a major step forward, but beware of the pitfalls. Lung Cancer 2005; 47:151.

127. Brodin O, Nou E, Mercke C, et al. Comparison of induction chemotherapy before radiotherapy with radiotherapy only in patients with locally advanced squamous cell carcinoma of the lung. The Swedish Lung Cancer Study Group. Eur J Cancer 1996; 32A:1893.

128. Jeremic B, Shibamoto Y, Acimovic L, Djuric L. Randomized trial of hyperfractionated radiation therapy with or without concurrent chemotherapy for stage III non-small-cell lung cancer. J Clin Oncol 1995; 13:452.

129. Marino P, Preatoni A, Cantoni A. Randomized trials of radiotherapy alone versus combined chemotherapy and radiotherapy in stages IIIa and IIIb nonsmall cell lung cancer. A meta-analysis. Cancer 1995; 76:593.

130. N/A. Chemotherapy in non-small cell lung cancer: a meta-analysis using updated data on individual patients from 52 randomised clinical trials. Non-small Cell Lung Cancer Collaborative Group. BMJ 1995; 311:899.

131. Pritchard RS, Anthony SP. Chemotherapy plus radiotherapy compared with radiotherapy alone in the treatment of locally advanced, unresectable, non-small-cell lung cancer. A meta-analysis. Ann Intern Med 1996; 125:723.

132. Sause W, Kolesar P, Taylor SI, et al. Final results of phase III trial in regionally advanced unresectable non-small cell lung cancer: Radiation Therapy Oncology Group, Eastern Cooperative Oncology Group, and Southwest Oncology Group. Chest 2000; 117:358.

133. Jett JR. Current treatment of unresectable lung cancer. Mayo Clin Proc 1993; 68:603.

134. Kurup A, Hanna NH. Treatment of small cell lung cancer. Crit Rev Oncol Hematol 2004; 52:117.

135. Lu C, Soria JC, Tang X, et al. Prognostic factors in resected stage I non-small-cell lung cancer: a multivariate analysis of six molecular markers. J Clin Oncol 2004; 22:4575.

136. Janssen-Heijnen ML, Smulders S, Lemmens VE, Smeenk FW, van Geffen HJ, Coebergh JW. Effect of comorbidity on the treatment and prognosis of elderly patients with non-small cell lung cancer. Thorax 2004; 59:602.

137. Potosky AL, Saxman S, Wallace RB, Lynch CF. Population variations in the initial treatment of non-small-cell lung cancer. J Clin Oncol 2004; 22:3261.

138. Guadagnoli E, Weitberg A, Mor V, Silliman RA, Glicksman AS, Cummings FJ. The influence of patient age on the diagnosis and treatment of lung and colorectal cancer. Arch Intern Med 1990; 150:1485.

139. Monfardini S, Yancik R. Cancer in the elderly: meeting the challenge of an aging population. J Natl Cancer Inst 1993; 85:532.

140. Satariano WA. Comorbidity and functional status in older women with breast cancer: implications for screening, treatment, and prognosis. J Gerontol 1992; 47 Spec No:24.

141. Wei JY. Cardiovascular comorbidity in the older cancer patient. Semin Oncol 1995; 22:9.

142. Damhuis RA, Schutte PR. Resection rates and postoperative mortality in 7,899 patients with lung cancer. Eur Respir J 1996; 9:7.

143. Ginsberg RJ, Hill LD, Eagan RT, et al. Modern thirty-day operative mortality for surgical resections in lung cancer. J Thorac Cardiovasc Surg 1983; 86:654.

144. Osaki T, Shirakusa T, Kodate M, Nakanishi R, Mitsudomi T, Ueda H. Surgical treatment of lung cancer in the octogenarian. Ann Thorac Surg 1994; 57:92.

145. Thomas P, Sielezneff I, Ragni J, Giudicelli R, Fuentes P. Is lung cancer resection justified in patients aged over 70 years? Eur J Cardiothorac Surg 1993; 7:246; discussion 50.

146. Battafarano RJ, Piccirillo JF, Meyers BF, Hsu HS, Guthrie TJ, Cooper JD, Patterson GA. Impact of comorbidity on survival after surgical resection in patients with stage I non-small cell lung cancer. J Thorac Cardiovasc Surg 2002; 123:280.

147. Firat S, Bousamra M, Gore E, Byhardt RW. Comorbidity and KPS are independent prognostic factors in stage I non-small-cell lung cancer. Int J Radiat Oncol Biol Phys 2002; 52:1047.

148. Firat S, Byhardt RW, Gore E. Comorbidity and Karnofksy performance score are independent prognostic factors in stage III non-small-cell lung cancer: an institutional analysis of patients treated on four RTOG studies. Radiation Therapy Oncology Group. Int J Radiat Oncol Biol Phys 2002; 54:357.

149. Piccirillo JF, Tierney RM, Costas I, Grove L, Spitznagel EL Jr. Prognostic importance of comorbidity in a hospital-based cancer registry. JAMA 2004; 291:2441.

150. Tammemagi CM, Neslund-Dudas C, Simoff M, Kvale P. Impact of comorbidity on lung cancer survival. Int J Cancer 2003; 103:792.

151. Tammemagi CM, Neslund-Dudas C, Simoff M, Kvale P. In lung cancer patients, age, race-ethnicity, gender and smoking predict adverse comorbidity, which in turn predicts treatment and survival. J Clin Epidemiol 2004a; 57:597.

152. Read WL, Tierney RM, Page NC, Costas I, Govindan R, Spitznagel EL, Piccirillo JF. Differential prognostic impact of comorbidity. J Clin Oncol 2004; 22:3099.

153. Tammemagi CM, Neslund-Dudas C, Simoff M, Kvale P. Smoking and lung cancer survival: the role of comorbidity and treatment. Chest 2004b; 125:27.

154. Batevik R, Grong K, Segadal L, Stangeland L. The female gender has a positive effect on survival independent of background life expectancy following surgical resection of primary non-small cell lung cancer: a study of absolute and relative survival over 15 years. Lung Cancer 2005; 47:173.

155. Xie L, Ugnat AM, Morriss J, Semenciw R, Mao Y. Histology-related variation in the treatment and survival of patients with lung carcinoma in Canada. Lung Cancer 2003; 42:127.

156. Jemal A, Chu KC, Tarone RE. Recent trends in lung cancer mortality in the United States. J Natl Cancer Inst 2001; 93:277.

157. Bach PB, Kelley MJ, Tate RC, McCrory DC. Screening for lung cancer: a review of the current literature. Chest 2003; 123:72S.

158. Diederich S, Wormanns D. Impact of low-dose CT on lung cancer screening. Lung Cancer 2004; 45 Suppl 2:S13.

159. Henschke CI. Experts are cautious, optimistic about detecting lung cancers earlier. J Natl Cancer Inst 1999; 91:1606.

160. Marcus PM. Lung cancer screening: an update. J Clin Oncol 2001; 19:83S.

161. Patz EF Jr, Swensen SJ, Herndon JE 2nd. Estimate of lung cancer mortality from low-dose spiral computed tomography screening trials: implications for current mass screening recommendations. J Clin Oncol 2004; 22:2202.

162. Sone S, Takashima S, Li F, et al. Mass screening for lung cancer with mobile spiral computed tomography scanner. Lancet 1998; 351:1242.

163. Stanzel F. Fluorescent bronchoscopy: contribution for lung cancer screening? Lung Cancer 2004; 45 Suppl 2:S29.

164. Deppermann KM. Lung cancer screening – where we are in 2004 (take home messages). Lung Cancer 2004; 45 Suppl 2:S39.

165. Kennedy TC, Hirsch FR. Using molecular markers in sputum for the early detection of lung cancer: a review. Lung Cancer 2004; 45 Suppl 2:S21.

166. Travis K. Lung cancer screening for all? Not yet, panel says. J Natl Cancer Inst 2004; 96:900.

Screening Programs for Lung Cancer

2

Gerold Bepler and Melvyn Tockman

Contents

2.1   Introduction

Lung cancer continues to be a disease of epidemic proportion. This year alone, it is estimated that 172,570 people will be newly diagnosed with the disease and 163,510 will die in the USA (ACS, Cancer Facts & Figures 2005; http://www.cancer.org/docroot/STT/stt_0.asp). Thus, more people will die from lung cancer than from breast cancer (40,870), colorectal cancer (56,290), and prostate cancer (30,250) combined. Lung cancer alone is responsible for 28.7% of cancer death in the USA. The magnitude of the problem is similar in Europe. Because of an increasing prevalence of cigarette smoking in most parts of the world, it is anticipated that the annual lung cancer mortality may exceed 10 million by 2030. It is estimated that one-third of all deaths in people between the ages of 35 and 69 years are attributable to cigarette smoking in the USA. The relative risk for lung cancer in current smokers is between 10- and 80-fold greater than for those who have never smoked, increasing with the amount smoked and with earlier age of smoking initiation. Almost half of lung cancers currently diagnosed in the USA occur in people with a prior history of cigarette use who successfully quit years before. In addition, lung cancer in those who have never smoked in their life, defined as having smoked less than 100 cigarettes, is on the rise, and estimated to contribute to approximately 16,000 cases per year.

The World Health Organization's international histopathologic classification of lung cancer was last revised in 1999 [1]. The term "lung cancer" comprises all malignant neoplasms of the lung. The current terminology has evolved over the last century and is based on distinct light-microscopy criteria. Squamous and glandular differentiation were the first recognized patterns, followed by the description of "oat-celled sarcoma of the mediastinum" as a lung cancer by Barnard in 1926, and the "bronchogenic large-cell carcinoma" as a lung cancer without squamous or glandular features by Patton in 1951. These four major histologic lung cancer types account for approximately 31% (squamous cell carcinoma), 21% (small cell carcinoma), 35% (adenocarcinoma), and 11% (large cell carcinoma) of cases respectively (SEER data 1983–1992; http://seer.cancer.gov). The remaining cases are other histopathologic lung cancer entities that include adenosquamous carcinomas, adenoid cystic carcinomas, mucoepidermoid carcinomas, carcinoid tumors, malignant mesotheliomas, and others. From a cell biological perspective, carcinoids and mesotheliomas are clearly distinct from adeno-, squamous, and large-cell carcinomas. Adenocarcinomas, squamous carcinomas, and large-cell carcinomas, hereafter referred to as non-small-cell lung cancers (NSCLC), are closely interrelated, share common risk factors and epidemiology, are frequently found simultaneously in tumor specimens, and are uniformly approached with common therapeutic interventions.

The 5-year survival from lung cancer has kept pace with the improvement in 5-year survival from all cancers over the last 40 years. Yet, it remains disappointingly low at approximately 15%. This improvement in 5-year survival is a result of heightened awareness, better technology for detection, better selection of patients for various therapeutic options, and the selective use of palliative interventions. However, lung cancer mortality remains extraordinarily high, and it is the benchmark by which future generations will judge our success in effectively combatting this disease.

Survival of patients with lung cancer is predominantly a function of disease stage, and it declines with increasing stage [2]. For patients with stages I and II NSCLC, long-term survival (≥5 years) can be achieved by surgery with or without systemic therapy. For patients with stage III disease, long-term survival is less likely (15–25% 5-year survival), and the mainstay for treatment is radiation in combination with systemic therapy if possible. Patients with stage IV disease rarely live beyond 5 years, and treatment predominantly consists of systemic therapy given with the goal of palliation.

For lung cancer patients, achieving 5-year survival most often (approximately 95% of cases) means that the disease will not recur and thus not cause mortality. It is exactly this observation that forms the basis for the lung cancer screening hypothesis, that implementation of a methodology that allows for detection of the disease at a point in time when it is surgically resectable rather than when it is unresectable will result in cure and consequently a decrease in mortality.

This hypothesis sets the stage for the primary outcome parameters by which studies that test lung cancer screening modalities must be judged. These are a stage shift: a reduction in the number of people with unresectable disease in the screened group compared to an unscreened group and mortality (i.e., a reduction in the number of people who die in the screened group compared to an unscreened group). In successful screening, demonstration of a stage shift precedes demonstration of a mortality reduction.

Other parameters are often considered as measures of screening efficacy. The two most frequently used are an increase in 5-year survival and an increase in the number of resectable cases. Both of these outcome parameters are necessary, but insufficient antecedents of a mortality reduction. They are insufficient indicators of a screening benefit because an increase in the number of resectable cases and improved 5-year survival may also result for lead-time and length-time bias. These biases, inherent to screening of asymptomatic subjects, prevent consideration of either the number of resectable cases or an improved survival as surrogate indicators of mortality, and cannot ultimately serve to assess the success of a screening program. Both biases are well explained in recent reviews [3–5].

Among the methodologies available for lung cancer screening, radiography has been most extensively studied. Other methods include cytomorphology, and more recently, molecular assays.

2.2   Standard Chest Radiography

Three large randomized trials were coordinated by the United States National Cancer Institute (the NCI Collaborative Lung Cancer Trials) during the 1960s and 1970s [6–8]. These trials differed from earlier screening trials conducted in Europe [9] by testing whether sputum cytology plus chest radiography (CXR) would lead to a greater reduction in lung cancer mortality than CXR alone. A similar trial was conducted in Czechoslovakia in the 1970s [10]. People without symptoms for lung cancer had CXR two to three times per year for up to 6 years. The results are summarized in Table 2.1. In all trials, more cancers were surgically resectable, and 5-year survival rates were better in the screened groups compared to the control groups. However, mortality rates from lung cancer, overall mortality, and the number of unresectable cases were not significantly reduced on final evaluation. As a result, professional organizations currently do not recommend using CXR for lung cancer screening. Interestingly, in all these trials, the more intensely screened arms had more lung cancer cases. Had these excess cases appeared early during screening followed by equalization of case numbers later on, the excess might be explained by lead- or length-time bias. Because the excess cases persisted after several years of screening, they are more likely the result of overdiagnosis. Overdiagnosis is an extreme form of length-time bias, where asymptomatic persons are diagnosed with the disease as a result of screening; however, the disease would have not impacted on their lives. In addition, contamination of the control groups may have contributed to these disappointing results, since many persons in the control groups actually had CXR more frequently (approximately every 24 months in the Mayo study) than would be expected in a healthy population.

2.3   Computed Tomography of the Chest

Computed tomography (CT) of the chest has several distinct advantages over standard CXR as a tool for lung cancer screening. First, CT sensitivity is superior to CXR in the detection of pulmonary lesions that may represent lung cancer [11], a finding that was confirmed in two screening trials that compared low-dose CT with CXR in the same people (27 lung cancers detected by CT vs 7 by CXR in one study; 13 by CT vs 5 by CXR in the other study) [12, 13]. Second, images on CT are acquired digitally, which facilitates automated image analysis. CT technology has advanced to a level whereby high-resolution imaging studies of the chest can be performed in seconds, thus reducing the inconvenience to the subjects. However, CT screening also has disadvantages. These include high cost, high radiation exposure, and the high rate of detection of lung abnormalities that may not be neoplastic.

The actual economic cost for lung cancer screening is unknown, but it has been suggested that it is between US$ 116,000 and US$ 2,300,000 per quality-adjusted life-year gained if screening by CT is done on a population of current and former smokers over the age of 60 years

Table 2.1. Overview of lung cancer screening randomized trials with chest radiography application

Autor	Trial characteristics								Prevalence screening			Incidence screening					Lung cancer mortality	
	Country	Year	Number of subjects	Number of subjects screened	Intervention	Men/Women	Age (years)	% Subjects ever smokers	% Subjects with lung cancer by CXR (N)	Patients with resectable lung cancer	Patients with unresectable lung cancer	No subjects with lung cancer (screen/control)	Screening-detected lung cancer in screening group	Interval lung cancer in screening group	Patients with resectable lung cancer (screen/control)	Patients with unresectable lung cancer (screen/control)	Screening group (N)	Control group (N)
Brett et al. [9]	UK	1968	55034	29416	q 6 months ×3 years	all/none	≥40	88%	0.09% (51)	31	20	101/76	65	36	44/22	57/54	0.28% (82)	0.27% (68)
Fontana et al. [8]*	USA	1986	10933	4618	q 4 months ×6 years	all/none	≥45	100%	0.68% (74)	33	41	206/160	90	116	94/51	112/109	2.64% (122)	1.82% (115)
Kubik et al. [10]*	Czeckoslovakia	1990	6364	3171	q 6 months ×3 years	all/none	≥40	100%	0.30% (19)			36/19	26	10	19/4	17/15	2.68% (85)	2.10% (67)

* The trial also used sputum cytology in addition to CXR.

[14]. Other economic analyses have suggested lower cost. Clear data on the impact of excess radiation exposure from frequent CT imaging on a potential lung cancer screening population are not available. However, it has been suggested that the number of lung cancers would increase by 1.8% if 50% of current and former cigarette smokers between the ages 50 and 75 years would have annual low-dose CT screening on single-slice scanners in the USA [15].

Abnormalities in the lung found on CT that may represent lung cancer can have a variety of features. Among these, noncalcified pulmonary nodules (NCPNs) are the most well defined and consistently described in the literature. Ground-glass opacities are another frequently encountered abnormality. In published CT screening trials, NCPNs were found in 5–50% of people screened [16, 17], suggesting that a significant number of subsequent tests will be required to follow and differentiate the detected abnormalities.

To date, results from randomized lung cancer screening trials using CT are not available. However, several large, single-arm trials have been reported. Pertinent results from 8 trials that included at least 500 subjects are summarized in Table 2.2, and all were reported since 1999 [12, 13, 16–23].

All eight trials used age as the key criterion to enrich for people at increased risk for lung cancer. In fact, when the results from four trials [13, 16, 19, 21] were analyzed for lung cancer detection by age cohorts, there was a near doubling in lung cancer risk from decade to decade [24]. Past or present cigarette smoking was a requirement for participation in five trials [12, 17–19, 23]. One trial required evidence of asbestos exposure [23], and another initially required evidence of obstructive pulmonary disease for enrollment [18]. Three trials were done in the USA [12, 17, 18], three in Japan [13, 16, 21], and two in Europe [19, 23]. Thus despite similar study hypotheses and designs, substantial population differences are present among these trials, making a direct comparison difficult.

On first screening, referred to as the prevalence screening, the overwhelming number of lung cancers were detected at potentially resectable stages (134 out of a total of 163; 82%). In the older screening studies, the proportion of resectable lung cancers on prevalence screening was substantially lower (64 out of a total of 125; 51%). Although this historical comparison is not conclusive, it is consistent with studies that directly compared CT with CXR in the same individuals [12, 13] and demonstrated that CT screening is more sensitive for lung cancer detection than CXR, resulting in the detection of more resectable cancers. However, 29 of the prevalence detected lung cancers were in advanced stages. In the CT screening study conducted at the Mayo clinic, 4 out of 1,520 patients (0.26%) had advanced-stage lung cancer compared to 41 out of 10,933 (0.38%) in the earlier CXR-based Mayo screening trial.

Preliminary results on follow-up screening CTs, referred to as incidence screening, are summarized in Table 2.2. The published data are incomplete and do not allow for a comprehensive assessment of the efficacy of CT as a screening tool. However, some important knowledge has been gained. In the USA trials, annual CT screening uncovered the development of NCPNs in 5–15% of participants per year, and the emergence of lung cancer in 0.4 to ≥0.9% of participants per year. Data from the Japanese trials suggest that the annual rate of lung cancer is below 0.4% in populations undergoing screening in Japan. European data are not available. Incidence-detected lung cancers are predominantly in resectable disease stages (80 out of a total of 100; 80%). These numbers are better than those reported from the older CXR-based screening trials (157 out of a total of 343; 46%). However, 20 of the incidence-detected lung cancers were in advanced stages, and only two of the six trials with reported incidence data included interval lung cancers in their reports [20, 22]. Interval cases are those that occur in the time that elapses between two screening studies and are not detected as part of the screening evaluation. In the CXR-based screening trials, 28–56% of all lung cancers in the screened group were interval cases. In the CT screening study conducted at the Mayo clinic, 6 advanced lung cancers occurred during 2,916 screening encounters (0.21%) [22]. In the Cornell study, 3 advanced lung cancers occurred during 1,184 screening encounters (0.25%) [20]. In the CXR-based Mayo clinic screening trial, 112 advanced lung cancers occurred during approximately 62,500 screening encounters (0.18%; total of 18 incident CXRs per subject over 6 years, with a 75% compliance rate) [8].

The positive predictive value (proportion of lung cancers among those with suspicious lesions) of CT-detected abnormalities for lung cancer is approximately 0.02–0.12, and it is thus in a range comparable to that of mammography or fecal occult blood testing in breast and colorectal cancer screening, respectively [25, 26]. Neither the specificity nor the sensitivity of CT scanning for lung cancer detection can be assessed because the proportion of individuals "truly negative" for lung cancer at the time of testing is unknown.

Whether CT-based lung cancer screening will result in a reduction of disease-specific mortality cannot be answered with certainty at this time. In the USA a randomized trial of annual CT versus CXR screening is ongoing in persons at risk for the disease [27]. This trial completed its enrollment and prevalence-screening phase in February of 2004. Incidence screening is ongoing, and it is hoped that the trial will generate more conclusive data on the true value of chest CT on lung cancer mortality reduction.

2.4 Developing Methods for Lung Cancer Screening

2.4.1 Cytomorphology

Papanicolaou and Saccomanno pioneered cytomorphology for the early detection of lung cancer, demonstrating that premalignant cytological changes can be detected several years prior to the clinical diagnosis of lung cancer [28, 29]. Evaluation of sputum specimens for cytomorphologic changes consistent with cancer was part of the NCI Collaborative Lung Cancer Screening Trials described earlier. They found no mortality benefit from morphologic evaluation of sputum specimens [8, 30, 31]. The trials observed that malignant cytomorphology was often associated with occult central lesions on CXR, most of which were squamous cell carcinomas [6, 7 32]. However, in a CXR-screened population, only 14% of lung cancers are radiographically occult [31]. A recent evaluation of sputum morphology demonstrated a relative lung cancer risk of 3.3 in individuals with moderate or higher-grade sputum atypia when compared to matched controls with normal sputum cytology [33]. Although insensitive for early lung cancer detection, sputum cytomorphologic assessment is part of most of the CT-based screening trials summarized in Table 2.2. As a result, microscope imaging and molecular techniques are now being explored as novel methods for early lung cancer detection on these easily and noninvasively collectable biospecimens [34, 35].

The nuclear features of epithelial cells have been investigated in sputum specimens from the CXR-based NCI Collaborative Lung Cancer Screening trials [36]. Seventy-three sputum slides were restained with a modified Feulgen method followed by automated image cytometry [37]. The investigators examined 40 slides from 9 patients in whom squamous carcinoma had developed, and 33 slides from 11 patients in whom no cancer had developed during a follow-up period of ≥5 years. Using nuclear features based on DNA distribution, a correct classification of nuclei was possible in 74% of the cases without human review of the material and without the use of visually abnormal nuclei. The receiver operating characteristic curve demonstrated 40% sensitivity at 90% specificity. A substantial number of patients with squamous cell cancer was detected in these 20-year-old slides without requiring a pathologist to recognize visually abnormal nuclei. This demonstrates that it is possible to detect subjects with early lung cancers even in the absence of malignant cells in the sputum.

Most recently, this group of investigators conducted a prospective study to evaluate whether automated quantitative image cytometry (AQC) of sputum cells can be conducted to improve the lung cancer detection rate [35]. A total of 561 current or former smokers ≥50 years of age with a ≥30 pack-year smoking history were studied. Among these, 423 were found to have ≥5 cells with abnormal DNA content by AQC. Of the 14 lung cancers in this study cohort, AQC detected 13 (sensitivity 92.8%) and chest CT detected 11 (sensitivity 71.4%). However, AQC identified 410 persons as abnormal who did not have lung cancer, resulting in a specificity of only 25% [35]. For a lung cancer screening test, a high specificity is crucial in order to avoid a costly and inconvenient subsequent work-up with its inevitable morbidity and mortality for those who are "false positive".

2.4.2 Molecular Assays

The basis for the development of molecular assays for lung cancer screening is the observation that the majority of lung cancers carry somatic genetic alterations that are not present in the normal constitutional germline DNA. However, several important aspects of existing knowledge have to be considered in the development of molecular assays for the purpose of detection of resectable lung cancer.

First, the process of lung cancer development from its normal cellular counterpart in the airways is thought of as a gradual evolutionary process with multiple intermediate steps that can be identified by morphologic or molecular parameters. From completely sectioned autopsy specimens, three progressive grades of histologic abnormality have been recognized in the bronchial epithelium: hyperplasia (an increase in the number of cell rows), metaplasia (loss of cilia), and dysplasia (presence of atypical cells) [38, 39]. In addition, an association between the frequency of carcinoma-in-situ and the frequency of smoking was noted, from 0% in nonsmokers to 11% in heavy smokers (≥2 packs per day).

Second, the precise molecular progression of normal airway epithelium to lung cancer is only rudimentarily understood. As a result, many somatic genetic alterations found in lung cancer are also present in morphologically premalignant lesions of the airways, and often in morphologically normal epithelial cells.

Third, widespread morphological damage exists in the aerodigestive tract of current and former smokers (field cancerization) [40]. Field cancerization implies that the entire bronchial epithelium is at increased risk of developing neoplastic lesions, and detection of premalignant or malignant lesions in one area may occur synchronously or metachronously to a similar process in one or more other regions of the airways.

Fourth, although enormous progress has been made in the development of technology required for precise molecular investigations, most of it has been developed

Table 2.2. Overview of large (more than 500 persons), single-arm only, lung cancer screening trials

Author	Trial characteristics					Prevalence screening					
	Intervention	Men/women	Age (years)	% Subjects ever smokers	Smoking packs×years	Number of subjects	% Subjects with NCPNs	No subjects with lung cancer (%)	Stage I & II (N)	Stage III (N)	Stage IV (N)
Henschke et al. [12]	CT & CXR×1, CT q12 m no limit	540/460	≥60	100%	≥10	1000	23.3%	27 (2.7%)	24	3	0
Sone et al. [16]	CT q 12 m×3	2971/2512	≥40	46%	not required	5483	5.1%	23 (0.4%)	23	0	0
Diederich et al. [19]	CT×1	588/229	≥40	100%	≥20	817	50.1%	11 (1.4%)	8	3	0
Nawa et al. [21]	CT q 12 m×2	6319/1637	≥50	62%	not required	7956	26.4%	36 (0.5%)	35	1	0
Sobue et al. [13]	CT, CXR, Sputum q 6 m no limit	1415/196	40–80	86%	not required	1611	11.5%	13 (0.8%)	10	3	0
Swensen et al. [22]	CT & Sputum q 12 m×4	785/735	≥50	100%	≥20	1520	51.4%	21 (1.4%)	17	4	0
Tiitola et al. [23]	CT & CXR x1	591/11	38–81	97%	≥10	602	18.4%	5 (0.8%)	1	2	2
Clark et al. [18]	CT & Sputum q 12 m×5	684/467	≥45	100%	≥30	1151	35.3%	27 (2.3%)	16	6	5

Author	Intervention	First incidence screening					
		Number of subjects	% Subjects with NCPNs	No subjects with lung cancer (%)	Stage I & II (N)	Stage III (N)	Stage IV (N)
Henschke et al. [12]		841					
Sone et al. [16]	*# interval cases not given	4425	3.9%	27 (0.6%)*	25	2	0
Nawa et al. [21]	*# interval cases not given	5568		4 (0.0007%)*	4	0	0
Sobue et al. [13]	*# interval cases not given	1180	7.1%	3 (0.3%)*			
Swensen et al. [22]	**new nodules only	1478	14.0%**				
Clark et al. [18]	*# interval cases not given	930	25.3%	8 (0.9%)*			

Second incidence screening

	Number of subjects	% Subjects with NCPNs	No subjects with lung cancer (%)	Stage I & II (N)	Stage III (N)	Stage IV (N)
Henschke et al. [12]	343					
Sone et al. [16]	3878	3.5%	10 (0.3%)*	9	0	1
Sobue et al. [13]	891	6.5%	5 (0.6%)*			
Swensen et al. [22]	1438	9%**				
Clark et al. [18]	612	22.4%	7 (1.1%)*			

*# interval cases not given (Sone et al. [16])
*# interval cases not given (Sobue et al. [13])
**new nodules only (Swensen et al. [22])
*# interval cases not given (Clark et al. [18])

3rd incidence screening

	Number of subjects	% Subjects with NCPNs	No subjects with lung cancer (%)	Stage I & II (N)	Stage III (N)	Stage IV (N)
Henschke et al. [12]	not reported					
Sobue et al. [13]	774	9.8%	2 (0.3%)*			
Swensen et al. [22]	not reported					
Clark et al. [18]	356	22.8%	2 (0.6%)*			

*# interval cases not given (Sobue et al. [13])
*# interval cases not given (Clark et al. [18])

4th incidence screening

	Number of subjects	% Subjects with NCPNs	No subjects with lung cancer (%)	Stage I & II (N)	Stage III (N)	Stage IV (N)
Henschke et al. [12]	not reported					
Sobue et al. [13]	669	10.2%	4 (0.6%)*			
Clark et al. [18]	140	15.7%	1 (0.7%)*			

*# interval cases not given (Sobue et al. [13])
*# interval cases not given (Clark et al. [18])

Incidence screening (all)

	Number of CTs	% CTs with NCPNs	No subjects with lung cancer	Stage I & II (N)	Stage III (N)	Stage IV (N)
Henschke et al. [12]	1184	5.3%**	9 (0.8%)***	6	3	0
Sone et al. [16]	8303	3.7%	37 (0.4%)*	34	2	1
Nawa et al. [21]	5568		4 (0.0007%)*	4	0	0
Sobue et al. [13]	7891	9.1%	19 (0.2%)*	16	2	1
Swensen et al. [22]	2916	11.5%**	13 (0.4%)****	7	5	1
Clark et al. [18]	2038	23.3%	18 (0.9%)*	13	2	3

**new nodules only; ***includes 2 interval cases (Henschke et al. [12])
*# interval cases not given (Sone et al. [16])
*# interval cases not given (Nawa et al. [21])
*# interval cases not given (Sobue et al. [13])
**new nodules only; ****includes 2 interval cases and 1 case detected by sputum cytology only (Swensen et al. [22])
*# interval cases not given (Clark et al. [18])

for molecular laboratory studies or for the application to clinical specimens with a known morphological diagnosis. Thus, most available molecular methods perform excellently in the environment for which they were designed; however, if applied to the environment of early detection of clinically meaningful disease (i.e., the detection of resectable lung cancer), their performance may be inadequate. For example, if the presence or absence of a nucleotide mutation or epigenetic alteration is used as a marker for lung cancer, then the methodology used for detection of such a change should not be able to generate such alterations during the assay process (i.e., generation of false-positive results). As another example, the presence or absence of a nucleotide mutation or epigenetic alteration must be specific to the disease under investigation (i.e., resectable lung cancer), and should not be present in clinically untreatable precursor lesions.

Some examples of molecular markers under development are aneuploidy, allele loss, microsatellite instability, and DNA methylation.

2.4.1.1 Aneuploidy

Sputum specimens from 33 cases and matched controls were investigated for aneusomy (nondiploid chromosome content) with a DNA fluorescence in situ hybridization assay. In specimens collected within 12 months prior to the lung cancer diagnosis, aneusomy was more frequent among cases (41%) than controls (6%; $p = 0.04$), and it was not associated with cytologic atypia. Combining aneusomy with cytology, any abnormality was found in 83% of the cases and 20% of the controls ($p = 0.0004$), suggesting that aneusomy improves the sensitivity of cytology as a predictor of lung cancer [41].

2.4.1.2 Allele Loss

An increasing frequency of allele loss in specific chromosomal regions has been described with increasing severity of histopathological changes in bronchial epithelium [42]. This genetic damage is widespread throughout the airways, even in areas of normal-appearing epithelium, and persists long after removal of the insult. As a result, these genetic changes could serve as markers of carcinogenesis and may be useful in the selection of populations with defined risks for lung cancer. In addition, the pattern of allele loss may be specific for certain types of cancer and the level of progression during tumor development. A high incidence of allele loss on chromosomes 3, 5, 8, 9, 10, 11, 17, and 20 has been described in lung cancer specimens [43–45], although the role of these changes in carcinogenesis is not yet known. Perhaps it is the cumulative effect of these genetic injuries that is important. It has recently been shown that genetic alterations at selected loci can

be recognized in sputum cells prior to clinical lung cancer [46]. Unfortunately, the results show a low sensitivity, perhaps due to dilution by the large numbers of inflammatory cells frequently seen in the sputum of smokers. European investigators have reported success by analyzing sputum for allele loss at multiple loci [47].

2.4.1.3 Microsatellite Instability

Microsatellites are di-, tri-, or tetranucleotide polymorphisms that are distributed throughout the genome, have a high degree of heterozygosity, and usually occur in multiple alleles. Expansion and reduction in the number of repeats has been observed in epithelial malignancy, and they are thought to arise from inefficient repair of physiologic mistakes that occur during DNA replication of such repeats (polymerase slippage). The presence of multiple new alleles in tumor specimens as a result of this process has been termed microsatellite instability (MSI). Thus the detection of MSI can potentially serve as a molecular marker of lung cancer. However, while widespread MSI was first reported in colorectal tumors [48], it is rarely observed in lung cancers. In addition, MSI can be observed as a false-positive result of the in vitro polymerase chain reaction that is performed with DNA polymerase for the purpose of generating sufficient amounts of DNA from a minute amount of target for detection. Thus, it is unlikely that MSI analysis will gain general acceptance as a molecular assay for the early detection of lung cancer. However, in a blinded study, microsatellite changes matching those in the tumor were detected in the urine sediment of 19 out of 20 patients (95%) who were diagnosed with bladder cancer, whereas standard urine cytopathology detected cancer cells in samples from only 9 out of 18 patients (50%) [49]. The specificity was 100% (in five noncancer cases). The NCI Early Detection Research Network is currently validating microsatellite analysis for the detection of bladder cancer in a multicenter trial.

2.4.1.4 *Kras* Mutations

Mutation of the *Kras* oncogene is one of the most commonly occurring genetic lesions in colorectal cancer [50], and it is mutated in approximately one-third of lung cancers [51]. Specific mutations have been detected in nonmalignant sputum specimens in advance of clinical lung cancer [52]. The study demonstrated that 8 out of 15 patients (53%) with adenocarcinoma or large-cell carcinoma of the lung could be detected by mutations in sputum cells from 1 to 13 months prior to clinical diagnosis. The ability to identify specific gene abnormalities is limited by the need to know the specific mutation sequence with which to probe the sputum specimens. In the study quoted above, the mutation sequence was determined from the resected tumor. This approach is obviously not practical for screening undiagnosed individuals at present. Perhaps with future advances in gene-chip technology, it might become feasible to probe for all possible mutations of common oncogenes and tumor suppressor genes in the sputum specimens of asymptomatic individuals.

2.4.1.5 Abnormal DNA Methylation

Methylation of the cytosine in so-called CpG islands is a physiologic process that results in activation or inactivation of DNA segments. This can lead to transcriptional silencing of genes that may serve important functions in the maintenance of a normal cellular phenotype [53]. Examples include the *CDKN2A* gene, which encodes p16^{INK4A} and p14^{ARF}, and the *ras*-association domain family 1 (*RASSF1*) gene. Both are silenced in many cancers through aberrant promoter hypermethylation [54, 55]. Hypermethylation of the CpG islands of the *p16* gene has been demonstrated in sputum from lung cancer patients [56]. The investigators suggest that detection of *p16* hypermethylation might be useful in the prediction of individuals at risk for the disease. Investigators from the Johns Hopkins and Colorado Lung Cancer SPOREs have conducted a nested case-control study to determine whether a panel of methylation markers could be developed to predict risk and/or detect lung cancer early. Methylation of the *p16*, *MGMT*, *RASSF1A*, *H-cadherin*, *PAX5-alpha*, *PAX5-beta*, *GATA5*, and *DAPK* genes was assessed in sputum specimens. Individual odds ratios (ORs) ranged from 1.0 to 2.2 for detecting methylation of a specific gene in cases versus controls. These studies suggest that while the presence of any one of these methylation markers in sputum confers a marked increase in the relative risk (OR = 4.0) for lung cancer, investigators are unlikely to be able to detect promoter hypermethylation within the developing tumor through the analysis of sputum [34]. The greater potential of sputum methylation markers will be to assess the relative risk of cancer by detecting field cancerization through quantifying the number of hypermethylated loci rather than detecting cancer by recognizing hypermethylation of specific genes.

Key Points

- The benchmark for any cancer screening technology is a reduction in disease-specific mortality and a reduction in incurable disease.
- Lung cancer screening with chest radiography (CXR) does not reduce overall or disease-specific mortality. Chest computed tomography (CT) detects more lung cancers in early and resectable stages than CXR-based screening. The smallest diameter of detectable lesions is below 3 mm. The positive predictive value of CT-detected abnormalities for lung cancer is approximately 0.02–0.12.

- Whether CT-based lung cancer screening will achieve these goals can not be answered at present.
- The evaluation of sputum specimens with currently available technology does not add to the present status of early detection of lung cancer. However, sputum is an easily accessible biospecimen that may become useful in future studies both for early detection and for risk assessment and stratification.
- All methods of early detection of lung cancer must be used within a controlled and approved clinical research initiative.

References

1. Travis WD, Colby TV, Corrin B, et al. World Health Organization Classification of Lung and Pleural Tumors. Springer-Verlag, Berlin, 1999.
2. Mountain C. Revisions in the International System for Staging Lung Cancer. Chest 1997; 111:1710.
3. Eddy DM. Screening for lung cancer. Ann Intern Med 1989; 111: 232.
4. Patz E, Goodman P, Bepler G. Screening for lung cancer. N Engl J Med 2000; 343:1627.
5. Strauss GM. The Mayo Lung Cohort: a regression analysis focusing on lung cancer incidence and mortality. J Clin Oncol 2002; 20:1973.
6. Frost JK, Ball WC, Levin ML, et al. Early lung cancer detection: results of the initial (prevalence) radiologic and cytologic screening in the Johns Hopkins study. Am Rev Respir Dis 1984; 130:549.
7. Flehinger BJ, Melamed MR, Zaman MB, et al. Early lung cancer detection: results of the initial (prevalence) radiologic and cytologic screening in the Memorial Sloan-Kettering study. Am Rev Respir Dis 1984; 130:555.
8. Fontana RS, Sanderson DR, Woolner LB, et al. Screening for lung cancer. A critique of the Mayo Lung Project. Cancer 1991; 67:1155.
9. Brett GZ. The value of lung cancer detection by six-monthly chest radiographs. Thorax 1968; 23:414.
10. Kubik A, Polak J. Lung cancer detection. Results of a randomized prospective study in Czechoslovakia. Cancer 1986; 57:2427.
11. Milla N, Ito K, Ikeda M, et al. Fundamental and clinical evaluation of chest computed tomography imaging in detectability of pulmonary nodule. Nagoya J Med Sci 1994; 57:127.
12. Henschke CI, McCauley DI, Yankelevitz DF, et al. Early Lung Cancer Action Project: overall design and findings from baseline screening. Lancet 1999; 354:99.
13. Sobue T, Moriyama N, Kaneko M, et al. Screening for lung cancer with low-dose helical computed tomography: anti-lung cancer association project. J Clin Oncol 2002; 20:911.
14. Mahadevia PJ, Fleisher LA, Frick KD, et al. Lung cancer screening with helical computed tomography in older adult smokers: a decision and cost-effectiveness analysis. J Am Med Assoc 2003; 289:313.
15. Brenner DJ. Radiation risks potentially associated with low-dose CT screening of adult smokers for lung cancer. Radiology 2004; 231:440.
16. Sone S, Li F, Yang ZG, Honda T, et al. Results of three-year mass screening programme for lung cancer using a mobile low-dose spiral computed tomography scanner. Br J Cancer 2001; 84:25.

17. Swensen SJ, Jett JR, Sloan JA, et al. Screening for lung cancer with low-dose spiral computed tomography. Am J Respir Crit Care Med 2002; 165:508.

18. Clark RA, Hazelton TR, Coppage L, et al. Screening for lung cancer with CT: a preliminary cost-effectiveness analysis. Radiology 2005; in press.

19. Diederich S, Wormanns D, Semik M, et al. Screening for early lung cancer with low-dose spiral CT: prevalence in 817 asymptomatic smokers. Radiology 2002; 222:773.

20. Henschke CI, Naidich DP, Yakelevitz DF, et al. Early lung cancer action project: initial findings on repeat screenings. Cancer 2001; 92:153.

21. Nawa T, Nakagawa T, Kusano S, et al. Lung cancer screening using low-dose spiral CT: results of baseline and 1-year follow-up studies. Chest 2002; 122:15.

22. Swensen SJ, Jett JR, Hartman TE, et al. Lung cancer screening with CT: Mayo Clinic experience. Radiology 2003; 226:756.

23. Tiitola M, Kivisaari L, Huuskonen MS, et al. Computed tomography screening for lung cancer in asbestos-exposed workers. Lung Cancer 2002; 35:17.

24. Bepler G, Carney DG, Djulbegovic B, et al. A systematic review and lessons learned from early lung cancer detection trials using low-dose computed tomography of the chest. Cancer Control 2003; 10:306.

25. Eddy D. Screening for colorectal cancer. Ann Intern Med 1990; 113:373.

26. Eddy DM. Screening for breast cancer. Ann Intern Med 1989; 111:389.

27. Gohagan J, Marcus P, Fagerstrom R, et al. Baseline findings of a randomized feasibility trial of lung cancer screening with spiral CT scan vs chest radiograph: the Lung Screening Study of the National Cancer Institute. Chest 2004; 126:114.

28. Cromwell HA, Papanicolaou GN. Use of the cytologic method in industrial medicine with special reference to tumors of the lung and the bladder. A M A Arch Ind Hyg Occup Med 1952; 5:232.

29. Saccomanno G, Saunders RP, Ellis H, et al. Concentration of carcinoma or atypical cells in sputum. Acta Cytol 1963; 63:305.

30. Melamed MR, Flehinger BJ, Zaman MB, et al. Screening for early lung cancer. Results of the Memorial Sloan-Kettering study in New York. Chest 1984; 86:44.

31. Tockman MS. Screening (lung cancer). Chest 1986; 89:324S.

32. Fontana RS, Sanderson DR, Taylor WF, et al. Early lung cancer detection: results of the initial (prevalence) radiologic and cytologic screening in the Mayo Clinic study. Am Rev Respir Dis 1984; 130:561.

33. Prindiville SA, Byers T, Hirsch FR, et al. Sputum cytological atypia as a predictor of incident lung cancer in a cohort of heavy smokers with airflow obstruction. Cancer Epidemiol Biomarkers Prev 2003; 12:987.

34. Belinsky SA. Gene-promoter hypermethylation as a biomarker in lung cancer. Nat Rev Cancer 2004; 4:707.

35. McWilliams A, Mayo J, MacDonald S, et al. Lung cancer screening: a different paradigm. Am J Respir Crit Care Med 2003; 168:1167.

36. Payne PW, Sebo TJ, Doudkine A, et al. Sputum screening by quantitative microscopy: a reexamination of a portion of the National Cancer Institute Cooperative Early Lung Cancer Study. Mayo Clin Proc 1997; 72:697.

37. Zhang Y, LeRiche JC, Jackson SM, et al. An automated image cytometry system for monitoring DNA ploidy and other cell features of radiotherapy and chemotherapy patients. Radiat Med 1999; 17:47.

38. Auerbach O, Stout AP, Hammond EC, et al. Changes in bronchial epithelium in relation to cigarette smoking and in relation to lung cancer. N Engl J Med 1961; 265:253.

39. Auerbach O, Hammond EC, Garfinkel L. Changes in bronchial epithelium in relation to cigarette smoking, 1955–1960 vs. 1970–1977. N Engl J Med 1979; 300:381.

40. Slaughter DP, Southwick HW, Smejkal W. Field cancerization in oral stratified squamous epithelium; clinical implications of multicentric origin. Cancer 1953; 6:963.

41. Varella-Garcia M, Kittelson J, Schulte AP, Vu KO, et al. Multi-target interphase fluorescence in situ hybridization assay increases sensitivity of sputum cytology as a predictor of lung cancer. Cancer Detect Prev 2004; 28:244.

42. Wistuba I, Behrens C, Milchgrub S, et al. Sequential molecular abnormalities are involved in the multistage development of squamous cell lung carcinoma. Oncogene 1999; 18:643.

43. Bepler G, Garcia-Blanco MA. Three tumor-suppressor regions on chromosome 11p identified by high-resolution deletion mapping in human non-small-cell lung cancer. Proc Natl Acad Sci U S A 1994; 91:5513.

44. Mao L, Lee JS, Kurie JM, et al. Clonal genetic alterations in the lungs of current and former smokers. J Natl Cancer Inst 1997; 89:857.

45. Xu LH, Bonacum J, Wu L, et al. Identification of frequently altered microsatellite markers for clinical detection of non-small cell lung cancer. Proc Annu Meet Am Assoc Cancer Res 1997; 38:329.

46. Tockman MS, Mulshine JL. The early detection of occult lung cancer. Chest Surg Clin N Am 2000; 10:737.

47. Arvanitis DA, Papadakis E, Zafiropoulos A, et al. Fractional allele loss is a valuable marker for human lung cancer detection in sputum. Lung Cancer 2003; 40:55.

48. Peinado MA, Malkhosyan S, Velazquez A, et al. Isolation and characterization of allelic losses and gains in colorectal tumors by arbitrarily primed polymerase chain reaction. Proc Natl Acad Sci U S A 1992; 89:10065.

49. Mao L, Schoenberg MP, Scicchitano M, et al. Molecular detection of primary bladder cancer by microsatellite analysis. Science 1996; 271:659.

50. Bos JL, Fearon ER, Hamilton SR, et al. Prevalence of ras gene mutations in human colorectal cancers. Nature 1987; 327:293.

51. Rodenhuis S, van de Wetering ML, Mooi WJ, et al. Mutational activation of the K-ras oncogene. A possible pathogenetic factor in adenocarcinoma of the lung. N Engl J Med 1987; 317:929.

52. Mao L, Hruban RH, Boyle JO, et al. Detection of oncogene mutations in sputum precedes diagnosis of lung cancer. Cancer Res 1994; 54:1634.

53. Jones PA, Baylin SB. The fundamental role of epigenetic events in cancer. Nat Rev Genet 2002; 3:415.

54. Dammann R, Li C, Yoon JH, et al. Epigenetic inactivation of a RAS association domain family protein from the lung tumour suppressor locus 3p21.3. Nat Genet 2000; 25:315.

55. Merlo A, Herman JG, Mao L, et al. 5′ CpG island methylation is associated with transcriptional silencing of the tumour suppressor p16/CDKN2/MTS1 in human cancers. Nat Med 1995; 7:686.

56. Belinsky S, Nikula K, Palmisano W, Michels R, et al. Aberrant methylation of p16(INK4a) is an early event in lung cancer and a potential biomarker for early diagnosis Proc Natl Acad Sci U S A 1998; 95:11891.

Biology of Tobacco and Smoking

Christine C. Maurer and Konstantinos N. Syrigos

Contents

3.1   Introduction

More than 40 years ago, the causal relationship between smoking and lung cancer was recognized by the US Surgeon General [1]. Over the years, an accumulation of epidemiological data and laboratory animal studies has established that there is indeed a link. However, it is the precise mechanistic steps between exposures to carcinogens to the development of lung cancer that scientists are enigmatically probing. With the integrated efforts of molecular biology, scientists have indeed uncovered sufficient mechanistic possibilities linking the two. We may never entirely map out this complex process, but the accumulated data has given us very little doubt as to what these carcinogens are capable of doing. Indeed, additional studies are constantly abating the gaps.

It has been estimated that the latency between the onset of smoking and the development of lung cancer is from 15 to 50 years [2–4]. The risks, of course, have been correlated with several factors including the quantity of cigarettes smoked per year and even the age of onset [5, 6]. Of the one billion smokers in the world, fewer than 20% will eventually develop lung cancer [7]. These observations are indicative of the impact of the amount and length of exposure to tobacco smoke and its carcinogens on the multifaceted progression to tobacco-related lung cancer. The constant exposure to these substances contributes to increased levels of circulating carcinogenic metabolites and permanent DNA damage. Various other factors, such as genetic variations in the processing or detoxifying of enzymes, are calculated into the equation of actual carcinogenic exposure influencing tumorigenesis.

Nicotine plays an integral role in the vicious circle between the continuous use of tobacco and a steady level of carcinogenic exposure. This constant exposure to carcinogens may contribute to a constant level of circulating active metabolites, which may expose the body to a continuous adduct burden. The entire process may be influenced by variants of genotypic enzymes. From activation, metabolites can either be deactivated through various detoxification pathways, the rate of clearance of which may also be determined genotypically, or remain active, causing direct or indirect damage to DNA, RNA, and proteins (for example, formation of adducts or point mutations). Critical genes may be affected, leading to the activation of various oncogenes or deactivation of tumor-suppressor genes. Loss of cell cycle control, cell signaling, and a saturated detoxification/repair system under this constant exposure may result in a selective clonal expansion.

3.2   The Carcinogens

There are several carcinogens in tobacco smoke. According to the International Agency for Research on Cancer, they can be categorized according to their putative carcinogenic potential (see Table 3.1) [8–10].

The International Agency for Research on Cancer has documented the existence of 55 carcinogens in mainstream tobacco smoke that have been evaluated as having "sufficient evidence of carcinogenicity" [11]. The criteria used are based upon the presence of these agents in cigarette smoke, known human or animal carcinogenicity, epidemiological data, and any mechanistic evidence indicating a positive carcinogenic outcome in either tobacco

Table 3.1. Carcinogens in tobacco smoke

Group 1: carcinogenic to humans	Group 2 A: probably carcinogenic to humans	Group 2 B: possibly carcinogenic to humans	Group 3: not classifiable as carcinogenic to humans (limited evidence)
4-Aminobiphenyl Benzene Cadmium Chromium Formaldehyde 2-Naphthylamine Nickel Vinyl Chloride Tobacco products, smokeless Involuntary smoking Tobacco smoking	Benz[a]anthracene Benzo[a]pyrene 1,3-Butadiene Dibenz[a,h]anthracene N-Nitrosodiethylamine N-Nitrosodimethylamine ortho-Toluidine	Acetaldehyde Acrylonitrile Benzo[b]fluoranthene Benzo[j]fluoranthene Benzo[k]fluoranthene Dibenz[a,h]acridine Dibenz[a,j]acridine 7H-Dibenzo[c,g]carbazole Dibenzo[a,e]pyrene Dibenzo[a,h]pyrene Dibenzo[a,l]pyrene Dibenzo[a,i]pyrene 1,1-Dimethylhydrazine Hydrazine Indeno[1,2,3-cd]pyrene Lead 5-Methylchysene 2-Nitropropane N-Nitrosodiethanolamine 4-(N-Nitrosomethylamino)- 1-(3-pyridyl)-1-butanone N-Nitrosomethylethylamine N-Nitrosomorpholine N-Nitrosonornicotine N-Nitrosopyrrolidine Ethyl carbamate	Acrolein Chrysene Crotonaldehyde Furfural Methyl chloride N-Nitrosoanabasine N-Nitrosoanatabine

smoke condensates as a whole or the individual carcinogen and their metabolites. Positive tumor development in one species of animal and not another may lead to a characterization of limited carcinogenicity.

Mainstream tobacco smoke is the smoke that is inhaled through the tobacco column and exits through the mouthpiece with each puff, whereas sidestream smoke is what is emitted between puffs. Environmental tobacco smoke (ETS) is defined as mainstream and sidestream smoke plus any exhaled smoke.

Mainstream smoke is an aerosol that contains 10^{10} particles/ml [12]. This complex aerosol consists of minute liquid droplets, denoted the particulate phase, suspended within a mixture of nitrogen, oxygen, and carbon dioxide gases and semi-volatile compounds [13]. Carcinogens and about 4,000 other compounds are present in the particulate phase of the cigarette smoke [12, 14, 15]. It has been estimated that approximately 80% of inhaled particles from cigarette mainstream smoke are deposited in the respiratory tract, mainly the tracheobronchial region [14].

The composition of tobacco smoke is affected by many factors, including the type of tobacco product, the properties of the tobacco, the blend of tobacco, any chemical additives, smoking pattern, pH, type of paper and filter used, and ventilation [14–17].

Although there are many compounds that are common to mainstream smoke and sidestream smoke, differences do exist between the two [15]. The concentrations and ratios of compounds between these two are outlined in the Table 3.2 [18–30]. Sidestream smoke is formed at lower temperatures than mainstream smoke (600 °C versus 900 °C), in an oxygen-deficient environment, and is rapidly diluted and cooled upon diffusing into the air [31]. Mainstream smoke is formed through the tobacco column at higher temperatures and in the presence of oxygen. These conditions are in favor of the formation of smaller particulates in sidestream smoke (0.01–0.1 μm) compared to mainstream smoke (0.1–1 μm) [31]. Sidestream smoke appears to contain higher concentrations of ammonia (40- to 170-fold), nitrogen oxides (4- to 10-fold), and chemical carcinogens (e.g., benzene 10-fold, N-nitrosamines 6- to 100-fold, and aniline 30-fold) than mainstream smoke [14]. However, their dilution with the air makes passive uptake far less for the nonsmoker than for the smoker, the risk of developing lung cancer is therefore also relatively lower for the nonsmoker [32].

Table 3.2. Known concentrations of carcinogens. *ND* Not detected

Group/Carcinogen	Amount in (mainstream) tobacco smoke ng/cigarette	Sidestream/mainstream ratio
Group 1: carcinogenic to humans		
4-Aminobiphenyl [18]	0.2–4.6 (unfiltered)	30.4 (unfiltered)
	0.2–23 (filtered)	6.1 (filtered)[a]
Benzene [19]	5,900–75,000	8.7[b]
Cadmium [20]	1,700	7.2 [21]
Chromium [22]	0.2–500	
Formaldehyde [23]	3,400–283,000	
2-Naphthylamine [24]	1.5–14.1 and 35	1.9–4.8[c]
Nickel [22]	0–510	13–30
Vinyl Chloride [22]	1.3–15.8	
Group 2A: probably carcinogenic to humans		
Benzo[*a*]anthracene [23]	Trace–80	
Benzo[*a*]pyrene [23]	4–108	2.5–3.5 [21]
1,3-Butadiene [25]	400,000	~1[d]
Dibenz[*a,h*]anthracene [23]	4–76	
N-Nitrosodiethylamine [26]	<8.3	0.96–8.8[e]
N-Nitrosodimethylamine [23,27]	13–65 (unfiltered)	~12 unfiltered
	5.7–43 (filtered)	~41 filtered[f]
	ND–1,620	
Group 2B: possibly carcinogenic to humans		
Benzo[*b*]fluoranthene [7]	4–22	
Benzo[*j*]fluoranthene [7]	6–21	
Benzo[*k*]fluoranthene [7]	6–12	
Dibenz[*a,h*]acridine* [28]	0.1	
Dibenz[*a,j*]acridine* [28]	2.7	
7H-Dibenzo[*c,g*]carbazole [28]	0.7 (in tar)	
Dibenzo[*a,i*]pyrene [7]	1.7–3.2	
Hydrazine* [29]	32,000	
Indeno[1,2,3-*cd*]pyrene [7]	4–20	
5-Methylchysene [7]	0.6	
NNK [30]	20–4,200	3.7[g]
Ethyl carbamate [7]	20–38	

* Exact source of extraction not specified, values may be higher than expected.
[a] Data estimated by the concentration of sidestream smoke at 140 ng/cigarette.
[b] Data estimated at 75,000 ng in mainstream smoke to 653,000 ng in sidestream smoke.
[c] Based on 14.1 and 35 ng per cigarette and sidestream smoke of 67 ng/cigarette.
[d] Based on sidestream smoke of 400,000 ng/cigarette.
[e] Based on sidestream smoke of 8–73 ng/cigarette.
[f] Based on upper level detection of sidestream smoke (823 ng unfiltered, 1,770 ng filtered).
[g] Based on sidestream smoke of 15,700 ng/cigarette.

3.2.1 Polycyclic Aromatic Hydrocarbons

One group of carcinogenic agents present in cigarette smoke is the polycyclic aromatic hydrocarbons, or PAHs, which have been well studied. There are no known uses for PAHs, but they are used in the fields of biochemistry, biomedicine, and cancer research; they are generally not produced for commercial use. PAHs are the products of the incomplete combustion of organic compounds. Their presence in air is due to the burning of wood or fuel (for heating). They are found in motor vehicle exhaust, open fires, industrial soot and smoke, and charcoal-broiled foods as well as in cigarette/cigar smoke and tar [28].

Strong evidence has linked these carcinogens to a variety of cancers. The IARC has documented sufficient conclusive evidence of carcinogenicity as a result of animal studies [33]. Evidence collected by the US Department of Health and Human Services as well as the IARC of different PAHs is listed in Table 3.3 [28, 34, 35]. Evidence of respiratory tumorigenicity in multianimal models (via the same route of exposures) is a compelling argument for lung cancer development. This is

Table 3.3. Polycyclic aromatic hydrocarbons in tobacco smoke

Polycyclic aromatic hydrocarbon	Animal model	Routes of exposure	Respiratory tumorigenicity	Extrapulmonary tumorigenicity in animal models; routes not specified
Benzo[a]anthracene	Mice	Oral, subcutaneous	Pulmonary adenomas and adenocarcinomas	Forestomach and skin Papillomas Hepatomas Bladder carcinomas
Benzo[b]fluoranthane	Mice			Skin tumors, sarcomas
Benzo[j]fluoranthane	Rats	Interpulmonary	Pulmonary squamous cell carcinoma	Skin papillomas Carcinomas Subcutaneous sarcomas
Benzo[k]fluoranthane	Rats	Interpulmonary	Pulmonary squamous cell carcinoma	Skin tumors
Benzo[a]pyrene	Mice	Oral	Lung adenomas	Malignant and benign forestomach tumors
	Hamsters Rats Subhuman primates	Subcutaneous, Intraperitoneal Inhalation Intratrachea instillation Intratracheal instillation Inhalation Intrabronchial implantation Intratracheal instillation	Tracheal papillomas, tracheal carcinomas Tracheobronchial tumors Lung tumors (unspecified) Pulmonary squamous cell carcinoma Local tumors Pulmonary squamous cell carcinoma	Mammary tumors Skin carcinomas and papillomas Hepatomas Abdominal fibrosarcomas Uterine carcinomas Offspring tumors
Dibenz[a,h]acridine	Mice	Intravenous	Lung tumors	Skin tumors, sarcomas
Dibenz[a,j]acridine	Mice	Subcutaneous	Lung tumors	Skin Tumors, sarcomas
Dibenz[a,h]anthracene	Mice	Oral	Alveologenic carcinoma of the lung	Forestomach squamous cell carcinomas and papillomas
	Rats	Intratracheal	Pulmonary squamous cell carcinomas	Hemangioendotheliomas
	Newborn mice	Subcutaneous Interpulmonary	Lung adenomas increased Lung adenomas	Mammary carcinomas Sarcomas Renal adenocarcinomas
7H–Dibenzo[c,g]carbazole	Hamsters	Intratracheal	Respiratory tract tumors	Forestomach papillomas and carcinomas Benign and malignant hepatomas
Dibenzo[a,e]pyrene	Mice			Skin tumors, sarcomas
Dibenzo[a,h]pyrene	Mice, Rats			Skin tumors, sarcomas
Dibenzo[a,i]pyrene	Mice Hamsters			Skin tumors, sarcomas
Dibenzo[a,l]pyrene	Mice			Sarcomas
Indeno[1,2,3-cd]pyrene	Mice			Sarcomas
5-Methylchrysene	Mice			Sarcomas

remarkably characteristic for benzo[a]pyrene (BaP). A tendency for the development of squamous cell carcinoma should also be noted.

BaP has been studied extensively and evidence of its presence in cigarette smoke is well established [11, 14]. BaP is more carcinogenic than the benzofluoranthenes or indeno[1,2,3-cd]pyrene [36]. It also overshadows other PAHs in studies, but other more potent carcinogens such as dibenz[a,h]anthracene, 5-methylchrysene, and dibenzo[a,i]pyrene are recognized even though their content in cigarette smoke is lower [37, 38].

In skin carcinogenesis studies on mice, BaP was consistently found to be associated with the development of more tumors in a shorter period of time than other PAHs; the exception was with dibenzo[a,h]anthracene. In a dose–response study involving subcutaneous injection in mice, the minimal dose at which carcinogenicity was detected was higher for BaP than for dibenz-[a,h]anthracene [34]. The latent periods were consistently shorter for BaP than for dibenz[a,h]anthracene. In studies using intratracheal administration in hamsters, BaP appeared to be less effective than 7H-dibenzo[c,g]carbazole.

Dibenz[*a,h*]anthracene has been shown to produce tumors following different routes of administration in a variety of animal species including mice, rats, guinea pigs, frogs, pigeons, and chickens. It has conclusively demonstrated both local and systemic carcinogenic effects [34].

In a dose–response study involving the subcutaneous administration of carcinogens, dibenz[*a,h*]anthracene, BaP, and 3-methylcholanthrene, were compared and evaluated. It was shown that dibenz[*a,h*]anthracene was a more effective carcinogen at a lower dose than either BaP or 3-methylcholanthrene [34]; however, its latent period was longer. Dibenz[*a,h*]anthracene induced the development of local sarcomas and increased the incidence of lung adenomas following a single injection via a subcutaneous route in newborn mice at dose levels that were ineffective with 3-methylcholanthrene [34]. In comparison with BaP, 7*H*-dibenzo[*c,g*]carbazole appears to be a stronger respiratory tract carcinogen for the hamster [34].

Both dibenz[*a,h*]acridine and 7H-dibenzo[*c,g*]carbazole are known pulmonary tumorigens. It appears that the activity of dibenz[*a,h*]acridine is significantly lower than that of BaP, while the activity of 7H-dibenzo[*c,g*]-carbazole is greater than that of BaP. The levels of both compounds compared to BaP in cigarette smoke are relatively low [34, 35].

3.2.2 *N*-Nitrosamines

The cancer-causing potential of nitrosamines is well established and well documented. Most nitrosamines that are present in tobacco smoke have been categorized as group 2 compounds by the IARC. The carcinogenic effects on animals of *N*-nitrosodiethylamine, *N*-nitrosodimethylamine, and 4-(*N*-nitrosomethylamino)-1-(3-pyridyl)-1-butanone (NNK) are presented in Table 3.4 [26, 27, 30].

N-Nitrosodiethylamine and *N*-nitrosodimethylamine, which are known to be present in tobacco smoke, are volatile oils that rapidly undergo photolytic degradation under ultraviolet illumination, whereas NNK is a crystalline solid with a melting point of around 64 °C [26, 27, 30]. Some nitrosamines such as NNK, *N*-nitrosonornicotine (NNN), *N*-nitrosoanatabine, and *N*-nitrosoanabasine are compounds that form naturally from the tobacco plant [10]. *N*-Nitrosodiethylamine and *N*-nitrosodimethylamine are used in several industries such as in the rubber or plastic industries, and have been detected as contaminants in food, beverages, and alcohol [26, 27]. *N*-Nitrosodiethylamine has even been found in baby pacifiers and baby bottle teats [26].

N-Nitrosodiethylamine, when administered to hamsters by inhalation, has been shown to produce tumors of the trachea, bronchi, and lungs; however, in rats, it produced only liver tumors [26]. On the other hand, another such inhalation study with *N*-nitrosodiethylamine has documented the development of lung tumors in both mice and rats [27].

NNK is formed naturally by the oxidation and nitrosation of nicotine during tobacco processing and by smoking [30]. Studies on endogenous nicotine metabolism suggest that the breakdown of nicotine in the liver can be linked to NNK [39]. The total dose accumulated over a lifetime of smoking is considered to be as close to the lowest total dose shown to induce lung tumors in rats [40]. One study showed that the concentration of NNK can be significantly decreased, by up to 73%, if the use of a filter is implemented [30].

NNK is not only considered to be a potent pulmonary carcinogen, but it has a remarkable tendency to develop adenocarcinomas and adenomas [30, 40]. NNK was the only nitrosamine that repeatedly exhibited pulmonary tumorigenicity in all three animal models used (rats, hamsters, and mice), whereas for *N*-nitrosodiethylamine, evidence of pulmonary tumorigenicity was apparent in two (hamsters and mice). The IARC Working Group interpreted the results of the studies as demonstrating that NNK induced the development of tumors in a dose-dependent manner [30].

3.2.3 Other Carcinogens and Chemicals

Although several carcinogenic agents in tobacco smoke are listed as having a possible link to cancer in humans and animals, studies have not yet evolved to complete this connection directly to lung tumorigenesis. With the help of epidemiological, mechanistic, and animal model studies, some conclusions about these compounds arise:

1. Acrylonitrile was shown to be correlated with lung cancer in workers exposed and observed for a period of 20 years [41].
2. 4-Aminobiphenyl has been strongly linked to cancer of the bladder, forming DNA adducts as seen in bladder tumors, and hemoglobin adducts as seen in red blood cells [42]. This arylamine, emits toxic fumes when heated, has been shown to cause genetic damage, cell transformation, and inhibition of DNA repair capacity in cultured mammalian cells as well as in mice [18]. Activation to its reactive metabolite requires *N*-hydroxylation (and detoxified via *N*-acetylation). It has been shown that smokers who were slow acetylators (due to variants in *N*-acetyltransferase) had higher levels of adducts than those who were rapid acetylators [43].
3. Benzene has been shown to produce lung tumors in mice of both sexes [19].
4. Cadmium, on the other hand, has been shown via inhalation studies to cause lung tumors (adenocarcinoma) in rats and various other lung tumors in mice

Table 3.4. *N*-Nitrosamines in tobacco smoke

N-Nitrosamines	Animal models	Routes of exposure	Respiratory tumorigenicity	Extrapulmonary sites
N-Nitrosodiethylamine	Rats Pregnant rats	Inhalation Oral Intraperitoneal Intravenous Intrarectal Subcutaneous	Nasal cavity tumors	Liver tumors Liver tumors, kidney tumors, esophageal tumors Liver tumors Kidney tumors Hepatocellular carcinomas Kidney and mammary tumors in offspring
	Hamsters Pregnant hamsters	Inhalation Subcutaneous Intraperitoneal Intradermal Subcutaneous	Tumors of the trachea, bronchi and lungs Respiratory tract tumors Respiratory tract tumors Nasal cavity papillomas Tracheal and respiratory tract tumors in offspring	Forestomach and esophageal tumors Liver tumors
	Mice Pregnant mice	Oral Topical Subcutaneous Intraperitoneal Subcutaneous	Lung tumors Nasal cavity tumors Increased lung tumors Lung tumors Pulmonary adenomas	Liver tumors, esophageal tumors, forestomach tumors Liver tumors Liver, esophageal and fore-stomach tumors in offspring
N-Nitrosodimethylamine	Rats	Oral Inhalation Intramuscular Intraperitoneal	Lung tumors, nasal cavity tumors Nasal cavity tumors	Kidney, bile duct tumors Liver, kidney tumors Kidney, liver tumors Hepatocellular carcinoma, bile duct tumors
	Hamsters	Oral Intramuscular	Nasal cavity tumors	Hemangiosarcoma of liver, bile duct tumors
	Mice	Oral Inhalation Intramuscular Intraperitoneal	Lung tumors Lung tumors Lung tumors (lung adenomas in newborn) Lung tumors	Hemangiomas of liver, hepato-cellular carcinoma, kidney tumors Liver, kidney tumors Liver tumors Liver, kidney tumors
4-(*N*-Nitrosomethyl-amino)-1-(3-pyridyl)-1-butanone	Rats	Multiple subcutaneous	Nasal cavity tumors (neuroblastomas, rhabdomyosarcomas, esthesioneuroepitheliomas, squamous cell carcinomas, anaplastic carcinomas, spindle cell sarcomas) Lung tumors (adeno-carcinomas and adeno-squamous cell carcinomas)	Liver tumors (hepatocellular carcinomas and hemangio-sarcomas)
	Hamsters	Multiple and single subcutaneous	Nasal cavity tumors (pleomorphic carcinomas) Tracheal tumors Lung tumors (adenocarcinomas)	
	Mice	Intraperitoneal	Lung tumors (adenomas and carcinomas)	

but not in hamsters [20]. It is also a known human carcinogen. In general it is the ionic form of cadmium that is responsible for genetic damage, including cell transformation. In addition, the sensitivity of cells to insults by cadmium appears to be related to their ability to produce metallothionein (MT). The difference in the carcinogenicity of cadmium between rats and mice is their ability to produce MT. Similar studies reiterate this [44].

5. 1,3-Butadiene has been shown to cause both benign and malignant tumors of the lung in mice but not in rats [45]. Genetic alterations in the K-*ras* genes and *p53* tumor-suppressor genes are observed. Active metabolites form guanine adducts [25].

6. Chromium compounds, which are known to be human carcinogens, have been shown to cause benign lung tumors in mice via inhalation, but intratracheal instillation did not induce tumors in hamsters, guinea pigs, or rabbits [46, 47]. Chromosomal aberrations, sister chromatid exchange, and aneuploidy have been observed in workers exposed to chromium [46].

7. Ethyl carbamate has been shown to cause lung cancer in mice but not in other species [48].

8. Squamous cell carcinoma of the nasal cavity was seen in rats following inhalation exposure to formaldehyde. However, carcinogenicity could not be established in hamsters and mice using the same method [49].

9. 2-Naphthylamine has been strongly associated with bladder cancer; however, further studies are needed to link it with smoking. Active metabolites of this arylamine have shown to form blood–serum adducts like hemoglobin [50].

10. Nickel compounds are known to be carcinogenic to humans. Cohort studies have shown that workers exposed to nickel compounds have an increase in the risk of lung cancer and nasal cancer [47]. In studies with rats and mice, inhalation or intratracheal exposure to compounds of nickel led to a dose-related induction of benign and malignant lung tumors [47, 51, 52].

11. Epidemiological studies indicate that vinyl chloride causes cancer in humans by its association with a rare tumor of the liver, angiosarcoma. It has been shown in mice to cause cancer in other sites, like the lungs [53, 54]. One of the metabolites of vinyl chloride is chloroethylene oxide, which can spontaneously rearrange to become an aldehyde [54]. Both form DNA adducts. Associated mutations in the *p53* tumor-suppressor gene and the *ras* proto-oncogene have been detected. Most of the mutations, which are most likely due to the etheno adducts, occur at A:T base pairs [55].

In addition to carcinogens, several other chemicals that are present in cigarette smoke act as respiratory irritants, such as ammonia, acetaldehyde, formaldehyde, and sulfur dioxide [7, 14, 49]. Acrolein, hydrogen cyanide, and formaldehyde affect mucociliary function, and at higher concentrations can inhibit smoke clearance from the lungs [14, 56]. Substantial levels of cocarcinogens are also present in cigarette smoke, including catechol, methylcatechols, pyrogallol, decane, undecane, pyrene, benzo[e]pyrene, and fluoranthene [7, 57].

Nicotine, although toxic and addictive, is not considered to be carcinogenic [58]. Studies on the metabolism of nicotine by p450 cytochromes in the liver have suggested that even though 80% of nicotine is converted to cotinine (its inactive metabolite, which is excreted in the urine), a smaller percentage may be converted to carcinogenic metabolites [39, 59]. In any case, its role in addiction links the tobacco user to a constant exposure of carcinogens and their consequences.

3.3 Chemical Carcinogenesis

Carcinogenesis occurs in two stages: initiation and promotion. A well-know experiment using BaP painted on the skin of mice resulted in no skin tumor growth. However, if the application of the carcinogen was followed by croton oil applications, many tumors developed. Croton oil alone did not develop skin tumors. In this case, BaP was the initiator, which apparently involved DNA modification and/or mutations. Croton oil acted as the promoter, which encouraged continued growth [60–62]. Although this case appears to suggest two very distinct processes from two very distinct compounds, most carcinogens are capable of acting as both initiators and promoters.

Chemical carcinogenesis is a complex, multifaceted process that ultimately results in tumorigenesis. Activation of the carcinogen is usually the first step. Some carcinogens do not require prior activation in order to exert their effects on their target molecules (direct carcinogens). However, many "procarcinogens" require metabolic activation, whereby one or more enzyme-catalyzed reactions is needed to covert the inactive procarcinogen to an active carcinogen. Any intermediate compounds are labeled proximate carcinogens, and the final compound, which reacts with the cellular components (such as DNA), is termed the ultimate carcinogen. In general, ultimate carcinogens are usually more reactive and electrophilic, readily attacking nucleophilic groups in DNA, RNA, and proteins.

The mechanism of activation of the xenobiotic or procarcinogen involves the known phase 1 and phase 2 reactions of xenobiotic metabolism. Phase 1 involves hydroxylation catalyzed by a group of enzymes referred to as monooxygenases or cytochrome p450s (CYPs). In addition to hydroxylation, other reactions involving deamination, dehalogenation, desulfuration, epoxidation, peroxygenation, and reduction can take place. Hydrolytic reactions and certain other non-p450-catalyzed reactions can also occur. The cytochrome p450 enzymes are a large multigene family that is important in the phase 1 activation of procarcinogens. CYP1A1, CYP2E1, and CYP2A6, among others, are phase 1 genes and have been investigated in relation to lung cancer risk.

Phase 2 is characterized by converting phase 1 compounds to polar metabolites by conjugation with glutathione, glucuronic acid, sulfate, acetate or amino acids, or by methylation. Three phase 2 genes have received wide attention as metabolic markers: glutathione-S-transferase class 1, N-acetyltransferase (NAT)1, and NAT2 [63]. Several studies have examined differences in genotypes for these and many other genes thought to alter risks for lung and other tobacco-related cancers. The genetic basis for this variation has been examined in many individual studies and summarized through systematic meta-analyses [64–68].

The goal, in general, of the metabolism of xenobiotics is to render the compound more water-soluble and thus ready for excretion. However, instead of converting xenobiotics to inactive forms, some compounds, like procarcinogens, such as BaP, are made more active during phase 1. However, detoxification of these compounds, like some nitrosamines, can still occur as by glucuronidation at phase 2. The biologically effective doses of carcinogenic and mutagenic intermediates, which reflect the metabolism of the carcinogens, might be enhanced by inherited variants of phase 1 or phase 2 proteins. These variants may accelerate activation of a carcinogen or decrease its rate of detoxification, or both. The balance between activation and detoxification plays an integral role in carcinogenesis and tumorigenesis.

Following activation, chemical carcinogens may then go on to form adducts with DNA, RNA, or proteins. This covalent interaction causes a variety of damage, which may enter into a repair system or remain "unrepaired", further perpetuating carcinogenesis. This binding to DNA may be the first step in the initiation of a carcinogenic process [63].

Several studies have focused on DNA adduct formation, as well as the formation of other adducts, such as with hemoglobin, and their importance in identifying carcinogenic exposure. These biomarkers integrate the identification, exposure, dose, and susceptibility of an individual to carcinogenic agents. It has been proposed that these biomarkers can be found in several tissues, cells, blood, urine, and even saliva [69–71]. Adducts formed by the binding of carcinogens or their metabolites have been measured in smokers and nonsmokers [7].

Most chemical carcinogens are mutagenic, inducing transitions, transversions, and other mutations. Environmental tobacco smoke, sidestream smoke and its condensate, as well as a mix of sidestream and mainstream condensates have all been shown to cause genetic damage [31, 72]. Lung cancers have been estimated to experience up to 20 genetic changes before any individual clonal tumor emerges [73]. Alterations have to take place in a sequence before any individual clone becomes truly malignant. This process of mutational selection is one of the most important issues being investigated in cancer biology. Central to this idea is the incorporation of cancer genes studies. Inactivation of tumor-suppressor genes or activation of certain oncogenes via genomic manipulation by chemical insults allows the "gatekeepers and caretakers" to lose control [74, 75]. Cell transformation then follows at an accelerated rate [76].

Evidence of the following establishes possible mechanisms of a substance to be carcinogenic: ability of phase 1 or phase 2 enzymes to activate procarcinogens to become reactive metabolites, formation of reactive electrophiles (either direct or indirect via metabolites) with possible mutagenic effects, evidence of DNA, RNA, or protein modification, and/or the formation of adducts, and/or interruption of the cell cycle, and/or cell signaling. In addition, the self-protection processes of a cell against tumorigenesis (carcinogen detoxification, DNA repair capacity, and apoptosis) would have to be tainted.

An emerging area of research is focusing on understanding the position of individual variations in DNA repair with respect to lung cancer risks. Defective DNA repair is not a new area of study in relation to tumorigenesis (reviewed in [77]). Cheng and colleagues reportedly found reduced expression levels of nucleotide excision repair genes in lung cancer patients compared with controls [78]. They proposed that this reduced expression level fosters a gene–environment interaction that may play a role in increasing the risk of lung cancer. Substantial work is being carried out to find the precise gene alterations responsible for these interactions. Many novel DNA repair gene polymorphisms have been observed, but their phenotypic expression remains ambiguous [65, 66].

Research on carcinogens has still not brought the exact order of mechanisms leading to tumorigenesis, but sufficient evidence has been accumulated.

3.4   Nitrosamines: Model NNK

It has been established that tobacco-specific *N*-nitrosamines, such as NNK and NNN, and their metabolites, are potent carcinogens. Evidence of their activation and formation of adducts has been outlined, as has their interference in the cell cycle and cell signaling, all of which contribute to carcinogenesis and tumorigenesis.

Studies indicate the cytochromes responsible for the activation of NNK are CYP 2A13 [79] and CYP2A6 [80]. CYP2A6 is a known nicotine c-oxidase in the liver that converts 80% of nicotine to cotinine, which can be detected in urine. It has been suggested that the metabolism of nicotine to NNK via CYP2A6 is an endogenous mechanism for NNK generation [39]. CYP2A6 has a 93.5% amino acid similarity to CYP 2A13, but it appears to be less active [79]. The presence of CYP2A13 is indicated by its high concentration in the nasal mucosa, trachea, and lung, but it also is present in several other organs, which demonstrate its use in xenobiotic metabolism [81]. In general, considerable genetic polymorphism is seen, in general, with CYPs, which again reiterates the susceptibility of populations to lung cancer and even a tendency for a certain kind of lung cancer. It has been shown that variants of CYP2A13 have a decreased risk of adenocarcinoma of the lung, but this is not seen with squamous cell carcinoma [82].

Metabolic activation of NNK leads the evolution of chemically reactive electrophiles, which react with DNA, forming adducts, to initiate a possible carcinogenic response. Activation of NNK to its reactive metabolites is thought to be accomplished by a-hydroxylation of the carbon atoms adjacent to the nitroso moiety by the CYP [83]. Its main metabolite is 4-(methylnitrosamino)-1-(3-pyridyl)-1-butanol (NNAL), a potent intermediate.

Two types of adducts are formed by a-hydroxylation of NNK: methyl and pyridoxobutyl adducts. Some of the methylated or pyridyloxobutylated adducts produced after activation are O(6)-methylguanine, N7-methylguanine, and O(6)-[4-oxo-4-(3-pyridyl)butyl]guanine [7, 84]. O(6)-methylguanine plays an important role in tumorigenesis in mice, whereas pyridoxobutyl adducts are seen more frequently in rats [40]. Some pyrimidine adducts have also been discovered using stable precursors of the products of methyl hydroxylated NNK and NNAL [85].

NNK and NNN are metabolically activated to 4-oxo-4-(4-pyridyl)-1-butanediazohydroxide, which is known to pyridoxobutylate DNA [86]. Adducts specific to NNK are the result of covalent linkage between DNA and a pyridyloxobutyl group [87]. A proportion of these DNA adducts release 4-hydroxy-1-(3-pyridyl)-1-butanone (4-HPB). These 4-HPB-releasing DNA adducts have been detected in several target tissues treated with NNK and NNN as well as in the lung tissue of smokers [86]. Other 4-HPB-releasing adducts, which relate to the instability of the adduct formed, have been investigated. These 4-HPB-releasing adducts have been indicated as possible biomarkers for the presence of pyridoxobutylated DNA [87].

NNK has been shown to activate nuclear factor (NK)-$\kappa\beta$ (which inhibits apoptosis and increases cell survival) and cyclooxygenase (COX)-1 (known for its involvement in the development and progression of cancer) [88]. Inhibition of COX-1 is actually a novel therapy via nonsteroidal antiinflammatory drugs [88]. Inhibitors of COX, lipoxygenase, and β-adrenergic receptors all inhibited the growth of NNK-induced pulmonary adenocarcinoma [89]. In colon cancer, NNK increased COX-2, phospholipase A2, and prostaglandin E2, which was inhibited by β2-adrenoceptor blockers [90].

NNK has also been shown to increase the proliferation of non-small-cell lung cancer cells by activation of Akt-dependent proliferation, which was linked to cyclin D1 expression [91]. Activation of NK-$\kappa\beta$ was also noted. The combination increases cell survival and the possibility of the insensitivity of tumor cells to apoptosis, thereby inducing proliferation. It is believed that the mechanism of action of NNK in Akt-dependent proliferation is due to the a7 subunits of nicotinic acetylcholine receptors (nAChRs) [92, 93]. The affinity for this particular subunit of nAChRs by NNK has been reported in other studies on the activation of the serine/threonine kinase Akt [94]. Active Akt has been found not only in NNK-treated mice, but also in smokers. The maintenance of Akt activity is necessary for the survival of preneoplastic or transformed cells [95]. It is also seen in a variety of other cancers, like that of the pancreas. Activation of the catalytic subunit phosphatidylinositol 3-kinase, PIK3CA, in association with Akt was seen in a variety of pulmonary carcinomas. Its amplification was noted in 70% of squamous cell carcinomas, 67% of small-cell carcinomas, 38% of large-cell carcinomas, and 19% of adenocarcinomas in a study by Massion et al. [96].

Cyclin D is an important regulator of G1 progression of the cell cycle and regulates cell proliferation [62]. It also responds to growth factors and has the ability to act as a proto-oncogene [62]. In a study by Ho et al., it was reported that NNK encouraged cell proliferation via first activating NF-$\kappa\beta$, which in turn upregulated cyclin D1, thus increasing the phosphorylation of Rb Ser(795) [97]. These events promoted cells to enter the S phase of the cell cycle. Entering the S phase of the cell cycle discourages the repair of DNA, and possible damaged DNA replication follows. In addition, an inhibitor of extracellular-signal-related protein kinase (ERK)1/2 suppressed 1$\kappa\beta a$ phosphorylation induced by NF-$\kappa\beta$, thereby indicating the pathway used [97]. In vivo, mice that were treated with NNK had increased expressions of cyclin D1 and NF-$\kappa\beta$ [97].

The tumor-suppressor gene *p16 INK2a* has been shown to be inactivated in over 70% of non-small-cell lung carcinomas, either by homozygous deletion or by aberrant methylation of its promoter region [98–100]. *p16* is an inhibitor of the cyclin-dependent kinases encoded by MTS1 tumor-suppressor gene [62]. The role of *p16* is to inhibit cell-cycle proliferation at G1. It binds to cyclin-dependent kinase-4 (cdk4), inhibiting the permissive action of cdk4/cyclin D to allow progression to the S-phase [62]. The inactivation of *p16* induces a loss of inhibition of cell proliferation, and furthers mutational duplication. It has been observed that hypermethylation of the promoter region of *p16*, and thus inactivation, was observed in 94% of adenocarcinomas that were induced by NNK [100]. Inactivation of the *p16* gene has been found in over 70% of cell lines derived from human non-small-cell lung cancers [101]. In addition, inactivation by multiple mechanisms of this gene has been detected in approximately 50% of primary non-small-cell lung cancers [102–104].

NNK has been documented to increase the level of *raf-1*, an oncogene that encodes for protein-serine/threonine kinase and induces cell proliferation of small-cell lung cancer cells [93]. It acts through the mitogen-activated protein (MAP) kinase pathway, which results in phosphorylation of *c-myc* [93]. In addition, all appear to be inhibited by serotonin reuptake inhibitors, like imipramine, and by the selective α7 nAChR agonist, bungarotoxin [93]. The role of *c-myc* in carcinogenesis may be to maintain cell proliferation of the immortalized cells. However, alone, it is not an inducer. The presence of *c-myc* in lung carcinomas is well known [62].

In general, tobacco-specific *N*-nitrosamines, when they are metabolically activated, are known to induce K-*ras* oncogenes. Lesions of guanine adducts of NNK in K-*ras* genes have been shown to form preferentially at the second position of codon 12, where known mutations of G->A and G->T base substitutions are seen in smoking-induced tumors of the lung [84]. This has also been demonstrated in mice where the O(6) methylguanine route of NNK is dominant, resulting in a high level of GGT->GAT mutations in the same codon [40]. However, the mutations in mice are not found in rat lung tumors like those induced by NNK. K-*ras* genes encode guanine nucleotide binding proteins and their activity is G-protein-like, which is involved with relating extracellular signals intracellularly. It is believed that this oncogene is an early event allowing the induction of cell alteration to occur. Considerable data has shown the relationship between exposure to tobacco carcinogens and mutations of this oncogene. Mutations of the K-*ras* gene are known to occur at codons 12, 13, and 61 in adenocarcinomas of the lung, and these mutations significantly increase in individuals who smoke cigarettes [105–114]. Surprisingly, these mutations are not associated with the duration or intensity of smoking [114]. It appears that K-*ras* mutations occur early in the lifetime of the smoker, and the mutated clones of the gene may be later selected for continued growth by tobacco carcinogens.

The inactivation of death-associated protein (DAP)-kinase by aberrant methylation is seen in both adenocarcinoma of the lung and NNK-induced hyperplasia at an alarmingly similar frequency, 46% and 52%, respectively [115]. DAP-kinase inactivation appears to be an early event in the carcinogenesis of many cancers. The event encourages tumor growth and possibly metastatic capacity of the tumors. The role of DAP-kinase is to inhibit *c-myc* and E2F-induced oncogenic transformation via activation of the *p53* apoptotic pathway [115]. For the tumor, early deactivation means selective growth, whereby late deactivation encourages metastasis.

NNK also appears to activate *bcl-2* phosphorylation at Ser (70) and *c-myc* at Thr (58) and Ser (62) via ERK1/2 and protein kinase Cα [116]. It was further noted that their cooperation, which was induced by NNK, promoted cell survival and proliferation. If *c-myc* was deleted there appeared to be a delay in the G1/S cell cycle transition. In these *c-myc*-deleted cells, NNK-induced proliferation was blocked [116].

Detoxification of NNK's major potent carcinogen, NNAL, is said to be mediated by glucuronidation. UDP-

glucuronosyltransferases (UGT)-mediated O-glucuronidation is an important detoxification pathway for NNAL. UGT1A9 mRNAs, which provide evidence of NNAL-glucuronidating activity, were detected in liver specimens but not in the lung [117]. UGT2B7 mRNAs, however, were detected significantly in the liver and at lower levels in the lung. Both UGTs appeared to play a role in inactivating NNAL [117]. In another study, UGT1A4 in human liver specimens appeared to be the culprit [118]. Several oxidoreductases have also been identified as participating in initiating the detoxification of NNK [119].

Removing the DNA adducts formed by alkylating mutagens found in tobacco smoke is an important task for preventing the proliferation of tumorigenesis. O-methylguanine-DNA-methyltransferase (MGMT) is a DNA-repair protein that acts this way and has an increased sensitivity to the genetic damage induced by NNK. In a study in which variants of this gene were coded, it was found that those who inherited two single-nucleotide polymorphisms (cSNP) had significantly higher levels of NNK-induced chromosomal aberrations than those with no or only one cSNP [120]. In essence, alterations of the MGMT proteins may in fact allow damaged DNA to linger and a malfunctioning repair system to enhance carcinogenic potential. Lung tumors have been shown to have an aberrant methylation in the promoter region of MGMT, which may indicate its malfunction [121].

In addition to its highly suspected carcinogenic potential, NNK has also been shown to induce immunomodulatory effects that may overall induce a decreased immune response and may therefore play a role in precancerous events. NNK has been shown to inhibit tumor necrosis facto, macrophage inflammatory protein-1a, interleukin (IL)-12, and nitrous oxide (NO), and stimulate IL-10 and prostaglandin E2 (PGE2) in alveolar macrophages [122]. In another study, inhibition of natural killer cells were noted as well as an increase in IgM secretory cell number [123]. Proulx et al. noted inhibition of IL-8, IL-6, and macrophage chemotactic protein-1, and an increase in PGE2 by metabolites of NNK [124].

3.5   PAHs: Model BaP

Although several PAHs are present in cigarette smoke, BaP is the most extensively studied, although not the most potent of the PAHs. The major active metabolite of BaP is 7,8-diol-9,10-epoxide, also known as BPDE. BPDE-2, one of BaP's diol oxides, is considered to be the ultimate carcinogen, whereas, BPDE-1 appears to not be carcinogenic [125]. This indicates a role in promotion for PAHs.

There is convincing evidence that the activation of BaP occurs via cytochrome 1A1 (CYP 1A1). It has been demonstrated that cigarette smoke induces aryl hydrocarbon hydroxylase (AHH) activity [14]. AHH assays measure the conversion of BaP to 3-hydroxy BaP, which requires this cytochrome [126–128]. A correlation between smokers with elevated AHH and a higher conversion of BaP-7,8-diol to tetraols was found in lung tissue compared to nonsmokers and ex-smokers [129]. Furthermore, BPDE-DNA adduct levels where associated with AHH activity in the same samples [130]. Tetraols, which were released from BPDE-DNA adducts, were detected in lung tissue samples of individuals devoid of *GSTM1* gene [131], which is responsible for phase 2 reactions.

There are known variations of CYP 1A1. It has been demonstrated that in Japanese and other Asian populations, polymorphic variants of the *CYP1A1* gene are highly prevalent and have been associated repeatedly with higher risks of smoking-related lung cancers [132–137]. Although genetic variations may exist, this has not been consistent in other populations.

PAH-DNA adducts have been measured extensively in lung and other tissues as well as in blood, as markers of exposure to tobacco carcinogens [138–149]. Levels of these adducts in lung tissue are correlated with those in blood, which have shown to differ depending on smoking status. Current smokers have appreciably elevated PAH-DNA adducts in their lungs. As smokers quit, it is believed that the adduct burdens declines rapidly [149, 150]. Several studies indicate that these DNA adducts may be related to the risk of an individual to lung cancer [151–153]. Investigation of PAH-DNA adducts in the lungs of cancer patients has advocated that age at the initiation of smoking is an independent predictor of the overall DNA adduct burden measured at the time of surgery for lung cancer [150].

BPDE and other PAH diol epoxides can form adducts with hemoglobin and albumin [154, 155]. Quantitative analysis has revealed that levels of tetraols, which are formed by the hydrolysis of these adducts, are higher in smokers than in nonsmokers [156, 157]. BPDE has also been known to induce chromosomal aberrations at specific loci; BPDE-induced chromosome 3p21.3 aberrations have been observed [158].

Urinary metabolites of the noncarcinogen pyrene, such as 1-hydroxypyrene and its glucuronide, have been used as indicators of PAH uptake. It has been demonstrated that 1-hydroxypyrene levels in smokers are higher than in nonsmokers [159–161]. Other studies have investigated specific PAH metabolites in urine, for example 3-hydroxy BaP and tetraols, which are the result of hydrolysis of the metabolite BPDE [162–168]. However, the studies involved a small number of individuals.

PAH carcinogens and their metabolites have been known to result in an accumulation of *p53* gene product in human and mouse cells. The *p53* tumor-suppressor gene has been studied extensively in smokers. It has shown to have an unusual range of mutations that are mainly of the missense type. These *p53* mutations are common in lung cancer, and a large number of tumors have been examined and categorized on the IARC database [169]. Tobacco carcinogens have been associated in lung cancer with particular *p53* mutations at codons 157, 248, and 273 [170]. Transversion mutations (namely G->T) that occur frequently in lung cancers of smokers are of the same type as those observed in vitro growing cells are exposed to BPDE. Remarkably, Denissenko et al. [171, 172] have remarkably concluded that these transversions of *p53* are attributable to the presence of BPDE. BPDEs form adducts selectively at these CpG sites in the same codons (157, 248, and 273). Their studies also show that methylated CpG sites are targets of PAH intermediates, which bind preferentially to the *p53* gene at these sites [171–173]. This suggests strongly that BaP contributes to the common mutations of the *p53* gene found in people with lung cancer. However, other reactive compounds, like diol epoxides of other PAHs, pyridoxobutylating metabolites of NNK and NNN, hydroxylamines of the aromatic amines, and crotonaldehydes, acrolein, and 8-oxodeoxyguanosine, can also be candidates for these G->T transversions [174–179].

As stated earlier, K-*ras* oncogene activation is an early and frequent event in both human lung adenocarcinoma and in spontaneous and chemically induced lung tumors in mice. Adenocarcinomas associated with smoking and mouse lung tumors induced with the tobacco carcinogen BaP contain G->T mutations in the K-*ras* oncogene at codon 12, which is indicative of the base mispairing associated with the BBDE-DNA adduct [180, 181].

The *GSTM1* gene codes for the M class glutathione S-transferases that are important in detoxification of PAH diol epoxides. GSTM1 null has been found as a genotype in 40–50% of the human population [182]. Data suggest that there is an association between this particular null genotype and lung cancer [182–184]. Detoxification pathways are an integral part of the carcinogen potential and further studies are warranted.

The repair capacity of DNA is also indicative of the importance of further clearance of carcinogenic activity. BPDE-DNA adducts appear to be repaired by nucleotide excision repair [185]. It has also been shown that the repair of these adducts is dependent upon the adduct conformation [186]. It has been observed that *cis*-adducts of BPDE with N(2) of deoxyguanosine are repaired more rapidly than their *trans*-analogue (176h). Lingering damaged DNA is potentially tumorigenic.

3.6   Concluding Remarks

Carcinogens have clearly shown to be present in cigarette smoke. Their activation to highly reactive metabolites contributes to the potential insults to DNA, RNA, and proteins- altering a system of "gatekeepers and caretakers" and permitting cells to transform into clones that develop into a neoplasm. Alterations in the detoxification and repair capacity pathways contribute to the perpetuation of DNA damage to linger and burden the system. Further studies are needed to link carcinogens to their full responsibility in tumorigenesis in relation to tobacco. However, there is little doubt that they play an important role in the process.

Key Points

- There are several carcinogens in tobacco smoke. Based on epidemiological evidence, animal model studies, and mechanistic data, we can link them to the development of tobacco-related lung cancer.
- Investigation of mechanisms of polycyclic aromatic hydrocarbons (PAHs) and N-nitrosamines, such as 4-(N-nitrosomethylamino)-1-(3-pyridyl)-1-butanone, can serve as models for tumorigenesis.
- Variable activation of carcinogens can lead to active metabolites, which can lead to direct or indirect damage to DNA, RNA, and proteins.
- Detoxification of carcinogenic metabolites plays an important role in the clearance of carcinogens from the body, preventing damaged DNA from lingering.
- Damage to critical genes, like tumor-suppressor genes, can cause several outcomes, including loss of cell cycle control and cell signaling, leading to the perpetuation of clonal expansion.
- Repair capacity, which may be influenced by variations in genotype, may also lead to decreased apoptotic events and the progression to tumorigenesis.

References

1. US Department of Health, Education and Welfare, Smoking and Health. Report of the Advisory Committee to the Surgeon General of the Public Health Service. Washington: US Dept of HEW, Public Health Service, 1964. PHS Publ. No. 1103.
2. Doll R, Peto R, Wheatley K, Gray R, Sutherland I. Mortality in relation to smoking: 40 years' observations on male British doctors. BMJ 1994; 309:901.
3. Haldorsen T, Grimsrud TK. Cohort analysis of cigarette smoking and lung cancer incidence among Norwegian women. Int J Epidemiol 1999; 28:1032.
4. Lubin JH, Blot WJ. Assessment of lung cancer risk factors by histologic category. J Natl Cancer Inst 1984; 73:383.
5. Harris JE, Thun MJ, Mondul AM, Calle EE. Cigarette tar yields in relation to mortality from lung cancer in the cancer prevention study II prospective cohort, 1982–8. BMJ 2004; 328:72.
6. Sasco AJ, Secretan MB, Straif K. Tobacco smoking and cancer: a brief review of recent epidemiological evidence. Lung Cancer 2004; 45(Suppl 2):S3.
7. Hecht SS. Tobacco smoke carcinogens and lung cancer. J Natl Cancer Inst 1999; 91:1194.
8. International Agency for Research on Cancer. Overall Evaluations of Carcinogenicity. *http://www-cie.iarc.fr* (accessed August 29, 2005).
9. US Department of Health and Human Services. Reducing the health consequences of smoking: 25 years of progress. A report of the Surgeon General. USDHHS, Public Health Service, Centers for disease control, Center for chronic disease prevention and health promotion, Office on smoking and health. 1989, DHHS Pub No. (CDC) 89-8411.
10. Physicians for a Smoke-Free Canada. Tobacco smoke components: carcinogens. 1999. *www.smoke-free.ca/factsheet* (accessed August 10, 2005).
11. Hoffmann D, Hoffmann I. The changing cigarette, 1950–1995. J Toxicol Environ Health 1997; 50:307.
12. Hoffmann D, Hecht SS. Advances in tobacco carcinogenesis. In: Cooper CS, Grover PL (eds), Handbook of Experimental Pharmacology. Springer-Verlag, Heidelberg, Germany, 1990; 94/I:63.
13. Smith CJ, Perfetti TA, Garg R, Hansch C. IARC carcinogens reported in cigarette mainstream smoke and their calculated log P values. Food Chem Toxicol 2003; 41:807.
14. International Agency for Research on Cancer. Tobacco smoking. In: IARC Monographs on the Evaluation of the Carcinogenic Risk of Chemicals to Humans. IARC, Lyon, France, 1986; p 38.
15. California Environmental Protection Agency. Health effects of exposure to environmental tobacco smoke. Office of Environmental Health Hazard Assessment, 1997.
16. National Research Council. Environmental tobacco smoke. Measuring exposures and assessing health effects. Board on environmental studies and toxicology, committee on passive smoking. National Academy Press, Washington DC, 1986.
17. Vineis P, Caporaso N. Tobacco and cancer: epidemiology and the laboratory. Environ Health Perspect 1995; 103:156.
18. NTP. Substance Profiles:4-Aminobiphenyl, CAS No. 92-67-1. Report on Carcinogens, 11th Edition; U.S. Department of Health and Human Services, Public Health Service, National Toxicology Program. *http://ntp.niehs.nih.gov* (accessed August 29, 2005).
19. NTP. Substance Profiles. Benzene, CAS No 71-43-2, Report on Carcinogens, 11th Edition; U.S. Department of Health and Human Services, Public Health Service, National Toxicology Program. *http://ntp.niehs.nih.gov* (accessed August 29, 2005).
20. NTP. Substance Profiles: Cadmium (CAS No. 7440-43-9) and cadmium compounds. Report on Carcinogens, 11th Edition; U.S. Department of Health and Human Services, Public Health Service, National Toxicology Program. *http://ntp.niehs.nih.gov* (accessed August 29, 2005).
21. Guerin MR, Jenkins RA, Tomkins BA. The Chemistry of Environmental Tobacco Smoke: Composition and Management. Lewis Publishers, Chelsea, MA, 1992.
22. Smith CJ, Livingston SD, Doolittle OJ. An international literature survey of "IARC group I carcinogens" reported in mainstream cigarette smoke. Food Chem Toxicol 1997; 35:1107

23. Smith CJ, Perfetti TA, et al. IARC Group 2A carcinogens reported in cigarette mainstream smoke. Food Chem Toxicol 2000; 38:371.

24. NTP. Substance Profiles: 2-Naphthylamine CAS No. 91-59-8. Report on Carcinogens, 11th Edition; U.S. Department of Health and Human Services, Public Health Service, National Toxicology Program. *http://ntp.niehs.nih.gov* (accessed August 29, 2005).

25. NTP. Substance Profiles: 1,3-Butadiene, CAS No. 106-99-0. Report on Carcinogens, 11th Edition; U.S. Department of Health and Human Services, Public Health Service, National Toxicology Program. *http://ntp.niehs.nih.gov* (accessed August 29, 2005).

26. NTP. Substance Profiles: *N*-Nitrosodiethylamine, CAS No.55-18-5. Report on Carcinogens, 11th Edition; U.S. Department of Health and Human Services, Public Health Service, National Toxicology Program. *http://ntp.niehs.nih.gov* (accessed August 29, 2005).

27. NTP. Substance Profiles: *N*-Nitrosodimethylamine, CAS No. 62-75-9. Report on Carcinogens, 11th Edition; U.S. Department of Health and Human Services, Public Health Service, National Toxicology Program. *http://ntp.niehs.nih.gov* (accessed August 29, 2005).

28. NTP. Substance Profiles: Polycyclic aromatic hydrocarbons, 15 listings. Report on Carcinogens, Eleventh Edition; U.S. Department of Health and Human Services, Public Health Service, National Toxicology Program. *http://ntp.niehs.nih.gov* (accessed August 29, 2005).

29. NTP. Substance Profiles: Hydrazine and Hydrazine Sulfate CAS Nos. 302-01-2 and 10034-93-2. Report on Carcinogens, 11th Edition; U.S. Department of Health and Human Services, Public Health Service, National Toxicology Program. *http://ntp.niehs.nih.gov* (accessed August 29, 2005).

30. NTP. Substance Profiles: 4-(*N*-Nitrosomethylamino)-1-(3-pyridyl)-1-butanone, CAS No. 64091-91-4. Report on Carcinogens, 11th Edition; U.S. Department of Health and Human Services, Public Health Service, National Toxicology Program. *http://ntp.niehs.nih.gov* (accessed August 29, 2005).

31. NTP. Substance Profiles: Tobacco-related exposures: Report on Carcinogens, 11th Edition; U.S. Department of Health and Human Services, Public Health Service, National Toxicology Program. *http://ntp.niehs.nih.gov* (accessed August 29, 2005).

32. Blot WJ, McLaughlin JK. Passive smoking and lung cancer risk: what is the story now? [editorial]. J Natl Cancer Inst 1998; 90:1416.

33. International Agency for Research on Cancer. Certain polycyclic aromatic hydrocarbons and heterocyclic compounds. In: IARC Monographs on the Evaluation of Carcinogenic Risk of Chemicals to Man. IARC, Lyon, France, 1972; 3:45.

34. International Agency for Research on Cancer. Some polycyclic aromatic hydrocarbons and heterocyclic compounds. In: IARC Monographs on the Evaluation of the Carcinogenic Risk of Chemicals to Humans. IARC, Lyon, France, 1973; 3:229, 249, 271.

35. International Agency for Research on Cancer. Polynuclear aromatic amines, part 1. chemical, environmental and experimental data. In: IARC Monographs on the Evaluation of Carcinogenic Risk of Chemicals to Humans. IARC, Lyon, France, 1983; 32.

36. Deutsch-Wenzel RP, Brune H, Grimmer G, Dettbarn G, Misfeld J. Experimental studies in rat lungs on the carcinogenicity and dose–response relationships of eight frequently occurring environmental polycyclic aromatic hydrocarbons. J Natl Cancer Inst 1983; 71:539.

37. Sellakumar A, Shubik P. Carcinogenicity of different polycyclic hydrocarbons in the respiratory tract of hamsters. J Natl Cancer Inst 1974; 53:1713.

38. Nesnow S, Ross JA, Stoner GD, Mass MJ. Mechanistic linkage between DNA adducts, mutations in oncogenes and tumorigenesis of carcinogenic environmental polycyclic aromatic hydrocarbons in strain A/J mice. Toxicology 1995; 105:403.

39. Hecht SS, Hochalter JB, Villalta PW, Murphy SE. 2′-Hydroxylation of nicotine by cytochrome P450 2A6 and human liver microsomes: formation of a lung carcinogen precursor. Proc Natl Acad Sci U S A 2000; 97:12493.

40. Hecht SS. Biochemistry, biology, and carcinogenicity of tobacco-specific *N*-nitrosamines. Chem Res Toxicol 1998; 11:559.

41. International Agency for Research on Cancer. Some monomers, plastics, and synthetic elastomers, and acrolein. In: IARC Monographs on the Evaluation of Carcinogenic Risk of Chemicals to Humans. IARC, Lyon, France, 1979; 19:513.

42. Feng Z, Hu W, Rom WN, et al. 4-aminobiphenyl is a major etiological agent of human bladder cancer: evidence from its DNA binding spectrum in human p53 gene. Carcinogenesis 2002; 23:1721.

43. Vineis P. Epidemiology from exposure to arylamines. Environ Health Perspect 1994; 102(Suppl 6):7.

44. Oberdorster G, Cherian MG, Baggs RB. Importance of species differences in experimental pulmonary carcinogenicity of inhaled cadmium for extrapolation to humans. Toxicol Lett 1994; 72:339.

45. International Agency for Research on Cancer. Occupational exposures to mists and vapours from strong inorganic acids; and some other industrial chemicals. In: IARC Monographs on the Evaluation of the Carcinogenic Risk of Chemicals to Humans. IARC, Lyon, France, 1992; 54:237.

46. NTP. Substance Profiles: Chromium Hexavalent Compounds. Report on Carcinogens, 11th Edition; U.S. Department of Health and Human Services, Public Health Service, National Toxicology Program. *http://ntp.niehs.nih.gov* (accessed August 29, 2005).

47. International Agency for Research on Cancer. Chromium, nickel and welding. In: IARC Monographs on the Evaluation of the Carcinogenic Risk of Chemicals to Humans. IARC, Lyon, France, 1990; 49:677.

48. International Agency for Research on Cancer. Some antithyroid and related substances, nitrofurans and industrial chemicals. In: IARC Monographs on the Evaluation of the Carcinogenic Risk of Chemicals to Man. IARC, Lyon, France, 1974; 7:111.

49. NTP. Substance Profiles: Formaldehyde (gas), CAS No. 50-00-0. Report on Carcinogens, 11th Edition; U.S. Department of Health and Human Service, National Toxicology Program. *http://ntp.niehs.nih.gov* (accessed August 29, 2005).

50. Yu, MC, Skipper PL, Tannenbaum SR, et al. Arylamine exposures and bladder cancer risk. Mutat Res 2002; 506–507:21.

51. NTP. Toxicology and carcinogenesis studies of nickel oxide (CAS No. 1313-99-1) in F344 rats and B6C3F1 mice (inhalation studies). Technical Report Series No 451. Research Triangle Park, NC: National Toxicology Program. 1996a; 381.

52. NTP. Toxicology and carcinogenesis studies of nickel subsulfide (CAS No. 12035-72-2) in F344 rats and B6C3F1 mice (inhalation studies). Technical Report Series No 453. Research Triangle Park, NC: National Toxicology Program. 1996b; 365.

53. International Agency for Research on Cancer. Vinyl chloride. Overall Evaluations of Carcinogenicity. In: IARC

Monographs on the Evaluation of Carcinogenic Risk of Chemicals to Humans, Supplement 7. IARC, Lyon, France, 1987; Suppl 7:440.

54. NTP. Substance Profiles: Vinyl chloride, CAS No. 75-01-4. Report on Carcinogens, 11th Edition; U.S. Department of Health and Human Services, Public Health Service, National Toxicology Program. *http://ntp.niehs.nih.gov* (accessed August 29, 2005).

55. Kielhorn J, Melber C, Wahnschaffe U, et al. Vinyl chloride: still a cause for concern. Environ Health Perspect 2000; 108:579.

56. Battista SP. Ciliatoxic components of cigarette smoke. In: Wynder EL, Hoffman D, Gori GB (eds), Smoking and Health I Measurement in the Analysis and Treatment of Smoking Behavior. US Government Printing Office, Washington DC, 1973.

57. Hecht SS. Carcinogenic effects of cigarette smoke on the respiratory tract. In: Roth RA (ed) Comprehensive Toxicology: Toxicology of the Respiratory System. Elsevier Science, Oxford UK, 1997; 8:437.

58. Hecht SS. Tobacco carcinogens, their biomarkers and tobacco-induced cancer. Nat Rev Cancer 2003; 3:733.

59. Rao Y, Hoffmann E, Zia M et al. Duplications and defects in the CYP2A6 gene: identification, genotyping, and in vivo effects on smoking. Mol Pharmacol 2000 Oct; 58:747.

60. Berembaum, I Subik P. A new, quantitative approach to the study of the stages of chemical carcinogenesis in the mouse's skin. Br J Cancer 1947; 1:383.

61. Farber E. The multistep nature of cancer development. Cancer Res 1984; 44:4217.

62. Cooper, G. Role of oncogenes and tumor suppressor genes in the pathogenesis of neoplasms. In: Oncogenes. Jones and Bartlett Publishers, Boston, 1995.

63. Garte S, Zocchetti C, Taioli E. Gene-environment interactions in the application of biomarkers of cancer susceptibility in epidemiology. In: Toniolo P, Boffetta P, et al. (eds) Application of Biomarkers in Cancer Epidemiology. IARC, Lyon, France, 1997; 251.

64. d'Errico A, Malats N, Vineis P, Boffetta P. Review of studies of selected metabolic polymorphisms and cancer. IARC Scientific Publications 1999; (148):323.

65. Marcus PM, Hayes RB, et al. Cigarette smoking, *N*-acetyltransferase 2 acetylation status, and bladder cancer risk: a case-series meta analysis of a gene–environment interaction. Cancer Epidemiol Biomarkers Prev 2000; 9:461.

66. Marcus PM, Vineis P, Rothman N. NAT2 slow acetylation and bladder cancer risk: a meta-analysis of 22 case-control studies conducted in the general population. Pharmacogenetics 2000; 10:115.

67. Benhamou S, et al. Meta- and pooled analyses of the effects of glutathione S-transferase M1 polymorphisms and smoking on lung cancer risk. Carcinogenesis 2002; 23:1343.

68. Vineis P, Veglia F, et al. CYP1A1 T3801 C polymorphism and lung cancer: a pooled analysis of 2,451 cases and 3,358 controls. Int J Cancer 2003; 104:650.

69. International Agency for Research on Cancer. Tobacco Smoke. Overall Evaluations of Carcinogenicity In: IARC Monographs on the Evaluation of Carcinogenic Risk of Chemicals to Humans, Supplement 7. IARC, Lyon, France, 1987; Suppl 7:359.

70. International Agency for Research on Cancer. Cancer incidence in five continents. IARC, Lyon, France, 1992; 6.

71. Schulte PA, Perera FP (eds). Molecular Epidemiology: Principles and Practices. Academic Press, New York, 1993; 4.

72. International Agency for Research on Cancer. Tobacco smoke and involuntary smoking. In: IARC Monographs on the Evaluation of Carcinogenic Risks to Humans. IARC, Lyon, France, 2002; 83.

73. Harlow E. An introduction to the puzzle. Cold Spring Harbor Symposia on Quantitative Biology 1994; 59:709.

74. Shields PG, Harris CC. Cancer risk and low-penetrance susceptibility genes in gene–environment interactions. J Clin Oncol 2000; 18:2309.

75. Vogelstein B, Kinzler KW (eds). The Genetic Basis of Human Cancer. McGraw-Hill, New York, 1998.

76. Levitt NC, Hickson ID. Caretaker tumour suppressor genes that defend genome integrity. Trends Mol Med, 2002; 8:179.

77. Oesch F, Aulmann W, Platt KL, Doerjer G. Individual differences in DNA repair capacities in man. Arch Toxicol Suppl 1987; 10:172.

78. Cheng L, Spitz MR, Hong WK, Wei Q. Reduced expression levels of nucleotide excision repair genes in lung cancer: a case-control analysis. Carcinogenesis 2000; 21:1527.

79. He XY, Shen J, Ding X, Lu AY, Hong JY. Identification of critical amino acid residues of human CYP2A13 for the metabolic activation of 4-(methylnitrosamino)-1-(3-pyridyl)-1-butanone, a tobacco-specific carcinogen. Drug Metab Dispos 2004; 32:1516.

80. Nishikawa A, Mori Y, Lee IS, et al. Cigarette smoking, metabolic activation and carcinogenesis. Curr Drug Metab 2004; 5:363 (review).

81. Su T, Bao Z, Zhang QT, et al. Human cytochrome P450 CYP2A13: predominant expression in the respiratory tract and its high efficiency metabolic activation of a tobacco-specific carcinogen, 4-(methylnitrosamino)-1-(3-pyridyl)-1-butanone. Cancer Res 2000; 60:5074.

82. Wang H, Tan W, Bingtao Hao B, et al. Substantial reduction in risk of lung adenocarcinoma associated with genetic polymorphism in CYP2A13, the most active cytochrome p450 for the metabolic activation of tobacco-specific carcinogen NNK. Cancer Res 2003; 63:8057.

83. Jalas JR, Seetharaman M, Hecht SS, Murphy SE. Molecular modelling of CYP2A enzymes: application to metabolism of the tobacco-specific nitrosamine 4-(methylnitrosamino)-1-(3-pyridyl)-1-butanone (NNK). Xenobiotica 2004; 34:515.

84. Ziegel R, Shallop A, Jones R, Tretyakova N. K-ras gene sequence effects on the formation of 4-(methylnitrosamino)-1-(3-pyridyl)-1-butanone (NNK)-DNA adducts. Chem Res Toxicol 2003; 16:541.

85. Hecht SS, Villalta PW, Sturla SJ, et al. Identification of O₂-substituted pyrimidine adducts formed in reactions of 4-(acetoxymethylnitrosamino)-1-(3-pyridyl)-1-butanone and 4-(acetoxymethylnitros- amino)-1-(3-pyridyl)-1-butanol with DNA. Chem Res Toxicol 2004; 17:588.

86. Wang M, Cheng G, Sturla SJ, et al. Identification of adducts formed by pyridyloxobutylation of deoxyguanosine and DNA by 4-(acetoxymethylnitrosamino)-1-(3-pyridyl)-1-butanone, a chemically activated form of tobacco specific carcinogens. Chem Res Toxicol 2003; 16:616.

87. Sturla SJ, Scott J, Lao Y, et al. Mass spectrometric analysis of relative levels of pyridyloxobutylation adducts formed in the reaction of DNA with a chemically activated form of the tobacco-specific carcinogen 4-(methylnitrosamino)-1-(3-pyridyl)-1-butanone. Chem Res Toxicol 2005; 18:1048.

88. Rioux N, Castonguay A. The induction of cyclooxygenase-1 by a tobacco carcinogen in U937 human macrophages is correlated to the activation of NF-B. Carcinogenesis 2000; 21:1745.

89. Schuller, HM, Tithof PK, Williams M, Plummer H 3rd. The tobacco-specific carcinogen 4-(methylnitrosamino)-1-(3-pyridyl)-1-butanone is a beta-adrenergic agonist and stimulates DNA synthesis in lung adenocarcinoma via beta-adrenergic receptor-mediated release of arachidonic acid. Cancer Res 1999; 59:4510.

90. Wu WK, Wong HP, Luo SW, et al. 4-(Methylnitrosami-no)-1-(3-pyridyl)-1-butanone from cigarette smoke stimulates colon cancer growth via beta-adrenoceptors. Cancer Res 2005; 65:5272.

91. Tsurutani J, Castillo SS, Brognard J, et al. Tobacco components stimulate Akt-dependent proliferation and NFkappaB-dependent survival in lung cancer cells. Carcinogenesis 2005; 26:1182.

92. Plummer HK 3rd, Dhar M, Schuller HM. Expression of the alpha7 nicotinic acetylcholine receptor in human lung cells. Respir Res 2005; 6:29.

93. Jull BA, Plummer HK, Schuller HM. Nicotinic receptor-mediated activation by the tobacco-specific nitrosamine NNK of the Raf-1/MAP kinase pathway, resulting in phosphorylation of the c-myc in human small cell lung carcinoma cells and the pulmonary neuroendocrine cells. J Cancer Res Clin Oncol 2001; 127:707.

94. West KA, Brognard J, Clark AS et al. Rapid Akt activation by nicotine and a tobacco carcinogen modulates the phenotype of normal human airway epithelial cells. J Clin Invest 2003; 111:81.

95. West KA, Linnoila IR, Belinsky SA. Tobacco carcinogen-induced cellular transformation increases activation of the phosphatidylinositol 3′-kinase/Akt pathway in vitro and in vivo. Cancer Res 2004; 64:446.

96. Massion PP, Taflan PM, Shyr Y, et al. Early involvement of the phosphatidylinositol 3-kinase/Akt pathway in lung cancer progression. Am J Respir Crit Care Med 2004; 170:1088.

97. Ho YS, Chen CH, Wang YJ, et al. Tobacco-specific carcinogen 4-(methylnitrosamino)-1-(3-pyridyl)-1-butanone (NNK) induces cell proliferation in normal human bronchial epithelial cells through NFkappaB activation and cyclin D1 up-regulation. Toxicol Appl Pharmacol 2005; 205:133.

98. Merlo A, Herman JG, Mao L, et al. 5′ CpG island methylation is associated with transcriptional silencing of the tumour suppressor p16/CDKN2/MTS1 in human cancers. Nat Med 1995; 1:686.

99. Otterson GA, Kratzke RA, Coxon A, et al. Absence of p16^{INK4} protein is restricted to the subset of lung cancer lines that retains wildtype RB. Oncogene 1994; 9:3375.

100. Belinsky SA, Nikula KJ, Palmisano WA, et al. Aberrant methylation of p16^{INK4a} is an early event in lung cancer and a potential biomarker for early diagnosis. Proc Natl Acad Sci U S A 1998; 95:11891.

101. Kamb A, Gruis NA, Weaver-Feldhaus J, et al. A cell cycle regulator potentially involved in genesis of many tumor types. Science 1994; 264:436.

102. Kratzke RA, Greatens TM, et al. Rb and p16INK4a expression in resected non-small cell lung tumors. Cancer Res 1996; 56:3415.

103. Vonlanthen S, Heighway J, et al. Expression of p16INK4a/p16alpha and p19ARF/p16beta is frequently altered in non-small cell lung cancer and correlates with p53 overexpression. Oncogene 1998; 17:2779.

104. Sanchez-Cespedes M, Reed AL, et al. Inactivation of the INK4A/ARF locus frequently coexists with TP53 mutations in non-small cell lung cancer. Oncogene 1999; 18:5843.

105. Slebos RJ, Kibbelaar RE, et al. K-ras oncogene activation as a prognostic marker in adenocarcinoma of the lung. N Engl J Med 1990; 323:561.

106. Sugio K, Ishida T, et al. Ras gene mutations as a prognostic marker in adenocarcinoma of the human lung without lymph node metastasis. Cancer Res 1992; 52:2903.

107. Rosell R, Li S, et al. Prognostic impact of mutated K-ras gene in surgically resected non-small cell lung cancer patients. Oncogene 1993; 8:2407.

108. Silini EM, Bosi F, et al. K-ras gene mutations: an unfavorable prognostic marker in stage I lung adenocarcinoma. Virchows Arch 1994; 424:367.

109. Rosell R, Monzo M, et al. K-ras genotypes and prognosis in non-small-cell lung cancer. Ann Oncol 1995; 6(Suppl 3):S15.

110. Cho JY, Kim JH, et al. Correlation between K-ras gene mutation and prognosis of patients with nonsmall cell lung carcinoma. Cancer 1997; 79:462.

111. Fukuyama Y, Mitsudomi T, et al. K-ras and p53 mutations are an independent unfavorable prognostic indicator in patients with non-small-cell lung cancer. Br J Cancer 1997; 75:1125.

112. De Gregorio L, Manenti G, et al. Prognostic value of loss of heterozygosity and KRAS2 mutations in lung adenocarcinoma. Int J Cancer 1998; 79:269.

113. Kwiatkowski DJ, Harpole DH Jr, et al. Molecular pathologic substaging in 244 stage I non-small-cell lung cancer patients: clinical implications. J Clin Oncol 1998; 16:2468.

114. Nelson HH, Christiani DC, et al. Implications and prognostic value of K-ras mutation for early-stage lung cancer in women. J Natl Cancer Inst 1999; 91:2032.

115. Pulling LC, Vuillemenot BR, Hutt JA, et al. Aberrant promoter hypermethylation of the death-associated protein kinase gene is early and frequent in murine lung tumors induced by cigarette smoke and tobacco carcinogens. Cancer Res 2004; 64:3844.

116. Jin Z, Gao F, Flagg T, Deng X. Tobacco-specific nitrosamine 4-(methylnitrosamino)-1-(3-pyridyl)-1-butanone promotes functional cooperation of Bcl2 and c-Myc through phosphorylation in regulating cell survival and proliferation. J Biol Chem 2004; 279:40209.

117. Ren Q, Murphy SE, Zheng Z, and Lazarus P. O-Glucuronidation of the lung carcinogen 4-(methylnitrosamino)-1-(3-pyridyl)-1-butanol (NNAL) by human udp-glucuronosyltransferases 2B7 and 1A9. Drug Metab Dispos 2000; 28:1352.

118. Wiener D, Doerge DR, Fang JL, et al. Characterization of N-glucuronidation of the lung carcinogen 4-(methylnitrosamino)-1-(3-pyridyl)-1-butanol (NNAL) in human liver: importance of UDP-glucuronosyltransferase 1A4. Drug Metab Dispos 2004; 32:72.

119. Maser E. Significance of reductases in the detoxification of the tobacco-specific carcinogen NNK. Trends Pharmacol Sci 2004; 25:235.

120. Hill CE, Wickliffe JK, Wolfe KJ, et al. The L84F and the I143V polymorphisms in the O6-methylguanine-DNA-methyltransferase (MGMT) gene increase human sensitivity to the genotoxic effects of the tobacco-specific nitrosamine carcinogen NNK. Pharmacogenet Genomics 2005; 15:571.

121. Russo AL, Thiagalingam A, Pan H, et al. Differential DNA Hypermethylation of Critical Genes Mediates the Stage-Specific Tobacco Smoke-Induced Neoplastic Progression of Lung Cancer. Clin Cancer Res 2005; 11(7):2466.

122. Therriault MJ, Proulx LI, Castonguay A, Bissonnette EY. Immunomodulatory effects of the tobacco-specific carcinogen, NNK, on alveolar macrophages. Clin Exp Immunol 2003; 132:232.

123. Rioux N, Castonguay A. 4-(methylnitrosamino)-1-(3-pyridyl)-1-butanone modulation of cytokine release in U937 human macrophages. Cancer Immunol Immunother 2001; 49:663.

124. Proulx LI, Castonguay A, Bissonnette EY. Cytokine production by alveolar macrophages is down regulated by the alpha-methylhydroxylation pathway of 4-(methylnitrosamino)-1-(3-pyridyl)-1-butanone (NNK). Carcinogenesis 2004; 25:997.

125. Rubin H. Synergistic mechanisms in carcinogenesis by polycyclic aromatic hydrocarbons and by tobacco smoke: a biohistorical perspective with updates. Carcinogenesis 2001; 12:1903.

126. Yun CH, Shimada T, Guengerich FP. Roles of human liver cytochrome P4502C and 3A enzymes in the 3-hydroxylation of benzo[a]pyrene. Cancer Res 1992; 52:1868.

127. Bauer E, Guo Z, Ueng YF, Bell LC, Zeldin D, Guengerich FP. Oxidation of benzo[a]pyrene by recombinant human cytochrome P450 enzymes. Chem Res Toxicol 1995; 8:136.

128. Shou M, Korzekwa KR, Crespi CL, Gonzalez FJ, Gelboin HV. The role of 12 cDNA-expressed human, rodent, and rabbit cytochromes P450 in the metabolism of benzo[a]pyrene and benzo[a]pyrene trans-7,8-dihydrodiol. Mol Carcinog 1994; 10:159

129. Rojas M, Camus AM, Alexandrov K, Husgafvel-Pursiainen K, Anttila S, Vainio H, et al. Stereoselective metabolism of (-)-benzo[a]pyrene-7,8-diol by human lung microsomes and peripheral blood lymphocytes: effect of smoking. Carcinogenesis 1992; 13:929.

130. Alexandrov K, Rojas M, Geneste O, et al. An improved fluorometric assay for dosimetry of benzo[a]pyrene diol-epoxide-DNA adducts in smokers' lung: comparisons with total bulky adducts and aryl hydrocarbon hydroxylase activity. Cancer Res 1992; 52:6248.

131. Rojas M, Alexandrov K, Cascarbi I, Brockmoller J, Likhachev A, Pozharisski K, et al. High benzo[a]pyrene diol-epoxide DNA adduct levels in lung and blood cells from individuals with combined CYP1A1 MspI/MspI-GSTM1*0/*0 genotypes. Pharmacogenetics 1997; 8:109.

132. Kawajiri K, Nakachi K, et al. Identification of genetically high risk individuals to lung cancer by DNA polymorphisms of the cytochrome P450IA1 gene. FEBS Lett 1990; 263:131.

133. Hayashi S, Watanabe J, Nakachi K, Kawajiri K. Genetic linkage of lung cancer-associated MspI polymorphisms with amino acid replacement in the heme binding region of the human cytochrome P450IA1 gene. J Biochem 1991; 110:407.

134. Nakachi K, Imai K, Hayashi S, et al. Genetic susceptibility to squamous cell carcinoma of the lung in relation to cigarette smoking dose. Cancer Res 1991; 51:5177.

135. Nakachi K, Hayashi S, Kawajiri K, Imai K. Association of cigarette smoking and CYP1A1 polymorphisms with adenocarcinoma of the lung by grades of differentiation. Carcinogenesis 1995; 16:2209.

136. Okada T, Kawashima K, Fukushi S, et al. Association between a cytochrome P450 CYPIA1 genotype and incidence of lung cancer. Pharmacogenetics 1994; 4:333.

137. Kawajiri K, Eguchi H, Nakachi K, et al. Associate of CYP1A1 germ line polymorphisms with mutations of the p53 gene in lung cancer. Cancer Res 1996; 56:72.

138. Chacko M, Gupta RC. Evaluation of DNA damage in the oral mucosa of tobacco users and non-users by 32P-adduct assay. Carcinogenesis 1988; 9:2309.

139. Phillips DH, Hewer A, Martin CN, et al. Correlation of DNA adduct levels in human lung with cigarette smoking. Nature 1988; 336:790.

140. Foiles PG, Miglietta LM, Quart AM, et al. Evaluation of 32P-postlabeling analysis of DNA from exfoliated oral mucosa cells as a means of monitoring exposure of the oral cavity to genotoxic agents. Carcinogenesis 1989; 10:1429.

141. Randerath E, Miller RH, Mittal D, et al. Covalent DNA damage in tissues of cigarette smokers as determined by ^{32}P-postlabeling assay. J Natl Cancer Inst 1989; 81:341.

142. Garner RC, Cuzick J, Jenkins D, et al. Linear relationship between DNA adducts in human lung and cigarette smoking. IARC Scientific Publications 1990; 104:421.

143. van Schooten FJ, Hillebrand MJ, van Leeuwen FE, et al. Polycyclic aromatic hydrocarbon-DNA adducts in lung tissue from lung cancer patients. Carcinogenesis 1990; 11:1677.

144. Routledge MN, Garner RC, Jenkins D, Cuzick J. ^{32}P-postlabelling analysis of DNA from human tissues. Mutat Res 1992; 282:139.

145. Bartsch H, Castegnaro M, Camus AM, et al. Analysis of DNA adducts in smokers' lung and urothelium by ^{32}P-postlabelling:metabolic phenotype dependence and comparisons with other exposure markers. IARC Scientific Publications 1993; 124:331.

146. Shields PG, Bowman ED, Harrington AM, et al. Polycyclic aromatic hydrocarbon-DNA adducts in human lung and cancer susceptibility genes. Cancer Res 1993; 53:3486.

147. Weston A, Bowman ED, Shields PG, et al. Detection of polycyclic aromatic hydrocarbon-DNA adducts in human lung. Environ Health Perspect 1993; 99:257.

148. Degawa M, Stern SJ, Martin MV, et al. Metabolic activation and carcinogenic-DNA adduct detection in human larynx. Cancer Res 1994; 54:4915.

149. Wiencke JK, Kelsey KT, Varkonyi A, et al. Correlation of DNA adducts in blood mononuclear cells with tobacco carcinogen-induced damage in human lung. Cancer Res 1995; 55:4910.

150. Wiencke JK, Thurston SW, Kelsey KT, et al. Early age at smoking initiation and tobacco carcinogen DNA damage in the lung. J Natl Cancer Inst 1999; 91:614.

151. Rudiger HW, Nowak D, Hartmann K, Cerutti P. Enhanced formation of benzo[a]pyrene: DNA adducts in monocytes of patients with a presumed predisposition to lung cancer. Cancer Res 1985; 45:5890.

152. Cheng YW, Chen CY, Lin P, et al. DNA adduct level in lung tissue may act as a risk biomarker of lung cancer. Euro J Cancer 2000; 36:11381.

153. Vulimiri SV, Wu X, Baer-Dubowska W, et al. Analysis of aromatic DNA adducts and 7,8-dihydro-8-oxo-2'-deoxyguanosine in lymphocyte DNA from a case-control study of lung cancer involving minority populations. Mol Carcinog 2000; 27:34.

154. Brunmark P, Harriman S, Skipper PL, et al. Identification of subdomain IB in human serum albumin as a major binding site for polycyclic aromatic hydrocarbon epoxides. Chem Res Toxicol 1997; 10:880.

155. Melikian AA, Sun P, Pierpont C, et al. Gas chromatographic-mass spectrometric determination of benzo[a]pyrene and chrysene diol epoxide globin adducts in humans. Cancer Epidemiol Biomarkers Prev 1997; 6:833.

156. Pastorelli R, Restano J, Guanci M, Maramonte M, Magagnotti C, Allevi R, et al. Hemoglobin adducts of benzo[a]pyrene diolepoxide in newspaper vendors: association with traffic exhaust. Carcinogenesis 1996; 17:2389.

157. Melikian AA, Sun P, Coleman S, Amin S, Hecht SS. Detection of DNA and globin adducts of polynuclear aromatic hydrocarbon diol epoxides by gas chromatography-mass spectrometry and [^{3}H]CH$_3$I postlabeling of released tetraols. Chem Res Toxicol 1996; 9:508.

158. Zhu Y, Spitz MR, Zheng YL, et al. BPDE-induced lymphocytic 3p21.3 aberrations may predict head and neck carcinoma risk. Cancer 2002; 95:563.

159. Jongeneelen FJ. Methods for routine biological monitoring of carcinogenic PAH-mixtures. Sci Total Environ 1997; 199:141.

160. Strickland P, Kang D, Sithisarankul P. Polycyclic aromatic hydrocarbon metabolites in urine as biomarkers of exposure and effect. Environ Health Perspect 1996; 104 Suppl 5:927.

161. Sithisarankul P, Vineis P, Kang D, Rothman N, Caporaso N, Strickland P. The association of 1-hydroxypyrene-glucuronide in human urine with cigarette smoking and

broiled or roasted meat consumption. Biomarkers 1997; 2:217.

162. Ariese F, Verkaik M, Hoornweg GP, van de Nesse RJ, Jukema-Leenstra SR, Hofstraat JW, et al. Trace analysis of 3-hydroxy benzo[a]pyrene in urine for the biomonitoring of human exposure to polycyclic aromatic hydrocarbons. J Anal Toxicol 1994; 18:195.

163. Grimmer G, Jacob J, Dettbarn G, Naujack KW. Determination of urinary metabolites of polycyclic aromatic hydrocarbons (PAH) for the risk assessment of PAH-exposed workers. Int Arch Occup Environ Health 1997; 69:231.

164. Mumford JL, Li X, Hu F, Lu XB, Chuang JC. Human exposure and dosimetry of polycyclic aromatic hydrocarbons in urine from Xuan Wei, China, with high lung cancer mortality associated with exposure to unvented coal smoke. Carcinogenesis 1995; 16:3031.

165. Becher G, Bjorseth A. Determination of exposure to polycyclic aromatic hydrocarbons by analysis of human urine. Cancer Lett 1983; 17:301

166. Haugen A, Becher G, Benestad C, et al. Determination of polycyclic aromatic hydrocarbons in the urine, benzo(a)pyrene diol epoxide-DNA adducts in lymphocyte DNA, and antibodies to the adducts in sera from coke oven workers exposed to measured amounts of polycyclic aromatic hydrocarbons in the work atmosphere. Cancer Res 1986; 46:4178.

167. Weston A, Bowman ED, Carr P, Rothman N, Strickland PT. Detection of metabolites of polycyclic aromatic hydrocarbons in human urine. Carcinogenesis 1993; 14:1053.

168. Bowman ED, Rothman N, Hackl C, Santella RM, Weston A. Interindividual variation in the levels of certain urinary polycyclic aromatic hydrocarbon metabolites following medicinal exposure to coal tar ointment. Biomarkers 1997; 2:321.

169. Hainaut P, Hernandez T, Robinson A, et al. IARC Database of p53 gene mutations in human tumors and cell lines: updated compilation, revised formats and new visualisation tools. Nucleic Acids Research 1998; 26:205.

170. Bennett WP, Hussain SP, Vahakangas KH, et al. Molecular epidemiology of human cancer risk: gene-environment interactions and p53 mutation spectrum in human lung cancer. J Pathol 1999; 187:8.

171. Denissenko MF, Pao A, Jang M, Pfeifer GP. Preferential formation of benzo[a]pyrene adducts at lung cancer mutational hotspots in P53. Science 1996; 274:430.

172. Denissenko MF, Chen JX, Tang MS, Pfeifer GP. Cytosine methylation determines hot spots of DNA damage in the human P53 gene. Proc Natl Acad Sci U S A 1997; 94:3893.

173. Chen JX, Zheng Y, West M, Tang M. Carcinogens preferentially bind at methylated CpG in the p53 mutational hot spots. Cancer Res 1998; 58:2070.

174. Delclos KB, Kadlubar FF. Carcinogenic aromatic amines and amides. In: Guengerich FP (ed) Comprehensive Toxicology: Chemical Carcinogens and Anticarcinogens. Elsevier Science, Oxford, UK, 1997; 12:141.

175. Shukla R, Liu T, Geacintov NE, Loechler EL. The major, N^2-dG adduct of (+)-anti-B[a]PDE shows a dramatically different mutagenic specificity (predominantly, G->A) in a 5'-CGT-3' sequence context. Biochem 1997; 36:10256.

176. Moriya M, Zhang W, Johnson F, Grollman AP. Mutagenic potency of exocyclic DNA adducts: marked differences between Escherichia coli and simian kidney cells. Proc Natl Acad Sci U S A 1994; 91:11899.

177. Moriya M. Single-stranded shuttle phagemid for mutagenesis studies in mammalian cells: 8-oxoguanine in DNA induces targeted G.C->T.A transversions in simian kidney cells. Proc Natl Acad Sci U S A 1993; 90:1122.

178. Ronai ZA, Gradia S, Peterson LA, Hecht SS. G to A transitions and G to T transversions in codon 12 of the Ki-ras oncogene isolated from mouse lung tumors induced by 4-(methylnitrosamino)-1-(3-pyridyl)-1-butanone (NNK) and related DNA methylating and pyridyloxobutylating agents. Carcinogenesis 1993; 14:2419.

179. Burcham PC, Marnett LJ. Site-specific mutagenesis by a propanodeoxyguanosine adduct carried on an M13 genome. J Biol Chem 1994; 269:28844.

180. Belinsky SA, Devereux TR, Maronpot RR, et al. Relationship between formation of promutagenic adducts and the activation of the K-ras protooncogene in lung tumors from A/J mice treated with nitrosamines. Cancer Res 1989; 49:5305.

181. You M, Cabdrian U, Maronpot RR, et al. Activation of the K-ras protooncogene in spontaneously occurring and chemically induced lung tumors of the strain A mouse. Proc Natl Acad Sci U S A 1989; 86:3070.

182. Spivack SD, Fasco MJ, Walker VE, Kaminsky LS. The molecular epidemiology of lung cancer. Crit Rev Toxicol 1997; 27:319.

183. McWilliams JE, Sanderson BJ, Harris EL, et al. Glutathione S-transferase M1 (GSTM1) deficiency and lung cancer risk. Cancer Epidemiol Biomarkers Prev 1995; 4:589.

184. Rebbeck TR. Molecular epidemiology of the human glutathione S-transferase genotypes GSTM1 and GSTT1 in cancer susceptibility. Cancer Epidemiol Biomarkers Prev 1997; 6:733.

185. Tang MS, Pierce JR, Doisy RP, et al. Differences and similarities in the repair of two benzo[a]pyrene diol isomers induced DNA adducts by uvrA, uvrB, and uvrC gene products. Biochemistry 1992; 31:8429.

186. Hess MT, Gunz D, Luneva N, et al. Base pair conformation-dependent excision of benzo[a]pyrene diol epoxide-guanine adducts by human nucleotide excision repair enzymes. Mol Cell Biol 1997; 17:7069.

Section II:
Preclinical Investigation of Lung Cancer

Laboratory Models of Lung Cancer

4

Jiang Liu and Michael R. Johnston

Contents

4.1   Introduction

Lung cancer is a devastating disease that is associated with significant morbidity and mortality. Most patients die of progressive metastatic disease despite aggressive local and systemic therapies [1]. The pathogenesis of lung cancer remains highly elusive due to its aggressive biologic nature and considerable heterogeneity as compared to other cancers. These circumstances substantially impede study of the disease in humans and necessitate the use of experimental models that can be used under more uniform, controlled conditions than those achievable in clinical settings. The development of animal models of lung cancer may aid in our understanding of lung tumor biology and facilitate the development and testing of novel therapeutic approaches and methods for early diagnosis. To this end, animal models should mimic both the genetic alterations found in human lung tumors and their histological characteristics.

Humans are one of only a few species that are susceptible to the spontaneous development of lung cancer. Lung tumors in domestic animals were periodically observed by veterinarians, but Livingood's histologic description 100 years ago of a papillary tumor in a mouse [2] initiated the idea of using animals as experimental

tools. There are currently several types of animal models that are widely used for experimental lung cancer research. These include chemically induced lung tumors, transgenic mouse models, and human tumor xenografts.

A single model system that faithfully reflects the whole process of lung cancer carcinogenesis and progression is unlikely to be developed. Lung cancer models that accurately reflect the different aspects of the disease are necessary to properly investigate its myriad of complexities. Tumorigenesis, proliferation, invasion, angiogenesis, metastasis, prevention, and therapy are all areas where specific models are required to ensure proper experimental design. To reflect the anticipated biological process being studied, model systems may require certain deviations from the human disease. Thus, we should interpret results of studies utilizing model systems with caution and with an appropriate understanding of their limitations. The purpose of this review is to summarize the various lung cancer model systems in use today and to define both their utility and limitations. As Siemann stated, it is best to "... choose the model to address the question rather than force the question on the tumor model" [3].

4.2   General Principles

Tumor–host interactions, including immunologic effects, vascular and stromal effects, and host-related pharmacologic and pharmacokinetic effects, are poorly modeled in vitro. Animal models to study these areas can be broadly divided into spontaneous or induced tumors, and transplanted tumors. The former group consists of those induced by some extrinsic chemical or carcinogen and animals genetically modified to express genes that lead to lung tumor development. The latter group includes the widely used heterograft and xenograft models. We will briefly describe all of these models and provide a more detailed description of the orthotopic lung cancer xenograft models.

In general, the spontaneous or chemical-induced tumor models [4, 5] most closely mimic the clinical situation. The advantage offered by these models is that they mimic the natural events leading to the development of lung cancer. Several studies have shown that lung tumors developed in mice or rats are quite similar in histology, molecular characteristics, and histogenesis to human lung cancer [6–9]. Unfortunately, these tumors are usually measurable only late in their course, their metastatic pattern is not uniform, and their response to therapy is generally poor. Because of these limitations, spontaneous and chemical-induced model systems are usually reserved for studies of carcinogenesis and cancer prevention [10].

The advent of transgenic technology has significantly improved the ability to define the role of specific genes in the process of transformation and disease progression. Targeting regulatory genes to the lungs in a cell-specific fashion by transgenic technology has produced a variety of mouse lung cancer models. The conventional transgenic mouse models for lung cancer constitutively expressed regulatory genes in the pulmonary epithelium. Subsequent generations of transgenic mouse models have further enhanced the ability to clarify specific molecular mechanisms by allowing for cell-specific-regulated expression or ablation of genes in the lung. Gene transfer technology has also rapidly advanced gene therapy. These genetically engineered models can be exploited to define the molecular events that contribute to the pathogenesis and progression of this disease.

Transplanted animal tumor models and human tumor xenografts are widely used in experimental therapeutics. Since malignant cells or tissue are directly inoculated into the host animal, effects on early events, such as initiation and carcinogenesis, are not well suited for study. Tumor development uniformly follows inoculation with predictable growth and metastatic pattern, and so areas amenable for investigation include tumor growth, invasion, and metastasis. Testing of new therapeutic approaches and screening strategies are also particularly well suited for these models.

4.3   Lung Cancer Animal Models

4.3.1   Chemical-Induced Lung Cancer Models

In our daily lives we are constantly exposed to potentially harmful mixtures of chemical and physical agents. The laboratory environment allows controlled administration of environmental and other toxins to animals [11]. Chemical- or carcinogen-induced lung tumors have been described in a variety of species, including dogs, cats, hamsters, mice, and ferrets; however, the mouse is most widely used. Specific inbred strains of mice susceptible to the development of spontaneous lung tumors, such as A/J and SWR, are also sensitive to chemically induced lung tumors [12]. This observation

has led to the development of quantitative carcinogenicity bioassays [13], and screening systems for the efficacy of chemopreventative agents [14]. If a newborn inbred A/J mouse is given a single intraperitoneal injection of ethyl carbamate (urethane), it will develop dozens of benign lung adenomas within a few months [13]. Some of these induced tumors eventually progress to adenocarcinomas that are histopathologically indistinguishable from human adenocarcinoma [15].

Strain A mice are also used extensively as a murine lung tumor bioassay to assess the carcinogenic activity of chemicals and environmental agents, including urethane, benzopyrene, metals, aflatoxin, and constituents of tobacco smoke such as polyaromatic hydrocarbons and nitrosamines [13, 16, 17]. These agents can act as initiators and/or promoters of pulmonary tumorigenesis by accelerating tumor onset and increasing tumor multiplicity. The most common environmental exposure contributing to human lung cancer is tobacco smoke, which contains over 4,000 chemicals, gases, and volatiles. Developing an animal model for tobacco-induced cancer has generally relied on carcinogenicity studies of single components such as N-nitrosamine 4-(methylnitrosamino)-1-(3-pyridyl)-1-butanone (NNK). If Male Balb/c and SWR mice are exposed to tobacco smoke for 5 months (6 h/day, 5 days/week; average concentration, 122 mg/m^3 of total suspended particulates) followed by a recovery period of 4 months, there is an increase in incidence and number of lung tumors in both strains [18]. Environmental tobacco smoke (ETS) also induced lung tumors in a series of studies in which strain A/J mice were exposed to a well-defined ETS atmosphere. These studies provide convincing evidence that ETS is a potent mouse carcinogen [19]. Studying the mechanisms underlying lung tumor development in these tobacco-induced models may provide valuable clues to sorting out the initiation of smoking-related lung cancer in humans.

In addition to chemicals, both radiation and viruses induce lung tumors in mice [20]. Although induction of lung tumors is highly reproducible [21], all chemical-induced lung tumors exhibit low metastatic potential. Table 4.1 summarizes data on some carcinogen-induced lung cancer models.

During tumor initiation and promotion, carcinogenesis is usually a result of changes in gene expression rather than structural alteration. The carcinogenic process is therefore still reversible, and a good opportunity for chemoprevention is potentially available. In addition to carcinogen detection, the strain A model has also been used to assess the ability of potential chemopreventive agents to protect against the development of carcinogen-induced lung tumors. A number of chemopreventive agents, including beta-naphthoflavone [22], butylated hydroxyanisole [23], ellagic acid [24], phenethyl isothiocyanate [25, 26], α-difluoromethylornithine combined with green tea, dexamethasone, and piroxi-

Table 4.1. Carcinogen-induced lung cancer models

Carcinogen	Route of administration	Phenotype	Reference
3-Methylcholanthrene	Transplacental	Pulmonary adenomas	Miller 1990
N-Nitrosobis-(2-chloroethyl) ureas	Topical	Squamous cell and adenosquamous carcinomas	Rehm 1991
Urethane	Intraperitoneal	Pulmonary adenomas	White 1970
Benzo(a)pyrene Diethylnitrosamine Ethylnitrosourea Dimethylhydrazine	Intraperitoneal	Pulmonary adenomas	Stoner 1984

cam [27], green tea and black tea [28–31] were shown to inhibit chemical-induced lung tumors in strain A mice. In most instances, inhibition of lung tumorigenesis was correlated with the effects of the chemopreventive agents on metabolic activation and/or detoxification of carcinogens.

Various anti-inflammatory drugs inhibit mouse lung tumorigenesis. These include nonsteroidal anti-inflammatory drugs, such as indomethacin, sulindac, and aspirin [32, 33]. Those that induce regression of benign colonic polyps in humans are modestly effective at lowering lung tumor incidence and multiplicity in mice [33]. The density of apoptotic cell bodies increased 2.9-fold in lung adenomas in A/J mice treated with indomethacin [34]. Studies have also shown that selective inhibition of cyclooxygenase (COX)-2 can reduce lung and regional lymph node metastasis in an in vivo lung cancer model [7, 15, 35]. However, in some murine lung tumor models, celecoxib, a selective COX-2 inhibitor, was ineffective in suppressing tumor development [36]. In a recent study, prostacyclin synthase overexpression significantly decreased both the lung tumor incidence and multiplicity in a tobacco-induced lung cancer model, providing additional evidence that manipulation of prostaglandin production distal to COX may be an attractive lung cancer chemopreventive strategy [37].

Two hamster models are used by the United States National Cancer Institute (NCI) Chemoprevention Branch to evaluate efficacy against respiratory tract cancers; the N-methyl-N-nitrosourea (MNU)-induced tracheobroncheal squamous cell carcinomas and the N-nitrosodiethylamine (DEN)-induced lung adenocarcinomas [38]. In the DEN model [39, 40], twice-weekly subcutaneous injections of 17.8 mg DEN/kg for 20 weeks starting at age 7–8 weeks produced lung tumors in 40–50% of male Syrian hamsters. Serial sacrifice studies demonstrate that most lung tumors originate from the respiratory Clara and endocrine cells [40]. This model may be appropriate for examining the chemopreventive activity of chemical agents in small-cell lung cancer (SCLC), a tumor that originates from neuroendocrine cells.

Since tumorigenesis in chemical-induced lung cancer is initiated by the investigator, each stage of neoplasia, such as hyperplasia, benign tumor formation, and the benign-to-malignant transition, can be studied independently. Thus, the molecular changes that precede the onset of hyperplastic foci and those during the evolution to malignancy can be distinguished from frank malignancy, and phenotypes identified that might be useful for early diagnosis.

Despite the usefulness of chemical- or carcinogen-induced lung cancer models, there are major disadvantages, including a heterogenous response to the carcinogen with variable natural histories, a very low rate of spontaneous development, and a long incubation time. Spontaneous neoplasms of the lung in mice are primarily bronchiolar-alveolar carcinomas (BAC). SCLC and squamous cell carcinoma rarely occur in murine models. The major histological type induced by carcinogen exposure is BAC, and that from chemical exposure is adenocarcinoma, whereas squamous cell carcinoma is more common in animals exposed to high doses of radiation [41]. Mouse BAC has a long latency following carcinogen application [42] and varies according to the susceptibility of the mouse to the carcinogen. In more resistant mice, the few carcinomas that develop occupy only a small portion of the lung, and tumor-bearing mice can live a normal life span.

4.3.2 Transgenic Lung Cancer Models

The ability to integrate a gene of interest into the genome of an animal provides a novel approach for cancer investigation. Transgenic mouse technology has proved useful in creating models of tumor development, in cloning immortalized cellular subpopulations, and in testing experimental therapeutic approaches [43–45]. Gene transfection can be achieved with microinjection [46–48], retroviral infection, or embryonic stem cell transfer [49–52]. Transgenic mice are excellent models for studying the consequences of oncogene expression in animals, the effect of oncogenes on growth and differentiation, and their potential for cellular transformation. Conventionally, the transgene DNA construct is generated by the fusion of a cell-specific promoter to direct transcription of the gene of interest. This transgene DNA is subsequently microinjected into fertilized oocytes, and the transgene is integrated into the host genome. The viable oocytes are then transferred into pseudopregnant mothers, and the DNA obtained from progeny is assessed for integration of the transgene into the mouse genome [53, 54]. Using this technology, gene expression has been directed in a cell-specific fashion to the lung. The first oncogene targeted specifically to the lung was the Simian virus large T antigen (TAg). TAg was targeted with both the surfactant protein C, SP-C [55], and Clara cell secretory protein, CCSP [56], promoters. Both models resulted in adenocarcinoma of the lung.

When mutated H-ras (retrovirus-associated DNA sequences), p53 or SV40 (Simian virus 40) T antigen are used as transgenes and integrated into the host genome, lung tumors develop in mice soon after birth, resulting in early death of the animal. These genes may be nonspecifically expressed throughout the body or linked to lung-specific promoters so that their expression is selective for Clara cells or alveolar type II pneumocytes [57–60]. Animals such as these are used to investigate molecular events in the progression of lung cancer. However, the rapid progression and early onset of cancer makes investigation of early events difficult [61]. When either new genetic material is added to the genome, or genes, such as tumor-suppressor genes, are removed from the genome (knock-out), the effects can occur immediately and continue throughout the lifespan of the animal. Thus, mice develop tumors early in life and usually have a shortened life span. Human lung cancers often have mutations of both the retinoblastoma (Rb)- and p53-suppressor genes. When transgenic mice are created with the same mutations, they develop bronchial hyperplasia, but die of other neoplasms, including islet cell carcinoma, before progression to lung cancer can occur [62].

Currently, the most effective regulatory systems for conditional transgenic mice are the ligand-inducible binary transgenic systems that confer regulated expression of the desired gene [63, 64]. These systems consist of using at least two transgene constructs, a regulator transgene, and a target transgene. The target transgene is silent until the regulator transgene is activated by the administration of an exogenous compound. An example is a bitransgenic model, such as the tetracycline transactivator-inducible system [65] in which mice are produced with two separate mutations that are activated or deactivated by tetracycline. This system has two major advantages over conventional transgenic mice. First, the transgene can be turned on at any time by administering tetracycline, and thus resembles a somatic mutation. Second, regulated loss of expression (turning off the transgene by withdrawing tetracycline) can be used to determine whether the transgene is required to maintain the growth and proliferation of the tumor.

A transgenic mouse model of lung adenocarcinoma with expression of a mutant active K-ras transgene was developed using this regulatory transgenic technology [66]. Tumors rapidly regress as a result of apoptosis when doxycycline, a tetracycline analogue, is withdrawn. This is a clear demonstration of the role of K-ras in lung tumorigenesis. Several other lung cancer mouse models are also described with conditional activation of oncogenic K-ras [26, 67, 68]. The use of regulatory transgenic systems such as this are valuable tools for identifying targets for future drug development strategies.

An animal model of SCLC has been particularly difficult to develop. Recently, Meuwissen et al. established an animal model of SCLC with remarkable similarity to the human disease [69]. This model utilizes mice carrying Cre-LoxP-based conditional alleles of the Rb and p53 tumor-suppressor genes. Deletion of these genes in cells of the lung was achieved through intrabronchial injection of a recombinant adenovirus expressing the Cre recombinase. This method reproducibly resulted in the development of lung tumors with the histology, immunohistochemistry, and metastatic behavior of human SCLC. Most of these tumors spread diffusely through the lung and gave rise to extrapulmonary metastases at multiple sites, including bone, brain, adrenal gland, ovary, and liver. This model system exhibits several other important similarities to human SCLC. First, the coexistence of SCLC and non-small-cell lung cancer (NSCLC) imitates a common clinical occurrence of both histologies present within the same tumor. Second, immunostaining revealed that most lesions are positive for the neuroendocrine marker synaptophysin and the neural cell adhesion molecule Ncam1 (CD 56), indicating neuroendocrine differentiation. If the model exhibits an autocrine growth signal similar to human SCLC, it may be of value in developing therapies directed at blocking this signal. Tables 4.2 and 4.3 summarize some useful information concerning conventional and conditional transgenic lung cancer models.

4.3.3 Human Lung Tumor Xenografts

Transplanting human tumor tissue into rodents and maintaining the histological and biological identity of tumor cells through successive passages in vivo has revolutionized cancer research, and drug development in particular [70, 71]. Since human neoplasms are rejected when implanted into another species, the host animal must be immunosuppressed. Irradiation, thymectomy, splenectomy, and corticosteroids were initially used to blunt acquired immunity. With the successful breeding of hairless nude mouse mutants (nu/nu homozygotes), severe combined immunodeficient (SCID) mice and Rowett nude rats, laboratory animals are now readily available for the transplantation of human tumors.

Subcutaneous implantation in nude mice is the most common method of transplanting human tumor materi-

Table 4.2. Conventional transgenic lung cancer models. *NE* Neuroendocrine, *CCSP* Clara cell secretory protein, *SP-C* surfactant protein C, *CaBP9K* vitamin-D-dependent calcium binding protein, *CC10* Clara cell secretory protein 10, *CGRP* calcitonin gene-related peptide, *EGF* epidermal growth factor, *TAg* Simian virus large T antigen, *hASH1* human achaete-scut homolog 1

Model Design	Transgene/Gene knockout/knock-in	Promoter	Phenotype	Reference
Viral oncogene	TAg	CCSP	Multifocal early onset bronchioloalveolar hyperplasias progressing to adenocarcinomas	DeMayo 1991
	TAg	SP-C	Adenocarcinomas including papillary, solid and bronchioloalveolar subtypes	Wikenheiser et al. 1992
	TAg	CaBP9K	Lung adenocarcinomas	Chailley-Heu 2001
Signaling/kinase	Myc	SP-C	Pulmonary tumors ranging from bronchioloalveolar adenomas to adenocarcinomas. Phenotype shows incomplete penetrance.	Ernhardt 2001
	c-Raf-1	SP-C	Lung adenomas	Kerkhoff 2000
	c-Raf-1-BxB	SP-C	Lung adenomas	Kerkhoff 2000
	H-Ras	CGRP	Pulmonary NE hyperplasia and non-NE adenocarcinomas	Sunday 1999
Growth factor receptor	RON	SP-C	Adenomas and adenocarcinomas	Chen 2002
Growth factor	IgEGF	SP-C	Alveolar hyperplasia	Ernhardt 2001
	IgEGF x Myc	SP-C	Accelerated tumor progression	Ernhardt 2001
Transcription factor	hASH1	CC10	Airway hyperplasia and bronchioloalveolar metaplasia	Linnoila 2000
	hASH1 x TAg	CC10	Adenocarcinoma with NE features	Linnoila 2000

Table 4.3. Conditional transgenic lung cancer models. *FGF* Fibroblast growth factor, *UASG* gal 10 upstream activating sequence

Model Design	Transgene	Promoter	Phenotype	Reference
Tumor suppressors	Rb, p53	Knock-in	Small-cell lung carcinoma	Meuwissen et al. 2003
	p53	Knock-in	Adenocarcinoma	Meuwissen et al. 2003
Signaling/kinases	LSL-K-ras G12D	Knock-in	Adenocarcinoma and epithelial hyperplasia of the bronchioles	Jackson et al. 2001
	K-ras4b G12D rtTA	Tet-O CCSP	Adenocarcinomas that regress upon removal of doxycycline	Fisher et al. 2001
	K-ras V12	β-actin	Adenocarcinomas	Meuwissen et al. 2001
Growth factor	FGF-3	UASG	Alveolar macrophage infiltration and alveolar type II cell hyperplasia	Zhao 2001
	GLp65	SP-C		

al. The procedure is straightforward and the site, usually the dorsal lateral flank, is easily accessible. Studies have shown that subcutaneous xenograft models can emulate clinical behavior [72–74], although recently some authors have questioned the accuracy of this data when applied to human drug trials [75]. These models have some disadvantages, however, including: (1) a low tumor take-rate for fresh clinical specimens [72, 76], (2) tumor growth in an unusual tissue compartment (the subcutis), the microenvironment of which might influence study results, and (3) the lack of consistent invasion and metastasis [72, 77, 78], properties that are closely linked to clinical outcome in humans.

In orthotopic models, human tumors are implanted in the laboratory animal directly into the appropriate organ or tissue of origin. Advantages include improved tumor take-rates, along with enhanced invasive and metastatic properties [77, 79, 80]. The metastatic phenotype of many tumors is expressed after orthotopic implantation; for example, colon carcinoma cells grown in the cecal wall, bladder carcinoma in the bladder, renal cell carcinoma cells under the renal capsule, and melanomas implanted subdermally all yield metastases at a much higher frequency than when grown subcutaneously [81, 82]. An organ-specific site presumably provides tumor cells with the most appropriate milieu for local growth and metastasis, thereby supporting Paget's hypothesis that metastasis is not a random phenomenon. Rather, he concluded, malignant cells have special affinity for growth in the environment of their origin, the familiar seed and soil theory [83]. Although orthotopic tumors are more virulent and animal survival is shortened, the models in general are more complex and more costly than subcutaneous models.

4.3.4   Orthotopic Lung Cancer Models

Orthotopic lung cancer models are described using endobronchial, intrathoracic, or intravenous injection of tumor cell suspensions [9, 28–31, 84, 85] and by surgical implantation of fresh tumor tissue [27–31, 86]. McLemore et al. [85] developed the first orthotopic lung cancer model by implanting lung cancer cell lines and disaggregated lung tumors into the lung of nude mice by endobronchial injection. The tumors grew more extensively within the lung than the same tumors implanted subcutaneously; however, most of the tumors stayed within the lung, resulting in only 3% metastasis to lymph nodes, liver, or spleen [85]. A second model was developed by McLemore et al. [87] by percutaneously injecting lung tumor cells into the pleural space. This model gave high tumor take-rates, reproducible growth, and a mortality endpoint as a result of local disease progression; however, few metastases were seen. Since cancer cells are seeded into the pleural space rather than within the pulmonary parenchyma or bronchi, its comparison to human lung cancer is suspect.

Our laboratory also used endobronchial implantation to grow non-small cell (A549, NCI-H460, and NCI-H125) and small-cell (NCI-H345) lung tumors, but in nude rats rather than mice [84]. Metastasis to mediastinal lymph nodes is frequently seen in these models, but systemic metastases are rare. Subsequently, we described a systemic metastatic model by endobronchial implantation of tumor fragments derived from orthotopic lung tumors grown from the H460 cell line. This H460 nude rat model has a 100% primary tumor take-rate in the lung, with a rapid and reproducible growth rate to about 4 g over a 32- to 35-day period. It also metastasizes at a consistent rate to both regional mediastinal lymph nodes and distant systemic sites, including bone, brain, kidney, and the contralateral lung. This is the first human lung cancer model to show extensive systemic metastasis from a primary lung site [9].

Several other intrathoracic human lung cancer models have been described, all using immunocompromised mice. One is the traditional intravenous model in which the lung is colonized with tumor cells after tail vein injection [88, 89]. In another, the tumor grows in a subpleural location from either tumor cell inoculation or fragments sewn onto the surface of the left lung [28–31, 90]. Recently, a SCID lung cancer model was described that develops lymphatic metastasis following percutaneous injection of cancer cells into the mouse lung [91]. None of these models grow from a primary endobronchial site and none develop a consistent metastatic pattern in extrathoracic locations.

The H460 orthotopic rat model has several advantages over the mouse models: (1) primary tumors originate within the bronchial tree, similar to most human lung cancers, (2) primary tumors are confined to the

right caudal lobe; this makes it unlikely that metastases arise from mechanical spread of the implanted tumor material, and (3) a ten-fold larger size of the rat facilitates surgical manipulations, such as cannulation, and allows implantation of tumor fragments that are too large for the mouse bronchus.

Fresh human lung tumor tissue or tissue from metastatic lesions are also implanted orthotopically [92]. Such models putatively maintain intact critical stromal epithelial relationships, even though the source of most stromal tissue is probably from the host rather than the xenograft [93]. Wang et al. [28–31] implanted human small cell lung cancer tissue into mouse lung. Metastases were found in the contralateral lung and mediastinal lymph nodes. Two tumor lines derived from fresh human NSCLC were established in our laboratory by endobronchial implantation in nude rats (unpublished data). Interestingly, one tumor line developed contralateral lung metastases that were very similar in appearance to metastases in the patient from whom the tumor line originated. Table 4.4 provides a summary of orthotopic lung cancer models.

4.3.5   Useful Models for the Study of Lung Cancer Metastasis

Over 85% of lung cancer patients harbor overt or subclinical metastases at diagnosis, thus accounting for the poor prognosis associated with this disease. Unfortunately, little is known about the molecular pathways responsible for tumor progression to metastasis. Appropriate animal models to study these sequences may help us understand these complex pathways.

Entry of tumor cells into the circulation is a critical first step in the metastatic cascade, and although assayed in various ways [94–96], it has not been observed directly. Novel approaches to specifically "mark" the tumor cell hold promise. For example, one can engineer tumor cells to express the green fluorescence protein (GFP) for in vivo fluorescence imaging. In order to understand the metastatic pattern of NSCLC, Yang et al. developed a high-expression GFP transductant of the human lung cancer cell line H460 (H460-GFP), which visualized widespread skeletal metastases when implanted orthotopically in nude mice [97]. It can reveal the microscopic stages of tumor growth and metastatic seeding as real-time visualization of micrometastases, even down to the single-cell level. This makes it possible to directly study tumor growth and metastasis as well as tumor angiogenesis and gene expression.

Neoplasms are biologically heterogeneous and contain genotypically and phenotypically diverse subpopulations of tumor cells, each of which have the potential to complete some, but not all of the steps in the metastatic process [98–105]. Recent studies using in situ hy-

Table 4.4. Orthotopic lung cancer models. *SCID* Severe combined immunodeficient

Author	Animal	Tumor material	Inoculation method	Take rate	Regional metastatic sites	Distant metastatic sites	Average growth time
McLemore et al. 1987	Nude mice	H125, H358, H460, A549	Endobronchial	90%	Trachea 2%, peritracheal 6%, Lymph node 90%	Left lung, liver, spleen 3%	9–61 days
Howard et al. 1991	Nude rats	H125,H460, A549, H345	Endobronchial	100%, 83%, 90%	Regional lymph nodes	H-125, A549 to contralateral lung	H460 (3 weeks) A549 (5 weeks) H125 (10 weeks)
Wang et al. 1992	SCID mice Nude mice	Tumor fragment from A549 subcutaneous tumor	Thoracotomy	3/5	Chest wall	Contralateral lung	N/A
Wang et al. 1992	SCID mice Nude mice	Human SCLC tumor fragment	Thoracotomy	100%	Mediastinum, chest wall lymph nodes	Contralateral lung	18.5–62 days
Cuenca et al. 1996	SCID mice	Human NSCLC biopsy specimens	Anterior thoracotomy	31%	N/A	Metastasis rate 50%; Contralateral lung 37.5%	4–6 months
Nagamachi et al. 1998	Nude mice	A549, H23, H441, H157, Lu65, Lu99A PC9, PC14	Intrapleural	100% except H23	Mediastinum, lymph nodes	Contralateral lung	Depends on specific cell line, PC14 within 30 days
Howard et al. 1999	Nude rats	Tumor fragment derived from H460 lung tumors	Endobronchial	100%	Lymph node 100%	Bone, brain, kidney, contralateral lung, soft tissue	32–35 days
Miyoshi et al. 2000	SCID mice	Ma-44	Percutaneous intrapulmonary	N/A	Lymph node 52%	Contralateral lung 52%	17.5±6.0 days
Kozaki et al. 2000	SCID mice KSN nude mice	H460-LNM35	Endobronchial	SCID 67%; KSN nude mice 86%	100%	N/A	28 days
Liu et al. 2004	Nude rats	H460SM	Endobronchial	100%	Lymph node 100%	Bone, brain, kidney, contralateral lung, soft tissue	32–40 days

bridization and immunohistochemical staining show that the expression of genes and proteins associated with proliferation, angiogenesis, cohesion, motility, and invasion vary among different regions of a neoplasm [106]. In general, metastasis favors the survival and growth of a few subpopulations of cells that preexist within the parent neoplasm. In addition, metastases may have a clonal origin, with different metastases originating from the proliferation of different single cells. Therefore, the search for those metastasis-associated genes and proteins cannot be conducted by an indiscriminate and nonselective processing of tumor tissues. Isolating these clones from other cell populations in the parent neoplasm provides a powerful tool with which to study those properties that distinguish metastatic from nonmetastatic cells [99, 107–110].

One method to separate these cell populations is to develop cell variants through in vivo propagation and selection. By selectively harvesting tumor cells from mediastinal lymph nodes in our H460 orthotopic lung cancer model and subjecting them to several cycles of in vitro and in vivo orthotopic passage, we have established a clonal H460SM variant cell line that spontaneously produces widespread systemic metastases following orthotopic implantation [102]. In contrast to the two-step NCI-H460 metastatic model mentioned previously [9], the one-step metastatic model with the H460SM cell line provides a simpler system with which to characterize the molecular mechanisms leading to nodal and systemic metastasis. To our knowledge, the H460SM orthotopic model represents the first lung cancer rodent model derived from a human lung cancer cell line that closely mimics the spectrum of common metastatic sites observed in NSCLC patients. We are currently examining the behavior of H460SM cells in SCID mice. A schematic diagram of the developmental strategy used for the H460SM cell variant and its associated lung cancer model is illustrated in Fig. 4.1.

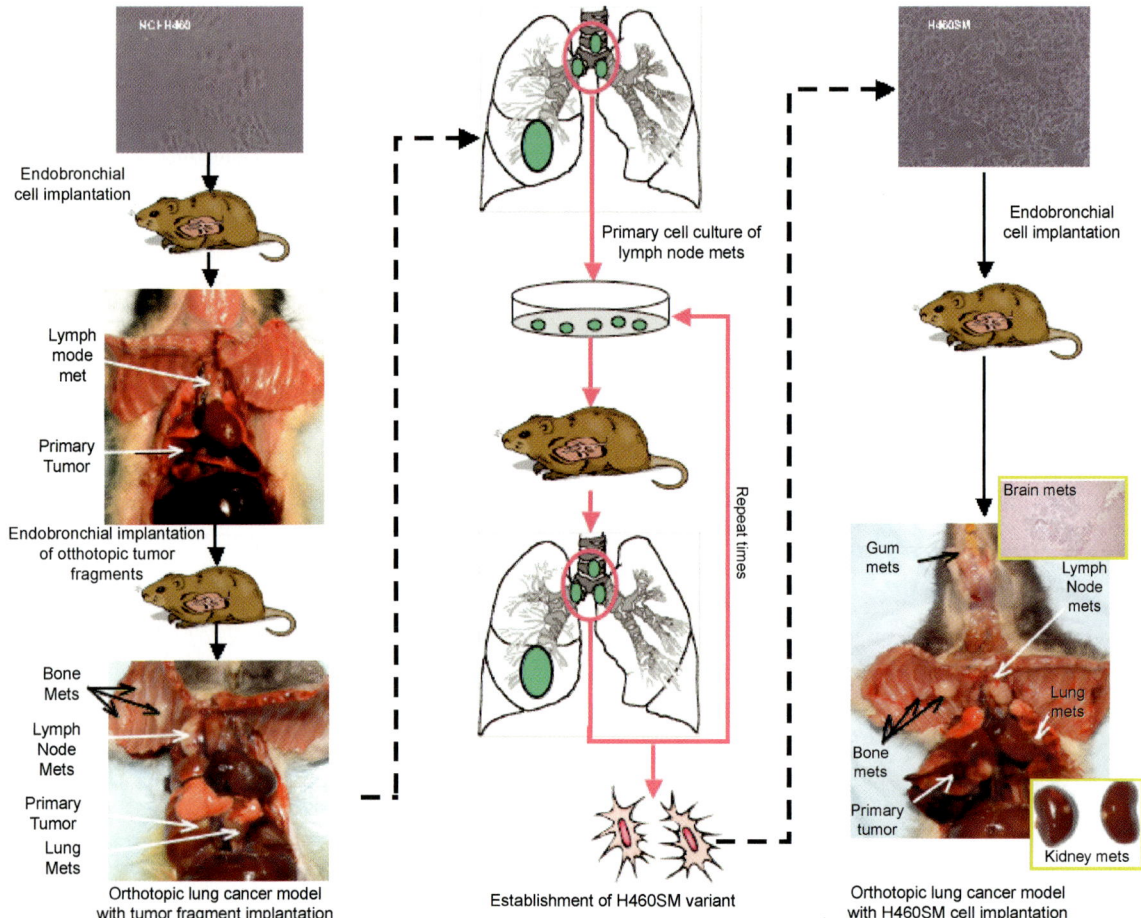

Fig. 4.1. Schematic diagram of the developmental strategy used for the H460SM cell variant and its associated lung cancer model. *Mets* Metastases

Kozaki et al. [101] also used the NCI-H460 cell line as a basis to establish a lymphatic metastasis model of NSCLC. In their model, the H460-LNM35 cell line was established following serial in vivo selection steps that included two rounds of implantation into the abdominal wall of nude mice and culturing of cells from the lung metastatic nodules. Cells were then passaged through the subcutaneous tissue, and the LNM35 cell line was established from metastatic tumor cells in the axillary lymph node. When implanted subcutaneously, the LNM35 cell line gave rise to axillary lymph node metastases in 100% of animals. Following endobronchial (orthotopic) implantation of LNM35 cells into the lungs of nude mice, mediastinal lymph node metastases were also noted in 100% of the animals. In contrast to the H460SM model, neither subcutaneous nor orthotopic implantation of the LNM35 cell line resulted in systemic metastases.

The H460SM and H460-LNM35 variant cell lines show a higher incidence of metastasis when implanted in immunocompromised rodents compared to the parent cell line. Such paired parent and variant cell lines

constitute a useful model for the discovery of genes involved in lung cancer metastasis. By comparing microarray data from each cell line, parent and variant, genes suspected of expressing the metastatic phenotype can be identified and investigated further [102].

4.4 Lung Cancer Models in Preclinical Cancer Drug Development

Despite advances in basic cancer biology, animal models, especially human tumor xenografts, will remain pivotal to preclinical cancer drug discovery and development. The value of such models depends upon their validity, selectivity, predictability, reproducibility, and cost [111, 112].

Initially, lung tumor xenografts were intended to facilitate patient-specific chemotherapy. In this scenario, a patient's tumor is implanted as a xenograft in nude mice and the animals then treated with various chemotherapy agents. By learning the drug responsiveness of the xenograft, treatment of the patient can then be individualized. Unfortunately, variations in take-rate, the time required for the xenografts to grow and the expense incurred, make this strategy untenable.

Early drug-screening systems utilized the L1210 mouse lymphoma or P388 mouse leukemia models. Anticancer agents had to prove themselves in these murine models before passing on to further in vivo animal model testing. However, only 2% of drugs active in the L1210 or P388 models were subsequently shown to have in vivo activity in Lewis lung or colon 38 adenocarcinoma models [10]. This persuaded the United States NCI to shift from a compound-oriented to a disease-oriented screening system. A high-throughput in vitro screening method capable of screening 20,000 compounds per year was developed using a panel of 60 cell lines, representing all of the major human solid tumors (*http:// dtp.nci.nih.gov/branches/btb/ivclsp.html*). Drugs found to have a favorable activity profile to a particular tumor histology or site are further tested in appropriate xenografts. The xenografts are used as a secondary screening system to judge efficacy prior to considering a drug for early phase human studies [113].

Primary lung tumors in mice can be used for screening effective single drugs and drug combinations prior to clinical testing. For example, cisplatin, administered by itself and in combination with indomethacin, decreased the sizes of NNK-induced carcinomas [114].

Subcutaneous xenograft models have a long history in the pharmaceutical industry because of their utility, ease of use and economy. Models are selected to demonstrate a specific cytotoxic effect of a drug or biological agent, such as xenografts that reflect the chemosensitivities of their tumors of origin. For instance, the growth of SCLC xenografts is inhibited by cisplatin, etoposide, cyclophosphamide, doxorubicin, and vincristine, whereas NSCLC grafts are much less responsive to those same agents [78].

Although the subcutaneous xenograft model is widely employed as an in vivo drug screen, the more complicated orthotopic models may be better suited for preclinical studies. Since orthotopic rodent tumors mimic biological aspects of clinical cancer (e.g., disease progression and metastasis), they are likely to provide more relevant pharmacokinetic and pharmacodynamic information than subcutaneous tumors [115]. Carcinogen-induced and genetically modified murine lung cancer models that have been shown to mimic the human disease, either histologically or in terms of gene expression, may also provide predictive models for performing preclinical testing of therapeutic efficacy. Genetically modified murine cancer models are used to examine the efficacy of some targeted therapeutics. For example, farnesyl transferase inhibitors (FTIs), which act to inhibit *Ras* signaling, have been tested in several models where upregulation of *ras* signaling results in tumor development. These studies demonstrated that FTIs are often effective in causing regression or preventing progression of tumor growth [116].

A range of methods are used to evaluate drug effects on tumors in animal models. Tumor size and tumor weight or volume changes are simple and easily reproducible parameters in subcutaneous xenograft models, but are more difficult, except at necropsy, in most orthotopic models. We used a mammographic imaging technique to assess both primary tumor growth and metastases in our orthotopic model [117]. Miniaturized human imaging methods, such as computed tomography, magnetic resonance imaging, and positron emission tomography, are now available for laboratory use. Morphologic changes and alterations in tumor immunogenicity or invasiveness are other markers of response. Survival, perhaps the ultimate parameter, is a valid endpoint only if clinically relevant tumor progression, such as systemic metastasis, is responsible for the animal's demise, a parameter better assessed in orthotopic than subcutaneous models.

To accurately evaluate anticancer activity in an animal model system, validation of the model is critical. This entails the design of studies aimed at assessing tumor response to drugs or other agents known to have efficacy in patients with the particular type of cancer represented by the model. We validated our H460 orthotopic lung cancer model [1] by treating tumor-bearing nude rats with one of four chemotherapy agents: doxorubicin, mitomycin, cisplatin, and the novel matrix metalloproteinase inhibitor, batimastat. The model showed consistent responses in the form of tumor weight, metastatic pattern, and longevity to cisplatin and mitomycin treatment. The other two agents, for the most part, were ineffective, which accurately reflects drug sensitivity patterns in NSCLC and the H460 cell line. The model also detected cisplatin toxicity, as assessed by body weight changes and kidney damage. A similar study was performed using two human lung cancers implanted into the pleural cavity of nude mice [118]. Both studies show that selective cytotoxic agents may reduce primary tumor burden and prolong the survival of tumor-bearing animals. However, none of these agents were capable of completely eradicating the tumor, reflecting the resistance of this disease to standard chemotherapy.

The orthotopic site may be crucial to a clinically relevant drug response. An orthotopic model of human SCLC demonstrates sensitivity to cisplatin and resistance to mitomycin C, reflecting the clinical situation [89]. However, the same tumor xenograft implanted subcutaneously responded to mitomycin and not to cisplatin, thus failing to match the clinical behavior of SCLC. Similar phenomena have been observed that underscore the effect of the microenvironment on drug sensitivity [119].

Several orthotopic models have been developed as in vivo preclinical screens for novel therapies that target invasion, metastasis, and angiogenesis [120–124]. Our own studies in the H460 orthotopic lung cancer model include the matrix metalloproteinase inhibitors batimastat and prinomastat (AG3340), the integrin-linked kinase inhibitor, KP-392, and the anti-invasive agent, swainsonine [1, 125, 126]. Assessment of multiple endpoints, such as tumor weight, metastatic pattern, and survival, appears to improve the sensitivity of the model system to demonstrate a treatment effect. By describing patterns of response in a model system, the results may also suggest mechanisms of action or the biological properties of a particular agent. For instance, batimastat was found to significantly increase length of survival, despite the fact that it showed no consistent effect on tumor size or on the incidence of metastases. Thus, the drug may be slowing, but not eradicating, the metastatic process.

In preclinical drug development the orthotopic model also takes into account the role of the microenvironment, which is biologically unique for each organ system. For instance, endothelial cells in the vasculature of various organs express different cell-surface receptors [127] and growth factors that may influence the phenotype of primary tumors or metastases developing in these organs [128]. Therapeutic efficacy can depend on multiple interactions between the tumor cells and their microenvironment. Therefore, therapy should be targeted not only against the cancer cells themselves, but also against the specific homeostatic factors that promote tumor-cell growth, survival, angiogenesis, invasion, and metastasis.

A concern in testing anticancer agents with animal models derived from human cell lines is the potential loss of tumor heterogeneity [81, 129]. In other words, does serial passage of cell lines over months and years select out and propagate only certain specific clonal elements of a tumor? Studies have shown that the molecular characteristics of both breast and lung cancer cell lines closely match their original human tumor [130, 131]. From a phenotypic perspective, the H460 cell line used in our studies continues to exhibit consistent invasive and metastatic properties and has maintained its drug sensitivity profile for over 10 years and in thousands of experimental animals. However, other important characteristics, such as cytokine production or still unknown gene expressions, may be lost or muted through serial passaging. And so, as mentioned at the outset, it behooves the investigator to understand both the strengths and limitations of the tumor model chosen for lung cancer studies.

4.5   Summary

Many lung cancer models are available, but none accurately reflect every aspect of human lung cancer. Each has its own advantages and disadvantages that should be understood and evaluated before their use. In selecting the best model system, consideration should be given to the genetic stability and heterogeneity of the transplanted cell line, its immunogenicity within the host animal, and the appropriate biologic endpoints. There is increasing pressure on the research community to reduce, or even eliminate the use of animals in research. However, relevant animal model systems provide the appropriate interface between the laboratory bench and a patient's bedside for continued progress in cancer research and drug development. As in many other diseases, even more sophisticated lung cancer models will be needed in the future, as the complexities of this devastating disease are slowly unraveled.

Key Points

- This chapter provides an overview of animal lung cancer models established by chemical induction, transgenic technologies, and human tumor transplantation. It also defines the utility and limitations of each. Areas of lung tumor modeling research that should be more intensively explored to assist translational research are listed below.
- A better understanding of carcinogenesis; for instance the failure of certain oncogene mutations to uniformly result in lung epithelial cells developing hyperplastic foci that then progress to lung tumor formation may provide a biological basis for spontaneous regression, and possibly yield insights into novel therapeutic development.
- More comparative genomic studies using microarray and other emerging technologies. These may delineate specific genes or combination of genes associated with carcinogenesis and metastasis and result in novel chemopreventive strategies or new combinations of molecular-targeted therapies.
- Studies aimed at understanding the heterogeneous response to therapy by tumors with a similar genetic make-up. The biochemical mechanisms underlying these phenotypes may lead to improved results with both chemotherapy and radiation therapy treatment protocols.

References

1. Johnston MR, Mullen JB, Pagura M, Howard RB. Validation of an orthotopic model of human lung cancer with regional and systemic metastases. Ann Thorac Surg 2001; 71:1120.
2. Livingood LE. Tumors in the mouse. Johns Hopkins Bull 1896; 66/67:177.
3. Siemann DW. Modification of chemotherapy by nitroimidazoles. Int J Radiat Oncol Biol Phys 1984; 10:1585.
4. Corbett TH, Griswold DP, Roberts BJ, Peckham JC, Schabel FM. Tumor induction relationships in development of transplantable cancers of the colon in mice for chemotherapy assays, with a note on carcinogen structure. Cancer Res 1975; 35:2434.
5. Corbett TH, Roberts BJ, Leopold WR, Peckham JC, Wilkoff LJ, Griswold DP, Schabel FM. Induction and chemotherapeutic response of two transplantable ductal adenocarcinomas of the pancreas in C57BL/6 mice. Cancer Res 1984; 44:717.
6. Balmain A, Harris CC. Carcinogenesis in mouse and human cells: parallels and paradoxes. Carcinogenesis 2000; 21:371.
7. Malkinson AM. Primary lung tumors in mice as an aid for understanding, preventing, and treating human adenocarcinoma of the lung. Lung Cancer 2001; 32:265.
8. Hoffman RM. Orthotopic metastatic mouse models for anticancer drug discovery and evaluation: a bridge to the clinic. Invest New Drugs 1999; 17:343.
9. Howard RB, Mullen JB, Pagura ME, Johnston MR. Characterization of a highly metastatic, orthotopic lung cancer model in the nude rat. Clin Exp Metastasis 1999; 17:157.
10. Curt GA. The use of animal models in cancer drug discovery and development. Stem Cells 1994; 12:23.
11. Malkinson AM, Belinsky SA. The use of animal models in preclinical studies. In: Pass HI, Mitchell JB, Johnson DH, Turrisi AT (eds) Lung Cancer – Principle and Practice. Lippincott-Raven, Philadelphia, 1996; p 273.
12. Tuveson DA, Jacks T. Modeling human lung cancer in mice: similarities and shortcomings. Oncogene 1999; 18:5318.
13. Shimkin MB, Stoner GD. Lung tumors in mice: application to carcinogenesis bioassay. Adv Cancer Res 1975; 21:1.
14. Stoner GD, Adam-Rodwell G, Morse MA. Lung tumors in strain A mice: application for studies in cancer chemoprevention. J Cell Biochem 1993; Suppl 17F:95.
15. Malkinson AM. Primary lung tumors in mice: an experimentally manipulable model of human adenocarcinoma. Cancer Res 1992; 52:2670s.
16. Kim SH, Lee CS. Induction of benign and malignant pulmonary tumors in mice with benzo(a)pyrene. Anticancer Res 1996; 16:465.
17. Stoner GD. Lung tumors in strain A mice as a bioassay for carcinogenicity of environmental chemicals. Exp Lung Res 1991; 17:405.
18. Witschi H, Espiritu I, Dance ST, Miller MS. A mouse lung tumor model of tobacco smoke carcinogenesis. Toxicol Sci 2002; 68:322.
19. Bogen K, Witschi H. Lung tumors in A/J mice exposed to environmental tobacco smoke: estimated potency and implied human risk. Carcinogenesis 2002; 23:511.
20. Rapp UR, Todaro GJ. Generation of oncogenic mouse type C viruses: in vitro selection of carcinoma-inducing variants. Proc Natl Acad Sci U S A 1980; 77:624.
21. Malkinson AM. The genetic basis of susceptibility to lung tumors in mice. Toxicology 1989; 54:241.
22. Anderson LM, Priest LJ. Reduction in the transplacental carcinogenic effect of methylcholanthrene in mice by prior treatment with beta-naphthoflavone. Res Commun Chem Pathol Pharmacol 1980; 30:431.
23. Wattenberg LW. Inhibition of chemical carcinogen-induced pulmonary neoplasia by butylated hydroxyanisole. J Natl Cancer Inst 1973; 50:1541.
24. Lesca P. Protective effects of ellagic acid and other plant phenols on benzo[a]pyrene-induced neoplasia in mice. Carcinogenesis 1983; 4:1651.
25. Morse MA, Eklind KI, Hecht SS, et al. Structure-activity relationships for inhibition of 4-(methylnitrosamino)-1-(3-pyridyl)-1-butanone lung tumorigenesis by arylalkyl isothiocyanates in A/J mice. Cancer Res 1991; 51:1846.
26. Jackson EL, Willis N, Mercer K, et al. Analysis of lung tumor initiation and progression using conditional expression of oncogenic K-ras. Genes Dev 2001; 15:3243.
27. Gunning WT, Kramer PM, Lubet RA, Steele VE, Pereira MA. Chemoprevention of vinyl carbamae-induced lung tumors in strain A mice. Exp Lung Res 2000; 26:757.
28. Wang X., Fu X, Hoffman RM. A new patient-like metastatic model of human lung cancer constructed orthotopically with intact tissue via thoracotomy in immunodeficient mice. Int J Cancer 1992; 51:992.
29. Wang X, Fu X, Hoffman RM. A patient-like metastasizing model of human lung adenocarcinoma constructed via thoracotomy in nude mice. Anticancer Res 1992; 12:1399.
30. Wang X, Fu X, Kubota T, Hoffman RM. A new patient-like metastatic model of human small-cell lung cancer constructed orthotopically with intact tissue via thoracotomy in nude mice. Anticancer Res 1992; 12:1403.
31. Wang ZY, Hong JY, Huang MT, Reuhl KR, Conney AH, Yang CS. Inhibition of N-nitrosodiethylamine- and 4-(methylnitrosamino)-1-(3-pyridyl)-1-butanone-induced tumorigenesis in A/J mice by green tea and black tea. Cancer Res 1992; 52:1943.
32. Jalbert G, Castonguay A. Effects of NSAIDs on NNK-induced pulmonary and gastric tumorigenesis in A/J mice. Cancer Lett 1992; 66: 21.
33. Duperron C, Castonguay A. Chemopreventive efficacies of aspirin and sulindac against lung tumorigenesis in A/J mice. Carcinogenesis 1997; 18:1001.
34. Moody TW, Leyton J, Zakowicz H, et al. Indomethacin reduces lung adenoma number in A/J mice. Anticancer Res 2001; 21:1749.
35. Kozaki K, Koshikawa K, Tatematsu Y, et al. Multi-faceted analyses of a highly metastatic human lung cancer cell line NCI-H460-LNM35 suggest mimicry of inflammatory cells in metastasis. Oncogene 2001; 20:4228.
36. Kisley LR, Barrett BS, Dwyer-Nield LD, Bauer AK, Thompson DC, Malkinson AM. Celecoxib reduces pulmonary inflammation but not lung tumorigenesis in mice. Carcinogenesis 2002; 23:1653.
37. Keith RL, Miller YE, Hudish TM, et al. Pulmonary prostacyclin synthase overexpression chemoprevents tobacco smoke lung carcinogenesis in mice. Cancer Res 2004; 64:5897.
38. Steele VE, Moon RC, Lubet RA, et al. Preclinical efficacy evaluation of potential chemopreventive agents in animal carcinogenesis models: methods and results from the NCI chemoprevention drug development program. J Cell Biochem 1994; 20:32.
39. Moon RC, Rao KV, Detrisac CJ, Kelloff GJ. Hamster lung cancer model of carcinogenesis and chemoprevention. Adv Exp Med Biol 1992; 320:55.
40. Schuller HM, McMahon JB. Inhibition of N-nitrosodiethylamine-induced respiratory tract carcinogenesis by piperonylbutoxide in hamsters. Cancer Res 1985; 45:2807.
41. Hahn FF, Lundgren DL. Pulmonary neoplasms in rats that inhaled cerium-144 dioxide. Toxicol Pathol 1992; 20:169.
42. Kauffman SL. Histogenesis of the papillary Clara cell adenoma. Am J Pathol 1981; 103:174.
43. Adams JM, Cory S. Transgenic models of tumor development. Science 1991; 254:1161.

44. Fowlis DJ, Balmain A. Oncogenes and tumour suppressor genes in transgenic mouse models of neoplasia. Eur J Cancer 1993; 29A:638.

45. Thomas H, Balkwill F. Assessing new anti-tumour agents and strategies in oncogene transgenic mice. Cancer Metastasis Rev 1995; 14:91.

46. Brinster RL, Chen HY, Trumbauer ME, Yagle MK, Palmiter RD. Factors affecting the efficiency of introducing foreign DNA into mice by microinjecting eggs. Proc Natl Acad Sci U S A 1985; 82:4438.

47. Hogan. Manipulating the mouse embryo: a laboratory manual. In: Hanahan D (ed) Cold Spring Harbor Laboratory Manual. Cold Spring Harbor, New York, 1986.

48. Gordon JW, Ruddle FH. Gene transfer into mouse embryos: production of transgenic mice by pronuclear injection. Methods Enzymol 1983; 101: 411.

49. Jaenisch R. Retroviruses and embryogenesis: microinjection of Moloney leukemia virus into midgestation mouse embryos. Cell 1980; 19:181.

50. Jaenisch R, Jahner D, Nobis P, Simon I, Lohler J, Harbers K, Grotkopp D. Chromosomal position and activation of retroviral genomes inserted into the germ line of mice. Cell 1981; 24:519.

51. Jahner D, Jaenisch R. Integration of Moloney leukaemia virus into the germ line of mice: correlation between site of integration and virus activation. Nature 1980; 287:456.

52. Soriano P, Jaenisch R. Retroviruses as probes for mammalian development: allocation of cells to the somatic and germ cell lineages. Cell 1986; 46:19.

53. Dosaka-Akita H, Cagle PT, Hiroumi H, et al. Differential retinoblastoma and p16(INK4A) protein expression in neuroendocrine tumors of the lung. Cancer 2000; 88:550.

54. Ehrhardt A, Bartels T, Geick A, Klocke R, Paul D, Halter R. Development of pulmonary bronchiolo-alveolar adenocarcinomas in transgenic mice overexpressing murine c-myc and epidermal growth factor in alveolar type II pneumocytes. Br J Cancer 2001; 84:813.

55. Fijneman RJ, de Vries SS, Jansen RC, Demant P. Complex interactions of new quantitative trait loci, Sluc1, Sluc2, Sluc3, and Sluc4, that influence the susceptibility to lung cancer in the mouse. Nat Genet 1996; 14:465.

56. Fong KM, Sekido Y, Minna JD. Molecular pathogenesis of lung cancer. J Thorac Cardiovasc Surg 1999; 18:1136.

57. Suda Y, Aizawa S, Hirai S, Inoue T, Furuta Y, Suzuki M, Hirohashi S, Ikawa Y. Driven by the same Ig enhancer and SV40 T promoter ras induced lung adenomatous tumors, myc induced pre-B cell lymphomas and SV40 large T gene a variety of tumors in transgenic mice. EMBO J 1987; 6:4055.

58. Maronpot RR, Palmiter RD, Brinster RL, Sandgren EP. Pulmonary carcinogenesis in transgenic mice. Exp Lung Res 1991; 17:305.

59. Wikenheiser KA, Clark JC, Linnoila RI, Stahlman MT, Whitsett JA. Simian virus 40 large T antigen directed by transcriptional elements of the human surfactant protein C gene produces pulmonary adenocarcinomas in transgenic mice. Cancer Res 1992; 52:5342.

60. Sandmoller A, Halter R, Suske G, Paul D, Beato M. A transgenic mouse model for lung adenocarcinoma. Cell Growth Differ 1995; 6:97.

61. Zhao B, Magdaleno S, Chua S, et al. Transgenic mouse models for lung cancer. Exp Lung Res 2000; 26:567.

62. Macleod KF, Jacks T. Insights into cancer from transgenic mouse models. J Pathol 1999; 187:43.

63. DeMayo FJ, Tsai SY. Targeted gene regulation and gene ablation. Trends Endocrinol Metab 2001; 12:348.

64. Lewandoski M. Conditional control of gene expression in the mouse. Nat Rev Genet 2001; 2:743.

65. Shockett PE, Schatz DG. Diverse strategies for tetracycline-regulated inducible gene expression. Proc Natl Acad Sci U S A 1996; 93:5173.

66. Fisher GH, Wellen SL, Klimstra D, et al. Induction and apoptotic regression of lung adenocarcinomas by regulation of a K-Ras transgene in the presence and absence of tumor suppressor genes. Genes Dev 2001; 15:3249.

67. Meuwissen R, Linn SC, van d V, Mooi WJ, Berns A. Mouse model for lung tumorigenesis through Cre/lox controlled sporadic activation of the K-Ras oncogene. Oncogene 2001; 20:6551.

68. Johnson L, Mercer K, Greenbaum D, Bronson RT, Crowley D, Tuveson DA, Jacks T. Somatic activation of the K-ras oncogene causes early onset lung cancer in mice. Nature 2001; 410:1111.

69. Meuwissen R, Linn SC, Linnoila RI, Zevenhoven J, Mooi WJ, Berns A. Induction of small cell lung cancer by somatic inactivation of both Trp53 and Rb1 in a conditional mouse model. Cancer Cell 2003; 4:181.

70. Povlsen CO, Rygaard J. Heterotransplantation of human adenocarcinomas of the colon and rectum to the mouse mutant Nude. A study of nine consecutive transplantations. Acta Pathol Microbiol Scand 1971; 79:159.

71. Sharkey FE, Fogh J, Hajdu S, et al. Experience in surgical pathology with human tumor growth in the nude mouse. In: Fogh J, Giovanella B (eds) The Nude Mouse in Experimental and Clinical Research. Academic, New York, 1978; p 188.

72. Mattern J, Bak M, Hahn EW, Volm M. Human tumor xenografts as model for drug testing. Cancer Metastasis Rev 1988; 7:263.

73. Boven E, Winograd B, Berger DP, et al. Phase II preclinical drug screening in human tumor xenografts: a first European multicenter collaborative study. Cancer Res 1992; 52:5940.

74. Steel GG, Courtenay VD, Peckham MJ. The response to chemotherapy of a variety of human tumour xenografts. Br J Cancer 1983; 47:1.

75. Takimoto CH. Why drugs fail: of mice and men revisited. Clin Cancer Res 2001; 7:229.

76. Fodstad O. Representativity of xenografts for clinical cancer. Tumor and host characteristics as variables of tumor take rate. In: Winograd B, Peckham MJ, Pinedo HM (eds) Human Tumor Xenografts in Anticancer Drug Development. Springer-Verlag, Berlin, 1988; p 15.

77. Fidler IJ. Rationale and methods for the use of nude mice to study the biology and therapy of human cancer metastasis. Cancer Metastasis Rev 1986; 5:29.

78. Shoemaker RH, McLemore TL, Abbott BJ, et al. Human tumor xenograft models for use with an in vitro-based, disease-oriented antitumor drug screening program. In: Winograd B, Peckham MJ, Pinedo HM (eds) Human Tumor Xenografts in Anticancer Drug Development. Springer-Verlag, Berlin, 1988:115.

79. Fidler IJ, Naito S, Pathak S. Orthotopic implantation is essential for the selection, growth and metastasis of human renal cell cancer in nude mice. Cancer Metastasis Rev 1990; 9:149.

80. Fidler IJ. Orthotopic implantation of human colon carcinomas into nude mice provides a valuable model for the biology and therapy of metastasis. Cancer Metastasis Rev 1991; 10:229.

81. Manzotti C, Audisio RA, Pratesi G. Importance of orthotopic implantation for human tumors as model systems: relevance to metastasis and invasion. Clin Exp Metastasis 1993; 11:5.

82. Kerbel RS, Cornil I, Theodorescu D. Importance of orthotopic transplantation procedures in assessing the effects of transfected genes on human tumor growth and metastasis. Cancer Metastasis Rev 1991; 10:201.

83. Paget S. Secondary growths of cancer of breast. Lancet 1889; 1:571.
84. Howard RB, Chu H, Zeligman BE, et al. Irradiated nude rat model for orthotopic human lung cancers. Cancer Res 1991; 51:3274.
85. McLemore TL, Liu MC, Blacker PC, et al. Novel intrapulmonary model for orthotopic propagation of human lung cancers in athymic nude mice. Cancer Res 1987; 47:5132.
86. Rashidi B, Yang M, Jiang P. A highly metastatic Lewis lung carcinoma orthotopic green fluorescent protein model. Clin Exp Metastasis 2000; 18:57.
87. McLemore TL, Eggleston JC, Shoemaker RH, et al. Comparison of intrapulmonary, percutaneous intrathoracic, and subcutaneous models for the propagation of human pulmonary and nonpulmonary cancer cell lines in athymic nude mice. Cancer Res 1988; 48:2880.
88. Kuo TH, Kubota T, Watanabe M, et al. Orthotopic reconstitution of human small-cell lung carcinoma after intravenous transplantation in SCID mice. Anticancer Res 1992; 12:1407.
89. Kuo TH, Kubota T, Watanabe M. Site-specific chemosensitivity of human small-cell lung carcinoma growing orthotopically compared to subcutaneously in SCID mice: the importance of orthotopic models to obtain relevant drug evaluation data. Anticancer Res 1993; 13: 627.
90. Nagamachi Y, Tani M, Shimizu K, Tsuda H, Niitsu Y, Yokota J. Orthotopic growth and metastasis of human non-small cell lung carcinoma cell injected into the pleural cavity of nude mice. Cancer Lett 1998; 127:203.
91. Miyoshi T, Kondo K, Ishikura H, Kinoshita H, Matsumori Y, Monden Y. SCID Mouse lymphogenous metastatic model of human lung cancer constructed using orthotopic inoculation of cancer cells. Anticancer Res 2000; 20:161.
92. Cuenca RE, Takita H, Bankert R. Orthotopic engraftment of human lung tumours in SCID mice for the study of metastasis. Surg Oncol 1996; 5:85.
93. Van Weerden WM, Romijn JC. Use of nude mouse xenograft models in prostate cancer research. Prostate 2000; 43:263.
94. Glaves D. Detection of circulating metastatic cells. Prog Clin Biol Res 1986; 212:151.
95. Butler TP, Gullino PM. Quantitation of cell shedding into efferent blood of mammary adenocarcinoma. Cancer Res 1975; 35:512.
96. Liotta LA, Kleinerman J, Saidel GM. Quantitative relationships of intravascular tumor cells, tumor vessels, and pulmonary metastases following tumor implantation. Cancer Res 1974; 34:997.
97. Yang M, Hasegawa S, Jiang P, et al. Widespread skeletal metastatic potential of human lung cancer revealed by green fluorescent protein expression. Cancer Res 1998; 58:4217.
98. Clark EA, Golub TR, Lander ES, Hynes RO. Genomic analysis of metastasis reveals an essential role for RhoC. Nature 2000; 406:532.
99. Naito S, Walker SM, Fidler IJ. In vivo selection of human renal cell carcinoma cells with high metastatic potential in nude mice. Clin Exp Metastasis 1989; 7:381.
100. Khanna C, Prehn J, Yeung C, Caylor J, Tsokos M, Helman L. An orthotopic model of murine osteosarcoma with clonally related variants differing in pulmonary metastatic potential. Clin Exp Metastasis 2000; 18:261.
101. Kozaki K, Miyaishi O, Tsukamoto T, Tatematsu Y, Hida T, Takahashi T, Takahashi T. Establishment and characterization of a human lung cancer cell line NCI-H460-LNM35 with consistent lymphogenous metastasis via both subcutaneous and orthotopic propagation. Cancer Res 2000; 60:2535.
102. Liu J, Blackhall F, Seiden-Long I, et al. (2004) Modeling of lung cancer by an orthotopically growing H460SM variant cell line reveals novel candidate genes for systemic metastasis. Oncogene 2004; 23:6316.
103. Fidler IJ, Hart IR. Biological diversity in metastatic neoplasms: origins and implications. Science 1982; 217:998.
104. Nicolson GL. Generation of phenotypic diversity and progression in metastatic tumor cells. Cancer Metastasis Rev 1984; 3:25.
105. Fidler IJ, Poste G. The cellular heterogeneity of malignant neoplasms: implications for adjuvant chemotherapy. Semin Oncol 1985; 12:207.
106. Fidler IJ. The organ microenvironment and cancer metastasis. Differentiation 2002; 70:498.
107. Morikawa K, Walker SM, Jessup JM, Fidler IJ. In vivo selection of highly metastatic cells from surgical specimens of different primary human colon carcinomas implanted into nude mice. Cancer Res 1988; 48:1943.
108. Dinney CP, Fishbeck R, Singh RK, et al. Isolation and characterization of metastatic variants from human transitional cell carcinoma passaged by orthotopic implantation in athymic nude mice. J Urol 1995; 154:1532.
109. Chu LW, Pettaway CA, Liang JC. Genetic abnormalities specifically associated with varying metastatic potential of prostate cancer cell lines as detected by comparative genomic hybridization. Cancer Genet Cytogenet 2001; 127:161.
110. Khanna C, Khan J, Nguyen P, et al. Metastasis-associated differences in gene expression in a murine model of osteosarcoma. Cancer Res 2001; 61:3750.
111. DeVita VT, Schein PS. The use of drugs in combination for the treatment of cancer: rationale and results. N Engl J Med 1973; 288:998.
112. Zubrod CG. Chemical control of cancer. Proc Natl Acad Sci U S A 1972; 69:1042.
113. Khleif SN, Curt GA. Animal models in drug development. In: Holland JF, Bast RC, Morton DL, Weichselbaum RR (eds) Cancer Medicine. Williams and Wilkins, Baltimore, 1997; p 855.
114. Belinsky SA, Stefanski SA, Anderson M W. The A/J mouse lung as a model for developing new chemointervention strategies. Cancer Res 1993; 53:410.
115. Mulvin DW, Howard RB, Mitchell DH, et al. Secondary screening system for preclinical testing of human lung cancer therapies. J Natl Cancer Inst 1992; 84:31.
116. Van Dyke T, Jacks T. Cancer modeling in the modern era: progress and challenges. Cell 2002; 108:135.
117. Zeligman BE, Howard RB, Marcell T, Chu H, Rossi RP, Mulvin D, Johnston MR. Chest roentgenographic techniques for demonstrating human lung tumour xenografts in nude rats. Lab Anim 1992; 26:100.
118. Kraus-Berthier L, Jan M, Guilbaud N, Naze M, Pierre A, Atassi G. Histology and sensitivity to anticancer drugs of two human non-small lung cell lung carcinomas implanted in the pleural cavity of nude mice. Clin Cancer Res 2002; 6:297.
119. Wilmanns C, Fan D, O'Brian CA, Bucana CD, Fidler IJ. Orthotopic and ectopic organ environments differentially influence the sensitivity of murine colon carcinoma cells to doxorubicin and 5-fluorouracil. Int J Cancer 1992; 52:98.
120. Davies B, Brown PD, East N, Crimmin MJ, Balkwill FR. A synthetic matrix metalloproteinase inhibitor decreases tumor burden and prolongs survival of mice bearing human ovarian carcinoma xenografts. Cancer Res 1993; 53:2087.
121. Marincola FM, Da Pozzo LF, Drucker BJ, Holder WD. Adoptive immunotherapy of human pancreatic cancer with lymphokine-activated killer cells and interleukin-2 in a nude mouse model. Surgery 1990; 108:919.

122. Russell PJ, Ho SI, Boniface GR, Izard ME, Philips J, Raghavan D, Walker KZ. Growth and metastasis of human bladder cancer xenografts in the bladder of nude rats. A model for intravesical radioimmunotherapy. Urol Res 1991; 19:207.

123. Schuster JM, Friedman HS, Archer GE, Fuchs HE, McLendon RE, Colvin OM, Bigner DD. Intraarterial therapy of human glioma xenografts in athymic rats using 4-hydroperoxycyclophosphamide. Cancer Res 1993; 53:2338.

124. Furukawa T, Kubota T, Watanabe M, Kitajima M, Hoffman RM. A novel "patient-like" treatment model of human pancreatic cancer constructed using orthotopic transplantation of histologically intact human tumor tissue in nude mice. Cancer Res 1993; 53:3070.

125. Johnston MR, Mullen JB, Pagura M, Appelt K, Shalinsky D. AG3340, a novel matrix metalloprotease (MMP) inhibitor, inhibits the growth of human large cell lung cancer tumors orthotopically implanted into the lung of athymic nude rats. Proc Am Assoc Cancer Res 1998; 39:A2060

126. Johnston MR, Mullen JB, Pagura M, Brekken J, Zou H, Shalinsky DR. AG3340 and carboplatin increase survival in an orthotopic nude rat model of primary and metastatic human lung cancer. Proc Am Assoc Cancer Res 1999; 40:A1946.

127. Pasualini R, Ruoslahti E. Organ targeting in vivo using phage display peptide libraries. Nature 1996; 380:364.

128. Uehara H, Kim SJ, Karashima T, et al. Effects of blocking platelet-derived growth factor-receptor signaling in a mouse model of experimental prostate cancer bone metastases. J Natl Cancer Inst 200395:458.

129. Price JE. Analyzing the metastatic phenotype. J Cell Biochem 1994; 56:16.

130. Gazdar AF, Kurvari V, Virmani A, et al. Characterization of paired tumor and non-tumor cell lines established from patients with breast cancer. Int J Cancer 1998; 78:766.

131. Wistuba II, Bryant D, Behrens C, Milchgrub S, Virmani AK, Ashfaq R, Minna JD, Gazdar AF. Comparison of features of human lung cancer cell lines and their corresponding tumors. Clin Cancer Res 1999; 5:991.

Genetics of Lung Cancer: Current Thinking on Genetic Predisposition to the Disease and Response to Treatment

5

Tim Benepal, Athena Matakidou, Ying Zee, Richard Houlston, and Tim Eisen

Contents

5.1 Introduction

Lung cancer is the most common cancer in the world, representing a major public health problem. In the United Kingdom it accounts for ~19% of all cancers and ~29% of all cancer deaths, being the commonest cause of cancer death in men, and is second only to breast cancer in women. Tobacco smoking is undoubtedly the major etiological risk factor, the risk being around ten times higher in long-term smokers compared with nonsmokers [1]. Only around 16% of people who smoke develop the disease [2], raising the possibility that individuals may have differing susceptibilities to developing lung cancer when exposed to the same carcinogens, which may in part be genetically defined. Here we review the evidence for a genetic predisposition to lung cancer, the possible molecular basis of an inherited susceptibility, and prediction of response to treatment.

5.2 The Multistep Evolution of Lung Cancer

Multiple morphological steps are well recognized in lung carcinogenesis [3]. In the development of squamous cell carcinoma, normal epithelial cells progress through hyperplasia, metaplasia, and dysplasia (premalignant stages) into carcinoma in situ and eventually frank malignancy. Adenocarcinoma is also considered to develop at least in part from premalignant precursor lesions such as atypical adenomatous hyperplasia. These preneoplastic changes are frequently detected in association with lung cancers and in the respiratory mucosa of smokers. Molecular biological studies have demonstrated that cancers carry multiple genetic and epigenetic changes, indicating inactivation of tumor-suppressor genes and activation of dominant oncogenes [4]. To date, relatively little is known about the molecular events preceding the development of lung carcinomas and the underlying genetic basis of tobacco-related lung carcinogenesis. However, recent studies have provided evidence of a multistep accumulation of genetic and epigenetic alterations, which often accompany the sequential morphological changes (Fig. 5.1) [5, 6]. The genetic alterations accompanying lung carcinogenesis are thought to result in perturbation of the integrity of integrated signaling networks, which positively or negatively regulate various cellular processes to maintain the homeostasis of the lung, leading to the carcinogenesis and progression of lung cancer. The accumulated genetic and epigenetic alterations are thought to confer various capabilities upon lung cancer cells, including an escape from growth inhibitory signals and senescence events, resistance to apoptosis, sustained stimuli for proliferation and angiogenesis, and invasive and meta-

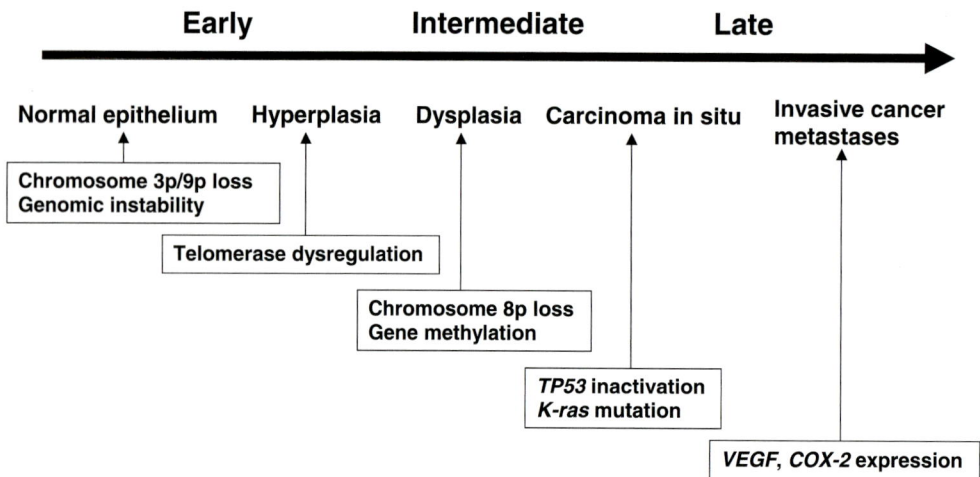

Fig. 5.1. Accumulation of alterations in the multistep progression of lung cancer carcinogenesis. *VEGF* Vascular endothelial growth factor, *COX-2* cyclooxygenase-2

static characteristics. The chronological order and catalogue of genes required to fully transform normal epithelial cells may vary among histological types of lung cancer or even within a given histological subtype.

5.3   Evidence for Inherited Susceptibility to Lung Cancer

5.3.1   Case-Control and Cohort Studies

Epidemiological case-control and cohort studies have consistently shown that relatives of lung cancer cases have a two-fold increased risk of developing the disease [7, 8]. However, as most studies have been based on cases who smoked, familial aggregation of smoking habits could explain the excess risk of lung cancer in case families relative to control families. Some investigators have attempted to address this issue by taking into account the smoking habits of the family members. Tokuhata and Lilienfeld found an excess risk of lung cancer in case relatives compared to control relatives, irrespective of the case or control relative's smoking history [9]. To minimize the impact of shared tobacco habits in families, several studies have estimated familial risks associated with nonsmoker status [10–13]. Although the familial risks obtained from three out of these four studies were nonsignificant, pooling the data does provide statistically significant support for an association between family history and lung cancer in nonsmokers (odds ratio, OR = 1.4; 95% confidence interval, CI = 1.0–1.9).

5.3.2   Twin Studies

Twin studies have reported nearly equal values of familial relative risks in monozygotic (MZ) and dizygotic (DZ) pairs among males [14–16]. This would suggest a strong environmental effect shared by twins (i.e., smoking behavior) rather than a genetic component. Such data has been cited widely to counter the proposition that an inherited basis exists for lung cancer. Twin studies have, however, consistently shown greater concordance for smoking behavior in MZ than DZ twins, suggesting that genetic factors as well as environmental exposure is being confounded in this study paradigm [17]. Yet, paradoxically, this concordance difference in smoking behavior is not reflected in a concordance difference for lung cancer. A study of United States male twins found a greater concordance in smoking for MZ versus DZ twins, yet no difference in concordance for lung cancer [18]. On the other hand, lung cancer among female twins [16], where the prevalence is much lower, did appear to follow a more conventional genetic pattern, with risks in MZ being greater than in DZ twins, indicating a genetic predisposition.

5.3.3   Cancer Syndromes Predisposing to Lung Cancer

To date, the only direct evidence of a genetic predisposition is provided by the increased risk of lung cancer associated with several rare Mendelian cancer syndromes. An increased lung cancer risk is observed in germ-line carriers [19] and retinoblastoma gene mutations [20], as well as in patients with xeroderma pigmentosum [21], Bloom's syndrome [22], and Werner's syndrome [23].

5.4   Genetic Models of Lung Cancer Susceptibility

Formal statistical modeling of the familial aggregation of lung cancer has suggested that the pattern of inheritance is best explainable by a model of the codominant inheritance of a rare autosomal gene predisposing to the disease. Sellers et al. estimated that such a gene mutation could be responsible for 69% of lung cancers occurring at the age of 50 years, falling to 22% of cases at age 70 years [24]. In an analogous situation to *BRCA1* and breast cancer, such a gene would be rare and would not account for much of the excess lung cancer risk seen in relatives of cases. However, if present it would be associated with a large relative risk, giving rise to multigenerational families. Such highly penetrant mutations can be detected through genetic linkage (the assessment of segregation of genetic markers with disease in families). Unfortunately, very few large lung cancer families in which multiple generations are affected have been described, and to date no genetic linkage has been established.

A polygenic mechanism might provide a more plausible explanation for the remaining familial risk. Under such a model, a large number of alleles, each conferring a small genotypic risk (perhaps of the order of 1.5–2.0), combine additively or multiplicatively to confer susceptibility. More than 100 such variants might contribute to susceptibility. Individuals carrying few such alleles would be at reduced risk, while those with many might suffer a lifetime risk as high as 50%. Such alleles will rarely cause multiple-case families, and their detection is reliant on association studies (comparison of the frequency of genotypes in cases with controls). Why may this be important? Firstly it may provide candidates suitable for enrollment in smoking cessation therapy, and secondly may identify individuals suitable for screening programs.

5.5   Candidate Loci for Lung Cancer Susceptibility Genes

There are more than 60 carcinogens in cigarette smoke [25]. Among these, tobacco-specific nitrosamines (such as 4-*N*(methylnitrosamino)-1-(3-pyridyl)-1-butanone, or NNK), polycyclic aromatic hydrocarbons (such as benzo(a)pyrene), and aromatic amines probably play an important role in the development of cancer [26]. In addition, cigarette smoke is a rich source of reactive oxygen species (free radicals), which may also contribute to lung cancer pathogenesis [27].

Figure 5.2 shows a depiction of the relationship between tobacco smoke and lung cancer. Nicotine addiction causes continual cigarette smoking and chronic exposure to carcinogens. Carcinogens such as NNK and polycyclic aromatic hydrocarbons are metabolically activated to intermediates that react with DNA, forming covalently bound products known as DNA adducts. Competing with this is the metabolic detoxification of carcinogens to harmless excreted products. If the DNA adducts are repaired by cellular repair enzymes, DNA is returned to its normal undamaged state. However if the adducts persist during DNA replication, miscoding can occur, resulting in a permanent mutation in the DNA sequence. Cells with damaged DNA may be removed by apoptosis. If a mutation occurs in a critical region of an oncogene (*RAS*, *MYC*) or tumor-suppressor gene (*TP53*), it can lead to activation or deactivation of this gene. Multiple events of this type lead to aberrant cells with loss of normal cellular growth-control regulation and, ultimately, to lung cancer development.

Any inherited susceptibility to lung cancer is likely to be mediated through biological differences in the bioactivation or degradation of carcinogens or cellular response to damage (e.g., DNA repair, cell-cycle control). It is almost inevitable that the loci currently considered as candidate low-penetrance susceptibility al-

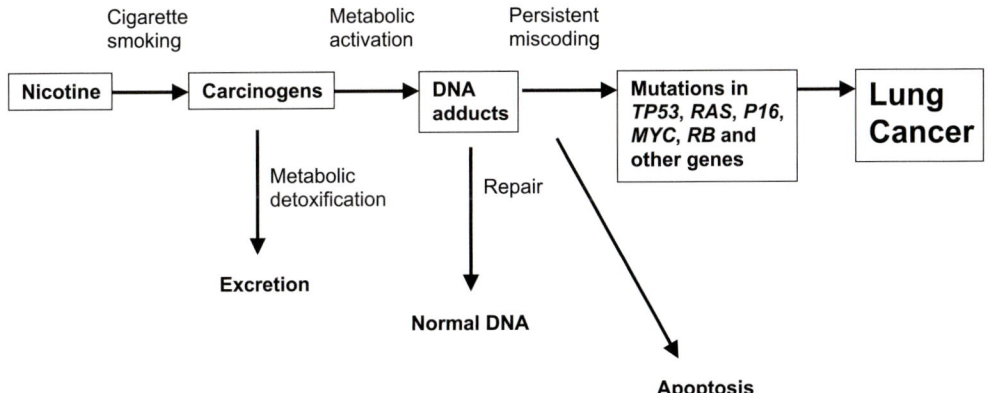

Fig. 5.2. Scheme linking nicotine addiction and lung cancer via tobacco smoke carcinogens, and their induction of multiple mutations in critical genes. *RB* Retinoblastoma

leles are based on preconceptions of cancer biology, and it is likely that other, as yet unrecognized genes may influence tumor development. The number of candidate loci will inevitably increase with advances in cancer biology.

Table 5.1 summarizes the genes implicated to date in lung cancer predisposition. Despite considerable research effort, few definite lung cancer susceptibility alleles have been identified. As with many other diseases, many positive associations have been reported, but few of the initial positive results have been replicated by subsequent studies. The most likely explanation for this has been the inadequate sample size of most, but not all, existing studies. The inherent statistical uncertainty of case-control studies involving just a few hundred cases and controls limits their ability to reliably identify genetic determinants of modest, but potentially important impact. Hence, most of the small case-control studies on the role of genetic polymorphisms and cancer risk have provided inconsistent results. The feasibility of identifying low-penetrance genes through association analyses is contingent on the ascertainment and collection of a large series of lung cancer cases and controls. One such DNA collection and epidemiological database, called the Genetic Lung Cancer Predisposition Study, is under construction in the UK. This study has already collected DNA and epidemiological data from over 5,000 patients with lung cancer and a similar number of controls.

5.6   Predictors of Response to Lung Cancer Therapy

Platinum agents, particularly cisplatin, remain the cornerstone of combination chemotherapy for non-small-cell lung cancer (NSCLC). Many cytotoxics induce DNA damage similar to that produced by carcinogens. The covalent binding of cytotoxic drug or carcinogen results in the formation of a chemically altered base in DNA that is termed an adduct [28]. Cisplatin has the structure of two labile chloro and two stabile amine ligands around a platinum core. Like other cytotoxics, cisplatin needs to be converted to a reactive form. This occurs nonenzymatically in solution with water, where displacement reactions result in stepwise exchange of labile chloro ligands with water molecules. The chloro-monoaquo species interacts with DNA at physiological pH. Carboplatin is a more stable molecule for which the aquation reaction is much slower. The monoaquated form of cisplatin reacts immediately with a DNA base to form a monofunctional adduct. The remaining chloride ligand is linked to platinum and then hydrolyzed, the resulting aquated species interacting with a second nucleophilic site to form DNA crosslinks [29]. It is these crosslinks are targeted by DNA repair pathways, which

Table 5.1. Genes implicated in or with an established role in lung cancer. *PAH* Polycyclic aromatic hydrocarbon

	Gene	Mechanism relevant to cancer
Carcinogen metabolism	*CYP1A1* *CYP2D6* *CYP2E1* *CYP2C9* *CYP2A6* *CYP2C19*	Bioactivation of tobacco procarcinogens
	NAT1 *NAT2*	Activation and inactivation of tobacco-derived aromatic amines
	GSTM1 *GSTM4* *GSTM3* *GSTT1* *GSTTP1*	Detoxification of PAH carcinogens
	SULT1A1	Bioactivation of aromatic amines
	mEH	Bioactivation of PAHs
	MPO	Activation of benzo(a)pyrene
	NQO1	Activation of nitrosamines
Methylation	*MTHFR* *DNMT3B*	Changes in DNA methylation (transcriptional activation/ silencing)
Nucleotide excision repair	*XPA* *XPD* *XPG* *XPC*	Repair of tobacco-related DNA adducts
Homologous recombination	*XRCC3* *DNA ligase I* *Poly(ADP)-ribose*	Repair of DNA strand breaks generated by reactive oxygen species in tobacco smoke
Base excision repair	*OGG1* *XRCC1* *APE/ref1*	Repair of DNA damage due to reactive oxygen species in tobacco smoke
Free-radical system	*hGPX1* *NE* *MNSOD* *MMP-1* *ADH3*	Detoxification of tobacco smoke-related free radicals
Apoptosis	*TP53* *TP73* *TP21*	Mediation of cellular responses to genotoxic insults by tobacco carcinogens
Proto-oncogene	*HRAS-VNTR* *L-MYC*	Control of cell growth and differentiation
Other genes	*AGT*	Repair of DNA adducts induced by the tobacco-specific nitrosamine NNK
	RAGE	Regulation of invasive process extension and cell migration in tumor cells
	DRD2	Role in smoking status and addiction
	TNFB	Host inflammatory response to lung cancer

in themselves are a common denominator for both carcinogenesis and platinum resistance.

Excision repair cross-complementation group 1 (ERCC1) and xeroderma pigmentosum group D (XPD) play a vital role in DNA repair. This section aims to describe the genetics and function of these genes, and to review the current literature on their relation to the risk of lung cancer and its response to treatment with chemotherapy.

5.6.1 ERCC1

The *ERCC1* gene is located at chromosome 19q13.2-q13.3. It comprises ten exons and spans approximately 16,300 base pairs. The ERCC1 gene product is essential for nucleotide excision repair (NER), which is an important mechanism for correcting abnormal DNA structures arising from DNA damage, replication errors or recombination processes [30]. This repair pathway involves specific damage recognition, dual incision of the damaged strand, followed by lesion removal, gap filling and eventually, strand ligation [31]. Damage recognition and strand incision in mammalian cells require several NER-specific enzymes. The *ERCC1* gene product is a single-stranded DNA endonuclease that forms a tight heterodimer with xeroderma pigmentosum complementation group F (XPF). The ERCC1/XPF complex incises the 5' side of DNA lesions [32]. The absence of ERCC1 is incompatible with life [33].

Tobacco carcinogens cause DNA damage, and reduced DNA repair capacity has been shown to be associated with lung cancer risk [34]. However, few studies have evaluated the role of expression of DNA repair genes like *ERCC1* in the etiology of lung cancer. A pilot case-control study measuring the relative expression levels of five NER genes [*ERCC1*, xeroderma pigmentosa (XB) group B (*XPB*)/*ERCC3*, *XPG*/*ERCC5*, Cochayne Syndrome complementary (*CSB*)/*ERCC6*, and *XPC*) in phytohemagglutinin-stimulated peripheral lymphocytes obtained from 75 lung cancer patients and 95 controls observed an 8.3% decrease in the baseline expression levels of *ERCC1* in cases compared with controls, although these differences were not statistically significant ($P=0.091$). Comparison of cases and controls with low *ERCC1* expression showed an adjusted OR of 1.76 with a 95% CI of 0.93–3.33. This study did find that individuals whose expression levels of *XPG*/*ERCC5* and *CSB*/*ERCC6* are reduced may be at higher risk of lung cancer [35].

5.6.1.1 Response to Treatment with Chemotherapy

Platinum compounds are commonly used in combination with chemotherapeutic agents such as gemcitabine and vinorelbine in the treatment of advanced NSCLC. Randomized trials have failed to identify major differences in survival between any of the standard doublets, but toxicity profiles do vary [36, 37]. Although platinum-based therapy has heralded a major advance in treatment and survival in NSCLC, incorporation of genetic analysis to help predict response to treatment may further improve the outcome of this disease.

Cisplatin activity is mediated through the formation of cisplatin DNA adducts that block replication and inhibit transcription. Removal of these adducts leads to chemoresistance, is largely carried out through NER, and NER-deficient cells are hypersensitive to cisplatin. High *ERCC1* expression has been associated with resistance to cisplatin [38]. Conversely, low *ERCC1* expression correlates with prolonged survival in advanced NSCLC patients treated with combination cisplatin chemotherapy [39]. Single-nucleotide polymorphisms in any of the NER genes may alter DNA repair capacity and contribute to individual variations in chemotherapy response. Two common polymorphisms of *ERCC1*, codon 118 and C8092A, have been reported [40]. The C/C genotype in codon 118 of *ERCC1* has been shown to be a surrogate marker for predicting better survival in NSCLC patients treated with cisplatin combination chemotherapy [41, 42]. A study of 128 advanced NSCLC patients treated with platinum-based chemotherapy showed a statistically significant association between the C8092A polymorphism and overall survival ($P=0.006$), with median survival times of 22.3 months (C/C genotype) and 13.4 months (C/A or A/A genotypes), respectively. This is the first study demonstrating that the *ERCC1* C8092A polymorphism may be a useful predictor of overall survival in advanced NSCLC patients treated with platinum-based chemotherapy [43].

5.6.2 XPD

The *XPD* gene, also called the *ERCC2* gene, is located at chromosome 19q13.3. It comprises 23 exons and spans approximately 54,000 base pairs [44]. The *XPD* gene product is a protein of 760 amino acids with a molecular weight of 86,900 and adenosine triphosphate-dependent 5'–3' DNA helicase activity. The XPD protein is a component of the core transcription factor IIH, which is a nine-protein complex that is essential for NER activity [45]. Once the DNA lesion has been recognized, the helicase activity of XPD, together with the XPB helicase, unwinds the DNA in the 5'–3' direction so that the damaged strand can be cut and the damaged piece of DNA excised. XPD activity is essential for life and total absence of the *XPD* gene results in embryonic lethality [46].

Two common polymorphisms of *XPD*, 751 A → C and 312 G → A, have been studied in relation to lung cancer risk. A meta-analysis of the published data from nine individual case-control studies of 3,725 lung cancer cases and 4,152 controls supports the hypothesis that both the *XPD* 751 C and 312 A are risk alleles and individuals with the *XPD* 751 CC and 312 AA genotypes are at higher risk of developing lung cancer [47]. However, a more recent meta-analysis looking at a total of 3,374 cases and 3,880 controls for the *XPD* 751 polymorphism (7 studies) and 2,886 cases and 3,085 controls for the *XPD* 312 polymorphism (6 studies) found no overall evidence of an association with lung cancer [48].

5.6.2.1 Response to Treatment with Chemotherapy

With its vital role in NER, *XPD* polymorphism has been related to lower DNA repair capacity and enhanced cisplatin sensitivity in patients with advanced NSCLC [49]. Conversely, high *XPD* expression is related to selective cisplatin resistance and reduced overall survival in patients with advanced NSCLC [50]. Rosell et al. observed that time to disease progression was significantly higher in gemcitabine+cisplatin treated patients with the Lys751Gln genotype (9.6 months) than in those with the Lys751Lys genotype (4.2 months; $P = 0.03$). However, in patients treated with vinorelbine+cisplatin, patients with the Lys751Lys genotype had a longer time to progression. When docetaxel was added to gemcitabine+cisplatin, patients with that genotype also had better survival [51]. These findings indicate that NER status can help to decide between gemcitabine+cisplatin and docetaxel+cisplatin.

5.6.3 Predicting Response to Epidermal Growth Factor Receptor Inhibition

The epidermal growth factor receptor (EGFR) is a 170-kD plasma membrane glycoprotein that is made up of an extracellular ligand-binding domain, a lipophilic transmembrane segment, and an intracellular protein kinase domain with a regulatory carboxyl terminal segment [52, 53]. It is part of a group that includes the following four distinct receptors: EGFR/ErbB-1, Her-2/ErbB-2, Her-3/ErbB-3, and Her-4/ErbB-4. There are several identified ligands that bind with high affinity to these receptors, and EGFR ligands include epidermal growth factor and transforming growth factor-alpha [54]. Binding of the ligand to the extracellular domain induces receptor homo- or heterodimerization, followed by internalization of the receptor–ligand complex and autophosphorylation. Tyrosine kinase (TK) signal transduction pathways are then activated, and these regulate cell function [55]. It is now accepted that the EGFR signal transduction network is an important factor in cell proliferation, survival, apoptosis, angiogenesis, adhesion, and motility, all factors related to the development of metastasis [56]. In addition, EGFR is expressed in many epithelial cancers, including 40–80% of NSCLC [57]. Following activation of the receptor, several down-stream signal-transduction cascades are activated, including Ras/Raf, mitogen-activated protein kinase, and phosphatidylinositol-3-kinase [58, 59]. Specific inhibition of EGFR signaling, therefore, seemed a logical target for anticancer therapy. Gefitinib (ZD1839, Iressa) is an oral, selective EGFR-TK inhibitor EGFR-TKI), which targets the ATP cleft within the receptor [60]. Erlotinib (OSI-774, Tarceva) is also a selective EGFR-TKI that is currently under evaluation. However, this review will concentrate on the published genetic data relative to gefitinib.

Preclinical in vitro studies indicate that gefitinib potently inhibits TK activity at low concentrations, whilst not affecting other kinases. Both as a single agent and in combination with several cytotoxics in vitro, a greater than additive effect was observed in several cell lines [61]. In vivo, a supra-additive effect was seen in combination with a number of cytotoxics including cisplatin, carboplatin, and paclitaxel [62]. Phase I trials included a total of 100 patients with NSCLC in whom a 10% response rate was observed [63, 64]. These factors led to the rapid clinical development of gefitinib. Gefitinib was tested in chemotherapy-nave patients in two large, randomized phase III studies (INTACT-1 and INTACT-2) in which 2,130 patients were treated with carboplatin and paclitaxel, or cisplatin and gemcitabine ± gefitinib. Neither study demonstrated a benefit in terms of overall survival, progression-free survival, or time to worsening symptoms for the addition of gefitinib to either chemotherapy regimen [65, 66].

Two studies of gefitinib monotherapy at 2 different doses (250 mg vs. 500 mg o.d.) were conducted in patients who had received at least 1 previous platinum-based chemotherapy regimen (IDEAL-1, 210 patients [67]), or a minimum of 2 chemotherapy regimens including platinum-based therapy and taxotere (IDEAL-2, 221 patients [68]). Similar response rates were seen in both studies at each dose level of gefitinib (18% for 250 mg and 19% for 500 mg; IDEAL-1, 9% for 250 mg; IDEAL-2, 12% for 500 mg), with a disease control rate (complete response + partial response + stable disease) of 52% [67], and a symptomatic improvement of approximately 40% [68].

More recently, a large, randomized study of more than 1,700 patients randomized to gefitinib versus placebo, whilst showing a significantly improved response rate for the gefitinib arm, showed no survival advantage for gefitinib versus best supportive care (Astra Zeneca – press release). A recent randomized phase III study of erlotinib versus placebo following chemotherapy, however, has demonstrated a statistically significant improvement in progression-free survival (2.23 months vs. 1.84 months, $P < 0.001$) and overall survival (6.7 months vs. 4.7 months, $P = 0.001$) for patients receiving erlotinib versus placebo [69].

Although disappointing overall, one consistent observation throughout these clinical trials has been that there appears to be an increased response rate in particular subsets of patients. Although only 10–19% of patients responded in the two large monotherapy studies, significantly higher response rates were observed in Japanese versus European patients (27.5% vs. 10.4%) and in females versus men (50% vs. 31%) with adenocarcinomas versus other subtypes (13% vs. 4%) [67, 68]. More recently, a high response rate has also been observed in chemotherapy pretreated Taiwanese patients (26–36%) [70, 71], and in chemonaive patients from Taiwan the response rate was even higher (56.5%) [72]. There has been no proven correlation between EGFR protein expression and response to gefitinib [73]. It has been widely observed, however, that patients responding to EGFR inhibition show a striking correlation between development of a cutaneous rash and drug response [74]. This may be due to genetic differences among individuals. One study has demonstrated that single-sequence polymorphisms in intron 1 of the *EGFR* gene can mediate response to EGFR inhibitors. In a panel of squamous cell carcinoma cell lines and patient tumor specimens, a lower number of CA-single-sequence repeat polymorphisms in intron 1 of the EGFR gene was associated with greater response to erlotinib as well as increased expression of EGFR mRNA and protein expression [75].

Further studies have demonstrated a significant correlation between EGFR mutations and response. Lynch and colleagues analyzed tumor specimens from 16 patients treated with gefitinib, 9 of whom responded [76]. Through sequencing of the entire coding region of the *EGFR* gene, heterozygous mutations were observed in eight out of nine responding patients. Matched normal tissue was obtained from four of the patients showing only the wild-type sequence, indicating that the mutations had arisen somatically. No mutations were observed in any of the seven nonresponding patients [76]. Paez and colleagues also searched for somatic *EGFR* gene mutations in 119 primary NSCLC tumors, consisting of 58 Japanese and 61 American patients, 70 adenocarcinomas and 49 other NSCLC pathologies, none of whom had received gefitinib [77]. The observed mutations showed a striking correlation with the observed patient characteristics. Mutations occurred more frequently in patients with adenocarcinomas (15/70, 21%) rather than other NSCLC pathologies (1/49, 2%), women (9/45, 20%) rather than men (7/74, 9%), and Japanese (15/58, 26%) rather than patients from the USA (1/61, 2%). Japanese women with adenocarcinomas demonstrated the highest frequency of *EGFR* mutations (8/14, 57%). Further analysis was then performed on a nine more patients who had been treated with gefitinib, of whom five responded and four did not respond to treatment. No mutations were observed in the four patients whose disease progressed while on gefitinib, but all five responding patients were identified as having EGFR kinase domain mutations [77].

Huang and colleagues analyzed 101 untreated patients with NSCLC (69/101 with adenocarcinomas) and 16 patients treated with gefitinib. Mutations in the kinase domain of the *EGFR* gene were identified in 39/101 (38.6%) patients, all but one with adenocarcinoma. Of the 69 adenocarcinoma patients, the mutation rate was 38/69 (55%). Of the 16 treated patients, 7 of the 9 responding patients and 1 of the 7 nonresponding mutations had EGFR kinase domain mutations ($P = 0.041$) [78]. Little work is published on the expression of downstream markers of response, but a smaller, immunohistochemical study examining phosphorylated-Akt (p-Akt) and phosphorylated-Erk (p-Erk) has demonstrated that overexpression of p-Akt is positively, and p-Erk negatively associated with response [79]. Similar work with erlotinib is ongoing and results are awaited. It remains uncertain, however, whether response is a good marker of benefit in terms of survival, nonprogression, and symptomatic benefit in this disease.

5.7 Conclusion

Recent technological developments have accelerated the search for genes predisposing to a variety of multifactorial diseases, including lung cancer. The completion of the human genome project has provided a vast amount of information regarding interindividual variability at the genomic level and is providing an increasing number of candidate susceptibility loci. Recent technological advances make high-throughput genotyping possible [80]. This allows rapid and highly reliable association studies to be initiated. These developments promise to advance our knowledge on lung cancer predisposition and allow the construction of individual lung cancer risk profiles. Identification of individuals at high risk of lung cancer will allow targeted screening, leading to improvements in early diagnosis, intervention strategies for treatment of preneoplasia and neoplasia, and continued improvements in public health policy.

It is important to note that such low-penetrance susceptibility alleles will need to be considered in the context of other risk factors. In lung cancer, the risk of any low-penetrance gene studied should be taken in the context of the risks of smoking. Smoking cessation clearly reduces lung cancer risk, but also reduces mortality and morbidity due to nonmalignant (e.g., cardiovascular) complications. Genetic risk may therefore be modified, so patients should not assume that they cannot affect their risk because of inheritance.

ERCC1 and *XPD* play pivotal roles in DNA repair. There are therefore significant theoretical implications with regard to these genes and lung cancer risk, as well as response to treatment with chemotherapy. Overall, there has been no statistically significant evidence to support an association between *ERCC1* and lung cancer risk, and two meta-analyses on *XPD* and lung cancer risk demonstrated conflicting results. However, most analyses to date have been restricted to one or two polymorphisms. It may be that only the joint effect of multiple polymorphisms within the gene provides information about an association with lung cancer [48]. Therefore, it is likely that the defining feature of future epidemiologic studies will be the simultaneous analysis of large numbers of polymorphisms in candidate genes in much larger samples of cases and controls [81, 82]. Indeed, a recent study has indicated that lung cancer risk is only moderately increased by single DNA repair gene variants, but it is considerably enhanced by specific combinations of variant alleles [83].

The first suggestions of a relationship between *ERCC1* or *XPD* expression and differential sensitivity to chemotherapy are now emerging. The results of ongoing and future studies into the roles of *ERCC1* and *XPD* may validate their respective predictive survival values. What is currently known serves to highlight the possibilities of individually tailored chemotherapy.

There is an emerging subset of patients with certain EGFR somatic mutations that have impressive and predictable responses to treatment following failure of standard combination chemotherapy in a disease which for most patients ultimately results in death.

Key Points

- Technological advances have made high-throughput genotyping possible, allowing high-powered, case-control analyses to be performed to help identify predisposition loci.
- DNA repair mechanisms may help define lung cancer predisposition as well as predicting response to therapy.
- Epidermal growth factor receptor mutations are associated with increased response to small molecule tyrosine kinase inhibitors, and development of a reliable/reproducible screening method may better identify patients who may respond to treatment.

References

1. Doll R, Peto J. The cause of cancer. London, Oxford University Press, London, 1981; p 1221.
2. Peto R, Darby S, Deo H, Silcocks P, Whitley E, Doll R. Smoking, smoking cessation, and lung cancer in the UK since 1950: combination of national statistics with two case-control studies. BMJ 2000; 321:323.
3. Colby TV, Wistuba, II, Gazdar A. Precursors to pulmonary neoplasia. Adv Anat Pathol 1998; 5:205.
4. Sekido Y, Fong KM, Minna JD. Progress in understanding the molecular pathogenesis of human lung cancer. Biochem Biophys Acta 1998; 1378: F21.
5. Osada H, Takahashi T. Genetic alterations of multiple tumor suppressors and oncogenes in the carcinogenesis and progression of lung cancer. Oncogene 2002; 21:7421.
6. Wistuba II, Mao L, Gazdar AF. Smoking molecular damage in bronchial epithelium. Oncogene 2002;21(48):7298.
7. Lee PN. Epidemiological Studies relating family history of lung cancer to risk of the disease. Indoor Environ 1993; 2:129.
8. Houlston RS, Peto J. Genetics of common cancers. In: Eeles RA, Ponder B, Easton DE, Horwich A (eds) Inherited Predisposition to Cancer. Chapman Hall, New York, 1996; p 208.
9. Tokuhata GK, Lilienfeld AM. Familial aggregation of lung cancer in humans. J Natl Cancer Inst 1963; 30:289.
10. Schwartz AG, Yang P, Swanson GM. Familial risk of lung cancer among nonsmokers and their relatives. Am J Epidemiol 1996; 144:554.
11. Wang TJ, Zhou BS, Shi JP. Lung cancer in nonsmoking Chinese women: a case-control study. Lung Cancer 1996; 14 Suppl 1: S93.
12. Wu AH, Fontham ET, Reynolds P, et al. Family history of cancer and risk of lung cancer among lifetime nonsmoking women in the United States. Am J Epidemiol 1996; 143:535.
13. Mayne ST, Buenconsejo J, Janerich DT. Familial cancer history and lung cancer risk in United States nonsmoking men and women. Cancer Epidemiol Biomarkers Prev 1999; 8:1065.
14. Braun MM, Caporaso NE, Page WF, Hoover RN. Genetic component of lung cancer: cohort study of twins. Lancet 1994; 344:440.
15. Braun MM, Caporaso NE, Page WF, Hoover, RN. A cohort study of twins and cancer. Cancer Epidemiol Biomarkers Prev 1995; 4:469.
16. Lichtenstein P, Holm NV, Verkasalo PK, et al. Environmental and heritable factors in the causation of cancer – analyses of cohorts of twins from Sweden, Denmark, and Finland. N Engl J Med 2000; 343:78.
17. Risch A, Wikman H, Thiel S, et al. Glutathione-S-transferase M1, M3, T1 and P1 polymorphisms and susceptibility to non-small-cell lung cancer subtypes and hamartomas. Pharmacogenetics 2001; 11:757.
18. Goldgar DE, Easton DF, Cannon-Albright LA, Skolnick MH. Systematic population-based assessment of cancer risk in first-degree relatives of cancer probands. J Natl Cancer Inst 1994; 86:1600.
19. Hwang SJ, Cheng LS, Lozano G, Amos CI, Gu, X, Strong LC. Lung cancer risk in germline p53 mutation carriers: association between an inherited cancer predisposition, cigarette smoking, and cancer risk. Hum Genet 2003; 113:238.
20. Sanders BM., Jay M, Draper GJ, Roberts EM. Non-ocular cancer in relatives of retinoblastoma patients. Br J Cancer 1989; 60:358.
21. Swift M, Chase C. Cancer in families with xeroderma pigmentosum. J Natl Cancer Inst 1979; 62:1415.

22. Takemiya M, Shiraishi S, Teramoto T, Miki Y. Bloom's syndrome with porokeratosis of Mibelli and multiple cancers of the skin, lung and colon. Clin Genet 1987; 31:35.

23. Yamanaka A, Hirai T, Ohtake Y, Kitagawa M. Lung cancer associated with Werner's syndrome: a case report and review of the literature. Jpn J Clin Oncol 1997; 27:415.

24. Sellers TA, Chen PL, Potter JD, Bailey-Wilson JE, Rothschild H, Elston RC. Segregation analysis of smoking-associated malignancies: evidence for Mendelian inheritance. Am J Med Genet 1994; 52:308.

25. International Agency for Research on Cancer. Tobacco smoke and involuntary smoking. IARC Monographs on the evaluation of carcinogenic risks to humans 2002; p 83.

26. Hecht SS. Tobacco carcinogens, their biomarkers and tobacco-induced cancer. Nat Rev Cancer 2003; 3:733.

27. Pryor WA, Stone K. Oxidants in cigarette smoke. Radicals, hydrogen peroxide, peroxynitrate, and peroxynitrite. Ann N Y Acad Sci 1993; 686:27.

28. Phillips, DH. The formation of DNA adducts. In: Alison MR (ed) The Cancer Handbook. Nature Publishing Group, London, 2002; p 293.

29. Siddik ZH. Mechanisms of action of cancer chemotherapeutic agents: DNA-interactive alkylating agents and antitumor platinum based drugs. In: Alison MR (ed) The Cancer Handbook. Nature Publishing Group, London, 2002; 1295.

30. Sancar A. DNA repair in humans. Annu Rev Genet 1995; 29:69.

31. Hoeijmakers JH. Human nucleotide excision repair syndromes: molecular clues to unexpected intricacies. Eur J Cancer 1994; 30A:1912.

32. Huang JC, Hsu DS, Kazantsev A, Sancar A. Substrate spectrum of human excinuclease: repair of abasic sites, methylated bases, mismatches, and bulky adducts. Proc Natl Acad Sci U S A 1994; 91:12213.

33. Wilson MD, Ruttan CC, Koop BF, Glickman BW. ERCC1: a comparative genomic perspective. Environ Mol Mutagen 2001; 38:209.

34. Wei Q, Cheng L, Hong WK, Spitz MR. Reduced DNA repair capacity in lung cancer patients. Cancer Res 1996; 56:4103.

35. Cheng L, Spitz MR, Hong WK, Wei Q. Reduced expression levels of nucleotide excision repair genes in lung cancer: a case-control analysis. Carcinogenesis 2000; 21:1527.

36. Martoni A, Marino A, Sperandi F, et al. Multicentre randomised phase III study comparing the same dose and schedule of cisplatin plus the same schedule of vinorelbine or gemcitabine in advanced non-small cell lung cancer. Eur J Cancer 2005; 41:81.

37. Schiller J, Harrington D, Belani PC, et al. Comparison of four chemotherapy regimens for advanced non-small-cell lung cancer N Engl J Med 2002; 346:92.

38. Furuta T, Ueda T, Aune G, Sarasin A, Kraemer KH, Pommier Y. Transcription-coupled nucleotide excision repair as a determinant of cisplatin sensitivity of human cells. Cancer Res 2002; 62:4899.

39. Lord RV, Brabender J, Gandara D, et al. Low ERCC1 expression correlates with prolonged survival after cisplatin plus gemcitabine chemotherapy in non-small cell lung cancer. Clin Cancer Res 2002; 8:2286.

40. Sturgis EM, Dahlstrom KR, Spitz MR, Wei Q. DNA repair gene ERCC1 and ERCC2/XPD polymorphisms and risk of squamous cell carcinoma of the head and neck. Arch Otolaryngol Head Neck Surg 2002; 128:1084.

41. Isla D, Sarries C, Rosell R, et al. Single nucleotide polymorphisms and outcome in docetaxel-cisplatin-treated advanced non-small-cell lung cancer. Ann Oncol 2004; 15:1194.

42. Ryu JS, Hong YC, Han HS, et al. Association between polymorphisms of ERCC1 and XPD and survival in non-small-cell lung cancer patients treated with cisplatin combination chemotherapy. Lung Cancer 2004; 44:311.

43. Zhou W, Gurubhagavatula S, Liu G, et al. Excision repair cross-complementation group 1 polymorphism predicts overall survival in advanced non-small cell lung cancer patients treated with platinum-based chemotherapy. Clin Cancer Res 2004; 10:4939.

44. Weber CA, Salazar EP, Stewart SA, Thompson LH. ERCC2: cDNA cloning and molecular characterization of a human nucleotide excision repair gene with high homology to yeast RAD3. EMBO J 1990; 9:1437.

45. Schaeffer L, Moncollin V, Roy R, et al. The ERCC2/DNA repair protein is associated with the class II BTF2/TFIIH transcription factor. EMBO J 1994; 13:2388.

46. Friedberg EC. DNA damage and repair. Nature 2003; 421:436.

47. Hu Z, Wei Q, Wang X, Shen H. DNA repair gene XPD polymorphism and lung cancer risk: a meta-analysis. Lung Cancer 2004; 46:1.

48. Benhamou S, Sarasin, A. ERCC2/XPD gene polymorphisms and lung cancer: a huge review. Am J Epidemiol 2005; 161:1.

49. Camps C, Sarries C, Roig B, et al. Assessment of nucleotide excision repair XPD polymorphisms in the peripheral blood of gemcitabine/cisplatin-treated advanced non-small-cell lung cancer patients. Clin Lung Cancer 2003; 4:237.

50. Gurubhagavatula S, Liu G, Park S, et al. XPD and XRCC1 genetic polymorphisms are prognostic factors in advanced non-small-cell lung cancer patients treated with platinum chemotherapy. J Clin Oncol 2004; 22:2594.

51. Rosell R, Taron M, Camps C, Lopez-Vivanco G. Influence of genetic markers on survival in non-small cell lung cancer. Drugs Today (Barc) 2003; 39:775.

52. Lemmon MA, Schlessinger J. Regulation of signal transduction and signal diversity by receptor oligomerization. Trends Biochem Sci 1994; 19:459.

53. Klapper LN, Kirschbaum MH, Sela M, Yarden Y. Biochemical and clinical implications of the ErbB/HER signaling network of growth factor receptors. Adv Cancer Res 2000; 77:25.

54. Jones JT, Akita RW, Sliwkowski MX. Binding specificities and affinities of egf domains for ErbB receptors. FEBS Lett 1999; 447:227.

55. Wells A. EGF receptor. Int J Biochem Cell Biol 1999; 31:637.

56. Hanahan D, Weinberg RA. The hallmarks of cancer. Cell 2000; 100:57.

57. Arteaga CL. ErbB-targeted therapeutic approaches in human cancer. Exp Cell Res 2003; 284:122.

58. Weinstein-Oppenheimer CR, Blalock WL, Steelman LS, Chang F, McCubrey JA. The Raf signal transduction cascade as a target for chemotherapeutic intervention in growth factor-responsive tumors. Pharmacol Ther 2000; 88:229.

59. Vivanco I, Sawyers CL. The phosphatidylinositol 3-Kinase AKT pathway in human cancer. Nat Rev Cancer 2002; 2:489.

60. Wakeling AE, Guy SP, Woodburn JR, Ashton SE, Curry BJ, Barker AJ, Gibson KH. ZD1839 (Iressa): an orally active inhibitor of epidermal growth factor signaling with potential for cancer therapy. Cancer Res 2002; 62:5749.

61. Ciardiello F, Caputo R, Bianco R, et al. Antitumor effect and potentiation of cytotoxic drugs activity in human cancer cells by ZD-1839 (Iressa), an epidermal growth factor receptor-selective tyrosine kinase inhibitor. Clin Cancer Res 2000; 6:2053.

62. Sirotnak FM, Zakowski, MF, Miller VA, Scher HI, Kris MG. Efficacy of cytotoxic agents against human tumor xenografts is markedly enhanced by coadministration of

ZD1839 (Iressa), an inhibitor of EGFR tyrosine kinase. Clin Cancer Res 2000; 6:4885.

63. Baselga J, Rischin D, Ranson M, et al. Phase I safety, pharmacokinetic, and pharmacodynamic trial of ZD1839, a selective oral epidermal growth factor receptor tyrosine kinase inhibitor, in patients with five selected solid tumor types. J Clin Oncol 2000; 20:4292.

64. Herbst RS, Maddox AM, Rothenberg ML, et al. Selective oral epidermal growth factor receptor tyrosine kinase inhibitor ZD1839 is generally well-tolerated and has activity in non-small-cell lung cancer and other solid tumors: results of a phase I trial. J Clin Oncol 2002; 20:3815.

65. Giaccone G, Herbst RS, Manegold C, et al. Gefitinib in combination with gemcitabine and cisplatin in advanced non-small-cell lung cancer: a phase III trial – INTACT 1. J Clin Oncol 2004; 22:777.

66. Herbst RS, Giaccone G, Schiller JH, et al. Gefitinib in combination with paclitaxel and carboplatin in advanced non-small-cell lung cancer: a phase III trial – INTACT 2. J Clin Oncol 2004; 22:785.

67. Fukuoka M, Yano S, Giaccone G, et al. Multi-institutional randomized phase II trial of gefitinib for previously treated patients with advanced non-small-cell lung cancer (The IDEAL 1 Trial) [corrected]. J Clin Oncol 2003; 21:2237.

68. Kris MG, Natale ,RB, Herbst RS, et al. Efficacy of gefitinib, an inhibitor of the epidermal growth factor receptor tyrosine kinase, in symptomatic patients with non-small cell lung cancer: a randomized trial. JAMA 2003; 290:2149.

69. Shepherd FA, Pereira J, Ciuleanu TE, et al. A randomized placebo-controlled trial of erlotinib in patients with advanced non-small cell lung cancer (NSCLC) following failure of 1st line or 2nd line chemotherapy. A National Cancer Institute of Canada Clinical Trials Group (NCIC CTG) trial. J Clin Oncol 2004; 22:7022.

70. Tsai C, Chiu C, Chen Y. Gefitinib in patients with advanced non-small-cell lung cancer: a relationship between drug toxicity and tumor response. Thoracic Med 2003; 18:93.

71. Wu MF, Fahn HJ, Wu TC. Experience of gefitinib (Iressa) for previously treated patients with advanced non-small cell lung cancer. Thoracic Med 2003; 18:203.

72. Chen K, Chang GC, Yang TY. A comparison of gefitinib monotherapy and chemotherapy with cisplatin and gemcitabine in chemonaive patients with advanced non-small cell lung cancer: a case control study. Thoracic Med 2003; 18:218.

73. Bailey R, Kris M, Wolf M. Gefitinib ('Iressa', ZD1839) monotherapy for pre-treated advanced non-small cell lung cancer in IDEAL-1 and 2: tumor response is not clinically relevantly predictable from tumor EGFR membrane staining alone. Lung Cancer 2004; 41:71.

74. Perez-Soler R, Chachoua A, Hammond LA, et al. Determinants of tumor response and survival with erlotinib in patients with non-small-cell lung cancer. J Clin Oncol 2004; 22:3238.

75. Amador ML, Oppenheimer D, Perea S, et al. An epidermal growth factor receptor intron 1 polymorphism mediates response to epidermal growth factor receptor inhibitors. Cancer Res 2004; 64:9139.

76. Lynch TJ, Bell DW, Sordella R, et al. Activating mutations in the epidermal growth factor receptor underlying responsiveness of non-small-cell lung cancer to gefitinib. N Engl J Med 2004; 350:2129.

77. Paez JG, Janne PA, Lee JC, et al. EGFR mutations in lung cancer: correlation with clinical response to gefitinib therapy. Science 2004; 304:1497.

78. Huang S, Armstrong EA, Benavente S, Harari PM. Dual agent molecular targeting of the EGFR: combining anti-EGFR antibody with tyrosine kinase inhibitor. Cancer Res 2004; 64:8195.

79. Han SW, Hwang PG, Chung DH, et al. Epidermal growth factor receptor (EGFR) downstream molecules as response predictive markers for gefitinib (Iressa, ZD1839) in chemotherapy-resistant non-small cell lung cancer. Int J Cancer 2005; 113:109.

80. Lander ES. Array of hope. Nat Genet 1999; 21(1 Suppl):3.

81. Brennan P. Gene-environment interaction and aetiology of cancer: what does it mean and how can we measure it? Carcinogenesis 2002; 23:381.

82. Caporaso NE. Why have we failed to find the low penetrance genetic constituents of common cancers? Cancer Epidemiol Biomarkers Prev 2002; 11:1544.

83. Popanda O, Schattenberg T, Phong CT, et al. Specific combinations of DNA repair gene variants and increased risk for non-small cell lung cancer. Carcinogenesis 2004; 25:2433.

Molecular Biology of Lung Cancer

6

Ignacio I. Wistuba, Zhongxing Liao
and Luka Milas

Contents

6.1 Introduction

The understanding of lung cancer pathogenesis has advanced as molecular technologies have brought insight to its biology. That we now know that lung cancers detected in the clinic are the product of numerous and complex genetic and epigenetic changes that inactivate tumor-suppressor genes (TSGs) and activate oncogenes is the result of recent work in molecular biology. These abnormalities, while bearing distinctions and similarities to those described in other cancers, can be organized under the "hallmarks of cancer," as proposed by Hanahan and Weinberg [1], which has proved a useful rubric for discussion of molecular studies [2].

Lung cancer comprises four major histologic types, including small-cell lung cancer (SCLC) and the three non-small-cell lung cancers (NSCLC): squamous cell carcinoma, adenocarcinoma, and large-cell carcinoma. Molecular differences between different lung cancer types are being identified and used for the development of more rational targeted therapy. In addition, work

identifying clonal genetic lesions that occur in smoking-damaged respiratory epithelia and lead to lung cancer development is intensifying [3]. The advancement of clinical applications for lung cancer risk assessment, prevention, early diagnosis, and treatment is the result of close integration of the molecular research efforts of several laboratories with clinical investigations.

6.2 Molecular Epidemiology

Eighty to ninety percent of lung cancer cases arise in cigarette smokers, and most are caused by tobacco smoking [4]. Tobacco smoking is the most important cause of lung cancers, and a lifetime smoker has a risk of developing lung cancer that is 20- to 30-fold higher than that of a lifetime nonsmoker [5]. There are major geographic, racial, and gender differences in incidence, and some reports suggest that women may be at increased risk of lung cancer from exposure to tobacco smoke carcinogens [4]. Smoking cessation results in decreased risk after a lag of about 7 years [6]; however, this decreased risk never reaches baseline levels, and about 50% of lung cancer cases in the USA occur in former smokers.

Tobacco contains more than 20 known lung-cancer-specific carcinogens. Approximately 11% of tobacco smokers develop lung cancer, which suggests that genetic factors influence the risk for lung cancer among those who are exposed to carcinogens [5]. Tobacco-smoke-prompted carcinogenesis is a process that involves activation of procarcinogens that lead to adduct formation and possible failure of DNA repair, which should normally remove these adducts. The polymorphisms that affect each of these steps can be inherited [5]. Molecular epidemiology has shown differences in smoking-related risk based on the interactions between tobacco carcinogens, genetic polymorphisms involved in activating and detoxifying these carcinogens, and host-cell efficiency in monitoring and repairing tobacco-carcinogen-caused DNA damage [7]. Epidemiologic studies show an approximately 2.5-fold increased risk attributable to a family history of lung cancer after controlling for tobacco smoke, suggesting the presence of a rare autosomal dominant gene predisposing to lung cancer [5]. A recent linkage analysis, under a simple autosomal dominant model, of 52 families with three or more individuals affected by lung, throat, and laryngeal cancers yielded a major susceptibility locus influencing lung cancer risk in the 6q23-25 chromosomal region [8].

A case-control study suggested that suboptimal DNA repair capacity (DRC) measured in peripheral lymphocytes is associated with increased risk of NSCLC, and DRC may modulate the risk of lung cancer associated with smoking [9]. Recently, studies have provided molecular epidemiologic evidence linking defects in cell-cycle checkpoints and DNA damage/repair capacity to elevated lung cancer risk [10]. The ultimate relevance of these epidemiology molecular studies will require careful consideration of the relative role of multiple low-penetrant genes in determining individual lung cancer risk, and translation of this knowledge to lung cancer risk assessment and prevention.

6.3   Hallmarks of Lung Cancer

The genetic and molecular changes involved in the carcinogenic process of epithelial tumors, including those of the lung, are notably diverse and complex; however, they can be systematically reviewed using Hanahan and Weinberg's hallmarks of cancer [1, 2] (Fig. 6.1). These changes include: (1) self-sufficiency in growth signaling, (2) insensitivity to antigrowth signals, (3) ability to evade apoptosis, (4) limitless replicative potential, (5) ability to sustain angiogenesis, and (6) tissue invasion and metastasis. Lung cancer histology types, SCLC and the three major forms of NSCLC, share many of these hallmarks of cancer; however, they may also be differentiated by specific genetic abnormalities and molecular pathways (Table 6.1) [11].

Table 6.1. Major differences in the genetic characteristics of small cell lung cancer and non-small-cell lung cancer pathogenesis. Adapted from Fong et al. (2003) [2]. *GRP* Gastrin-releasing peptide, *HGF* hepatocyte growth factor, *MET* MET proto-oncogene, *SCF* stem cell factor, *KIT* KIT proto-oncogene, *NDF* neu differentiation factor, *ERBB* neuregulin receptor, *EGFR TK* epidermal growth factor receptor tyrosine kinase, *BCL2* BCL2 antiapoptotic proto-oncogene, *IHC* immunohistochemistry, *LOH* loss of heterozygosity, *RB* or *rb* retinoblastoma, *PTEN* phosphatase and tensin homologue deleted on chromosome 10, *MMAC1* mutated in multiple advanced cancers, *TSG* tumor suppressor gene, *RAR* retinoic acid receptor

Gene/Characteristic	Small-cell lung cancer	Non-small-cell lung cancer
Frequency	20–25%	80–85%
Neuroendocrine cells	Yes	No
Putative autocrine loop	GRP/GRP receptor	HGF/MET
	SCF/KIT	NDF/ERBB
EGFR TK domain mutations	No	10–40% (adenocarcinomas)
RAS mutations	<1%	15–20% (adenocarcinomas)
MYC amplification	18–31%	8–20%
BCL2 (IHC)	75–95%	10–35%
TP53 abnormalities		
LOH	90%	65%
Mutation	75%	~50%
p53 (IHC)	40–70%	40–60%
RB abnormalities		
LOH	67%	31%
rb abnormalities (IHC)	90%	15–30%
P16 abnormalities		
LOH	53%	66%
Mutation	<1%	10–40%
P16 (IHC)	0–10%	30–70%
PTEN/MMAC1 loci LOH	91%	41%
TSG101 abnormal transcripts	~100%	0%
DMBT1 abnormal expression	100%	43%
3p LOH various regions	>90%	>80%
4p LOH various regions	50%	~20%
4q LOH various regions	80%	30%
8p2123 LOH	80–90%	80–100%
Other specific LOH regions	1q23, 9q22-32, 10p15, 13q34	13q11, Xq22.1
Microsatellite instability	35%	22%
Promoter hypermethylation		
RASSF1 gene	>90%	~40%
RARβ gene	72%	41%
Other genes	Not studied	10–40% various genes[a]

[a] P16, death-associated protein kinase, glutathione S transferase P1, and O6-methylguanine-DNA methyltransferase

Hallmarks of Lung Cancer

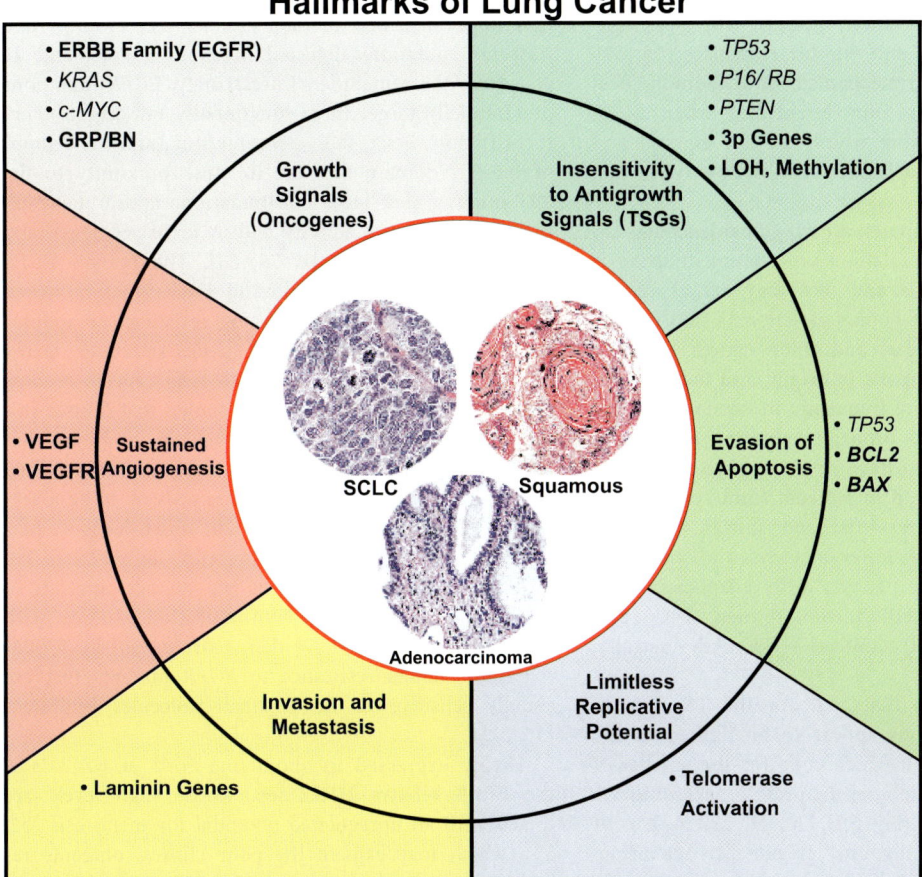

Fig. 6.1. The genetic and molecular changes involved in lung carcinogenesis are notably diverse and complex, and they can be reviewed systematically using the hallmarks of cancer defined by Hanahan and Weinberg [1]. The major molecular changes identified as important in small-cell lung cancer (*SCLC*) and non-small-cell lung cancer (adenocarcinoma and squamous cell carcinoma) for each hallmark are represented.

EGFR Epidermal growth factor receptor, *GRP/BN* gastrin-releasing peptide/bombesin-like peptide, *TSGs* tumor-suppressor genes, *VEGF* vascular endothelial growth factor, *VEGFR* vascular endothelial growth factor receptor, *LOH* loss of heterozygosity, *PTEN* phosphatase and tensin homolog deleted on chromosome 10

6.3.1 Self-sufficiency in Growth Signaling: Proto-oncogenes

Many growth factors and their receptors are abnormally expressed by lung cancer cells and adjacent stromal cells, producing autocrine and paracrine growth stimulation loops [12]. Several of those factors and receptors are encoded by proto-oncogenes that become activated by various mechanisms during the development of lung cancer [12].

Stimulating this growth, especially in NSCLCs, is a potential growth stimulatory loop made up of the ERBB family, including four transmembrane receptor tyrosine kinases (TKs) together with their cognate ligands [13–15]. ERBB neuregulin receptors are composed of an extracellular ligand-binding domain, a transmembrane segment, and an intracellular TK domain followed by a

regulatory C-terminal segment [16]. To induce TK activation and receptor transphosphorylation, ERBB receptors, on ligand bindings, homodimerize or heterodimerize, initiating intracellular signal transduction cascades including Ras, phophatidylinositol-3-kinase, and Akt, the Stat pathways, and mitogen-activated protein kinases [13–15]. The activation of these pathways sets off transcription events that influence apoptosis, angiogenesis, cell motility, invasion, adhesion, and repair [16]. Significant in lung cancer are the epidermal growth factor receptor (EGFR) and HER2/neu.

Because of the important role in cancer pathogenesis of EGFR-mediated effects, their blockade should theoretically arrest the growth of tumor cells. Although several targeted approaches have been investigated, the most advanced clinical application in lung cancer is the use of quinazoline, a small-molecule reversible TK inhibitor [13, 17]. Several preclinical and clinical trials have shown that EGFR TK inhibitor treatment appears to be promising for advanced NSCLC, with some patients having dramatic and durable responses [13, 17–19]. However, the main mechanism of antitumor effect or drug sensitivity was only established when *EGFR* gene mutations, occurring within the TK domain and predicting sensitivity to EGFR TK inhibitors, were discovered [20, 21].

Since those initial reports, a body of evidence has indicated that *EGFR* TK mutations are present in approximately 20% of NSCLCs and that they are absent in other common types of human carcinomas [22] including, among others, breast and colon cancer [22, 23]. *EGFR* mutations are somatic in origin, and they are observed significantly more frequently in adenocarcinoma with and without the bronchioloalveolar component (44–55%), in those who have never smoked (51–68%), in women (42–62%), and in patients from countries in Asia, such as Japan (30–44%) and Taiwan (30–50%) [22, 24–27]. In contrast, lower incidences of mutations have been detected in patients with adenocarcinoma who have ever smoked (10%), who are men, (14%), and who are from Western countries (USA and Australia, 8%) [22].

Of the seven exons that code for the TK domain (exons 18–24), mutations appear to be limited to the first four (exons 18–21), which code for the smaller N lobe and part of the C lobe of the protein, including the crucial activating loop (Fig. 6.2) [20, 21, 22, 24–27]. At least three types of mutations, presumably activating, have been identified, including in-frame deletions in exon 19, a single missense mutation in exon 20 (L858R), and in-frame duplications/insertions in exon

20. These three mutations account for nearly 95% of the mutations identified to date [20, 21, 22, 24–27]. Rare missense mutations detected in exons 18, 20, and 21 constitute the remainder. Interestingly, *EGFR* mutations preferentially target three functionally important structures (the αC helix, the activation loop, and the P-loop) of the TK domain that are in close proximity to the ATP-binding cleft [16]. The mutations appear to result in enhanced kinase activity and in increased sensitivity to TK inhibitors [20, 21, 26, 28]. The mutant *EGFR* genes selectively activate Akt and STAT signaling, which promote cell survival by inducing resistance to apoptosis [28,29]. Thus, mutant *EGFR* genes selectively transduce the survival signals to which lung cancers become dependent. However, it has been shown that despite initial responses to EGFR small-molecule inhibitors, patients eventually progress by mechanisms of acquired resistance. One of those mechanisms seems to be a secondary *EGFR* mutation in exon 20, which leads to substitution of methionine for threonine at position 790 (T790M) in the kinase domain. Biochemical analyses of transfected cells and growth-inhibition studies with lung cancer cell lines have demonstrate that the T790M mutation confers resistance to *EGFR* mutants that are usually sensitive to EGFR small-molecules inhibitors [30, 31].

Highly expressed in about one-third of NSCLCs is the ERBB relative HER2/neu, whose high levels are linked with an upregulated potential for metastasis [32, 33], which may explain the poor clinical outcome reported by some investigators [34, 35]. Recently, mutations affecting *HER2/neu* TK have been also identified in lung cancers, but at a lower frequency (4%) than the

EGFR Mutations in Lung Adenocarcinoma

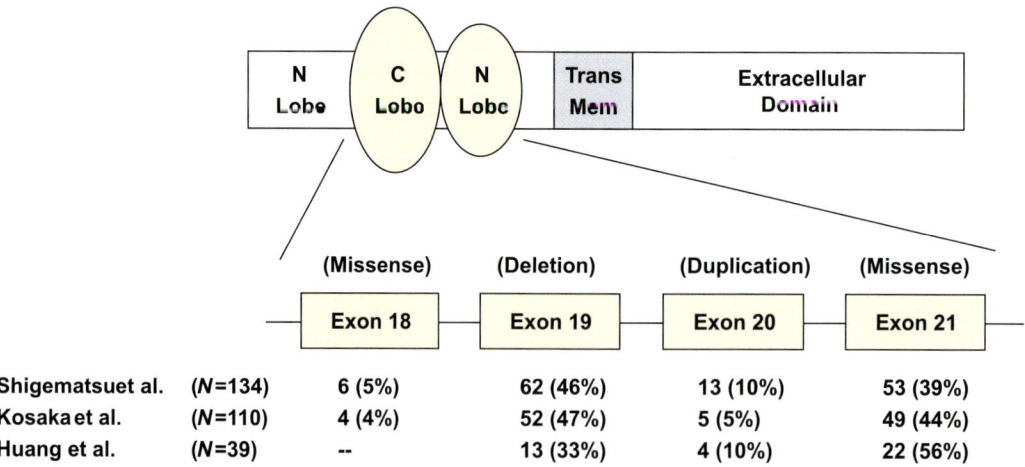

		Exon 18 (Missense)	Exon 19 (Deletion)	Exon 20 (Duplication)	Exon 21 (Missense)
Shigematsu et al.	(N=134)	6 (5%)	62 (46%)	13 (10%)	53 (39%)
Kosaka et al.	(N=110)	4 (4%)	52 (47%)	5 (5%)	49 (44%)
Huang et al.	(N=39)	--	13 (33%)	4 (10%)	22 (56%)

Fig. 6.2. Summary of the *EGFR* mutation frequency distribution by exons reported in lung adenocarcinomas in three major studies: Shigematsu et al. [22], Kosaka et al. [25], and Huang et al. [24]. Nearly 90% of mutations occur in exons 19 and 21, which encompass the *EGFR* tyrosine kinase domain (C and N lobes). *Trans Mem* Transmembrane

EGFR TK mutations [36]. Of interest, although uncommon, is the finding that activating mutations of two key players of kinase pathway activation, such as *BRAF* (3%) [37] and *PIK3CA* (1%) [38] in NSCLC, may also identify a subset of tumors that are sensitive to targeted therapy.

The *RAS* proto-oncogenes (*HRAS*, *KRAS*, and *NRAS*) are components of an important signal transduction pathway. The *RAS* oncogenes, which acquire their transforming capacity by point mutations, encode a 21-kDa plasma membrane protein. In lung cancer, *RAS* mutations are usually detected in the *KRAS* member of the family and they preferentially target adenocarcinoma histology (20–30%) [2]. Often G->T transversions, *KRAS* mutations are associated with tobacco use [39]. In experiments with mice, Johnson found that somatic activation of *KRAS* by spontaneous recombination predisposes patients to adenocarcinoma and early-onset lesions [40]. Of interest is the finding that *KRAS* and *EGFR* mutations in lung adenocarcinomas are mutually exclusive [22], indicating the presence of at least two different pathogenic pathways leading to lung adenocarcinoma development.

RAS signaling activates nuclear proto-oncogene products like MYC, which transcriptionally activates downstream genes, thereby stimulating cell growth. The *MYC* proto-oncogene family includes *c-MYC*, *NMYC*, and *LMYC*, and encodes nuclear DNA-binding proteins, which are involved in transcriptional regulation [41]. Gene amplification or transcriptional dysregulation causes protein overexpression, which activates the *MYC* genes. In 18–31% of SCLCs, amplification of one or more *MYC* family member occurred; this compares with 8–20% of NSCLCs [11].

Many growth factors and their receptors are expressed by adjacent lung cancer cells or normal cells, leading to the development of several autocrine and paracrine growth-stimulatory loops [42]. The best-characterized autocrine systems involve gastrin-releasing peptide (noted in 20–60% of SCLCs but less frequently in NSCLCs) and other bombesin-like peptides (GRP/ BN). Other potential autocrine growth systems that are under analysis for their implications in lung cancer are insulin-like growth factor (IGF) I and IGFII, platelet-derived growth factor (PDGF) and its receptor (PDGFR), and the hepatocyte growth factor/receptor (HGF/c-Met) [2, 43–45].

6.3.2 Insensitivity to Antigrowth Signaling: Tumor-Suppressor Genes

In normal cell growth, TSGs provide two safety nets: not only do they generally inhibit tumorigenesis, but they also respond to and repair DNA damage. According to Knudson's hypothesis [46], loss of function of TSGs requires that both alleles have to be inactivated. One may be inactivated by mutation, methylation (epigenetic) changes, or other changes that target the individual TSG, whereas the other allele is usually inactivated as part of loss of many genetic markers by deletion, nonreciprocal translocation, or mitotic recombination in the chromosomal region. This is referred to as an "allele loss" or "loss of heterozygosity" (LOH).

Studies of LOH as a marker of TSG inactivation have shown that several chromosomal regions are lost in lung cancer cells, including 1q, 3p, 4p, 4q, 5q, 6p, 6q, 8p, 8q, 9p (*P16* locus), 9q, 10p, 10q, 11p, 13q (*retinoblastoma*, *RB* locus), 14q, 17p (*TP53* locus), 18q, and 22q [47–50]. Some of the novel sites will direct the search for new candidate TSGs. In addition, the presence of homozygously deleted chromosomal regions 2q33, 5p13-q14, 8, and X/Y in lung cancer provide further evidence that these regions harbor as yet unidentified TSGs [48]. So far, 17–22 hot spots of chromosomal loss have been identified in lung cancer cells through genome-wide LOH analyses, indicating some important differences between SCLC and NSCLC and providing additional evidence that SCLC and NSCLC differ significantly in the TSGs that are inactivated during their pathogenesis [47].

The very frequent loss of alleles on chromosome 3p in both SCLC (>90%) and NSCLC (>80%) [51] provides strong evidence for the existence of one or more TSGs on this chromosomal arm. Several distinct 3p regions have been identified by high-density allelotyping, including 3p25-26, 3p24, 3p21.3-22 (several sites), 3p14.2 (fragile histidine triad, or *FHIT*, gene), and 3p12 (U2020 deletion site), suggesting that there are several different TSGs located on chromosome 3p. The 3p21.3 region has been examined extensively for putative TSGs, and several candidate TSGs have been identified [51]. One candidate TSG is the *FHIT* at the 3p14.2 region, which encompasses approximately 1 Mbase of genomic DNA, which includes the human common fragile site (FRA3B). *FHIT* is a candidate TSG for lung cancer on the basis of frequent 3p14.2 allele loss in lung cancer (100% of SCLCs and 88% of NSCLCs) and homozygous deletion in several lung cancer cell lines [52, 53]. Although almost all lung cancer cells express very low levels of wild-type FHIT transcripts, only 40–80% express abnormal mRNA transcripts of *FHIT* [52, 53]. While *FHIT* point mutations are rare, lung cancer cells frequently express abnormal mRNA transcripts of *FHIT*, and hypermethylation of the promoter region of the *FHIT* gene is a frequent event, occurring in 64% of SCLC and NSCLC cell lines and 37% of noncultured NSCLC primary tumors [54]. What is of importance is that in immunohistochemistry studies, most lung cancers expressed undetectable or very low levels of *FHIT* mRNA and exhibited loss of *FHIT* protein expression [55, 56]. In nude mice, researchers may have succeeded in suppressing tumorigenesis of all lung cancer cell lines by reintroducing exogenous *FHIT* [57, 58].

Also of interest in the 3p21 region are the genes *SEMA3B*, *FUS1*, *RASSF1A*, and *DUTT1/ROBO1*, and the retinoic acid receptor (*RAR*) *β*. Located in the 3p21 region with 5 kbase and 50 kbase, respectively, are the *SEMA3B* [59, 60] and *FUS1* [61–64] genes. In vitro and in vivo studies have demonstrated tumor-suppression activity for both. While allelic loss and promoter region methylation (40–50%) are important mechanisms for *SEMA3B* inactivation in NSCLC [60], a recent study shows that a novel mechanism, protein myristoylation, is required for *FUS1*-mediated tumor-suppressing activity in lung cancer and plays a role in deficient posttranslational modification in tumor suppressor-gene-mediated carcinogenesis [64]. N-myristoylation is a protein-modification process in which a 14-carbon myristoyl group is cotranslationally and covalently added to the NH2-terminal glycine residue of the nascent polypeptide. Another, perhaps more familiar, candidate TSG at the 3p21.3 region is *RASSF1A*, the splicing isoform of the *RASSF1* gene. Like other candidates in this region, it appears, when reintroduced into lung cancers, to suppress the tumorigenic phenotype [51]. Promoter hypermethylation costs this gene its expression in 60% of NSCLCs and almost 90% of SCLCs [65, 66], and investigators have demonstrated that demethylation of lung cancer cells with 5-aza-2′deoxycytidine restores its expression [65]. Only rarely is its loss of expression owed to mutation. When activated, *RASSF1A* can downregulate cyclin D1 expression at a posttranscriptional level as well as inhibit DNA synthesis. Finally, located at 3p22–24 and 3p12 deletion regions, respectively, are two other candidate TSGs, *RAR β*, which is a frequent victim of LOH and promoter of methylation in NSCLCs (41%) and SCLC (72%), and the gene *DUTT1/ROBO1* [67, 68].

As in other cancers, known TSGs, including *TP53* (17p13), *RB* (13q12), *P16* (9p21), and phosphatase and tensin homologue deleted on chromosome 10 (*PTEN*; 10q22), are found in lung cancer in regions of chromosomes characterized by allelic loss [2]. Loss of p53 function allows inappropriate survival of genetically damaged cells, setting the stage for the accumulation of multiple mutations and the subsequent evolution of a cancer cell [69]. Mutant p53 protein, which accumulates to high levels when missense *TP53* mutations prolong the protein's half-life, is easily detected using immunochemistry. In fact, multiple studies have shown abnormal p53 protein expression is detected by immunohisto-

chemistry in 40–70% of lung cancers [48]. *TP53* abnormalities play a critical role in lung cancer pathogenesis. Chromosome 17p13 sequences, the site of the *TP53* locus, are frequently hemizygously lost in SCLC (90%) and NSCLC (65%) [70], and mutational inactivation of the remaining allele occurs in 50–75% of these neoplasms [71]. *TP53* mutations in lung tumors correlate with cigarette smoking and are mostly the G->T transversions expected of tobacco-smoke carcinogens, especially in female smokers [71]. There was no relationship between adenocarcinomas and squamous cell carcinomas, independent of gender. Furthermore, in lung cancers a relationship has been described between mutational hot spots at the *TP53* gene and adduct hot spots caused by benzo[a]pyrene metabolites in cigarette smoke [72].

Also mutated or altered in lung cancer, as in many cancers, is the P16-cyclin D1-CDK4-RB pathway, a regulatory pathway that controls the cell cycle's G1-S transition [48, 73]. In most SCLCs, this pathway is usually disrupted by *RB* gene inactivation, while *cyclin D1*, *CDK4*, and *P16* abnormalities are rare in SCLC but common in NSCLC (particularly *P16* abnormalities) [48]. The major growth-suppressing function of RB protein is to block G1-S progression. Inactivation of both *RB* alleles at chromosomal region 13q14 is common in SCLC [73], with protein abnormalities reported at frequencies of over 90% [74]. There is frequent loss of one of the *RB* 13q14 alleles [70]. Functional loss of the remaining *RB* allele can include deletion, nonsense mutations, or splicing abnormalities, leading to a truncated RB protein encoded by the remaining allele. Likewise, *P16* is not expressed in 30–50% of early-stage primary NSCLCs [75]. This happens in lung cancer, when *P16* (or CDKN2), located in the 9p21 region, becomes unable to inhibit CDK4 and CDK6 kinase activity, and thereby regulate RB function when it is inactivated by mutation, methylation, or heterozygous or homozygous loss [75, 76].

PTEN, also called "mutated in multiple advanced cancers" (*MMAC1*), has been identified and localized to chromosome region 10q23.3 [77]. Allelotyping analysis utilizing microsatellite markers in close proximity to the *PTEN*-gene have demonstrated high incidence of LOH in lung cancers, especially in SCLCs (91% LOH in SCLC, and 41% in NSCLC) [49]; however, *PTEN* mutations were detected in only 11% of lung cancers, including both SCLC and NSCLC tumors [78]. Although genetic alterations of the *PTEN* gene are rare in NSCLC, loss of PTEN protein is not an uncommon event in early-stage NSCLCs, occurring in 24% of cases. Lack of PTEN expression may be partially explained by promoter methylation (35%) [79].

These reports make it evident that methylation can be expected to execute the loss of TSG function, just as deletions or mutations do. Aberrant methylation of normally unmethylated CpG-rich areas, also known as CpG islands, which are located in or near the promoter region of many genes, has been associated with transcriptional inactivation of TSGs in human cancer [80, 81]. In primary lung cancer, as discussed above, several genes are frequently methylated, including, among others, adenomatous polyposis coli (*APC*), retinoic acid receptor *β*-2 (*RARβ*), H-cadherin (*CDH13*), *FHIT, RASSF1A, SEMA3B, PTEN*, tissue inhibitor of metalloproteinase-3 (*TIMP-3*), *P16*, death-associated protein kinase (*DAPK*), *p14ARF, GSTP1, Reprimo*, Wingless-type inhibitory factor-1 (*WIF-1*), *caveolin-1*, high in normal-1 (*HIN-1*), laminin-5 (*LN5*)-encoding genes, and target of methylation-induced silencing (*TMS1*) [82–91]. It has been demonstrated that SCLC, squamous cell carcinomas, adenocarcinomas, and carcinoids of the lung have unique profiles of aberrant methylation [92]. A significantly shorter disease-free survival for patients whose tumors were methylated for *DAPK* was reported by Tang et al. [93], and Burbee et al. [65] found a shorter overall survival for patients whose tumors were methylated for *RASSF1A*. Aberrant methylation can be reversed in vitro by drugs that block methylation, such as 5-aza-20-deoxycytidine, which results in gene reexpression and tumor growth inhibition [67].

The number of genes showing a high incidence of abnormal methylation in lung cancer is rapidly increasing. All these recent findings suggest that aberrant methylation of genes is a frequent abnormality in lung cancers and may have applications for risk assessment, diagnosis, and for development of novel therapeutic approaches. The mechanisms underlying the precise role of this hypermethylation in gene silencing must be further defined, as must the determinants of the hypermethylation changes themselves.

6.3.3 Ability to Evade Apoptosis

Tumor cells often escape the normal physiological response (programmed cell death or apoptosis) when challenged by cellular and DNA damage. Key players include the *TP53* gene and the *BCL2* proto-oncogene. BCL2 protects cells from apoptosis and is negatively regulated by *p53*. Immunohistochemical studies have shown that BCL2 protein is more frequently overexpressed in SCLCs (75–95%) than in NSCLCs, and its expression is higher in squamous cell carcinomas than in adenocarcinomas [94]. Of interest, some studies demonstrate a survival benefit for patients with BCL2-positive tumors [94, 95], but these findings are controversial [96, 97]. BAX is a BCL2-related protein that promotes apoptosis and is a downstream transcription target of *p53* [98]. *BAX* and *BCL2* expression are inversely related in neuroendocrine lung cancers; high *BCL2* and low *BAX* expression occurs in most SCLCs, which are usually *p53* deficient [98].

6.3.4 Limitless Replicative Potential

The ends of human chromosomes (telomeres) contain the hexameric TTAGGG tandem repeats. During normal cell division, the absence of telomerase activity is associated with progressive telomere shortening, leading to cell senescence and normal cell mortality [99]. On the contrary, germ cells, some stem cells, and most cancer cells have telomerase activity that results in replacing the hexameric repeats, therefore leading to potential cellular immortality [99]. The majority of SCLCs and about 80% of NSCLCs show high levels of telomerase activity [100, 101]. The mechanism for reexpression of the catalytic component human telomerase reverse transcriptase or the RNA component of telomerase in tumors is currently unknown.

6.3.5 Ability to Sustain Angiogenesis

Angiogenesis is important in neoplastic development and progression because both tumor growth and metastatic dissemination of tumor cells depend on vascular support [102]. Generally, tumors cannot grow beyond 2 mm in diameter without developing a vascular network [103]. A number of angiogenic factors, including inducers and inhibitors regulating endothelial cell proliferation and migration, have been identified in lung cancer. Angiogenic factors affect vasculature formation, permit growth of the primary tumor, and provide a pathway for migrating tumor cells to gain access to the systemic circulation and to establish metastases. Among these, vascular endothelial growth factor (VEGF) is the most potent and specific of the endothelial cell mitogens, acting both as an endothelial cell survival factor and mobilizing circulating endothelial cell precursors to nascent blood vessels [104, 105]. There are several isoforms of *VEGFR*. The expression ratio of the VEGF189 mRNA isoform has been shown to have a greater correlation with tumor angiogenesis, postoperative relapse time, and survival than the ratios for the VEGF121, VEGFR165, and VEGFR206 mRNA isoforms [106]. In NSCLC, the majority of studies support a correlation between *VEGF* expression, microvessel density (MVD), and poor prognosis [102]. In early, operable NSCLCs, a significantly higher level of MVD has been detected than is found in normal lung distal to the tumor or the inner tumor areas, which means it occurs in the invading front of the tumors and in the normal lung adjacent to the tumors [107]. In addition, it has been demonstrated that microvessel count is a highly significant adverse predictor of both overall and disease-free survival in patients with NSCLC, suggesting that the evaluation of tumor angiogenesis may be useful in the postsurgical staging of NSCLC [108].

6.3.6   Tissue Invasion and Metastasis

Lung cancer development and growth and subsequent tissue invasion and metastasis are the products of mutation, deletion, methylation, and other processes that have already been discussed. The same molecular biology that uncovered these processes is reexamining, employing such molecular proteins as laminins and integrins as key biomarkers of basement membrane invasion and eventual metastasis. In lung cancer, basement membrane fragmentation, the resulting proliferation of stromal elements, and cancer cell invasion have been attributed by some to often reduced laminin a chains ($a3$ and $a5$).

LN5, which is a heterotrimeric protein, consists of the $a3$ chain, the $\beta3$ chain (encoded by the LAMB3 gene), and the $\gamma2$ chain (encoded by the *LAMC2* gene). Researchers have found *LAMB3* expressed in NSCLC cells but not in SCLC cells [109]. A study demonstrated frequent loss of gene expression and epigenetic inactivation of LN5-encoding genes *LAMA3*, *LAMB3*, and *LAMC2* in lung cancers [85], with frequent losses of expression in NSCLC (20–60%) and SCLC (65–86%) cell lines. In addition, methylation of LN5-encoding genes was present more frequently in SCLC cell lines (60–80%) than in NSCLC cell lines (15–60%), and at least one gene was methylated in 95% of SCLC and 60% of NSCLC cell lines. Methylation was more frequent in SCLC tumors (58–77%) than in NSCLC tumors (22–42%) or carcinoids (13–33%), and at least one gene was methylated in 92% of SCLC tumors and 47% of NSCLC tumors.

6.4   Early Molecular Pathogenesis

Lung cancers are believed to arise after a series of progressive pathological changes (preneoplastic or precursor lesions) in the respiratory mucosa. While the sequential preneoplastic changes have been defined for centrally arising squamous carcinomas, they have been poorly documented for large-cell carcinomas, adenocarcinomas, and SCLCs [110]. Mucosal changes in the large airways that may precede or accompany invasive squamous cell carcinoma include hyperplasia (basal cell hyperplasia and goblet cell hyperplasia), squamous metaplasia, squamous dysplasia, and carcinoma in situ [110]. While hyperplasia and squamous metaplasia are considered reactive and reversible changes, dysplasia and carcinoma in situ are the changes most frequently associated with the development of squamous cell lung carcinomas. Adenocarcinomas may be accompanied by changes including atypical adenomatous hyperplasia (AAH) [110] in peripheral airway cells, although the malignant potential of these lesions has not been dem-

onstrated. For SCLC, no specific preneoplastic changes have been described in the respiratory epithelium. Currently available information suggests that lung preneoplastic lesions are frequently extensive and multifocal throughout the lung, indicating a field effect ("field cancerization"), by which much of the respiratory epithelium has undergone malignant change, presumably from exposure to carcinogens. Figure 6.3 illustrates progression in the pathogenesis of NSCLC and associated molecular changes.

6.4.1   Genetic Abnormalities in the Sequential Development of Lung Cancer

Although our knowledge of the molecular events underlying the development and progression of invasive lung cancer is relatively extensive, until recently we knew little about the sequence of events in preneoplastic lesions. A few studies have provided suggestions that molecular lesions can be identified at early stages of the pathogenesis of lung cancer (Table 6.2). Myc upregulation, cyclin D1 overexpression, p53 protein accumulation, and DNA aneuploidy have been detected in dysplastic epithelium adjacent to invasive lung carcinomas [111–113]. *KRAS* mutations have been also detected in AAH [114], which may be a potential precursor lesion of adenocarcinoma with bronchioalveolar features. Several molecular changes frequently present in adenocarcinomas are also present in AAH lesions, providing further evidence that they may represent true preneoplastic lesions [115]. *TP53* gene abnormalities (including mutations, deletions, and overexpression) have been demonstrated in the nonmalignant epithelium of lung specimens obtained from lung cancer patients [116–118]. Franklin et al. (1997) described an identical *TP53* gene mutation widely dispersed in normal and preneoplastic epithelium of a smoker without lung cancer [119]. Our recent studies allowed us to identify some of the genetic changes involved in the pathogenesis of lung cancer. Because the preneoplastic changes have been well established only for squamous cell carcinoma of the lung, most of our findings are related to this histologic type of lung cancer.

Several studies have demonstrated that in lung cancer the developmental sequence of molecular changes is not random, with allelic loss at one or more 3p regions (especially telomeric regions 3p21, 3p22-24 and 3p25) and 9p21 (*P16*), and to a lesser extent at 8p21 -23, 13q14 (*RB*) and 17p13 (*TP53*), being detected frequently very early in pathogenesis (histologically normal epithelium) [50, 120, 121]. Methylation of promoter regions has been demonstrated to be an early event in the pathogenesis of lung cancer [80]. The finding of *P16* methylation in the early stages of progression of squamous cell carcinoma of the lung supports a critical role

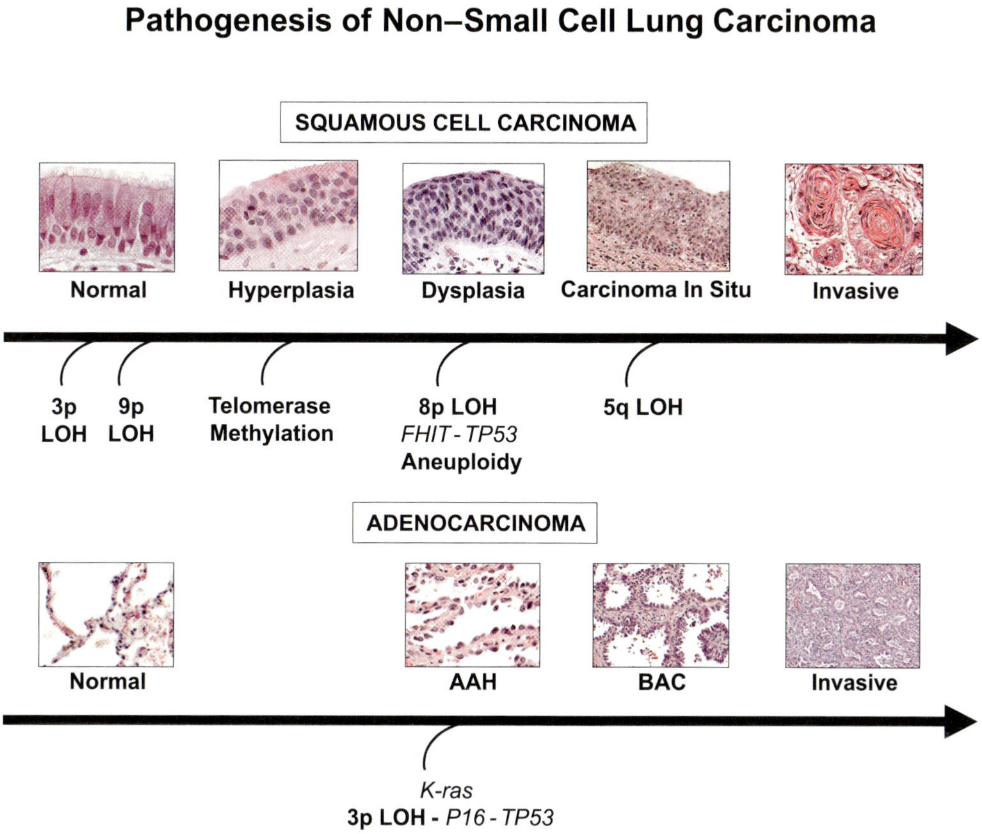

Pathogenesis of Non–Small Cell Lung Carcinoma

Fig. 6.3. Lung squamous cell carcinoma and adenocarcinoma pathogenesis. For squamous cell carcinoma, a defined sequence of histopathological lesions and molecular changes have been identified. Allelic losses (LOH) at chromosomes 3p and 9p are the earliest events, and occur in normal bronchial epithelium. For adenocarcinoma, atypical adenomatous hyperplasia (*AAH*) is the only identified preneoplastic lesion that could lead to bronchioloalveolar adenocarcinoma (*BAC*). *FHIT* Fragile histidine triad gene

Table 6.2. Summary of the histopathological and molecular abnormalities in the precursors of the major types of lung cancer. Adapted from Wistuba et al. (2002) [3]. *LOH* Loss of heterozygosity

Abnormalities	Small-cell lung cancer	Non-small-cell lung cancer	
		Squamous cell carcinoma	Adenocarcinoma
Histopathological			
Precursor	Unknown	Known	Probable
Lesion	Normal epithelium and hyperplasia?	Squamous dysplasia and carcinoma in situ	Adenomatous atypical hyperplasia?
Molecular			
Gene abnormalities	*MYC* overexpression	*TP53* LOH and mutation	*KRAS* mutation
	TP53 LOH and mutation		*EGFR* mutation
Loss of heterozygosity	High	Intermediate	Low
Frequency	90%	54%	10%
Chromosomal regions	5q21, 8p21-23, 9p21, 17p/*TP53*	8p21-23, 9p21, 17p/*TP53*	9p21, 17p/*TP53*
Genetic instability	High	Intermediate	Low
Frequency of instability	68%	10%	13%

for this molecular change [122]. *P16* methylation has been detected in 75% of carcinoma in situ adjacent to squamous cell carcinomas, and the frequency of this event increases during disease progression from basal cell hyperplasia (17%) to squamous metaplasia (24%) to carcinoma in situ lesions (50%). Recently, aberrant methylation of the *P16* and/or O6-methyl-guanine-DNA methyltransferase promoters have been detected in DNA from sputum in 100% of patients with squamous cell lung carcinoma up to 3 years before clinical diagnosis [123]. Although more studies need to be performed on lung cancer preneoplastic lesions, these findings suggest that aberrant gene methylation can be an early event in lung cancer and may constitute in this neoplasm a new marker for risk assessment, early detection, and monitoring in chemoprevention trials [80].

Telomerase also has been detected in preinvasive lesions in several tumor systems, including lung [124]. In the lung, low levels of telomerase activity have been detected in hyperplasia, dysplasia, and carcinoma in situ compared to invasive cancer, while weak telomerase RNA expression is detected in the basal layers of normal and hyperplastic epithelium from patients with lung cancer. Dysregulation of telomerase expression increases with tumor progression, with moderate to strong expression occurring throughout the multilayers of the epithelium in metaplasia, dysplasia, and carcinoma in situ [124].

6.4.2   Smoking-damaged Bronchial Epithelium

After smoking cessation, the risk of developing lung cancer decreases, but never reaches the baselines levels of those who have never smoked [125]. It has been established that advanced lung preneoplastic changes occur more frequently in smokers than in nonsmokers and increase in frequency with amount smoking, adjusted by age. Risk factors that identify normal and premalignant bronchial tissue at increased risk for malignant progression need to be better defined. However, only scant information is available about molecular changes in the respiratory epithelium of smokers without cancer. Two independent studies showed that the genetic changes found in invasive cancers and preneoplasia (LOH and microsatellite instability) can also be identified in bronchial epithelium from current or former smokers that appears to be morphologically normal and may persist for many years after smoking cessation [126, 167]. In general, such genetic changes are not found in the bronchial epithelium from individuals who never smoked. As observed in epithelial foci accompanying invasive lung carcinoma [121], allelic losses on chromosomes 3p and 9p were frequently detected. These findings support the hypothesis that identifying biopsy specimens with extensive or certain patterns of

allelic loss may provide new a method for assessing the risk in smokers of developing invasive lung cancer and for monitoring responses to chemoprevention. We have demonstrated that molecular changes (allelic loss and genomic instability) in the bronchial epithelium may persist long after smoking cessation [126, 127].

Recent results on the methylation analysis of several genes, including *RARβ-2*, *H-cadherin*, *APC*, *P16*, and *RASFF1* indicate that abnormal gene methylation is relatively frequent (at least one gene, 48%) in oropharyngeal and bronchial epithelial cells in heavy smokers with evidence of sputum atypia [128]. Methylation in one or more of three genes tested (*P16*, *GSTP1*, and *DAPK*) has been demonstrated in bronchial brush specimens in about one-third of smoker subjects [129]. Results from another study indicate that aberrant promoter hypermethylation of the *P16* gene, and to a lesser extent *DAPK*, occurs frequently in the bronchial epithelium of lung cancer cases and cancer-free controls, and persists after smoking cessation [130]. These findings indicate that methylation of gene promoter regions may be a useful marker for the assessment of lung cancer risk in smokers.

6.5   Molecular Profiling Studies in Lung Cancer

There is a belief that the pathogenesis and behavior of individual lung cancers cannot be completely understood through the analysis of individual or a small number of genes [12]. Recently, the use of molecular global profiling technologies, including cDNA microarrays and proteomics-based analyses, has led to a significant number of exciting new biological discoveries and important correlations between gene and protein expression patterns and disease states in lung cancer [131]. In lung cancer, cDNA microarray analysis has been used to simultaneously investigate thousands of RNA expression levels and has begun to identify patterns associated with biological and phenotypic characteristics [132, 133]. Oligonucleotide and cDNA microarrays can contain probes representing over 10,000 genes each. Supervised and unsupervised learning methods have been applied successfully to distinguish between classes of cancer and to discover new classes of genes, respectively. A variety of studies on gene expression profiles have sought to identify new molecular markers for different lung cancer histologies, including adenocarcinomas [132, 133].

Recently, it has been suggested that proteomics-based approaches complement the genomics initiatives and represent the next step in attempts to understand the biology of cancer. As mRNA expression is not always correlated with levels of protein expression, cDNA-based gene expression analysis cannot always indicate which proteins are expressed or how their activity might be modulated after translation [134]. Accordingly, comprehensive analysis of protein expression patterns in tissues might improve our ability to understand the molecular complexities of tumor cells. Among others, matrix-assisted laser desorption/ionization time-of-flight mass spectrometry (MALDI-TOF MS) can profile proteins in tissues [135]. This technology cannot only address peptides and proteins in sections of tumor tissues, but it also can be used for high-resolution imaging of individual biomolecules present in tissue sections [135]. Recently, proteomic pattern analysis using MALDI-TOF MS directly from small amounts of frozen lung tumor tissues was used to accurately classify and predict histological groups as well as nodal involvement and survival in resected NSCLCs [131]. If these data are confirmed in larger series, the resulting analysis could have great prognostic and therapeutic implications for patients with NSCLC.

Key Points

- Clinically evident lung cancers are the result of the accumulation of numerous genetic and epigenetic changes, including inactivation of tumor-suppressor genes and activation of oncogenes.
- Tobacco use causes 80–90% of lung cancers, and molecular epidemiology has shown interactions between tobacco carcinogens and the genetic polymorphisms involved in activating and detoxifying these carcinogens, and demonstrated that host-cell efficiency in monitoring and repairing tobacco carcinogen-prompted DNA damage affects smoking-related lung cancer risk.
- The ERBB (neuregulin receptor) family plays an important role in uncontrolled growth signaling in lung cancer through stimulation of cell proliferation, inhibition of apoptosis, and promotion of angiogenesis, invasion, and metastasis. Anti-growth signaling is also defective in lung cancer, and abnormal p53 expression has been detected in 40–70% of lung cancers.
- Loss of alleles (e.g., on chromosome 3p), loss of gene expression because of hypermethylation (RASSF1), cell-cycle pathway disruption, and other protein expression abnormalities, such as protein myristoylation (FUS1), are ways in which tumor-suppressor genes are rendered ineffectual.
- Attracting attention as potential keys to detection or treatment are the possible biomarkers laminins and integrins, a search for precursor lesions, and methylation analysis of gene promoter regions. In addition, continuing proteomics studies hold promise of correlations between protein expression patterns and lung cancer disease states.

References

1. Hanahan D, Weinberg RA. The hallmarks of cancer. Cell 2000; 100(1):57.
2. Fong KM, Sekido Y, Gazdar AF, Minna JD. Lung cancer. 9: Molecular biology of lung cancer: clinical implications. Thorax 2003; 58(10):892.
3. Wistuba II, Mao L, Gazdar AF. Smoking molecular damage in bronchial epithelium. Oncogene 2002; 21(48):7298.
4. Jemal A, Murray T, Ward E, et al. Cancer statistics, 2005. CA Cancer J Clin 2005; 55(1):10.
5. Amos CI, Xu W, Spitz MR. Is there a genetic basis for lung cancer susceptibility? Recent Results Cancer Res 1999; 151:3.
6. Peto R, Chen ZM, Boreham J. Tobacco the growing epidemic. Nat Med 1999; 5(1):15.
7. Xu H, Spitz MR, Amos CI, Shete S. Complex segregation analysis reveals a multigene model for lung cancer. Hum Genet 2005; 116(12):121.
8. Bailey-Wilson JE, Amos CI, Pinney SM, et al. A major lung cancer susceptibility locus maps to chromosome 6q23-25. Am J Hum Genet 2004; 75(3):460.
9. Shen H, Spitz MR, Qiao Y, et al. Smoking, DNA repair capacity and risk of nonsmall cell lung cancer. Int J Cancer 2003; 107(1):84.
10. Wu X, Roth JA, Zhao H, et al. Cell cycle checkpoints, DNA damage/repair, and lung cancer risk. Cancer Res 2005; 65(1):349.
11. Wistuba II, Gazdar AF, Minna JD. Molecular genetics of small cell lung carcinoma. Semin Oncol 2001; 28(2 Suppl 4):3.
12. Minna JD, Gazdar A. Focus on lung cancer. Cancer Cell 2002; 1:49.
13. Andratschke N, Kittmann K, Mason K, et al. Epidermal growth factor receptor as a target to improve treatment of lung cancer. Clin Lung Cancer 2004; 5:340.
14. Herbst RS. Review of epidermal growth factor receptor biology. Int J Radiat Oncol Biol Phys 2004; 59(2 Suppl):21.
15. Milas L, Fan Z, Mason K, Ang K. Role of epidermal growth factor receptor and its inhibition in radiotherapy. In: Nieder C, Milas L, Ang K (eds) Modification of Radiation Response: Cytokines, Growth Factors and Other Biological Targets. Springer-Verlag, Berlin – Heidelberg – New York; 2003; p 189.
16. Gazdar AF, Shigematsu H, Herz J, Minna JD. Mutations and addiction to EGFR: the Achilles 'heal' of lung cancers? Trends Mol Med 2004; 10(10):481.
17. Herbst RS, Sandler AB. Overview of the current status of human epidermal growth factor receptor inhibitors in lung cancer. Clin Lung Cancer 2004; 6 Suppl 1:S7.
18. Fukuoka M, Yano S, Giaccone G, et al. Multi-institutional randomized phase II trial of gefitinib for previously treated patients with advanced non-small-cell lung cancer (The IDEAL 1 Trial) [corrected]. J Clin Oncol 2003; 21(12):2237.
19. Herbst RS, Fukuoka M, Baselga J. Gefitinib a novel targeted approach to treating cancer. Nat Rev Cancer 2004; 4(12):956.
20. Lynch TJ, Bell DW, Sordella R, et al. Activating mutations in the epidermal growth factor receptor underlying responsiveness of non-small-cell lung cancer to gefitinib. N Engl J Med 2004; 350(21):2129.
21. Paez JG, Janne PA, Lee JC, et al. EGFR mutations in lung cancer: correlation with clinical response to gefitinib therapy. Science 2004; 304(5676):1497.
22. Shigematsu H, Lin L, Takahashi T, et al. Clinical and biological features of epidermal growth factor receptor mutations in lung cancers. J Natl Cancer Inst 2005; 97(5):339.

23. Lee JW, Soung YH, Kim SY, et al. Absence of EGFR mutation in the kinase domain in common human cancers besides non-small cell lung cancer. Int J Cancer 2005; 113(3):510.

24. Huang SF, Liu HP, Li LH, et al. High frequency of epidermal growth factor receptor mutations with complex patterns in non-small cell lung cancers related to gefitinib responsiveness in Taiwan. Clin Cancer Res 2004; 10(24):8195.

25. Kosaka T, Yatabe Y, Endoh H, Kuwano H, Takahashi T, Mitsudomi T. Mutations of the epidermal growth factor receptor gene in lung cancer: biological and clinical implications. Cancer Res 2004; 64(24):8919.

26. Pao W, Miller V, Zakowski M, et al. EGF receptor gene mutations are common in lung cancers from "never smokers" and are associated with sensitivity of tumors to gefitinib and erlotinib. Proc Natl Acad Sci U S A 2004; 101(36):13306.

27. Tokumo M, Toyooka S, Kiura K, et al. The relationship between epidermal growth factor receptor mutations and clinicopathologic features in non-small cell lung cancers. Clin Cancer Res 2005; 11(3):1167.

28. Amann J, Kalyankrishna S, Massion PP, et al. Aberrant epidermal growth factor receptor signaling and enhanced sensitivity to EGFR inhibitors in lung cancer. Cancer Res 2005; 65(1):226.

29. Sordella R, Bell DW, Haber DA, Settleman J. Gefitinib-sensitizing EGFR mutations in lung cancer activate anti-apoptotic pathways. Science 2004; 305(5687):1163.

30. Kobayashi S, Boggon TJ, Dayaram T, et al. EGFR mutation and resistance of non-small-cell lung cancer to gefitinib. N Engl J Med 2005; 352(8):786.

31. Pao W, Miller VA, Politi KA, et al. Acquired resistance of lung adenocarcinomas to gefitinib or erlotinib is associated with a second mutation in the EGFR kinase domain. PLoS Med 2005; 2(3):1.

32. Rachwal WJ, Bongiorno PF, Orringer MB, Whyte RI, Ethier SP, Beer DG. Expression and activation of erbB-2 and epidermal growth factor receptor in lung adenocarcinomas. Br J Cancer 1995; 72(1):56.

33. Yu D, Wang SS, Dulski KM, Tsai CM, Nicolson GL, Hung MC. c-erbB-2/neu overexpression enhances metastatic potential of human lung cancer cells by induction of metastasis-associated properties. Cancer Res 1994; 54(12):3260.

34. Brabender J, Danenberg KD, Metzger R, et al. Epidermal growth factor receptor and HER2-neu mRNA expression in non-small cell lung cancer is correlated with survival. Clin Cancer Res 2001; 7(7):1850.

35. Kern JA, Slebos RJ, Top B, et al. C-erbB-2 expression and codon 12 K-ras mutations both predict shortened survival for patients with pulmonary adenocarcinomas. J Clin Invest 1994; 93(2):516.

36. Stephens P, Hunter C, Bignell G, et al. Lung cancer: intragenic ERBB2 kinase mutations in tumours. Nature 2004; 431(7008):525.

37. Brose MS, Volpe P, Feldman M, et al. BRAF and RAS mutations in human lung cancer and melanoma. Cancer Res 2002; 62(23):6997.

38. Samuels Y, Wang Z, Bardelli A, et al. High frequency of mutations of the PIK3CA gene in human cancers. Science 2004; 304(5670):554.

39. Slebos RJ, Rodenhuis S. The ras gene family in human non-small-cell lung cancer. Monogr Natl Cancer Inst 1992; 13:23.

40. Johnson L, Mercer K, Greenbaum D, et al. Somatic activation of the K-ras oncogene causes early onset lung cancer in mice. Nature 2001; 410(6832):1111.

41. Grandori C, Eisenman RN. Myc target genes. Trends Biochem Sci 1997; 22(5):177.

42. Viallet J, Sausville EA. Involvement of signal transduction pathways in lung cancer biology. J Cell Biochem Suppl 1996; 24:228.

43. Jerome L, Shiry L, Leyland-Jones B. Deregulation of the IGF axis in cancer: epidemiological evidence and potential therapeutic interventions. Endocr Relat Cancer 2003; 10(4):561.

44. Jones AV, Cross NC. Oncogenic derivatives of platelet-derived growth factor receptors. Cell Mol Life Sci 2004; 61(23):2912.

45. Maulik G, Kijima T, Ma PC, et al. Modulation of the c-Met/hepatocyte growth factor pathway in small cell lung cancer. Clin Cancer Res 2002; 8(2):620.

46. Knudson AG. Hereditary cancers disclose a class of cancer genes. Cancer 1989; 63(1888):1888.

47. Girard L, Zochbauer-Muller S, Virmani AK, Gazdar AF, Minna JD. Genome-wide allelotyping of lung cancer identifies new regions of allelic loss, differences between small cell lung cancer and non-small cell lung cancer, and loci clustering. Cancer Res 2000; 60(17):4894.

48. Sekido Y, Fong KM, Minna JD. Progress in understanding the molecular pathogenesis of human lung cancer. Biochim Biophys Acta 1998; 1378(1):F21.

49. Virmani AK, Fong KM, Kodagoda D, et al. Allelotyping demonstrates common and distinct patterns of chromosomal loss in human lung cancer types. Genes Chromosomes Cancer 1998; 21(4):308.

50. Wistuba II, Behrens C, Virmani AK, et al. Allelic losses at chromosome 8p21-23 are early and frequent events in the pathogenesis of lung cancer. Cancer Res 1999; 59(8):1973.

51. Lerman MI, Minna JD. The 630-kb lung cancer homozygous deletion region on human chromosome 3p21.3: identification and evaluation of the resident candidate tumor suppressor genes. The International Lung Cancer Chromosome 3p21.3 Tumor Suppressor Gene Consortium. Cancer Res 2000; 60(21):6116.

52. Fong KM, Biesterveld EJ, Virmani A, et al. FHIT and FRA3B allele loss are common in lung cancer and preneoplastic bronchial lesions and are associated with cancer-related FHIT cDNA splicing aberrations. Cancer Res 1997; 57:2256.

53. Sozzi G, Veronese ML, Negrini M, et al. The FHIT gene 3p14.2 is abnormal in lung cancer. Cell 1996; 85(1):17.

54. Zochbauer-Muller S, Fong KM, Maitra A, et al. 5′ CpG island methylation of the FHIT gene is correlated with loss of gene expression in lung and breast cancer. Cancer Res 2001; 61(9):3581.

55. Geradts J, Fong KM, Zimmerman PV, Minna JD. Loss of Fhit expression in non-small-cell lung cancer: correlation with molecular genetic abnormalities and clinicopathological features. Br J Cancer 2000; 82(6):1191.

56. Sozzi G, Pastorino U, Moiraghi L, et al. Loss of FHIT function in lung cancer and preinvasive bronchial lesions. Cancer Res 1998; 58(22):5032.

57. Ji L, Fang B, Yen N, Fong K, Minna JD, Roth JA. Induction of apoptosis and inhibition of tumorigenicity and tumor growth by adenovirus vector-mediated fragile histidine triad (FHIT) gene overexpression [In Process Citation]. Cancer Res 1999; 59(14):3333.

58. Siprashvili Z, Sozzi G, Barnes LD, et al. Replacement of Fhit in cancer cells suppresses tumorigenicity. Proc Natl Acad Sci U S A 1997; 94(25):13771.

59. Castro-Rivera E, Ran S, Thorpe P, Minna JD. Semaphorin 3B (SEMA3B) induces apoptosis in lung and breast cancer, whereas VEGF165 antagonizes this effect. Proc Natl Acad Sci U S A 2004; 101(31):11432.

60. Kuroki T, Trapasso F, Yendamuri S, et al. Allelic loss on chromosome 3p21.3 and promoter hypermethylation of semaphorin 3B in non-small cell lung cancer. Cancer Res 2003; 63(12):3352.

61. Ito I, Ji L, Tanaka F, et al. Liposomal vector mediated delivery of the 3p FUS1 gene demonstrates potent antitumor activity against human lung cancer in vivo. Cancer Gene Ther 2004; 11(11):733.

62. Ji L, Nishizaki M, Gao B, et al. Expression of several genes in the human chromosome 3p21.3 homozygous deletion region by an adenovirus vector results in tumor suppressor activities in vitro and in vivo. Cancer Res 2002; 62(9):2715.

63. Kondo M, Ji L, Kamibayashi C, et al. Overexpression of candidate tumor suppressor gene FUS1 isolated from the 3p21.3 homozygous deletion region leads to G1 arrest and growth inhibition of lung cancer cells. Oncogene 2001; 20(43):6258.

64. Uno F, Sasaki J, Nishizaki M, et al. Myristoylation of the fus1 protein is required for tumor suppression in human lung cancer cells. Cancer Res 2004; 64(9):2969.

65. Burbee DG, Forgacs E, Zochbauer-Muller S, et al. Epigenetic inactivation of RASSF1A in lung and breast cancers and malignant phenotype suppression. J Natl Cancer Inst 2001; 93(9):691.

66. Dammann R, Li C, Yoon JH, Chin PL, Bates S, Pfeifer GP. Epigenetic inactivation of a RAS association domain family protein from the lung tumour suppressor locus 3p21.3. Nat Genet 2000; 25(3):315.

67. Virmani AK, Rathi A, Zochbauer-Muller S, et al. Promoter methylation and silencing of the retinoic acid receptor-beta gene in lung carcinomas. J Natl Cancer Inst 2000; 92(16):1303.

68. Xian J, Clark KJ, Fordham R, Pannell R, Rabbitts TH, Rabbitts PH. Inadequate lung development and bronchial hyperplasia in mice with a targeted deletion in the Dutt1/Robo1 gene. Proc Natl Acad Sci U S A 2001; 98(26):15062.

69. Harris CC. p53 Tumor suppressor gene: from the basic research laboratory to the clinic – an abridged historical perspective. Carcinogenesis 1996; 17:1187.

70. Wistuba II, Berry J, Behrens C, et al. Molecular changes in the bronchial epithelium of patients with small cell lung cancer. Clin Cancer Res 2000; 6(7):2604.

71. Toyooka S, Tsuda T, Gazdar AF. The TP53 gene, tobacco exposure, and lung cancer. Hum Mutat 2003; 21(3):229.

72. Denissenko MF, Pao A, Tang M-S, Pfeifer GP. Preferential formation of benz[a]pyrene adducts in lung cancer mutational hotspots in p53. Science 1996; 274:430.

73. Harbour JW, Sali SL, Whang-Peng J, Gazdar AF, Minna JD, Kaye FJ. Abnormalities in structure and expression of the human retinoblastoma gene in SCLC. Science 1988; 241(353):353.

74. Cagle PT, el-Naggar AK, Xu HJ, Hu SX, Benedict WF. Differential retinoblastoma protein expression in neuroendocrine tumors of the lung. Potential diagnostic implications. Am J Pathol 1997; 150(2):393.

75. Geradts J, Fong KM, Zimmerman PV, Maynard R, Minna JD. Correlation of abnormal RB, P16ink4a, and p53 expression with 3p loss of heterozygosity, other genetic abnormalities, and clinical features in 103 primary non-small cell lung cancers. Clin Cancer Res 1999; 5(4):791.

76. Toyooka S, Suzuki M, Maruyama R, et al. The relationship between aberrant methylation and survival in non-small-cell lung cancers. Br J Cancer 2004; 91(4):771.

77. Li J, Yen C, Liaw D, et al. PTEN, a putative protein tyrosine phosphatase gene mutated in human brain, breast and prostate cancer. Science 1997; 275:1943.

78. Forgacs E, Biesterveld EJ, Sekido Y, et al. Mutation analysis of the PTEN/MMAC1 gene in lung cancer. Oncogene 1998; 17(12):1557.

79. Soria JC, Lee HY, Lee JI, et al. Lack of PTEN expression in non-small cell lung cancer could be related to promoter methylation. Clin Cancer Res 2002; 8(5):1178.

80. Belinsky SA. Gene-promoter hypermethylation as a biomarker in lung cancer. Nat Rev Cancer 2004; 4(9):707.

81. Herman JG, Baylin SB. Gene silencing in cancer in association with promoter hypermethylation. N Engl J Med 2003; 349(21):2042.

82. Esteller M, Corn PG, Baylin SB, Herman JG. A gene hypermethylation profile of human cancer. Cancer Res 2001; 61(8):3225.

83. Herman JG. Epigenetics in lung cancer: focus on progression and early lesions. Chest 2004; 125(5 Suppl): 119S.

84. Mazieres J, He B, You L, et al. Wnt inhibitory factor-1 is silenced by promoter hypermethylation in human lung cancer. Cancer Res 2004; 64(14):4717.

85. Sathyanarayana UG, Toyooka S, Padar A, et al. Epigenetic inactivation of laminin-5-encoding genes in lung cancers. Clin Cancer Res 2003; 9(7):2665.

86. Shigematsu H, Suzuki M, Takahashi T, et al. Aberrant methylation of HIN-1 (high in normal-1) is a frequent event in many human malignancies. Int J Cancer 2005; 113(4):600.

87. Sunaga N, Miyajima K, Suzuki M, et al. Different roles for caveolin-1 in the development of non-small cell lung cancer versus small cell lung cancer. Cancer Res 2004; 64(12):4277.

88. Suzuki M, Shigematsu H, Takahashi T, et al. Aberrant methylation of Reprimo in lung cancer. Lung Cancer 2005; 47(3):309.

89. Toyooka S, Maruyama R, Toyooka KO, et al. Smoke exposure, histologic type and geography-related differences in the methylation profiles of non-small cell lung cancer. Int J Cancer 2003; 103(2):153.

90. Virmani A, Rathi A, Sugio K, et al. Aberrant methylation of TMS1 in small cell, non small cell lung cancer and breast cancer. Int J Cancer 2003; 106(2):198.

91. Zochbauer-Muller S, Fong KM, Virmani AK, Geradts J, Gazdar AF, Minna JD. Aberrant promoter methylation of multiple genes in non-small cell lung cancers. Cancer Res 2001; 61(1):249.

92. Toyooka S, Toyooka KO, Maruyama R, et al. DNA methylation profiles of lung tumors. Mol Cancer Ther 2001; 1(1):61.

93. Tang X, Khuri FR, Lee JJ, et al. Hypermethylation of the death-associated protein (DAP) kinase promoter and aggressiveness in stage I non-small-cell lung cancer. J Natl Cancer Inst 2000; 92(18):1511.

94. Pezzella F, Turley H, Kuzu I, et al. bcl-2 protein in non-small-cell lung carcinoma. N Engl J Med 1993; 329:690.

95. Fontanini G, Vignati S, Bigini D, et al. Bcl-2 protein: a prognostic factor inversely correlated to p53 in non-small-cell lung cancer. Br J Cancer 1995; 71(5):1003.

96. Anton RC, Brown RW, Younes M, Gondo MM, Stephenson MA, Cagle PT. Absence of prognostic significance of bcl-2 immunopositivity in non-small cell lung cancer: analysis of 427 cases. Hum Pathol 1997; 28(9):1079.

97. Bubb RS, Komaki R, Hachiya T, et al. Association of Ki-67, p53, and bcl-2 expression of the primary non-small-cell lung cancer lesion with brain metastatic lesion. Int J Radiat Oncol Biol Phys 2002; 53(5):1216.

98. Brambilla E, Negoescu A, Gazzeri S, et al. Apoptosis-related factors p53, Bcl2, and Bax in neuroendocrine lung tumors. Am J Pathol 1996; 149(6):1941.

99. Shay JW, Zou Y, Hiyama E, Wright WE. Telomerase and cancer. Hum Mol Genet 2001; 10(7):677.

100. Albanell J, Lonardo F, Rusch V, et al. High telomerase activity in primary lung cancers: association with increased cell proliferation rates and advanced pathologic stage. J Natl Cancer Inst 1997; 89(21):1609.

101. Hiyama E, Gollahon L, Kataoka T, et al. Telomerase activity in human breast tumors. J Natl Cancer Inst 1996; 88:116.

102. Sandler AB, Johnson DH, Herbst RS. Anti-vascular endothelial growth factor monoclonals in non-small cell lung cancer. Clin Cancer Res 2004; 10(12 Pt 2):4258s.

103. Folkman J. The role of angiogenesis in tumor growth. Semin Cancer Biol 1992; 3(2):65.

104. Asahara T, Takahashi T, Masuda H, et al. VEGF contributes to postnatal neovascularization by mobilizing bone marrow-derived endothelial progenitor cells. EMBO J 1999; 18(14):3964.

105. Ferrara N. Role of vascular endothelial growth factor in the regulation of angiogenesis. Kidney Int 1999; 56(3):794.

106. Yuan A, Yu CJ, Kuo SH, et al. Vascular endothelial growth factor 189 mRNA isoform expression specifically correlates with tumor angiogenesis, patient survival, and postoperative relapse in non-small-cell lung cancer. J Clin Oncol 2001; 19(2):432.

107. Koukourakis MI, Giatromanolaki A, Thorpe PE, et al. Vascular endothelial growth factor/KDR activated microvessel density versus CD31 standard microvessel density in non-small cell lung cancer. Cancer Res 2000; 60(11):3088.

108. Fontanini G, Lucchi M, Vignati S, et al. Angiogenesis as a prognostic indicator of survival in non-small-cell lung carcinoma: a prospective study. J Natl Cancer Inst 1997; 89(12):881.

109. Manda R, Kohno T, Niki T, et al. Differential expression of the LAMB3 and LAMC2 genes between small cell and non-small cell lung carcinomas. Biochem Biophys Res Commun 2000; 275(2):440.

110. Colby TV, Wistuba, II, Gazdar A. Precursors to pulmonary neoplasia. Adv Anat Pathol 1998; 5(4):205.

111. Betticher DC, Heighway J, Thatcher N, Hasleton PS. Abnormal expression of CCND1 and RB1 in resection margin epithelia of lung cancer patients. Br J Cancer 1997; 75(12):1761.

112. Nuorva K, Soini Y, Kamel D, et al. Concurrent p53 expression in bronchial dysplasias and squamous cell lung carcinomas. Am J Pathol 1993; 142:725.

113. Smith AL, Hung J, Walker L, et al. Extensive areas of aneuploidy are present in the respiratory epithelium of lung cancer patients. Br J Cancer 1996; 73:203.

114. Westra WH, Baas IO, Hruban RH, et al. K-ras oncogene activation in atypical alveolar hyperplasias of the human lung. Cancer Res 1996; 56:2224.

115. Kitamura H, Kameda Y, Ito T, Hayashi H. Atypical adenomatous hyperplasia of the lung. Implications for the pathogenesis of peripheral lung adenocarcinoma [see comments]. Am J Clin Pathol 1999; 111(5):610.

116. Ahrendt SA, Chow JT, Xu LH, et al. Molecular detection of tumor cells in bronchoalveolar lavage fluid from patients with early stage lung cancer. J Natl Cancer Inst 1999; 91(4):332.

117. Lang SM, Stratakis DF, Freudling A, et al. Detection of K-ras and p53 mutations in bronchoscopically obtained malignant and non-malignant tissue from patients with non-small cell lung cancer. Eur J Med Res 2000; 5(8):341.

118. Sundaresan V, Ganly P, Hasleton P, et al. p53 and chromosome 3 abnormalities, characteristic of malignant lung tumours, are detectable in preinvasive lesions of the bronchus. Oncogene 1992; 7:1989.

119. Franklin WA, Gazdar AF, Haney J, et al. Widely dispersed p53 mutation in respiratory epithelium. J Clin Invest 1997; 100:2133.

120. Wistuba II, Behrens C, Virmani AK, et al. High resolution chromosome 3p allelotyping of human lung cancer and preneoplastic/preinvasive bronchial epithelium reveals multiple, discontinuous sites of 3p allele loss and three regions of frequent breakpoints. Cancer Res 2000; 60(7):1949.

121. Wistuba II, Behrens C, Milchgrub S, et al. Sequential molecular abnormalities are involved in the multistage development of squamous cell lung carcinoma. Oncogene 1999; 18:643.

122. Belinsky SA, Nikula KJ, Palmisano WA, et al. Aberrant methylation of P16(INK4a) is an early event in lung cancer and a potential biomarker for early diagnosis. Proc Natl Acad Sci U S A 1998; 95(20):11891.

123. Palmisano WA, Divine KK, Saccomanno G, et al. Predicting lung cancer by detecting aberrant promoter methylation in sputum. Cancer Res 2000; 60(21):5954.

124. Yashima K, Litzky LA, Kaiser L, et al. Telomerase expression in respiratory epithelium during the multistage pathogenesis of lung carcinomas. Cancer Res 1997; 57(12):2373.

125. Peto R, Darby S, Deo H, Silcocks P, Whitley E, Doll R. Smoking, smoking cessation, and lung cancer in the UK since 1950: combination of national statistics with two case-control studies. BMJ 2000; 321(7257):323.

126. Mao L, Lee JS, Kurie JM, et al. Clonal genetic alterations in the lungs of current and former smokers. J Natl Cancer Inst 1997; 89:857–862.

127. Wistuba II, Lam S, Behrens C, et al. Molecular damage in the bronchial epithelium of current and former smokers. J Natl Cancer Inst 1997; 89:1366.

128. Zochbauer-Muller S, Lam S, Toyooka S, et al. Aberrant methylation of multiple genes in the upper aerodigestive tract epithelium of heavy smokers. Int J Cancer 2003; 107(4):612.

129. Soria JC, Rodriguez M, Liu DD, Lee JJ, Hong WK, Mao L. Aberrant promoter methylation of multiple genes in bronchial brush samples from former cigarette smokers. Cancer Res 2002; 62(2):351.

130. Belinsky SA, Palmisano WA, Gilliland FD, et al. Aberrant promoter methylation in bronchial epithelium and sputum from current and former smokers. Cancer Res 2002; 62(8):2370.

131. Yanagisawa K, Shyr Y, Xu BJ, et al. Proteomic patterns of tumour subsets in non-small-cell lung cancer. Lancet 2003; 362(9382):433.

132. Beer DG, Kardia SL, Huang CC, et al. Gene-expression profiles predict survival of patients with lung adenocarcinoma. Nat Med 2002; 8(8):816.

133. Bhattacharjee A, Richards WG, Staunton J, et al. Classification of human lung carcinomas by mRNA expression profiling reveals distinct adenocarcinoma subclasses. Proc Natl Acad Sci U S A 2001; 98(24):13790.

134. Wilkins-Haug L. The emerging genetic theories of unstable DNA, uniparental disomy, and imprinting. Curr Opin Obstet Gynecol 1993; 5:179.

135. Caprioli RM, Farmer TB, Gile J. Molecular imaging of biological samples: localization of peptides and proteins using MALDI-TOF MS. Anal Chem 1997; 69(23):4751.

Preneoplastic Lesions of the Lung

7

Ekaterini N. Politi and Konstantinos N. Syrigos

Contents

7.1   Introduction

Despite advances in therapy, the overall survival rate for lung cancer patients remains only 15%. This poor survival rate is probably due to the relatively advanced stage of the disease at diagnosis. To date, screening trials have had no significant impact on survival [1]. Screening can detect small (2–3 mm in size) asymptomatic nodules, but even these nodules may already be malignant, and therefore late in the course of the disease. Tumor cells have been found in the peripheral blood and bone marrow of patients with lung cancer of all sizes and stages [2, 3]. If lung cancer could be identified earlier – at a preneoplastic stage, before angiogenesis, invasion, and micrometastases occurs – we might have a greater chance of improving survival. Advances in computerized tomography (CT), bronchoscopy, and genomics technology raise the possibility that we may be able to detect these early lesions in vivo.

7.2   The Field Carcinogenesis Concept

Lung carcinoma arises after a series of morphological and genetic alterations, which lead to progression of normal bronchial epithelium to invasive squamous cell carcinoma [4]. Increasing evidence suggests that lung cancer, like other solid tumors, is the result of a multistep process rather than a sudden transformation of previously normal epithelium. Evidence for this hypothesis includes the frequent occurrence of multifocal synchronous or metachronous tumors and dysplasias found in the airways of patients with lung cancer. Squamous metaplasia or dysplasia is frequently found in association with invasive carcinomas of all histological types. It is thought that multiple intraepithelial lesions develop at various times in patients who have been exposed to carcinogens. This supports the idea that the entire bronchial mucosa is damaged by carcinogens. This phenomenon, first described in head and neck tumors, is referred to as the field carcinogenesis process.

Field carcinogenesis has two possible biological explanations. In one scenario, high exposure of respiratory epithelium to multiple carcinogens produces various, multiple genetic mutations at various, random sites in the airways. Alternatively, a single, mutated, progenitor epithelial clone may expand over time to populate widespread areas of the respiratory tract. Such a mechanism would result in the occurrence of a common mutation at multiple sites. Although the evidence collected so far appears contradictory, a combination of these molecular mechanisms may in fact be responsible for lung carcinogenesis. Cells harboring a single mutation would have a proliferative advantage over nonmutant bronchial cells. Expansion of this mutant cell population would subject it to further mutations, resulting in the transformation into an invasive tumor.

7.3   Definition

Morphologically speaking, the term preneoplasia is used to identify groups of phenotypically altered cells. Preneoplastic changes have been shown to consistently reflect sequential steps in carcinogenesis. They include specific alterations in the bronchial mucosa and epithelial alveolar layer. These lesions are visible microscopically. Preneoplastic lesions of the lung may start in the basal layer of the bronchial mucosa or in the bronchial mucus glands, as well as in the bronchioloalveolar epithelial layer (Clara cells and type 2 pneumocytes). They may also affect neuroendocrine cells, which are dispersed throughout the bronchial mucosa.

The World Health Organization (WHO) histological classification of tumors of the lung [5] lists three main forms of preinvasive lesions in the lung: (1) squamous dysplasia (SD) and carcinoma in situ (CIS), (2) atypical adenomatous hyperplasia (AAH), and (3) diffuse idiopathic pulmonary neuroendocrine cell hyperplasia (DIP-NECH). The first, SD and CIS, may be precursors to squamous cell carcinoma. The second, AAH, may be the progenitor lesion for adenocarcinoma (particularly peripheral), including bronchioloalveolar carcinoma. Finally, DIP-NECH may progress to a carcinoid. Additional possible preneoplastic lesions and conditions include: basal cell hyperplasia (BCH) and squamous metaplasia (progressing to SD and CIS), adenomatous hyperplasia (progressing to AAH), angiogenic squamous dysplasia (consisting of microscopic projections into the bronchial lumen, surfaced by squamous dysplasia), and pulmonary fibrosis.

No preneoplastic lesion has been clearly identified for small-cell carcinoma, but occasionally, SD/CIS can be seen in the adjacent airway mucosa. However, mucosa that appears normal but with significant genetic abnormalities is often found near small cell tumors. This suggests that these tumors arise without ever going through a stage of morphologically recognizable, preinvasive lesion [6].

7.4   Hyperplasia, Dysplasia and Carcinoma In Situ in the Bronchial Compartment of the Lung

7.4.1   Basal Cell Hyperplasia

BCH is present when the basal epithelial layer in the bronchial lining epithelium is more than three cells thick. BCH may be a precursor of a squamous metaplasia process. In some cases there are cells with atypical features in the zone of BCH. They should rather be considered as pseudoatypical changes that mimic atypia. There is a possibility that they may be produced by viral infections.

7.4.2   Squamous Metaplasia/Immature Squamous Metaplasia

The process of squamous metaplasia/dysplasia usually starts in a zone of preexisting BCH. In this zone, squamous differentiation may occur, but a differentiated ciliated epithelium may be preserved that masks the growing basal zone. This is called immature squamous metaplasia.

In some cases in the areas of squamous metaplasia there is an intensive angiogenic process. This "angiogenic squamous metaplasia/dysplasia" is usually present in the airways of high-risk smokers [7]. These changes may be visible with the aid of fluorescence fibroscopy as projections of capillary loops into the metaplastic/dysplastic epithelial layer.

7.4.3   Mild Dysplasia

Mild dysplasia occurs in an epithelium with squamous metaplasia. The architectural and cytological disturbance of the epithelium is minimal (an insignificant pleomorphism of a small number of cells having changed shape and size). Expansion in the basilar zone with cellular crowding is limited to the lower third of the epithelium and the cell nuclei are vertically oriented. Mitosis is absent.

7.4.4   Moderate Dysplasia

In moderate dysplasia, the architecture of the epithelial layer is minimally disturbed. Maturation of cells from the basal surface to the luminal surface shows only a partial progression, but a flattening of the superficial cells is still evident. The basilar zone occupies two-thirds of the epithelium and the cell nuclei are oriented vertically. In this grade of dysplasia there are more cytological disturbances (pleomorphism is more prominent, but cell nuclei still possess finely granular chromatin). Mitosis is present in the lower third of the zone.

7.4.5 Severe Dysplasia

The architecture of the squamous epithelial layer is not completely preserved in cases of severe dysplasia. In spite of little maturation, there is superficial cell flattening. The crowded basilar zone extends into the upper third with their cell nuclei located vertically. The prickle cell layer has almost disappeared. Severe dysplasia exhibits considerable cellular pleomorphism. Cell nuclei show abnormalities in size and shape, and have coarse, uneven chromatin. There is an increase in the nuclear: cytoplasmic ratio and an evident hyperchromatic chromatin pattern. Mitosis is present in the lower two-thirds.

7.4.6 Carcinoma In Situ

In situ squamous cell carcinoma usually arises near bifurcations in the segmental bronchi, extending proximally into the adjacent lobar bronchus and distally into subsegmental branches. The lesions are less frequent in the trachea. CIS is grossly visible in about half of cases [8]. It usually looks like minor irregularities in the bronchial mucosa with granularity, papillation, a loss of rugae and, rarely, a polypoid conformation. In the remaining cases, the site of the bronchial mucosa involved cannot be distinguished from normal tissue.

CIS may or may not be associated with epithelial thickening. Cytological aberrations are extreme – similar to those visible in invasive cancer. Mitosis occurs at all levels and maturation is absent such that if the epithelium were inverted, it would not look any different (Fig. 7.1). CIS often extends down the ducts of submucosal glands (pagetoid spreading), where subsequent invasion may began at this site [9]. Unless the cells clearly invade the adjacent stroma, however, the tumor is still considered in situ even if there is extensive submucosal gland involvement.

With conventional bronchoscopy, most of these pre-invasive lesions are not visible; their appearance in bronchial biopsy specimens is fortuitous. If fluorescence bronchoscopy techniques, such as lung imaging fluorescence endoscopy (LIFE) become more widely used, this situation may change [10, 11]. Such techniques greatly increase the sensitivity of bronchoscopy in detecting areas of abnormal epithelium, due to their tendency to show less autofluorescence than normal mucosa. Unfortunately, the specificity of this technique is not high.

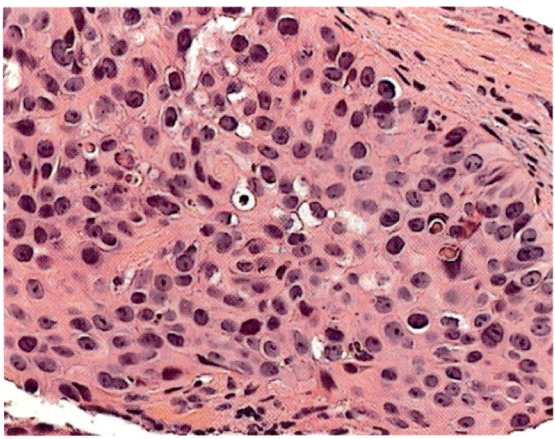

Fig. 7.1. Carcinoma in situ. Full-thickness severe cytological atypia with a chaotic appearance (magnification ×100)

Possibly only one-third of all biopsy specimens taken from areas signaled as abnormal during LIFE do indeed show any histological abnormality. In any case, histological normality does not guarantee the absence of genetic alterations in bronchial epithelial cells.

Little is known about the rate of progression from BCH to squamous metaplasia to SD and onward to CIS. Experimental studies suggest that all of these preneoplastic changes are reversible if the stimulus (the carcinogen) fails to act [12, 13]. In addition, not all cases of CIS of the bronchial tree are progressive. Some are even regressive. In any case, however, the aforementioned processes eventually do become irreversible and invasive cancer will result [14].

The initial changes in basal cell hyperplasia and in early squamous metaplasia represent a relatively acute response to injury. As a result of the irritation effected by chronic exposure (e.g., tobacco smoke), a subacute preneoplastic injury takes place (squamous cell metaplasia). This may lead to genetic abnormalities that appear morphologically as various degrees of dysplasia, including CIS [15].

Few clinical studies have looked at the outcome of preneoplastic lesions. Based on studies of epithelial dysplasia seen in sputum samples, it might take up to 10 years for invasion to occur [8]. Some studies have shown that when atypia is seen in the sputum, it may take 6–36 months for a lesion to be visible bronchoscopically [6]. In a study of patients who underwent fluorescence bronchoscopy at regular intervals for at least 6 months, progression to invasive cancer occurred in five out of nine patients with CIS. Neoplastic lesions were detected in four, but at other sites [16]. Another study followed a group of smokers without lung cancer for 4 years. Initially, 22 bronchial dysplastic lesions were detected. Ten lung cancers developed during follow-up, seven of which developed lesions that expressed p53. The authors suggested that p53 immunohistochemistry could be used to identify the bronchial preneoplastic lesions that will progress to lung cancer [17].

7.5 Hyperplastic and Dysplastic Lesions in the Respiratory Compartment of the Lung

7.5.1 Atypical Adenomatous Hyperplasia

Lesions in AAH are usually small, asymptomatic, and often incidental findings on a surgically resected lung. They are also radiologically invisible except with a spiral CT, which has a current resolution of about 3 mm. In the majority of cases of AAH, the size of the lesion ranges from less than 1 mm to up to 3 mm. Larger lesions may be grossly visible on the cut surface of the lung, or appear as ground glass lesions on a chest CT. Most of the AAH foci are very small and have been found incidentally by pathologists with suspicion of primary cancer or other pathological reasons. Lungs with very high numbers of AAH (>40) have been reported in conjunction with multiple synchronous peripheral primary adenocarcinomas or BAC [18–23]. Autopsy studies have reported AAH in 2–4% of non-cancer-bearing patients [24–26].

The origin of AAH cells is still unknown, but the differentiated phenotype derived from immunohistochemical and ultrastructural features suggests an alveolar origin. AAH cells are probably derived from a progenitor cell with a potential for both type II pneumocyte and Clara cell differentiation. AAH is a discrete parenchymal lesion that often arises in the centriacinar region, close to respiratory bronchioles (Fig. 7.2). Microscopically, it consists of a group of alveoli that are lined with cuboidal or columnar epithelial cells that are similar to type II pneumocytes or Clara cells with characteristic "hobnail" shapes. Excess collagen and/or lymphocytic infiltration might cause slight thickening of the alveolar septa. Rare cases have shown large amounts of scar tissue or heavy lymphocytic infiltration. In larger lesions, an increase in cytological atypia appears. The cells become tall with hyperchromatic nuclei and lose their hobnail features. Nuclear inclusions may also be observed and mitotic figures are extremely rare. In cases with atypia, the epithelial lining is usually more cellular.

AAH must be distinguished from reactive hyperplasia, secondary to parenchymal inflammation or fibrosis where the alveolar lining cells are not the dominant feature but are more diffusely distributed. In general, AAH cannot be identified in the presence of an inflammatory or fibrosing disease.

There is little information about the incidence of AAH in either smoking or nonsmoking populations. Autopsy studies of AAH cases are hampered by the

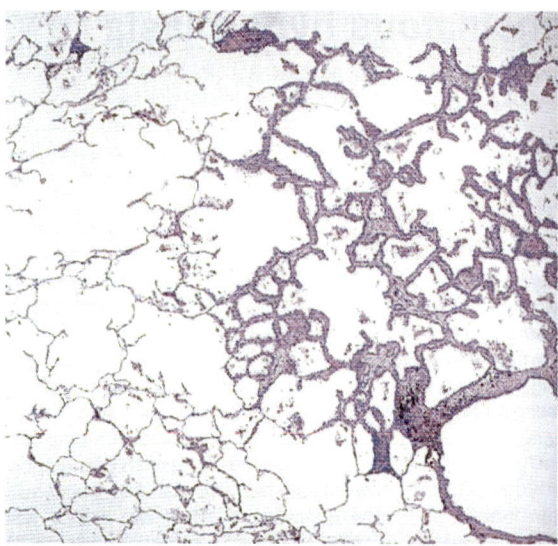

Fig. 7.2. Atypical adenomatous hyperplasia lesion found in the centriacinar zone and showing alveolar wall thickening and increased numbers of alveolar lining cells (magnification ×10)

presence of coincident pathologies such as pneumonia, obstructive pneumonitis, or fibrosis, which make AAH almost impossible to find [24, 25]. It is more common to find AAH in lungs resected for adenocarcinoma or large-cell undifferentiated carcinoma than for squamous carcinoma [19, 23]. The site, size, and visibility of AAH as revealed by most imaging methods makes longitudinal studies of AAH even more difficult than for bronchial dysplasia/CIS. The first descriptions of AAH in association with lung cancer were made in the 1980s [27, 28]. Overall figures for AAH incidence range from 4.4–9.6% in lungs removed for benign or metastatic disease, and 3.3–11.1% in lungs resected for squamous cell carcinoma, to 23.2–34.5% in lungs resected for adenocarcinoma [20, 23, 25].

Zones of AAH are sometimes seen around the tumor. Niho and colleagues determined that, the AAH lesions in seven patients with AAH and BAC were all monoclonal. In two cases, the BAC and contiguous AAH had identical monoclonality [29]. These findings support the idea that the AAH-like edge that is sometimes observed around a peripheral adenocarcinoma is evidence of the preexisting adenoma. In fact, as indicative in this and other studies, many patients had multiple AAH lesions and/or multiple synchronous primaries [20, 21, 30]. The multifocal nature of AAH may explain the multicentricity that is observed with some adenocarcinomas.

Despite the increasing amount of data that supports a progression toward malignancy at the morphological and molecular level, there is no data to suggest the risk of progression of AAH to invasive carcinoma. The impossible task of identifying these lesions before resection and the absence of an animal model for AAH rules out any longitudinal study [31]. Until then, evidence that AAH does progress through BAC to invasive adenocarcinoma will largely be based on observational and circumstantial evidence.

7.5.2 Neuroendocrine Cell Hyperplasia and Neuroendocrine Preneoplastic Lesions

These lesions may occur in the central as well as in the peripheral part of the lung. The histogenesis of neuroendocrine lung tumors is not well understood and remains to be discovered. Neuroendocrine lung tumors represent about 25% of all lung malignancies. According to the current WHO classification, small-cell lung carcinoma (SCLC), large-cell neuroendocrine carcinoma (LCNC), typical carcinoid (TC), and atypical carcinoid (AC) are included in this spectrum, as well as one neuroendocrine preinvasive lesion, DIPNECH. Although investigated for nearly half a century, neuroendocrine cell disorders remain very mysterious; their origin has yet to be determined and the nature of the stem cells of neuroendocrine neoplasms remains unclear. It is highly probable that they arise from an undifferentiated multipotential bronchial epithelial cell and not from well-differentiated neuroendocrine cells [32, 33].

Pulmonary neuroendocrine cells (PNECs) are nonciliated, and conical or spindle-shaped, and extend from the basement membrane to just below the airway lumen. They can be basally oriented dendritic cells that extend along the basement membrane between adjacent airway epithelial cells. Their most distinctive histological feature is the presence of basally oriented secretion granules, which are evident with the aid of a transmission electron microscope [34]. A receptor role of PNECs has been postulated; they appear to be involved in controlling bronchomotor and vasomotor tone in response to alterations in airway gas composition. Their secretory products (especially bombesin-releasing peptide) take part in airway differentiation and stimulate airway mucosal gland secretion [35]. Furthermore, they also serve as autocrine growth factors in SCLC. PNECs promote growth of the developing airway by stimulating proliferation [36].

The first PNEC secretory product to be recognized was serotonin, followed by bombesin. Other known human lung endocrine cell markers that are peptides and amines are: protein gene product 9.5, neuron-specific enolase, chromogranin, synaptophysin, leukocyte 7/human natural killer cell antigen, human small-cell carcinoma membrane protein, somatostatin, calcitonin gene-related peptide, enkephalin, bombesin/gastrin-releasing peptide, calcitonin, cholecystokinin, substance P, and neuroendocrine-specific protein A. Some of these factors may potentially be sensitive plasma markers of neuroendocrine tumors.

7.5.3 Pulmonary Neuroendocrine Cell Hyperplasia

There is evidence that living at high altitude (being exposed to hypoxia and hypercapnia) stimulates the proliferation of PNECs. It has been established that PNECs react to changes in the oxygen levels of the airways by releasing secretory substances. These substances affect their targets, which are most likely the bronchial smooth muscles and their associated nerves. Smoking also influences PNECs [37]. Some smokers (the susceptible ones) exhibit PNEC hyperplasia along with an increase in bombesin-releasing peptides as well as an increase in serum calcitonin levels. It is thought that these people are at higher risk of developing tobacco-related lung diseases [38]. Exposure to other airway irritants such as naphthalene and diethylnitrosamine can also cause PNEC hyperplasia. It is probable that PNEC hyperplasia associated with many inflammatory lung conditions is partly caused by the effects of tumor necrosis factor a (TNFa) on undifferentiated neuroendocrine cell precursors.

When the hyperplasia of the PNEC appears under the form of a small tumor, usually located in the distal part of the bronchial tree, the lesion is characterized as a carcinoid tumorlet (Fig. 7.3). If such a lesion exceeds more than 5 mm in diameter, it should be regarded as a typical carcinoid tumor. Hyperplasia of PNECs is also seen in the airway mucosa of lungs bearing typical (usually peripheral) carcinoid tumors [39]. This process may also occur in lungs exhibiting higher-grade neuroendocrine malignancy. The relationship between hyperplasia and the tumor, if any, is not currently understood.

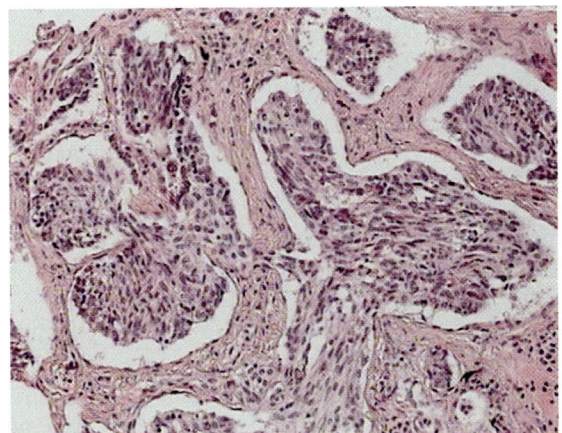

Fig. 7.3. Neuroendocrine tumourlet in the peripheral part of the lung. The bronchiolar epithelium is entirely replaced by proliferating neuroendocrine cells (magnification ×40)

7.5.4   Diffuse Idiopathic Pulmonary Neuroendocrine Cell Hyperplasia

DIPNECH is probably the most enigmatic pulmonary neuroendocrine disorder. The pathogenesis of this disorder is still unknown. Our only evidence that DIPNECH is a preneoplastic lesion is circumstantial. Essentially, it is based upon lungs found to have both carcinoid tumors and DIPNECH, of which most of the data is derived from case studies [39, 40]. DIPNECH is a lung disease diagnosed mostly in women in their 6th decade, but it has been also observed in much younger patients and in both sexes. Patients have no history of long-term smoking, living at a high altitude, or exposure to other airway irritants [41]. The history is noted as a dry cough accompanied by breathlessness, which slowly, often over many years, progressively worsens. It is often misdiagnosed as a mild bronchial asthma. Physical examination usually reveals no signs, but pulmonary function tests show an obstructive or mixed obstructive/restrictive pattern of impairment with reduced diffusing capacity. Chest X-ray is often normal, but tomographic scanning reveals a mosaic pattern of air trapping, sometimes with nodules and thickened bronchial and bronchiolar walls [42]. Multiple nodules corresponding to tumorlets or carcinoid tumors may be present. Open lung biopsy sampling reveals a diffuse hyperplasia and dysplasia of neuroendocrine cells, numerous neuroepithelial bodies, and neuroendocrine tumorlets, confined to the bronchial or bronchiolar epithelium and associated with airway-wall thickening and fibrosis [40]. These cells are immunoreactive for bombesin-like peptide and neuron-specific enolase. In contrast to neuroendocrine carcinomas, a high expression of neutral endopeptidase is observed in DIPNECH [43]. It is believed that hyperplastic neuroendocrine cells may cause airway disease. The airway fibrosis, perhaps due to the effects of a paracrine secretion, was presumed to be the cause of the widespread small airways obstruction. DIPNECH has a long history and low death rate, which can be ascribed to the counterbalancing effects of neutral endopeptidase over bombesin-like peptide [43]. It remains unclear whether DIPNECH can evolve into a neoplastic disorder accompanied by metastasis.

7.6   Molecular Genetics of Preneoplastic Lung Lesions

There is a general consensus that numerous genetic and molecular abnormalities occur at a very early stage of lung carcinogenesis, including hyperplasia and metaplasia. It is also seen in the normal-appearing bronchial epithelium of smokers [44, 45]. These abnormalities might be sequential, as their frequency and number appear to increase with atypia in both the metaplasia to dysplasia to CIS sequence, and the AAH to adenocarcinoma sequence. None of these isolated molecular abnormalities have been shown to predict a progression to cancer, but their accumulative rate may be associated with the risk of cancer in the bronchial tree [46].

7.6.1   P53 Expression

Many studies have found an increase in stainable p53, with an increasingly severe bronchial squamous dysplasia. The range in several studies varies from an average of 5% in low-grade dysplasia to 60.4% in high-grade dysplasia [47–53]. Studies of p53 expression in AAH have yielded similar results; they show an increase in p53 expression with increasing atypia. The overall levels, however, are somewhat lower in these preneoplastic lesions, indicating perhaps that the p53 mutation is a later event in peripheral adenocarcinogenesis than in squamous carcinogenesis [25, 54, 55]. In contrast, studies have found no staining in normal epithelium, and minimal staining in metaplasia. Brambilla and colleagues found p53 expression in all cases of SD/CIS from cancer-bearing lungs, but similar lesions from lungs without cancer showed no staining. This suggests that stabilization of p53 in the preinvasive lesion has a high predictive value for invasion [56].

7.6.2   Bcl-2 Expression

The protein bcl-2 inhibits apoptosis and therefore overexpression might provide survival advantage in a cell population. Overexpression of bcl-2 has been seen in preinvasive bronchial lesions with an associated increase in the degree of dysplasia [50, 51, 57]. Bcl-2 overexpression was associated with a downregulation of *bax* (an inducer of apoptosis) in preinvasive lesions that were later maintained during invasion [56]. Some authors conclude that bax/bcl-2 imbalance contributes to a clonal expansion during premalignant states [56].

7.6.3   K-ras Mutation

The *ras* genes play an important role in signal transduction and cellular proliferation, through the mitogen-activated protein kinase pathways. *K-ras* mutations have been found more commonly in AAH than in SD. The AAH lesions often have different base changes at codon 12 compared to the concurrent adenocarcinoma. This finding is consistent with the notion that AAH represents field cancerization in the lung periphery [58–60].

Several studies have shown that parenchymal tumors and AAH have *K-ras* mutations more frequently than bronchial adenocarcinoma. This finding supports the classification of adenocarcinomas into bronchial and parenchymal subtypes, and suggests the importance of AAH in the development of parenchymal cancers. The bronchial subtype might arise from bronchial epithelial dysplasia [61].

7.6.4 Fragile Histidine Triad Tumor-Suppressor Gene

Fragile histidine triad (*FHIT*) tumor-suppressor gene is found at chromosome 3p14.2, which spans the FRA3B fragile site. These fragile sites might be especially susceptible to carcinogenic damage. It has been suggested that the FHIT protein might play a role in cell death through apoptosis and/or affect cell proliferation. Its true function is still unknown; however, its role as a tumor-suppressor gene is reflected by the fact that most primary lung cancers show a loss of FHIT protein expression with aberrant RNA and altered FHIT genome DNA [62, 63]. Loss of FHIT protein is the most frequent alteration in non-small-cell lung carcinoma and precancerous lesions. The frequency of loss increases as the grade of dysplasia increases [64], and is almost universal in the severe SD/CIS stage. This loss is significantly more frequent in preneoplastic lesions of smokers than of nonsmokers [65, 68].

7.6.5 Telomerase Activation

Telomerase is activated and expressed in most human cancers. It may be one mechanism by which a progressive telomere shortening is prevented and, therefore, cellular senescence. This would confer immortality to tumor cell populations. Most adult somatic cells have inactive telomerase, but at some stage in the carcinogenic process it becomes reactivated. Using in situ hybridization, telomerase was demonstrated in as much as 95–100% of CIS and invasive carcinomas, in 70–80% of both hyperplastic and dysplastic bronchial epithelium, and in only 20% of normal epithelium. Preinvasive lesions, including CIS, had enzyme activity that was only three- to fourfold higher than normal. In an invasive disease, telomerase activity was 40 times greater. Yet, with alveolar cells and AAH, the detection of telomerase was negative [69].

7.7 Cell Proliferation Markers and Cell Cycle Regulators

Loss of cell cycle control and hyperproliferation seem to be early events in malignant transformation. Several studies have looked at different proliferation markers and cell cycle regulators in preneoplastic lesions. Proliferating cell nuclear antigen and ki-67 expression increases with increasing atypia in both squamous cell dysplasias and AAH [25, 48]. As atypia increases, the distribution of positively stained nuclei reflects the change in epithelial cytoarchitecture from the basal to the more superficial layer [70]. Several studies have found that the growth fraction in AAH is intermediate between normal lung tissue and adenocarcinoma [71, 72]. Of the cell cycle regulators, p16 expression was lost in moderate dysplasia (12%) and CIS (30%). This loss of expression was seen exclusively in lesions found in cancer-bearing lungs rather than non-cancer-bearing lungs [51]. Loss of p16 is rare in AAH and adenocarcinoma. Cyclins D1 and E are overexpressed in hyperplasia, metaplasia, dysplasia, CIS, and AAH. Increasing levels are seen with increasing grade. Levels are, however, lower in BAC. Loss of the retinoblastoma gene (*Rb*), which plays an important role in cell cycle regulation during the G0/G1 phase, has not been seen in preinvasive lesions of either type [51, 52, 73].

7.8 DNA Ploidy

Studies of the DNA content of cell nuclei, as a rough measure of chromosomal gain or loss, have been used to assess the degree of nuclear aberration in a malignant cell population. Studies of both squamous cell metaplasia/dysplasia and AAH have shown a progressive increase in aneuploidy with increasing atypia [27, 73, 74]. Some authors suggest that the development of aneuploidy is a relatively early event in the progression to malignancy. It is also indicative that the development of aneuploidy is dependent upon the preexistence of a hyperproliferative state in the bronchial epithelium [48].

7.9 Genomic Alterations and Loss of Heterozygosity Studies

Several chromosomal sites appear to be involved frequently in lung cancer. The most common and earliest changes in both squamous cell carcinoma and adenocarcinoma seem to involve allele-specific loss of genome at 3p, 9p, and perhaps 17q, among others [21, 75]. These changes coincide with increasing frequency with increasing atypia [75–82] and involve all regions of the respiratory tract, even with the normal-appearing bronchial epithelium of chronic smokers [44, 45, 83]. These deletions occur more frequently in squamous metaplasia/SD than in AAH, suggesting that they represent a later event in the pathogenesis of adenocarcinoma [80].

7.10 Gene Methylation

Recently, there has been increased interest in the significance of the methylation of genes and their promoters. Aberrant methylation of gene promoters can silence gene expression. With *p16INK4a*, *p53*, and *K-ras* promoters, hypermethylation has been demonstrated in human lung carcinomas. The methylation of *p16INK4a* has also been detected at early stages of squamous preinvasive lesions with a frequency that increases during the progression from BCH to squamous metaplasia to CIS [84]. Detection of such changes in sputum may be of predictive value in identifying smokers who are at an increased risk of developing lung cancer [85].

7.11 Other Possible Markers of Transformation

Many proteins have been found to have increased or decreased expression, correlating with increasing histopathologic abnormality. In the metaplasia → dysplasia → squamous cell carcinoma sequence, some of the proteins that may have increased expression include epidermal growth factor receptor [49, 86], vascular endothelial growth factor [87], HER2/neu [88], hyaluronan [89], calcyclin [90], cytokeratin 5/6 [91], thrombomodulin [92], fatty acid synthase [93], and epithelial cellular adhesion molecule [94]. Loss of *RAR-β* expression occurs very frequently in the bronchial epithelium of smokers [95, 96]. Type IV collagen staining highlights discontinuities in the basement membranes, which increase from BCH to SD, progressing to destruction in CIS and invasive carcinoma [97]. Changes also occur in matrix metalloproteinase (MMP) and tissue inhibitor of metalloproteinase (TIMP). Expressions of MMP and TIMP correspond to a progression in severity of dysplasia, CIS, and invasive carcinoma [97].

In the AAH → adenocarcinoma sequence, overexpressed proteins include: surfactant apoprotein A [73], carcinoembryonic antigen [73], MMPs [98], cytochrome p450 [73], cyclooxygenase 2 [99, 100], c-erbB-2 [54] and thyroid transcription factor-1 [5].

7.12 Pulmonary Preneoplastic Lesions: Clinical Relevance and Future Perspectives

Apart from the academic interest in the process of carcinogenesis, knowledge of pulmonary preinvasive lesions also has a relevant position in several clinical situations. The persistently high incidence of bronchial carcinomas and the high percentage of advanced tumor stages when presented as a feasibly clinical manifestation gravely indicate a need for new strategies of lung cancer detection and prevention. Although the main risk factors for lung cancer development, such as heavy smoking or asbestos exposure, are well known, prevention studies on populations at high risk have failed until now [101, 102]. If progress is ever to be made with screening for lung cancer, then more needs to be understood about its progenitor lesions. It is clear that detecting pulmonary neoplasia at a stage when invasion is already present is too late. To date, screening has been based largely upon examining sputum specimens for atypical cells, or mass radiography campaigns. Nowadays, screening using sputum cytology (and/or chest X-ray) has been abandoned, except in Japan and by some groups in the USA [103]. Morphology of sputum alone is not good enough to differentiate invasive from preinvasive bronchial disease. It remains to be seen whether any other specific marker can be found that can reliably identify exfoliated neoplastic cells. It is generally accepted that a tumor must be at least 1 cm in diameter and unobscured by rib, vascular, or mediastinal shadows to be reliably detectable on any plain chest radiograph. At 1 cm diameter, a tumor has already undergone about 30 doublings of its cell population, something that possibly took several years. Thus, a radiologically visible lung tumor is usually relatively late in reference to the history of the tumor. It may have already been invasive for months or years upon detection, and has possibly become metastasized. Newer technologies, such as LIFE, might increase the detection of SD/CIS lesions that are more or less invisible with standard visualization methods. However, we have little knowledge of how these lesions progress and currently, limited therapeutic options available. The clinical value of making these diagnoses is questionable. Their presence might help to persuade a patient to stop smoking, and their lesions may be subsequently treatable with photodynamic therapy. However, the real hope is that some form of chemopreventive intervention can be implemented with an ongoing surveillance using fluorescence bronchoscopy.

In general, the lung periphery is much harder to attain. Given the size and architecture of most lesions, they are invisible on plain chest X-ray or CT scans using standard resolution. High-resolution CT might provide a means of detecting relatively large lesions that can be excised, perhaps using stereotactic needle localization. New technologies, such as the rapidly developing microarray technology, may compliment the information that can be derived from the evaluation of surgical specimens, and may enhance the diagnostic armamentarium of the clinical pathologist. Overall, the main goal of our efforts is to identify any genetically altered lesions that predispose to malignant transformation and to develop the means to prevent this transformation.

Key Points

- The World Health Organization histological classification of tumors of the lung defines three separate lesions that are regarded as preinvasive neoplasia: (1) squamous dysplasia (SD) and carcinoma in situ, which may be precursors to squamous cell carcinoma; (2) atypical adenomatous hyperplasia, which may be the progenitor lesion for adenocarcinoma (particularly peripheral), including bronchioloalveolar carcinoma; (3) diffuse idiopathic pulmonary neuroendocrine cell hyperplasia, which may progress to become carcinoid.
- Alterations in chromosome structure and gene expression known to be associated with malignant transformation can be demonstrated in all of these lesions, but also in morphologically normal epithelium. These changes might be sequential, with their number and frequency increasing with atypia.
- Better understanding of preinvasive histomorphologic changes, and how these changes relate to molecular abnormalities may permit earlier diagnosis and more effective monitoring of chemoprevention trials. Advances in computerized tomography, bronchoscopy, and genomics technology raise the possibility that we may, some day, be able to detect these early lesions in vivo.

References

1. Patz E, Goodman P, Bepler G. Screening for lung cancer. N Engl J Med 2000; 343:1627.
2. Pantel K, Izbicki J, Passlick B, et al. Frequency and prognostic significance of isolated tumour cells in bone marrow of patients with non-small-cell lung cancer without overt metastases. Lancet 1996; 347:649.
3. Peck K, Sher Y, Shih J, Roffler S, Wu C, Yang P. Detection and quantitation of circulating cancer cells in the peripheral blood of lung cancer patients. Cancer Res 1998; 58:2761.
4. Vogelstein B, Kinzler KW. The multistep nature of cancer. Trends Genet 1993; 9:138.
5. Travis W, Brambilla E, Muller-Hemerlink K, Harris C. World Health Organization Classification of Tumours. Pathology and Genetics of Tumours of the Lung, Pleura, Thymus and Heart. IARC Press, Lyon, 2004.
6. Kerr K. Pulmonary preinvasive neoplasia. J Clin Pathol 2001; 54:257.
7. Franklin WA. Pathology of lung cancer. J Thorac Imaging 2000; 15:3.
8. Saccomanno G, Archer V, Auerbach O, Saunders R, Brennan L. Development of carcinoma of the lung as reflected in exfoliated cells. Cancer 1974; 33:256.
9. Carter D. Squamous cell carcinoma of the lung: an update. Semin Diagn Pathol 1985; 2:226.
10. Lam S, MacAulay C, Hung J, LeRiche J, Profio AE, Palcic B. Detection of dysplasia and carcinoma in situ with a lung imaging fluorescence endoscope device. J Thorac Cardiovasc Surg 1993; 105:1035.
11. George PJ. Fluorescence bronchoscopy for the early detection of lung cancer. Thorax 1999; 54:180.
12. Nettesheim P, Klein-Szanto A, Yarita T. Experimental models for the study of morphogenesis of lung cancer. In: Shimosato Y, Melamed M, Nettesheim P (eds) Morphogenesis of Lung Cancer. CRC Press, Boca Raton, 1982; 131.
13. Nasiell M, Auer G, Kato H. Cytological studies in men and animals on the development of bronchogenic carcinoma. In: McDowel E (ed.) Lung Carcinomas. Churchill Livingstone, Edinburgh, 1987; 207.
14. Willis R (ed). The Pathology of Tumors. Butterworths, London, 1967; 1.
15. Niklinski J, Niklinska W, Chyczewski L, Becker HD, Pluygers E. Molecular genetic abnormalities in premalignant lung lesions: biological and clinical implications. Eur J Cancer Prev 2001; 10:213.
16. Venmans B, van Boxem T, Smit E, Postmus P, Sutedja T. Outcome of bronchial carcinoma in situ. Chest 2000; 117:1572.
17. Ponticiello A, Barra E, Giani U, Bocchino M, Sanduzzi A. P53 immunohistochemistry can identify bronchial dysplastic lesions proceeding to lung cancer: a prospective study. Eur Respir J 2000; 15:547.
18. Miller RR. Bronchioloalveolar cell adenomas. Am J Surg Pathol 1990; 14:904.
19. Nakanishi K. Alveolar epithelial hyperplasia and adenocarcinoma of the lung. Arch Pathol Lab Med 1990; 114:363.
20. Weng S, Tsuchiya E, Kasuga T, Sugano H. Incidence of atypical bronchioloalveolar cell hyperplasia of the lung: relation to histological subtypes of lung cancer. Virchows Arch A Pathol Anat Histopathol 1992; 420:463.
21. Anami Y, Matsuno Y, Yamada T, et al. A case of double primary adenocarcinoma of the lung with multiple atypical adenomatous hyperplasia. Pathol Int 1998; 48:634.
22. Suzuki K, Takahashi K, Yoshida J, et al. Synchronous double primary lung carcinomas associated with multiple atypical adenomatous hyperplasia. Lung Cancer 1998; 19:131.
23. Chapman A, Kerr K. The association between atypical adenomatous hyperplasia and primary lung cancer. Br J Cancer 2000; 83:632.
24. Sterner D, Mori M, Roggli V, Fraire A. Prevalence of pulmonary atypical alveolar cell hyperplasia in an autopsy population: a study of 100 cases. Mod Pathol 1997; 10:469.
25. Yokose T, Ito Y, Ochiai A. High prevalence of atypical adenomatous hyperplasia of the lung in autopsy specimens from elderly patients with malignant neoplasms. Lung Cancer 2000; 29:125.
26. Yokose T, Doi M, Tanno K, Yamazaki K, Ochiai A. Atypical adenomatous hyperplasia of the lung in autopsy cases. Lung Cancer 2001; 33:155.
27. Kodama T, Biyajima S, Watanabe S, Shimosato Y. Morphometric study of adenocarcinomas and hyperplastic

epithelial lesions in the peripheral lung. Am J Clin Pathol 1986; 85:146.

28. Miller R, Nelems B, Evans K, Muller N, Ostrow D. Glandular neoplasia of the lung. A proposed analogy to colonic tumors. Cancer 1988; 61:1009.

29. Niho S, Yokose T, Suzuki K, Kodama T, Nishiwaki Y, Mukai K. Monoclonality of atypical adenomatous hyperplasia of the lung. Am J Pathol 1999; 154:249.

30. Dohmoto K, Fujita J, Ohtsuki Y, et al. Synchronous four primary lung adenocarcinoma associated with multiple atypical adenomatous hyperplasia. Lung Cancer 2000; 27:125.

31. Sone S, Takashima S, Li F, et al. Mass screening for lung cancer with mobile spiral computed tomography scanner. Lancet 1998; 351:1242.

32. Muller NL, Miller RR. Neuroendocrine carcinomas of the lung. Semin Roentgenol 1990; 25:96.

33. Addis BJ. Neuroendocrine differentiation in lung carcinoma. Thorax 1995; 50:113.

34. Johnson DE, Georgieff MK. Pulmonary neuroendocrine cells. Their secretory products and their potential roles in health and chronic lung disease in infancy. Am Rev Respir Dis 1989; 140:1807.

35. Lundgren JD, Baraniuk JN, Ostrowski NL, et al. Gastrin-releasing peptide stimulates glycoconjugate release from feline trachea. Am J Physiol 1990; 258:L68.

36. Pearse AG, Takor T. Embryology of the diffuse neuroendocrine system and its relationship to the common peptides. Fed Proc 1979; 38:2288.

37. Aguayo SM. Pulmonary neuroendocrine cells in tobacco-related lung disorders. Anat Rec 1993; 236:122.

38. Tabassian AR, Nylen ES, Linnoila RI, Snider RH, Cassidy MM, Becker KL. Stimulation of hamster pulmonary neuroendocrine cells and associated peptides by repeated exposure to cigarette smoke. Am Rev Respir Dis 1989; 140:436.

39. Miller R, Muller N. Neuroendocrine cell hyperplasia and obliterative bronchiolitis in patients with peripheral carcinoid tumors. Am J Surg Pathol 1995; 19:653.

40. Aguayo S, Miller Y, Waldron J, et al. Brief report: idiopathic diffuse hyperplasia of pulmonary neuroendocrine cells and airways disease. N Engl J Med 1992; 327:1285.

41. Johnson JE. Idiopathic hyperplasia of pulmonary neuroendocrine cells. N Engl J Med 1993; 328:581.

42. Lee JS, Brown KK, Cool C, Lynch DA. Diffuse pulmonary neuroendocrine cell hyperplasia: radiologic and clinical features. J Comput Assist Tomogr 2002; 26:180.

43. Cohen AJ, King TE Jr, Gilman LB, Magill-Solc C, Miller YE. High expression of neutral endopeptidase in idiopathic diffuse hyperplasia of pulmonary neuroendocrine cells. Am J Respir Crit Care Med 1998; 158:1593.

44. Mao L, Lee J, Kurle J, et al. Clonal genetic alterations in the lungs of current and former smokers. J Natl Cancer Inst 1997; 89:857.

45. Wistuba I, Lam S, Behrens C, et al. Molecular damage in the bronchial epithelium of current and former smokers. J Natl Cancer Inst 1997; 89:1366.

46. Jeanmart M, Lantuejoul S, Fievet F, et al. Value of immunohistochemical markers in preinvasive bronchial lesions in risk assessment of lung cancer. Clin Cancer Res 2003; 9:2195.

47. Bennett W, Colby T, Travis W, et al. p53 protein accumulates frequently in early bronchial neoplasia. Cancer Res 1993; 53:4817.

48. Hirano T, Franzen B, Kato H, Ebihara Y and Auer G. Genesis of squamous cell lung carcinoma. Sequential changes of proliferation, DNA ploidy, and p53 expression. Am J Pathol 1994; 144:296.

49. Rusch V, Klimstra D, Linkov I, Dmitrovsky E. Aberrant expression of p53 or the epidermal growth factor receptor is frequent in early bronchial neoplasia and coexpression precedes squamous cell carcinoma development. Cancer Res 1995; 55:1365.

50. Katabami M, Dosaka-Akita H, Honma K, et al. p53 and Bcl-2 expression in pneumoconiosis-related pre-cancerous lesions and lung cancers: frequent and preferential p53 expression in pneumoconiotic bronchiolar dysplasias. Int J Cancer 1998; 75:504.

51. Brambilla E, Gazzeri S, Moro D, et al. Alterations of Rb pathway (Rb-p16INK4-cyclin D1) in preinvasive bronchial lesions. Clin Cancer Res 1999; 5:243.

52. Lonardo F, Rusch V, Langenfeld J, et al. Overexpression of cyclins D1 and E is frequent in bronchial preneoplasia and precedes squamous cell carcinoma development. Cancer Res 1999; 59:2470.

53. Chyczewski L, Chyczewska E, Niklinski J, et al. Morphological and molecular aspects of cancerogenesis in the lung. Folia Histochem Cytobiol 2001; 39:149.

54. Kerr K, Carey F, King G, Lamb D. Atypical alveolar hyperplasia: relationship with pulmonary adenocarcinoma, p53, and c-erbB-2 expression. J Pathol 1994; 174:249.

55. Slebos R, Baas I, Clement M, et al. p53 alterations in atypical alveolar hyperplasia of the human lung. Hum Pathol 1998; 29:801.

56. Brambilla E, Gazzeri S, Lantuejoul S, et al. p53 mutant immunophenotype and deregulation of p53 transcription pathway (Bcl2, Bax, and Waf1) in precursor bronchial lesions of lung cancer. Clin Cancer Res 1998; 4:1609.

57. Walker C, Robertson L, Myskow M, Dixon G. Expression of the BCL-2 protein in normal and dysplastic bronchial epithelium and in lung carcinomas. Br J Cancer 1995; 72:164.

58. Sugio K, Kishimoto Y, Virmani A, et al. K-ras mutations are a relatively late event in the pathogenesis of lung carcinomas. Cancer Res 1994; 54:5811.

59. Westra W, Baas I, Hruban R, et al. K-ras oncogene activation in atypical alveolar hyperplasias of the human lung. Cancer Res 1996; 56:2224.

60. Sagawa M, Saito Y, Fujimura S, Linnoila R. K-ras point mutation occurs in the early stage of carcinogenesis in lung cancer. Br J Cancer 1998; 77:720.

61. Cooper C, Carby F, Bubb V, et al. The pattern of K-ras mutation in pulmonary adenocarcinoma defines a new pathway of tumour development in the human lung. J Pathol 1997; 181:401.

62. Ong ST, Fong KM, Bader SA, et al. Precise localization of the FHIT gene to the common fragile site at 3p14.2 (FRA3B) and characterization of homozygous deletions within FRA3B that affect FHIT transcription in tumor cell lines. Genes Chromosomes Cancer 1997; 20:16.

63. Sozzi G, Tornielli S, Tagliabue E, et al. Absence of Fhit protein in primary lung tumors and cell lines with FHIT gene abnormalities. Cancer Res 1997; 57:5207.

64. Sozzi G, Pastorino U, Moiraghi L, et al. Loss of FHIT function in lung cancer and preinvasive bronchial lesions. Cancer Res 1998; 58:5032.

65. Fong K, Biesterveld E, Virmani A, et al. FHIT and FRA3B 3p14.2 allele loss are common in lung cancer and preneoplastic bronchial lesions and are associated with cancer-related FHIT cDNA splicing aberrations. Cancer Res 1997; 57:2256.

66. Sozzi G, Sard L, De Gregorio L, et al. Association between cigarette smoking and FHIT gene alterations in lung cancer. Cancer Res 1997; 57:2121.

67. Huebner K, Druck T, Siprashvili Z, et al. The role of deletions at the FRA3B/FHIT locus in carcinogenesis. Recent Results Cancer Res 1998; 154:200.

68. Tseng J, Kemp B, Khuri F, et al. Loss of Fhit is frequent in stage I non-small cell lung cancer and in the lungs of chronic smokers. Cancer Res 1999; 59:4798.

69. Yashima K, Litzky L, Kaiser L, et al. Telomerase expression in respiratory epithelium during the multistage pathogenesis of lung carcinomas. Cancer Res 1997; 57:2373.

70. Pendleton N, Dixon GR, Burnett HE, et al. Expression of proliferating cell nuclear antigen (PCNA) in dysplasia of the bronchial epithelium. J Pathol 1993; 170:169.

71. Carey F, Wallace W, Fergusson R, Kerr K, Lamb D. Alveolar atypical hyperplasia in association with primary pulmonary adenocarcinoma: a clinicopathological study of 10 cases. Thorax 1992; 47:1041.

72. Kurasono Y, Ito T, Kameda Y, Nakamura N, Kitamura H. Expression of cyclin D1, retinoblastoma gene protein, and p16 MTS1 protein in atypical adenomatous hyperplasia and adenocarcinoma of the lung. An immunohistochemical analysis. Virchows Arch 1998; 432:207.

73. Mori M, Tezuka F, Chiba R, Funae Y, Watanabe M, Nukiwa T, Takahashi T. Atypical adenomatous hyperplasia and adenocarcinoma of the human lung: their heterology in form and analogy in immunohistochemical characteristics. Cancer 1996; 77:665.

74. Smith A, Hung J, Walker L, Rogers T, Vuitch F, Lee E, Gazdar A. Extensive areas of aneuploidy are present in the respiratory epithelium of lung cancer patients. Br J Cancer 1996; 73:203.

75. Sozzi G, Miozzo M, Donghi R, et al. Deletions of 17p and p53 mutations in preneoplastic lesions of the lung. Cancer Res 1992; 52:6079.

76. Chung G, Sundaresan V, Hasleton P, et al. Sequential molecular genetic changes in lung cancer development. Oncogene 1995; 11:2591.

77. Hung J, Kishimoto Y, Sugio K, et al. Allele-specific chromosome 3p deletions occur at an early stage in the pathogenesis of lung carcinoma. JAMA 1995; 273:1908.

78. Kishimoto Y, Sugio K, Hung J, et al. Allele-specific loss in chromosome 9p loci in preneoplastic lesions accompanying non-small cell lung cancers. J Natl Cancer Inst 1995; 87:1224.

79. Endo C, Sagawa M, Sato M, et al. Sequential loss of heterozygosity in the progression of squamous cell carcinoma of the lung. Br J Cancer 1998; 78:612.

80. Kohno H, Hiroshima K, Toyozaki T, et al. p53 mutation and allelic loss of chromosome 3p, 9p of preneoplastic lesions in patients with nonsmall cell lung carcinoma. Cancer 1999; 85:341.

81. Nishisaka T, Takeshima Y, Inai K. Evaluation of p53 gene mutation and loss of heterozygosity of 3p, 9p and 17p in precancerous lesions of 29 lung cancer patients. Hiroshima J Med Sci 2000; 49:109.

82. Yamasaki M, Takeshima Y, Fujii S, et al. Correlation between genetic alterations and histopathological subtypes in bronchiolo-alveolar carcinoma and atypical adenomatous hyperplasia of the lung. Pathol Int 2000; 50:778.

83. Wistuba I, Behrens C, Virmani A, et al. High resolution chromosome 3p allelotyping of human lung cancer and preneoplastic/preinvasive bronchial epithelium reveals multiple, discontinuous sites of 3p allele loss and three regions of frequent breakpoints. Cancer Res 2000; 60:1949.

84. Belinsky S, Nikula K, Palmisano W, et al. Aberrant methylation of p16(INK4a) is an early event in lung cancer and a potential biomarker for early diagnosis. Proc Natl Acad Sci U S A 1998; 95:11891.

85. Belinsky SA, Palmisano WA, Gilliland FD, et al. Aberrant promoter methylation in bronchial epithelium and sputum from current and former smokers. Cancer Res 2002; 62:2370.

86. Kurie JM, Shin HJ, Lee JS, et al. Increased epidermal growth factor receptor expression in metaplastic bronchial epithelium. Clin Cancer Res 1996; 2:1787.

87. Fisseler-Eckhoff A, Rothstein D, Muller K. Neovascularization in hyperplastic, metaplastic and potentially preneoplastic lesions of the bronchial mucosa. Virchows Arch 1996; 429:95.

88. Franklin WA, Veve R, Hirsch FR, et al. Epidermal growth factor receptor family in lung cancer and premalignancy. Semin Oncol 2002; 29:3.

89. Fisseler-Eckhoff A, Prebeg M, Voss B, Muller K. Extracellular matrix in preneoplastic lesions and early cancer of the lung. Pathol Res Pract 1990; 186:95.

90. Kayser K, Andre S, Bovin N, Zeng F, Gabius H. Preneoplasia-associated expression of calcyclin and of binding sites for synthetic blood group A/H trisaccharide – exposing neoglycoconjugates in human lung. Cancer Biochem Biophys 1997; 15:235.

91. Anderson M, Sladon S, Michels R, et al. Examination of p53 alterations and cytokeratin expression in sputa collected from patients prior to histological diagnosis of squamous cell carcinoma. J Cell Biochem Suppl 1996; 25:185.

92. Tolnay E, Wiethege T, Muller K. Expression and localization of thrombomodulin in preneoplastic bronchial lesions and in lung cancer. Virchows Arch 1997; 430:209.

93. Piyathilake C, Frost A, Manne U, et al. The expression of fatty acid synthase (FASE) is an early event in the development and progression of squamous cell carcinoma of the lung. Hum Pathol 2000; 31:1068.

94. Piyathilake C, Frost A, Weiss H, et al. The expression of Ep-CAM (17-1A) in squamous cell cancers of the lung. Hum Pathol 2000; 31:482.

95. Martinet N, Alla F, Farre G, et al. Retinoic acid receptor and retinoid X receptor alterations in lung cancer precursor lesions. Cancer Res 2000; 60:2869.

96. Toyooka S, Maruyama R, Toyooka KO, et al. Smoke exposure, histologic type and geography-related differences in the methylation profiles of non-small cell lung cancer. Int J Cancer 2003; 103:153.

97. Galateau-Salle FB, Luna RE, Horiba K, et al. Matrix metalloproteinases and tissue inhibitors of metalloproteinases in bronchial squamous preinvasive lesions. Hum Pathol 2000; 31:296.

98. Kumaki F, Matsui K, Kawai T, et al. Expression of matrix metalloproteinases in invasive pulmonary adenocarcinoma with bronchioloalveolar component and atypical adenomatous hyperplasia. Am J Pathol 2001; 159:2125.

99. Hosomi Y, Yokose T, Hirose Y, et al. Increased cyclooxygenase 2 (COX-2) expression occurs frequently in precursor lesions of human adenocarcinoma of the lung. Lung Cancer 2000; 30:73.

100. Wardlaw S, March T and Belinsky S. Cyclooxygenase-2 expression is abundant in alveolar type II cells in lung cancer-sensitive mouse strains and in premalignant lesions. Carcinogenesis 2000; 21:1371.

101. Kayser K, Becker C, Seeberg N, Gabius HJ. Quantitation of asbestos and asbestos-like fibers in human lung tissue by hot and wet ashing, and the significance of their presence for survival of lung carcinoma and mesothelioma patients. Lung Cancer 1999; 24:89.

102. Kayser K, Seemann C, Andre S, et al. Association of concentration of asbestos and asbestos-like fibers with the patient's survival and the binding capacity of lung parenchyma to galectin-1 and natural alpha-galactoside- and alpha-mannoside-binding immunoglobulin G subfractions from human serum. Pathol Res Pract 2000; 196:81.

103. Bechtel JJ, Kelley WR, Petty TL, Patz DS, Saccomanno G. Outcome of 51 patients with roentgenographically occult lung cancer detected by sputum cytologic testing: a community hospital program. Arch Intern Med 1994; 154:975.

Pathology of Lung Cancer

Ignacio I. Wistuba and Adi F. Gazdar

8

Contents

8.1 Introduction

Lung cancer is the leading cause of cancer deaths in the USA and worldwide [1]. The high mortality associated with this disease is due primarily to the fact that the majority of the lung cancers are diagnosed at advanced stages when the options for treatment are mostly palliative. When diagnosed, the majority of patients have either locally advanced unresectable lung cancer (44%) or metastatic lung cancer (35%), for which chemotherapy is the standard treatment [2]. Accurate pathologic classification of lung cancer is essential for patients to receive appropriate therapy. Although classification of the vast majority of lung cancers is straightforward, areas of controversy and diagnostic challenges remain. From histopathological and biological perspectives, lung cancer is a highly complex neoplasm [2]. Lung cancer comprises several histological types, the most frequently occurring being small-cell lung carcinoma (SCLC, 15%) and the non-small-cell lung carcinoma (NSCLC) types squamous cell carcinoma (30%), adenocarcinoma (including the noninvasive type of bronchioloalveolar carcinoma, BAC; 45%), and large-cell carcinoma (9%) [3].

Advances in molecular technologies are providing insight into the biology involved in the pathogenesis of lung cancer. Recent findings indicate that clinically evident lung cancers are the result of the accumulation of numerous genetic and epigenetic changes, including abnormalities of the inactivation of tumor-suppressor genes and the activation of oncogenes [2]. All of these molecular abnormalities involve the "hallmarks of cancer", including abnormalities in self-sufficiency of growth signals, insensitivity to antigrowth signals, sustained angiogenesis, evading apoptosis, limitless replicative potential, and tissue invasion and metastasis [4, 5]. Recent molecular advances have provided unique opportunities for rational targeted therapies for lung cancer that have led to an emerging and exciting new area of therapy, which takes advantage of cancer-specific molecular defects that render the cancer cells more likely to respond to specific agents [6, 7]. In this setting, the analysis of molecular abnormalities of lung cancers is becoming increasingly important, and represents an interesting challenge for adequate integration of routine pathological and molecular examination for the diagnosis, classification, and choice of therapy options.

Although many molecular abnormalities have been described in clinically evident lung cancers, relatively little is known about the molecular events preceding the development of lung carcinomas and the underlying genetic basis of lung carcinogenesis [8]. In the last decade, several studies have provided information regarding the molecular characterization of the preneoplastic changes involved in the pathogenesis of lung cancer, especially squamous cell carcinoma and adenocarcinoma [8, 9]. Many of these molecular changes have been detected in the histologically normal respiratory mucosa of smokers [8].

In this chapter we will describe the most important histological types of lung cancer, with brief references to their molecular and genetic characteristics. In addition, we will review the current concepts regarding the early pathogenesis and progression of lung cancer.

8.2   General Pathology Features

Almost all lung cancers are carcinomas, with other histologies comprising less than 1%. Data available from 2002 indicate that SCLC comprises about 20% of cases and large-cell carcinomas about 9% [10]. For the other major histological types, squamous cell carcinoma and adenocarcinoma, the proportions differ significantly according to gender [11]. While adenocarcinomas represent 28% of lung cancers in men and 42% in women, squamous cell carcinomas comprise 44% of cases in men and 25% in women. Interestingly, in East Asian countries the adenocarcinoma incidence in males exceeds that of squamous carcinoma, and is highly predominant in females (72% in Japan, 65% in Korea, and 61% in Singapore). Shifts in lung cancer histological type frequency in the last decades have resulted in adenocarcinoma surpassing squamous cell carcinoma as the most common type of lung cancer, with the incidence of SCLC is steadily decreasing. It is believed that these gender- and geographical-location-related differences in histological profiles are strongly influenced by the evolution of the epidemic of smoking-related lung cancer over time. Other factors, such as the use of low-tar and filter-tip cigarettes, may contribute to the increasing frequency of peripherally located carcinomas.

The pathologic diagnosis of lung cancer can be established by examination of cytologic or surgical pathology specimens. The location of the tumor, its stage, and the medical condition of the patient may influence the type of specimen that can be obtained. Histological specimens may be obtained from bronchoscopic or needle biopsy sampling (fine-needle aspiration, and core biopsy sampling), or open biopsy procedures such as thoracoscopy, excisional wedge biopsy, lobectomy, or pneumonectomy.

In lung cancer the stage of the disease is important for prognosis and treatment decisions. The internationally accepted "Tumor, Nodes, Metastases" (TNM) staging system is widely used [12]. The pathological staging of NSCLCs is based on the pathological evaluation of sampled tumor tissues (tumor size, distance of the invasion to the main bronchus carina, pleural invasion, atelectasis or obstructive pneumonitis, mediastinal organs or chest wall invasion, malignant pleural effusion, and separate tumor nodule in the same lobe), lymph node stations (numbered 1–14 depending on their location), and presence of distant metastases. In contrast, SCLC is usually staged as either limited or extensive disease [13]. Limited SCLC disease is restricted to one hemithorax with regional lymph node metastases, including hilar, mediastinal, supraclavicular ipsilateral and contralateral lymph node involvement, and ipsilateral pleural effusion. Extensive SCLC disease includes all patients with sites of the disease beyond the definition of limited disease.

8.3   Precursor Lesions

Lung cancers are believed to arise after a series of progressive pathological changes (preneoplastic or precursor lesions) in the respiratory mucosa. The recent 2004 World Health Organization (WHO) International Association for the Study of Lung Cancer (IASLC) histological classification of preinvasive lesions of the lung lists three main morphologic forms of preneoplastic lesions in the lung [3]: (1) squamous dysplasia and carcinoma in situ (CIS; Fig. 8.1), (2) atypical adenomatous hyperplasia (AAH; Fig. 8.2), and (3) diffuse idiopathic pulmonary neuroendocrine cell hyperplasia (DIPNECH).

While the sequential preneoplastic changes have been defined for centrally arising squamous carcinomas, they have been poorly documented for large-cell carcinomas, adenocarcinomas, and SCLCs [14, 15]. Mucosal changes in the large airways that may precede invasive squamous cell carcinoma include squamous dysplasia and CIS [14, 15]. Adenocarcinomas may be preceded by morphological changes including AAH in peripheral airway cells [9, 14]. While DIPNECHs are thought to be precursors lesions for lung carcinoids, no specific preneoplastic changes have been identified for SCLC.

8.3.1   Squamous Cell Carcinoma Preneoplastic Lesions

Mucosal changes in the large airways that may precede or accompany invasive squamous cell carcinoma include hyperplasia, squamous metaplasia, squamous dysplasia, and CIS (Fig. 8.1) [14, 15]. Dysplastic squamous lesions may be of different intensities (i.e., mild, moderate, or severe); however, these lesions represent a continuum of cytologic and histologic atypical changes that may show some overlapping between categories. Little is known about the rate and risks of progression of squamous dysplasia to CIS and ultimately to invasive squamous cell carcinoma.

The current working model of the sequential molecular abnormalities in the pathogenesis of squamous cell lung carcinoma indicates that:

1. Genetic abnormalities commence in histologically normal epithelium and increase with increasing severity of histologic change [16].

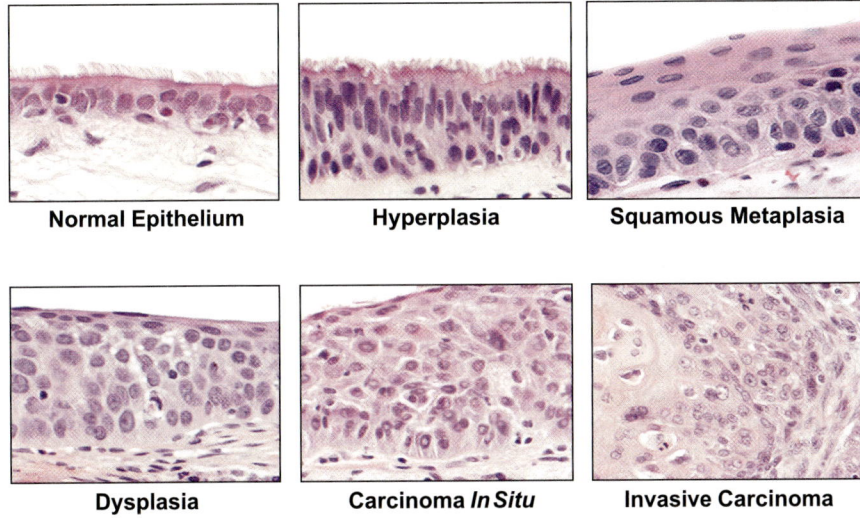

Fig. 8.1. Histopathological sequence of squamous cell carcinoma pathogenesis (hematoxylin and eosin staining, ×400 magnification). Mucosal changes that precede squamous cell carcinoma include hyperplasia, squamous metaplasia, squamous dysplasia and carcinoma in situ. Dysplastic squamous lesions may be of different intensities [14, 15]

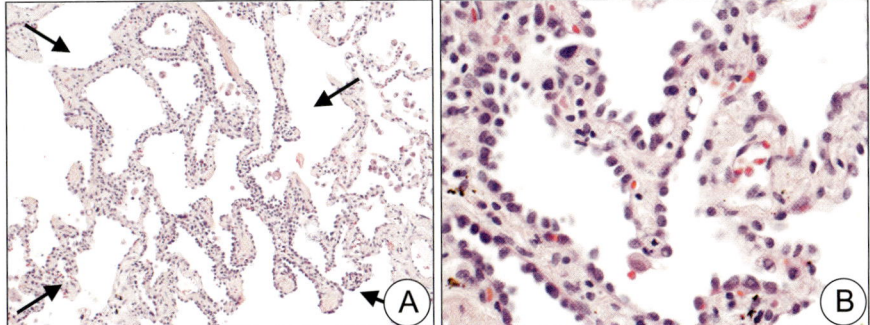

Fig. 8.2. Atypical adenomatous hyperplasia (AAH). **A** This 4-mm-sized lesion (demarcated by *arrows*) is characterized by mild thickening of the alveolar wall and proliferation of bronchioloalveolar cells. **B** AAH maintains an alveolar structure lined by rounded, cuboidal or low columnar cells with various degrees of cell atypia (**A** and **B**, hematoxylin and eosin staining, ×100 and ×400 magnifications, respectively) [9, 14]

2. Mutations follow a sequence, with progressive allelic losses at multiple 3p (3p21, 3p14, 3p22-24 and 3p12) chromosome sites and 9p21 ($p16^{INK4a}$) as the earliest detected changes. Later changes include 8p21-23, 13q14 (retinoblastoma, *RB*) and 17p13 (*TP53*) (16-18). $p16^{INK4a}$ methylation has been also detected at an early stage of squamous preinvasive lesions with a frequency that increases during histopathologic progression (24% in squamous metaplasia and 50% in CIS) [19].

3. Molecular changes in the respiratory epithelium are extensive and multifocal throughout the bronchial tree of smokers and lung cancer patients, indicating a field effect (field cancerization), resulting in widespread mutagenesis of the respiratory epithelium, presumably from exposure to tobacco-related carcinogens [16–18, 21].

4. Multiple clonal and subclonal patches of molecular abnormalities, including allelic losses and genomic instability, not much larger in size than the average bronchial biopsy specimen obtained by fluorescence bronchoscopy, estimated to contain approximately 40,000–360,000 cells, can be detected in the normal and slightly abnormal bronchial epithelium of patients with lung cancer [22].

8.3.2 Adenocarcinoma Precursor Lesions

It has been suggested that adenocarcinomas are preceded by AAH in peripheral airway cells (Fig. 8.2) [9, 14]; however, the respiratory structures and the specific epithelial cell types involved in the origin of most lung adenocarcinomas are unknown. AAH is considered a putative precursor of adenocarcinoma [9, 14]. AAH is a discrete parenchymal lesion arising in the alveoli, close to terminal and respiratory bronchioles. Because of their size, AAHs are usually incidental histological findings, but they may be detected grossly, especially if they are 0.5 cm or larger. The increasing use of high-resolution CT scans for screening purposes has led to an increasing awareness of this entity, as it remains one of the most important differential diagnoses of air-filled peripheral lesions (called "ground-glass opacities"). AHH maintains an alveolar structure lined by rounded, cuboidal, or low columnar cells. The postulated progression of AAH to adenocarcinoma with BAC features, apparent from the increasingly atypical morphology, is supported by morphometric, cytofluorometric, and molecular studies [9, 15]. Distinction between highly atypical AAH and nonmucinous BAC is sometimes difficult. Somewhat arbitrarily, BACs are considered generally >10 mm in size, with more cell atypia than their AAH counterparts. The origin of AAH remains unknown, but the differentiation phenotype derived from immunohistochemical and ultrastructural features suggests an origin from the progenitor cells of the peripheral airways, such as Clara cells and type II pneumocytes [23, 24].

There is an increasing body of evidence to support the concept of AAH as precursor of at least a subset of adenocarcinomas. AAH is most frequently detected in lungs from patients bearing lung cancers (9–20%), especially adenocarcinomas (up to 40%) compared to squamous cell carcinomas (11%) [15, 25–28]. By contrast, autopsy studies have reported AAH in ~3% of noncancer patients [29].

Several molecular changes that frequently present in lung adenocarcinomas are also present in AAH lesions, and they are further evidence that AAH may represent true preneoplastic lesions [23]. The most important finding is the presence of *K-ras* (codon 12) mutations in up to 39% of AAHs, which are also a relatively frequent alteration in lung adenocarcinomas [9, 30]. Other molecular alterations detected in AAH are overexpression of cyclin D1 (~70%), p53 (ranging from 10% to 58%), survivin (48%), and HER2/neu (7%) proteins [9, 31, 32]. Of great interest, epidermal growth factor receptor gene (*EGFR*) mutations have recently been detected in some cases of atypical AAH accompanying resected peripheral adenocarcinomas, providing further evidence that they represent precursor lesions of peripheral adenocarcinomas arising from the stem cells of the peripheral airways (the so-called terminal respiratory unit) [33].

8.3.3 Precursor Lesions of Neuroendocrine Tumors

As stated above, the precursor lesions for the most common type of neuroendocrine carcinoma of the lung, the SCLC, are unknown [14, 15]. However, a rare lesion, DIPENECH, has been associated with the development of other neuroendocrine tumors of the lung, typical and atypical carcinoids [14, 34, 35]. DIPENECH lesions include local extraluminal proliferations in the form of tumorlets. Carcinoid tumors are arbitrarily separated from tumorlets if the neuroendocrine proliferation is 0.5 cm or larger.

The findings of more widespread and more extensive genetic damage present in normal and hyperplastic bronchial epithelium in patients with SCLC compared to NSCLC [36], suggest that SCLC arises directly from histologically normal or from mildly abnormal epithelium, without passing through a more complex histologic sequence.

8.4 Pathology of Lung Cancers

8.4.1 Adenocarcinoma

Lung adenocarcinoma accounts for nearly 40% of all lung cancers. According to the 2004 WHO classification, adenocarcinoma can be subclassified into five major

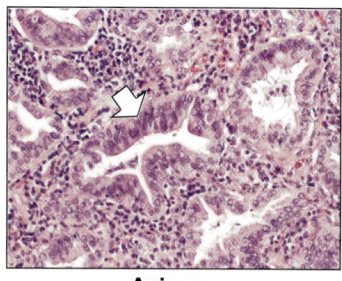   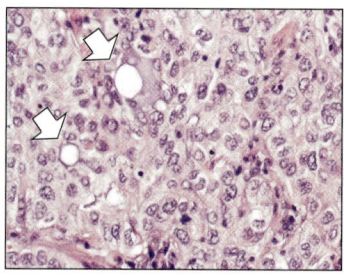

Acinar   **Papillary**   **Solid with Mucin**

Fig. 8.3. Although most adenocarcinomas of the lung are heterogeneous, consisting of two or more of the histological subtypes (mixed adenocarcinomas), the most important histological patterns include acinar, papillary, solid with mucin produc-tion, and bronchioloalveolar (BAC, Fig. 8.4). *Arrows* indicate a gland formation in the acinar type, papillae in the papillary type, and mucin production in the solid type of adenocarcinoma (hematoxylin and eosin staining, ×200 magnification) [3]

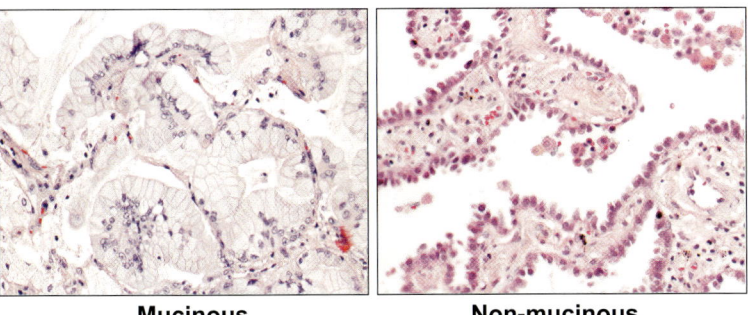

Mucinous   **Non-mucinous**

Fig. 8.4. Mucinous and nonmucinous subtypes of BAC. Mucinous BAC showing proliferation of well-differentiated mucinous tumor epithelial cells growing along alveolar walls. Non-mucinous BAC is characterized by columnar-shaped cells growing along alveolar walls in a lepidic fashion (hematoxylin and eosin staining, ×200 magnification) [3, 38]

subtypes: acinar, papillary, solid with mucin production, BAC, and mixed adenocarcinomas (Figs. 8.3 and 8.4) [3]. Most adenocarcinomas are heterogeneous, consisting of two or more of the histological subtypes; thus, most adenocarcinomas fall into the mixed subtype (80%) [37]. When tumor cells grow in a purely lepidic fashion without evidence of invasion, they are regarded as BAC (Fig. 8.4) [38]. Unfortunately, this strict definition of BAC as a true noninvasive tumor is not uniformly applied, with pathologists frequently labeling mixed tumors with varying degrees of lepidic growth as either BAC tumors or adenocarcinomas with BAC features. This inconsistency of terminology has led to considerable confusion. Solid adenocarcinomas with mucin formation resemble large-cell carcinomas, except for the production of intracytoplasmic mucin in tumor cells (Fig. 8.3). Well, moderate, and poorly differentiated histologies are recognized among acinar and papillary tumors (Fig. 8.3). While the BAC pattern is usually well differentiated, the solid adenocarcinoma pattern is, by definition, poorly differentiated.

Adenocarcinomas of the lung may be single or multiple, and range widely in size. The most common macroscopic pattern is peripheral lung localization with pleural invasion [39]. Other localization patterns include central or endobronchial sites, diffuse pneumonia-like bilateral disease (typical of mucinous BAC), bilateral widespread nodules (varying from minute to large), and tumors preferentially invading and extensively disseminated along visceral pleura, mimicking malignant mesothelioma [40]. Adenocarcinoma may develop in a background of underlying fibrosis; however, adenocarcinoma of the lung arising in association with a focal scar is uncommon [41]. The current notion is that most of the scars associated with adenocarcinomas of the lung are caused by tumor growth [40].

While adenocarcinomas of the lung spread primarily by lymphatic and hematogenous routes, aerogeneous dissemination often occurs in BAC, and is characterized by spread of tumor cells through the airways, forming lesions separate from the main mass [40].

8.4.1.1 Bronchioloalveolar Carcinoma

BAC is defined as an adenocarcinoma of the lung that grows in a lepidic fashion along the alveolar septae without invasion of stroma, blood vessels, or pleura [40]. BAC has been subclassified in three types: nonmucinous, mucinous, and mixed mucinous and nonmucinous (Fig. 8.4). Nonmucinous BAC consists of varying mixtures of type II pneumocytes and Clara cells. Although a BAC-like pattern of spread is common at the edge of conventional adenocarcinomas, histologically pure BAC is uncommon, comprising only 3% of all lung cancers [38].

BAC and mixed-subtype adenocarcinomas with a BAC component have been recognized to have several gross pathologies in the lung, including a solitary peripheral nodule, multiple nodules, and lobar consolidation [38]. When multiple nodules occur, they may be unilateral or bilateral [42]. It has been shown that while small peripheral lung adenocarcinomas with a pure BAC pattern and no invasion have 100% 5-year survival, patients with mixed BAC and invasive components have a 5-year survival of 75%, in contrast to those with a purely invasive growth pattern who had a 5-year survival of 52% [43].

BAC also may consist of a large dominant mass with satellite nodules within the same lobe, or multiple nodules in more than one lobe [44, 45]. The lobar consolidation pattern shows a diffuse parenchymal infiltration that is difficult to distinguish grossly from lobar pneumonia. While lung BACs presenting with multicentric nodules and lobar consolidation may represent a different clinical problem because they have fallen into a more advanced stage, the histologic patterns encountered are similar. Diffuse or multicentric growth patterns can be seen with both nonmucinous and mucinous BAC, but multicentricity is more characteristic of mucinous tumors [44, 45]. Detailed pathologic study of these tumors is more problematic because they are unresectable and are often diagnosed from small biopsy or cytology specimens. Because of the limited sampling, it is difficult to make an accurate pathologic assessment of the subtype or state of invasion.

8.4.1.2 Molecular Pathology

The genetic abnormalities of lung adenocarcinomas include point mutations of dominant oncogenes, such as *K-ras*, *BRAF*, and *EGFR*, and tumor-suppressor genes such as *TP53* and *p16*^{Ink4} [2, 46–49]. In lung cancer, activating *K-ras* mutations preferentially target adenocarcinoma histology (20–30%) [2]. Most *K-ras* mutations in lung cancer are G->T transversions and they affect exons 12 (~90% of mutations), 13, and 61. These types of *K-ras* mutation have been associated with tobacco-related carcinogens [50]. Activation of *BRAF* gene mutations, a Raf serine-threonine kinase pathway component, has also been detected in lung adenocarcinoma cell lines (11%) [47] and primary tumors (3%) [46].

Recently, a body of evidence has indicated that *EGFR* mutations affecting the tyrosine kinase domain of the gene (exons 18–21) are present in approximately 20–55% of adenocarcinomas, and that they are almost entirely absent in other types of lung carcinomas [48]. *EGFR* mutations are somatic in origin, and they occur significantly more frequently in adenocarcinomas in patients who have never smoked (51–68%), women (42–62%), and patients from countries in East Asia (30–50%) [48, 51–54]. In addition, although infrequent (3%), *HER-2/neu* gene mutations have been detected predominantly in lung adenocarcinoma histology and patients with an East Asian ethnic background [49]. The remarkable similarities of mutations in *EGFR* and *HER2/neu* genes involving adenocarcinoma histology type, mutation type, gene location (tyrosine kinase domain), and the specific patient subpopulations targeted are unprecedented and suggest similar etiologic factors. Of great interest *EGFR*, *HER2/neu*, and *K-ras* mutations are mutually exclusive, suggesting different pathways to lung cancer in smokers and never smokers.

TP53 mutations are frequent in lung adenocarcinomas, with different patterns detected depending upon gender and smoking status [55]. *P16*^{Ink4} inactivation by multiple mechanisms occurs frequently in adenocarcinomas and may be smoking related [2]. In addition, gene methylation studies have showed that the methylation rates of the *APC*, *CDH13*, and *RARβ* genes are significantly higher in adenocarcinomas than in the other major NSCLC histology, squamous cell carcinoma [56, 57]. Among other chromosomal abnormalities, localized chromosome 3p deletions are also frequently detected in lung adenocarcinoma [58].

8.4.2 Squamous Cell Carcinoma

Squamous cell carcinoma accounts for approximately 30% of all lung cancers. Intercellular bridges, squamous pearl formation, and individual cell keratinization characterize squamous differentiation in this tumor type (Fig. 8.5). While all of these features are very apparent in well-differentiated squamous cell carcinomas, they are difficult to find in poorly differentiated tumors. The histologic subtypes described include basaloid, small cell, papillary, and clear cell types [3].

Most squamous cell carcinomas (~70%) of the lung present as central lung tumors [59]. The tumor may grow to a large size and then cavitate, and most cavitating lung cancers are squamous cell carcinomas [45]. Central squamous cell carcinomas may form intraluminal polypoid masses and may occlude the bronchial lumen. Similar to other lung cancer types, squamous cell carcinomas spread primarily by lymphatic and hematogenous routes. In addition, squamous cell carcinomas may directly invade mediastinal lymph nodes and other mediastinal structures by extending through the peribronchial tissues [59]. Thus, locoregional recurrence after surgical resection is more common in squamous cell carcinomas than other cell types [60]. There are no squamous cells normally present in the respiratory mucosa, and they arise from metaplastic cells as a result of tobacco exposure.

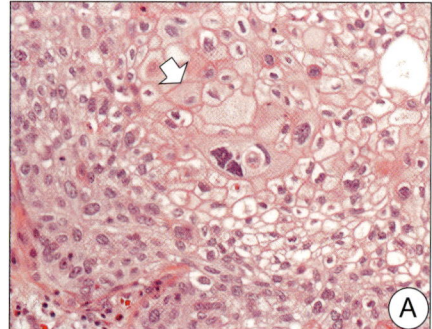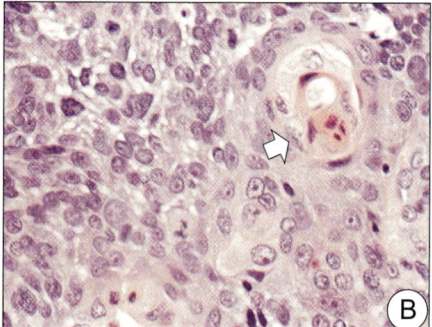

Fig. 8.5. Squamous cell carcinoma of the lung. Squamous differentiation is characterized by the evident keratinization of tumor cells (indicated by an *arrow* in **A**) and squamous keratin pearl formation (indicated by an *arrow* in **B**; hematoxylin and eosin staining, ×200 magnification)

8.4.2.1 Molecular Pathology

Squamous cell carcinomas demonstrate most of the genetic abnormalities commonly present in lung NSCLCs, excluding *K-ras* and *EGFR* gene mutations, which occur more frequently in adenocarcinomas [2]. However, squamous cell carcinoma is characterized by a very high frequency (84%) of EGFR expression by immunohistochemical methods [61]. Disruption of *TP53* and *RB* gene pathways are frequently observed in squamous cell carcinomas [2]. Most tumors exhibit large segments of chromosome 3p deletions [58].

8.4.3 Adenosquamous Carcinoma

Adenosquamous carcinoma of the lung is characterized by the presence of squamous cell carcinoma and adenocarcinoma with each comprising at least 10% of the tumor [62]. They are usually located in the periphery of the lung and may contain a central scar. Spreading and metastasis is similar to the other NSCLC types. There are no specific studies reporting molecular abnormalities in adenosquamous carcinomas of the lung, although they have been included in NSCLC studies.

8.4.4 Large-Cell Carcinoma

Large cell carcinoma is an undifferentiated carcinoma that lacks the features of squamous cell carcinoma, adenocarcinoma, or SCLC [64]. Thus, it is a diagnosis of exclusion. They account for approximately 9% of all lung cancers, and they represent a spectrum of morphology, and most large-cell carcinomas consist of large cells with abundant cytoplasm and large nuclei with prominent nucleoli (Fig. 8.6) [45]. They also include some specific variants, including large-cell neuroendocrine carcinomas (LCNECs), basaloid carcinomas, lymphoepithelioma-like carcinomas, clear-cell carcinomas, and large-cell carcinomas with rhabdoid component [63]. LCNEC demonstrates neuroendocrine differentiation [64]. Lymphoepithelioma-like carcinoma is characterized by dense lymphocytic infiltration and the presence of Epstein-Barr virus (EBV) viral sequences [65, 66]. Many poorly differentiated squamous cell carcinomas and adenocarcinomas may show a component of large-cell carcinomas; however the tumors are classified according to their best-differentiated component.

Most large-cell carcinomas are usually large, peripheral masses [63]. The tumor usually invades the visceral pleura, chest wall, or adjacent structures. LCNECs are often peripheral. Basaloid variants of large-cell carcinoma are usually central tumors with exophytic bronchial growth pattern. The pattern of spread of large-cell carcinomas is usually similar to other NSCLCs.

8.4.4.1 Large-Cell Neuroendocrine Carcinoma

This tumor types is defined by the presence of large undifferentiated cells with prominent nucleoli, a neuroendocrine pattern of growth, high mitotic rate, and neurocrine differentiated, as demonstrated using immunohistochemistry (Fig. 8.6) [64]. They are usually peripheral, nodular masses, with necrosis. LCNEC is considered an aggressive malignancy with a prognosis similar to that of SCLC [64]. The term combined LCNEC is used for tumors associated with other better-differentiated types of NSCLC, mostly adenocarcinomas [63].

Few molecular studies have focused on large-cell carcinomas, mostly due to the fact that the diagnosis is usually of exclusion. Large-cell carcinomas share the molecular and genetic abnormalities commonly seen in NSCLCs, including *TP53* and *RB* pathway disruptions

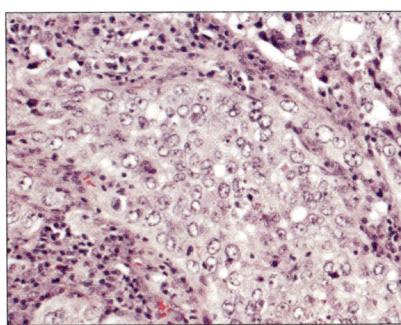
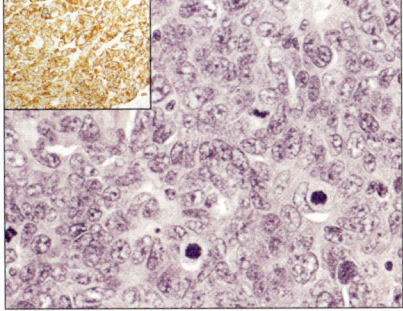

Large-Cell Carcinoma

Large-Cell Neuroendocrine Carcinoma

Fig. 8.6. Large-cell carcinoma of the lung is characterized by large tumor cells with abundant cytoplasm, large and vesicular nuclei, and prominent nucleoli. No glandular, squamous or neuroendocrine differentiation (hematoxylin and eosin staining, ×200 magnification). Large-cell neuroendocrine carcinoma (LCNEC) shows large cells, large nuclei with prominent nucleoli, numerous mitosis, and histological and immunohistochemical neuroendocrine differentiation (hematoxylin and eosin staining, ×200 magnification). The smaller picture (×20 magnification) shows chromogranin immunostaining of tumor LCNEC cells as an indication of neuroendocrine differentiation [45, 65]

[67, 68]. Lymphoepithelioma-like carcinoma, like other histologically similar tumors arising in other organs, has been associated to EBV infection [65, 66].

8.4.5 Sarcomatoid Carcinomas

Sarcomatoid carcinomas of the lung are a group of poorly differentiated NSCLCs that contain a component of sarcoma or sarcoma-like (spindle and/or giant cell) differentiation [69]. Currently, five variants have been identified: pleomorphic carcinoma, spindle-cell carcinoma, giant-cell carcinoma, carcinosarcoma, and pulmonary blastoma [69, 70]. Sarcomatoid carcinomas are rare tumors (0.3–1.3%) [37, 69]. They can arise in the central or peripheral lung. Peripheral tumors are usually large masses, and they invade the chest wall [71]. Pleomorphic carcinoma is a poorly differentiated type of NSCLC (squamous cell carcinoma, adenocarcinoma, or large-cell carcinoma) containing at least 10% of spindle or giant cells (Fig. 8.7) [69]. Spindle-cell carcinoma is a NSCLC consisting exclusively of spindle-shaped tumor cells, which resemble the spindle cells found in sarcomas (Fig. 8.7) [69]. Giant-cell carcinomas are composed entirely of highly pleomorphic and multinucleated tumor giant cells [69]. Carcinosarcoma is defined as a tumor with a mixture of usual NSCLC (large-cell carcinoma, squamous cell carcinoma, and adenocarcinoma), and sarcomatous elements, such as malignant cartilage (chondrosarcoma), bone (osteosarcoma), and muscle (rhabdomyosarcoma) [69]. Pulmonary blastoma is a mixed tumor containing a primitive epithelial component that may resemble well-differentiated fetal adenocarcinoma and a primitive mesenchymal stroma, with some sarcomatous components [69]. Sarcomatoid carcinoma cells, namely spindle and giant cells, which are present in pleomorphic, spindle-, and giant-cell sarcomatoid carcinomas, exhibit epithelial differentiation, as demonstrated by immunohistochemical and ultra-structural studies [70, 72]. Therefore, those three sarcomatoid carcinoma variants are exclusively composed of epithelial tumor cells. In contrast, the sarcomatoid element present in carcinosarcoma and pulmonary blastoma are truly sarcomatous, and those subtypes represent mixed epithelial and mesenchymal malignancies.

For some of these tumors, molecular analyses have demonstrated that phenotypically epithelial and sarcomatous elements exhibit similar acquired genetic changes [73]. The molecular profiles of these tumors are not unlike those of other NSCLCs; however, more studies are needed.

8.4.6 Small-Cell Carcinoma

SCLC accounts for approximately 15% of all lung cancers [74]. They are characterized by consisting of small epithelial tumor cells with finely granular chromatin and absent or inconspicuous nucleoli (Fig. 8.8) [74]. Necrosis is frequent and extensive and the mitotic count is high. Although there is not a precise upper limit for small-cell size, it has been suggested that the cells should measure approximately the diameter of two or three small mature lymphocytes [75]. It has been shown that SCLC tumor cells appear larger (and better preserved) in surgical biopsy and resection specimens than in small, frequently crushed needle or bronchoscopic biopsy specimens. The latter often demonstrate artifactual phenomena probably related to handling and formalin fixation [75]. While SCLCs can be diagnosed with the aid of a light microscope, electron microscopy shows neuroendocrine granules in at least two-thirds of cases and immunohistochemistry for neuroendocrine markers (chromogranin and synaptophysin) is positive in most (~ 90%) cases [74, 76]. Less than 10% of SCLCs present as a combined entity, termed combined SCLCs, comprising a mixture including NSCLC histologic types, usually adenocarcinoma, squamous cell carcinoma, or large-cell carcinoma [74].

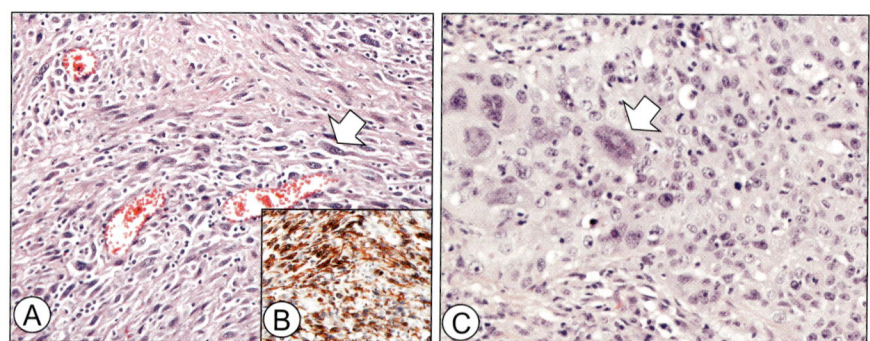

Fig. 8.7. Two histologic patterns of sarcomatoid carcinomas of the lung: Spindle cell (**A**; ×10 magnification) and pleomorphic carcinoma with giant cells (**C**; indicated by *arrows*, hematoxylin and eosin staining, ×200 magnification). The smaller picture (**B**; ×10 magnification) shows cytokeratin staining of the cytoplasm in spindle tumor cells, indicating epithelial differentiation [69]

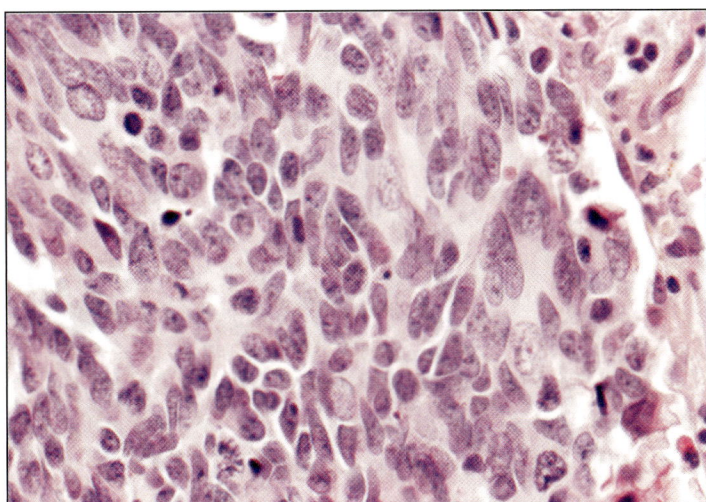

Fig. 8.8. Small-cell lung carcinoma (SCLC). Tumor cells are small, densely packed and have scant cytoplasm. Nuclei exhibit finely granular chromatin and absence of nucleoli (×100 magnification). Mitosis occurs frequently [74]

Mixed histologies may be more often present in samples obtained after initial cytotoxic therapy.

Most SCLCs present as a perihilar mass. SCLCs are typically situated in a peribronchial location with infiltration of the bronchial submucosa and peribronchial tissue [74]. Extensive lymph node metastases are common [77]. The tumors are large masses with extensive necrosis. Diagnosis is usually made by bronchoscopy, bronchial and transbronchial lung biopsy sampling, and cytology; it is highly unusual to encounter SCLC as a surgical specimen [75]. Approximately 5% of SCLCs present as peripheral small lesions [74]. The tendency of widespread dissemination at presentation has led to SCLC being staged as a limited versus extensive disease, rather than using the TNM system.

8.4.6.1 Molecular Pathology

The etiology of SCLC is strongly tied to cigarette smoking, and now there is considerable information concerning the molecular abnormalities involved in its pathogenesis [2, 78, 79]. Autocrine growth factors such as neuroendocrine regulatory peptides (e.g., bombesin/gastrin-releasing peptide) are prominent in SCLC [79]. Dominant oncogenes of the Myc family are frequently overexpressed (and may be amplified) in both SCLC and NSCLC, while the *K-ras* oncogene is never mutated in SCLC, although it is in 30% of NSCLCs. *TP53* is mutated in more than 90% of SCLCs, and the *RB* gene is inactivated in over 90% of SCLCs. In contrast to NSCLCs, $p16^{INK4a}$, the other component of the retinoblastoma/p16 pathway, is almost never abnormal in SCLC. A genome-wide allelotyping study using approximately 400 polymorphic markers distributed at around 10 centiMorgan (cM; recombination units) resolution across the human genome found that, on average, loss of heterozygosity was observed at 17 loci in individual SCLCs and at 22 loci in NSCLC, with an average size of loss of 50–60 cM, and an average frequency of microsatellite abnormalities of 5 per tumor [80]. There were 22 different "hot spots" for loss of heterozygosity, 13 with a preference for SCLC, 7 for NSCLC, and 2 affecting both. This provides clear evidence on a genome-wide scale that SCLC and NSCLC differ significantly with regard to the tumor-suppressor genes that are inactivated during their pathogenesis [81]. In addition, differences in gene methylation profiles have been detected between SCLC and NSCLC tumors [81].

8.4.7 Carcinoid Tumors

Lung tumors with neuroendocrine morphology and differentiation include the low-grade typical carcinoid, intermediate-grade atypical carcinoid, and the high-grade LCNEC and SCLC [82]. Carcinoid tumors are characterized by an organoid growth pattern, uniform cytologic features, and immunohistochemical expression of neuroendocrine markers, such as chromogranin and synaptophysin [83]. Carcinoid tumors have been divided into two categories, typical and atypical types, based on their clinical behavior and pathologic features, with atypical carcinoids having more malignant histologic and clinical features [84]. Typical and atypical carcinoids are also referred to as low- and intermediate-grade neuroendocrine carcinomas, respectively. Histologically, typical carcinoids show fewer than two mitoses per 2 mm^2 and lack necrosis, while atypical carcinoids show 2–10 mitoses per 2 mm^2 and/or foci of necrosis (Fig. 8.9) [83].

Typical carcinoids are distributed uniformly throughout the lungs, whereas atypical carcinoids are more commonly peripheral tumors [85]. Compared to typical carcinoids, atypical carcinoids have a larger tu-

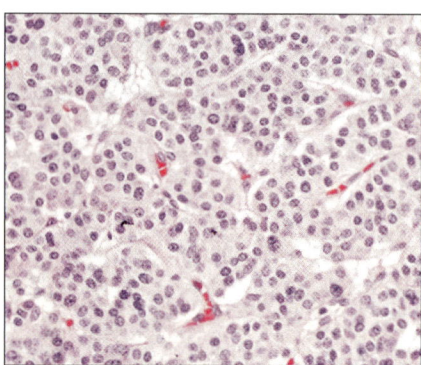
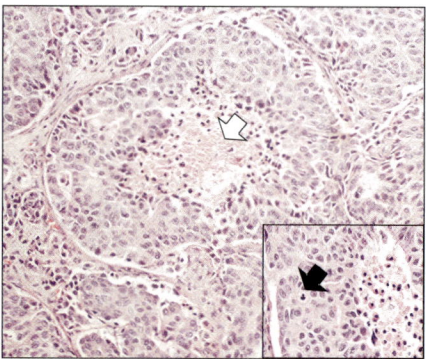

Typical Carcinoid   **Atypical Carcinoid**

Fig. 8.9. Carcinoid tumors are characterized by growth patterns that suggest neuroendocrine differentiation. Tumor cells have uniform cytological features and eosinophilic cytoplasm. A typical carcinoid (*left*; ×40 magnification) shows organoid patterns of growth. Atypical carcinoids (*right*; ×20 magnification) show some cytological atypia, foci of necrosis (*open arrow*) and mitosis (*closed arrow* in smaller picture) [83]

mor size, a higher rate of metastases, and their survival is significantly reduced [85]. At presentation, approximately 10–15% of typical and 40–50% of atypical carcinoids have already metastasized to regional lymph nodes, and 5–20% to distant sites such as bone and liver [83].

Carcinoid tumors are derived from neuroendocrine cells that are known to exist in normal airways. However, in contrast to most other lung cancers, they show no relationship to smoke exposure. Carcinoid tumors share certain molecular abnormalities with SCLCs and NSCLCs [67, 86]. In general, typical and atypical carcinoids have a similar pattern of molecular changes, with the latter exhibiting more extensive changes [67, 87]. Allelic losses at chromosome 3p sites and the *RB* locus at 13p14 are rare in typical carcinoids, but occur with higher frequencies in atypical tumors (20% and 40%, respectively) [67]. A distinctive feature of carcinoids not found in other lung cancers is the frequent presence of mutation in the *MEN1* gene and absence of its protein (menin) [86]. The mutation is accompanied by allelic loss at the *MEN1* locus at 11p13. Except for *RASFF1A* (located at 3p21.3) and *Caspase-8* genes, methylation occurs infrequently in carcinoid tumors compared to other lung cancer types [81].

8.5   Concluding Remarks

In contrast to most other organs, the lungs are prone to a very wide range of epithelial tumors, varying in their location and histology. These tumors show varying degrees of relationship to smoke exposure, with the central carcinomas showing the greatest relationship. The molecular lesions found in these tumors share certain common elements and exhibit characteristic changes. Their precursor lesions also differ, with some being well defined and others being poorly understood because of the difficulty of identifying them prior to surgical resection of an existing tumor. Thus, their natural history is also poorly understood. The advent of newer diagnostic procedures such as fluorescence bronchoscopy and high-resolution CT scanning will aid in their diagnosis and permit us to study their natural history.

Key Points

- In contrast to most other organs, the lungs demonstrate a very wide range of epithelial tumors, varying in their location and histology, the most frequent being small-cell lung carcinoma (15%) and the non-small-cell lung carcinoma types squamous cell carcinoma (30%), adenocarcinoma (including the noninvasive type of bronchioloalveolar carcinoma; 45%), and large-cell carcinoma (9%).
- Accurate pathologic classification of lung cancer is essential if patients are to receive appropriate therapy. Although classification of the vast majority of lung cancers is straightforward, areas of controversy and diagnostic challenges remain.
- Although many molecular abnormalities have been described in clinically evident lung cancers, relatively little is known about the molecular events preceding the development of lung carcinomas and the underlying genetic basis of lung carcinogenesis.

References

1. Jemal A, Murray T, Ward E, et al. Cancer statistics, 2005. Ca Cancer J Clin 2005; 55:10.
2. Minna JD, Gazdar A. Focus on lung cancer. Cancer Cell 2002; 1:49.
3. Travis WD, Brambilla E, Muller-Hermelink HK, Harris CC. Tumours of the lung. In: Travis WD, Brambilla E, Muller-Hermelink HK, Harris CC (eds.) Pathology and Genetics: Tumours of the Lung, Pleura, Thymus and Heart. IARC Press, Lyon, 2004; p 9.
4. Hanahan D, Weinberg RA. The hallmarks of cancer. Cell 2000; 100:57.
5. Fong KM, Sekido Y, Gazdar AF, Minna JD. Lung cancer. Molecular biology of lung cancer: clinical implications. Thorax 2003; 58:892.
6. Herbst RS, Sandler AB. Overview of the current status of human epidermal growth factor receptor inhibitors in lung cancer. Clin Lung Cancer 2004; 6(Suppl 1):S7.
7. Herbst RS, Onn A, Sandler A. Angiogenesis and lung cancer: prognostic and therapeutic implications. J Clin Oncol 2005; 23:3243.
8. Wistuba, II, Mao L, Gazdar AF. Smoking molecular damage in bronchial epithelium. Oncogene 2002; 21:7298.
9. Westra WH. Early glandular neoplasia of the lung. Respir Med 2000; 1:163.
10. Parkin MD, Whelan SL, Ferlay J, et al. Cancer incidence in five continents. IARC Press, Lyon, 2002.
11. Travis WD, Lubin J, Ries L, Devesa S. United States lung carcinoma incidence trends: declining for most histologic types among males, increasing among females. Cancer 1996; 77:2464.
12. Mountain CF. Revisions in the International System for Staging Lung Cancer. Chest 1997; 111:1710.
13. Argiris A, Murren JR. Staging and clinical prognostic factors for small-cell lung cancer. Cancer J 2001; 7:437.
14. Colby TV, Wistuba, II, Gazdar A. Precursors to pulmonary neoplasia. Adv Anat Pathol 1998; 5:205.
15. Kerr KM. Pulmonary preinvasive neoplasia. J Clin Pathol 2001; 54:210.
16. Wistuba II, Behrens C, Milchgrub S, et al. Sequential molecular abnormalities are involved in the multistage development of squamous cell lung carcinoma. Oncogene 1999; 18:643.
17. Wistuba, II, Behrens C, Virmani AK, et al. Allelic losses at chromosome 8p21-23 are early and frequent events in the pathogenesis of lung cancer. Cancer Res 1999; 59:1973.
18. Wistuba, II, Behrens C, Virmani AK, et al. High resolution chromosome 3p allelotyping of human lung cancer and preneoplastic/preinvasive bronchial epithelium reveals multiple, discontinuous sites of 3p allele loss and three regions of frequent breakpoints. Cancer Res 2000; 60:1949.
19. Belinsky SA, Nikula KJ, Palmisano WA, et al. Aberrant methylation of p16(INK4a) is an early event in lung cancer and a potential biomarker for early diagnosis. Proc Natl Acad Sci U S A 1998; 95:11891.
20. Wistuba II, Lam S, Behrens C, et al. Molecular damage in the bronchial epithelium of current and former smokers. J Natl Cancer Inst 1997; 89:1366.
21. Mao L, Lee JS, Kurie JM, et al. Clonal genetic alterations in the lungs of current and former smokers. J Natl Cancer Inst 1997; 89:857.
22. Park IW, Wistuba, II, Maitra A, et al. Multiple clonal abnormalities in the bronchial epithelium of patients with lung cancer. J Natl Cancer Inst 1999; 91:1863.
23. Kitamura H, Kameda Y, Ito T, Hayashi H. Atypical adenomatous hyperplasia of the lung. Implications for the pathogenesis of peripheral lung adenocarcinoma [see comments]. Am J Clin Pathol 1999; 111:610.
24. Osanai M, Igarashi T, Yoshida Y. Unique cellular features in atypical adenomatous hyperplasia of the lung: ultrastructural evidence of its cytodifferentiation. Ultrastruct Pathol 2001; 25:367.
25. Weng SY, Tsuchiya E, Kasuga T, Sugano H. Incidence of atypical bronchioloalveolar cell hyperplasia of the lung: relation to histological subtypes of lung cancer. Virchows Arch A Pathol Anat Histopathol 1992; 420:463.
26. Nakanishi K. Alveolar epithelial hyperplasia and adenocarcinoma of the lung. Arch Pathol Lab Med 1990; 114:363.
27. Chapman AD, Kerr KM. The association between atypical adenomatous hyperplasia and primary lung cancer. Br J Cancer 2000; 83:632
28. Koga T, Hashimoto S, Sugio K, et al. Lung adenocarcinoma with bronchioloalveolar carcinoma component is frequently associated with foci of high-grade atypical adenomatous hyperplasia. Am J Clin Pathol 2002; 117:106.
29. Yokose T, Doi M, Tanno K, et al. Atypical adenomatous hyperplasia of the lung in autopsy cases. Lung Cancer 2001; 33:155.
30. Westra WH, Baas IO, Hruban RH, et al. K-ras oncogene activation in atypical alveolar hyperplasias of the human lung. Cancer Res 1996; 56:2224.
31. Tominaga M, Sueoka N, Irie K, et al. Detection and discrimination of preneoplastic and early stages of lung adenocarcinoma using hmRNP B1, combined with the cell cycle-related markers p16, cyclin D1, and Ki-67. Lung Cancer 2003; 40:45.
32. Nakanishi K, Kawai T, Kumaki F, et al. Survivin expression in atypical adenomatous hyperplasia of the lung. Am J Clin Pathol 2003; 120:712.
33. Yatabe, Y., Kosaka, T., Takahashi, T. & Mitsudomi, T. EGFR mutation is specific for terminal respiratory unit type adenocarcinoma. Am J Surg Pathol 2005; 29:633.
34. Aguayo SM, Miller YE, Waldron JA, et al. Brief report: idiopathic diffuse hyperplasia of pulmonary neuroendocrine cells and airways disease [see comments]. N Engl J Med 1992; 327:1285.
35. Armas OA, White DA, Erlanson RA, Rosai J. Diffuse idiopathic pulmonary neuroendocrine cell proliferation presenting as interstitial lung disease. Am J Surg Pathol 1995; 19:963.
36. Wistuba, II, Berry J, Behrens C, et al. Molecular changes in the bronchial epithelium of patients with small cell lung cancer. Clin Cancer Res 2000; 6:2604.
37. Brambilla E, Travis WD, Colby TV, et al. The new World Health Organization classification of lung tumours. Eur Respir J 2001; 18:1059.
38. Travis WD, Garg K, Franklin WA, et al. Evolving concepts in the pathology and computed tomography imaging of lung adenocarcinoma and bronchioloalveolar carcinoma. J Clin Oncol 2005; 23:3279.
39. Shimosato Y, Suzuki A, Hashimoto T, et al. Prognostic implications of fibrotic focus (scar) in small peripheral lung cancers. Am J Surg Pathol 1980; 4:365.
40. Colby TV, Noguchi M, Henschke C, et al. Tumours of the lung. Adenocarcinoma. In: Travis WD, Brambilla E, Muller-Hermelink HK, Harris CC (eds.) Pathology and Genetics: Tumours of the Lung, Pleura, Thymus and Heart. IARC Press, Lyon, 2004; p 35.
41. Noguchi M, Shimosato Y. The development and progression of adenocarcinoma of the lung. Cancer Treat Res 1995; 72:131.
42. Sabloff BS, Truong MT, Wistuba, II, Erasmus JJ. Bronchioloalveolar cell carcinoma: radiologic appearance and dilemmas in the assessment of response. Clin Lung Cancer 2004; 6:108.

43. Noguchi M, Morikawa A, Kawasaki M, et al. Small adeno-carcinoma of the lung. Histologic characteristics and prognosis. Cancer 1995; 75:2844.

44. Clayton F. The spectrum and significance of bronchioloal-veolar carcinomas. Pathol Annu 1988; 2:361.

45. Colby TV, Koss MN, Travis WD. Tumors of the lower respiratory tract, 3rd. series, Fascicle 13. Washington, DC: Armed Forces Institute of Pathology, 1995; p 1.

46. Brose MS, Volpe P, Feldman M, et al. BRAF and RAS mutations in human lung cancer and melanoma. Cancer Res 2002; 62:6997.

47. Davies H, Bignell GR, Cox C, et al. Mutations of the BRAF gene in human cancer. Nature 2002; 417:949.

48. Shigematsu H, Lin L, Takahashi T, et al. Clinical and biological features associated with epidermal growth factor receptor gene mutations in lung cancers. J Natl Cancer Inst 2005; 97:339.

49. Shigematsu H, Takahashi T, Nomura M, et al. Somatic mutations of the HER2 kinase domain in lung adenocarcinomas. Cancer Res 2005; 65:1642.

50. Slebos RJ, Rodenhuis S. The ras gene family in human non-small-cell lung cancer. Monogr Natl Cancer Inst 1992; 13:23.

51. Huang SF, Liu HP, Li LH, et al. High frequency of epidermal growth factor receptor mutations with complex patterns in non-small cell lung cancers related to gefitinib responsiveness in Taiwan. Clin Cancer Res 2004; 10:8195.

52. Kosaka T, Yatabe Y, Endoh H, et al. Mutations of the epidermal growth factor receptor gene in lung cancer: biological and clinical implications. Cancer Res 2004; 64:8919.

53. Pao W, Miller V, Zakowski M, et al. EGF receptor gene mutations are common in lung cancers from "never smokers" and are associated with sensitivity of tumors to gefitinib and erlotinib. Proc Natl Acad Sci U S A 2004; 101:13306.

54. Tokumo M, Toyooka S, Kiura K, et al. The relationship between epidermal growth factor receptor mutations and clinicopathologic features in non-small cell lung cancers. Clin Cancer Res 2005; 11:1167.

55. Toyooka S, Tsuda T, Gazdar AF. The TP53 gene, tobacco exposure, and lung cancer. Hum Mutat 2003; 21:229.

56. Toyooka S, Maruyama R, Toyooka KO, et al. Smoke exposure, histologic type and geography-related differences in the methylation profiles of non-small cell lung cancer. Int J Cancer 2003; 103:153.

57. Toyooka S, Suzuki M, Maruyama R, et al. The relationship between aberrant methylation and survival in non-small-cell lung cancers. Br J Cancer 2004; 91:771.

58. Wistuba, II, Behrens C, Virmani AK, et al High resolution chromosome 3p allelotyping of human lung cancer and preneoplastic/preinvasive bronchial epithelium reveals multiple, discontinuous sites of 3p allele loss and three regions of frequent breakpoints Cancer Res 2000; 60:1949.

59. Hammar SP, Brambilla C, Pugatch B, et al. Tumours of the Lung. Squamous cell carcinoma. In: Travis WD, Brambilla E, Muller-Hermelink HK, Harris CC (eds.) Pathology and Genetics: Tumours of the Lung, Pleura, Thymus and Heart. IARC Press, Lyon, 2004; p 26

60. Jang KM, Lee KS, Shim YM, et al. The rates and CT patterns of locoregional recurrence after resection surgery of lung cancer: correlation with histopathology and tumor staging. J Thorac Imaging 2003; 18:225.

61. Hirsch FR, Varella-Garcia M, Bunn PA, Jr., et al. Epidermal growth factor receptor in non-small-cell lung carcinomas: correlation between gene copy number and protein expression and impact on prognosis. J Clin Oncol 2003; 21:3798.

62. Brambilla C, Travis WD. Tumours of the lung. Adenosquamous carcinoma. In: Travis WD, Brambilla E, Muller-Hermelink HK, Harris CC (eds.) Pathology and Genetics:

Tumours of the Lung, Pleura, Thymus and Heart. IARC Press, Lyon, 2004; p 51.

63. Brambilla C, Pugatch B, Geisinger K, et al. Tumours of the lung. Large cell carcinoma. In: Travis WD, Brambilla E, Muller-Hermelink HK, Harris CC (eds.) Pathology and Genetics: Tumours of the Lung, Pleura, Thymus and Heart. IARC Press, Lyon, 2004; p 45.

64. Takei H, Asamura H, Maeshima A, et al. Large cell neuroendocrine carcinoma of the lung: clinicopathologic study of eighty-seven cases. J Thorac Cardiovasc Surg 2002; 124:285.

65. Pittaluga S, Wong MP, Chung LP, Loke SL. Clonal Epstein-Barr virus in lymphoepithelioma-like carcinoma of the lung. Am J Surg Pathol 1993; 17:678.

66. Kobayashi M, Ito M, Sano K, et al. Pulmonary lymphoepithelioma-like carcinoma: predominant infiltration of tumor-associated cytotoxic T lymphocytes might represent the enhanced tumor immunity. Intern Med 2004; 43:32.

67. Onuki N, Wistuba, II, Travis WD, et al. Genetic changes in the spectrum of neuroendocrine lung tumors. Cancer 199; 85:600.

68. Przygodzki RM, Finkelstein SD, Langer JC, et al. Analysis of p53, K-ras-2, and C-raf-1 in pulmonary neuroendocrine tumors. Correlation with histological subtype and clinical outcome. Am J Pathol 1996; 148:1531.

69. Corrin B, Chang YL, Rossi G, et al. Tumors of the lung. Sarcomatoid carcinoma. In: Travis WD, Brambilla E, Muller-Hermelink HK, Harris CC (eds.) Pathology and Genetics: Tumours of the Lung, Pleura, Thymus and Heart. IARC Press, Lyon, 2004; p 53.

70. Rossi G, Cavazza A, Sturm N, et al. Pulmonary carcinomas with pleomorphic, sarcomatoid, or sarcomatous elements: clinicopathologic and immunohistochemical study of 75 cases. Am J Surg Pathol 2003; 27:311.

71. Wick MR, Ritter JH, Humphrey PA. Sarcomatoid carcinomas of the lung: clinicopathologic review. Am J Clin Pathol 1997; 108:40.

72. Ro JY, Chen JL, Lee JS, et al. Sarcomatoid carcinoma of the lung. Immunohistochemical and ultrastructural studies of 14 cases. Cancer 1992; 69:376.

73. Nishida K, Kobayashi Y, Ishikawa Y, et al. Sarcomatoid adenocarcinoma of the lung: clinicopathological, immunohistochemical and molecular analyses. Anticancer Res 2002; 22:3477.

74. Travis WD, Nicholson S, Hirsch F, et al. Tumours of the lung. Small cell carcinoma. In: Travis WD, Brambilla E, Muller-Hermelink HK, Harris CC (eds.) Pathology and Genetics: Tumours of the Lung, Pleura, Thymus and Heart. IARC Press, Lyon, 2004; p 31.

75. Nicholson SA, Beasley MB, Brambilla E, et al. Small cell lung carcinoma (SCLC): clinicopathologic study of 100 cases with surgical specimens. Am J Surg Pathol 2002; 26:1184.

76. Guinee DG, Jr., Fishback NF, Koss MN, et al. The spectrum of immunohistochemical staining of small-cell lung carcinoma in specimens from transbronchial and open-lung biopsies. Am J Clin Pathol 1994; 102:406.

77. Abrams J, Doyle LA, Aisner J. Staging, prognostic factors, and special considerations in small cell lung cancer. Semin Oncol 1988; 15:261.

78. Wistuba, II, Gazdar AF. Molecular pathology of lung cancer. Verh Dtsch Ges Pathol 2000; 84:96.

79. Wistuba, II, Gazdar AF, Minna JD. Molecular genetics of small cell lung carcinoma. Semin Oncol 2001; 28:3.

80. Girard L, Zochbauer-Muller S, Virmani AK, et al. Genome-wide allelotyping of lung cancer identifies new regions of allelic loss, differences between small cell lung cancer and non-small cell lung cancer, and loci clustering. Cancer Res 2000; 60:4894.

81. Toyooka S, Toyooka KO, Maruyama R, et al. DNA methylation profiles of lung tumors. Mol Cancer Ther 2001; 1:61.

82. Flieder DB. Neuroendocrine tumors of the lung: recent developments in histopathology. Curr Opin Pulm Med 2002; 8:275.

83. Beasley MB, Thunissen FB, Hasleton PS, et al. Tumours of the lung. Carcinoid tumor. In: Travis WD, Brambilla E, Muller-Hermelink HK, Harris CC (eds.) Pathology and Genetics: Tumours of the Lung, Pleura, Thymus and Heart. IARC Press, Lyon, 2004; p 59.

84. Travis WD, Rush W, Flieder DB, et al. Survival analysis of 200 pulmonary neuroendocrine tumors with clarification of criteria for atypical carcinoid and its separation from typical carcinoid. Am J Surg Pathol 1998; 22:934.

85. Beasley MB, Thunnissen FB, Brambilla E, et al. Pulmonary atypical carcinoid: predictors of survival in 106 cases. Hum Pathol 2000; 31:1255.

86. Debelenko LV, Brambilla E, Agarwal SK, et al. Identification of MEN1 gene mutations in sporadic carcinoid tumors of the lung. Hum Mol Genet 1997; 6:2285.

87. Kobayashi Y, Tokuchi Y, Hashimoto T, et al. Molecular markers for reinforcement of histological subclassification of neuroendocrine lung tumors. Cancer Sci 2004; 95:334.

Section III:
Clinical Evaluation of Lung Cancer

Clinical Presentation of Lung Cancer

9

Spyros A. Papiris and Charis Roussos

Contents

9.1   Introduction

Lung cancer is usually recognized late in its natural history. Late recognition, which is the case in 80% of newly diagnosed patients with lung cancer, relates to disseminated and unresectable disease at presentation. Actually, despite major advances in biomedical technology the 5-year mortality rate from the day of its presentation approximates 87–90% [1–3]. The clinical presentation of lung cancer usually relates to the development of a new, or worsening of a preexisting clinical symptom or sign and, less frequently, to an abnormal chest roentgenographic shadow in an asymptomatic patient. Indeed, more than 90% of patients with lung cancer are symptomatic at presentation. Lung cancer symptoms are multiple and variable and can be the result of: (1) the local growth of the primary tumor, (2) its extension to the adjacent intrathoracic structures, (3) distant metastases, (4) nonspecific systemic effects, and (5) the immunologic response or the ectopic production of peptide proteins (hormones) by the same lung cancer or its metastases (paraneoplastic syndromes) [4, 5].

9.2   Symptoms and Signs due to Local Growth (Bronchopulmonary) of the Primary Tumor

Cough, hemoptysis, dyspnea, and chest discomfort are common presenting symptoms in patients with lung cancer [6]. Cough is by far the most common local manifestation of lung cancer and is usually mildly productive or even dry. In some patients it may present as paroxysmal, while in a minority, those affected by a secretory bronchoalveolar carcinoma may be associated with bronchorrhea. Most patients with lung cancer also present with a chronic productive cough due to chronic bronchitis, and in these patients the initial manifestation of lung cancer development is a change in the character of cough or the appearance of blood-tinged sputum. Hemoptysis is a common presenting symptom, but is rarely severe. It is

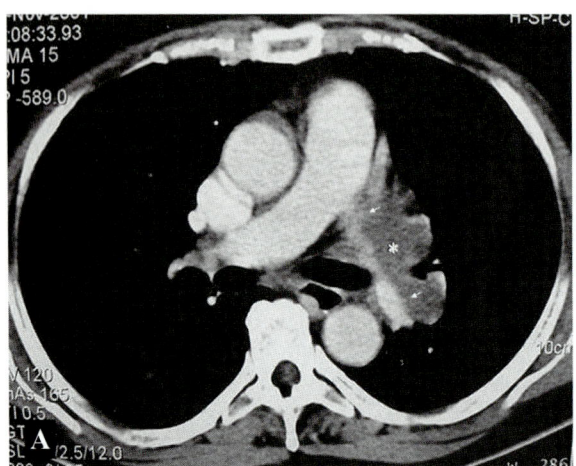
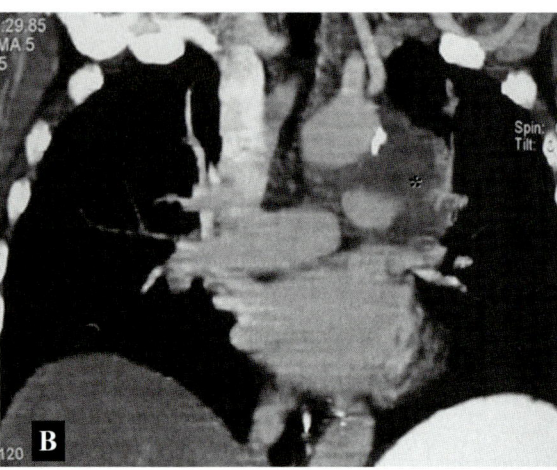

Fig. 9.1. A A contrast-enhanced spiral computed tomography (CT) scan showing the infiltration of the left pulmonary artery (*arrows*) by a central bronchogenic neoplasm (*asterisk*). **B** The coronary reconstruction film reveals better the encircling infiltration of the left pulmonary artery (*asterisk*). Reproduced courtesy of Dr. K. Malagari

an important sentinel sign in smokers and, if related to the development of lung cancer is usually associated with an abnormal chest roentgenogram. However, in the case of a normal chest roentgenogram, further diagnostic examinations are mandatory in the high-risk patient, including chest computed tomography (CT), bronchoscopy, and repetitive sputum cytology and close observation for several months [7]. In some patients the local development of lung cancer may lead to large mediastinal vessel invasion, including the pulmonary artery, its divisions, and others (Fig. 9.1 A and B). More frequently the local bronchial development of lung cancer leads to obstructive pneumonia. Many cases of obstructive pneumonia are sterile and the inflammatory reaction that leads to parenchymal consolidation is presumably due to retained secretions. However, the occurrence of fever is usually the result of a secondary infection and should be adequately treated. Pneumonia in high-risk patients, especially if it reoccurs, should be observed with suspicion for occult carcinoma and further diagnostic examinations should be requested. A local wheeze is a sign of localized bronchial stenosis and may be associated with unilateral hyperinflation in the chest roentgenogram obtained at full expiration. In such cases, further diagnostic examination is necessary to unmask the cancer. A recent appearance of dyspnea on exertion or even at rest may be related to the central (trachea or main bronchi) development of lung caner and in this case is commonly associated with wheeze. An ill-defined chest discomfort is not uncommonly associated with the development of lung cancer. Finally, in few cases the development of lung cancer heralds itself by the reactivation of old tuberculosis leading at the same time to diagnostic confusion and delay [8].

The local growth and the intrathoracic extension of the non-small-cell primary lung cancer according to the staging system developed by the American Joint commission on cancer classifies as follows [3, 9]: T (tumor) 1, tumor less than 3 cm in size, surrounded by lung or pleura; no tumor more proximal than the lobe bronchus; T2, tumor of more than 3 cm, involving the main bronchus at a distance greater than 2 cm from the carina, invading pleura, atelectasis or pneumonia extending to the hilum but not the entire lung; T3, tumor invading the chest wall, diaphragm, mediastinal pleura, pericardium, main bronchus at a distance of less than 2 cm from the carina, atelectasis or pneumonia of the entire lung; T4, tumor that invades the mediastinum, the heart, the great vessels, the trachea, the esophagus, the vertebral body, the carina (including separate tumor nodules), and malignant pleural effusion.

9.3 Symptoms and Signs due to the Intrathoracic Extension of the Primary Tumor

Intrathoracic extension of lung cancer, either directly by compression or invasion or via the lymphatics, produces a variety of symptoms and signs including the following characteristic syndromes.

9.3.1 Superior Pulmonary Sulcus Tumor, Pancoast Syndrome, and Horner's Syndrome

According to Pancoast's classic description, a lung cancer "at a definitive location at the thoracic inlet produces constant and characteristic phenomena of pain in the eight cervical and first and second thoracic trunk distribution, and Horner's syndrome" [10]. Pancoast tu-

Table 9.1. Common and rare conditions causing Pancoast's syndrome

Neoplasms	Infections	Miscellaneous
Lung cancer	*Staphylococcus aureus, Pseudomonas aeruginosa*	Cervical rib syndrome
Adenoid cystic carcinoma	Nocardiosis, Actinomycosis	Amyloidoma
Hemangiopericytoma	Tuberculosis	Thyroid cyst
Mesothelioma	*Pasteurella multocida*	Sympathetic dystrophy
Plasmocytoma	Hydatid cyst	
Lymphomatoid granulomatosis	Mucormycosis, Aspergilloma, *Cryptococcus neformans*	
Lymphoma non-Hodgkin	Mycotic aneurism	
Thyroid carcinoma		
Metastatic neoplasms		

mor is quite consistantly a lung cancer (other malignancies as well as inflammatory and infectious diseases are rare etiologic conditions; Table 9.1) [11] that develops peripherally at the apex of the upper lobes, at or near the superior pulmonary sulcus, and more commonly is a low-grade epidermoid bronchogenic carcinoma that grows slowly and metastasizes late (Fig. 9.2 A–C) [12]. Constrained by the narrow confines of the thoracic inlet, the developing carcinoma invades the lymphatics of the endothoracic fascia and involves by direct extension one or more of the following structures: the lower roots of the brachial plexus, the intercostals nerves, the stellate ganglion, the sympathetic chain, and the adjacent ribs and vertebrae. It's initial clinical presentation is pain localized to the shoulder and the vertebral border of the scapula; later the pain extends

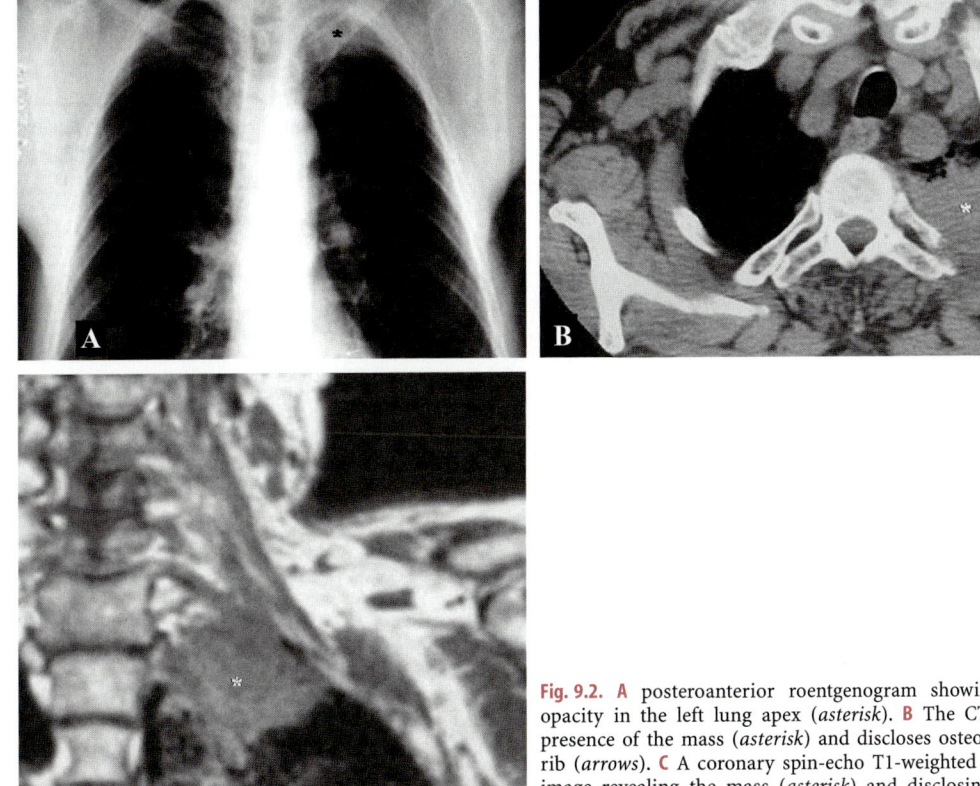

Fig. 9.2. A posteroanterior roentgenogram showing a homogeneous opacity in the left lung apex (*asterisk*). **B** The CT scan confirms the presence of the mass (*asterisk*) and discloses osteolysis of the adjacent rib (*arrows*). **C** A coronary spin-echo T1-weighted magnetic resonance image revealing the mass (*asterisk*) and disclosing the infiltration of the lower scalene muscle and brachial plexus. Reproduced courtesy of Dr. K. Malagari

down the arm toward the elbow, along the distribution of the ulnar nerve (T1 nerve root involvement) and subsequently to the ulnar surface of the forearm and the small ring fingers of the hand (C8 dermatome distribution). Weakness and atrophy of the muscles of the hand supervenes, as well as the loss of the triceps reflex. When the lung cancer invades the sympathetic chain and the stellate ganglion, Horner's syndrome (enophthalmos, pupillary constriction, palpebral ptosis, and anhidrosis) develops on the ipsilateral side of the face. Adjacent bone involvement increases the severity of pain. Furthermore, the invasion of the spinal canal and spinal cord leads to the signs and symptoms of spinal-cord compression syndrome. Infrequent manifestations include supraclavicular adenopathy, superior vena cava syndrome, and involvement of the phrenic or laryngeal nerves [11]. The vast majority of superior sulcus tumors are due to non-small-cell lung cancer and can be staged as T3N0M0 (stage IIB) or higher. T3 refers to the direct invasion of the chest wall and T4 to the direct invasion of the mediastinum, the great vessels, the esophagus, the trachea, the vertebral body, or the heart [13]. In a series reported from the MD Anderson Cancer Center at the University of Texas, 25% of patients with superior sulcus tumors were stage IIB (T3N0M0), 22% were stage IIIA (T1-3N2), and 53% stage IIIB (T4 or N3) [14]. Pretreatment evaluation in patients with Pancoast's lung cancer should include: (1) history and physical examination, (2) blood count and serum chemistries, (3) pulmonary function tests, (4) CT scan of the chest and the upper abdomen, (5) magnetic resonance imaging (MRI) in the case of brachial plexus symptomatology in order to assess local vessel involvement and determine resectability, (6) surgical as-

sessment of the mediastinum (mediastinoscopy), or alternatively, via fluorodeoxyglucose-positron emission tomography (PET) scan, (7) CT scan or MRI of the head, and eventually (8) whole-body PET scan to rule out distant metastasis [13, 15]. A combined-(tri)-modality therapeutic approach (chemotherapy, radiotherapy, and after restaging, surgical resection provided an experienced surgeon is available) should be attempted in patients with locally extensive disease.

9.3.2 Superior Vena Cava Syndrome

The superior vena cava is a 6- to 8-cm long, thin-walled, low-pressure vessel that drains venous blood from the head, neck, upper extremities, and upper thorax to the heart. It extends from the junction of the right and left innominate veins to the right atrium. It is located in the middle mediastinum and is surrounded by the sternum, trachea, right bronchus, aorta, pulmonary artery, and the perihilar and paratracheal nodes. Several space-occupying lesions developing in the middle mediastinum may compress or invade the vessel, leading to blood flow reduction or complete obstruction. In such conditions, intravascular thrombosis quite constantly coexists. Superior vena cava syndrome is the clinical syndrome resulting from the homonymous vessel obstruction or the severe reduction of venous return from the head, neck, and upper extremities [16]. Clinically, it presents with head, facial, neck, upper thorax, and upper extremity edema and venous distension, headache, cyanosis, and the formation of an extensive collateral circulation. Bending forward or lying down

Table 9.2. Common and rare conditions causing superior vena cava syndrome

Neoplasms	Infections	Vascular conditions	Miscellaneous
Lung Cancer	Histoplasmosis	Thromboembolism	Fibrosing mediastinitis
Lymphomas, non-Hodgkin, Hodgkin	Tuberculosis	Catheter-related: e.g., pacemakers, defibrillators	Encapsulated pleural effusion
Plasmocytomas	Syphilis	Pericarditis	Biermer's disease
Metastatic cancers	Actinomycosis	Budd-Chiari syndrome	Hirschprung's disease
Sarcomas	Nocardia species	Aortic aneurism	Mediterranean fever
Castleman's disease	Aspergillosis	Arterial-venous fistulas	Retrosternal goiter
Teratoma, amartoma	Zygomycosis	Vasculitis	Sarcoidosis
Dermoid cyst	HIV infection	Hyperhomocysteinemia	Cystic fibrosis
Cystic hygroma	Klebsiella pneumoniae	Right subclavian aneurism	Postsurgery
Thymoma	Hydatid cyst	Innominate artery aneurism	Mustard operation
Thyroid carcinoma		Behcet's disease	
Atrial myxoma		Leukocytoclastic vasculitis	
Paraganglioma		Heparin-induced thrombosis	
Choriocarcinoma		Thoracic outlet syndrome	
Melanoma			
Lymphangioma			
Neurogenic tumor			
Lymphocytic leukemia			
Esophageal melanotic-Schwannoma			

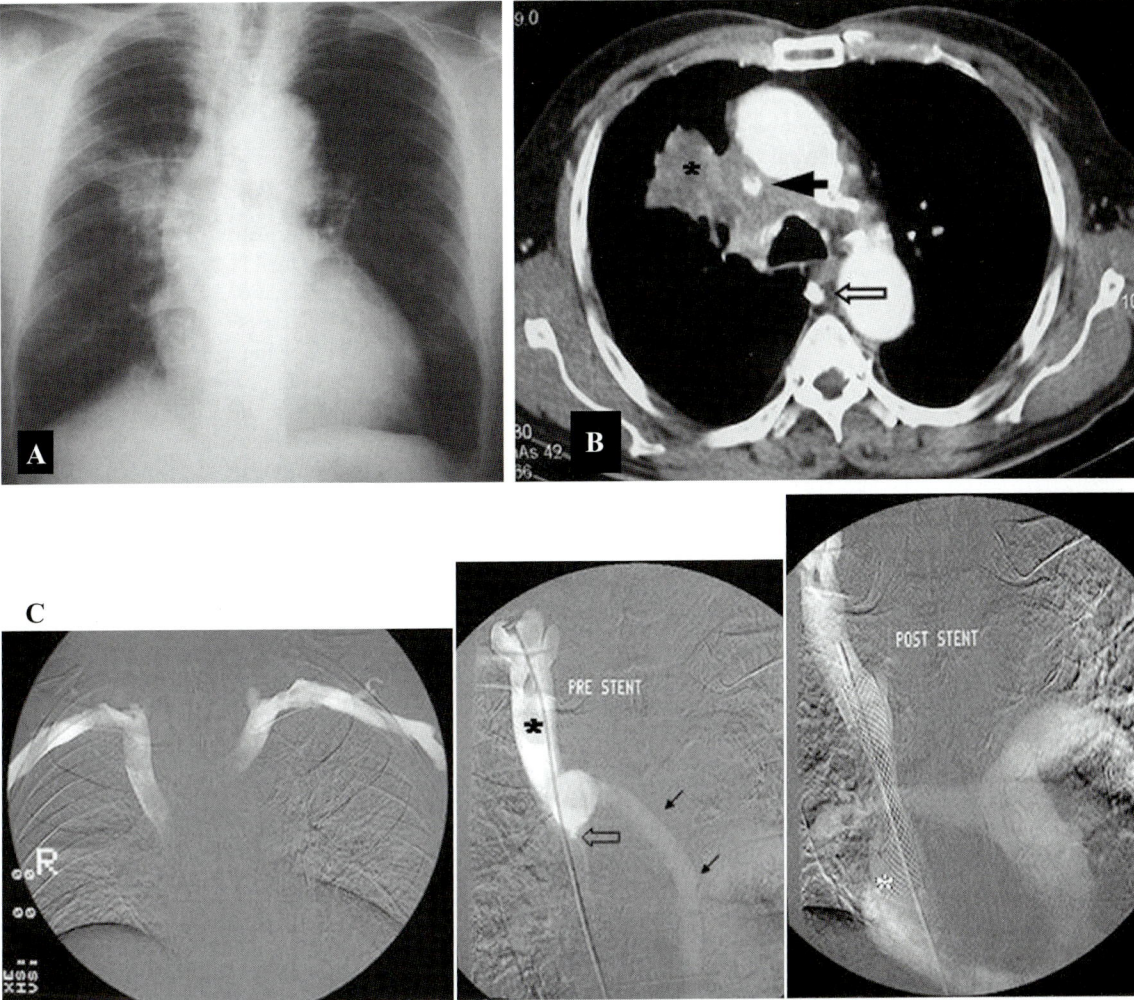

Fig. 9.3. A A posteroanterior chest roentgenogram showing an opacity of the right upper lobe with extensive basis in the mediastinum. **B** The contrast-enhanced spiral CT scan reveals a soft-tissue mass in the right upper lobe (*asterisk*) that circumscribes and compresses the superior vena cava (*arrow*). Also evident is the azygos dilation that is eventually related to the development of a collateral circulation (*open arrow*). **C** Sequential venous angiograms before (*left*), during (*middle*, *PRE STENT*), and after the placement of a stent (*right*, *POST STENT*). A subclavian venogram (*left*) reveals the complete obstruction of the superior vena cava (it is evident only in the lower course of the brachiocefalic veins). In the next image (*middle*) a balloon-tipped catheter has been introduced through the lower vena cava, the right atrium and the obstruc-tive portion of the superior vena cava in the right brachiocefalic vein (*asterisk*). The concentric obstruction of the superior vena cava is clearly evident (*open arrow*). Also evident is reverse flow in the azygos vein (*arrows*). In the next image (*right*) the patient underwent balloon dilatation of the superior vena cava stenosis followed by placement of a metallic mesh stent. The stent is positioned in the brachiocefalic vein and superior vena cava. The restoration of normal flow in the superior vena cava and opacification of the right atrium are clearly seen (*asterisk*), as is that of the central pulmonary arteries. Reverse flow is no longer evident in the azygos vein. The patient experienced marked symptomatic relief following endovascular therapy. Reproduced courtesy of Dr. K. Malagari

aggravates symptoms and signs. Laryngeal edema and, in severe cases, stupor and coma may ensue. Lung cancer is by far the most common cause of the syndrome (70%), although several other conditions have been described in its etiology (Table 9.2). Because of the localization of the causative process in the mediastinum, superior vena cava syndrome may coexist with other mediastinal syndromes such as dysphagia, vocal hoarseness, and dyspnea due to large airways obstruction.

The severity of superior vena cava syndrome depends upon the rapidity of occlusion and collateral vessel development; the more acute the occlusion, the more severe the syndrome. Collateral venous return to the heart, in the case of obstruction, occurs through four principal pathways: (1) the azygous venous system, which include the azygous vein, the hemiazygous vein, and the connecting intercostal veins, (2) the internal mammary venous system plus the tributaries and the secondary communications to the superior and inferior epigastric veins, and (3) and (4) the long thoracic venous system with its connections to the femoral and vertebral veins, respectively. In the absence of tracheal compression and airway compromise, superior vena cava syndrome is rarely an oncologic emergency [17]. In the majority of cases there is enough time to obtain an etiological diagnosis and decide upon adequate and specific management. Chemotherapy and radiotherapy are effective in relieving symptoms in lung-cancer-related superior vena cava syndrome. The insertion of stents may provide a more rapid relief from symptoms (Fig. 9.3 A–C) [18].

9.3.3   Recurrent Laryngeal and Phrenic Nerve Palsy

Compression, entrapment, or invasion of the recurrent laryngeal nerve by the primary cancer or its nodal metastases around the aortic arc, leads to hoarseness. Hoarseness is an uncommon sign at presentation and appears late in the natural history of the disease. Recurrent laryngeal nerve palsy predisposes to lung aspiration and is associated with ineffective ability to cough and expectorate. Rarely, recurrent laryngeal nerve palsy manifests with dysphagia both for solid and liquid foods, since this nerve contributes to the innervation of the cricoid muscles and the proximal esophagus.

Neoplastic involvement can also affect the phrenic nerve, leading to hemidiaphragmatic paresis or paralysis. Clinically, phrenic nerve palsy may be asymptomatic in patients with good respiratory reserve, or may manifest with dyspnea on exertion or even at rest in the respiratory-compromised patient. Chest roentgenogram shows hemidiaphragmatic elevation, while fluoroscopy or ultrasound examination during the sniff maneuver unequivocally poses the diagnosis by disclosing the paradoxical movement of the involved hemidiaphragm.

9.3.4   Chest Wall Invasion

Chest wall invasion refers to the direct involvement by the lung cancer in the rib cage, the vertebral bodies, the diaphragm, and the structures that form the anatomical limits of the superior pulmonary sulcus. Ribcage and vertebral-body invasion leads to pain in the involved area that is usually dull, intermittent, and aching, lasting from minutes to hours. The invasion of the central dome of the diaphragm manifests with pain in the ipsilateral shoulder. Superior pulmonary sulcus carcinoma leads to the characteristic Pancoast's syndrome, as mentioned above. Limited and circumscribed chest wall invasion belongs to the T3 category, which also includes invasion of the mediastinal pleura or the parietal

pericardium and is considered resectable by current surgical techniques (vertebral body invasion is considered T4 category).

9.3.5   Pleural Involvement

Lung cancer is the leading cause of malignant pleural effusion [19]. A pleural effusion is observed in 15% of patients at their first evaluation. However, during the course of the disease at least 50% of patients with disseminated disease will develop a pleural effusion. The mechanisms by which a lung cancer leads to pleural effusion are several and may be distinguished directly and indirectly [20]. Direct mechanisms include: (1) the pleural metastatic involvement that induces an increased pleural permeability, (2) the pleural metastatic involvement that induces obstruction of the lymphatic vessels and decreased pleural fluid drainage, (3) the mediastinal lymph node involvement that also leads to decrease pleural lymphatic drainage, (4) the thoracic duct interruption that leads to chylothorax, (5) the large bronchi obstruction that leads to atelectasis and decreases the intrapleural pressure, thus increasing fluid formation, and finally (6) the pericardial effusion that may increase hydrostatic pressures in both the systemic and pulmonary circulation. Indirect mechanisms of pleural effusion formation in lung cancer patients include: (1) hypoproteinemia, (2) postobstructive pneumonitis, (3) pulmonary embolism, and (4) postradiation therapy. When symptomatic, pleural involvement manifests itself with dyspnea, pain, and cough. In patients with lung cancer, pleural effusion is an exudate, and in the large majority of cases indicates that the patient is not curable with surgery [20]. In cytology-negative pleural effusions, a thoracoscopy and a CT scan of the chest to evaluate the mediastinal nodes are necessary to consider operability. Occasionally, pleural involvement in lung cancer may manifest with spontaneous pneumothorax.

9.3.6   Heart Involvement

The mechanisms by which lung cancer leads to pericardium and heart involvement are several and include: (1) retrograde lymphatic migration of tumor cells, (2) hematogenous dissemination, and (3) direct tumor invasion. The pericardial neoplastic involvement usually presents as pericardial effusion, cardiac tamponade, or constrictive pericarditis [21]. Malignant pericardial effusion is often asymptomatic and discovered by imaging or at autopsy. When clinically evident, it most commonly manifests with the onset of an arrhythmia (sinus tachycardia or atrial fibrillation) and enlargement of the cardiac shadow in the chest roentgenogram, or with signs of congestive heart failure or tamponade. Unlike pericardial neoplastic involvement, myocardial neoplastic involvement is more frequently silent and discovered only at autopsy or, less often, during surgery. Echocardiography is the primary imaging tool used to establish the presence of a pericardial effusion. It is also useful to quantify the volume of the neoplastic effusion and to evaluate its hemodynamic effects, particularly the presence of tamponade or constrictive pericarditis. Malignant pericardial effusion with mild hemodynamic compromise may be treated conservatively with careful monitoring, repeated echocardiography, fluid administration, and in the presence of a definitive histological diagnosis, specific therapy aimed at the underlying malignancy [22]. Cardiac tamponade and overt hemodynamic compromise requires removal of the fluid by percutaneous catheter pericardiocentesis [23, 24]. When the malignant pericardial effusion does not respond, substernal pericardiostomy or surgical-limited or radical pericardiectomy may be attempted [23].

9.3.7 Esophageal Involvement

Esophageal displacement and deformity is common in patients with lung cancer and may be related to the primary tumor or, more commonly, to its nodal metastases. However, displacement and deformity are not enough to lead to obstructive symptoms and clinically evident dysphagia. Esophageal invasion by the primary tumor, which more commonly occurs when this develops in the left main stem bronchus, is more likely to lead to obstruction, thus manifesting with dysphagia. In rare cases, a bronchoesophageal fistula may develop and manifests with cough upon swallowing or aspiration.

The American Joint Commission on Cancer staging system classifies the nodal involvement of the non-small-cell primary lung cancer as follows [3, 9]: N (node) 1, involvement of the ipsilateral peribronchial or hilar nodes and intrapulmonary nodes by direct extension; N2, involvement of ipsilateral mediastinal or subcarinal nodes; N3, involvement of contralateral lung nodes or any supraclavicular node.

9.4 Symptoms and Signs due to Distant Extrathoracic Spread of the Primary Tumor

Widespread hematogenous dissemination occurs early in lung cancer patients. Metastases may involve any organ or system [25], and are present in approximately one-third of these patients at presentation. Small-cell and poorly differentiated carcinomas present with a higher tendency to metastasize, followed by the adenocarcinomas, large-cell carcinomas, and squamous cell carcinomas. The most common sites of distant metastases are: (1) the brain, where metastases may manifest with symptoms and signs of increased intracranial pressure and/or neurologic deficits, (2) the bones, where symptoms include pain and pathological fractures, (3) the liver, where metastases may manifest with fever, biochemical abnormalities, pain, and general symptoms such as anorexia, weakness, and weight loss, (4) the spinal bones and the relative epidural tissues, where metastases manifest with spinal cord compression syndromes, and (5) the adrenal glands, which are clinically silent.

The distal metastases of the non-small-cell primary lung cancer according to the staging system developed by the American Joint commission on cancer are classified as stage IV disease [3, 9].

Summarizing the case for the non-small-cell lung cancer, the current classification states as: (1) local disease, IA if T1N0M0, IB if T2N0M0, and IIA if T1N1M0, (2) locally advanced disease, IIB, if T2, N1,M0 or T3N0M0, IIIA if T1N2M0, or T2N2M0, or T3N1M0, or T3N2M0 and IIIB if any TN3M0, and (3) advanced disease, IIIB if T4 any NM0, and IV if any T any NM1 [3, 9].

9.4.1 Nonspecific Systemic Effects Related to Lung Cancer

Systemic symptoms such as anorexia leading to weight loss and cachexia, and generalized malaise occur in at least 20% of patients with advanced disease and contribute considerably to poor performance status [26]. Tumor necrosis factor-a and related cytokines have been considered to be involved in the pathogenesis of this generalized tissue-wasting syndrome.

9.4.2 Paraneoplastic Endocrine Syndromes Associated with the Lung Cancer

A paraneoplastic syndrome is the constellation of symptoms and signs that appear in patients with malignancy unrelated to the local effects of the primary tumor or its metastases [5]. The pathogenetic mechanisms by which these syndromes occur are several and include the ectopic production of peptide proteins with hormonal activity, immunologic mechanisms, and other incompletely understood mechanisms. Paraneoplastic syndromes may affect virtually every organ system of the body, and in some cases herald the appearance or the recurrence of a cancer.

9.4.3   Ectopic Cushing's syndrome

A proportion estimated between 10 and 30% of Cushing's syndrome cases are caused by the ectopic production of adrenocorticotropic hormone (ACTH) by several neoplasms, and among them most commonly by lung cancer [5]. The normal human lung produces small amounts of the parent compound pro-opiomelanocortin (pro-OMCT), which is cleaved into several molecules including pro-ACTH and ACTH [27]. In the setting of the lung malignancy, most commonly in small-cell carcinoma or in carcinoid tumor, overexpression of the gene responsible for the production of the pro-OMCT may lead to clinically active levels of ACTH and the expression of the related syndromes. Clinically, ectopic Cushing's syndrome differs from the classic clinical expression of Cushing's disease (probably because of the presence of an aggressive malignancy) and manifests mainly with weight loss, peripheral edema, proximal myopathy, and moon face. Drowsiness, confusion, depression, and frank psychosis may also occur. Hypokalemia, alkalosis, and hyperglycemia are the most common biochemical abnormalities observed. Diagnostic validity for an ectopic Cushing's syndrome present the finding of elevated 24-h urinary free-cortisol levels, an elevated plasma cortisol level, and an elevated plasma ACTH that does not decrease after a high-dose dexamethasone suppression test, in the presence of malignancy. Ectopic Cushing's syndrome has been associated with decreased survival in lung cancer patients [28], decreased chemoresponsiveness, and an increase in chemotherapy-related complications including severe opportunistic infections [5]. Effective treatment of the underlying tumor may contribute to improvement of the clinical picture for these patients. If this is not feasible and the patients experience significant clinical effects or deterioration, steroid-synthesis inhibitors, such as aminoglutetimide, mitotane, metyrapone, and ketoconazole, or ACTH-production suppressors, such as the somatostatin analogue octreotide, may offer some benefit. Bilateral adrenalectomy has also been attempted in severe cases.

9.4.4   Syndrome of Inappropriate Antidiuretic Hormone

The antidiuretic hormone (ADH) that is produced in the hypothalamus and secreted by the posterior pituitary gland is involved in the maintenance of extracellular fluid homeostasis. The ectopic secretion of clinically significant levels of ADH by lung cancer (most commonly small-cell carcinoma) manifests with hyponatremia and "inappropriate" natriuresis. When severe enough, it presents clinically with mental status changes, confusion, lethargy, seizures, and coma [5, 29]. The syndrome of inappropriate ADH is diagnosed when hyponatremia and decreased plasma osmolality coexist with "inappropriate" urine osmolality, in the presence of continued urinary sodium excretion. The syndrome resolves with chemotherapy for small-cell lung cancer and reappears when the cancer reoccurs. Specific measures for the treatment of severe hyponatremia include fluid restriction and the administration of demeclocycline, a drug that interferes with the activity of ADH at the renal collecting duct. In the case of severe symptomatic hyponatremia the administration of hypertonic saline and furosemide may become necessary. The rapid correction of hyponatremia should be obviated since this may lead to central pontine myelinolysis.

9.4.5   Hypercalcemia

Hypercalcemia occurs in approximately 1% of patients with lung cancer at presentation, but may affect up to 40% of patients at some point in their clinical course [5]. Hypercalcemia is due to either osteolytic bone destruction or ectopic hormone production. Hormonal hypercalcemia is the most common paraneoplastic syndrome in lung cancer patients (mainly squamous cell) and is related to the ectopic production of parathyroid hormone-related peptide (PTHrP) by the tumor. PTHrP is a 141-amino-acid protein that has parathyroid-hormone-like action that is mediated through its N-terminal sequences, which show some limited sequence homology with the hormone. The clinical picture of the syndrome includes neurological and gastrointestinal manifestations as well as dehydration. Fatigue, irritability, confusion, headache, drowsiness, lethargy, and coma may simulate cerebral metastases. Abdominal pain, anorexia, nausea, and vomiting are related to the gastrointestinal effects of the ectopic hormone. Occasionally, renal tubular damage due to hypercalcemia may lead to hypokalemic alkalosis. The rapid onset as well as the absence of nephrocalcinosis and ectopic soft-tissue calcifications may help to distinguish this disorder from primary hyperparathyroidism. Treatment of cancer-related hypercalcemia is mandatory, regardless of symptoms, when serum calcium is above 3.5 mmol/l (14 mg/dl) and includes vigorous intravenous hydration with normal saline and after with volume repletion loop diuretics. Biphosphonates (pamidronate), which act by reducing osteoclastic bone resorption, is the most effective specific treatment. Alternative drugs include gallium nitrate, calcitonin, and plicamycin. Radical lung cancer resection may resolve hypercalcemia in some patients.

9.4.6   Carcinoid Syndrome

Carcinoid syndrome was first described 44 years ago [30] and since then several cases have been described, mainly in patients with small-cell or undifferentiated lung carcinoma. The neoplasm secretes either 5-hydroxytryptamine or 5-hydroxytryptophan, and high levels of 5-hydroxyindoleacetic acid can be detected in the urine. The syndrome is characterized clinically by episodes of explosive diarrhea, cutaneous flushing, tachycardia, anorexia, and weight loss. The expression of this syndrome coexists with the presence of multiple liver metastases, as is the case with the gastrointestinal and pulmonary carcinoid tumors.

9.4.7 Miscellaneous

Secretion of human chorionic gonadotropin accompanied with relative clinical signs and symptoms is rare in lung cancer patients and occurs mainly in large-cell carcinoma. Affected men present with gynecomastia, testicular atrophy, and a high-pitched voice. Calcitonin production is common in patients with lung cancer. It usually remains an asymptomatic biochemical abnormality.

9.4.8 Paraneoplastic Neurologic Syndromes

Paraneoplastic neurologic syndromes may affect any component of the nervous system from the central nervous system to the striated muscles and present with an extensive list of clinical syndromes. These syndromes may develop well before lung cancer is clinically and roentgenologically evident, and may present an independent clinical course from the primary disease. Most of the paraneoplastic neurological syndromes associated with lung cancer appear to share a common autoimmune pathogenetic mechanism related to the fact that lung cancer and the nervous system have common antigens and may become the target of autoantibodies [31]. In recent years several autoantibodies have been identified in patients with neurologic paraneoplastic syndromes recognizing nuclear and cytoplasmic antigens of neurons in the brain, spinal cord, and ganglia. The association between paraneoplastic neurologic syndrome and a specific antinuclear autoantibody, type-1 antineuronal nuclear antibody (ANNA-1, or anti-Hu) has been described in subacute sensory peripheral neuropathy and paraneoplastic encephalomyelitis. Autoantibodies against retinal antigens have been associated with cancer-associated retinopathy and autoantibodies against P/Q-type voltage-gated calcium channels have been associated with Lambert-Eaton myasthenic syndrome. Small-cell lung cancer is the most common type of lung cancer associated with these syndromes. After studying autoimmune-mediated paraneoplastic neurologic syndromes, it soon became evident that neither removal of the autoantibodies (e.g., by plasma exchange) nor suppression of the inflammation with specific cytotoxic drugs affected the clinical course of this neurological disorder. This might be related to the fact that damage is rapid and irreparable, or that autoantibodies are produced locally in the neural tissue and not removed by plasma exchange.

9.4.9 Paraneoplastic Encephalomyelitis and the Anti-Hu Antibody Syndrome

Encephalomyelitis may involve several areas of the nervous system, producing several neurological syndromes such as: (1) paraneoplastic limbic encephalitis due to involvement of the limbic region, presenting with mood and behavior changes, memory loss progressing to dementia, and seizures, (2) paraneoplastic cerebellar degeneration due to the involvement of the cerebellum, presenting with ataxia, nystagmus, dysarthria, and diplopia, and ends by limiting the ability of the patient to ambulate, (3) autonomic neuropathy due to the involvement of the autonomic nervous system, presenting with symptoms of autonomic dysfunction such as orthostatic hypotension, neurogenic bladder, and intestinal pseudo-obstruction (Ogilvies's syndrome), and (4) opsoclonus-myoclonus paraneoplastic syndrome. Anti-Hu antibody syndrome is known as the encephalomyelitis and sensory neuropathy syndrome associated with the type-1 antineuronal nuclear autoantibody ANNA-type1 or anti-Hu.

9.4.10 Cancer-Associated Retinopathy

Cancer-associated retinopathy is rare and presents with rapid vision loss, night blindness, color loss, and central or ring scotomas. It is associated with autoantibodies against several retinal proteins.

9.4.11 Lambert-Eaton Myasthenic Syndrome

Lambert-Eaton myasthenic syndrome is the most common and the better-studied neurologic paraneoplastic syndrome, with a prevalence of 3% in patients with small-cell lung cancer. This syndrome is mainly characterized clinically by proximal muscle weakness that is more prevalent in the lower extremities, fatigue, and depression of the deep tendon reflexes. Lambert-Eaton myasthenic syndrome is associated with autoantibodies against P/Q-type voltage-gated calcium channels. A transient increase in strength with repetitive action, lack of palpebral muscle involvement, and failure to improve with the administration of anticholinesterases help in the differential diagnosis from myasthenia gravis.

9.4.12 Cutaneous Paraneoplastic Manifestations

Lung cancer is occasionally associated with a variety of cutaneous paraneoplastic manifestations including: (1) acquired hypertrichosis lanuginosa, an excess growth of fine lanugo hair on the hair-bearing surfaces of the body, (2) Bazex's disease, an erythematous hyperkeratosis with scales and pruritus on the palms and soles, (3) erythema gyratus repens, consisting of a marbled erythematous swirling and a thin covering of scale over the trunk, axilla, and groin, (4) Leser-Trelat syndrome, which is characterized by the sudden appearance of a large crop of hyperpigmented seborrhoeic keratoses, (5) acanthosis nigricans, a bilaterally symmetric hyperkeratosis and hyperpigmentation of the skin that mainly involves the flexural and intertriginous areas, and several other, less commonly occurring manifestations [2, 4, 32]. Cutaneous paraneoplastic manifestations may coincide, follow, or antedate the diagnosis of lung cancer, or herald its recurrence. Since they may be the presenting sign of an occult carcinoma, recognition of their features is of paramount importance for early detection, although their presence is often associated with a poor prognosis.

9.4.13 Coagulopathies and Hematologic Manifestations

Several hematologic manifestations may occur during the natural history of lung cancer, including: (1) normochromic, normocytic or hypochromic, microcytic anemia, (2) neutrophilic leukocytosis and lymphocytopenia, (3) leukemoid reactions, (4) peripheral eosinophilia either associated or not with eosinophilic pulmonary infiltrates (eosinophilic pneumonia), (5) thrombocytosis, (6) thrombocytopenia and purpura, and (7) hemolytic anemia associated with disseminated intravascular coagulation.

Migratory thrombophlebitis (Trousseau's sign) and thromboembolic disease have been well documented in patients with lung cancer [33]. Thrombophlebitis is typically migratory, may involve any vessel including unusual sites, and tends to be resistant to anticoagulant treatment. Occasionally, thrombophlebitis, either with or without pulmonary embolism, constitutes the first manifestation of an occult lung carcinoma.

Thrombotic nonbacterial (marantic) endocarditis is a rare and late manifestation in lung cancer. It involves mainly the valves of the left side of the heart and presents with emboli to the brain or other organs.

9.4.14 Paraneoplastic Rheumatic Syndromes

Lung cancer is occasionally associated with a variety of rheumatological syndromes, including dermatomyositis/polymyositis, vasculitis, and carcinoma polyarthritis [34, 35]. Paraneoplastic rheumatic syndromes may coincide, follow, or antedate the diagnosis of lung cancer, or herald its recurrence [36].

9.4.15 Renal Manifestations

Both glomerulonephritis and nephrotic syndromes have occasionally been associated with lung cancer and are recognized as paraneoplastic syndromes.

9.4.16 Pierre Marie-Bamberger syndrome (Secondary Hypertrophic Osteoarthropathy)

Hypertrophic osteoarthropathy is characterized by the coexistence of finger clubbing, subperiosteal new bone formation, mainly along the long bones of the extremities, and arthritis. Finger clubbing can occur as an isolated manifestation in lung cancer patients. Hypertrophic osteoarthropathy is one of the most commonly occurring paraneoplastic syndromes in lung cancer and is usually observed in squamous cell and adenocarcinomas, while it is extremely rare in the small-cell carcinoma. Finger clubbing is related to the local vascular neoformation in the nail bed and the volar pad of the distal phalanx of the digits. The pathogenesis of hypertrophic pulmonary osteoarthropathy is associated with the presence of megakaryocytes and platelet clumps that find access at the distal arterial (digital) circulation through right to left shunting within the pulmonary circulation. Localized neovascular formation and proliferation is associated with platelet-induced endothelial activation and the production in the local circulation of growth factors such as platelet-derived growth factor and others [37, 38]. Joint manifestations vary from arthralgia to painful arthritis involving the knees, ankles, and wrists. Isolated clubbing is usually asymptomatic and is often first noted by the physician. In order to effectively identify clubbing, a value of the digital profile angle greater than $180°$ and a phalangeal depth ratio greater than 1 are necessary [39]. Roentgenologic findings include periosteal thickening of the long bones, soft-tissue swelling, and high radioactive tracer uptake along the involved bones (Fig. 9.4). The bony alterations at the distal phalanxes and on the periostium of the long bones of the extremities may remain indelible several centuries after the death of the individual [40].

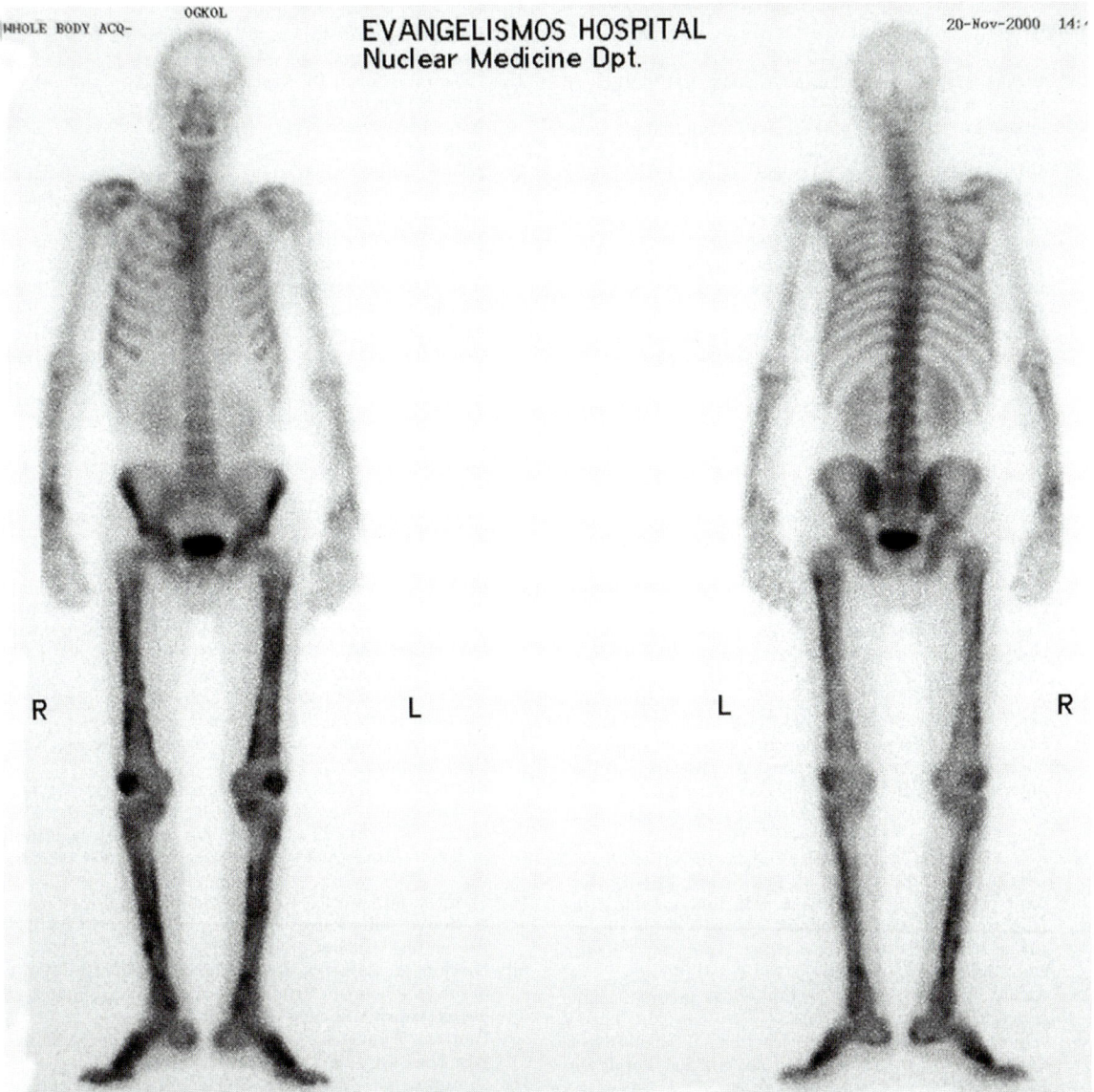

Fig. 9.4. Pierre Marie-Bamberger syndrome (secondary hypertrophic osteoarthropathy) in a patient with squamous lung cancer. The high uptake of radioactive tracer is clearly seen along the long bones of the extremities and the pelvis. *R* Right side, *L* left side. Reproduced courtesy of Dr. Ph. Rondogianni

Key Points

- Lung cancer is usually recognized late in its natural history. Late recognition relates to disseminated and unresectable disease at presentation.
- The clinical presentation of lung cancer usually relates to the development of a new, or worsening of a preexisting clinical symptom or sign and, less frequently, to an abnormal chest roentgenographic shadow in an asymptomatic patient.
- Lung cancer symptoms are multiple and variable and can be the result of the local growth of the primary tumor, its extension to the adjacent intrathoracic structures, or its distant metastases.
- Nonspecific systemic effects, and symptoms due to an immunologic response to or ectopic production of peptide proteins (hormones) by the same lung cancer or its metastases (paraneoplastic syndromes) may be present.
- Paraneoplastic syndromes may coincide, follow, or antedate the diagnosis of lung cancer, or herald its recurrence.

References

1. Beckles AM, Spiro SG, Colice GL, Rudd RM. Initial evaluation of the patient with lung cancer. Symptoms, signs, laboratory tests, and paraneoplastic syndromes. Chest 2003; 123:97S.
2. Scagliotti GV. Symptoms, signs and staging of lung cancer. Eur Respir Mon 2001; 17:86.
3. Spira A, Ettinger DS. Multidisciplinary management of lung cancer. N Engl J Med 2004; 350:379.
4. Fraser RS, Müller NL, Colman N, Paré PD. Fraser and Paré's Diagnosis of Diseases of the Lung. WB Saunders, Philadelphia, 1999.
5. Gerber RB, Mazzone P, Arroliga AC. Paraneoplastic syndromes associated with bronchogenic carcinoma. Clin Chest Med 2002; 23(1):257.
6. Grippi MA. Clinical aspects of lung cancer. Semin Roentgenol 1990; 25:12.
7. Santiago SM, Lehrman S, Williams AJ. Bronchoscopy in patients with haemoptysis and normal chest roentgenograms. Br J Dis Chest 1987; 81(2):186.
8. Snider GL, Placik B. The relationship between pulmonary tuberculosis and bronchogenic carcinoma: a topographic study. Am Rev Respir Dis 1969; 99(2):229.
9. Mountain CF, Dresler CM. Regional lymph node classification for lung cancer staging. Chest 1997; 111:1718.
10. Pancoast HK. Superior pulmonary sulcus tumor: tumor characterized by pain, Horner's syndrome, destruction of bone and atrophy of hand muscles. JAMA 1932; 99:1391.
11. Arcasoy SM, Jett JR. Superior pulmonary sulcus tumors and Pancoast syndrome. N Engl J Med 1997; 337:1370.
12. Paulson DL. Treatment of superior sulcus carcinoma. In: Fishmans AP (ed.) Update: Pulmonary Diseases and Disorders. McGrow and Hill, New York, 1982; p 318.
13. Jett JR. Superior sulcus tumors and Pancoast's syndrome. Lung Cancer 2003; 42:S17.
14. Komaki R, Roth JA, Walsh GL, Putnam JB, Vaporciyan A, Lee JS, Fossella FV, Chasen M, Delclos ME, Cox JD. Outcome predictors for 143 patients with superior sulcus tumors treated by multidisciplinary approach at the University of Texas MD Anderson Cancer Center. Int J Radiat Oncol Biol Phys 2000; 48:347.
15. Archie VC, Thomas CR. Superior sulcus tumors: a mini review. Oncologist 2004; 9:550.
16. Yellin A, Rosen A, Reichert N, Lieberman Y. Superior vena cava syndrome: the myth – the facts. Am Rev Respir Dis 1990; 141:1114.
17. Wudel LJ, Nesbitt JC. Superior vena cava syndrome. Curr Treat Options Oncol 2001; 2(1):77.
18. Rowel NP, Gleeson FV. Steroids, radiotherapy, chemotherapy and stents for superior vena caval obstruction in carcinoma of the bronchus: a systematic review. Clin Oncol (R Coll Radiol) 2002; 14:338.
19. Light RW. Pleural Diseases, 4th edn. Lippincott, Williams and Wilkins, Philadelphia, 2001.
20. Rodriguez-Panadero F. Lung cancer and ipsilateral pleural effusion. Ann Oncol 1995; 6:S25.
21. Wilkes JD, Fidias, P, Vaickus, L, Perez, RP. Malignancy-related pericardial effusion. 127 cases from the Roswell Park Cancer Institute. Cancer 1995; 76:1377.
22. Laham RJ, Cohen DJ, Kuntz RE, Baim DS, Lorell BH, Simons M. Pericardial effusion in patients with cancer: outcome with contemporary management strategies. Heart 1996; 75:67.
23. Allen KB, Faber LP, Warren WH, Shaar CJ. Pericardial effusion: subxiphoid pericardiostomy versus percutaneous catheter drainage. Ann Thorac Surg 1999; 67:437.
24. Tsang TSM, Freeman WK, Sinak LJ, Seward JB. Echocardiographically guided pericardiocentesis: evolution and state-of-the-art technique. Mayo Clin Proc 1998; 73(7):647.
25. Pauzner R, Istomin V, Segal-Lieberman G Matetzky S, Farfel Z. Bilateral patellar metastases as the clinical presentation of bronchogenic adenocarcinoma. J Rheum 1996; 23:939.
26. Andersen HA, Prakash UBS. Diagnosis of symptomatic lung cancer. Semin Respir Med 1982; 3:165.
27. Mendelsohn G, Baylin SB. Ectopic hormone production: biological and clinical implications. Prog Clin Biol Res 1984; 142:291.
28. Dimopoulos AM, Fernandez JF, Samaan NA Holoye PY, Vassilopoulou-Sellin R. Paraneoplastic Cushing's syndrome as an adverse prognostic factor in patients who die early with small cell lung cancer. Cancer 1992; 69:66.
29. Johnson BE, Chute JP, Rusdin J, Williams J, Le PT, Venzon D, Richardson GE. A prospective study of patients with lung cancer and hyponatremia of malignancy. Am J Respir Crit Care Med 1997; 156(5):1669.
30. Williams ED, Azzopardi JG. Tumours of the lung and the carcinoid syndrome. Thorax 1960; 15:30.
31. Posner JB, Dalmau J. Paraneoplastic syndromes. Curr Opin Immunol 1997; 9:723.
32. Kurzrock R, Cohen PR. Cutaneous paraneoplastic syndromes in solid tumors. Am J Med 1995; 99(6):662.
33. Rickles FR, Edwards RL. Activation of blood coagulation in cancer: Trousseau's syndrome revisited. Blood 1983; 66; 14.
34. Masin N, Buchard PA, Gerster JC. Polymyalgia rheumatica et cancer pulmonaire: syndrome paraneoplastique. Rev Rheum Mal Osteoartic 1992; 59:153.
35. Naschitz JE, Rosner I, Rozenbaum M, Zuckerman E, Yeshurun D. Rheumatic syndromes: clues to occult neoplasia. Semin Arthritis Rheum 1999; 29(1):43.
36. Fam AG. Paraneoplastic rheumatic syndromes. Baillieres Best Pract Res Clin Rheumatol 2000; 14(3):515.
37. Dickinson CJ, Martin JF. Megakaryocytes and platelet clumps as the cause of finger clubbing. Lancet 1987; 2:1434.
38. Dickinson CJ. The aetiology of clubbing and hypertrophic osteoarthropathy. Eur J Clin Invest 1993; 23(6):330.
39. Meyers KA, Farquhar DR. The rational clinical examination. Does this patient have clubbing? JAMA 2001; 286(3):341.
40. Martinez-Lavin M. Hypertrophic osteoarthropathy. Curr Opin Rheumatol 1997; 9(1):83.

The Role of Bronchoscopy and the Diagnosis and Staging of Lung Cancer

10

Pallav L. Shah

Contents

10.1 Introduction

Bronchoscopy is one of the key investigations in the diagnosis and staging of patients with suspected lung cancer. It should be utilized in conjunction with a clinical assessment and radiological evaluation of the patient. The symptoms and signs that should prompt further assessment are listed in Table 10.1. We advocate a low threshold for performing a chest radiograph in patients with clinical features suspicious of neoplasia, and computed tomography (CT) of the thorax and abdomen in patients with a significant suspicion of lung cancer. Bronchoscopy compliments the assessment of these patients and allows visual examination of the vocal cords, trachea, and endobronchial tree down to the subsegmental level. Specimens can also be obtained during flexible bronchoscopy.

Table 10.1. Clinical features suspicious of neoplasia

Symptoms
- hemoptysis
- persistent cough
- recurrent infections

Signs
- stridor
- unexplained paralysis of vocal cords
- unexplained paralysis of hemidiaphragm
- localized monophonic wheeze
- unexplained pleural effusion
- segmental or lobar collapse

10.2 Equipment

The flexible bronchoscope consists of a flexible tube, the distal end of which can be angulated through 160° by a lever at the head of the scope. There are bundles of fibers within the tube that carry light to the distal end, illuminating the airways, and a further bundle to transmit the image to the eyepiece. There is also an instrument channel that allows procedures such as biopsy sampling to be performed. This channel also functions as a suction channel. A variety of instruments are available with different-sized instrument channels and various external diameters. These characteristics influence the use of the bronchoscope; for example, bronchoscopes with larger instrument channels are more suitable for interventional procedures. Videobronchoscopes are also becoming more widespread; these have a charged couple device (CCD chip) at the distal end, which allows the image to be projected onto a monitor. The latest system utilizes high-definition TV technology and produces high-quality, full-screen images, which significantly enhance diagnosis.

10.3 Patient Preparation and Procedure

Flexible bronchoscopy is usually performed with or without conscious sedation as an outpatient procedure. Verbal and written instructions should be given to the patients. They should be specifically advised not to eat or drink for at least 4 h before the procedure. Patients who are sedated should have an escort to accompany them home and ide-

Table 10.2. Preparation for bronchoscopy

- Patient information; verbal and written
- Informed consent
- Full blood count and clotting prior to transbronchial lung biopsy
- Baseline ECG if history of cardiac disease
- Spirometry if oxygen saturations less than 95%
- Arterial blood gases if oxygen saturation less than 95%
- Intravenous access
- Consider bronchodilators if evidence of bronchospasm
- Prophylactic antibiotics if asplenia, heart valve prosthesis, cardiac murmur, or history of endocarditis

ally have supervision for a 24-h period. Appropriate radiology (chest radiographs and ideally CT of the thorax) should be available for review prior to the procedure. A full blood count and coagulation study should be performed on all patients being considered for a transbronchial lung biopsy procedure. Arterial blood gases and spirometry should be performed if the patient is dyspneic and oxygen saturations are less than 95% on air, or if hypercapnea is suspected (Table 10.2). During the procedure, arterial oxygenation is monitored by pulse oximetry and patients are given supplemental oxygen to maintain oxygen saturations above 90%. Continuous ECG monitoring should be performed in all patients with a history of cardiac disease or where the hypoxia cannot be corrected.

10.4   Diagnosis of Lung Cancer

10.4.1   Central Lesions

Flexible bronchoscopy enables visual inspection and biopsy sampling from the main airways down to the segmental levels for diagnostic purposes. The external diameter of the bronchoscope determines the size of the airways that can be reached. The endobronchial appearance of bronchial neoplasia ranges from exophytic polypoid lesions through to subtle mucosal irregularities (Fig. 10.1). In submucosal disease there may be thickening of the airway and changes in the mucosal folds. Tumor masses and enlarged lymph nodes may also lead to extrinsic compression of the airway.

Where an exophytic lesion is visible, pathological confirmation should be achieved in over 90% of patients. A combination of techniques can be used to obtain samples for diagnosis. Bronchial washing involves the instillation of 20-ml aliquots of normal saline around the site of the abnormality. The success rates associated with bronchial washing alone is around 31–50% [1, 2]. Biopsy forceps can be inserted through the instrument channel of the bronchoscope and pinch biopsies obtained under direct vision. Several biopsy specimens should be obtained in order to ensure that adequate tissue has been obtained for diagnosis. A cytology brush can also be used to scrape some cells from the surface of any abnormal areas. For submucosal lesions, a transbronchial fine needle can also be inserted through the mucosa into the lesion and a few cells aspirated for a cytological analysis [3].

A recent review evaluated 30 studies where the yield from the different bronchoscopic techniques was evaluated in at least 50 patients with suspected lung cancer [4]. The sensitivity from cytological techniques such as bronchial washing was 48% (range 21–76%), that from bronchial brushing was 59% (range 23–93%), and that from endobronchial fine-needle aspiration of mucosal lesions was around 56% (range 23–90%). A higher yield was obtained from endobronchial biopsy procedures, with an overall sensitivity of 74% (range 4–97%). The collective sensitivity when all the modalities are used is 88% (range 67–97%) for central lesions that are visible at bronchoscopy.

Bronchial biopsy specimens can either be first rinsed in saline or rolled onto a glass slide in order to further increase the diagnostic yield. The latter is known as imprint cytology, where any loose cells from the biopsy specimen are fixed onto a glass slide and may allow cytological analysis [5]. However, this technique may damage the biopsy specimen and impair its histological

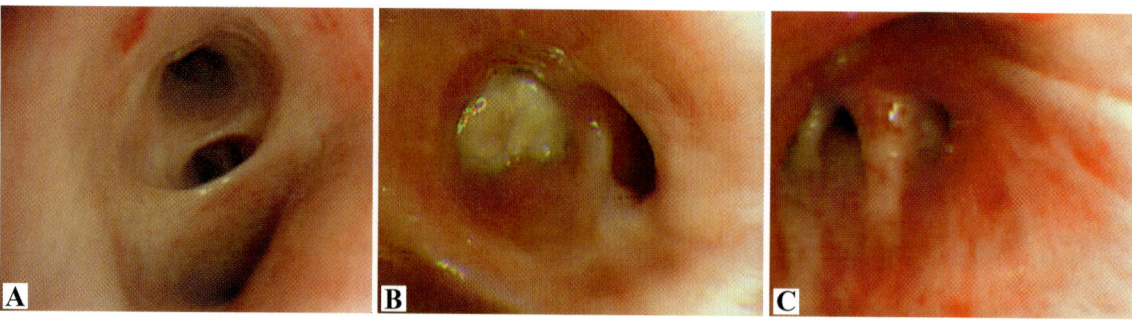

Fig. 10.1. Videbronchoscopy appearance of normal endobronchial airway at the segmental level (**A**), a polypoid exophytic tumor (**B**), and a submucosal lesion (**C**)

analysis. The former technique is simple and involves placing the biopsy samples first in saline solution and then transferring them at the end of the procedure into formalin. The saline solution may contain some cells that can be evaluated by cytology [6]. This technique has been shown to improve the diagnostic yield, and in one study four additional patients were identified from a total of 93 patients (added yield of 4.8%).

Review of a recent CT scan prior to flexible bronchoscopy significantly improves the yield from the procedure. A study by Laroche [7] randomized 171 patients who were being evaluated for suspected lung cancer. All patients had a CT scan performed prior to the procedure, but in one group the scans were reviewed before the procedure, whereas in another group the procedure was performed without any knowledge of the CT findings (control group). The yield for the procedure was 73% in the group where the CT scan was reviewed prior to the procedure, compared to 54% in the control group. Furthermore, fewer investigations were required in the group where the CT scan was reviewed compared to the group without CT review prior to procedure. Hence, it is more cost-effective for a scan to be performed and reviewed prior to bronchoscopy. We advocate this for all patients undergoing assessment for possible lung cancer. It also allows additional staging procedures such as transbronchial needle aspiration (TBNA; see below) to be performed at the same time as the initial diagnostic bronchoscopy.

10.4.2   Peripheral Lesions

Where abnormalities are beyond the reach of the bronchoscope, the segment involved can be determined from the CT scan. The bronchoscope is then wedged into the appropriate segment and 60-ml aliquots of saline are instilled into the segment. The aspirate is then sent off for cytological analysis. This technique has an overall yield of 43% (range 12–65%) [8, 9]. Selective brushing of the affected segment is more effective and has a greater yield (52%, range 21–84%).

For selected lesions it is possible to use two-dimensional fluoroscopic guidance to sample lesions that are just beyond the visibility of the bronchoscope. The yield is dependent on the size and location of the abnormality. The diagnostic yield for lesions greater than 20 mm in diameter is between 30 and 50%, whereas the yield for nodules less than 20 mm is less than 10%. TBNA can also be utilized with fluoroscopic guidance for selected peripheral lesions [10]. The yield is marginally better than with forceps biopsy. The diagnostic yield of peripheral lesions improves when these techniques are performed in combination. The main limitation of these techniques is that it is still difficult to be certain that the forceps or needle have reached the lesion.

10.4.3   Endobronchial Ultrasound-Guided Peripheral Lung Biopsy

Two new bronchoscopic techniques promise improved sensitivity in the diagnosis of peripheral pulmonary lesions. The first utilizes a miniature vascular ultrasound probe with a guide sheet, in conjunction with fluoroscopy. The guide sheet and probe are inserted through the instrument channel of the bronchoscope, advanced until there is resistance, and then withdrawn slightly and the site scanned with the radial ultrasound probe. Normal lung does not produce an ultrasonic image, but when the tumor is reached the ultrasound image demonstrates a solid lesion. The probe is then withdrawn whilst maintaining the position of the guide sheet. Aspiration needles and biopsy forceps can then be inserted through the sheet to a marked distance and samples obtained. Where no signal is detected, the probe is replaced with an angulated curette and this is then maneuvered under fluoroscopic guidance into an alternate bronchial segment. A further attempt can then be made with the ultrasound probe to locate the lesion. A recent study has evaluated this technique in 150 patients with a peripheral lesion and a definitive diagnosis was obtained in 116 patients (sensitivity of 77%) [11]. The yield is higher in lesions greater than 30 mm in size.

10.4.4   Magnetic-Navigation-Guided Lung Biopsy

Magnetic positional tip technology can also be utilized with bronchoscopy to improve the diagnostic yield in peripheral lesions. A spiral CT with 1.5- to 3-mm reconstructions is required; a catheter with a magnetic tracking device is then inserted through the instrument channel (SuperDimensions Bronchus) and the catheter tip position calibrated at 3–6 points with the aid of a CT scan. The system can then be used to guide the catheter and magnetic tracking device to the target lesion. Once the target is reached the tracking device is removed, the biopsy forceps or needle is inserted through the catheter, and appropriate samples can be obtained for diagnosis.

10.5   Staging

Staging information is also obtained at routine bronchoscopy. Tumors are staged as T3 where there is infiltration within 1 cm of the carina or T4 where there is infiltration into the trachea.

10.5.1   Transbronchial Fine-Needle Aspiration

This is a technique that provides both diagnostic and staging information in patients suspected of lung cancer. In over 25% of procedures it is also the sole diagnostic modality. Once again, the technique is dependent upon the availability of a recent CT scan of the thorax prior to bronchoscopy. Virtually all mediastinal and hilar lymph nodes greater than 10 mm in cross-section can be sampled by TBNA. A variety of TBNA needles are available and the basic principle involves appropriate planning of the site of needle insertion from the CT scan. The TBNA needle is then inserted through the bronchoscopic channel at the appropriate point through the airway. It is then pushed all the way through and suction is applied to the other end with a 20-ml syringe. A jabbing action during the procedure allows cytological material to be aspirated into the needle. The sample obtained is then spread on to slides or injected into a liquid medium and sent for cytological analysis. TBNA is performed prior to inspection of the airways so as not to contaminate the samples and minimize the risk of false-positive results. This is important as TBNA in this context provides both diagnostic and staging information. On-site cytological analysis appears to enhance the diagnostic yield of TBNA and reduces the number of samples that are required for diagnosis [12]. Negative TBNA results do not exclude neoplastic disease and should be followed up by further investigations such as mediastinoscopy in appropriate cases. TBNA is a very safe and effective technique. Complications are rare and consist of pneumothorax, pneumomediastinum, and bleeding. [13]. However, despite the potential benefits and relative safety, this technique is underutilized [14].

10.5.2   Endobronchial-Ultrasound-Guided TBNA

Endobronchial ultrasound may be utilized to prove the diagnostic yield for TBNA [15]. This is performed using a 20-mHz radial vascular mini ultrasound probe enclosed in a water-filled balloon sheet. This produces excellent images of the mediastinum and hilar structures and can provide information on vascular invasion and involvement of the different bronchial layers from the submucosa to the adventitia.

Prototype bronchoscopes have been developed that have a linear-array ultrasound probe integrated into a videobronchoscope, which allow simultaneous ultrasound and conventional bronchoscopic imaging. This integrated bronchoscope can be used to accurately assess the mediastinum and significantly improves the diagnosis and staging of patients with suspected lung cancer. The linear-array probe is applied against the tracheal wall and the mediastinum assessed for lymph nodes. Abnormal lymph nodes are visible as hypoechoic lesions. The Doppler mode allows these to be distinguished from blood vessels. The bronchoscope has a dedicated needle that can be inserted through the instrument channel of the bronchoscope and TBNA performed with real-time ultrasound imaging. A preliminary study in 70 patients has demonstrated a high sensitivity (95.7%) and accuracy (97.1%) in patients with suspected malignancy [16]. Furthermore, abnormal nodes as small as 5 mm in diameter can be identified [17]. This technique has the promise to replace mediastinoscopy.

10.6   Early Diagnosis of Lung Cancer

The vast majority of lung cancers are detected at an advanced stage and hence are only amenable to palliative therapy. The early detection of cancers may improve the proportion that are amenable to curative treatment and the overall prognosis of the disease. Fluorescence bronchoscopy utilizes the principle that normal tissue emits a green fluorescence when illuminated by a light in the blue wavelength, whereas dysplastic or cancerous tissue absorbs this fluorescence and appears reddish-brown in color [18]. The intensity is low and not visible with the unaided eye, but it can be visualized with the use of appropriate filters and image enhancement [19]. Several commercial systems are now available: the LIFE system from Xillix technologies, The SAFE-1000 from Pentax, and the Storz system.

Early studies have shown that the sensitivity of fluorescence bronchoscopy in comparison to conventional white light bronchoscopy is 6.3 (55.9% vs. 8.8%, respectively) [20]. False-positive results are still the main problem with this technique. Fluorescence bronchoscopy is unlikely to become the first step in a screening program, as that would require considerable resources in bronchoscopist, histopathologist, and nursing time, and equipment. It is more likely to be a second-line investigation in patients with abnormal molecular markers during initial screening and as a research tool. In a Japanese study, patients with sputum cytology that was suspicious for malignancy were evaluated with white light and fluorescence bronchoscopy [21]. Similar numbers of patients with invasive cancer were detected with the two techniques, but a much higher proportion of patients with invasive carcinoma or dysplasia were detected in patients who underwent fluorescence bronchoscopy ($p < 0.005$).

References

1. Govert JA, Kopita JM, Matchar D, Kussin PS, Samuelson WM. Cost-effectiveness of collecting routine cytologic specimens during fiberoptic bronchoscopy for endoscopically visible lung tumor. Chest 1996; 109:451.
2. Mak VHF, Johnston IDA, Hetzel MR, Grubb C. Value of washings and brushings in fibreoptic bronchoscopy in the diagnosis of lung cancer. Thorax 1990; 45:373.
3. Dasgupta A, Jain P, Minai OA, Sandur S, Meli Y, Arroliga AC, Mehta AC. Utility of transbronchial needle aspiration in the diagnosis of endobronchial lesions. Chest 1999; 115:1237.
4. Schreiber G, McCrory DC. Performance characteristics of different modalities for diagnosis of suspected lung cancer: summary of published evidence. Chest 2003; 123(1 Suppl):115S.
5. Popp W, Rauscher H, Ritska L, et al. Diagnostic sensitivity of different techniques in the diagnosis of lung tumors with the flexible fiberoptic bronchoscope. Comparison of brush biopsy, imprint cytology of forceps biopsy, and histology of forceps biopsy. Cancer 1991; 67:72.
6. Rosell A, Monso E, Lores L, Vila X, Llatjos M, Ruiz J, Morera J. Cytology of bronchial biopsy rinse fluid to improve the diagnostic yield for lung cancer. Eur Respir J 1998; 12:1415.
7. Laroche C, Fairbairn I, Moss H, Pepke-Zaba J, Sharples L, Flower C, Coulden R. Role of computed tomographic scanning of the thorax prior to bronchoscopy in the investigation of suspected lung cancer. Thorax 2000; 55:359.
8. Lam WK, So SY, Hsu C, et al. Fibreoptic bronchoscopy in the diagnosis of bronchial cancer: comparison of washings, brushings and biopsies in central and peripheral tumours. Clin Oncol 1983; 9:35.
9. Reichenberger F, Weber J, Tamm M, Bolliger CT, Dalquen P, Perruchoud AP, Soler M. The value of transbronchial needle aspiration in the diagnosis of peripheral pulmonary lesions. Chest 1999; 116:704.
10. Gasparini S, Zuccatosta L, Zitti P, Bichi Secchi E, Ferretti M, Gusella P. Integration of TBNA and TCNA in the diagnosis of peripheral lung nodules. Influence on staging. Ann Ital Chir 1999; 70:851.
11. Kurimoto N, Miyazawa T, Okimasa S, Maeda A, Oiwa H, Miyazu Y, Murayama M. Endobronchial ultrasonography using a guide sheath increases the ability to diagnose peripheral pulmonary lesions endoscopically. Chest 2004; 126:959.
12. Davenport RD. Rapid on-site evaluation of transbronchial aspirates. Chest 1990; 98:59.
13. Harrow EM, Abi-Saleh W, Blum J, et al. The utility of transbronchial needle aspiration in the staging of bronchogenic carcinoma. Am J Respir Crit Care Med 2000; 161(2):601.
14. Prakash UB, Offord KP, Stubbs SE. Bronchoscopy in North America: the ACCp Survey. Chest 1991; 100:1668.
15. Herth FJ, Becker HD, Ernst A. Ultrasound-guided transbronchial needle aspiration: an experience in 242 patients. Chest 2003; 123:604.
16. Yasufuku K, Chiyo M, Sekine Y, Chhajed PN, Shibuya K, Iizasa T, Fujisawa T. Real-time endobronchial ultrasound-guided transbronchial needle aspiration of mediastinal and hilar lymph nodes. Chest 2004; 126:122.
17. Krasnik, M., Vilmann, P., Larsen, S. S., and Jacobsen, G. K. Preliminary experience with a new method of endoscopic transbronchial real time ultrasound guided biopsy for diagnosis of mediastinal and hilar lesions. Thorax 2003; 58(12):1083.
18. Hung J, Lam S, LeRiche JC, Palcic B. Autofluorescence of normal and malignant bronchial tissue. Lasers Surg Med 1991; 11(2):99.
19. Lam S, MacAulay C, Palcic B. Detection and localization of early lung cancer by imaging techniques. Chest 1993; 103(1 Suppl):12S.
20. Lam S, Kennedy T, Unger M, et al. Localization of bronchial intraepithelial neoplastic lesions by fluorescence bronchoscopy. Chest 1998; 113(3):696.
21. Shibuya K, Fujisawa T, Hoshino H, et al. Fluorescence bronchoscopy in the detection of preinvasive bronchial lesions in patients with sputum cytology suspicious or positive for malignancy. Lung Cancer 2001; 32(1):19.

Radiological Diagnosis and Staging of Lung Cancer

11

Simon Padley

Contents

11.1   Epidemiology

Lung cancer is the most frequently encountered malignancy worldwide, with 1.2 million new cases annually, causing 17.8% of all cancer deaths [1]. Four major cell types exist, accounting for 95% of lung cancers. The first three are squamous cell carcinoma (SCC), adenocarcinoma, and large-cell carcinoma, which are collectively known as non-small-cell lung cancer (NSCLC). The fourth major cell type, small-cell lung cancer (SCLC), is grouped separately. Currently there is a 3:1 male to female predominance. In women, breast cancer is currently more common, but lung cancer causes more deaths; in some Scandinavian countries female lung cancer deaths surpass those in males.

Smoking tobacco significantly increases the likelihood of developing lung cancer, the relative risk increasing 20- to 30-fold in smokers as compared to non-smokers. Passive smokers are also at an approximately 24% increased risk of developing lung cancer [2]. Other risk factors for developing lung cancer include occupational exposure to asbestos and several other carcinogens, pulmonary fibrosis, and radiotherapy.

Late presentation is one of the factors that has impaired significant improvements in survival rates over the past 30 years, despite advances in detection methods and treatments. Median survival from diagnosis has remained at 6–12 months, and overall 5-year survival is approximately 5% [3]. No study has described definite benefit from screening for lung cancer. Recent large computed tomography (CT) studies have demonstrated increased lung cancer detection in at-risk populations, but many questions remain unanswered. Most importantly, there is no current evidence that screening confers a disease-specific survival benefit. In an effort to provide definitive evidence, a large-scale trial, the National Lung Cancer Screening Trial (USA), is currently underway. This will study the overall and comparative utility of chest radiography and spiral CT for lung cancer screening and has recruited 50,000 patients. This trial commenced in 2002 and is due to continue until 2009, after which the findings will be reported.

11.2   Presentation and Diagnosis

11.2.1   Symptoms

Overall, approximately 10% of patients with lung cancer are asymptomatic at presentation [4, 5], the diagnosis usually arising incidentally from a radiograph undertaken for other reasons. In symptomatic patients the underlying disease may cause cough, hemoptysis or pain. Mediastinal invasion can lead to symptoms of hoarseness, Horner's syndrome, phrenic nerve paralysis, dysphagia, and superior vena cava obstruction [6]. Large pleural effusions may cause breathlessness. In addition, symptoms may be constitutional (e.g., malaise, weight loss) or directly related to metastatic deposits (e.g., pain from skeletal metastases). Other manifestations include paraneoplastic phenomena such as hypertrophic osteoarthropathy, Lambert Eaton Syndrome, and inappropriate antidiuretic hormone secretion.

Symptoms are often nonspecific, but their first-line investigation often includes chest radiography, which may identify the presence of the tumor. Cross-sectional imaging with CT is then usually undertaken to confirm the nature of the mass.

11.2.2   Chest Radiography

It is rare that a lung cancer is identified on chest radiography unless it is greater than 1 cm in diameter [7–11]. Furthermore, it has been reported that 85% of missed lung cancers are peripheral, <2 cm in size, of low contrast density, and are in areas of anatomical overlap (e.g., between the ribs and clavicle) [12]. Although small lung cancers (<1 cm) are difficult to detect, optimal viewing conditions and systematic analysis with particular attention to review areas (apices, retrocardiac, hilar, and diaphragmatic areas) have been found to aid detection [13]. Once a suspicious lesion is identified it is important to undertake comparison with any previous radiographs. If the lesion was present previously but is unchanged over a 2-year interval it can be presumed to be benign [14, 15]. In circumstances where no old films are available, CT is usually employed to characterize the lesion further [16].

11.2.3   Computed Tomography

CT is useful in further classification of nodules identified on chest radiography. Lung cancers on CT typically appear as soft-tissue-density mass lesions within the lung parenchyma, but occasionally they may appear as focal ground-glass opacities (especially in adenocarcinoma). Other imaging findings include:
1. Air bronchograms (typically in adenocarcinoma).
2. Calcification (rarely seen on chest radiography, seen in up to 10% of cases on CT) is found predominantly in tumors greater than 5 cm in diameter, but amorphous or cloud-like calcification may be seen in small peripheral tumors [17]. Cancers may engulf a preexisting calcified focus.
3. Cavitation, most typically a feature of SCC [18, 19], is normally eccentric and can occur in tumors of any size. The cavity is normally thick-walled and may contain fluids and necrotic tumor fragments. In

rare cases an air-crescent may be seen within the cavity outlining the tumor mass [20].
4. Nodules (≤3 cm) that contain mixed soft-tissue and ground-glass densities carry greater risk of malignancy than purely solid nodules and are more commonly associated with bronchioalveolar cell carcinoma (BAC) [21]. The histology of mixed nodules was found to differ from that of purely solid nodules, and is more commonly associated with BAC histology [21].

Other findings on chest radiography and CT that raise the suspicion of malignancy include:
1. The radiographic 'S' sign of Golden (seen as a bulging fissure deviated around a central tumor mass, typically in the right upper zone), which implies a proximal lung tumor causing distal lung collapse.
2. Large lesions. The likelihood of malignancy of a lesion identified on CT is increased with increasing size (up to 80% of nodules with a diameter greater than 2 cm are malignant [22, 23].
3. Localized consolidation confined to one lobe that persists for longer than 2 weeks or recurs in the same lobe, especially if there is no associated loss of volume or air bronchograms. It is generally held that complete resolution of a consolidation excludes an underlying obstructing mass.
4. Consolidation confined to one lobe in a patient >35 years old associated with volume loss, mucus-filled bronchi ,and absence of air bronchograms. Mucus-filled dilated airways seen within collapsed lobes (better appreciated on postcontrast images) should prompt the search for a centrally obstructing tumor [17]. Careful analysis of CT images may reveal an endobronchial mass.
5. Unilateral hilar enlargement. This may be the only radiographic feature of a lung malignancy [24–28] and may reflect a proximal tumor, lymphadenopathy, consolidated lung, or a combination of all three. CT scanning is useful in this scenario to differentiate these from vascular causes (e.g., poststenotic dilatation of the pulmonary artery).
6. Lesion margins. The tumor margin may be lobulated, which is thought to reflect differential growth rates within the tumor. Alternatively, the tumor may be spiculated due to local extension or incitement of a fibrotic response in the surrounding lung. Although prominent spiculation significantly increases the likelihood of a solitary pulmonary nodule being malignant, it is not highly specific [17].
7. Differential enhancement. Several studies have examined the enhancement characteristics of benign and malignant lung masses. Nodules that fail to enhance to ≤15 Hounsfield Units (HU) after a standard dose of intravenous contrast, were found to be benign [29]. Despite this test having a high sensitivity for

benign lesions, it is not highly specific for excluding malignancy.

Signs associated with benignity include:

1. The presence of fat (–40 HU to –120 HU) within a lesion. The presence of fat or calcification, or a combination of the two was shown to correctly identify 30/46 hamartomas (benign tumors) in one series [30].
2. Calcification in soft-tissue lung lesions. This should be interpreted with caution in masses >3 cm, however, as the tumor may engulf granulomata leading to an eccentric pattern of calcification within the mass.
3. The enhancing rim sign. A homogenously low-density, centered nodule that has a minimal enhancing rim (<15 HU) has been associated with an increased probability of benignity [31].

Using imaging to differentiate between histological varieties of lung cancer is not often rewarding, but some features may aid in the differential diagnosis.

11.2.4   Adenocarcinoma

Adenocarcinoma tends to present as smoothly marginated round or oval nodules or mass in the periphery of the lung [17], but in up to 35% of cases may present as a pulmonary mass with associated mediastinal nodal enlargement [32]. Lesions rarely calcify [16] or cavitate [33]. BAC is a subtype of adenocarcinoma that may present as solitary or multiple lesions [34], but most (60%) usually manifest as a well-circumscribed nodule

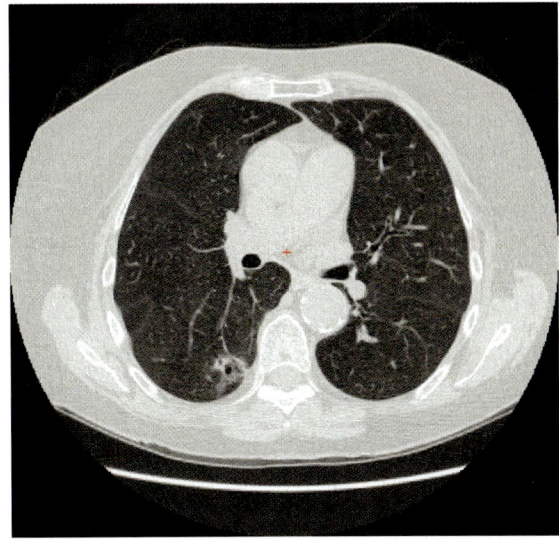

Fig. 11.1. Computed tomography (CT) section (imaged on lung window settings) demonstrating a predominantly ground-glass mass in the posterior right lung. Histological analysis revealed this to be a bronchoalveolar cell carcinoma

in the lung periphery. BAC may have multiple peripheral focal areas of low-attenuation cystic spaces or air bronchograms within it (Fig. 11.1) [16]. Multifocal BAC may manifest as multiple well-defined nodules of varying size or multiple poorly defined or ground-glass opacities that coalesce and resemble pneumonia or reticulonodular opacities. Other features include pleural effusions, atelectasis, and (rarely) pneumothorax.

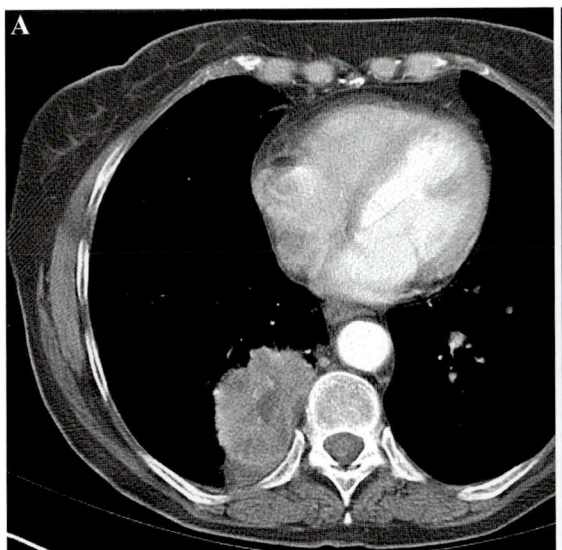

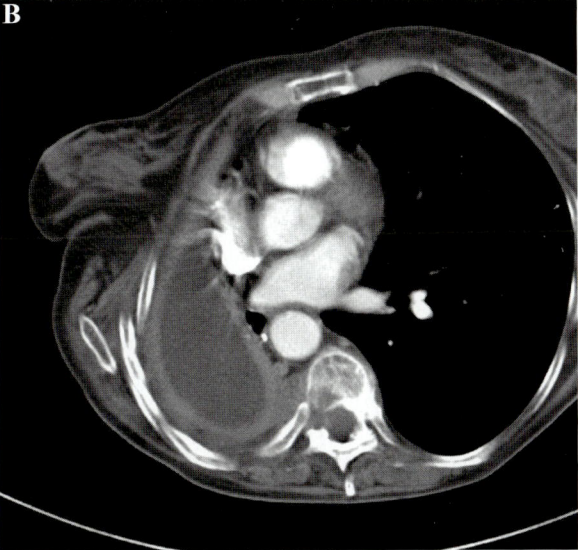

Fig. 11.2. A Large peripheral squamous cell tumor in the posterior aspect of the right lung. **B** Follow-up scan taken 1 year postpneumonectomy showing recurrence at the site of the original tumor, with invasion into the adjacent vertebral body

11.2.5   Squamous Cell Carcinoma

SCC is relatively slow growing and commonly arises from lobar or segmental bronchi, causing occlusion of a central lumen of the bronchus and distal collapse. Thus it may present with the same radiological features as an episode of infective pneumonia. Alternatively, there may be hemoptysis or signs related to invasion of adjacent structures, such as recurrent laryngeal nerve palsy [17]. Peripheral tumors may be asymptomatic until they have grown to a substantial size (Fig. 11.2 A) when they may also cavitate in up to 20% of cases [33].

11.2.6   Large-Cell Carcinoma

Large-cell carcinoma typically presents as large peripheral masses with irregular margins. Cavitation and calcification are rare [16].

11.2.7   Small-Cell Lung Cancer

SCLC most commonly arises from the main airways, but is associated with rapid invasion into vascular and lymphatic tissues, resulting in a high rate of metastatic lymph node involvement. Even though the primary lesion may be small and unidentified on chest radiography there may be bulky hilar and mediastinal lymph node enlargement.

11.2.8   Subsequent Patient Investigation

After an initial working diagnosis of a lung carcinoma, further work will be required for confirmation of the diagnosis and to establish disease stage. If the imaging features of the lesion suggest a low likelihood of malignancy, follow-up scanning may be performed to detect changes in lesion characteristics and to confirm lack of interval change. Whilst it may be sufficient to undertake serial chest radiographs, in some cases it is more usual to employ CT for this purpose. Accurate assessment of growth allows calculation of tumor doubling time. The doubling time is calculated from the increase in tumor volume over a known period. A 25% increase in diameter is approximately equivalent to a doubling in volume [17]. It is generally accepted that doubling times in lung cancer range from 30 to 490 days, but owing to this wide range, considerable overlap exists between the doubling times of benign and malignant nodules. Very rapid nodule doubling times (<7 days) should suggest an infective etiology. However, this method of analysis is not without its own problems.

One study of the reliability of observer measurements of nodule size on CT using electronic calipers suggested that measurements may be so variable between multiple observations by single or multiple observers that results are misleading and could lead to unnecessary invasive investigations or to malignant growth being missed [35]. However, the advent of multidetector CT (MDCT) scanners with automated volume analysis software has been shown to more accurately assess nodule size [36]. Overall, it is generally held that stability or regression in the size of a nodule with no significant changes in overall morphology for a period of 2 years is required to confirm a nonmalignant etiology [37].

11.2.9   Biopsy

In cases where the probability of malignancy is high, early histological confirmation may become the preferred course of action. In practice, a tissue diagnosis is obtained, where feasible, to help guide further treatment. Sputum cytology is often performed but has varying yields. Only 1.9% cases were diagnostic in one series of patients in whom a diagnosis of lung cancer was established by other means [13], whereas in a further series (of high-risk patients screened for lung cancer with chest radiograph or CT and sputum cytology), sputum cytology detected cancer cells in all 251 patients studied, many of whom had no evidence of lung cancer on imaging at that time [38]. If a pleural effusion is present then thoracocentesis should be performed. In patients with a possible extrathoracic metastasis, biopsy of that lesion is of the greatest prognostic value.

Staging using CT can be of great utility for biopsy planning and may help to predict the likelihood of obtaining a positive tissue diagnosis by any particular method. CT is an invaluable guide to the bronchoscopist, with successful biopsy sampling being more likely if one or more of the following CT features are present: ill-defined lesion margins, endobronchial soft-tissue component, a large airway leading directly to the lesion, and the lesion lying <4 cm from the nearest lobar bronchus [39].

Percutaneous biopsy sampling can be performed under CT or ultrasound guidance, and is the preferred method in peripheral lesions. Percutaneous biopsy sampling is relatively contraindicated in patients with a single lung. Other relative contraindications include bleeding diathesis, vascular malformations, severe obstructive lung disease, pulmonary arterial hypertension, and an inability to cooperate. Potential complications include hemoptysis, pneumothorax, air embolus, and tumor implantation. Hemoptysis occurring as a result of focal pulmonary hemorrhage occurs in approximately

10% of cases, and major bleeding is the commonest cause of death as a complication of lung biopsy [40]. To reduce this risk, bleeding diatheses should be corrected, major vessels should be avoided, and perihilar lesions carefully assessed for vascular anatomy prior to biopsy procedures. To reduce the incidence of pneumothorax, reported in 17.9–44% of case series [40], the coaxial biopsy technique and avoidance of interlobar fissures is preferred to reduce the number of pleural surfaces punctured. Tumor implantation and dissemination as a result of percutaneous biopsy sampling are very rare.

11.2.10 Positron Emission Tomography

Positron emission tomography (PET) has made a significant contribution to range of tools available to assess possible lung cancer. A full description of PET is beyond the scope of this chapter. However in brief, fluorine-18 (^{18}F) is attached to deoxyglucose to produce fluorodeoxyglucose (FDG). This is used to assess cellular glucose metabolism. Tumor cells and inflammatory processes are characterized by a higher than normal level of glucose metabolism. The amount of FDG trapped within tumor cells can be identified by imaging ^{18}F decay using a PET camera. Detection is most commonly measured semiquantitatively using a standard uptake value (SUV). This is the ratio of tracer uptake by the lesion corrected for body weight and serum glucose and compared with background. Lesions with SUV values greater than 2.5 are generally regarded as malignant [41]. The use of PET in Europe has increased dramatically in the past 5 years, but remains limited by lack of availability. To help assess whether a detected lung nodule is benign or malignant, PET can be used to assess metabolic activity and thus help gauge whether further action is required. Those lesions that appear to be metabolically inert are probably benign and may be followed up radiologically. However, caveats to this exist. Although the sensitivity of PET in detecting primary NSCLC is generally reported as 95% for lesions ≥3 cm [42, 43], the spatial resolution of PET does not allow such high sensitivities for lesions <1 cm [44]. In a recent study of 136 nodules, 20 were <1 cm in diameter; all were negative on PET despite 8 being malignant on final histology [45]. False-negative results have been reported most commonly in BAC and carcinoid tumors, which are histologically relatively well differentiated. In contrast, false-positive results may be seen in several infective and inflammatory conditions, notably in tuberculosis, sarcoidosis, histoplasmosis, and rheumatoid nodules. Furthermore, the serum glucose concentration at the time of scanning is an important factor in image quality and if raised, causes reduced FDG uptake into tumor cells, resulting in reduced tumor conspicuity [46].

A less widely employed nuclear medicine technique relies on the fact that most malignant lung tumor cells express somatostatin receptors. The radionuclide ^{99}mTc depreotide, which binds to somatostatin receptors, can help in the differentiation of cancerous from benign lung nodules. In one study of 114 patients, 85 out of 88 malignant nodules and 19 out of 26 benign lesions were correctly identified [47]. At present no comparative studies of PET and somatostatin receptor radionucleotides have been published.

11.3 Staging

11.3.1 Staging of NSCLC

Lung cancer staging provides information about the anatomical extent and histological nature of disease, which helps to optimize therapy, informs on prognosis, and allows assessment for possible resection. In those in whom surgery is not deemed appropriate, assessment of disease burden aids the oncologist to plan radiotherapy and chemotherapeutic regimens and assists in the assessment of response to therapy.

11.3.1.1 The International Staging System

The current staging system for NSCLC is based on the Tumor, Nodal, Metastasis (TNM) classification (Tables 11.1 and 11.2) [48]. Stage I tumors are confined to the lung parenchyma (Fig. 11.3). They do not breach the parietal pleura and are not associated with metastatic spread. IA tumors are ≤3 cm in size; five-year survival in this group ranges from 61 to 67%. IB tumors are >3 cm in size; five-year survival in this group ranges from 38 to 57%.

Stage II tumors are divided into those that are ≤3 cm in size but are associated with metastasis to ipsilateral hilar nodes (IIA) and those that are >3cm and are either associated with metastasis to ipsilateral hilar nodes or have invaded the adjacent mediastinum, diaphragm, or chest wall (IIB). Stage IIB may extend along main bronchi for up to 2 cm from the carina and remain suitable for surgical resection. For stage IIA disease, 5-year survival is 34–55%, whereas for stage IIB disease it is 22–24% for clinically staged disease or 38–39% for pathologically staged disease. It can be seen, therefore, that clinical staging tends to underestimate the stage of disease as compared to pathological staging.

Stage III tumors include those patients with extensive but resectable disease (IIIA) and those with disease deemed irresectable by conventional surgical techniques (IIIB). Tumors that are classified as IIIA include tumors that have N2 nodal spread with no distant metastases

Table 11.1. The Tumor, Nodal, Metastasis (TNM) Classification of tumor extent

Primary tumor (T)	
Tx	Primary tumor cannot be assessed Or Tumor cells identified on bronchial washings but not visible on imaging or bronchoscopy
T0	No evidence of primary tumor
Tis	Carcinoma in situ
T1	Tumor 3 cm in greatest dimension, surrounded by lung or visceral pleura without bronchoscopic evidence of invasion more proximal than the lobar bronchus (i.e., not in the main bronchus)
T2	Tumor with any of the following features of size or extent: <3 cm in greatest dimension; involves the main bronchus, 2 cm distal to the carina; invades the visceral pleura; associated with atelectasis or obstructive pneumonitis that extends to the hilar region but does not involve the entire lung
T3	Tumor of any size that directly invades any of the following: chest wall (including superior sulcus tumor), diaphragm, mediastinal pleura, parietal pericardium; tumor in the main bronchus <2 cm distal to the carina, but without involvement of the carina; associated atelectasis or obstructive pneumonitis of the entire lung
T4	Tumor of any size that invades any of the following: mediastinum, heart, great vessels, trachea, esophagus, vertebral body, carina; tumor with a malignant pleural or pericardial effusion (provided that evidence for malignancy as the cause of effusion is cytopathologically confirmed), or satellite tumor nodule(s) within the ipsilateral primary-tumor lobe of the lung

Regional lymph nodes (N)	
NX	Regional lymph nodes cannot be assessed
N0	No regional lymph nodes
N1	Metastases to ipsilateral peribronchial and/or ipsilateral hilar lymph nodes, and intrapulmonary nodes invaded by the most distant extension of the primary tumor
N2	Metastases to ipsilateral mediastinal and/or subcarinal lymph nodes(s)
N3	Metastases to contralateral mediastinal, contralateral hilar, ipsilateral or contralateral scalene, or supraclavicular lymph node(s)

Distant metastases (M)	
MX	Distant metastases cannot be assessed
M0	No distant metastases
M1	Distant metastases are present

Table 11.2. Staging with respect to TNM grouping

Stage:	Definition (via TNM grouping):
IA	T1 N0 M0
IB	T2 N0 M0
IIA	T1 N1 M0
IIB	T2 N1 M0 or T3 N0 M0
IIIA	T3 N1 M0 or T1 N2 M0 or T2 N2 M0 or T3 N2 M0
IIIB	T4 N0 M0 or T4 NI M0 or T4 N2 M0 or T1 N3 M0 or T2 N3 M0 or T3 N3 M0 or T4 N3 M0
IV	Any T, any N, M1

and those T3 tumors where spread is only to hilar nodes. Stage IIIB tumors include any T4 tumor or any N3 nodes (Fig. 11.4). Although not usually surgical candidates, stage IIIB tumors may be considered for extended procedures after neoadjuvant chemotherapy [49]. Five-year survival for patients with stage IIIA tumors ranges from 9 to 13% for clinically staged disease or from 23 to 25% for pathologically staged disease; that for stage IIIB tumors is 1–8% for clinically staged disease.

Stage IV represents all tumors with M1 disease (Fig. 11.5). Five-year survival in this group is 1%.

11.3.1.2 Staging of the Primary Tumor

CT is the most commonly used tool in evaluation of the primary tumor. Defining the primary tumor in terms of T staging enables prediction of resectability. This definition may not be straightforward, as distinction from the adjacent collapsed lung may be impossible and thus lead to an overestimation of tumor size. Differentiation of central lung cancer from distal collapse can sometimes be achieved on CT using bolus contrast enhancement. The collapsed lung tends to enhance to a greater extent than the adjacent tumor. This difference in enhancement is most marked 40 s to 2 min postinjection of the contrast medium [50]. Despite this, contrast differences between the tumor and the adjacent lung are not always readily identifiable [50–52]. T1 and T2 tumors are most amenable to surgical resection using standard techniques. T3 tumors that involve the chest wall or mediastinum to a limited extent may also be candidates for surgical resection, albeit with more complex techniques. T4 tumors are irresectable.

Chest radiography is of little use when assessing mediastinal invasion. However, phrenic nerve involvement may be inferred by the presence of "new" diaphragmatic elevation. Imaging of diaphragmatic movement with ultrasound or fluoroscopy can produce similar information [53]. Noninvasive assessment of an extensive mediastinal tumor is usually provided by CT. Borderline invasion by less extensive disease is unreliable [54].

Historically, Glazer et al. described three features that predicted resectability: (1) less than 3 cm of mediastinal contact, (2) intact fat plane between the tumor and mediastinum, and (3) <90° circumferential contact with the aorta [55]. The utility of these described criteria can, however, be limited. For example, loss of fat plane identified on CT may be due to motion artifact, inflammation, or tumor infiltration. Newer, faster, MDCT scanners can reduce the effect of motion artifact and partial volume averaging, improving radiological accuracy. However, no reliable method of noninvasive differentiation of local inflammatory reaction from direct malignant invasion has yet been developed. Thus, without clear evidence of invasion tumors tend to be understaged to prevent denying the patient the chance of a curative resection [56].

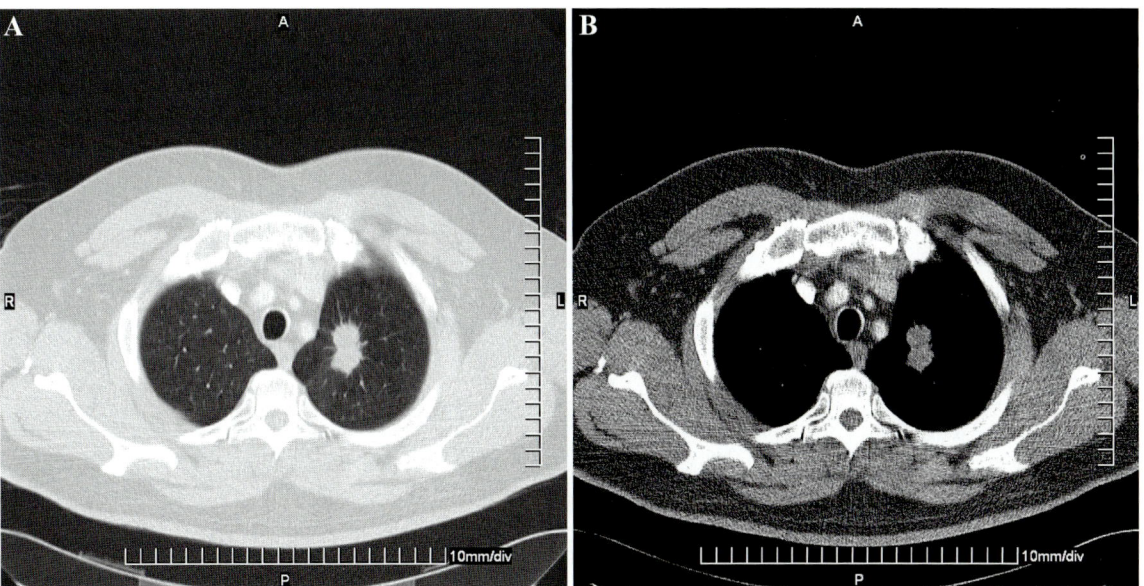

Fig. 11.3. T2 N0 M0 tumor. CT sections (with lung and mediastinal window settings, **A** and **B**, respectively) demonstrate a large (> 3 cm) solid spiculated mass in the left upper lobe

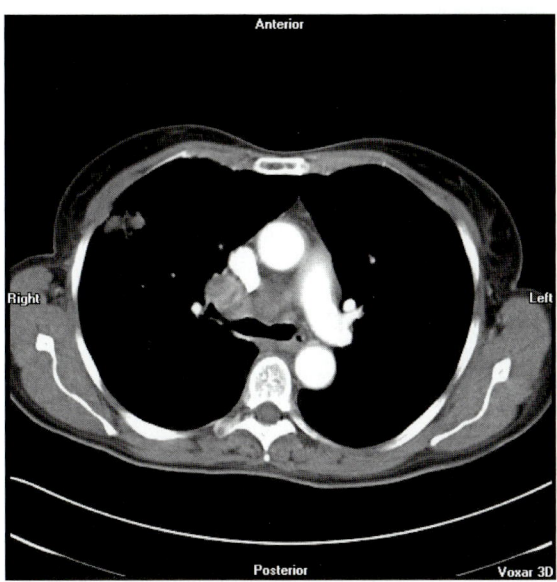

Fig. 11.4. CT section demonstrating a small peripheral (T1) tumor with large hilar and mediastinal (N3) nodal enlargement

Magnetic resonance imaging (MRI) may be employed to clarify issues regarding invasion of local structures. The integrity of the mediastinal or extrapleural fat stripe allows more accurate assessment of tumor transgression [57]; in addition, MRI may demonstrate endoluminal tumor extension and infiltration of the pericardium and heart (T4) better than CT. The arguments regarding the superior capability of MRI for multiplanar imaging have now been largely superseded by MDCT (Fig. 11.6) [58]. However, in one recent study

contrast-enhanced magnetic resonance angiography was shown to demonstrate mediastinal and hilar invasion with a sensitivity of up to 90%, a specificity of up to 87%, and an accuracy of up to 88%, values that are higher than those for CT and standard T1-weighted MRI [59]. Another comparison of the two modalities (CT and MRI) showed no significant differences in their sensitivities or specificities other than superior MRI assessment of myocardial invasion and extension of tumor into the left atrium via the pulmonary veins. Therefore, these authors did not recommend routine use of MRI in patients who initially present for evaluation for mediastinal dissemination [57]. At present, the role of MRI in the investigation of mediastinal invasion remains one of a problem-solving tool in selected cases [60].

Current PET scanners do not offer the anatomical detail provided by CT and MRI; however, they do allow accurate identification of involved nodes or direct mediastinal extension, especially when undertaken as part of a combined CT/PET study (Fig. 11.7). PET can also be used to confirm direct invasion of a tumor into the left recurrent laryngeal nerve, as in these circumstances it can reveal increased uptake in the internal laryngeal muscles on the right side, owing to their compensatory increased use [61].

11.3.1.3 Chest-Wall Invasion

Local chest-wall invasion is not an absolute contraindication to surgery, but it does require alteration of surgical technique. Currently, local chest-wall pain remains a more specific a marker of chest-wall invasion than any

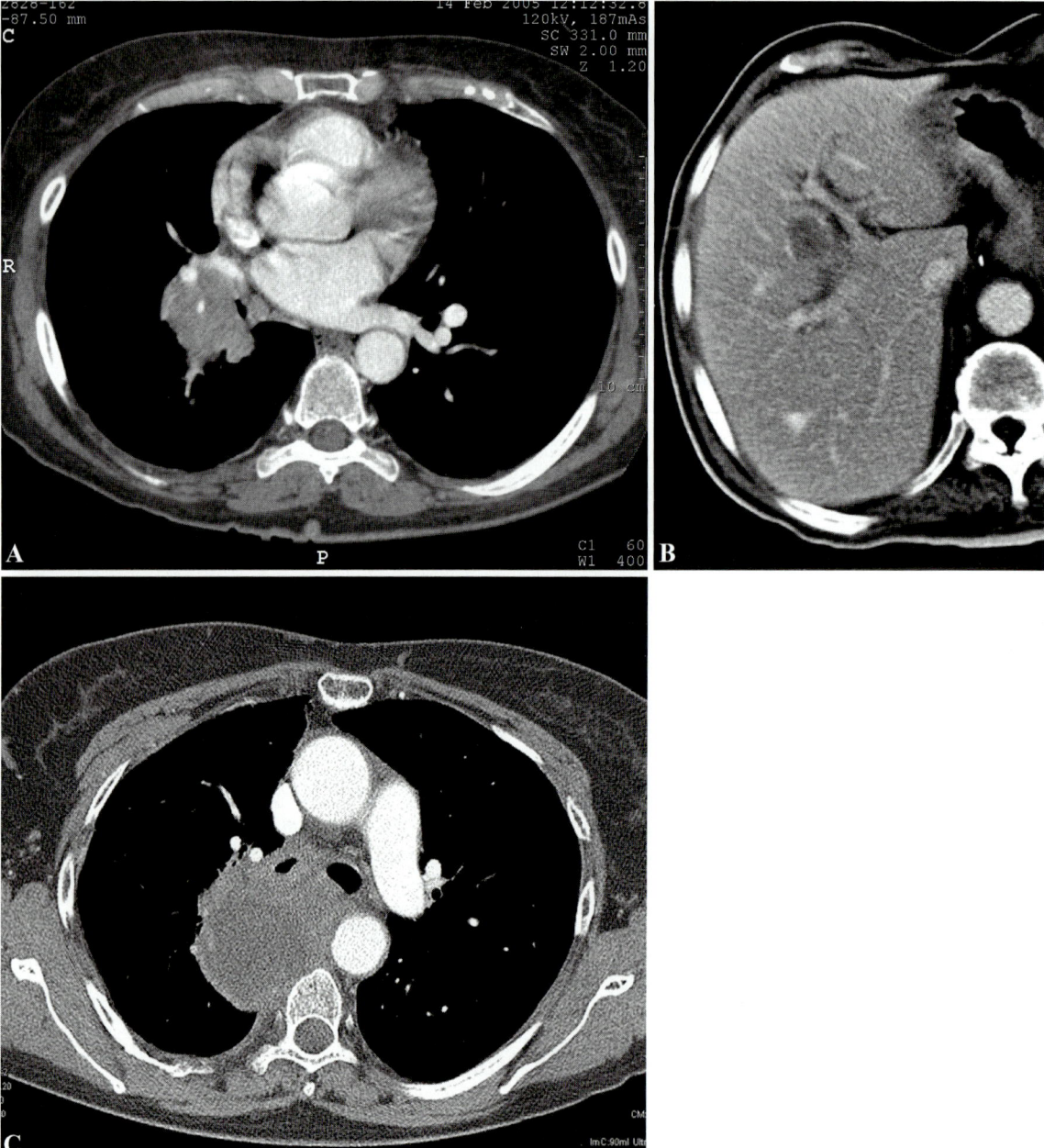

Fig. 11.5. A CT section demonstrating a right hilar (T3) tumor. **B** CT section through the liver (of the same patient) revealing a low-density deposit consistent with a metastasis (stage 4 dis-ease). **C** A large soft-tissue mass (in another patient) at the level of the right hilum encasing vessels and extending into the mediastinum at that level (stage 4 tumor)

imaging test [62]. Chest radiography is relatively insensitive in the detection of chest-wall invasion. Although advanced rib destruction can be identified, more subtle changes are not.

CT can be used to detect cortical bone destruction, but is not as sensitive as radionuclide bone scanning for this purpose (Fig. 11.8). Chest wall soft-tissue involvement is identified on CT by the presence tumor extending through the intercostal muscles, beyond the

line of the ribs or into the extrapleural fat. More subtle invasion is less confidently assessed [62–64]. Described signs of pleural invasion on CT include: an obtuse angle of contact between the tumor and chest wall, obliteration of extrapleural fat, pleural thickening, and the presence of extrapleural soft tissue. Once again the presence of inflammatory changes causing false-positive signs reduces the specificity of this method. However, obliteration of the extrapleural fat with a large degree

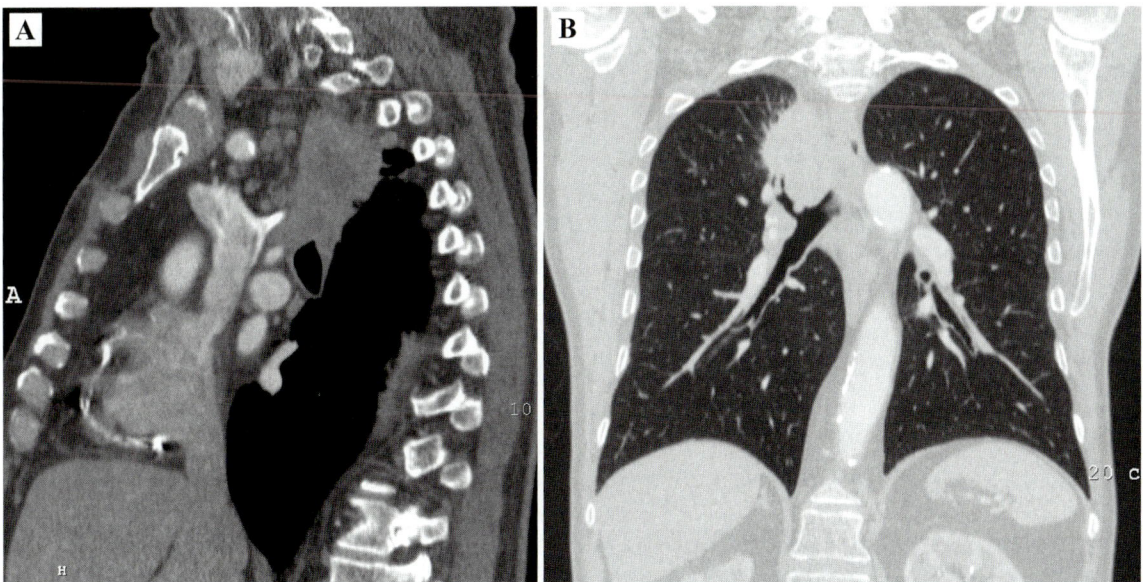

Fig. 11.6. Right upper lobe tumor. CT transverse (**A**) and coronal sections (**B**) with multiplanar reformation on mediastinal (**A**) and lung window settings (**B**) demonstrating a tumour mass in the right upper lobe abutting the mediastinum and encasing the azygos and superior pulmonary veins. Inspection of the right upper lobe bronchus on the coronal section shown in **B** reveals a soft tissue nodule within its wall, consistent with an endobronchial metastasis

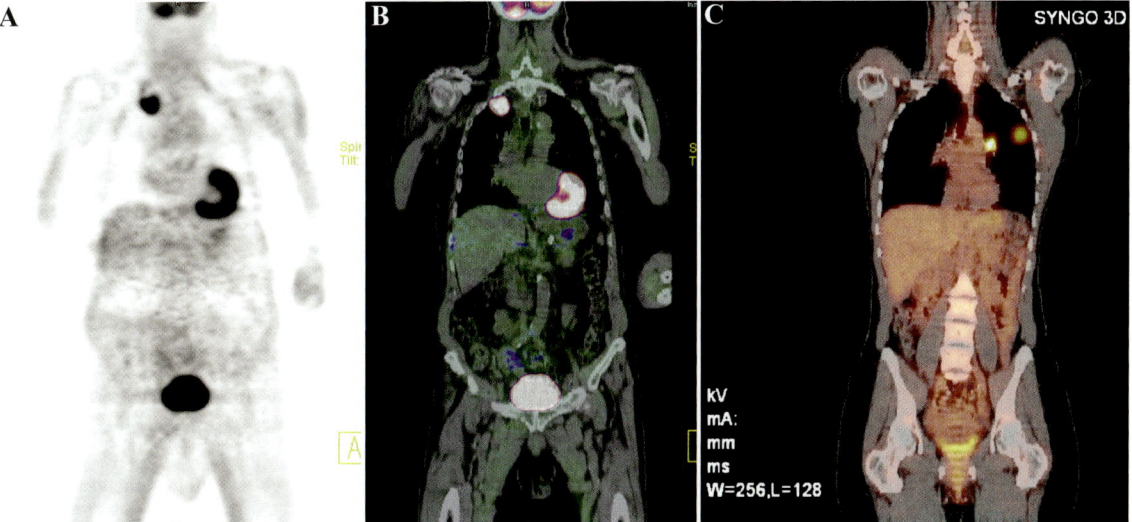

Fig. 11.7. B Coronal positron emission tomography (PET) image demonstrating a focus of tracer uptake in the right upper lobe (note normal uptake in the heart). **B** PET-CT image of the same patient at the same level, highlighting the improved anatomical resolution with this technique. **B** PET-CT image of another patient with a left upper lobe tumor. A second focus of tracer uptake is identified at the left hilum, consistent with the tumor involving lymph nodes at this site

of pleural contact and extensive pleural thickening have been described as CT signs that make pleural invasion very likely [65].

Techniques such as diagnostic pneumothorax, which have also been used in the assessment of mediastinal invasion, have been utilized in attempts to improve the accuracy of differentiation between visceral and parietal invasion and have shown some benefit but have not gained general acceptance. Furthermore, use of dynamic expiratory MDCT (viewed on cine loop) has been reported to be 100% accurate for chest-wall and mediastinal fixation when compared to pathological examination, but has likewise not become a common technique [66].

There are similar difficulties in the differentiation between benign and malignant pleural adhesion using

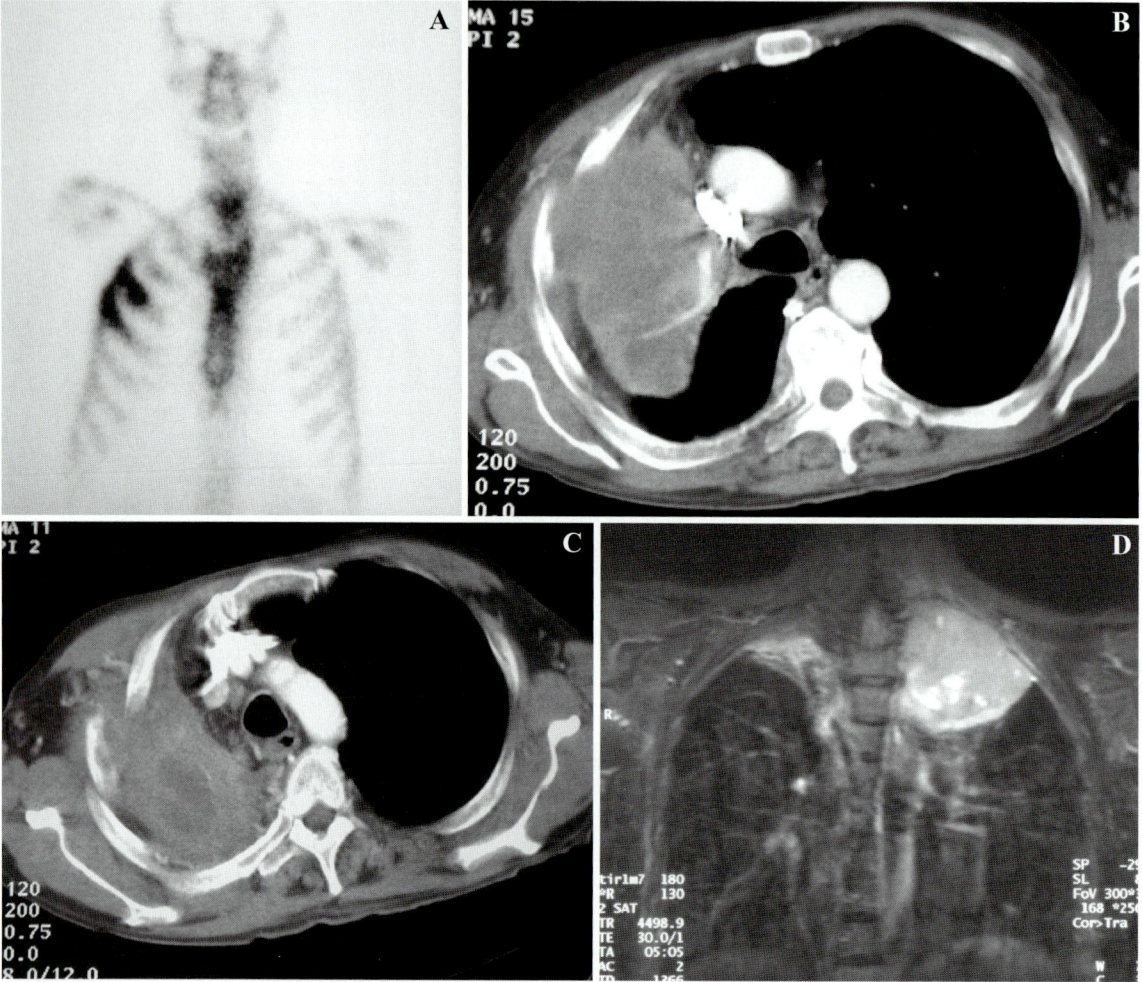

Fig. 11.8. A A bone scan image demonstrating tracer uptake in the right third and fourth ribs. **B, C** CT sections demonstrating chest-wall invasion in the same patient, with destruction of the adjacent ribs. **D** Coronal magnetic resonance imaging section from another patient demonstrating local chest-wall invasion from a superior sulcus tumor

both CT and MRI [57]. However, in one study of 34 patients, the presence of low-intensity material (identical signal to the tumor) encroaching into the high-intensity extrapleural fat (on T1-weighted images) identified invasion with 85% sensitivity and 100% specificity [67].

Assessment of superior sulcus tumors with MRI has been shown to be superior to CT, which suffers from considerable image degradation from shoulder streak artifact. Older studies in which MRI was found to have a 94% correlation with surgical and clinical findings and CT had an accuracy of 63% are now outdated due to the advent of MDCT [68]. MRI reliably diagnoses chest-wall invasion and extension into the root of the neck, with the added benefit of visualization of vascular and neural structures.

Several reports, mainly from Japan, have demonstrated that ultrasound can be used to assess chest-wall invasion. Disruption of the continuous pleural line has been thought to represent a useful sign of invasion, with lack of movement of the tumor during respiration implying adherence. In one report this technique was superior to CT, with >95% sensitivity and specificity for invasion [69]. Another report suggested that biopsy sampling was necessary for optimal accuracy [70].

A recent study of PET reported 100% sensitivity, 71% specificity, and a negative predictive value of 100% in detecting malignant pleural disease, whereas CT was found to be indeterminate in 71% of cases but had 100% specificity and negative predictive value [71]. In a further study examining lone pleural effusion, PET was found to have 95% sensitivity for detecting malignancy [72], whereas it is known that thoracocentesis may not prove malignancy in up to 40% of patients with truly malignant effusions [73].

11.3.1.4   Nodal Staging

Lung cancers normally spread to the ipsilateral hilar nodes, then ipsilateral mediastinal, contralateral mediastinal, and supraclavicular nodes. Although nodal spread is most often sequential, metastases to the mediastinal nodes in the absence of hilar nodes is seen in 33% of cases [74].

11.3.1.5   Detection of Nodal Enlargement

Chest radiography is generally insensitive for nodal staging. However, the presence of enlarged hilar or paratracheal nodes has been shown to be specific (92%) for N2-N3 disease [57].

In a recent study, it was found that use of ultrasound (with or without fine-needle aspiration, FNA) had three times the sensitivity of clinical palpation for the detection of involved supraclavicular nodes. The detection of these nodes establishes an N3 nodal stage, placing the patient in an inoperable category (Fig. 11.9). Previous studies have reported a prevalence of 12% for involved supraclavicular nodes when evaluated by palpation alone; on postmortem, however, their presence has been reported in up to 37.5% of cases [75]. Thus routine use of ultrasound and FNA to detect supraclavicular adenopathy has been suggested as a method to improve the accuracy of preoperative staging and reduce the overall number of staging investigations required.

Lymph node assessment on CT is achieved primarily by measuring lymph node size. Currently, the short-axis diameter is considered the most useful predictor of metastatic nodal involvement [76, 77]. However, the use of size as a discriminator of metastatic lymph node involvement has several pitfalls. Firstly, there is a normal variation of lymph node size throughout the mediastinum; thus, standardization of an upper limit of normal is inherently inaccurate. Secondly, the diameter of individual nodes varies with orientation to scan plane. Furthermore, the presence of enlargement is not diagnostic of metastasis and may be due to reactive hyperplasia, infection, or coincidental inflammatory conditions. In addition, normal-sized nodes do not preclude the presence of metastases, especially in cases of adenocarcinoma where up to 25% of resected normal-sized nodes have been demonstrated to contain metastases [78]. Despite these problems the use of lymph node size as a staging tool is standard CT practice. A 1-cm short-axis diameter is used as the upper limit of normal and has been found to be associated with 64% sensitivity and 62% specificity for detecting malignancy based on a station-by-station surgical/radiological correlation [79]. The negative predictive value of this measurement is in the order of 85%.

The accuracy of MRI, despite its improved contrast resolution, is limited by the same constraints of overlap of features of benign and malignant causes of node enlargement. Although it is generally felt that an MRI sig-

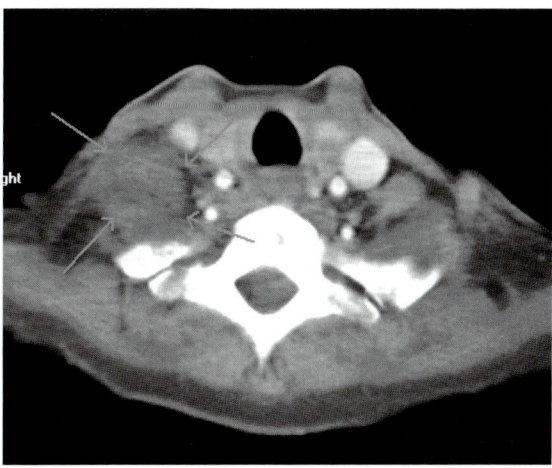

Fig. 11.9. Right supraclavicular lymphadenopathy. CT section demonstrating (arrows) a lymph node mass in the right supraclavicular fossa

nal within nodes is not a useful predictor of involvement, a recent study has reported that short-tau inversion-recovery imaging produces a sufficient signal difference between normal and pathological nodal tissue to detect metastases with 93% sensitivity and 87% specificity [80]. The previously cited advantage of MRI over CT in nodal detection due to the ability to distinguish small nodes from vessels without the use of intravenous contrast medium has been effectively negated by the advent of MDCT.

Many studies have examined the efficacy of PET in nodal staging of lung cancer. In a meta-analysis of 29 studies encompassing 2,226 patients, PET was found to have a mean sensitivity of 79% and mean specificity of 91% for malignant nodal involvement [80]. Accuracy for mediastinal lymph node staging has been reported as 85–96% [81, 82]. It has also been suggested that whole-body PET demonstrates all lymph node stations and so may obviate the need for mediastinoscopy in some cases. This is because the negative predictive value of PET for N3 disease is identical to that for mediastinoscopy (96%) [83]. Thus, patients with a negative PET result could proceed directly to surgical resection, whereas those with a positive PET result should undergo mediastinal lymph node sampling [84].

One study comparing conventional workup and conventional workup with the addition of PET in 188 patients demonstrated that significantly more patients in the non-PET group underwent a "futile" thoracotomy. Futile thoracotomy was defined as thoracotomy for benign stage IIIA-N2 disease or stage III disease, or patients with recurrence or death within 1 year of surgery. In this study, 42% of the conventional workup group underwent a futile thoracotomy, compared with only 21% in the PET group. In most cases, PET detected N2 and N3 disease that was otherwise not apparent [85]. A further large meta-analysis of PET, CT, and endoscopic ultrasound (EUS) has shown that the sensitivity and specificity of PET for mediastinal staging is greater than for the other two modalities [86]. However, another study showed PET to be inferior to EUS with FNA [87].

EUS is a relatively new technique that visualizes aortopulmonary, subcarinal, and posterior mediastinal nodes. Anterior mediastinal and paratracheal nodes are not as well demonstrated due to the presence of air in the trachea. Endosonographic features of neoplastic involvement include round rather than oval nodal shape, sharp nodal borders, and inhomogeneous hypoechoic internal echo texture [88]. EUS also allows FNA to be performed through the endoscope, and can also assess the operability of the primary tumor and of nodal metastases. In one study the sensitivity of EUS was found to be similar to that of PET but its specificity was far greater (100% for EUS and 72% for PET) [87].

At the present time mediastinoscopy and mediastinotomy remain the most widely employed techniques for mediastinal lymph node sampling. They have a high sensitivity and specificity for detecting malignant disease and, although invasive, are indicated prior to thoracotomy when other forms of imaging suggest nodal involvement.

11.3.1.6   Extrathoracic Staging

Lung cancer is commonly associated with widespread hematogenous dissemination at the time of presentation. Detection of metastatic disease precludes surgical resection of the primary tumor. Disease quantification at extrathoracic sites is useful to assess the response to therapy on sequential scans. Currently, there is a lack of consensus regarding whether or not to perform extrathoracic screening in patients who otherwise have potentially operable disease. The frequency of extrathoracic occult metastases in one study was reported as 18% overall [89]. However, the accuracy of the imaging modality in question, the effectiveness of laboratory and clinical screening at excluding disseminated disease, and the requirement for further confirmatory tests that have repercussions on economic and logistic considerations are all factors that influence practice.

Some staging protocols take into account the histological type of the tumor. At presentation, SCLC is commonly widely disseminated, whereas SCC is less likely to have detectable metastases than any other histology for any given TN stage [90–92].

Most patients with lung cancer in the UK have initial staging with contrast-enhanced CT of the thorax, which is routinely continued down to include the liver and adrenals. If suspicious lesions are seen at the time of scanning a delayed-phase scan may be performed. If identified later, the patient may return for a further CT or MRI characterization.

11.3.1.7   Liver Metastases

Up to 12% of patients with lung cancer have been reported to have asymptomatic liver metastases at initial work-up [93]. Whilst clinical assessment and laboratory tests are known to have a low positive predictive value for liver metastases, deposits are usually detected on contrast-enhanced CT (Fig. 11.5). CT detects colorectal tumor metastases in the liver with an accuracy of 85% when compared with postmortem studies. Conventional ultrasound is significantly less sensitive than CT for detection of hepatic deposits. MRI is at least as good (and probably better) than CT, but the cost and limited access to MRI tend to confine its role to characterization of previously identified lesions.

11.3.1.8   Adrenal Metastases

Incidental nonfunctioning adenomas of the adrenal glands are present in 2–10% of the adult population. Adrenal metastases were present in 6.9% of patients with NSCLC in one meta-analysis [94]. Thus, in patients with NSCLC the presence of a small (<3 cm) solitary adrenal nodule presents a reasonably commonplace diagnostic difficulty. Overall incidental adrenal masses have been shown to be more commonly due to adenoma than metastasis with ratio of 68% (17/25) to 32% (8/25) [95]. However, for lesions >3 cm in size the converse is true. Adenomas are normally well circumscribed, homogenous, and have a density of ≤10 Hounsfield Units (HU) on unenhanced CT owing to high lipid content. Following administration of intravenous contrast they display little enhancement. Several useful algorithms for characterization of incidental adrenal masses have been developed (Fig. 11.10).

When CT has failed to characterize an adrenal nodule, then MRI may be undertaken and can be used to characterize a nodule as an adenoma on the basis of signal characteristics that reflect high adenoma lipid content. In one study this technique was demonstrated to have 100% sensitivity and 81% specificity [96].

PET has been shown to have high sensitivity (100%) and specificity (80–100%) for adrenal metastases of more than 1 cm in size. Adrenal masses smaller than 1 cm are not reliably assessed with this technique. In addition, some PET-positive benign adrenal adenomas have also been reported [97].

11.3.1.9   Brain Metastases

Brain metastases are more frequent when the primary tumor is greater than 3 cm in diameter [98]. Isolated central nervous system metastases are uncommon in NSCLC and are generally associated with abnormal neurological examination [99, 100]. Truly asymptomatic brain metastases are thought to occur in 2.7–9.7% patients [16] and are more common with SCLC and adenocarcinoma than with SCC [95, 101, 102]. MRI is more

Imaging management of adrenal incidentalomas

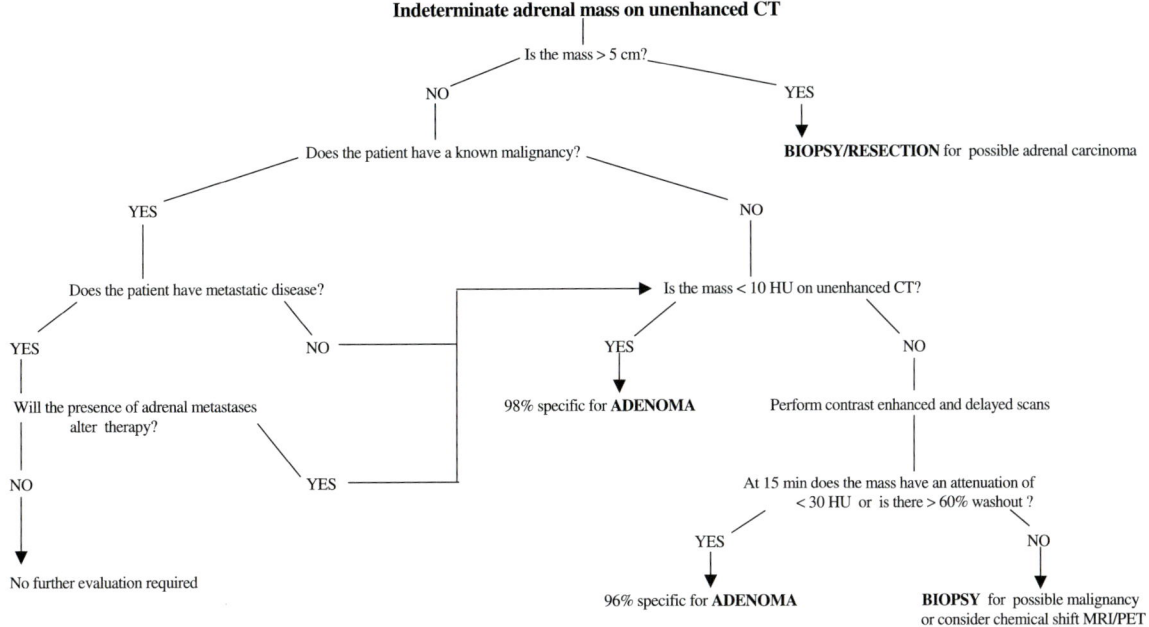

Fig. 11.10. Diagnostic flow diagram outlining a proposed system for management of incidental adrenal masses. Adapted from Dunnick and Korobkin 2002 [109]. *HU* Hounsfield units, *MRI* magnetic resonance imaging

sensitive than CT for the detection of brain metastases and is the modality of choice for brain imaging when available (Fig. 11.11).

Screening for brain metastases is contentious. One study compared a standardized clinical neurological examination with CT of the brain and concluded that CT was not indicated in patients with a normal clinical examination [103]. In a further study, gadolinium-enhanced MRI detected occult brain metastases in 6 out of 29 patients with lung tumors greater than 3 cm in diameter on CT [98]. These MRI findings were deemed to have altered the treatment and follow-up, and this study suggests that for primary tumors of more than 3 cm in diameter (especially if adenocarcinoma or large-cell carcinoma) MRI of the brain may be indicated as part of the routine staging. PET imaging does not alter this conclusion since normal brain has substantial metabolic activity, and focal abnormal cerebral accumulation of labeled glucose due to metastasis is unreliable, with a sensitivity of only 60%. Thus, it should not replace traditional imaging modalities for this purpose.

11.3.1.10 Bone Metastases

The frequency of otherwise occult bony metastases detected on initial work-up is reported to be between 3.4 and 15% (Figs. 11.12 and 11.13) [93]. In patients with symptomatic disease, a radionuclide bone scan (which detects osteoblastic activity) is often utilized as an ini-

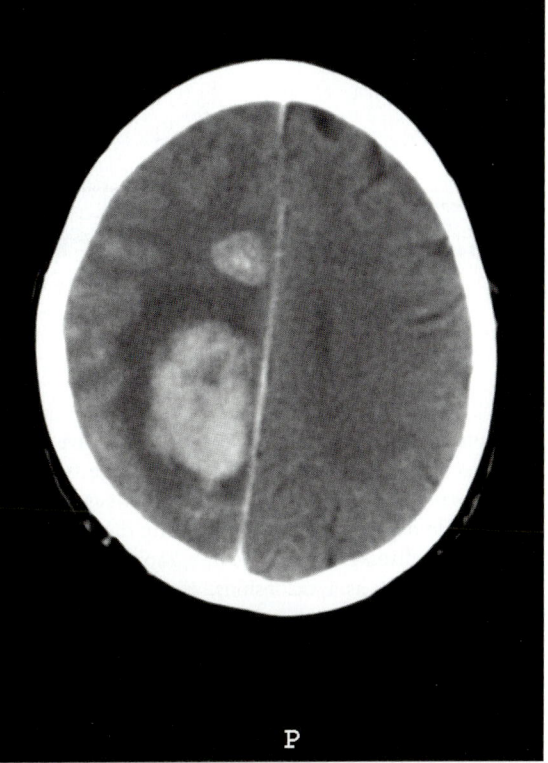

Fig. 11.11. Brain metastases. Contrast-enhanced CT section demonstrating two metastases in the right cerebral hemisphere. Note the halo of low attenuation around the lower of the two metastases, consistent with vasogenic edema

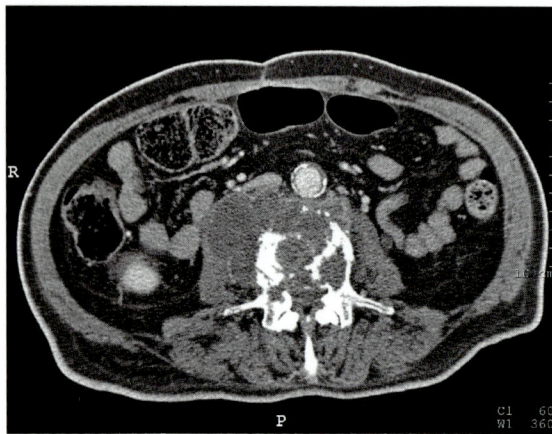

Fig. 11.12. Bone metastasis. CT section showing destruction of vertebral body and replacement of normal bone with tumor

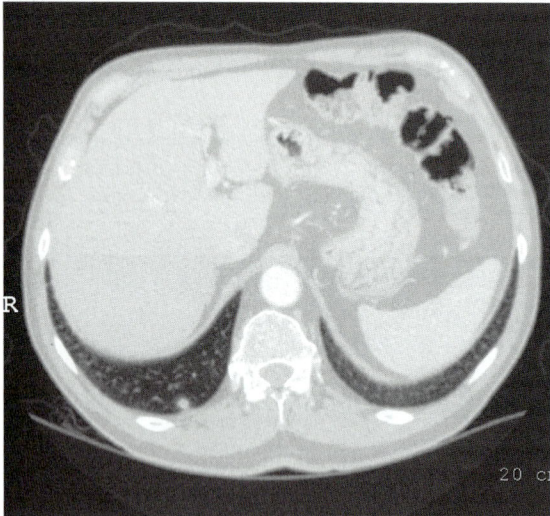

Fig. 11.13. Lung metastasis. CT section through the base of the lungs demonstrating a small nodule at the right base, consistent with a metastasis

tial investigation. Although it is 95% sensitive, false positives from coexistent degenerative disease occur in many cases. Plain film radiography is then suggested to differentiate degenerative from metastatic disease. Metastatic bone disease on plain radiography most commonly manifests as lytic lesions. However, significant loss of bone is required before plain radiography detects these metastases.

Screening for asymptomatic bony metastases with radionuclide scintigraphy is not currently recommended owing to its high false-positive rate. Whole-body MRI could also be employed as a staging tool, but despite interesting studies of the potential for whole-body MRI to replace scintigraphy having been published, this technique is not yet widely employed.

PET has been found to be 92% sensitive and 99% specific for bone metastases compared to bone scintigraphy (which has a specificity of 50% and sensitivity of 92%). However, as standard CT and PET studies do not include the lower limbs, they do not provide a full skeletal survey. Some would argue that if PET replaced radionuclide bone scanning, whole-body studies would be required [84]. However, isolated metastases below the knees are distinctly uncommon and distal metastases are usually part of more widely disseminated disease.

11.3.1.11 Lung Metastases

These are not common at presentation but are seen in approximately 20% of cases at postmortem. However, in one retrospective study it was found that at presentation, up to 52% of patients with lung cancer had multiple lung nodules, which in most patients (78%) numbered greater than 50. The size also varied from 2 mm to 30 mm (80% were <10 mm). The primary associated histology was pulmonary adenocarcinoma and the survival rate was commensurate with stage IV disease [104].

As pulmonary metastases indicate stage IV disease and render the patient inoperable, preoperative detection is important. In these days of MDCT, nodule detection is usually not problematic. More frequently the problem is accurate assessment of the nature of a possible metastatic nodule. Characteristic benign calcification within such a lesion is the exception. Most lesions are of soft-tissue density and studies that have tried to further evaluate these lesions have lead to inconsistent results. PET scanning may be useful to assess the likelihood of metastatic malignancy or a second primary in indeterminate cases.

11.3.2 Staging of SCLC

SCLC is normally regarded as a systemic disease. At the time of presentation surgical resection is viable in less than 5% of cases, as up to 80% cases have already metastasized [105, 106]. Classification is based on a two-stage system proposed by the Veteran's Administration Lung Cancer Study Group, which divides patients into limited and extensive disease groups [105]. Patients with limited-stage disease are conferred a survival advantage.

Limited disease is defined as that which is confined to one hemithorax (but including ipsilateral and contralateral mediastinal, and supraclavicular nodes). To assess disease stage in these patients chest radiography is supplemented with CT of the chest, liver and adrenals, and brain. Bone scintigraphy and bone marrow aspiration to evaluate medullary disease are also performed. Liver and bone metastases are present in up to 30% of patients and brain metastases in up to 15% of patients. The use of PET has not been extensively examined in SCLC. In one series, apparently limited disease was upstaged to extensive disease in 7 out of 24 patients [107].

Extensive disease is that which extends outside the boundaries of a single radiotherapy field. MRI of the brain, body, spine, abdomen, and pelvis has been shown to compare favorably to conventional techniques for the detection of extensive disease. In addition, it has been found to delineate bone metastases not detected by bone marrow aspiration or bone scintigraphy. The disadvantage of whole-body MRI, however, remains the length of acquisition time and cost.

Isolated bone metastases are uncommon. When other extrathoracic metastases are found then radionuclide bone scanning or bone marrow aspiration or MRI are indicated [16].

Central nervous system metastases are common at presentation and are a common site of disease. Routine CT evaluation of the brain is indicated as approximately 5% of patients with brain metastases are asymptomatic, and aggressive treatment with chemotherapy and radiotherapy can improve prognosis and decrease morbidity if the brain is the only site of extrathoracic disease [106].

An alternative approach, to avoid an exhaustive search for extensive disease, is to allow clinical symptoms to direct imaging, terminating on the discovery of extensive disease.

To this approach could be added MRI scanning in cases of superior sulcus tumor, and PET scanning to help assess nodal staging in difficult cases and to help differentiate cancer from an adjacent collapsed/consolidated lung. PET also has a role to play in the more difficult issue of detecting important asymptomatic metastases that, if discovered, would divert patients from a futile attempt at curative surgery.

Key Points

- The diagnosis of lung cancer may occur during coordinated investigation of symptoms or incidentally on imaging performed for other reasons.
- Once identified the tumor should be staged using the TNM system.
- Currently diagnosis and staging rely predominantly on chest radiography and computed tomography (CT) scanning.
- Use of positron emission tomography for staging disease is increasing in concert with availability.
- Use of magnetic resonance imaging remains confined to problem-solving in cases of uncertainty on CT (e.g., superior sulcus tumors).

11.4 Conclusion

The diagnosis and staging of lung cancer is a multiphase process. The initial diagnosis may arise following investigation of associated clinical symptoms or, as is often the case, may be an incidental finding on chest radiography performed for another reason. Once detected, the tumor should be graded according to the TNM system and then staged using the International Staging System.

Currently, the British Thoracic Society and Society of Cardiothoracic Surgeons of Great Britain and Ireland Working Party [108] guidelines for preoperative suitability assessment for patients with lung cancer are:

1. All patients being considered for surgery should have a plain chest radiograph and a CT scan of the thorax including the liver and adrenal glands.
2. Confirmatory diagnostic percutaneous needle biopsy in patients presenting with peripheral lesions is not mandatory in patients who are otherwise fit, particularly if there are previous chest radiographs showing no evidence of a lesion.
3. Patients with mediastinal nodes with a short-axis diameter greater than 1 cm in short axis diameter on the CT scan should undergo biopsy sampling by staging mediastinoscopy, anterior mediastinotomy, or needle biopsy, as appropriate.

References

1. Spiro S, Porter C. Lung cancer –Where are we today? Am J Respir Crit Care Med 2002; 166:1166.
2. Hackshaw AK, Law MR, Wald NJ. The accumulated evidence on lung cancer and environmental tobacco smoke. BMJ 1997; 315:980.
3. Janssen-Heijnen M, Gatta G, Forman D, Capocaccia R, Coebergh J, and the Eurocare Working Group: variation in survival of patients with lung cancer in Europe, 1985–1989. Eur J Cancer 1998; 34:2191.
4. Filderman A, Shaw C, Matthay R. Lung cancer. Part I: etiology, pathology, natural history, manifestations and diagnostic techniques. Invest Radiol 1986; 21:80.
5. Ferguson M. Diagnosing and staging of non-small cell lung cancer. Hematol Oncol Clin North Am 1990; 4:1053.
6. Jett J, Cortese D, Fontana R. Lung cancer current concepts and prospects. Cancer 1983; 33:74.
7. Steele JD. The solitary pulmonary nodule. Report of a cooperative study of resected asymptomatic solitary pulmonary nodules in males. J Thorac Cardiovasc Surg 1963; 46:21.
8. Goldmeier E. Limits of visibility of bronchogenic carcinoma. Am Rev Respir Dis 1965; 91:232.
9. Theros E. Varying manifestations of peripheral pulmonary neoplasms: a radiologic-pathologic correlative study. AJR Am J Roentgenol 1977; 128:893.
10. Kundel HL. Predictive value and threshold detectability of lung tumors. Radiology 1981; 139:25.
11. Muhm JR, Miller WE, Fontana RS, Sanderson DR, Uhlenhopp MA. Lung cancer detected during a screening program using four-month chest radiographs. Radiology 1983; 148:609.

12. Woodring J. Pitfalls in the radiologic diagnosis of lung cancer. AJR Am J Roentgenol 1990; 154:609.
13. Gomersall L, Olson S. Imaging in lung cancer. Imaging 2004; 16:1.
14. Good C, Wilson T. The solitary circumscribed pulmonary nodule. JAMA 1958; 166:210.
15. Yankelevitz D, Henschke C. Does 2-year stability imply pulmonary nodules are benign? AJR Am J Roentgenol 1997; 168:325.
16. Patz EF, Jr. Imaging bronchogenic carcinoma. Chest 2000; 117:90, 23.
17. Armstrong P. Neoplasms of the lungs, airways and pleura. In: Armstrong P, Wilson A, Dee P, Hansell D (eds.) Imaging Diseases of the Chest. Mosby (Harcourt), London, 2000; p 305.
18. Stewart J, MacMahon H, Viborny C, Pollak E. Dystrophic calcification in carcinoma of the lung: demonstration by CT. AJR Am J Roentgenol 1987; 148:29.
19. Mahoney M, Shipley R, Corcoran H, Dickson B. CT demonstration of calcification in carcinoma of the lung. AJR Am J Roentgenol 1990; 154:255.
20. Felson B, Wiot J. Some less familiar roentgen manifestations of carcinoma of the lung. Semin Roentgenol 1977; 12:187.
21. Henschke C, Yankelevitz D, Mirtcheva R, McGuiness G, McCauley D, Miettinen S, ELCAP Group. CT screening for lung cancer: frequency and significance of part-solid and nonsolid nodules. AJR Am J Roentgenol 2002; 178:1053.
22. Henschke C, McCauley D, Yankelevitz D, et al. Early lung cancer action project: overall design and findings from baseline screening. Lancet 1999; 354:99.
23. Hasegawa M, Sone S, Takashima S, et al. Growth rate of small lung cancers detected on mass CT screening. Radiology 2000; 73:1252.
24. Lehar TJ, Carr DT, Miller WE, Payne WS, Woolner LB. Roentgenographic appearance of bronchogenic adenocarcinoma. Am Rev Respir Dis 1967; 96:245.
25. Byrd RB, Miller WE, Carr DT, Payne WS, Woolner LB. The roentgenographic appearance of small cell carcinoma of the bronchus. Mayo Clin Proc 1968; 43:337.
26. Byrd RB, Miller WE, Carr DT, Payne WS, Woolner LB. The roentgenographic appearance of large cell carcinoma of the bronchus. Mayo Clin Proc 1968; 43:333.
27. Byrd RB, Miller WE, Carr DT, Payne WS, Woolner LB. The roentgenographic appearance of squamous cell carcinoma of the bronchus. Mayo Clin Proc 1968; 43:327.
28. Byrd RB, Carr DT, Miller WE, Payne WS, Woolner LB. Radiographic abnormalities in carcinoma of the lung as related to histologic cell type. Thorax 1969; 24:573.
29. Erasmus J, Patz E, McAdams H, et al. Evaluation of adrenal masses in patients with bronchogenic carcinoma using 18F-fluorodeoxyglucose positron emission tomography. AJR Am J Roentgenol 1997; 168:1357.
30. Siegelman S, Khouri N, Leo F, Fishman E, Baverman R, Zerhouni E. Solitary pulmonary nodules: CT assessment. Radiology 1986; 160:307.
31. Muhm J, McCullough A. The enhancing rim: a new sign of a benign pulmonary nodule. Mayo Clin Proc 2003; 78:1092.
32. Quinn D, Gianlupi A, Broste S. The changing radiographic presentation of bronchogenic carcinoma with reference to cell types. Chest 1996; 110:1474.
33. Chaudhuri M. Primary pulmonary cavitating carcinomas. Thorax 1973; 28:354.
34. Matthews M. Morphology of lung cancer. Semin Oncol 1974; 1:175.
35. Revel M, Bissery A, Bienvenu M, Aycard L, Lefort C, Frija G. Are two-dimensional CT measurements of small noncalcified pulmonary nodules reliable? Radiology 2004; 231:453.
36. Revel M, Lefort C, Bissery A, et al. Pulmonary nodules: preliminary experience with three-dimensional evaluation. Radiology 2004; 231:459.
37. Nathan M, Collins V, Adams R. Differentiation of benign and malignant pulmonary nodules by growth rate. Radiology 1962; 79:221.
38. Sato M, Saito Y, Endo C, Sakurada A, Feller-Kopman D, Ernst A, Kondo T. The natural history of radiographically occult bronchogenic squamous cell carcinoma: a retrospective study of overdiagnosis bias. Chest 2004; 126:108.
39. Bungay H, Pal C, Davies C, Davies R, Gleeson F. An evaluation of computed tomography as an aid to diagnosis in patients undergoing bronchoscopy for suspected bronchial carcinoma. Clin Radiol 2000; 55:560.
40. Murphy J, Gleeson F, Flower C. Percutaneous needle biopsy of the lung and its impact on patient management. World J Surg 2001; 25:373.
41. Baldwin D, Birchall J, Ganatra R, Pointon K. Evaluation of the solitary pulmonary nodule: clinical management, role of CT and nuclear medicine. Imaging 2004; 16:22.
42. Dwamena B, Sonnad S, Angobaldo J, Wahl R. Metastases from non-small cell lung cancer: mediastinal staging in the 1990s – meta-analytic comparison of PET and CT. Radiology 1999; 213:530.
43. Pieterman R, van Putten J, Meuezelaar J, et al. Preoperative staging of non-small cell lung cancer with positron emission tomography. New Eng J Med 2000; 343:254.
44. Erasmus J, McAdams, HP, Patz E, Goodman, PC, Coleman R. Thoracic FDG PET: state of the art. Radiographics 1998; 18:5.
45. Nomori H, Watanabe K, Ohtsuka M, et al. Evaluation of F-18 fluoro-deoxy-glucose (FDG) PET scanning for pulmonary nodules less than 3 cm in diameter, with special reference to the CT images. Lung Cancer 2004; 45:19.
46. Langen K, Braun U, Rota Kops E, et al. The influence of plasma glucose levels on fluorine-18-fluorodeoxyglucose uptake in bronchial carcinomas. J Nucl Med 1993; 34:355.
47. Blum J, Handmaker H, Lister-James J, Rinne N. A multicenter trial with a somatostatin analog 99mTc Depreotide in the evaluation of solitary pulmonary nodules. Chest 2000; 117:1232.
48. Mountain CF. Revisions in the International System for Staging Lung Cancer. Chest 1997; 111:1710.
49. Grunenwald D, Mazel C, Girard P, Berthiot G, Dromer C, Baldeyrou P. Total vertebrectomy for en bloc resection of lung cancer invading the spine. Ann Thorac Surg 1996; 61:723.
50. Onitsuka H, Tsukuda M, Araki A, Murakami J, Torii Y, Masuda K. Differentiation of central lung tumor from postobstructive lobar collapse by rapid sequence computed tomography. J Thorac Imaging 1991; 6:28.
51. Tobler J, Levitt RG, Glazer HS, Moran J, Crouch E, Evens RG. Differentiation of proximal bronchogenic carcinoma from post-obstructive lobar collapse by magnetic resonance imaging. Comparison with computed tomography. Invest Radiol 1987; 22:538.
52. Kono M, Adachi S, Kusumoto M, Sakai E. Clinical utility of Gd-DTPA-enhanced magnetic resonance imaging in lung cancer. J Thorac Imaging 1993; 8:18.
53. Houston JG, Fleet M, McMillan N, Cowan MD. Ultrasonic assessment of hemidiaphragmatic movement: an indirect method of evaluating mediastinal invasion in non-small cell lung cancer. Br J Radiol 1995; 68:695.
54. Martini N, Heelan R, Westcott J, et al. Comparative merits of conventional, computed tomographic, and magnetic resonance imaging in assessing mediastinal involvement in surgically confirmed lung carcinoma. J Thorac Cardiovasc Surg 1985; 90:639.
55. Glazer HS, Kaiser LR, Anderson DJ, Molina PL, Emami B, Roper CL, Sagel SS. Indeterminate mediastinal invasion in

bronchogenic carcinoma: CT evaluation. Radiology 1989; 173:37.

56. Musset D, Grenier P, Carette MF, et al. Primary lung cancer staging: prospective comparative study of MR imaging with CT. Radiology 1986; 160:607.

57. Webb WR, Gatsonis C, Zerhouni EA, Heelan RT, Glazer GM, Francis IR, McNeil BJ. CT and MR imaging in staging non-small cell bronchogenic carcinoma: report of the Radiologic Diagnostic Oncology Group. Radiology 1991; 178:705.

58. Mayr B, Lenhard M, Fink U, Heywang-Kobrunner SH, Sunder-Plassmann L, Permanetter W. Preoperative evaluation of bronchogenic carcinoma: value of MR in T- and N-staging. Eur J Radiol 1992; 14:245.

59. Ohno Y, Adachi S, Motoyama A, et al. Multiphase ECG-triggered 3D contrast-enhanced MR angiography: utility for evaluation of hilar and mediastinal invasion of bronchogenic carcinoma. J Magn Resonance Imaging 2001; 12:215.

60. Pugatch RD. Radiologic evaluation in chest malignancies. A review of imaging modalities. Chest 1995; 107:294S.

61. Kamel EM, Goerres GW, Burger C, von Schulthess GK, Steinert HC. Recurrent laryngeal nerve palsy in patients with lung cancer: detection with PET-CT image fusion – report of six cases. Radiology 2002; 224:153.

62. Glazer HS, Duncan-Meyer J, Aronberg DJ, Moran JF, Levitt RG, Sagel SS. Pleural and chest wall invasion in bronchogenic carcinoma: CT evaluation. Radiology 1985; 157:191.

63. Pennes DR, Glazer GM, Wimbish KJ, Gross BH, Long RW, Orringer MB. Chest wall invasion by lung cancer: limitations of CT evaluation. AJR Am J Roentgenol 1985; 144:507.

64. Pearlberg JL, Sandler MA, Beute GH, Lewis JW, Jr., Madrazo BL. Limitations of CT in evaluation of neoplasms involving chest wall. J Comput Assist Tomogr 1987; 11:290.

65. Ratto GB, Piacenza G, Frola C, et al. Chest wall involvement by lung cancer: computed tomographic detection and results of operation. Ann Thorac Surg 1991; 51:182.

66. Murata K, Takahashi M, Mori M, et al. Chest wall and mediastinal invasion by lung cancer: evaluation with multisection expiratory dynamic CT. Radiology 1994; 191:251.

67. Padovani B, Mouroux J, Seksik L, et al. Chest wall invasion by bronchogenic carcinoma: evaluation with MR imaging. Radiology 1993; 187:33.

68. Heelan RT, Demas BE, Caravelli JF, et al. Superior sulcus tumors: CT and MR imaging. Radiology 1989; 170:637.

69. Suzuki N, Saitoh T, Kitamura S. Tumor invasion of the chest wall in lung cancer: diagnosis with US. Radiology 1993; 187:39.

70. Nakano N, Yasumitsu T, Kotake Y, Morino H, Ikezoe J. Preoperative histologic diagnosis of chest wall invasion by lung cancer using ultrasonically guided biopsy. J Thorac Cardiovasc Surg 1994; 107:891.

71. Schaffler GJ, Wolf G, Schoellnast H, et al. Non-small cell lung cancer: evaluation of pleural abnormalities on CT scans with 18F FDG PET. Radiology 2004; 231:858.

72. Erasmus JJ, McAdams HP, Rossi SE, Goodman PC, Coleman RE, Patz EF. FDG PET of pleural effusions in patients with non-small cell lung cancer. AJR Am J Roentgenol 2000; 175:245.

73. Light RW, Erozan YS, Ball WC Jr. Cells in pleural fluid. Their value in differential diagnosis. Arch Intern Med 1973; 132:854.

74. Tateishi M, Fukuyama Y, Hamatake M, Kohdono S, Ishida T, Sugimachi K. Skip mediastinal lymph node metastasis in non-small cell lung cancer. J Surg Oncol 1994; 57:139.

75. van OH, Brakel K, Heijenbrok MW, van Kasteren JH, van de Moosdijk CN, Roldaan AC, van Gils AP, Hansen BE.

Metastases in supraclavicular lymph nodes in lung cancer: assessment with palpation, US, and CT. Radiology 2004; 232:75.

76. Glazer GM, Gross BH, Quint LE, Francis IR, Bookstein FL, Orringer MB. Normal mediastinal lymph nodes: number and size according to American Thoracic Society mapping. AJR Am J Roentgenol 1985; 144:261.

77. Quint LE, Glazer GM, Orringer MB, Francis IR, Bookstein FL. Mediastinal lymph node detection and sizing at CT and autopsy. AJR Am J Roentgenol 1986; 147:469.

78. Kerr KM, Lamb D, Wathen CG, Walker WS, Douglas NJ. Pathological assessment of mediastinal lymph nodes in lung cancer: implications for non-invasive mediastinal staging. Thorax 1992; 47:337.

79. McLoud TC, Bourgouin PM, Greenberg RW, et al. Bronchogenic carcinoma: analysis of staging in the mediastinum with CT by correlative lymph node mapping and sampling. Radiology 1992; 182:319.

80. Ohno Y, Hatabu H, Takenaka D, et al. Metastases in mediastinal and hilar lymph nodes in patients with non-small cell lung cancer: quantitative and qualitative assessment with STIR turbo spin-echo MR imaging. Radiology 2004; 231:872.

81. Steinert HC, Hauser M, Allemann F, Engel H, Berthold T, von Schulthess GK, Weder W. Non-small cell lung cancer: nodal staging with FDG PET versus CT with correlative lymph node mapping and sampling. Radiology 1997; 202:441.

82. Antoch G, Stattaus J, Nemat AT, et al. Non-small cell lung cancer: dual-modality PET/CT in preoperative staging. Radiology 2003; 229:526.

83. Gdeedo A, Van SP, Corthouts B, Van MF, Van MJ, Van ME. Prospective evaluation of computed tomography and mediastinoscopy in mediastinal lymph node staging. Eur Respir J 1997; 10:1547.

84. Marom EM, McAdams HP, Erasmus JJ, et al. Staging non-small cell lung cancer with whole-body PET. Radiology 1999; 212:803.

85. van OH, Hoekstra OS, Smit EF, et al. Effectiveness of positron emission tomography in the preoperative assessment of patients with suspected non-small-cell lung cancer: the PLUS multicentre randomised trial. Lancet 2002; 359:1388.

86. Toloza EM, Harpole L, McCrory DC. Noninvasive staging of non-small cell lung cancer: a review of the current evidence. Chest 2003; 123:137S.

87. Fritscher-Ravens A, Davidson BL, Hauber HP, et al. Endoscopic ultrasound, positron emission tomography, and computerized tomography for lung cancer. Am J Respir Crit Care Med 2003; 168:1293.

88. Potepan P, Meroni E, Spagnoli I, et al. Non-small-cell lung cancer: detection of mediastinal lymph node metastases by endoscopic ultrasound and CT. Eur Radiol 1996; 6:19.

89. Smith RA. Evaluation of the long-term results of surgery for bronchial carcinoma. J Thorac Cardiovasc Surg 1981; 82:325.

90. Feld R, Rubinstein LV, Weisenberger TH. Sites of recurrence in resected stage I non-small-cell lung cancer: a guide for future studies. J Clin Oncol 1984; 2:1352.

91. Sider L, Horejs D. Frequency of extrathoracic metastases from bronchogenic carcinoma in patients with normal-sized hilar and mediastinal lymph nodes on CT. AJR Am J Roentgenol 1988; 151:893.

92. Kormas P, Bradshaw JR, Jeyasingham K. Preoperative computed tomography of the brain in non-small cell bronchogenic carcinoma. Thorax 1992; 47:106.

93. Salvatierra A, Baamonde C, Llamas JM, Cruz F, Lopez-Pujol J. Extrathoracic staging of bronchogenic carcinoma. Chest 1990; 97:1052.

94. Silvestri GA, Littenberg B, Colice GL. The clinical evaluation for detecting metastatic lung cancer. A meta-analysis. Am J Respir Crit Care Med 1995; 152:225.

95. Oliver TW Jr, Bernardino ME, Miller JI, Mansour K, Greene D, Davis WA. Isolated adrenal masses in non-small-cell bronchogenic carcinoma. Radiology 1984; 153:217.

96. Korobkin M, Lombardi TJ, Aisen AM, et al. Characterization of adrenal masses with chemical shift and gadolinium-enhanced MR imaging. Radiology 1995; 197:411.

97. Schrevens L, Lorent N, Dooms C, Vansteenkiste J. The role of PET scan in diagnosis, staging, and management of non-small cell lung cancer. Oncologist 2004; 9:633.

98. Earnest F, Ryu JH, Miller GM, Luetmer PH, Forstrom LA, Burnett OL, Rowland CM, Swensen SJ, Midthun DE. Suspected non-small cell lung cancer: incidence of occult brain and skeletal metastases and effectiveness of imaging for detection–pilot study. Radiology 1999; 211:137.

99. Hooper RG, Tenholder MF, Underwood GH, Beechler CR, Spratling L. Computed tomographic scanning of the brain in initial staging of bronchogenic carcinoma. Chest 1984; 85:774.

100. Klein JS, Webb WR. The radiologic staging of lung cancer. J Thorac Imaging 1991; 7:29

101. Newman SJ, Hansen HH. Proceedings: Frequency, diagnosis, and treatment of brain metastases in 247 consecutive patients with bronchogenic carcinoma. Cancer 1974; 33:492.

102. Kormas P, Bradshaw JR, Jeyasingham K. Preoperative computed tomography of the brain in non-small cell bronchogenic carcinoma. Thorax 1992; 47:106.

103. Colice GL, Birkmeyer JD, Black WC, Littenberg B, Silvestri G. Cost-effectiveness of head CT in patients with lung cancer without clinical evidence of metastases. Chest 1995; 108:1264.

104. Marom EM, Patz EF, Jr., Swensen SJ. Radiologic findings of bronchogenic carcinoma with pulmonary metastases at presentation. Clin Radiol 1999; 54:665.

105. Osterlind K, Hansen M, Hansen HH, Dombernowsky P. Influence of surgical resection prior to chemotherapy on the long-term results in small cell lung cancer. A study of 150 operable patients. Eur J Cancer Clin Oncol 1986; 22:589.

106. Abrams J, Doyle LA, Aisner J. Staging, prognostic factors, and special considerations in small cell lung cancer. Semin Oncol 1988; 15:261.

107. Schumacher T, Brink I, Mix M, et al. FDG-PET imaging for the staging and follow-up of small cell lung cancer. Eur J Nucl Med 2001; 28:483.

108. British Thoracic Society guidelines: guidelines on the selection of patients with lung cancer for surgery. Thorax 2001; 56:89.

109. Dunnick N, Korobkin M. Imaging of adrenal incidentalomas: current status. AJR Am J Roentgenol 2002; 179:559.

Surgical Staging of Non-Small-Cell Lung Cancer

12

Ricardo Bello and Steven M. Keller

Contents

12.1   Introduction

Accurate intraoperative assessment of disease extension is an essential component of surgery for non-small-cell lung cancer (NSCLC). Although the size of the primary tumor and invasion of adjacent structures (T descriptor) may be readily determined by the surgeon and pathologist, the presence or absence of tumor within the intrathoracic lymph nodes (N descriptor) can be ascertained only by microscopic examination. Histologic staging relies on the quality of the specimens that are submitted to the pathologist. Thus, care must be taken to ensure that the appropriate specimens are obtained and properly handled. In order to appreciate the technical aspects of the staging procedures, an understanding of pulmonary lymphatic drainage and intrathoracic metastatic patterns is necessary. The information that is derived from the surgical/pathologic staging process is important for three reasons. First, it allows optimal decisions regarding the need for additional therapy. Second, it provides prognostic information. Third, it provides a reproducible method for comparison of different treatment strategies.

12.2   Patterns of Lymphatic Drainage and Metastases

The classic description of the mediastinal lymph nodes in the human adult is found in Anatomie des Lymphatiques de l'Homme, in which meticulous postmortem dissection was combined with dye injection of the lymphatics to identify common drainage pathways. An in vivo radionuclide investigation of pulmonary drainage patterns was performed in 179 patients who had no evidence of lymph node metastases [1]. ^{99m}Tc-labeled antimony sulfide or rhenium colloid was injected submucosally under bronchoscopic guidance into each segmental bronchus. A total of 192 lymphoscintigraphies were performed. The results are summarized in Fig. 12.1. The apical and posterior segments of the right upper lobe drained to the ipsilateral scalene nodes via the hilum, tracheobronchial angle, and upper paratracheal nodes. The anterior segment of the right upper lobe drained via three dominant pathways. Approximately half of the patients drained via the same pathway as the other right upper lobe segments. The remainder drained via the subcarinal nodes, continuing to the pretracheal, right paratracheal (left paratracheal rarely), and right scalene nodes, or alternatively to the left scalene nodes by way of the innominate vein and left anterior mediastinal nodes. The middle lobe and superior segment of the lower lobe exhibited similar drainage patterns. In both cases, the preferential pathway was to the right scalene nodes through the pathways described above. However, a minority drained to the left scalene nodes via the subcarinal and left paratracheal nodes. The basal segments of the right lung ultimately drained to the right scalene nodes via the subcarinal and right paratracheal nodes.

Drainage patterns observed in the left lung were more variable. The dominant pathway of the apical-posterior segment of the left upper lobe was to the subcarinal nodes, continuing along either the vagus nerve to the scalene nodes or along the recurrent laryngeal nerve to the mediastinal nodes. The lingula and anterior segments of the left upper lobe shared a similar

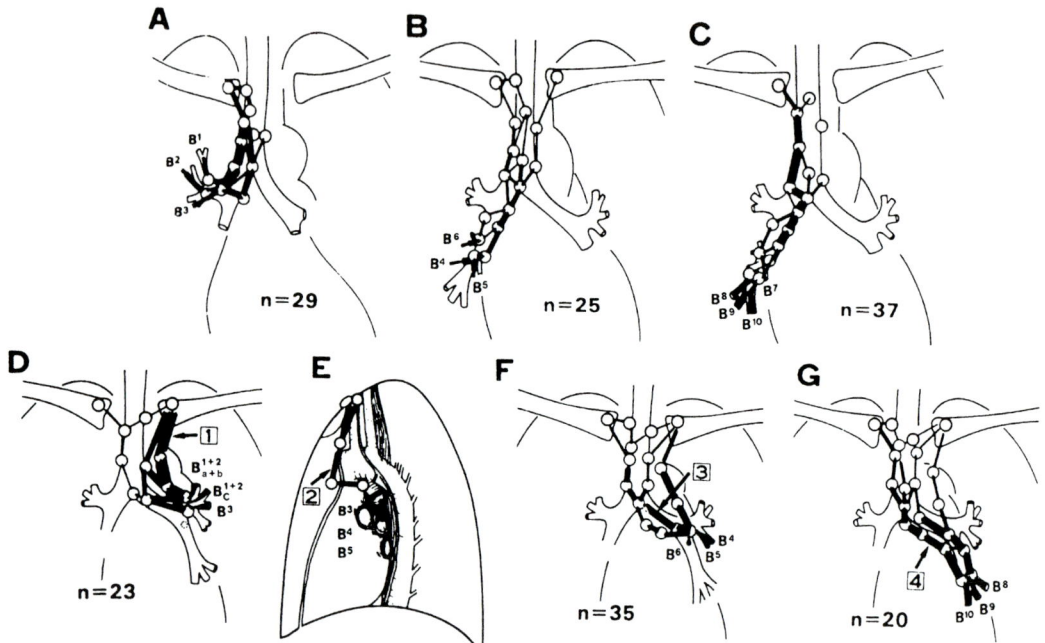

Fig. 12.1. Patterns of metastases to the mediastinal lymph nodes. The width of each *arrow* corresponds to the relative metastases via the indicated pathways. **A** The apical and dorsal segments of the right upper lobe. **B** The middle lobe and superior segment of the right lower lobe. **C** The basal segments of the right lower lobe. **D** The apicoposterior segment of the left upper lobe. **E** The anterior segment of the left upper lobe and lingula. **F** The superior segment of the left lower lobe. **G** The basal segments of the left lower lobe. B^1–B^{10} Mediastinal lymph nodes groups, *boxed numbers 1–4* main drainage pathways. Reproduced by permission from Hata et al. [1]

pattern, draining along the phrenic nerve to the para-aortic and left scalene nodes. The basal segments of the lower lobe drained primarily through the subcarinal, pretracheal, and right (occasionally left) paratracheal nodes to the right scalene nodes. The superior segment of the lower lobe exhibited the most variability, draining by all of the above pathways.

Whereas Hata et al. [1] outlined the lymphatic drainage patterns of patients without lymph node metastases, several investigators have studied the metastatic patterns in patients with biopsy-proven nodal involvement. Borrie [2] documented the patterns of dissemination within the intrapulmonary lymphatics of resected specimens from 92 patients. He found that tumors in all lobes of the right lung metastasized to the lymph nodes situated between the upper lobe and the middle lobe bronchi. Similarly, tumors of both lobes of the left lung commonly metastasized to the lymph nodes between the lobar bronchi (sumps of Borrie). The mediastinal lymph nodes were not studied.

Nohl-Oser [3, 4] confirmed these findings and supplemented them with his own results regarding metastasis to the mediastinal nodes. Lymph nodes harvested by mediastinoscopy, scalene node biopsy, or mediastinal lymph node dissection from 749 patients with stage I–IV NSCLC were analyzed. Right upper lobe tumors frequently spread to the ipsilateral mediastinum, but rarely to the subcarinal nodes or the contralateral mediastinum. Right lower lobe tumors commonly metastasized to the subcarinal nodes and ipsilateral mediastinum, but were unlikely to spread to the contralateral mediastinum. He could not draw conclusions regarding tumors originating in the right middle lobe, due to an insufficient number of cases. Tumors of the left upper and lower lobe seemed to metastasize to the subcarinal and contralateral mediastinal nodes.

In a study of 166 patients with biopsy-proven N2 NSCLC, Asamura et al. [5] described metastatic patterns with some similarities to those described above. Tumors in all lobes appeared to metastasize to the mediastinum by way of the interlobar and hilar nodes. Right upper lobe tumors most commonly spread to the lower pretracheal nodes (74%). Metastases to the subcarinal nodes were much less frequent (13%). Right middle lobe tumors involved the subcarinal nodes most frequently (88%), followed by the lower pretracheal nodes (75%). Right lower lobe tumors involved the ipsilateral paratracheal nodes as well as the upper and lower pretracheal nodes (76%), and the subcarinal nodes less often (58%). Left upper lobe tumors, collectively, spread most commonly to the aortopulmonary window (59%) and para-aortic nodes (32%). Subcarinal nodes were less frequently involved (21%), but were the most common site for tumors of the lingula. Left lower lobe tumors

Table 12.1. Pattern of intrathoracic metastases in patients with N2 lymph node involvement. Right upper lobe tumors tended to metastasize to the right paratracheal and lower pretracheal nodes. Right and left lower lobe tumors predominantly metastasized to the lower mediastinal and subcarinal nodes. Left upper lobe tumors spread to the aortopulmonary window, pretracheal, and left paratracheal nodes. Centrally located tumors on both sides frequently involved the subcarinal nodes. Central tumors are not classified into a particular lobe and thus are considered separately

Primary location	n	N2 Nodal levels								
		1	2	3	4	5	6	7	8	9
Right upper lobe	17	1	2	9	13			1	1	
Right middle lobe	2				1			1		
Right lower lobe	12	1	1		1			5	7	2
Right central	23		5	10	12			13	4	2
Left upper lobe	19		2	5		16	1	1		1
Left lower lobe	9			1	1			4	4	2
Left central	41		2	10		20	11	16	2	1

most commonly metastasized to the subcarinal nodes (58%). Superior mediastinal or aortic nodes were also involved quite frequently (58%).

Kotoulas et al. [6] conducted a retrospective review of 557 patients who underwent pulmonary resection and lymph node dissection. Their results are summarized in Table 12.1 and are in general agreement with the findings of Nohl-Oser [4] and Asamura et al. [5]. In addition, centrally located tumors from all lobes were more likely to metastasize to the subcarinal nodes than peripherally located tumors. This may explain the unexpected findings of Watanabe et al. [7], who described frequent metastasis from the right upper lobe to the subcarinal nodes.

12.3   Intraoperative Staging

12.3.1   Lymph Node Dissection

A precise definition of the operative technique and staging system is crucial to the conduct of multi-institutional trials and comparison of investigational results. In general, "sampling" refers to the removal of any lymph nodes that are obviously abnormal. "Systematic sampling" indicates that routine biopsy is performed at the specified lymph node stations. "Complete mediastinal lymph node dissection" refers to removal of all lymph-node-bearing tissue at the specified levels [8–10].

Because of its dependence on visual and tactile identification of abnormal lymph nodes, sampling is considered inferior to both systematic sampling and complete mediastinal lymph node dissection. In a study of 95 consecutive patients, Gaer and Goldstraw [11] compared intraoperative assessment by the surgeon to histopathologic examination of the resected lymph nodes. All patients underwent mediastinal lymph node dissection following pulmonary resection of NSCLC. Samples taken from 287 nodal levels were examined by the surgeon prior to submission for microscopic examination. Assessment by the surgeon had a sensitivity of only 71% and a positive predictive value of only 64%. These results are not surprising, as micrometastases would not be expected to change the texture or appearance of the lymph nodes. Had the surgeon examined the lymph nodes through an unopened pleura, the sensitivity would presumably have been even poorer.

Further evidence for the unreliable nature of sampling for precise staging comes from a study by Haiderer et al. [12]. Lymph nodes harvested from 102 patients who underwent pulmonary resection and mediastinal lymph node dissection were examined histologically. Enlarged lymph nodes were noted in 41% of the patients, but metastatic disease was identified in only 56% of this group. Moreover, in the patients with normal-appearing lymph nodes, 4.1% were found to have evidence of metastasis. Bollen et al. [13] reviewed a series of 155 patients with NSCLC, 85 of whom underwent complete mediastinal lymph node dissection and 70 of whom had lymph nodes removed if they appeared or felt abnormal. N2 disease was 2.1 times (95% confidence interval 1.04–4.2) more likely to be detected in patients who had undergone either systematic sampling or complete mediastinal lymph node dissection than in those who underwent sampling. Several studies have demonstrated that systematic sampling and complete mediastinal lymph node dissection are equally efficacious for diagnosing N2 disease [13–16]. However, complete mediastinal lymph node dissection will demonstrate more levels of N2 disease.

In addition to the superior diagnostic ability suggested by the aforementioned studies, several studies have reported a survival benefit in patients who underwent mediastinal lymph node dissection. In a prospective randomized trial of 169 patients, Izbicki et al. [17] demonstrated that mediastinal lymph node dissection tended to improve survival ($p = 0.058$) and prolong disease-free survival ($p = 0.037$) in patients with pN1 or limited (single node) pN2 disease. In a prospective non-randomized trial of 373 patients with stages II and IIIa,

Keller et al. [10] found that systematic sampling and complete mediastinal lymph node dissection diagnosed N2 disease equally well. However, complete mediastinal lymph node dissection detected disease in significantly more N2 lymph node stations compared to systematic sampling (30% vs. 12%, $p = 0.001$). Complete mediastinal lymph node dissection also conferred a survival advantage compared to systematic sampling (57.5 vs. 29.2 months median survival, $p = 0.004$) in patients with tumors of the right lung. Wu et al. [18] conducted a prospective randomized trial of 532 patients with stages I–IIIa NSCLC who underwent pulmonary resection and either complete mediastinal lymph node dissection or sampling. The 5-year overall survival was 48% in the mediastinal lymph node dissection group and 37% in the sampling group ($p = 0.0001$). A survival benefit in patients who underwent mediastinal lymph node dissection was also seen when the patients were compared by stage ($p = 0.0104$, $p = 0.028$, and $p = 0.024$ for stage I, II, and IIIa, respectively). In addition, mediastinal lymph node dissection reduced the rate of local recurrence and distant metastasis. The American College of Surgeons – Oncology Group has completed, but not yet analyzed, a trial (Z0030) designed to compare the diagnostic and survival differences between systematic sampling and complete mediastinal lymph node dissection.

12.3.2   Sentinel Node Mapping

Micrometastases to intrathoracic lymph nodes can be difficult to detect by routine microscopic analysis. Falsely identifying lymph nodes to be free of disease can lead to understaging and decreased survival [19, 20]. Highly sensitive methods, such as immunohistochemistry or polymerase chain reaction, have been used to detect micrometastatic disease. However, routine application of these methods to all nodes harvested during a lymph node dissection can be a formidable task. Sentinel lymph node mapping provides a way to identify the first lymph node(s) in the lymphatic drainage pathway for a given primary tumor. Theoretically, the sentinel node(s) should be the first site of nodal involvement if metastases have occurred. Immunohistochemistry or polymerase chain reaction can be used to selectively examine this node(s), which is most likely to contain metastases, while the remaining nodes can be examined with routine methods. Identification of the sentinel node(s) should, therefore, improve staging accuracy and prognosis.

Sentinel node mapping is a relatively simple procedure that is performed at the time of pulmonary resection. Either preoperatively by computed tomography (CT) guidance or upon entering the chest, a small amount of dye or radioactive tracer is injected with a fine needle into or around the primary tumor. If a dye

is used, the hilar and mediastinal pleura are opened to allow for better visualization of the underlying structures. While allowing time (at least 10–15 min) for dye or tracer dispersion, the hilar dissection can be performed. Dissection around the bronchus should be limited, as the majority of lymphatics are found in this area. The sentinel node(s) is sought by visual inspection or with the aid of a gamma counter. Once identified, it is removed intact and its nodal level noted.

Liptay et al. [21] reported 91 patients with resectable NSCLC who underwent sentinel lymph node mapping (^{99m}Tc sulfur colloid), anatomic resection, and complete mediastinal lymph node dissection. A sentinel lymph node was found in 78 (86%) patients. In 21 out of 78 (27%), the sentinel node was found to contain metastatic disease, and in 9 patients it was the only positive node. Serial sectioning or immunohistochemistry was required to detect the disease in seven of the nine patients, and all seven were subsequently upstaged. Interestingly, the sentinel node was found in the mediastinum (N2) in 16 patients with an identifiable sentinel node, without concomitant disease in the intrapulmonary lymph nodes (N1). In 9 out of 78 (15%) of patients the sentinel node was declared to be free of tumor in the presence of disease in other lymph nodes.

Schmidt et al. [22] studied 31 patients with clinical stage I or II NSCLC who underwent sentinel lymph node mapping (^{99m}Tc sulfur colloid and/or isosulfan blue), pulmonary resection, and complete mediastinal lymph node dissection. Sentinel nodes were sought only in the mediastinum and were identified in 25 patients. The sentinel node was commonly demonstrated by both methods, but occasionally the sentinel node contained only dye or radiotracer. Thus, it appears that using both dye and radiotracer increases the likelihood of finding a sentinel node. In three patients a tumor was found in the sentinel node; two of these patients also had a tumor in the hilar lymph nodes. One patient demonstrated skip metastases. No immunohistochemistry or serial sectioning was employed, so it is not known whether the 22 negative sentinel nodes contained micrometastases; however, in those cases no tumor was found in the more distant mediastinal nodes. The authors concluded that the presence of a mediastinal sentinel node(s) free of disease may obviate the need for a mediastinal lymph node dissection.

Investigations by Melfi et al. [23], Faries et al. [24], and Nomori et al. [25] in patients with clinical stage I NSCLC resulted in similar conclusions. A sentinel lymph node was identified in 81–100% of patients when a radiotracer was used for detection. The presence of bulky tumors or emphysema disrupted intrapulmonary lymphatic drainage sufficiently to preclude detection of a sentinel node in every case. The sentinel node(s) was found to be free of disease when, in fact, metastases were detected in other nonsentinel nodes in only 2.3–3.8% of patients. Tumor was present in the sentinel lymph node in 18–36% of patients and skip metastases were observed in 13–28%. All three studies suggest that patients without disease in the hilar and mediastinal sentinel lymph nodes may not require a complete mediastinal lymph node dissection. Data regarding long-term survival in patients undergoing sentinel lymph node mapping to determine the need for mediastinal lymph node dissection are not available. The efficacy of this procedure has yet to be proven in randomized trials and, as such, is still considered an experimental procedure. The Cancer and Leukemia Group B has opened a multicenter study (protocol 140203) to investigate the role of sentinel lymph node mapping in the treatment of early stage NSCLC

12.4   Evolution of the Staging System

Ample data support the conclusion that long-term survival varies with the location of tumor-bearing lymph nodes. This has led to the development of standardized lymph node maps, which in turn serve as a basis for the definition of the N categories. The map proposed by Naruke et al. (Fig. 12.2) [26] and accepted by the American Joint Committee on Cancer Staging and End Results Reporting (AJCC) became the international standard. Due to the lack of precise anatomic definitions, interpretations among investigators and institutions have varied [27]. For example, the limits of the aortic (levels 5–6) and superior mediastinal (levels 1–4) nodes were not clearly delineated. Thus, some investigators reported single-level metastases, whereas others reported multilevel nodal involvement. However, it is the definition of the hilar (level 10) lymph nodes and their categorization as N1 vs. N2 nodes that has drawn the most attention. The controversy stems from the fact that Naruke et al. [26] defined their location with reference to the tracheobronchial tree. In subsequent revisions of the staging system, their location relative to the pleural reflection was taken into account. Several studies have been conducted to address this issue; however, the results have not been consistent [28–31].

The American Thoracic Society (ATS) attempted to ameliorate the confusion by issuing an official statement in which the definitions offered by Naruke were replaced with detailed descriptions of each nodal level. This classification was based on constant anatomic structures that were easily identified in the operating room [32]. The issue regarding the classification of level 10 as N1 or N2 remained unresolved. Although they were used widely, the AJCC did not officially adopt these definitions.

The Lung Cancer Study Group initially used the AJCC nodal definitions, but later adopted the modified ATS definitions. In this scheme, level 10 nodes were categorized as N2 nodes. In 1986, the staging system was revised by Mountain [28] and gained acceptance by the international community. Both the AJCC and the Union International Contre le Cancer adopted this system in which the nodal level definitions remained unchanged, but the components of the N2 group were modified. In addition, the N3 group, which included disease in the supraclavicular, scalene, and contralateral mediastinal lymph nodes, was created.

This system remained in use until 1997 when new definitions for the lymph node level definitions were created (Figs. 12.3 and 12.4, Table 12.2) [33, 34]. In contrast to the ATS definitions, which were based on anatomic structures identified in the operating room, the new definitions referred to structures identifiable by CT scan. Several definitions referenced structures in the mediastinum, thus rendering the intraoperative identification of those levels more difficult.

12.5   Mediastinal Lymph Node Dissection

The earliest mention of mediastinal lymph node dissection performed at the time of a pulmonary resection for lung cancer appeared in an article by Brock [35]. However, it wasn't until several years later that Cahan et al. [36] and Weinberg [37] independently published a highly detailed description of their methods. As discussed earlier in this chapter, there are three broad categories of techniques for harvesting lymph nodes from the ipsilateral hemithorax: sampling, systematic sampling, and complete mediastinal lymph node dissection. Another approach, extended lymphadenectomy, entails removal of scalene, supraclavicular, jugular, and contralateral lymph nodes, and necessitates additional incisions (median sternotomy and cervical collar) and maneuvers (mobilization of the aortic arch and division of the ligamentum arteriosum).

Mediastinal lymph node dissection is easily accomplished via posterolateral or muscle-sparing thoracotomy using single-lung ventilation. Although typically performed after the pulmonary resection, mediastinal lymph node dissection may be performed first if the presence of tumor within the lymph nodes will alter the operative procedure. Lymph nodes harvested from the different levels must be labeled appropriately and sent from the operating room as discrete specimens. Improper handling of the specimens can negate the value of the most meticulous lymph node dissection.

12.5.1   Right Hemithorax

Entry to the chest through the fourth or fifth interspace provides access to the necessary lymph node levels. The superior mediastinum, encompassed by the superior

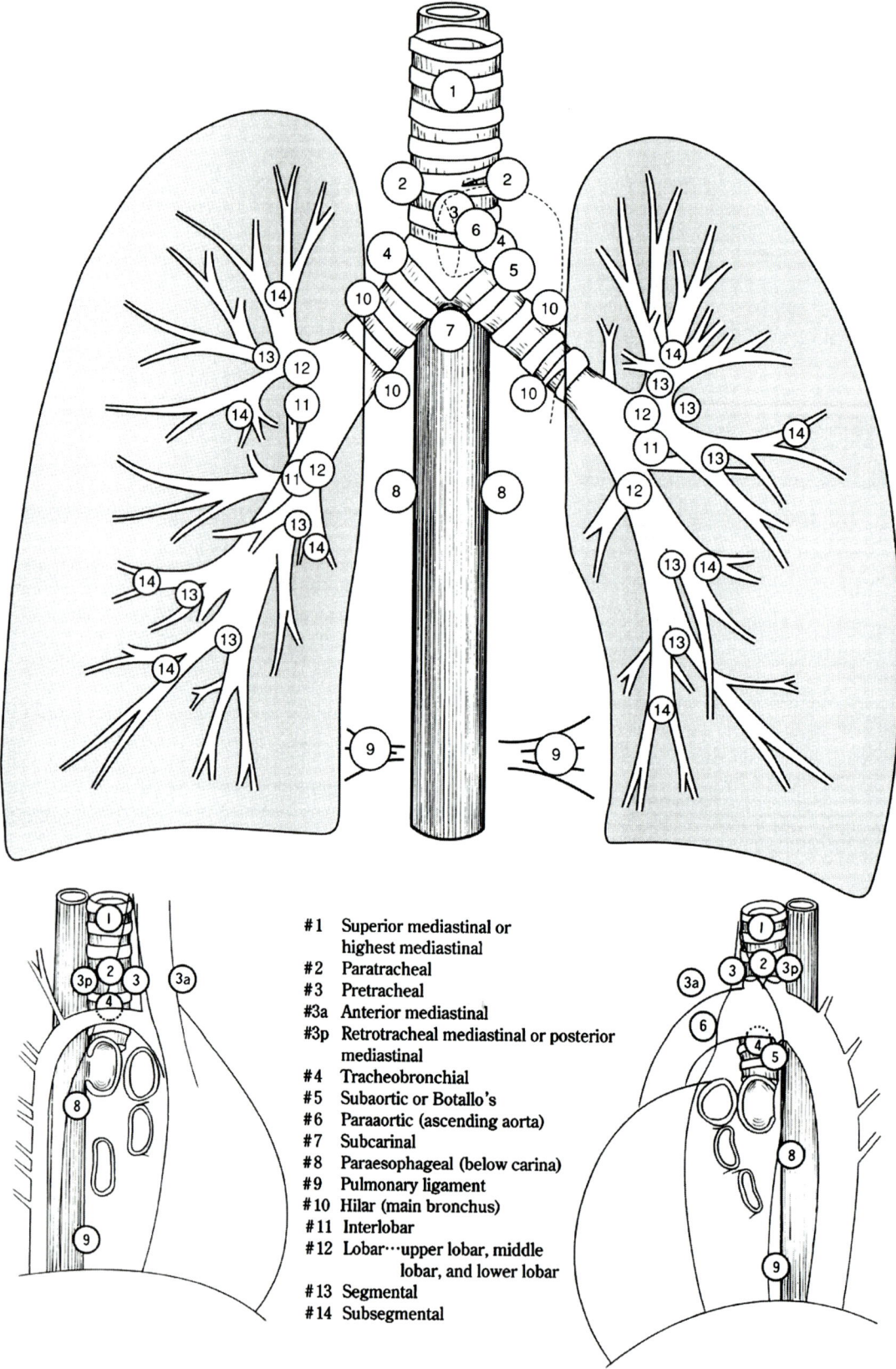

#1   Superior mediastinal or
      highest mediastinal
#2   Paratracheal
#3   Pretracheal
#3a   Anterior mediastinal
#3p   Retrotracheal mediastinal or posterior
      mediastinal
#4   Tracheobronchial
#5   Subaortic or Botallo's
#6   Paraaortic (ascending aorta)
#7   Subcarinal
#8   Paraesophageal (below carina)
#9   Pulmonary ligament
#10   Hilar (main bronchus)
#11   Interlobar
#12   Lobar···upper lobar, middle
               lobar, and lower lobar
#13   Segmental
#14   Subsegmental

Fig. 12.2. Lymph node map originally proposed by Naruke et al. [26]

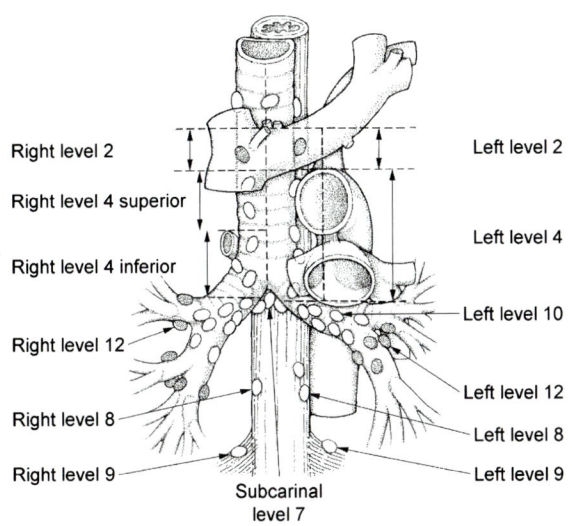

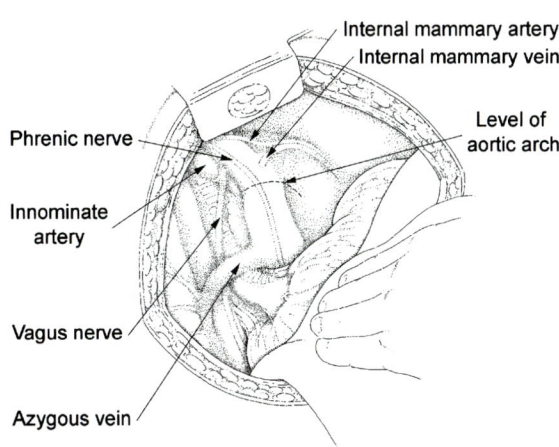

Fig. 12.5. Exposure of the right superior mediastinum with the pleura intact

Fig. 12.3. Schematic representation of intrapulmonary and mediastinal nodal levels according to American Joint Committee on Cancer Staging and End Results Reporting (AJCC) and Union International Contre le Cancer (UICC) 1996 definitions

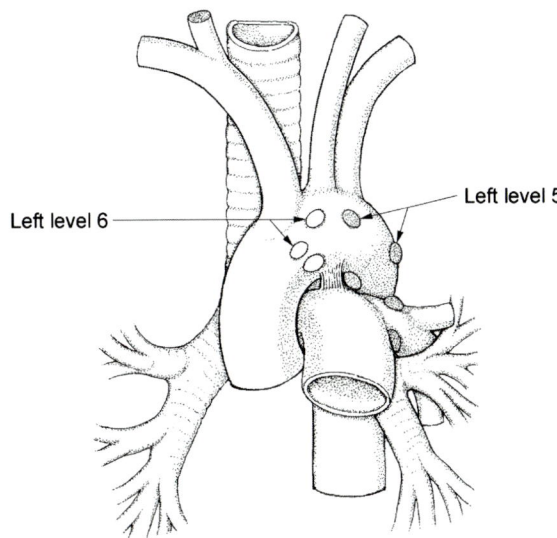

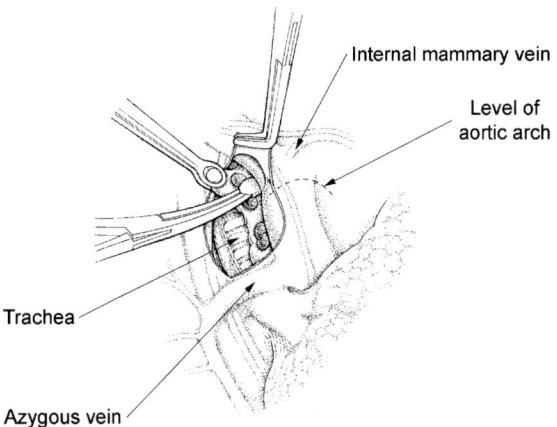

Fig. 12.6. Dissection of the right level 2 lymph nodes. Because the aortic arch is not visible from the right hemithorax, the juncture of the internal mammary vein and the superior vena cava can be used as a surrogate marker to distinguish between level 2 and level 4 superior lymph nodes

Fig. 12.4. Schematic representation of subaortic and para-aortic nodal levels according to AJCC and UICC 1996 definitions

vena cava, trachea, and azygous vein, is exposed by retracting the lung caudally (Fig. 12.5). The phrenic nerve is identified on the lateral aspect of the superior vena cava. The vagus nerve can be visualized through the unopened pleura more posteriorly. The mediastinal pleura, cephalad to the azygous vein and between the trachea and superior vena cava, is elevated with forceps and incised to the level of the innominate artery. The pleural edge overlying the trachea is retracted and the mediastinal fat pad is bluntly dissected off the anterolateral aspect of the trachea using a peanut sponge on a clamp. Similarly, the pleural edge over the superior vena

cava is placed on traction and the mediastinal fat pad is dissected from the junction of the superior vena cava and the azygous vein to the level of the innominate artery. A small vein is frequently seen draining from this fat pad into the superior vena cava and should be ligated. Nonmagnetic clips are applied liberally to small blood vessels and lymphatics. Level 2 lymph nodes are those located between the cephalad border of the innominate vein and the cephalad border of the aortic arch (Fig. 12.6). Lymph nodes lying between the cephalad border of the aortic arch and the cephalad border of the azygous vein (Fig. 12.7) are level 4 superior. The azygous vein is elevated with a vein retractor. The lymph nodes located between the cephalad border of the azygous vein and the origin of the right upper lobe bronchus (Fig. 12.8) are removed and labeled as level 4 inferior. During this part of the dissection, care must be taken not to injure the pulmonary artery.

Table 12.2. American Joint Committee on Cancer and Union International Contre le Cancer 1996 intrapulmonary and medi- astinal lymph node level definitions. Reproduced with permission from Mountain and Dresler [34]

Nodal station		Anatomic landmarks
N2 nodes: All N2 nodes lie within the mediastinal pleural envelope		
1	Highest mediastinal nodes	Nodes lying above a horizontal line at the upper rim of the bracheocephalic (left innominate) vein where it ascends to the left, crossing in front of the trachea at its midline
2	Upper paratracheal nodes	Nodes lying above a horizontal line drawn tangential to the upper margin of the aortic arch and below the inferior boundary of No. 1 nodes
3	Prevascular and retrotracheal nodes	Prevascular and retrotracheal nodes may be designated 3A and 3P; midline nodes are considered to be ipsilateral
4	Lower paratracheal nodes	The lower paratracheal nodes on the right lie to the right of the midline of the trachea between a horizontal line drawn tangential to the upper margin of the arch and a line extending across the right main bronchus at the upper margin of the upper lobe bronchus, and contained within the mediastinal pleural envelope; the lower paratracheal nodes on the left lie to the left of the midline of the trachea between a horizontal line drawn tangential to the upper margin of the aortic arch and a line extending across the left main bronchus at the level of the upper margin of the left upper lobe bronchus, medial to the ligamentum arteriosum and contained within the mediastinal pleural envelope Researchers may wish to designate the lower paratracheal nodes as No. 4s (superior) and No. 4i (inferior) subsets for study purposes; the No. 4s nodes may be defined by a horizontal line extending across the trachea and drawn tangential to the cephalic border of the azygos vein; the No. 4i nodes may be defined by the lower boundary of No. 4s and the lower boundary of No. 4, as described above
5	Subaortic (aortopulmonary window)	Subaortic nodes are lateral to the ligamentum arteriosum or the aorta or left pulmonary artery and proximal to the first branch of the left pulmonary artery and lie within the mediastinal pleural envelope
6	Para-aortic nodes (ascending aorta or phrenic)	Nodes lying anterior and lateral to the ascending aorta and the aortic arch or the innominate artery, beneath a line tangential to the upper margin of the aortic arch
7	Subcarinal nodes	Nodes lying caudal to the carina of the trachea, but not associated with the lower lobe bronchi or arteries within the lung
8	Paraesophageal nodes (below carina)	Nodes lying adjacent to the wall of the esophagus and to the right or left of the midline, excluding subcarinal nodes
9	Pulmonary ligament nodes	Nodes lying within the pulmonary ligament, including those in the posterior wall and lower part of the inferior pulmonary vein
N1 nodes: All N1 nodes lie distal to the mediastinum		
10	Hilar nodes	The proximal lobar nodes, distal to the mediastinal pleural reflection and the nodes adjacent to the bronchus intermedius on the right; radiographically, the hilar shadow may be created by enlargement of both hilar and interlobar nodes
11	Interlobar nodes	Nodes lying between the lobar bronchi
12	Lobar nodes	Nodes adjacent to the distal lobar bronchi
13	Segmental nodes	Nodes adjacent to the segmental bronchi
14	Subsegmental nodes	Nodes around the subsegmental bronchi

Dissection between the esophagus and membranous portion of the trachea at a level cephalad to the azygous vein will reveal the level 3 posterior nodes. Level 3 anterior nodes are found anterior and medial to the superior vena cava at the insertion of the azygous vein (Fig. 12.9). Level 10 nodes are seen along the anterior border of the bronchus intermedius, distal to the pleural reflection, and are exposed by retracting the lung posteriorly and the pulmonary artery anteriorly (Fig. 12.10). Level 11 lymph nodes are found in the sump of Borrie between the lobar bronchi. Exposure is provided by posterior retraction of the lung. Level 12 lymph nodes are situated at the distal aspect of the lobar bronchi and are resected with the specimen (Fig. 12.11). Clips should be avoided in this area if a stapling device is to be used for division of the bronchus.

Exposure of the level 7 nodes is gained by retracting the lung anteriorly and incising the pleura. The pleural edge overlying the esophagus is placed on traction and the esophagus is retracted posteriorly (Fig. 12.12). A ring clamp is used to grasp the subcarinal fat pad and

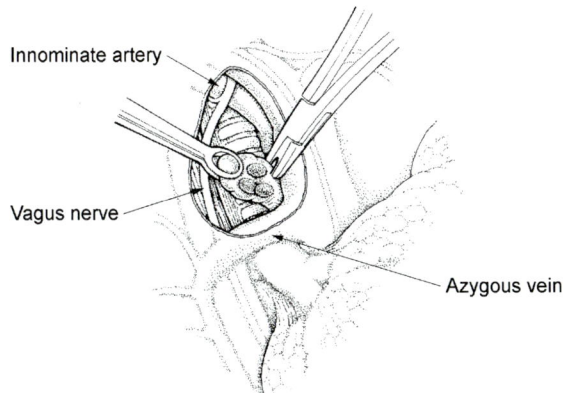

Fig. 12.7. Dissection of right level 4 superior lymph nodes

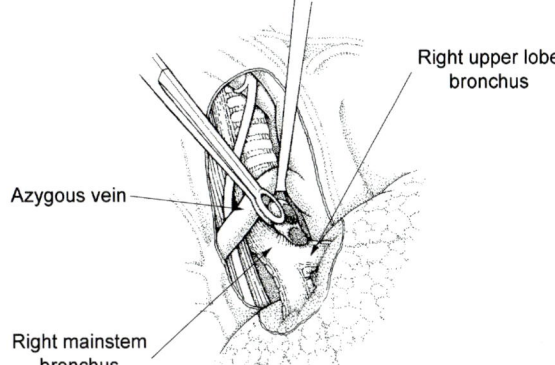

Fig. 12.8. Dissection of the right level 4 inferior lymph nodes. A small vein, frequently seen draining into the superior vena cava, must be ligated

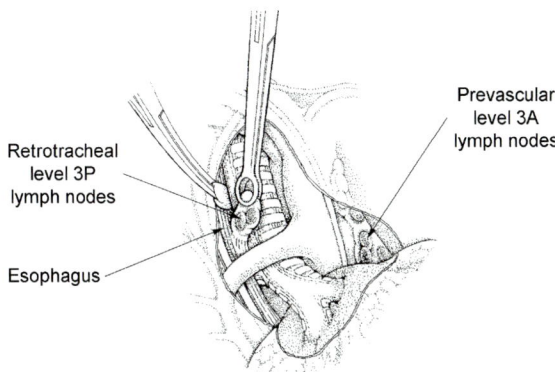

Fig. 12.9. Dissection of the level 3 anterior and level 3 posterior lymph nodes. The phrenic and vagus nerves, as well as the membranous portion of the trachea must be identified prior to the application of clips

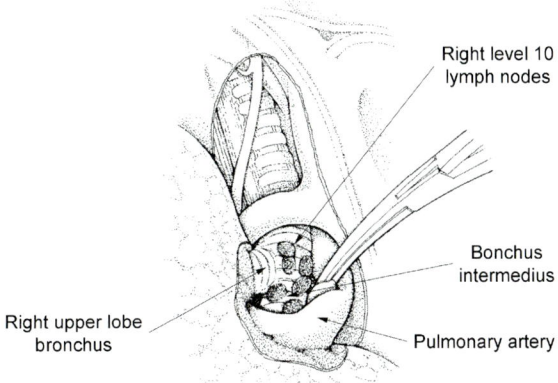

Fig. 12.10. Exposure of the level 10 lymph nodes is accomplished by retracting the pulmonary artery anteriorly

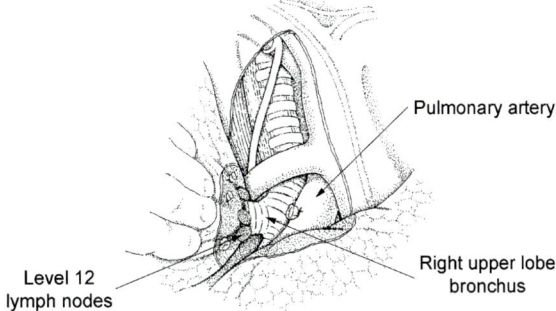

Fig. 12.11. Dissection of the right level 12 lymph nodes. Use cautery rather than clips to avoid interference with the application of a stapling device

elevate it from the pericardium. Attachments to the right and left mainstem bronchi are clipped and the vessels entering from the area of the anterior carina ligated. Level 9 lymph nodes are found in the inferior pulmonary ligament and are readily resected using clips or cautery. Level 8 nodes may or may not be present.

12.5.2 Left Hemithorax

The lung is retracted anteriorly to expose the aortopulmonary window. The phrenic and vagus nerves are identified. The pleura overlying the aortopulmonary window is elevated and incised in a cephalad direction midway between the phrenic and vagus nerves. The ligamentum arteriosum is identified by palpation. Level 6 lymph nodes are located in the fat pad anterior to the ligamentum arteriosum, whereas level 5 lymph nodes can be found posterior to the ligamentum arteriosum (Fig. 12.13). Only blunt dissection should be performed and clips rather than cautery utilized for hemostasis. The recurrent laryngeal and proximal vagus nerves

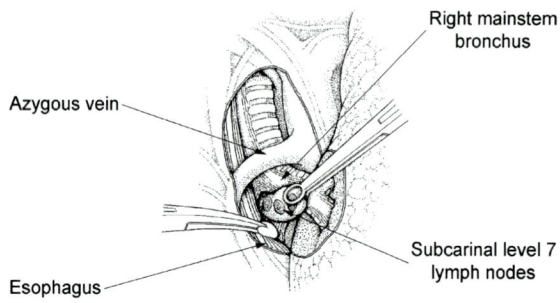

Fig. 12.12. Dissection of the level 7 lymph nodes from the right hemithorax. The esophagus and membranous portion of the mainstem bronchi must not be injured

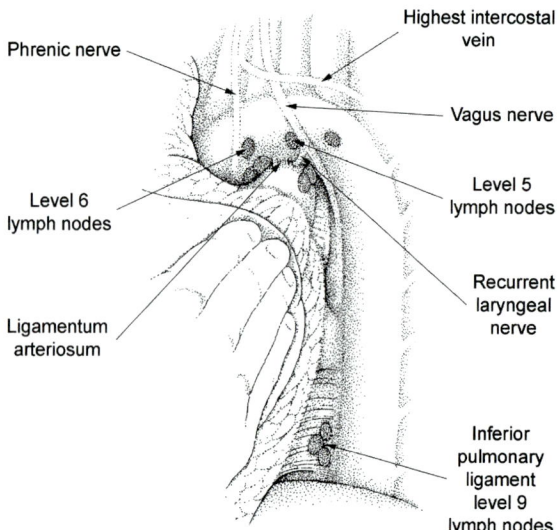

Fig. 12.13. Exposure of the level 5, level 6, and left level 9 lymph nodes. Exposure of the left level 2 and level 4 lymph nodes would require mobilization of the aortic arch

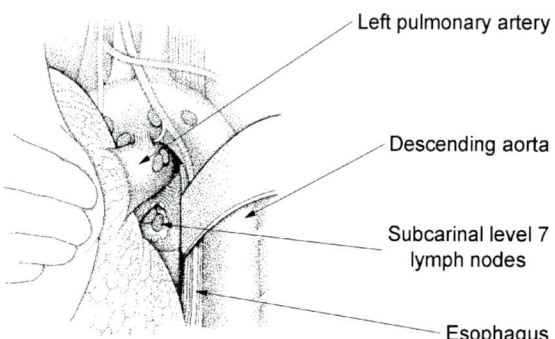

Fig. 12.14. Exposure of the level 7 lymph nodes from the left hemithorax. A malleable retractor is used to retract the aorta and esophagus posteriorly

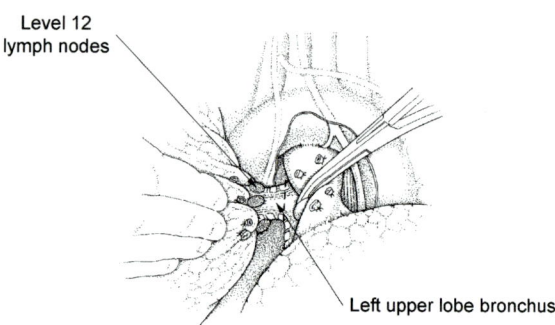

Fig. 12.15. Dissection of the left level 12 lymph nodes

must be avoided to prevent the rare, but serious complication of vocal cord paralysis.

The level 7 nodes are exposed by incising the posterior pleural reflection anterior to the aorta. The aorta and esophagus are retracted posteriorly and the left mainstem bronchus is identified inferomedial to the pulmonary artery (Fig. 12.14). The subcarinal fat pad is grasped with a ring forceps. Attachments to the left and right mainstem bronchi are clipped. Vessels entering from the region of the carina are ligated. Level 11 nodes are located distal to the pleural reflection between the lobar bronchi and are exposed by retracting the pulmonary artery posteriorly. Level 12 nodes are situated along the distal aspect of the lobar bronchus and are usually removed with the specimen (Fig. 12.15). Level 9 lymph nodes can be identified in the inferior pulmonary ligament and are removed with clips or cautery. Injury to the esophagus must be avoided.

12.6   Complications

Some surgeons are hesitant to perform a complete mediastinal lymph node dissection for fear of complications that might arise from either interrupting the blood supply to the bronchial stump or from removal of a large portion of the intrathoracic lymphatics. In a study of 155 patients who had either no sampling or sampling, systematic sampling, or complete mediastinal lymph node dissection, Bollen et al. [13] found no difference in the intraoperative blood loss or transfusion requirement. There was increased chest tube drainage in patients who underwent systematic sampling or complete mediastinal lymph node dissection compared to the other two groups. Recurrent laryngeal nerve injury was reported in three (5%) patients and chylothorax was reported in two patients who underwent complete mediastinal lymph node dissection. Bronchopleural fistulas were reported in two patients who did not undergo any lymph node dissection. Hata et al. [1] reported 2 recurrent laryngeal nerve paralyses and one phrenic injury among 55 patients who underwent extended lymphadenectomy.

In a prospective randomized trial of 182 patients who underwent either systematic sampling or complete mediastinal lymph node dissection, Izbicki et al. [38] noted no difference in blood loss, mortality, need for reoperation, chest tube drainage, or length of stay. One chylothorax occurred in each group. Recurrent laryngeal nerve injury was reported in six patients who underwent systematic sampling and five patients who underwent complete mediastinal lymph node dissection. Complete mediastinal lymph node dissection extended the procedure by 20 min.

In a prospective nonrandomized trial of 373 patients, Keller et al. [10] found no difference in blood loss, transfusion requirement, or duration of operation between patients who underwent either systematic sampling or complete mediastinal lymph node dissection. These conclusions were confirmed in a randomized prospective trial conducted by the American College of surgery Oncology Group (Z0030) in which 1,111 patients were randomized to either systematic sampling or complete mediastinal lymph node dissection. There was no difference in morbidity, mortality, or hospital length of stay. Complete mediastinal lymph node dissection was associated with a statistically significant, but clinically insignificant, increase in blood loss (18 ml), chest tube drainage (48 ml), and operating room time (14 min.; M. Allen, personal communication).

12.7   Thoracoscopic Lymph Node Dissection

The use of the thoracoscope in the diagnosis and treatment of chest diseases was introduced by Jacobaeus [39]. In contrast to open thoracotomy, video-assisted thoracoscopic surgery (VATS) is performed through multiple small port sites using specially designed instruments. Occasionally, a minithoracotomy is used (without spreading the ribs) in addition to the port sites so that traditional instruments can be introduced into the thorax. Although the reported advantages of VATS include smaller incisions, decreased blood loss, decreased postoperative pain, improved postoperative immunologic and pulmonary function, decreased length of stay, and decreased hospital costs, skepticism remains regarding the oncologic adequacy and safety of this technique [40–45]. Several retrospective reviews can be found in the literature. However, only two small prospective trials have been conducted directly comparing VATS and thoracotomy approaches with regard to mediastinal lymph node dissection.

In a prospective randomized trial of 100 consecutive patients with clinical stage I NSCLC, Sugi et al. [46] compared lobectomy by VATS (VATS group) and open thoracotomy (open group). Fifty patients were assigned to each arm, however, 2 patients randomized to the VATS arm required conversion to thoracotomy. The number of lymph nodes harvested did not differ, with a mean of 8 hilar and 13 mediastinal lymph nodes being removed in both groups. Actuarial 5-year survival was 85% and 90% for the open and VATS groups, respectively. Locoregional recurrence occurred in 19% and 10% for the open and VATS groups, respectively. These results were not significantly different.

In another prospective trial, Sagawa et al. [47] studied 35 patients with clinical stage I lung cancer who underwent VATS lobectomy with mediastinal lymph node dissection through two port sites and a small thoracotomy. After the thoracoscopic part of the procedure, a different surgeon performed a thoracotomy to assess the completeness of the lymph node dissection. Lobectomy could not be completed thoracoscopically in 6 of the 35 patients. An average of 40.3 lymph nodes were harvested by VATS from the right hemithorax and an additional 1.2 (range 0–6) were removed by thoracotomy. An average of 37.1 lymph nodes were removed by VATS from the left hemithorax and an additional 1.2 (range 0–4) were resected by thoracotomy. Survival and recurrence data were not presented.

VATS mediastinal lymph node dissection is technically difficult. Limited data regarding nodal staging and long-term survival suggest that the results achieved with this technique, when performed by surgeons with VATS skills, approach that of open thoracotomy. Nevertheless, before the thoracoscopic approach to mediastinal lymph node dissection can be accepted as the standard of care, it must withstand the scrutiny of a prospective randomized trial.

Key Points

- The common patterns of lymphatic drainage and metastases must be recognized so that that the principles of surgical staging can be properly applied.
- Familiarity with the various revisions of the staging system is necessary to correctly interpret published results.
- Complete mediastinal lymph node dissection or systematic sampling via thoracotomy is currently considered the standard of care and should be performed in all patients undergoing curative surgery. Both procedures can be performed in a short time and the benefit of more accurate staging far outweighs the risks incurred by performing either technique. Complete mediastinal lymph node dissection may be associated with improved survival.
- Sentinel lymph node mapping and the thoracoscopic approach to surgical staging should be considered experimental procedures.

References

1. Hata E, Hayakawa K, Miyamoto H, Hayashida R. Rationale for extended lymphadenectomy for lung cancer. Theor Surg 1990; 5:19.
2. Borrie J. Primary carcinoma of the bronchus; prognosis following surgical resection: a clinico-pathological study of 200 patients. Ann R Coll Surg Engl 1952; 10:165.
3. Nohl HC. An investigation into the lymphatic and vascular spread of carcinoma of the bronchus. Thorax 1956; 11:172.
4. Nohl-Oser HC. An investigation of the anatomy of the lymphatic drainage of the lungs as shown by the lymphatic spread of bronchial carcinoma. Ann R Coll Surg Engl 1972; 51:157.
5. Asamura H, Nakayama H, Kondo H, Tsuchiya R, Naruke T. Lobe-specific extent of systematic lymph node dissection for non-small cell lung carcinomas according to a retrospective study of metastasis and prognosis. J Thorac Cardiovasc Surg 1999; 117:1102.
6. Kotoulas CS, Foroulis CN, Kostikas K, et al. Involvement of lymphatic metastatic spread in non-small cell lung cancer accordingly to the primary cancer location. Lung Cancer 2004; 44:183.
7. Watanabe Y, Shimizu J, Tsubota M, Iwa T. Mediastinal spread of metastatic lymph nodes in bronchogenic carcinoma. Chest 1990; 97:1059.
8. Naruke T. Mediastinal lymph node dissection. In: Shields TW (ed.) General Thoracic Surgery. Williams and Wilkins, Baltimore, 1994; p 469.
9. Abolhoda A, Keller S. Surgical staging of the mediastinum. In: Pass HI, Mitchell JB, Johnson DH, Minna JD, Turris AT (eds.) Lung Cancer: Principles and Practice. Lippincott, Williams and Wilkins, Philadelphia, 2000; p 28.
10. Keller SM, Adak S, Wagner H, Johnson DH. Mediastinal lymph node dissection improves survival in patients with stages II and IIIa non-small cell lung cancer. Eastern Cooperative Oncology Group. Ann Thorac Surg 2000; 70:358.
11. Gaer JA, Goldstraw P. Intraoperative assessment of nodal staging at thoracotomy for carcinoma of the bronchus. Eur J Cardiothorac Surg 1990; 4:207.
12. Haiderer O, Wustinger E, Lexer G, Weitensfelder W. [Mediastinal lymphadenectomy. Anatomical basis and its surgical relevance in central bronchus carcinoma]. Wien Med Wochenschr 1990; 140:422.
13. Bollen EC, van Duin CJ, Theunissen PH, vt Hof-Grootenboer BE, Blijham GH. Mediastinal lymph node dissection in resected lung cancer: morbidity and accuracy of staging. Ann Thorac Surg 1993; 55:961.
14. Izbicki JR, Knoefel WT, Passlick B, Habekost M, Karg O, Thetter O. Risk analysis and long-term survival in patients undergoing extended resection of locally advanced lung cancer. J Thorac Cardiovasc Surg 1995; 110:386.
15. Sugi K, Nawata K, Fujita N, et al. Systematic lymph node dissection for clinically diagnosed peripheral non-small-cell lung cancer less than 2 cm in diameter. World J Surg 1998; 22:290.
16. Gajra A, Newman N, Gamble GP, Kohman LJ, Graziano SL. Effect of number of lymph nodes sampled on outcome in patients with stage I non-small-cell lung cancer. J Clin Oncol 2003; 21:1029.
17. Izbicki JR, Passlick B, Pantel K, Pichlmeier U, Hosch SB, Karg O, Thetter O. Effectiveness of radical systematic mediastinal lymphadenectomy in patients with resectable non-small cell lung cancer: results of a prospective randomized trial. Ann Surg 1998; 227:138.
18. Wu Y, Huang ZF, Wang SY, Yang XN, Ou W. A randomized trial of systematic nodal dissection in resectable non-small cell lung cancer. Lung Cancer 2002; 36:1.
19. Kubuschok B, Passlick B, Izbicki JR, Thetter O, Pantel K. Disseminated tumor cells in lymph nodes as a determinant for survival in surgically resected non-small-cell lung cancer. J Clin Oncol 1999; 17:19.
20. Osaki T, Oyama T, Gu CD, et al. Prognostic impact of micrometastatic tumor cells in the lymph nodes and bone marrow of patients with completely resected stage I non-small-cell lung cancer. J Clin Oncol 2002; 20:2930.
21. Liptay MJ, Grondin SC, Fry WA, et al. Intraoperative sentinel lymph node mapping in non-small-cell lung cancer improves detection of micrometastases. J Clin Oncol 2002; 20:1984.
22. Schmidt FE, Woltering EA, Webb WR, Garcia OM, Cohen JE, Rozans MH. Sentinel nodal assessment in patients with carcinoma of the lung. Ann Thorac Surg 2002; 74:870.
23. Melfi FM, Chella A, Menconi GF, et al. Intraoperative radioguided sentinel lymph node biopsy in non-small cell lung cancer. Eur J Cardiothorac Surg 2003; 23:214.
24. Faries MB, Bleicher RJ, Ye X, Essner R, Morton DL. Lymphatic mapping and sentinel lymphadenectomy for primary and metastatic pulmonary malignant neoplasms. Arch Surg 2004; 139:870.
25. Nomori H, Watanabe K, Ohtsuka T, Naruke T, Suemasu K. In vivo identification of sentinel lymph nodes for clinical stage I non-small cell lung cancer for abbreviation of mediastinal lymph node dissection. Lung Cancer 2004; 46:49.
26. Naruke T, Suemasu K, Ishikawa S. Lymph node mapping and curability at various levels of metastasis in resected lung cancer. J Thorac Cardiovasc Surg 1978; 76:832.
27. Watanabe S, Ladas G, Goldstraw P. Inter-observer variability in systematic nodal dissection: comparison of European and Japanese nodal designation. Ann Thorac Surg 2002; 73:245.
28. Mountain CF. A new international staging system for lung cancer. Chest 1986; 89:225S.
29. Asamura H, Suzuki K, Kondo H and Tsuchiya R. Where is the boundary between N1 and N2 stations in lung cancer? Ann Thorac Surg 2000; 70:1839.
30. Ueda K, Kaneda Y, Saeki K, Fujita N, Zempo N, Esato K. Hilar lymph nodes in N2 disease: survival analysis of patients with non-small cell lung cancers and regional lymph node metastasis. Surg Today 2002; 32:300.
31. Rea F, Marulli G, Callegaro D, Zuin A, Gobbi T, Loy M, Sartori F. Prognostic significance of main bronchial lymph nodes involvement in non-small cell lung carcinoma: N1 or N2? Lung Cancer 2004; 45:215.
32. Tisi GM, Friedman PJ, Peters RM. Clinical staging of primary lung cancer. Am Rev Respir Dis 1983; 127:659.
33. Mountain CF. Revisions in the system for staging lung cancer. Chest 1997; 111:1710.
34. Mountain CF, Dresler CM, Mountain CF. Regional lymph node classification for lung cancer staging. Chest 1997; 111:1718.
35. Brock RC. Bronchial carcinoma. Br Med J 1948; 2:737.
36. Cahan WG, Watson WL, Pool JL. Radical pneumonectomy. J Thorac Surg 1951; 22:449.
37. Weinberg JA. Identification of regional lymph nodes in the treatment of bronchogenic carcinoma. J Thorac Surg 1951; 22:517.
38. Izbicki JR, Thetter O, Habekost M, et al. Radical systematic mediastinal lymphadenectomy in non-small cell lung cancer: a randomized controlled trial. Br J Surg 1994; 81:229.
39. Jacobaeus HC. The practical importance of thoracoscopy in surgery of the chest. Surg Gynecol Obstet 1922; 34:289.
40. Ohbuchi T, Morikawa T, Takeuchi E, Kato H. Lobectomy: video-assisted thoracic surgery versus posterolateral thoracotomy. Jpn J Thorac Cardiovasc Surg 1998; 46:519.

41. Inaoka M, Obama T, Kawaharada N. [Video-assisted mini-thoracotomy versus conventional posterolateral thoracotomy for performing lobectomy of lung carcinomas]. Kyobu Geka 2000;53:18.

42. Yim AP, Wan S, Lee TW, Arifi AA. VATS lobectomy reduces cytokine responses compared with conventional surgery. Ann Thorac Surg 2000; 70:243.

43. Nakajima J, Takamoto S, Kohno T, Ohtsuka T. Costs of videothoracoscopic surgery versus open resection for patients with of lung carcinoma. Cancer 2000; 89:2497.

44. Nagahiro I, Andou A, Aoe M, Sano Y, Date H, Shimizu N. Pulmonary function, postoperative pain, and serum cytokine level after lobectomy: a comparison of VATS and conventional procedure. Ann Thorac Surg 2001; 72:362.

45. Nomori H, Horio H, Naruke T, Suemasu K. What is the advantage of a thoracoscopic lobectomy over a limited thoracotomy procedure for lung cancer surgery? Ann Thorac Surg 2001; 72:879.

46. Sugi K, Kaneda Y, Esato K. Video-assisted thoracoscopic lobectomy reduces cytokine production more than conventional open lobectomy. Jpn J Thorac Cardiovasc Surg 2000; 48:161.

47. Sagawa M, Sato M, Sakurada A, Matsumura Y, Endo C, Handa M, Kondo T. A prospective trial of systematic nodal dissection for lung cancer by video-assisted thoracic surgery: can it be perfect? Ann Thorac Surg 2002; 73:900.

Molecular Staging of Non-Small-Cell Lung Cancer

13

Yuhchyau Chen and David Gandara

Contents

13.1   Introduction

Staging of non-small-cell lung cancer (NSCLC) is currently evolving. The conventional TNM system was first proposed in 1946 by Denoix and is an anatomically structured system [1]. It provides information about the size and local extension of the primary tumor (T stage), the regional lymph node metastasis (N stage), and distant hematogenous cancer spread (M stage). The TNM staging system also groups tumors of various TNM stage into subgroups I, II, III, and IV. Such division not only provides prognostic information, but also directs therapeutic decisions for tumors of different grouping categories. TNM staging was adapted by the American Joint committee for Cancer Staging (AJCC) in 1974 [2], and has been through further revisions in 1986 [3] and 1997 [4]. The staging is based on clinical information including physical examination findings, endoscopic examination findings, histologic examination of biopsy specimens, and imaging information from computed tomography (CT) scans, magnetic resonance imaging (MRI) scans, bone scans, and in the recent years, positron emission tomography (PET) scans.

While TNM staging remains the current standard staging system, clinical experience has revealed a portion of patients in each group whose prognoses defy the assigned stage grouping. For example, patients with stage I, the earliest stage NSCLC, had a 5 year survival rate of only 60–70% after complete surgical removal of chest tumor [5]. This highlights the portion of patients (30–40% of stage I NSCLC) who have biologically more virulent tumors that are not adequately staged by the anatomical staging of TNM. In clinical practice, such deviation from predicted prognosis has often been observed in individual cancer patients of all stage groups. Additional prognostic information that will complement the TNM staging is needed. In the past 2 decades, the refinement of immunohistochemical (IHC) staining techniques and the advancement of molecular technology have contributed to significant discoveries in the diagnosis and treatment of lung cancer. New molecular techniques have markedly improved the sensitivity and specificity of diagnosing molecular markers. The genetic abnormalities of particular genes may be detected by identifying specific mutations using direct sequencing or single-strand conformational polymorphism [6]. Other assays such as reverse-transcriptase polymerase chain reaction (RT-PCR) [7, 8], in-situ hybridization, and enzyme-linked immunosorbent assay (ELISA) are also being applied to the analyses of molecular markers. Our knowledge of molecular markers has furthered our understanding of the pathobiology, etiology, and natural history of lung cancer, with the potential to lead to breakthroughs in early detection, screening, identifying molecular targets for therapy and intervention, and molecular staging of lung cancer [9].

13.2   Molecular Markers for Staging

There are three different approaches or mechanisms by which molecular markers can potentially be applied to the molecular staging of lung cancer:

1. Identifying molecular markers of prognostic value in the primary tumors or regional lymph nodes. These include markers for tumor antigen, oncogenes, gene promoter methylation, cell proliferation, tumor-suppressor genes, angiogenesis, telomerase, growth factor receptors, extracellular matrix, cell motility, proteolytic enzyme, adhesion molecules, and other markers for cancer invasion and metastasis.
2. Applying sensitive molecular techniques to detect occult regional lymph node metastasis not discernable by standard hematoxylin and eosin (HE) stains. These generally apply to the markers for epithelial cells such as cytokeratins, or oncogene markers such as p53 and or *Ras*.
3. Applying sensitive molecular techniques to detect occult distant macrometastasis using markers for epithelium, DNA, oncogenes, or angiogenesis in the bone marrow or in the patient's blood. On example of this type of markers is the cytokeratins, which are present in 70–80% of tumors, but are not normally present in lymph nodes, bone marrow, or serum [10–12].

This chapter summarizes the published work in the application of molecular markers to the staging of NSCLC.

13.3   Molecular Prognostic Markers in Primary Tumors or Regional Lymph Nodes: Oncogenes and Tumor-Suppressor Genes

13.3.1   *Ras* Oncogenes/p21

The *ras* oncogene family encodes guanosine-triphosphate-binding proteins with a 21-kDa (p21) molecular weight. The proteins are localized at the inner surface of the cell membrane and are involved in the transduction of growth signals. There are three well-characterized members of the *ras* oncogene family: H-*ras*, K-*ras*, and N-*ras* [13]. The oncogenic potential of *ras* genes is triggered by point mutations occurring mainly in codon 12, 13, or 61. A *ras* gene mutation is detected in 10–30% of NSCLC cases, and 80–90% of *ras* mutations occur at codon 12 of the K-*ras* gene [14–17]. *Ras* mutations are frequently observed in smokers but not nonsmokers, are more frequent in adenocarcinoma than in squamous cell carcinoma, and are absent in small-cell lung cancer [16, 18, 19]. Several investigators have reported that *ras* mutations are a poor prognostic factor in NSCLC. Slebos et al. [15] found that the K-*ras* codon-12 point mutation was a strong and unfavorable prognostic factor for disease-free survival and for cancer-specific mortality in stage I, II, and IIIA tumors after complete resection. Mitsudomi et al. reported that *ras* gene mutations in NSCLC are associated with shortened survival irrespective of treatment [16]. Sugio et al. [17] reported *ras* gene mutation as an unfavorable prognostic marker in adenocarcinoma of the human lung without lymph node metastasis. Fukuyama et al. [20] reported that K-*ras* mutation at codon 12 was an independent unfavorable prognostic indication in patients with adenocarcinoma but not squamous cell carcinoma of NSCLC. Similarly, out of four molecular markers investigated (p53, K-*ras*, and the metastasis-suppressor genes *MRP-/CD9* and *KA11/CD82*), Miyake and colleagues reported that K-*ras* mutation as well as *MRP-1/CD9* status significantly impacted on poorer prognosis [21]. Rosell et al. reported that K-*ras* mutation at codon 12 was a strong unfavorable predictive factor for tumor recurrence and death independently of tumor stage and histology [22]. Kwiatkowski et al. investigated multiple clinical, pathological, and molecular factors in stage I NSCLC and found that K-*ras* codon 12 mutation as well as the absence of H-*ras* p21 expression were among the nine independent predictors for recurrence [23]. A different approach to characterizing K-*ras* mutation was accomplished by IHC using a monoclonal antibody against protein *ras* p21 [24]. Harada and colleagues found that surgical specimens stained negative for p21 correlated with better survival. This was independent of histological type, stage of disease, tumor or node status, or the resectability of tumors. On the other hand, a few studies did not find a significant prognostic value of the K-*ras* gene mutation or protein expression using surgical specimens [19, 25].

13.3.2   p53 Tumor-Suppressor Gene

p53 is a tumor-suppressor gene encoding a 53-kDa nuclear phosphoprotein with a transcriptional activator, which controls cell proliferation by regulating a G-S checkpoint before DNA synthesis, through the cyclin-dependent kinase (CDK) pathway [26]. In response to DNA damage by ionizing radiation and a variety of chemical agents or carcinogens, p53 induces cells to repair damage or promotes apoptosis [27–29]. Mutations of the p53 gene are the most common findings in human cancer cells of all types [30]. Investigations of p53 as a prognostic factor have been conducted either by gene mutation studies (DNA sequencing or single-strand conformation polymorphism) or protein expression (by IHC staining) in tumor tissues.

p53 mutation has been observed in approximately 45% of NSCLC tumors, while overexpression has been observed in approximately 50%. The prognostic significance remains unclear, since some studies have demonstrated p53 overexpression or mutation as a favorable prognostic factor, some have shown an unfavorable correlation, and others reported no differences. These conflicting findings may be attributed to the analysis of mutation versus protein expression, differences in laboratory techniques or scoring criteria, differences in the monoclonal antibodies applied in each study, or differences in the population of tumors examined. For the most part, studies conducted by investigating gene alterations (point mutations or deletions) have revealed p53 mutation to be an unfavorable marker, with few studies in disagreement. Point mutation or allelic deletion has been observed in 36–58% of NSCLC tumors. Huang et al. found p53 point mutations in 36.8% of 96 tumors from stage I, II, and III NSCLC [31]. Patients with p53 mutations at exon 8 had worse survival for both adenocarcinoma and squamous cell carcinoma. Mitsudomi et al. detected 43% p53 point mutations in 120 tumor specimens from all cancer stages of NSCLC. p53 mutation is associated with significantly shorter survival of stages IIIA–IV diseases, but not stage I and II diseases [32]. The study by Horio et al. found 49% point mutation and allelic deletion. Point mutation was an unfavorable prognostic factor for NSCLC, while allelic deletion showed a trend toward being an unfavorable factor without reaching significance [33]. Fukuyama et al. found that p53 mutation was an unfavorable prognostic factor in early stage disease of stages I and II NSCLC. p53 was an unfavorable prognostic factor for adenocarcinoma but not for squamous cell carcinomas

[20]. Ahrendt et al. [34] detected p53 mutations in 55% of resected tumors of stage I, II, and IIIA disease, and found mutation of p53 an unfavorable factor for survival only in stage I NSCLC.

Several studies have carried out both mutation and protein expression (IHC) analyses of p53. Tomizawa et al. [35] investigated mutation and IHC of 103 resected stage I NSCLC tumors. They found a 48% positivity of p53 mutation and 40% IHC staining in 103 stage I NSCLC tumors. The concordance rate between mutations and protein overexpression was 69%. p53 mutation, but not expression was significantly associated with a shortened survival. Carbone et al. [36] found a 51% mutation rate and 67% positivity of p53 in 85 resected NSCLC tumors. The concordance rate was 67%. There was a negative survival correlation with p53-protein-positive stain, but not with the gene mutation.

Greatens and colleagues [19] performed analyses with both p53 mutation and protein overexpression by IHC. They found a 40% mutation rate and a 47% rate for p53 overexpression in 101 tumor specimens. p53 mutation predicted a significantly shorter survival, while p53 overexpression did not significantly predict survival. In this study, 28 out of 48 (58%) grade 2+ immunopositive tumors were also positive for p53 mutations. Top and colleagues [37] investigated both p53 gene mutation and protein accumulation in 54 NSCLC specimens. They found that patients with p53 alteration in their tumors tended to have a better prognosis than those without a p53 alteration (mutation or overexpression). Vega et al. [38] found that 46.9% of IHC p53-positive and 44.7% of p53-immunopositive tumors exhibited p53 mutations. A shorter survival was found in patients with p53 mutations but not those with p53 positivity.

Many studies have investigated protein expression using IHC staining. Approximately half of those studies found p53 protein overexpression to be an unfavorable factor [24, 36, 39–46], the other half of the studies found p53 protein overexpression with no prognostic significance [19, 35, 38, 47–53], while some studies showed an association with better prognosis [54, 55].

In an attempt to resolve the controversy of the prognostic value of p53, meta-analyses based on published literature on p53 and NSCLC have been conducted. There are at least three published works on p53 meta-analysis. Mitsudomi et al. [56] performed a meta-analysis of 43 articles. p53 alteration was detected either by overexpression of the protein or as mutation in DNA studies. They found that the incidence of p53 alteration in DNA studies to be 37% (381/1031) and the incidence of protein overexpression to be 48% (1725/3579). The incidence of p53 overexpression and mutation in adenocarcinoma (36% and 34%, respectively) was lower than that in squamous cell carcinoma (54% and 52%, respectively). p53 alteration had a significant negative prognostic effect for adenocarcinomas but not for squamous cell carcinomas. Mitsudomi et al. concluded that p53 alteration either by protein overexpression or by DNA mutation was a significant marker of poor prognosis in patients with pulmonary adenocarcinoma [56]. Steels et al. [57] carried out a meta-analysis of 74 eligible papers. The studies were categorized by histology, disease stage, treatment, and laboratory technique. Combined hazard ratios suggest that an abnormal p53 status had an unfavorable impact on survival for all tumor stages (I–IV) and for both squamous cell carcinoma and adenocarcinoma. Huncharek et al. [58] published a meta-analysis of 8 studies investigating p53 mutations involving a total of 829 patients; they did not find p53 mutation to be a prognostic marker in NSCLC, and felt that selection bias, smoking history, race, geographic location of the study, and socioeconomic status may have been the confounding factors.

13.3.3   c-erB-1 (Epidermal Growth Factor Receptor)

c-erB-1 (EGFR) is the proto-oncogene encoding the protein for epidermal growth factor receptor (EGFR). EGFR is a member of the erB family of tyrosine kinase receptor proteins, which also includes erb-B2 (HER-2/neu), erb-B3, and erb-B4 [59]. Intracellular signaling is triggered by the binding of ligands, such as epidermal growth factor, resulting in the dimerization of EGFR molecules or heterodimerization with other closely related receptors, such as HER2/neu. Phosphorylation of the receptors through their tyrosine kinase domains leads to intracellular signal transduction and the activation of proliferative signals and DNA synthesis [60, 61]. In NSCLC, EGFR is more commonly overexpressed than HER2/neu, and has been observed in 40–80% of cancer specimens [59, 62, 63]. EGFR overexpression has also been demonstrated in premalignant bronchial epithelium, suggesting a role in lung carcinogenesis [64–66]. Similar to p53 overexpression data, the prognostic value of EGFR overexpression as analyzed by IHC stains in lung cancer has been a controversial issue. Greatens et al. [19] found that c-erbB-1 protein expression was not correlated with survival. Some other reports have indicated that EGFR overexpression is associated with a poor prognosis [67–69], while others shave shown no prognostic association [19, 40, 52, 70–72]. Despite the controversy of EGFR overexpression assessed using IHC stains, Hirsch et al. has reported analyses of the gene copy number of EGFR using the fluorescence in situ hybridization technique as well as protein expression using IHC staining [73]. In that report, EGFR protein overexpression was observed more frequently in squamous cell carcinoma than in non-squamous-cell carcinoma (82% vs. 44%, respectively) and in 80% of the bronchioloalveolar carcinomas. In addition, EGFR overexpression or high gene copy number per se had no significant influence as independent prognostic factors. Hirsch et al. found, however, that EGFR overexpression was correlated with increased gene copy number

per cell. Poor prognosis was observed in tumors with high gene copy numbers combined with low EGFR score, using IHC.

Despite the lack of prognostic value of protein overexpression and gene copy number as independent predictors, somatic mutation of the EGFR gene in the tyrosine kinase domain was found to be predictive for tumor response to treatment by gefitinib (Iressa), an EGFR tyrosine kinase inhibitor. Response to gefitinib was seen in approximately 10% of patients. Most of theses patients were female nonsmokers and those with bronchioloalveolar tumors [74, 75]. Lynch et al. found that a subgroup of patients who had mutations in the EGFR gene by either in-frame deletions or amino acid substitutions around the ATP-binding pocket of the tyrosine kinase domain also had clinical responsiveness to gefitinib [76]. Likewise, Paez et al. found somatic mutation in the kinase domain (exons 18 through 24) in five out of five patients who responded to gefitinib, and none in four patients who did not respond to gefitinib. In addition, somatic mutations of EGFR were more frequent in adenocarcinomas (21%) than in other NSCLCs (2%), more frequent in women (20%) than in men (9%), and more frequent in patients from Japan (26%) than in patients from the USA (2%). The highest fraction of EGFR mutations were found in Japanese women with adenocarcinomas (57%) [77]. These two studies support the concept of molecular targeting by specific markers in terms of tumor response, but do not address the impact on survival.

13.3.4   c-erbB-2 (HER-2/neu)

The c-erbB-2 (HER-2/neu) proto-oncogene shares approximately 80% homology with c-erbB-1 and encodes a p185 protein [78]. It is a membrane-bound receptor with tyrosine kinase activity [79, 80]. Several reports have demonstrated that overexpression of this protein product is associated with an adverse outcome, particularly in adenocarcinomas. Kern et al. [81] examined 55 NSCLC tumors and found overexpression of p185[neu] in 31% of squamous cell carcinomas and in 35% of adenocarcinomas, but not in large-cell carcinomas. Patients with adenocarcinoma and overexpression of p185[neu] had a significantly poorer survival than those who did not. p185[nue] expression did not influence survival for squamous histology, however [81]. Shi et al. reported that 59% of 114 NSCLC tumor specimens expressed p185[neu] protein. The rate of expression was 81% in adenocarcinomas and 44% in squamous cell carcinomas. They found that p185[neu] expression was significantly associated with clinical stage of the tumors [82]. Harpole et al. found that 21% of 271 resected stage I NSCLC tumors expressed p185[neu] (14% in adenocarcinomas, 41% in large-cell carcinomas, 26% in squamous cell carcinomas, and 8% in alveolar cell carcinomas). They determined that erbB-2 expression was an independent factor that adversely impacted on the cancer-free survival and overall survival rates [40, 43]. Tateishi et al. examined c-erbB-2 protein expression in 119 adenocarcinomas and 84 squamous cell carcinoma tumors. They found 28% positivity in adenocarcinomas and 2% positivity in squamous cell cancers. p185^{neu} expression adversely impacted on the survival outcome at 5 years (30% vs. 52%) [83]. Contrary to these observations, Pfeiffer et al. [71] did not find c-erB-2 of significant prognostic value. Likewise, Pastorino et al. reported a 16% rate of c-erbB-2 expression in 485 tumor specimens. Similar to their finding with c-erbB-1, the expression of c-erbB-2 did not predict prognosis [52]. Greatens et al. [19], Kwiatkowski et al. [23], and Hilbe et al. [84], who analyzed multiple markers simultaneously, did not find that c-erbB-2 protein expression was of prognostic value.

13.4   Markers of Cell Proliferation and Cell-Cycle-Related Proteins

13.4.1   Ki-67

Ki-67 nuclear antigen is one of the proliferation indexes for cells, and as such is a marker for rapidly dividing tumors. It is a nonhistone nuclear protein that is expressed near the mitotic phase of cell cycle. IHC staining of Ki-67 has been utilized to determine the growth fraction of tumors. Hommura and colleagues [85] performed Ki-67 IHC on 215 surgically resected NSCLC. They found that a high Ki-67 labeling index (LI) (>30%) was significantly associated with male gender, squamous cell carcinoma histology, and smoking. In 109 NSCLC tumors of stages I and II, those with high Ki-67 LI survived for a significantly shorter time than patients with a low Ki-67 LI (<5%), the 5-year survival rates being 48% vs. 78%, respectively. Harpole et al. [86] found that a Ki-67 proliferation index of >7% significantly predicts for survival, with a 5-year survival rate of 68% for a Ki-67 index of 7% and 57% for a Ki-67 index of >7%. Pence et al. [87] reported a significant inverse association between patient survival and Ki-67 indexes. Patients with a tumor Ki-67 index of less than 3.5 survived significantly longer than those with higher Ki-67 indexes. Contrary to these findings, D'Amico et al. [40] and Hilbe et al. [84] found that Ki-67 was not significantly associated with survival.

13.4.2   Proliferating Cell Nuclear Antigen

Proliferating cell nuclear antigen (PCNA) is a nuclear protein that binds to DNA polymerase δ. Similar to Ki-67, IHC staining of PCNA is also utilized as a marker of cell proliferation. Ishida et al. [88] investigated IHC PCNA staining in 125 resected stage I tumors. PCNA positivity (>5% positive tumor cells) correlated with cell cycle fraction, the peak of S-phase, and the survival of cancer patients. Fontanini et al. [89] investigated 40 resected peripheral node-negative NSCLCs using IHC. Positivity was seen in all samples and was confined to the nuclei of cancer cells, but not to the surrounding, tumor-negative cells. Its frequency ranged from 0 to 70% (mean 15%). Tumors expressed either a low (0–25%) or intermediate (26–75%) proliferative activity. PCNA (intermediate vs. low immunoactivity) was a significant predictor of survival. Fukuse et al. [90] investigated the expression of PCNA in both primary and lymph node metastases of pathologic stage III A (N2) NSCLC and found a significant correlation between PCNA LI in the primary tumor and that in lymph node metastases. Patients with PCNA-negative primary tumors had a 5-year survival rate of 66.0%, compared with 21.5% for those with PCNA-positive primary tumors. The PCNA-negative nodal metastasis had a 5-year survival rate of 65%, compared with 30% for the node-positive patients. Volm et al. [91] analyzed IHC of 21 molecular markers of tumors from stage I–IIIA NSCLC and found that PCNA was associated with a decrease in survival. On the other hand, Hirata et al. [92] investigated adhesion molecule CD44 and PCNA IHC in stage I NSALC. They found PCNA-positive tumors with more frequent CD44v6 (a variant of CD44) positivity, but the expression of PCNA was not a statistically significant prognostic indicator. Likewise, Esposito et al. [93] found no predictive significance of PCNA for survival.

13.4.3   Cyclins

Progression of the cell cycle is governed by the CDKs, which are modulated by the binding of positive effectors, the cyclins [94, 95] and by negative regulators, the CDK inhibitors [96, 97]. Several classes of cyclins are up- and downregulated at specific points during the cell cycle [24]. Müller-Tidow et al. [98] investigated the gene expression (m-RNA) of cyclins from fresh-frozen biopsy specimens of resected NSCLC tumors of stages I–IIIA using quantitative real-time RT-PCR. They found that among the makers tested, cyclin A1, A2, E, and E2, only cyclin E had a significant prognostic value, with a mean survival time of 69.4 months for those with low cyclin E and 47.2 months for those with high cyclin E. Cyclins A1, A2, and E2 did not have prognostic relevance for survival. Fukuse et al. [99] examined the expression of cyclin E in 242 resected NSCLC tumors with pathological stages I, II, and IIIA. They found cyclin E to be an independent prognostic indicator. When cyclin E and PCNA are combined, the cases negative for both had a significantly better prognosis than the other cases. Dosaka-Akita et al. [100] performed IHC of cyclin D1, cyclin E, Ki-67, and *ras* p21 of 217 resected NSCLC tumors. Cylin E was found to be an independent unfavorable prognostic factor, while cyclin D1 was not. Caputi et al. [101] performed IHC in 135 resected NSCLC specimens for cyclin D1 and found that cyclin D1 overexpression was associated with higher tumor proliferation rate as measured by PCNA, as well as being a negative prognostic marker for patient survival. Volm et al. [91] found that the reduction in cyclin A as well as another four markers (FOS, JUN, ERBB1, or PCNA) was associated with long-term survival. Jin et al. [102] performed IHC for cyclin D1 in tissue from patients with stage I and II NSCLC. They found that patients with positive cyclin D1 had significantly poorer survival prognoses than those with negative cyclin D1.

13.4.4   p27KIP1

p27 KIP1 is a member of the cip/kip family of CDK inhibitors. It plays a pivotal role in cell cycle regulation from the G1 to S phase by inhibiting CDK4/6-cyclin D1 and CDK2-cyclin E [96]. A reduction or lack of p27 has been reported to correlate with shorter survival or to be a negative prognostic factor in many types of tumors including NSCLC [103]. Hommura et al. [85] performed IHC of resected NSCLC tumors for p27KIP1 protein (p27) expression. In 109 NSCLC tumors of stages I and II, patients with tumors lacking p27 expression survived for a significantly shorter time than those with tumors expressing p27, with a 5-year survival rate of 38% vs. 68%, respectively. Catzavelos and colleagues [104] investigated p27KIP1 expression using IHC and found reduced levels of p27 in 86% of cases and a statistically significant inverse correlation between p27 levels and tumor grade. All patients with high p27 levels were alive at the time of study follow-up. Yatabe et al. [105] investigated p27KIP1 expression in resected NSCLC and found that reduced expression of p27KIP1 was significantly associated with better survival.

13.4.5   *Rb* Tumor-Suppressor Gene

The retinoblastoma gene (Rb) family consists of a group of genes sharing a high percentage of sequence homology. At present there are pRb/p105, p107, and pRb2/p130 identified. Each of the Rb family members is a tumor suppressor gene as well as a nuclear phosphoprotein that regulates G1 progression to the S phase of the cell cycle [106]. They are also involved in various forms of differentiation (growth suppression in a cell-type dependent manner), and are critical targets for inactivation by transforming oncoproteins of DNA tumor viruses [107, 108]. Xu et al. [109] investigated Rb pro-

tein expression in 101 resected early stage NSCLCs. They found a 24% loss of Rb protein expression. The median survival for Rb-positive patients was significantly longer at 32 months, and was 18 months for those with Rb-negative tumors. Caputi et al. [110] evaluated the IHC expression of pRb2/p130 in 135 lung cancer specimens, and performed Western-blot analysis in a subset of 30 corresponding tumor lysates. They found that the loss or reduced expression of pRb2/p130 was associated with a shorter overall survival. On the other hand, D'Amico et al. [40] investigated multiple molecular markers of stage I resected NSCLC by IHC and found no prognostic value of Rb protein expression. Kwiakowski et al. [23] performed IHC of multiple markers of 317 resected stage I NSCLCs and found no prognostic significance of Rb expression. Jin et al. [102] performed IHC of RB of tumors from patients with stages I and II NSCLC. They did not find a significant prognostic value of pRb. Chen et al. [111] performed IHC of p16 and pRb in 107 NSCLC tumors. They also found no statistically significant prognostic values of pRb.

13.4.6   p21 waf1/cip1

p21 waf1/cip1 is the gene product of WAF/CIP1/SD11, and is an inhibitor of the CDK complexes [112–114]. Activated through p53-dependent or p53-independent pathways, it plays an important role in the regulation of the cell cycle, especially in G1 arrest [112, 115]. Caputi et al. [116] performed IHC on 60 surgically resected NSCLC tumors and found that p21 protein was expressed in both normal and neoplastic tissues. In normal tissue, p21 was detected in a low percentage of well-differentiated cells. p21 immunostain was positive in 80% of tumors and was overexpressed in 73% of tumors. Median survival time of p21-positive patients was 36 months, and was 14 months for p21-negative patients, with a 5-year survival rate of 38% versus 10%, respectively. Shoji et al. [117] conducted IHC on 233 resected NSCLC tumors of stages I–IIIA. Expression of p21 was positive in 120 patients (51.5%). The 5-year survival rate of p21-positive patients was 74%, significantly higher than that of p21 negative patients (61%). Multivariate analysis confirmed p21 positivity to be a significant favorable prognostic factor. There was no significant correlation between p21 expression and p53 status, proliferative activity, or incidence of apoptosis.

13.4.7   p16

p16 is the gene product of p16^{INK4a}/CDKN2/MTS1, which is a CDK inhibitor. The protein controls the transition from the G1 phase to the S phase in the cell cycle by inhibiting the phosphorylation of the *Rb* gene product. Kratzke et al. [118] performed IHC staining of p16 and pRb in 101 resected NSCLC tumors. Abnormal p16 and pRb protein expression was found in 51% and 15% of tumors, respectively. There was an inverse correlation between pRb and p16. Tumors with aberrant expression of p16 were associated with a significantly worse survival. Taga et al. [119] found negative p16 staining in 27% of 115 NSCLC specimens. The frequency of negative p16 expression was higher in squamous cell carcinoma (39.5%) than in adenocarcinoma (20.3%). Patients with negative p16 expression had a significantly shorter survival period than those with positive p16 expression. González-Quevedo et al. [120] investigated p16 expression by Western-blot analysis in 98 resected NSCLC tumor specimens. They found that p16 positivity was associated with significantly better survival of patients with stage I and stage II disease. Jin et al. [102] performed IHC on p16 in tumors from patients with stage I and II NSCLC. p16-positive patients had significantly better prognoses than p16-negative patients. Esposito and colleagues [93] investigated four cell cycle regulator marker proteins (p21, p16, p53, and PCNA) and found only p16 to be a significant predictor for survival by multivariate analysis. On the contrary, Chen et al. [111] performed IHC of p16 and pRb in 107 NSCLC tumors. They found no reciprocal correlation between p16 and pRb. They also found no statistically significant prognostic value of p16.

13.5 Markers for Angiogenesis

Tumor-induced neovascularization (i.e., angiogenesis) is important in neoplastic development, local cancer invasion, and metastasis to distant sites [121]. There are different markers for tumor angiogenesis, including vascular endothelial growth factor (VEGF) and microvessel density (MVD) measurement by IHC staining for factor VIII, CD31 (platelet/endothelial cell adhesion molecule), and CD34 (endothelial cell marker). Imoto et al. [122] assayed expression of VEGF and MVD by assessing anti-factor-VIII IHC in 91 resected NSCLC tumors. They found expression of VEGF to be an important prognostic factor, while microvessel count was not. D'Amico and colleagues [40] examined 10 molecular markers in 408 stage I NSCLC patients and found factor VIII positivity to be one of the 5 significant prognostic molecular markers, the other 4 being p53, erb-b2, adhesion molecule CD-44, and RB, The 5-year survival was 56% for patients who were factor VIII positive, and 70% for patients who were factor VIII negative. Fontanini et al. [72, 123] investigated MVD using an anti-CD34 monoclonal antibody, which was specific for endothelial cells. They found that MVD was significantly associated with a worse prognosis. Koukourakis et al. [124] investigated the expression of VEGF using IHC, standard MVD assay, and

VEGF/KDR complex (VEGF and VEGF receptor 2 complex)-activated MVD. All three measurements were significant prognostic factors for survival, and VEGF/KDR was the most potent prognosticator. Harpole et al. [86] examined angiogenesis in 275 tumors from patients with stage I NSCLC. They found a significant survival advantage for low-level expression of microvessel count. Volm et al. [125] investigated angiogenesis in 143 resected NSCLC specimens of stage I, II and IIIA tumors. The expression of both VEGF and angiostatin, a potent inhibitor of angiogenesis, was found to have prognostic value. Patients with the angiostatin-positive and VEGF-negative carcinomas had significantly longer survival than patients with tumors that stained positive for other combinations of angiostatin and VEGF. Baillie et al. [126] examined VEGF expression and vascularity in 81 NSCLC archival specimens by IHC staining. They found that mean survival times were shorter in patients with high VEGF expression, but their finding was not statistically significant. However, high VEGF expression was associated with significantly poorer survival in patients who also had high vascularity. Han et al. [127] investigated VEGF expression, intratumoral MVD, and angiolymphatic invasion in 85 resected stage I NSCLC tumors. They found that patients with low VEGF expression had a significantly higher survival rate than those with high VEGF expression (80% vs. 48%, respectively). Patients with high MVD also had a significantly lower survival rate than those with low MVD (46% vs. 73%, respectively). Volm et al. [128] investigated expression of basic fibroblast growth factor (bFGF), a cytokine involved in proliferation, differentiation, and angiogenesis [129], and its receptor (FGFR-1) by IHC. They found that patients with high FGFR-1 expression had significantly shorter survival times than patients with weak or moderate expression. There was no significant correlation between bFGF expression and patient survival. Ohta et al. [130] investigated mRNA expression of VEGF in 42 cases of primary lung cancer tissues. They found a significant association with poor survival for tumors with high VEGF expression than tumors with low VEGF expression (16.7% vs. 77.9%, respectively).

13.6 Tumor Invasion and Metastasis Markers

13.6.1 Plasmin

Several proteolytic enzymes are involved in the degradation of the extracellular matrix, leading to tumor invasion or metastasis. Among these enzymes are the collagenases, metalloproteases, and serine proteases, including plasmin [131]. Pedersen et al. [132] investigated the prognostic value of urokinase-type plasminogen activator (uPA), uPA receptor (uPAR), and plasminogen activator inhibitor (PAI)-1 in tumor extracts from 84 patients with squamous cell lung carcinoma and 38 patients with large-cell lung carcinoma using ELISAs. High uPAR levels were significantly associated with short overall survival in patients with squamous cell lung carcinomas, while no statistically significant prognostic impact of uPA and PAI-1 was found. Yoshino et al. [133] examined the expression of uPA, uPAR, and PAI-1 and PAI-2 in 105 tumors using IHC and RT-PCR techniques. The expression of uPA, uPAR, and PAI-1 was detected in approximately 80% of primary lung cancers, whereas detectable PAI-2 expression was observed only 50% of cases. They found that a diminished expression level of PAI-2 was significantly correlated with lymph node metastasis and poor prognosis.

13.6.2   Cathepsin B

Cathepsin B is a lysosomal cysteine proteinase that is involved in the catabolism of various intracellular proteins in lysosomes and is implicated in the direct or indirect degradation of the extracellular matrix in tumor cells [134]. It is thought to play a role in the complex process of tumor invasion and metastasis. Sukoh and colleagues [135] examined the IHC expression of cathepsin B in the resected tumors of 108 patients with NSCLC. They found that higher expression of cathepsin B was associated significantly with shorter survival for stage I NSCLC. Inoue and colleagues [136] examined cathepsin B expression by IHC and found the 5-year survival rates of patients with high and low cathepsin B expressions were 26% and 77%, respectively, including 45% and 94% for patients with stage I disease, respectively, and 15% and 60% for those with stage IIIB disease, respectively.

13.6.3   Laminin

Laminin is a glycoprotein component of basement membrane, which is an important barrier against tumor invasion and metastasis [137]. Mori et al. [138] investigated protein expression of both laminin and cathepsin B by IHC in resected tumor tissues of 31 stage I NSCLC patients. Neither laminin nor cathepsin B was associated with survival of patients. Pastorino and colleagues [52] also found laminin to be of no prognostic value.

13.6.4   Adhesion Molecules

Adhesion molecules are involved in cell-to-cell and cell-to-extracellular matrix interactions, thus they may be involved in the metastatic spread of tumors. Hirata et

al. [92] examined standard CD44 and an isoform of CD44 (the variant CD44 v6) in pathological stage I NSCLC. They found that CD44v6 was correlated with adverse prognosis, but standard CD44 was not. The 5-year survival rate of stage I NSCLC was 50% for CD44v6-positive tumors and 88% for those with CD44v6-negative tumors. D'Amico et al. [40] investigated the prognostic significance of CD44 among ten molecular markers and found a 5-year survival of 54% in CD44-positive patients and 67% in CD44-negative patients. Kase et al. [139] investigated expression of E-cadherin, a calcium-dependent cell-cell adhesion molecule, as well as $\alpha/\beta/r$-catenin expression, a group of undercoat proteins that bind the E-cadherin complex to the actin cytoskeleton. They found that E-cadherin expression was not correlated with the prognosis, but reduced β-catenin expression was significantly correlated with a poor prognosis. The prognosis was significantly unfavorable when both E-cadherin and β-catenin were reduced.

13.6.5   Motility-Related Protein-1

Motility-related protein-1 (MRP-1/CD9) is a transmembrane glycoprotein that is identical to the CD9 antigen. MRP-1/CD9 causes low motility and diminished metastatic potential to the lung [140]. Using RT-PCR, Higashiyama et al. [141] investigated the gene expression of MRP-1/CD9 in 109 NSCLC tumors. They found 67/109 (61.5%) tumors that were positive for MRP-1/CD9 expression. The survival rate was significantly higher than among patients with positive tumors than among those whose tumors had reduced gene expression (62.3% 34.9%, respectively). MRP-1/CD9, along with 3 other molecular markers (K-*ras*, p53, and KA11/CD82) were investigated in tumors from 187 NSCLC patients by Miyaki et al. [21]. Only MRP-1/CD9 and K-*ras* status were found to be significant factors for prognosis.

13.6.6   KA11/CD82

KA11/CD82 is a transmembrane protein that is known to suppress tumor metastasis of prostate cancer. Adachi et al. [142] investigated 151 NSCLC tumors using RT-PCR. They found 35/151 (23%) tumors with conserved KA11/CD82 expression, while the remaining tumors had reduced gene expression. The overall survival rate of patients with KA11/CD82-positive tumors was significantly higher than that of patients with KA11/CD82-negative tumors (77.4% vs. 38.5%, respectively). Miyaki and colleague [21] found no prognostic value of KA11/CD82 in tumors from 187 NSCLC patients.

13.7   Other Molecular Markers

13.7.1   Bcl2

Bcl2 encodes for a protein product that inhibits apoptosis. Pezzella et al. [143] investigated bcl-2 protein expression in 122 resected stage I and II NSCLC tumors by IHC. They reported a better survival for bcl-2-positive tumors, and the better survival reached statistical significance for squamous cell histology. Fontanini et al. [47] analyzed bcl-2 protein expression in 91 resected NSCLC tumors. The mean bcl-2 expression was significantly lower among those who developed metastatic disease. Patients with positive bcl-2 survived significantly longer. Despite these two positive studies, none of the other studies that have investigated bcl-2 expression in early stage, resected NSCLC, in which multiple molecular markers were assessed simultaneously in large sample sizes, reported a significant prognostic value of bcl-2 expression [19, 23, 40, 52, 84].

13.7.2   Blood Group Antigens

The cancer cells from various human cancers frequently lose their blood-group A and B antigens [144]. It was hypothesized that the loss of blood-group antigens may be associated with metastatic spread of tumors. Lee et al. [145] investigated 164 resected tumor specimens of NSCLC stained for A and B antigens using monoclonal antibodies, and stained for H antigen (precursor antigen) with Ulex europaeus agglutinin I. They found a significantly worse survival for 28 patients who were type A or AB and whose tumors had lost type A antigen. Expression of blood-group antigen B or H I in tumor cells did not correlate with survival. Kwiatkowski and colleagues investigated seven molecular markers including blood group A antigen [23] and did not find a prognostic significance of blood group A antigen. D'Amico et al. [40] investigated the prognostic significance of blood group A antigen among 10 molecular markers in 408 stage I NSCLC patients, and found no prognostic significance of this marker. Likewise, Pastorino and colleagues [53] did not find prognostic significance for blood group A antigen among multiple other molecular markers by studying IHC staining of 515 stage I NSCLC tumor specimens. Miyake et al. [146] investigated the precursor of blood cell antigen H and H-related antigens in resected NSCLC tumors. They used MIA-15-5 (a monoclonal antibody that inhibits the motility and metastatic potential of tumor cells) to stain for the precursor antigens H/Le^y/Le^b of 149 resected NSCLC tumors. They found that 91 patients with MIA-positive tumors had significantly lower 5-year survival than the 58 patients with MIA-negative tumors (survival

rate 20.9% vs. 58.6%, respectively). The difference in survival between patients with MIA-positive and MIA-negative tumors was significant among patients with blood groups A and AB, but not among those with blood groups B or O.

13.7.3   CpG Hypermethylation

CpG hypermethylation is a feature of human cancers that silences the expression of tumor-suppressor genes or other cancer-associated genes. DNA methylation may be an alternative mechanism to mutation or deletions of gene function. Aberrant gene methylation has been found frequently in NSCLC, including the *p16*, O^6-methylguanine-DNA methyltransferase (*MGMT*), death-associated protein kinase (*DAPK*), retinoic acid receptor-*β* (*RARβ*), *Ras* association domain family 1A (*RASSF1A*), and adenomatous polyposis coli (*APC*) genes [147–154]. Chan et al. [155] used methylation-specific polymerase chain reaction (MSP) to analyze methylation of *p16*, *RARβ*, *DAPK*, and *MGMT* genes in 75 NSCLC tumors and 68 bronchoalveolar lavage samples (BAL). They found an 84% aberrant methylation in at least one of these genes. Wang et al. [156] investigated 119 resected NSCLC tumors from stage I/II to stage IIIA for *p16^{INK4a}* and *RASSF1A* by MSP. Hypermethylation of the p16^{INK4a} and *RASSF1A* promoters was found in 49% and 39% tumors, respectively. Hypermethylation of both gene promoters was observed in 25% of tumors. In patients with stage I/II tumors, only *p16^{INK4a}* promoter hypermethylation was associated with a poor 5-year survival rate. In patients with stage IIIA disease, *RASSF1A* promoter hypermethylation was a stronger predictor of a poor 5-year survival rate than *p16^{INK4a}* promoter hypermethylation. Tang et al. [149] reported that *DAPK* promoter methylation was associated with a significantly decreased survival at 5 years after surgery. Brabender et al. [157] found that patients with low *APC* methylation status in the tumor had a significantly longer survival among patients with NSCLC.

13.7.4   Telomerase

Telomerase is a ribonucleoprotein enzyme that lengthens telomeres, which are specialized chromosome ends that have been shortened during successive cycles of cell division [158]. In humans and other vertebrates, telomeric DNA consists of tandem repeats of the G-rich sequence TTAGGG. Its activation plays a critical role in tumorigenesis by sustaining cellular immortality. Taga et al. [159] studied 103 NSCLC specimens using a polymerase chain reaction based on a telomeric repeat amplification assay. They found 82.5% telomerase positivity in the tumor tissues and none in the paired normal lung tissue specimens. Telomerase positivity was seen more frequently in advanced disease and in poorly differentiated tumors. It was not correlated with histologic type or other characteristics. Patients with telomerase-positive tumors survived for a significantly shorter period than those with a telomerase-negative tumor. Telomerase was identified as an independent prognostic factor. González-Quevedo et al. [120] investigated 98 tumor specimens for telomerase activity as well as *p16* expression. They also found a positive interaction between the two parameters, thus telomerase negativity appears to be a significant prognostic factor for better survival. Wang et al. [160] investigated the expression of human telomerase reverse transcriptase catalytic subunit (hTERT) as a prognostic marker in 153 stage I NSCLC specimens and found hTERT expression to be associated with shorter survival; hTERT was found to be an independent prognostic marker in multivariate analysis. Hara et al. [161] investigated the telomerase activity and hTERT expression of 62 lung cancer specimens. Telomerase activity and hTERT were detected in cancerous tissues (75.8% and 75.8%, respectively), and not in any noncancerous tissues. Patients with hTERT-positive tumors survived for a significantly shorter period than those with hTERT-negative tumors.

13.8   Multimarker and Multivariate Analyses

Individual molecular markers and their prognostic significance have been reported in the aforementioned studies. Since the malignant transformation and virulence of cancer involve complex interactions between cellular molecules and signals, it is likely that while single markers may be significant in predicting prognosis, they may be covariates to other markers. Likewise, single markers may not be significant in predicting prognosis, but some combinations of multiple factors may prove to be significant. Several investigators have therefore studied combinations of markers and analyzed their significance using multivariate analyses. Hilbe et al. [84] investigated 9 molecular markers with IHC for EGFR, c-erB-2, c-erB-3, CD82, Ki-67, p120, p53, bcl-2, and CD31 in 79 tumor specimens. None of the tested markers was significant in univariate survival analysis. However, cases expressing two or three of c-erbB3, p53, and MVD positivity showed a significantly lower survival probability than those expressing none or only one factor. Greatens and colleagues [19] investigated 6 molecular markers, including K-ras gene mutation, *p53* gene mutation, and p53 protein, bcl-2 protein, c-erbB-1 protein, c-erbB-2 protein, and MIA-15-5 antigen by IHC in surgical specimens of 101 patients of NSCLC. Among these markers, only MIA-15-5 antigen expression was correlated with improved survival (as assessed by uni-

variate and multivariate analysis). This finding was contrary to their original report, which showed a worse prognosis with MIA-15-5 expression. They concluded that the multiple cell markers are not clinically useful in predicting survival among patients undergoing surgery for NSCLC. Esposito and colleagues [93] examined IHC of four molecular markers, p21, p16, p53, and PCNA in 68 surgical specimens of NSCLC. They found that p21, p16, and p53 were significantly correlated with survival by univariate analysis, while only p16 expression remained as a significant predictor by multivariate analysis. Kwiatkowski and colleagues [23] investigated 7 molecular markers (p185[new] protein, p53 protein, Rb protein, bcl-2 protein, H-ras-p21 protein, blood group A, and K-ras mutation) in 244 stage I NSCLC patients. Only p53 expression, K-ras codon 12 mutation, and the absence of H-ras p21 expression were found to be independent predictors of recurrence, as assessed by multivariate analysis. D'Amico and colleagues [40] carried out IHC analysis of 406 stage I patients, using 10 molecular markers (EGFR, ereb-b2, p53, bcl-2, Rb, Ki-67, angiogenic marker factor VIII, adhesion molecule CD44, sialyl-Tn, and blood group A). Those who had five of these ten markers were associated with the risk of recurrence and death, representing independent metastatic pathways: p53, factor VIII, erb-b2, CD44, and Rb. Miyake and colleagues [21] investigated the expression of four molecular markers (*p53* mutations, K-*ras* mutations, *MRP-1/CD9* gene, and *KA11/CD82* gene) in 187 NSCLC tumor specimens. K-ras and *MRP-1/CD9* were significant factors for prognosis. Pastorino and colleagues [52] conducted IHC of multiple molecular markers (blood group A antigen and precursors of blood antigens, laminin receptor, c-erbB1/EGFR, and cerbB2/Neu, bcl2, p53), and angiogenesis in 515 patients with stage I NSCLC and concluded that IHC markers are of no prognostic value. Volm et al. [91] examined the expression of 21 molecular markers of tumor specimens in relationship to survival of 216 patients with NSCLC using IHC. Five of the 21 markers (FOS, JUN, ERBB1, cyclin A, and PCNA) were found to be associated with a decrease in survival. Esposito et al. [93] investigated expression of cell-cycle-related proteins p21, Rb-p16, p53, and PCNA in 68 NSCLC tumors by IHC. They found that only Rb-p16 influences survival (multivariate analysis). Fontanini et al. [72] evaluated 195 NSCLC tumors of stages I–IIIA for transforming growth factor alpha, amphiregulin (AR), CRIPTO, EGFR, erbB-2, erbB-3, and tumor angiogenesis. Apart from nodal status, only microvessel count and AR overexpression were independent molecular prognostic factors for survival.

13.9 Molecular Detection of Occult Metastasis

13.9.1 Detecting Occult Regional Metastasis in Lymph Nodes

Detecting micrometastasis in surgically removed regional lymph nodes negative for cancer (as assessed by HE stain) may allow early detection of regional cancer spread that is not achievable by imaging studies or traditional morphology-based methods. Studies on detecting occult metastasis have mostly focused on detecting epithelial cell markers such as cytokeratin, but have also been conducted with other markers. Vollmer et al. [162] reported IHC detection of occult lymph metastasis of specimens from Cancer and Leukemia Group B (CALGB) from clinically stage T1-2N0M0 NSCLC; 825 lymph nodes were studied. Routine HE staining detected 18 positive lymph nodes, while IHC using antibodies for cytokeratins (AE1/3) detected 45 positive lymph nodes. There were 28 occult metastases detectable only by IHC. Pantel et al. [163] performed IHC on lymph nodes from patients with NSCLC stage pT1-4N1-2M0 after surgery. Monoclonal antibody CK2 against cytokeratin polypeptide 18 (CK18) was used to stain the lymph nodes, and they found a 54.3% cytokeratin-positive rate for pathologic pN0 nodes. Maruyama et al. [10] stained 973 regional lymph nodes from 44 patients with stage I NSCLC using CAM-5.2 anti-cytokeratin monoclonal antibody. They found a 5.6% of 450 lymph nodes from T1N0M0 diseases were CAM-5.2 immunopositive, and of 523 lymph nodes from T2N0M0 diseases in which metastases were not detected by the routine HE stain, 12.6% were CAM-5.2 immunopositive. Disease-free survival duration was significantly shorter in those patients with micrometastases in the mediastinal lymph nodes than in patients with node-negative disease. Using the anti-keratin antibody stain, Chen et al. [164] stained 588 nodes of 60 patients with disease confined to the lung and a diagnosis of metastasis to some regional lymph nodes. They found that 63% of the 60 patients whose nodes appeared to be negative on examination by HE staining were anti-keratin immunopositive. Patients with occult lymph node metastasis had a median survival time shorter than that of patients whose nodes did not contain occult metastasis, but was longer than that of patients whose nodes contained metastases detectable on HE staining. Passlick et al. [165] stained for epithelial marker (Ber-Ep4 against epithelial surface glycoproteins of 34 kD and 49 kD) in lymph nodes and bone marrow in 391 lymph nodes of 72 patients. They found a total positivity of 15.2% for those considered pN0 by HE staining. The occult lymph node metastasis did not correlate with occult metastasis in the bone marrow, nor did it correlate with the size or grade of the primary tumor. Patients with occult lymph node metastasis had significantly shorter disease-free survival durations than node-negative patients. Ohta et al. [12] assessed occult micrometastasis by anti-cytokeratin IHC stain of resected lymph nodes. They detected 29% cytokeratin-positive cells in lymph nodes and found a significantly worse survival for those with occult micrometastasis than those without micrometastasis (57% vs. 83% at 3 years, respectively).

Several molecular markers other than cytokeratin staining have also been applied to detect occult metastasis in resected lymph nodes. Salerno et al. [166] used RT-PCR to detect mRNA transcripts for MUC1 (a cell-surface glycoprotein present in lung tissue but absent from normal lymph nodes). Occult metastasis was identified in 33 out of 88 lymph nodes determined to be free of tumor by HE stain. D'Cunha et al. [167] compared standard RT-PCR with quantitative RT-PCR to detect mRNA in 232 lymph nodes from 53 patients with stage I disease, which were negative according to histologic examination. The rate of detection of occult micrometastasis was 16.4% for standard RT-PCR and 25.4% for quantitative RT-PCR. The rate of upstaging stage I NSCLC was 43.4% for standard RT-PCR and 56.6% for quantitative RT-PCR. Maruyama et al. [168] detected occult lymph node metastasis using cytokeratin positivity in 43.9% of hilar nodes and 29.3% mediastinal nodes in stage I NSCLC. They also fond that *p53* alterations (mutation and overexpression) in the primary tumors were not correlated with occult lymph node metastases, while *p53* gene mutation was an unfavorable prognostic factor in patients with occult lymph node metastasis. Dobashi et al. [169] investigated 480 lymph nodes taken from 47 patients who underwent lung resection for NSCLC. The primary lesions were positive for p53 by IHC. They found that 8.3% of lymph nodes that were pathologically negative expressed *p53*. Ahrendt et al. [170] investigated p53 and K-*ras* mutation in the lymph nodes of resected stage I NSCLC by direct sequencing. They found a 28% rate of occult metastasis in the lymph nodes, which shared similar TP53 or K-*ras* mutations as the primary tumors. Their data showed that standard histopathologic assessment of regional lymph nodes failed to detect metastases at levels below 0.9% tumor-specific mutant p53 clones per node, supporting a much better sensitivity of molecular staging by DNA sequencing. However, there was no statistically significant difference in disease-specific or overall survival between patients with and without molecular lymph node metastasis. Wallace et al. [171] examined telomerase expression using RT-PCR methods in fine-needle-aspirated specimens of mediastinal lymph nodes of patients with NSCLC. They found that RNA was available from 87 of 100 lymph node aspirates, and 5 out of 18 (28%) patients with no pathologically evident mediastinal disease expressed telomerase in at least one lymph node. A counter-argument for using telomerase as a marker for occult lymph node metastasis was made by Ahrendt et al. [172]. In this study, resected lymph nodes were assessed for telomerase activity, *p53* mutation and K-*ras* mutation. They found that 8 out of 9 (89%) histologically positive lymph nodes were telomerase positive, and 26 out of 48 (54%) histopathologically negative lymph nodes were telomerase positive. Most of the nodes found to be positive by telomerase assay did not harbor the oncogene mutation markers (*p53* and K-*ras*) of the primary tumors, which led investigators to conclude that the high rate of false positives using telomerase analysis limits its role in staging lymph nodes for NSCLC. Gene promoter hypermethylation in the tumors and lymph nodes of stage I NSCLC was investigated by Harden et al. [173] using reverse-transcriptase MSP. Five gene promoters were investigated for hypermethylation, including *CDKN2A* (*p16*), *MGMT*, glutathione S-transferase P1 (*GSTP1*), *APC*, and *DAPK*. They found that 5/11(45%) patients with occult metastasis detected by methylation analysis have died compared with 17/62 (27%) patients with negative lymph nodes, although survival analysis did not reach statistical significance.

13.9.2 Detection of Occult Distant Metastasis in Bone Marrow

Detecting micrometastasis in the bone marrow before it becomes clinically evident has been made possible by the remarkable increase in sensitivity of molecular technology. This may provide early detection of distant cancer spread not hitherto achievable by imaging studies or traditional methods based on cell morphology. While under normal circumstances only hematopoietic cells exist in the bone marrow, studies in detecting occult metastasis have mostly been based on detecting epithelial cell markers, such as cytokeratins in the bone marrow. Pantel et al. [163] performed IHC on bone marrow from 139 patients with NSCLC (stage pT1-4N1-2M0) who showed no evidence of distant metastases by standard staging methods. Monoclonal antibody CK2 against CK18 was used for staining the 139 tumor specimens, as well as tissue from 215 patients without the diagnosis of epithelial tumors. They found a 59.7% positivity of cytokeratin at frequencies of 1 in 100,000 to 1 in 1,000,000 cells, and a 2.8% positive rate of the 215 control bone marrow samples. The presence of such isolated cells was a significant and independent predictor for clinical relapse in node-negative patients. Cote et al. [174] stained for cytokeratin positivity using monoclonal antibody AE-1 and CAM 5.2 in resected bone marrow from 43 patients with stage I/II–III NSCLC. They found a 33% positive rate for stage I disease and a 46% positive rate for stage III disease. Patients with positive cytokeratin cells in bone marrow had a signifi-

cantly shorter time to disease recurrence than those without occult metastasis (7.3 months vs. 35.1 months, respectively). Ohgami et al. [175] also stained for CK18-positive cells in the bone marrow from 39 patients with operable NSCLC. They found a 39% positivity among these patients, and noted that patients with CK18-positive cells in their bone marrow demonstrated a significantly earlier recurrence than those without such cells.

13.9.3 Detection of Occult Metastasis in Blood

Detection of occult metastasis in peripheral blood has also been reported. Attempts have been made to analyze epithelial markers, DNA markers, and markers of angiogenesis. Bearzatto et al. [176] investigated *p16^{INK4A}* promoter hypermethylation detected by fluorescence MSP in resected tumor tissue and plasma from 35 NSCLC patients in comparison with15 healthy donors. *p16^{INK4A}* hypermethylation was positive in 63% of tumors, 55% of the plasma of cancer patients, and none of the 15 healthy donors. Gautschi et al. [177] analyzed the total serum or plasma DNA of 185 patients with NSCLC. They found a significant correlation between increased plasma DNA concentrations and elevated lactate dehydrogenase levels, advanced tumor stage, and poor survival. Tumor progression after chemotherapy was significantly associated with increasing plasma DNA concentrations. Sozzi et al. [178] investigated hTERT in the plasma DNA of 100 NSCLC patients. They found that the median concentration of circulating plasma DNA in patients was almost eight times the value detected in controls, suggesting that high plasma DNA was a strong risk factor for lung cancer. Andriani et al. [179] investigated three plasma DNA markers in the tumor and plasma of cancer patients with NSCLC: *p53* mutations, fragile histidine triad gene (FHIT), and microsatellite alteration at location chromosome 3. They found *p53* mutations in the tumors of 40.6% (26/64) of the patients. Among patients with these mutated tumors, 73.1% (19/26) exhibited corresponding mutations in the plasma. With regard to FHIT, 39.3% (22/56) of the patients exhibited FHIT positivity in their tumor, 16.1% (9/56) exhibited FHIT positivity in their plasma. Of those with FHIT-positive tumors, 32% (7/22) exhibited corresponding changes in the plasma. Microsatellite alterations were found in tumors from 40 out of 64 (62.5%) patients, and in the plasma of 23 (35.9%) patients. Of those with microsatellite alterations in their tumor, 47.5% (19/40) exhibited corresponding changes in their plasma. An et al. [180] investigated *p16* hypermethylation in both the tumor and the plasma of 105 patients with NSCLC. They found that *p16* hypermethylation was present in 73.3% (77/105) of the plasma samples and 79.3% (73/92) of the tumor samples. Only patients whose tumor cells had hypermethylated *p16* gene exhibited aberrant methylation in their plasma samples, suggesting that *p16* hypermethylation is an excellent biomarker for early diagnosis and follow-up of patients. Tamura et al. [181] measured circulating levels of VEGF and intratumoral VEGF by ELISA in lung cancer patients in comparison to healthy controls. They found a significant correlation between plasma VEGF levels and MVD, and between plasma VEGF levels and intratumoral VEGF levels, suggesting that plasma VEGF in patients with lung cancer is an indicator of tumor angiogenesis. Brattström et al. [182] analyzed serum levels of VEGF and bFGF in patients with operable NSCLC. They found that VEGF levels correlated with tumor volume, platelet counts, and performance status, while b-FGF level correlated significantly with recurrent disease.

13.10 Conclusion

Investigations in molecular markers have made great strides in revealing the pathogenesis and natural history of cancer. The application of modern molecular techniques to study tumor specimens from NSCLC has provided further prognostic information that may change the algorithms for lung cancer staging in the future. So far, molecular staging has not been applied to clinical decision-making and management, but holds great promise. Accurately subcategorizing patients into different prognostic groups may allow for individualized therapies and prioritizing local therapy versus targeting distant disease for tumors of all stages. In addition, identifying specific tumor markers of individual tumors may offer the option of molecular targeted therapy for selected cancer patients who may have a better chance of responding to a particular type of targeted therapy, such as seen in lung cancer patients with specific *EGFR* mutation who were found to be responders to IRESSA treatment [76, 77].

While new discoveries from an array of molecular markers hold great promise, at present, TNM staging criteria remain the most powerful determinants of lung cancer survival. It is evident that the application of molecular markers to lung cancer staging will be a challenging task, as many confounding factors have been recognized. These include differences in molecular techniques, different types of monoclonal antibodies used for IHC, different study subpopulations of tumors such as tumor stage or histology, smoking history, race, geographic clusters of patients, and other potential demographic information. In addition, while several markers have been found to have prognostic value using univariate analysis, many were found to be not significant in multivariate analysis as discussed in 13.8. Studies investigating multiple molecular markers for prognostic values indeed support the complexity of this matter; further substantiating the intricate interactions of DNA and many cellular mole-

cules in signaling and malignant transformation. It may be necessary to establish a risk-stratification mode of NSCLC using different combinations of molecular markers, as suggested by Dosaka-Akita et al. [100].

As for detecting occult metastasis, although RT-PCR has markedly enhanced the sensitivity of assays for molecular markers, the specificity of RT-PCR methods maybe the limiting factor in the detection of occult metastasis. For example, when evaluating the utility of molecular markers in the detection of metastases in the lymph nodes and blood of breast cancer patients, Bostick et al. found that many noncancer patients had detectable mRNA for carcinoembryonic antigen (CEA), cytokeratin 19 (CK19), GA-733.2, and MUC-1, as assessed by RT-PCR [183]. Likewise, epithelial markers of glycoprotein-40, desmoplakin-1, CEA, erb-B2, erb-B3, and CK18 were found in normal bone marrow [184]. Ko et al. [185] reported limitations in detecting tumor cells in peripheral blood. In their report, CK19-positive cells were found in peripheral blood from healthy blood donors using RT-PCR, and reported a 29% false-positive rate. The future challenges in the application of molecular markers to the detection of occult metastasis of lung cancer will need to balance the sensitivity and specificity of each assay system for individual markers and should be accompanied by robust statistical supports. As for the concern of potential interactions among different molecular markers, the development of biomathematical models in integrating these various molecular markers may be necessary to sort out the biases from covariates as well as to define the mechanisms by which molecular staging can be a powerful addition to the TNM staging system.

Key Points

- While TNM staging remains the current standard staging system, clinical experience reveals a portion of patients in each group whose prognoses defy the assigned stage grouping. Additional prognostic information that will complement the TNM staging is needed.
- Recent refinement of immunohistochemical staining techniques and the advancement of molecular technology (such as sequencing, single-strand conformational polymorphism, reverse-transcriptase polymerase chain reaction, in situ hybridization, and enzyme-linked immunosorbent assay) have markedly improved the sensitivity and specificity of diagnosing molecular markers and have enabled discoveries about lung cancer.
- Our knowledge of molecular markers has furthered our understanding of the pathobiology, etiology, and natural history of lung cancer, with the potential to lead to breakthroughs in early detec-

tion, screening, identifying molecular targets for therapy and intervention, and molecular staging of lung cancer.

References

1. Denoix PF. [Enquete permanent dans les centres anticancereux]. Bull Inst Nat Hyg (Paris) 1946; 1:70.
2. Mountain CF. Carr DT. Anderson WA. A system for the clinical staging of lung cancer. Am J Roentgenol Radium Ther Nucl Med 1974; 120(1):130.
3. Mountain CF. A new International Staging System for Lung Cancer. Chest 1986; 89(4 Suppl):225S.
4. Mountain CF. Revisions in the International System for Staging Lung Cancer. Chest 1997; 111(6):1710.
5. Greene FL. AJCC Cancer Staging, 6th edn. Springer-Verlag, New York, 2002
6. Suzuki Y, Orita M, Shiraishi M, Hayashi K, Sekiya T. Detection of ras gene mutations in human lung cancers by single-strand conformation polymorphism analysis of polymerase chain reaction products. Oncogene 1990; 5(7):1037.
7. Saiki RK, Scharf S, Faloona F, Mullis KB, Horn GT, Erlich HA, Arnheim N. Enzymatic amplification of beta-globin genomic sequences and restriction site analysis for diagnosis of sickle cell anemia. Science 1985; 230(4732):1350.
8. Saiki RK, Gelfand DH, Stoffel S, Scharf SJ, Higuchi R, Horn GT, Mullis KB, Erlich HA. Primer-directed enzymatic amplification of DNA with a thermostable DNA polymerase. Science 1988; 239(4839):487.
9. Chen Y, Okunieff P, Ahrendt SA. Translational research in lung cancer. Semin Surg Oncol 2003; 21:205.
10. Maruyama R, Sugio K, Mitsudomi T, Saitoh G, Ishida T, Sugimachi K. Relationship between early recurrence and micrometastases in the lymph nodes of patients with stage I non-small-cell lung cancer. J Thorac Cardiovasc Surg 1997; 114(4):535.
11. Hashimoto T, Kobayashi Y, Ishikawa Y, et al. Prognostic value of genetically diagnosed lymph node micrometastasis in non-small cell lung carcinoma cases. Cancer Res 2000; 60(22):6472.
12. Ohta Y, Nozawa H, Tanaka Y, Oda M, Watanabe Y. Increased vascular endothelial growth factor and vascular endothelial growth factor-c and decreased nm23 expression associated with microdissemination in the lymph nodes in stage I non-small cell lung cancer. J Thorac Cardiovasc Surg 2000; 119(4 Pt 1):804.
13. Barbacid M. ras genes. Ann Rev Biochem 1987; 56:779.
14. Bos JL. ras oncogenes in human cancer: a review. Cancer Res 1989; 49(17):4682.
15. Slebos RJ, Kibbelaar RE, Dalesio O, et al. K-ras oncogene activation as a prognostic marker in adenocarcinoma of the lung. N Engl J Med 1990; 323(9):561.
16. Mitsudomi T, Steinberg SM, Oie HK, et al. ras gene mutations in non-small cell lung cancers are associated with shortened survival irrespective of treatment intent. Cancer Res 1991; 51(18):4999.
17. Sugio K, Ishida T, Yokoyama H, Inoue T, Sugimachi K, Sasazuki T. ras gene mutations as a prognostic marker in adenocarcinoma of the human lung without lymph node metastasis. Cancer Res 1992; 52(10):2903.
18. Rodenhuis S, Slebos RJ. Clinical significance of ras oncogene activation in human lung cancer. Cancer Res 1992; 52(9 Suppl):2665s.
19. Greatens TM, Niehans GA, Rubins JB, Jessurun J, Kratzke RA, Maddaus MA, Niewoehner DE. Do molecular markers predict survival in non-small-cell lung cancer? Am J Respir Crit Care Med 1998; 157:1093.
20. Fukuyama Y, Mitsudomi T, Sugio K, Ishida T, Akazawa K, Sugimachi K. K-ras and p53 mutations are an independent unfavourable prognostic indicator in patients with non-small-cell lung cancer. Br J Cancer 1997; 75(8):1125.
21. Miyake M, Adachi M, Huang C, Higashiyama M, Kodama K, Taki T. A novel molecular staging protocol for non-small cell lung cancer. Oncogene 1999; 18(14):2397.
22. Rosell R, Monzo M, Pifarre A, et al. Molecular staging of non-small cell lung cancer according to K-ras genotypes. Clin Cancer Res 1996; 2(6):1083.
23. Kwiatkowski DJ, Harpole DH Jr, Godleski J, et al. Molecular pathologic substaging in 244 stage I non-small-cell lung cancer patients: clinical implications. J Clin Oncol 1998; 16(7):2468.
24. Harada M, Dosaka-Akita H, Miyamoto H, Kuzumaki N, Kawakami Y. Prognostic significance of the expression of ras oncogene product in non-small cell lung cancer. Cancer 1992; 69(1):72.
25. Nemunaitis J, Klemow S, Tong A, et al. Prognostic value of K-ras mutations, ras oncoprotein, and c-erb B-2 oncoprotein expression in adenocarcinoma of the lung. Am J Clin Oncol 1998; 21(2):155.
26. Cordon-Cardo C. Mutations of cell cycle regulators. Biological and clinical implications for human neoplasia. Am J Pathol 1995; 147(3):545.
27. Yin Y, Tainsky MA, Bischoff FZ, Strong LC, Wahl GM. Wild-type p53 restores cell cycle control and inhibits gene amplification in cells with mutant p53 alleles. Cell 1992; 70(6):937.
28. Hartwell L. Defects in a cell cycle checkpoint may be responsible for the genomic instability of cancer cells. Cell 1992; 71(4):543.
29. Farmer G, Bargonetti J, Zhu H, Friedman P, Prywes R, Prives C. Wild-type p53 activates transcription in vitro. Nature 1992; 358(6381):83.
30. Greenblatt MS, Bennett WP, Hollstein M, Harris CC. Mutations in the p53 tumor suppressor gene: clues to cancer etiology and molecular pathogenesis. Cancer Res 1994; 54(18):4855.
31. Huang C, Taki T, Adachi M, Konishi T, Higashiyama M, Miyake M. Mutations in exon 7 and 8 of p53 as poor prognostic factors in patients with non-small cell lung cancer. Oncogene 1998; 16(19):2469.
32. Mitsudomi T, Oyama T, Kusano T, Osaki T, Nakanishi R, Shirakusa T. Mutations of the p53 gene as a predictor of poor prognosis in patients with non-small-cell lung cancer. J Natl Cancer Inst 1993; 85(24):2018.
33. Horio Y, Takahashi T, Kuroishi T, et al. Prognostic significance of p53 mutations and 3p deletions in primary resected non-small cell lung cancer. Cancer Res 1993; 53(1):1.
34. Ahrendt SA, Hu Y, Buta M, McDermott MP, Benoit N, Yang SC, Wu L, Sidransky D. p53 mutations and survival in stage I non-small cell lung cancer: results of a prospective study. J Natl Cancer Inst 2003; 95:961.
35. Tomizawa Y, Kohno T, Fujita T, et al. Correlation between the status of the p53 gene and survival in patients with stage I non-small cell lung carcinoma. Oncogene 1999; 18:1007.
36. Carbone DP, Mitsudomi T, Chiba I, et al. p53 immunostaining positivity is associated with reduced survival and is imperfectly correlated with gene mutations in resected non-small cell lung cancer. A preliminary report of LCSG 871. Chest 1994; 106:377S.
37. Top B, Mooi WJ, Klaver SG, et al. Comparative analysis of p53 gene mutations and protein accumulation in human non-small cell lung cancer. Int J Cancer 1995; 64:83.
38. Vega FJ, Iniesta P, Caldes T, et al. p53 exon 5 mutations as a prognostic indicator of shortened survival in non-small cell lung cancer Br. J Cancer 1997; 76:44.

39. Dalquen P, Sauter G, Torhorst J, et al. Nuclear p53 overexpression is an independent prognostic parameter in node-negative non-small cell lung carcinoma. J Pathol 1996; 178:53.

40. D'Amico TA, Massey M, Herndon JE 2nd, Moore MB, Harpole DH Jr. A biologic risk model for stage I lung cancer: immunohistochemical analysis of 408 patients with the use of ten molecular markers. J Thorac Cardiovasc Surg 1999; 117(4):736.

41. Ebina M, Steinberg SM, Mulshine JL, Linnoila RI. Relationship of p53 overexpression and up-regulation of proliferating cell nuclear antigen with the clinical course of non-small cell lung cancer. Cancer Res 1994; 54(9):2496.

42. Fujino M, Dosaka-Akita H, Harada M, Hiroumi H, Kinoshita I, Akie K, Kawakami Y. Prognostic significance of p53 and ras p21 expression in nonsmall cell lung cancer. Cancer 1995; 76(12):2457.

43. Harpole DH Jr, Herndon JE 2nd, Wolfe WG, Iglehart JD, Marks JR. A prognostic model of recurrence and death in stage I non-small cell lung cancer utilizing presentation, histopathology, and oncoprotein expression. Cancer Res 1995; 55(1):51.

44. Nishio M, Koshikawa T, Kuroishi T, et al. Prognostic significance of abnormal p53 accumulation in primary, resected non-small-cell lung cancers. J Clin Oncol 1996; 14(2):497.

45. Quinlan DC, Davidson AG, Summers CL, Warden HE, Doshi HM. Accumulation of p53 protein correlates with a poor prognosis in human lung cancer. Cancer Res 1992; 52(17):4828.

46. Xu HJ, Cagle PT, Hu SX, et al. Altered retinoblastoma and p53 protein status in non-small cell carcinoma of the lung: potential synergistic effects on prognosis. Clin Cancer Res 1996; 2:1169.

47. Fontanini G, Vignati S, Bigini D, Mussi A, Lucchi M, Angeletti CA, Basolo F, Bevilacqua G. Bcl-2 protein: a prognostic factor inversely correlated to p53 in non-small-cell lung cancer. Br J Cancer 1995; 71(5):1003.

48. Brambilla E, Gazzeri S, Moro D, et al. Immunohistochemical study of p53 in human lung carcinomas. Am J P 1993; 143(1):199.

49. McLaren R,. Kuzu I, Dunnill M, Harris A, Lane D, Gatter KC. The relationship of p53 immunostaining to survival in carcinoma of the lung. Br J Cancer 1992; 66(4):735.

50. Morkve O, Halvorsen OJ, Skjaerven R, Stangeland L, Gulsvik A, Laerum OD. Prognostic significance of p53 protein expression and DNA ploidy in surgically treated non-small cell lung carcinomas. Anticancer Res 1993; 13(3):571.

51. Ohsaki Y, Toyoshima E, Fujiuchi S. bcl-2 and p53 protein expression in non-small cell lung cancers: correlation with survival time. Clin Cancer Res 1996; 2:915.

52. Pastorino U, Andreola S, Tagliabue E, et al. Immunocytochemical markers in stage I lung cancer: relevance to prognosis. J Clin Oncol 1997; 15(8):2858.

53. Pappot H, Francis D, Brunner N, et al. p53 protein in non-small cell lung cancer as quantitated by enzyme-linked immunosorbent assay: relation to prognosis. Clin Cancer Res 1996; 2:1169.

54. Lee JS, Yoon A, Kalapurakal SK, et al. Expression of p53 oncoprotein in non-small-cell lung cancer: a favorable prognostic factor. J Clin Oncol 1995; 13(8):1893.

55. Passlick B, Izbicki JR. Riethmuller G. Pantel K. p53 in non-small-cell lung cancer. J Natl Cancer Inst 1994; 86(10):801.

56. Mitsudomi T, Hamajima N, et al. Prognostic significance of p53 alterations in patients with non-small cell lung cancer: a meta-analysis. Clin Cancer Res 2000; 6:4055.

57. Steels E, Paesmans M, et al. Role of p53 as a prognostic factor for survival in lung cancer: a systematic review of the literature with a meta-analysis. Eur Respir J 2001; 18:705.

58. Huncharek M, Kupelnick B, et al. Prognostic significance of p53 mutations in non-small cell lung cancer: a meta-analysis of 829 cases from eight published studies. Cancer Letters 2000; 153:219.

59. Franklin WA, Veve R, Hirsch FR, Helfrich BA, Bunn PA Jr. Epidermal growth factor receptor family in lung cancer and premalignancy. Sem Oncol 2002; 29(1 Suppl 4):3.

60. Yarden Y, Sliwkowski MX. Untangling the ErbB signalling network. Nature Rev Mol Cell Biol 2001; 2(2):127.

61. Jorissen RN, Walker F, Pouliot N, Garrett TP, Ward CW, Burgess AW. Epidermal growth factor receptor: mechanisms of activation and signalling. Exp Cell Res 2003; 284(1):31.

62. Arteaga CL. ErbB-targeted therapeutic approaches in human cancer. Exp Cell Res 2003; 284(1):122.

63. Berger MS, Gullick WJ, Greenfield C, Evans S, Addis BJ, Waterfield MD. Epidermal growth factor receptors in lung tumours. J Pathol 1987; 152(4):297.

64. Rusch V, Baselga J, Cordon-Cardo C, et al. Differential expression of the epidermal growth factor receptor and its ligands in primary non-small cell lung cancers and adjacent benign lung. Cancer Res 1993; 53(10 Suppl):2379.

65. Kurie JM, Shin HJ, Lee JS, et al. Increased epidermal growth factor receptor expression in metaplastic bronchial epithelium. Clin Cancer Res 1996; 2(10):1787.

66. Piyathilake CJ, Frost AR, Manne U, Weiss H, Bell WC, Heimburger DC, Grizzle WE. Differential expression of growth factors in squamous cell carcinoma and precancerous lesions of the lung. Clin Cancer Res 2002; 8(3):734.

67. Volm M, Rittgen W, Drings P. Prognostic value of ERBB-1, VEGF, cyclin A, FOS, JUN and MYC in patients with squamous cell lung carcinomas. Br J Cancer 1998; 77(4):663.

68. Ohsaki Y, Tanno S, Fujita Y, et al. Epidermal growth factor receptor expression correlates with poor prognosis in non-small cell lung cancer patients with p53 overexpression. Oncol Rep 2000; 7(3):603.

69. Cox G, Jones JL, O'Byrne KJ. Matrix metalloproteinase 9 and the epidermal growth factor signal pathway in operable non-small cell lung cancer. Clin Cancer Res 2000; 6(6):2349.

70. Rusch V, Klimstra D, Venkatraman E, Pisters PW, Langenfeld J, Dmitrovsky E. Overexpression of the epidermal growth factor receptor and its ligand transforming growth factor alpha is frequent in resectable non-small cell lung cancer but does not predict tumor progression. Clin Cancer Res 1997; 3(4):515.

71. Pfeiffer P, Clausen PP, Andersen K, Rose C. Lack of prognostic significance of epidermal growth factor receptor and the oncoprotein p185HER-2 in patients with systemically untreated non-small-cell lung cancer: an immunohistochemical study on cryosections. Br J Cancer 1996; 74(1):86.

72. Fontanini G, De Laurentiis M, Vignati S, et al. Evaluation of epidermal growth factor-related growth factors and receptors and of neoangiogenesis in completely resected stage I-IIIA non-small-cell lung cancer: amphiregulin and microvessel count are independent prognostic indicators of survival. Clin Cancer Res 1998; 4(1):241.

73. Hirsch FR, Varella-Garcia M, Bunn PA Jr, et al. Epidermal growth factor receptor in non-small-cell lung carcinomas: correlation between gene copy number and protein expression and impact on prognosis. J Clin Oncol 2003; 21(20):3798.

74. Kris MG, Natale RB, Herbst RS, et al. Efficacy of gefitinib, an inhibitor of the epidermal growth factor receptor tyrosine kinase, in symptomatic patients with non-small cell lung cancer: a randomized trial. JAMA 2003; 290(16):2149.

75. Fukuoka M, Yano S, Giaccone G, et al. Multi-institutional randomized phase II trial of gefitinib for previously treated patients with advanced non-small-cell lung cancer (The IDEAL 1 Trial). J Clin Oncol 2003; 21(12):2237.

76. Lynch TJ, Bell DW, Sordella R, et al. Activating mutations in the epidermal growth factor receptor underlying responsiveness of non-small-cell lung cancer to gefitinib. N Engl J Med 2004; 350(21):2129.

77. Paez JG, Janne PA, Lee JC, Tracy S, et al. EGFR mutations in lung cancer: correlation with clinical response to gefitinib therapy. Science 2004; 304(5676):1497.

78. Yamamoto T, Ikawa S, Akiyama T, Semba K, Nomura N, Miyajima N, Saito T, Toyoshima K. Similarity of protein encoded by the human c-erb-B-2 gene to epidermal growth factor receptor. Nature 1986; 319(6050):230.

79. Schechter AL, Hung MC, Vaidyanathan L, Weinberg RA, Yang-Feng TL, Francke U, Ullrich A, Coussens L. The neu gene: an erbB-homologous gene distinct from and unlinked to the gene encoding the EGF receptor. Science 1985; 229(4717):976.

80. Stern DF, Heffernan PA, Weinberg RA. p185, a product of the neu proto-oncogene, is a receptorlike protein associated with tyrosine kinase activity. Mol Cell Biol 1986; 6(5):1729.

81. Kern JA, Slebos RJ, Top B, Rodenhuis S, Lager D, Robinson RA, Weiner D, Schwartz DA. C-erbB-2 expression and codon 12 K-ras mutations both predict shortened survival for patients with pulmonary adenocarcinomas. J Clin Invest 1994; 93(2):516.

82. Shi D, He G, Cao S, Pan W, Zhang HZ, Yu D, Hung MC. Overexpression of the c-erbB-2/neu-encoded p185 protein in primary lung cancer. Mol Carcinogen 1992; 5(3):213.

83. Tateishi M, Ishida T, Mitsudomi T, Kaneko S, Sugimachi K. Prognostic value of c-erbB-2 protein expression in human lung adenocarcinoma and squamous cell carcinoma. Eur J Cancer 1991; 27(11):1372.

84. Hilbe W, Dirnhofer S, Oberwasserlechner F, et al. Immunohistochemical typing of non-small cell lung cancer on cryostat sections: correlation with clinical parameters and prognosis. J Clin Pathol 2003; 56:736.

85. Hommura F, Dosaka-Akita H, Mishina T, et al. Prognostic significance of p27KIP1 protein and ki-67 growth fraction in non-small cell lung cancers. Clin Cancer Res 2000; 6(10):4073.

86. Harpole DH Jr, Richards WG, Herndon JE 2nd, Sugarbaker DJ. Angiogenesis and molecular biologic substaging in patients with stage I non-small cell lung cancer. Ann Thorac Surg 1996; 61(5):1470.

87. Pence JC, Kerns BJ, Dodge RK, Iglehart JD. Prognostic significance of the proliferation index in surgically resected non-small-cell lung cancer. Arch Surg 1993; 128(12):1382.

88. Ishida T, Kaneko S, Akazawa K, Tateishi M, Sugio K, Sugimachi K. Proliferating cell nuclear antigen expression and argyrophilic nucleolar organizer regions as factors influencing prognosis of surgically treated lung cancer patients. Cancer Res 1993; 53(20):5000.

89. Fontanini G, Macchiarini P, Pepe S, et al. The expression of proliferating cell nuclear antigen in paraffin sections of peripheral, node-negative non-small cell lung cancer. Cancer 1992; 70(6):1520.

90. Fukuse T, Hirata T, Naiki H, Hitomi S, Wada H. Prognostic significance of proliferative activity in pN2 non-small-cell lung carcinomas and their mediastinal lymph node metastases. Ann Surg 2000; 232(1):112.

91. Volm M, Koomagi R, Mattern J, Efferth T. Expression profile of genes in non-small cell lung carcinomas from long-term surviving patients. Clin Cancer Res 2002; 8(6):1843.

92. Hirata T, Fukuse T, et al. Expression of CD44 variant exon 6in stage I non-small cell lung carcinoma as a prognostic factor. Cancer Res 1998; 58:1108.

93. Esposito V, Baldi A, Tonini G, et al. Analysis of cell cycle regulator proteins in non-small cell lung cancer. J Clin Pathol 2004; 57(1):58.

94. Morgan DO. Principles of CDK regulation. Nature 1995; 374(6518):131.

95. Sherr CJ. G1 phase progression: cycling on cue. Cell 1994; 79(4):551.

96. Sherr CJ, Roberts JM. Inhibitors of mammalian G1 cyclin-dependent kinases. Genes Dev 1995; 9(10):1149.

97. Reed SI, Bailly E, Dulic V, Hengst L, Resnitzky D, Slingerland J. G1 control in mammalian cells. J Cell Sci 1994; 18S:69.

98. Muller-Tidow C, Metzger R, Kugler K, Diederichs S, Idos G, Thomas M, Dockhorn-Dworniczak B, Schneider PM, Koeffler HP, Berdel WE, Serve H. Cyclin E is the only cyclin-dependent kinase 2-associated cyclin that predicts metastasis and survival in early stage non-small cell lung cancer. Cancer Res 2001; 61(2):647.

99. Fukuse T, Hirata T, Naiki H, Hitomi S, Wada H. Prognostic significance of cyclin E overexpression in resected non-small cell lung cancer. Cancer Res 2000; 60(2):242.

100. Dosaka-Akita H, Hommura F, Mishina T, Ogura S, Shimizu M, Katoh H, Kawakami Y. A risk-stratification model of non-small cell lung cancers using cyclin E, Ki-67, and ras p21: different roles of G1 cyclins in cell proliferation and prognosis. Cancer Res 2001; 61(6):2500.

101. Caputi M, Groeger AM, Esposito V, Dean C, De Luca A, Pacilio C, Muller MR, Giordano GG, Baldi F, Wolner E, Giordano A. Prognostic role of cyclin D1 in lung cancer. Relationship to proliferating cell nuclear antigen. Am J Respir Cell Mol Biol 1999; 20(4):746.

102. Jin M, Inoue S, Umemura T, Moriya J, Arakawa M, Nagashima K, Kato H. Cyclin D1, p16 and retinoblastoma gene product expression as a predictor for prognosis in non-small cell lung cancer at stages I and II. Lung Cancer 2001; 34(2):207.

103. Lloyd RV, Erickson LA, Jin L, Kulig E, Qian X, Cheville JC, Scheithauer BW. p27kip1: a multifunctional cyclin-dependent kinase inhibitor with prognostic significance in human cancers. Am J Pathol 1999; 154(2):313.

104. Catzavelos C, Tsao MS, DeBoer G, Bhattacharya N, Shepherd FA, Slingerland JM. Reduced expression of the cell cycle inhibitor p27Kip1 in non-small cell lung carcinoma: a prognostic factor independent of Ras. Cancer Res 1999; 59(3):684.

105. Yatabe Y, Masuda A, Koshikawa T, et al. p27KIP1 in human lung cancers: differential changes in small cell and non-small cell carcinomas. Cancer Res 1998; 58(5):1042.

106. Paggi MG, Baldi A, Bonetto F, Giordano A. Retinoblastoma protein family in cell cycle and cancer: a review. J Cell Biochem 1996; 62(3):418.

107. Stiegler P, Kasten M, Giordano A. The RB family of cell cycle regulatory factors. J Cell Biochem 1998; 30-31:30. correct?

108. Planas-Silva MD, Weinberg RA. The restriction point and control of cell proliferation. Curr Opin Cell Biol 1997; 9(6):768.

109. Xu HJ, Quinlan DC, Davidson AG, Hu SX, Summers CL, Li J, Benedict WF. Altered retinoblastoma protein expression and prognosis in early-stage non-small-cell lung carcinoma. J Natl Cancer Inst 1994; 86(9):695.

110. Caputi M, Groeger AM, Esposito V, De Luca A, Masciullo V, Mancini A, Baldi F, Wolner E, Giordano A. Loss of pRb2/p130 expression is associated with unfavorable clinical outcome in lung cancer. Clin Cancer Res 2002; 8(12):3850.

111. Chen JT, Chen YC, Chen CY, Wang YC. Loss of p16 and/or pRb protein expression in NSCLC. An immunohistochemical and prognostic study. Lung Cancer 2001; 31(2–3):163.

112. el-Deiry WS, Tokino T, Velculescu VE, et al. WAF1, a potential mediator of p53 tumor suppression. Cell 1993; Nov 19; 75(4):817.

113. Harper JW, Adami GR, Wei N, Keyomarsi K, Elledge SJ. The p21 Cdk-interacting protein Cip1 is a potent inhibitor of G1 cyclin-dependent kinases. Cell 1993; Nov 19; 75(4):805.

114. Xiong Y, Hannon GJ, Zhang H, Casso D, Kobayashi R, Beach D. p21 is a universal inhibitor of cyclin kinases. Nature. 1993; 366(6456):701.

115. Michieli P, Chedid M, Lin D, Pierce JH, Mercer WE, Givol D. Induction of WAF1/CIP1 by a p53-independent pathway. Cancer Res 1994; 154(13):3391.

116. Caputi M, Esposito V, Baldi A, et al. P21$^{waf1/cip1mda-6}$ expression in non-small cell lung cancer. Am J Respir Cell Mol Biol 1998; 18:213.

117. Shoji T, Tankka F, Takata T. et al. Clinical significance of p21 expression in non-small cell lung cancer. J Clin Oncol 2002; 20:3865.

118. Kratzke RA, Greatens TM, Rubins JB, Maddaus MA, Niewoehner DE, Niehans GA, Geradts J. Rb and p16INK4a expression in resected non-small cell lung tumors. Cancer Res 1996; 56(15):3415.

119. Taga S, Osaki T, Ohgami A, et al. Prognostic value of the immunohistochemical detection of p16INK4 expression in nonsmall cell lung carcinoma. Cancer 1997; 80(3):389.

120. Gonzalez-Quevedo R, Iniesta P, Moran A, et al. Cooperative role of telomerase activity and p16 expression in the prognosis of non-small-cell lung cancer. J Clin Oncol 2002; 20(1):254.

121. Folkman J. What is the evidence that tumors are angiogenesis dependent? J Natl Cancer Inst 1990; 82(1):4.

122. Imoto H, Osaki T, Taga S, Ohgami A, Ichiyoshi Y, Yasumoto K. Vascular endothelial growth factor expression in non-small-cell lung cancer: prognostic significance in squamous cell carcinoma. J Thorac Cardiovasc Surg 1998; 115(5):1007.

123. Fontanini G, Lucchi M, Vignati S, et al. Angiogenesis as a prognostic indicator of survival in non-small-cell lung carcinoma: a prospective study. J Natl Cancer Inst 1997; 89(12):881.

124. Koukourakis MI, Giatromanolaki A, Thorpe PE, et al. Vascular endothelial growth factor/KDR activated microvessel density versus CD31 standard microvessel density in non-small cell lung cancer. Cancer Res 2000; 60(11):3088.

125. Volm M, Mattern J, Koomagi R. Angiostatin expression in non-small cell lung cancer. Clin Cancer Res 2000; 6(8):3236.

126. Baillie R, Carlile J, Pendleton N, Schor AM. Prognostic value of vascularity and vascular endothelial growth factor expression in non-small cell lung cancer. J Clin Pathol 2001; 54(2):116.

127. Han H, Silverman JF, Santucci TS, et al. Vascular endothelial growth factor expression in stage I non-small cell lung cancer correlates with neoangiogenesis and a poor prognosis. Ann Surg Oncol 2001; 8(1):72.

128. Volm M, Koomagi R, Mattern J, Stammler G. Prognostic value of basic fibroblast growth factor and its receptor (FGFR-1) in patients with non-small cell lung carcinomas. Eur J Cancer 1997; 33(4):691.

129. Baird A, Klagsbrun M. The fibroblast growth factor family. Cancer Cells 1991; 3(6):239.

130. Ohta Y, Endo Y, Tanaka M, et al. Significance of vascular endothelial growth factor messenger RNA expression in primary lung cancer. Clin Cancer Res 1996; 2(8):1411.

131. Blasi F, Vassalli JD, Dano K. Urokinase-type plasminogen activator: proenzyme, receptor, and inhibitors. J Cell Biol 1987; 104(4):801.

132. Pedersen H, Brunner N, Francis D, et al. Prognostic impact of urokinase, urokinase receptor, and type 1 plasminogen activator inhibitor in squamous and large cell lung cancer tissue. Cancer Res 1994; 54(17):4671.

133. Yoshino H, Endo Y, Watanabe Y, Sasaki T. Significance of plasminogen activator inhibitor 2 as a prognostic marker in primary lung cancer: association of decreased plasminogen activator inhibitor 2 with lymph node metastasis. Br J Cancer 1998; 78(6):833.

134. Lah TT, Buck MR, Honn KV, Crissman JD, Rao NC, Liotta LA, Sloane BF. Degradation of laminin by human tumor cathepsin B. Clin Exp Metastasis 1989; 7(4):461.

135. Sukoh N, Abe S, Ogura S, Isobe H, Takekawa H, Inoue K, Kawakami Y. Immunohistochemical study of cathepsin B. Prognostic significance in human lung cancer. Cancer 1994; 74(1):46.

136. Inoue T, Ishida T, Sugio K, Sugimachi K. Cathepsin B expression and laminin degradation as factors influencing prognosis of surgically treated patients with lung adenocarcinoma. Cancer Res 1994; 54:6133.

137. Wetzels RH, van der Velden LA, Schaafsma HE, Manni JJ, Leigh IM, Vooijs GP, Ramaekers FC. Immunohistochemical localization of basement membrane type VII collagen and laminin in neoplasms of the head and neck. Histopathology 1992; 21(5):459.

138. Mori M, Kohli A, Baker SP, Savas L, Fraire AE. Laminin and cathepsin B as prognostic factors in stage I non-small cell lung cancer: are they useful? Mod Pathol 1997; 10(6):572.

139. Kase S, Sugio K, et al. Expression of E-cadherin and β-catenin in human non-small cell lung cancer and the clinical significance. Clin Cancer Res 2000; 6:4789.

140. Miyake M, Koyama M, Seno M, Ikeyama S. Identification of the motility-related protein (MRP-1), recognized by monoclonal antibody M31-15, which inhibits cell motility. J Exp Med 1991; 174(6):1347.

141. Higashiyama M, Taki T, Ieki Y, et al. Reduced motility related protein-1 (MRP-1/CD9) gene expression as a factor of poor prognosis in non-small cell lung cancer. Cancer Res 1995; 55(24):6040.

142. Adachi M, Taki T, Ieki Y, et al. Correlation of KA11/CD82 gene expression with good prognosis in patients with non-small cell lung cancer. Cancer Res 1996; 56, 1751.

143. Pezzella F, Turley H, Kuzu I, Tungekar MF, Dunnill MS, Pierce CB, Harris A, Gatter KC, Mason DY. bcl-2 protein in non-small-cell lung carcinoma. N Engl J Med 1993; 329(10):690.

144. Kovarik S, Davidsohn I, Stejskal R. ABO antigens in cancer: detection with the mixed cell agglutination reaction. Arch Pathol 1968; 86:12.

145. Lee JS, Ro JY, Sahin AA, et al. Expression of blood-group antigen A – a favorable prognostic factor in non-small-cell lung cancer. N Engl J Med 1991; 324(16):1084.

146. Miyake M, Taki T, et al. Correlation of expression of H/Le^y/Le^b antigens with survival in patients with carcinoma of the lung. N Engl J Med 1992; 327:14.

147. Belinsky SA, Nikula KJ, Palmisano WA, et al. Aberrant methylation of p16(INK4a) is an early event in lung cancer and a potential biomarker for early diagnosis. Proc Natl Acad Sci U S A 1998; 95(20):11891.

148. Esteller M, Hamilton SR, Burger PC, Baylin SB, Herman JG. Inactivation of the DNA repair gene O6-methylguanine-DNA methyltransferase by promoter hypermethylation is a common event in primary human neoplasia. Cancer Res 1999; 59(4):793.

149. Tang X, Khuri FR, Lee JJ, Kemp BL, Liu D, Hong WK, Mao L. Hypermethylation of the death-associated protein (DAP) kinase promoter and aggressiveness in stage I non-small-cell lung cancer. J Natl Cancer Inst 2000; 92(18):1511.

150. Virmani AK, Rathi A, Zochbauer-Muller S, et al. Promoter methylation and silencing of the retinoic acid receptor-beta gene in lung carcinomas. J Natl Cancer Inst 2000; 92(16):1303.

151. Palmisano WA, Divine KK, Saccomanno G, Gilliland FD, Baylin SB, Herman JG, Belinsky SA. Predicting lung cancer by detecting aberrant promoter methylation in sputum. Cancer Res 2000; 60(21):5954.

152. Burbee DG, Forgacs E, Zochbauer-Muller S, et al. Epigenetic inactivation of RASSF1A in lung and breast cancers and malignant phenotype suppression. J Natl Cancer Inst 2001; 93(9):691.

153. Zochbauer-Muller S, Fong KM, Virmani AK, Geradts J, Gazdar AF, Minna JD. Aberrant promoter methylation of multiple genes in non-small cell lung cancers. Cancer Res 2001; 61(1):249.

154. Usadel H, Brabender J, Danenberg KD, et al. Quantitative adenomatous polyposis coli promoter methylation analysis in tumor tissue, serum, and plasma DNA of patients with lung cancer. Cancer Res 2002; 62(2):371.

155. Chan EC, Lam SY, Tsang KW, et al. Aberrant promoter methylation in Chinese patients with non-small cell lung cancer: patterns in primary tumors and potential diagnostic application in bronchoalveolar lavage. Clin Cancer Res. 2002; 8(12):3741.

156. Wang J, Lee JJ, Wang L, Liu DD, Lu C, Fan YH, Hong WK, Mao L. Value of p16INK4a and RASSF1A promoter hypermethylation in prognosis of patients with resectable non-small cell lung cancer. Clin Cancer Res 2004; 10(18 Pt 1):6119.

157. Brabender J, Usadel H, Danenberg KD, et al. Adenomatous polyposis coli gene promoter hypermethylation in non-small-cell lung cancer is associated with survival. Oncogene 2001; 20:3528.

158. Greider CW, Blackburn EH. Identification of a specific telomere terminal transferase activity in Tetrahymena extracts. Cell 1985; 43(2 Pt 1):405.

159. Taga S, Osaki T, Ohgami A, et al. Prognostic impact of telomerase activity in non-small cell lung cancers. Ann Surg 1999; 230:715.

160. Wang L, Soria JC, Kemp BL, Liu DD, Mao L, Khuri FR. hTERT expression is a prognostic factor of survival in patients with stage I non-small cell lung cancer. Clin Cancer Res 2002; 8(9):2883.

161. Hara H, Yamashita K, Shinada J, Yoshimura H, Kameya T. Clinicopathologic significance of telomerase activity and hTERT mRNA expression in non-small cell lung cancer. Lung Cancer 2001; 34(2):219.

162. Vollmer RT, Herndon JE 2nd, D'Cunha J, et al. Cancer and Leukemia Group B Trial 9761. Immunohistochemical detection of occult lymph node metastases in non-small cell lung cancer: anatomical pathology results from Cancer and Leukemia Group B Trial 9761. Clin Cancer Res 2003; 9(15):5630.

163. Pantel K, Izbicki J, Passlick B, Angstwurm M, Haussinger K, Thetter O, Riethmuller G. Frequency and prognostic significance of isolated tumour cells in bone marrow of patients with non-small-cell lung cancer without overt metastases. Lancet 1996; 347(9002):649.

164. Chen ZL, Perez S, Holmes EC, Wang HJ, Coulson WF, Wen DR, Cochran AJ. Frequency and distribution of occult micrometastases in lymph nodes of patients with non-small-cell lung carcinoma. J Natl Cancer Inst 1993; 85(6):493.

165. Passlick B, Izbicki JR, Kubuschok B, et al. Immunohistochemical assessment of individual tumor cells in lymph nodes of patients with non-small-cell lung cancer. J Clin Oncol 1994a; 12(9):1827.

166. Salerno CT, Frizelle S, Niehans GA, Ho SB, Jakkula M, Kratzke RA, Maddaus MA. Detection of occult micrometastases in non-small cell lung carcinoma by reverse transcriptase-polymerase chain reaction. Chest 1998; 113(6):1526.

167. D'Cunha J, Corfits AL, Herndon JE 2nd, et al. Molecular staging of lung cancer: real-time polymerase chain reaction estimation of lymph node micrometastatic tumor cell burden in stage I non-small cell lung cancer – preliminary results of Cancer and Leukemia Group B Trial 9761. J Thorac Cardiovasc Surg 2002; 123(3):484.

168. Maruyama R, Sugio K, Fukuyama Y, Hamatake M, Sakada T, Saitoh G, Sugimachi K. Evaluation of p53 alterations in occult lymph node metastases. J Surg Oncol 2000; 73(3):143.

169. Dobashi K, Sugio K, Osaki T, Oka T, Yasumoto K. Micrometastatic P53-positive cells in the lymph nodes of non-small-cell lung cancer: prognostic significance. J Thorac Cardiovasc Surg 1997; 114(3):339.

170. Ahrendt SA, Yang SC, Wu L, et al. Molecular assessment of lymph nodes in patients with resected stage I non-small cell lung cancer: preliminary results of a prospective study. Journal of Thorac Cardiovasc Surg 2002; 123(3):466.

171. Wallace MB, Block M, Hoffman BJ, et al. Detection of telomerase expression in mediastinal lymph nodes of patients with lung cancer. American J Respir Crit Care Med 2003; 167(12):1670.

172. Ahrendt SA, Yang SC, Wu L et al. Comparison of oncogene mutation detection and telomerase activity for the molecular staging of non-small cell lung cancer. Clin Cancer Res 1997; 3:1207.

173. Harden SV, Tokumaru Y, Westra WH, et al. Gene promoter hypermethylation in tumors and lymph nodes of stage I lung cancer patients. Clin Cancer Res 2003; 9:1370.

174. Cote RJ, Beattie EJ, Chaiwun B, et al. Detection of occult bone marrow micrometastases in patients with operable lung carcinoma. Ann Surg 1995; 222(4):415.

175. Ohgami A, Mitsudomi T, Sugio K, et al. Micrometastatic tumor cells in the bone marrow of patients with non-small cell lung cancer. Ann Thorac Surg 1997; 64(2):363.

176. Bearzatto A, Conte D, Frattini M, et al. p16(INK4A) Hypermethylation detected by fluorescent methylation-specific PCR in plasmas from non-small cell lung cancer. Clin Cancer Res 2002; 8(12):3782.

177. Gautschi O, Bigosch C, Huegli B, et al. Circulating deoxyribonucleic Acid as prognostic marker in non-small-cell lung cancer patients undergoing chemotherapy. J Clin Oncol 2004; 22(20):4157.

178. Sozzi G, Conte D, Leon M, et al. Quantification of free circulating DNA as a diagnostic marker in lung cancer. J Clin Oncol 2003; 21(21):3902.

179. Andriani F, Conte D, Mastrangelo T, et al. Detecting lung cancer in plasma with the use of multiple genetic markers. Int J Cancer 2004; 108(1):91.

180. An Q, Liu Y, Gao Y, et al. Detection of p16 hypermethylation in circulating plasma DNA of non-small cell lung cancer patients. Cancer Lett 2002; 188(1-2):109.

181. Tamura M, Ohta Y, Kajita T, et al. Plasma VEGF concentration can predict the tumor angiogenic capacity in non-small cell lung cancer. Oncol Rep 2001; 8(5):1097.

182. Brattstrom D, Bergqvist M, Hesselius P, et al. Elevated preoperative serum levels of angiogenic cytokines correlate to larger primary tumours and poorer survival in non-small cell lung cancer patients. Lung Cancer 2002; 37(1):57.

183. Bostick PJ, Chatterjee S, Chi DD, Huynh KT, Giuliano AE, Cote R, Hoon DS. Limitations of specific reverse-transcriptase polymerase chain reaction markers in the detection of metastases in the lymph nodes and blood of breast cancer patients. J Clin Oncol 1998; 16(8):2632.

184. Zippelius A, Kufer P, Honold G, et al. Limitations of reverse-transcriptase polymerase chain reaction analyses for detection of micrometastatic epithelial cancer cells in bone marrow. J Clin Oncol 1997; 15(7):2701.

185. Ko Y, Grunewald E, Totzke G, et al. High percentage of false-positive results of cytokeratin 19 RT-PCR in blood: a model for the analysis of illegitimate gene expression. Oncology 2000; 59(1):81.

Clinical Prognostic Factors in Non-Small-Cell Lung Cancer

14

Maria Werner-Wasik and Merrill Solan

Contents

14.1 Prognostic Factors in Non-Small-Cell Lung Cancer

Identification of prognostic factors is critical in optimizing treatment for patients with cancer. The purpose of this chapter is to review the modern literature with regard to clinical prognostic factors for patients with non-small-cell lung cancer (NSCLC), taking into account ongoing advances in clinical evaluation, staging, surgery, radiation therapy, and chemotherapy, in this widely heterogeneous patient population.

14.2 TNM Staging of Lung Cancer

A primary goal of the Tumor, Nodes, Metastasis (TNM) staging system for lung cancer is to categorize patients based on prognostic variables that can be used to guide treatment decisions and facilitate comparisons between various treatment regimens. For NSCLC, the concept of curability has been linked to resectability, and the stag-

ing system seeks to group patients with similar expected outcome based on potential for surgical management. Tumors that fall into stage groupings IA and B, IIA and B, and IIIA are deemed potentially resectable for cure, while stage groupings IIIB and IV are generally accepted as surgically incurable.

In 1997, revisions of the International System for Staging Lung Cancer were adopted by the American Joint Committee on Cancer (AJCC) and the Union Internationale Contre le Cancer in an attempt to more accurately define stage grouping by prognostic factors with minimal disruption of the existing TNM classifications. The impetus for the revisions was the perceived "heterogeneity of end results existing for the TNM categories within stage groups and.... need for greater specificity in stage classification" [1]. The changes incorporated prognostic information gained from a collected database of 5,319 patients. Patients within each new stage grouping showed similar 5-year survival by both clinical (c) and pathological (p) staging criteria (Table 14.1). Minor changes within the individual TNM staging components were limited to the designation of satellite tumor nodules within the primary tumor lobe as T4 (stage IIIB) and synchronous tumor nodules in nonprimary ipsilateral lobes as M1 (stage IV).

Table 14.1. TNM stage grouping and survival. Modified from Mountain 1997 [1]. *cTNM* Clinical TNM stage, *pTNM* pathological TNM stage

Stage grouping	cTNM	%5-year survival	pTNM	%5-year survival
I A	T1N0M0	61	T1N0M0	67
I B	T2N0M0	38	T2N0M0	57
II A	T1N1M0	34	T1N1M0	55
II B	T2N1M0	24	T2N1M0	39
	T3N0M0	22	T3N0M0	38
III A	T3N1M0	9	T3N1M0	25
	T1-2-3N2M0	1	T1-2-3N2M0	23
III B	T4N0-1-2M0	7		
	T1-2-3N3M0	3		
IV	T1-2-3N1-2-3M1	1		

14.2.1 Deficiencies in TNM Staging

The 1997 staging revisions remain unchanged in the newest published staging guidelines (AJCC Cancer Staging Manual [2]), even though the database supporting those revisions derives from patients treated in an era during which neoadjuvant and adjuvant therapy was poorly established, and chemoradiation in nonsurgical patients was regarded as investigational (1975–1988). In addition, it is argued that there is no significant survival difference between patients with stage pIIIA and pIIIB disease, primarily because of heterogeneity within the T3 and T4 designations, and that a more appropriate classification of T3 and T4 subsets should be based on surgical curability [3]. This concept of surgical curability may be changing as reports emerge of prolonged survival for patients with locally advanced and even metastatic disease treated aggressively with trimodality therapy [4–6]. The T4 (stage IIIB) designation of satellite tumor nodules or pleural effusion is challenged by those who argue that patients with satellite nodules confined to the primary lobe may be amenable to surgical resection and long-term survival and that survival of patients with malignant pleural effusion is similar to those with stage IV disease [7–9]. In addition, documented poorer survival for patients with T3N2 NSCLC over T1–2N2 patients might warrant upstaging that subset, and special designation upstaging has been suggested for synchronous primary lung cancers [10].

Histologic cell type is a prognostic factor not addressed in the current staging system. Several studies have shown improved survival for squamous cell histology over adenocarcinoma or large-cell undifferentiated histology in patients treated both surgically and nonsurgically. Cox et al. evaluated patterns of failure and cause of death by cell type for patients irradiated for locally advanced lung cancer [11]. For all histologies, local failure was a significant finding. However, for squamous cell carcinoma, intrathoracic progression was the primary cause of death in about three-quarters of patients. While local failure also was significant for large-cell and adenocarcinoma histologies, death was related to distant metastatic spread. Lung Cancer Study Group (LCSG) trials in 1,121 surgically treated patients showed superior outcome for patients with squamous cell carcinoma over nonsquamous histology in all TN categories and for survival in all but stage III disease [12]. Five-year survival data comparing squamous cell vs. adenocarcinoma histology were 65% vs. 55%, respectively, and overall survival (OS) 64–83% vs. 52–69%, respectively, for stage I, 53% vs. 25%, respectively, for stage II, and 37–46% vs. 21–48%, respectively, for stage III patients. NSCLC with neuroendocrine differentiation, as assessed by immunohistochemistry, appears to have little impact on survival for surgical patients, but has been associated with improved survival in advanced inoperable NSCLC [13].

Patient-related prognostic factors such as comorbidity and performance status (PS) also are ignored in current TNM staging. Nonetheless, these factors play a significant role in clinical practice treatment decisions, with patients unfavorable according to these parameters usually selected for nonsurgical management and often ineligible for investigational protocols. Feinstein and Wells developed a Clinical-Severity Staging System for lung cancer consisting of five stages (A–E) denoting "a hierarchy of prognostic severity" to be coupled with the TNM anatomic staging for greater prognostic value [14]. Wigren and colleagues proposed a prognostic index for patients with inoperable lung cancer in 1977 based on the five variables, disease extent, Feinstein clinical symptom score, PS, tumor size, and hemoglobin level [15]. The authors confirmed the validity of the index in 1997 for patients managed in the modern treatment era [16]. Two-year survival of 52%, 36%, 9.8%, 1.8%, 0%, and 0% were seen depending on the number of risk factors present (0–5).

In an analysis of 77 prognostic factors in over 5,000 patients with inoperable NSCLC treated on Veterans Administration Lung Group protocols, the three most important for survival were Karnofsky Performance Score (KPS), extent of disease, and weight loss within the previous 6 months. Patients with a KPS of 100, no weight loss, and disease confined to one hemithorax survived for a median of 72 weeks, in contrast to patients with a KPS of 40–50, with supraclavicular disease, and >10% weight loss, whose median survival time was as short as 6–8 weeks [17]. Other comorbidity scoring scales include the Charlson Scale (Table 14.2) [18] and the Cumulative Illness Rating Scale for Geriatrics (CIRS-Gl; Table 14.3) [19]. Both attempt to quantify comorbidity and thereby allow an objective evaluation of impact on outcome.

Table 14.2. Charlson scale – weighted comorbidity indices. Modified from Charlson 1987 [18]

Comorbidity	Assigned Points
Myocardial infarction	1
Congestive heart failure	1
Peripheral vascular disease	1
Cerebrovascular disease	1
Dementia	1
Chronic pulmonary disease	1
Connective tissue disease	1
Ulcer disease	1
Mild liver disease	1
Diabetes	1
Diabetes with end-organ damage	2
Hemiplegia	2
Moderate or severe renal disease	2
Any tumor (nonmetastatic)	2
Leukemia	2
Lymphoma, multiple myeloma	2
Moderate or severe liver disease	3
Metastatic solid tumor	6
Acquired immunodeficiency syndrome	6

Table 14.3. Cumulative illness rating scale for geriatrics. Modified from Linn 1968 [19]

Scored Organ System	
Heart	
Vascular	
Hematopoietic	
Respiratory	
Eyes, ears, nose, throat	
Upper gastrointestinal tract	
Lower gastrointestinal tract	
Liver	
Renal	
Genitourinary	
Musculoskeletal/integument	
Neurologic	
Endocrine/metabolic and breast	
Psychiatric	
Rating Strategy	
No problem	0
Mild – does not interfere with normal activity; prognosis excellent	1
Moderate – interferes with normal activity; treatment necessary	2
Severe – disabling impairment, urgent treatment necessary; prognosis poor	3
Extremely severe – life-threatening; prognosis grave	4

The presence of significant comorbidity and KPS < 70 have been identified as independent negative prognostic variables in both stage I and stage III NSCLC treated by either surgery or radiation. Using the comorbidity scoring scales in their stage I surgical patients, Firat et al. [20, 21] found the presence of a CIRS-G score of 4 in at least 1 out of 13 categories resulted in 5-year OS of 15%m compared with 65% when not present. According to the Charlson severity index (SI) rating, 5-year survival was 58% vs. 32% for SI≤2 vs. SI≥2, respectively. Surgical stage I patients with KPS≥70 had a 5-year OS of 48%, compared with 8% for those with initial KPS < 70. Stage I patients treated with radiation therapy had a 3-year survival of 50% vs. 8% depending upon the absence or presence of a CIRS-G score of 4, respectively, 35% vs. 7% for SI < 2 vs. SI > 2, and 25% vs. 14% for KPS≥70 vs. < 70. Stage III patients treated with radiation therapy alone showed a 2-year survival of 24.7% vs. 7.4% depending upon the absence or presence of a CIRS-G score of 4, 33.9% vs. 5.6% by SI > 2 vs. ≤2, and 26.7% vs. 5.5% by KPS > 70 vs. ≤70 [20, 21]. While some studies have identified advanced age (> 70 years) as a negative prognostic factor for NSCLC, this may simply reflect the greater likelihood of comorbid conditions in the elderly. This theory appears to be validated by Langer et al., who determined that age did not negatively impact survival in "fit" elderly NSCLC patients treated with cisplatinum-based chemotherapy [22]. "Fit" elderly patients ≥70 years of age were similar to patients < 70 years of age in terms of response rate (23% vs. 21.5%, respectively), time to progression (4.30 vs. 4.37 months, respectively), median survival (8.53 vs.

9.05 months, respectively), 1-year survival (28% vs. 38%, respectively), and 2-year survival (12% vs. 14%, respectively). As expected, advanced age was associated with increased cardiovascular and pulmonary comorbidity. Modifications of the TNM system to include factors of comorbidity and PS have been suggested.

The current staging system based on anatomic extent of disease is geared toward the determination of operability, in spite of the fact that the majority of lung cancer patients are not treated surgically. While the TNM staging system for NSCLC has the most predictive value for surgical patients, however, it falls short as a prognostic tool for nonsurgical patients [23]. In 1973 the Radiation Therapy Oncology Group (RTOG) modified the then AJCC staging system (Table 14.4) primarily in its classification of chest-wall invasion and contralateral lymph node involvement. While no longer employed in clinical trials, the RTOG system does have prognostic value for nonoperative patients. Curran et al. compared the prognostic value of both staging systems among patients receiving hyperfractionated radiation therapy on RTOG protocol 83-11 and found them to be complementary [24]. Survival data supported the AJCC distinction of contralateral mediastinal or hilar adenopathy (AJCC IIIB vs. RTOG III) and the RTOG distinction of chest-wall invasion (RTOG IV vs. AJCC IIIA) in nonsur-

Table 14.4. Radiation Therapy Oncology Group Lung Cancer Staging

T1			
Tumor < 3 cm without pleural or mainstem involvement			
T2			
Tumor either > 3 cm, involvement of mainstem bronchus > 2 cm from carina or lobar atelectasis			
T3			
Tumor < 2 cm from carina, visceral pleural involvement, entire lung atelectasis, or negative cytology pleural effusion			
T4			
Tumor with chest wall, nerve, major vessel, heart or pericardium, vertebrae, or deep mediastinal structure invasion, positive cytology pleural effusion, or superior vena cava syndrome			
N1			
Ipsilateral peribronchial or hilar nodal involvement			
N2			
Metastasis in mediastinal lymph nodes			
N3			
Metastasis in supraclavicular lymph nodes			
Stage grouping			
Stage I	T1	N0	M0
Stage II	T1,2	N1	M0
	T2	N0	M0
Stage III	T1–3	N2	M0
	T3	N0–2	M0
Stage IV	T4	Any N	M0
	Any T	N3	M0
	Any T	Any N	M1

gical patients. RTOG stage III patients showed a 2-year survival of 26% vs. 4% when stratified into AJCC stages II/IIIA vs. IIIB, respectively. AJCC IIIA patients showed 2-year survival of 22% vs. 10% when stratified into RTOG stages II/III vs. IV, respectively.

Ball et al. examined the effect of T-stage on outcome in 231 NSCLC patients treated with radiation with or without chemotherapy and found no correlation with survival [25]. Jeremic et al. reviewed the pertinent literature for early stage NSCLC patients treated with radiation therapy [26], and suggest that T-stage may not be as important a prognostic indicator in irradiated patients in whom tumor size and volume of tissue irradiated (i.e., elective nodal irradiation) are of greater consequence than tumor location. Tumor size is relevant only for T1 disease (≤3 cm) within the current TNM system, with tumor location or local extension defining more advanced T categories. In contrast, basic tenets of radiobiology dictate that for tumors treated with radiation therapy, tumor size should be the more important predictor of curability than anatomic location.

Finally, Paci et al. argue that the rigid TNM staging rules ignore the needs of the individual patient, whose situation is characterized by plasticity and singularity, and suggest that the current staging system is especially lacking with regard to treatment and survival prospects for patients with locally advanced and metastatic disease [27]. The authors advocate an individualized approach to decision-making in NSCLC beyond current clinical staging procedures to include: functional evaluation, positron emission tomography (PET) and computed tomography (CT) of the brain, and histologic confirmation of N and M stage. In the authors' opinion, this "approach guarantees the reduction of the current overtreatment of patients with stage N3 or M-positive disease, without removing the possibility of increasing the survival of selected patients who are in advanced stages of disease."

Brundage and associates used the TNM staging system to stratify the widely heterogeneous population of patients with NSCLC into the three basic categories: resectable disease, locally advanced disease (nonmetastatic confined to the chest), and advanced disease (metastatic), and reviewed the available literature within each of these broad categories [28]. Within each category, prognostic factors could be defined depending on the treatment modality selected.

14.3   Resectable Disease

14.3.1   Patients Treated with Surgery

Bernard et al. identified the prognostic factors for surgical risk in 500 NSCLC patients [29]. The risk of significant postoperative complications or death increased in patients with forced expiratory volume in 1 s <80%,

comorbidity indices>4, and increasing extent of surgery (i.e., wedge resection, lobectomy, pneumonectomy, extended resection of thoracic structures, or bronchoplastic procedures). The authors propose a risk group system to facilitate decisions regarding operability.

In a retrospective review of 2,382 surgically treated patients, Naruke et al. relate the staging system to surgical treatment options (i.e., thoracoscopic lobectomy for T1N0 lesions, bilobectomy for T2 lesions, and bilobectomy or pneumonectomy for T3 lesions) [30]. Selection of stage IIIA patients appropriate for curative surgery is discussed, stressing the need for gross total resection of all involved nodal disease and/or disease involving chest wall, diaphragm, mediastinum, or pericardium. The TNM staging system lost prognostic significance in this study between stage IIIB and IV disease, with 5-year survival rates of 9% and 11.2%, respectively. Stage IV patients with intrapulmonary metastasis in the primary tumor lobe had a 5-year survival rate of 17.8%, compared with 8.3% for those with intrapulmonary metastasis in another ipsilateral lobe. Controversy arises when patients approach the "gray zone" of resectability, as with limited N2 disease, or extended surgical procedures in selected stage IIIB without N2 involvement or with squamous cell histology.

The LCSG correlated risk of recurrence in 392 resected Stage I NSCLC patients with pathologic nodal involvement, nonsquamous cell histology, visceral pleural invasion, and CEA≥2.5 [31]. Risk of death correlated with advanced age, poor PS, comorbidity, and visceral pleural invasion. Komaki and colleagues also found squamous cell histology prognostic for improved outcome in patients with pathologically staged N1 NSCLC. The authors looked at levels of apoptosis and mitosis in their surgical N1 population and found a direct correlation with incidence of metastasis for adenocarcinoma and large-cell carcinoma histologies [32].

Suzuki et al. examined 18 clinicopathologic prognostic factors within each pathologic TNM stage and determined significant stage-dependent differences in impact on survival [33]. For stage I patients, prognostic factors included tumor size, clinical N status, vascular invasion, and curativity (complete vs. incomplete resection). Five-year survival was 65% for stage I patients with tumors >4 cm, 82.5% with tumors 2–4 cm, and 92.5% with tumors ≤2 cm, and 82.5% with tumors 2–4 cm. The 65% survival rate of stage I patients with tumors >4 cm was similar to that for those with stage II disease. Complete surgical resection resulted in a 5-year survival of 83%, compared with 44% with incomplete resection. The survival rate was 85% versus 51% for cN0-1 versus cN2 disease. In contrast to other reports, adenocarcinoma histology was a favorable prognostic factor for patients with stage I disease, with survival of 86% for adenocarcinoma and 72% for squamous cell carcinoma histology. The presence of vascular invasion was a negative prognostic factor only in patients with stage I disease, with a 5-year survival of 90% without and 69% with vascular invasion. For patients with more advanced pathologic stage (II–IV), adenocarcinoma histology and incomplete surgical resection were as significant poor prognostic factors as tumor size and N stage. Survival for these patients was 55.5% versus 37.7% for squamous cell versus adenocarcinoma, 48.4% versus 20.9% for complete versus incomplete resection, 61% versus 35% for tumors ≤ 3 cm versus > 3 cm, and 49% versus 26% for cN0-1 versus cN2 disease. In this series, the ability to undergo curative resection was prognostic across all stages. Good prognostic indicators for stage IIIB patients included T4N0-N1 disease in this highly selective patient group, with a 5-year survival of 58% compared to 13% for patients with N2-3 disease.

It is clear that N2 lymph-node-positive NSCLC is a heterogeneous clinical entity, with vastly different survival rates following surgery depending on the extent of mediastinal lymph node involvement. A subclassification of stage IIIA (N2-positive) was proposed by Ruckdeschel et al. [34], dividing patients with stage IIIA into four subgroups, with the most favorable one comprising patients with N2 involvement discovered only at thoracotomy (after previous negative mediastinoscopy) and the least favorable one, those with bulky nodes found on the CT scan.

An important retrospective review of 702 N2 lymph-node-positive patients who underwent surgical resection [35] demonstrated different prognostic groups based on clinical versus microscopic nodal involvement, number of nodal levels involved, and delivery of preoperative chemotherapy. The best 5-year OS rates were achieved by patients with microscopic single nodal level involved (34%), followed by those with microscopic multinodal involvement (11%), and clinical nodal involvement (3–8%). The extent of mediastinal lymph node removal at surgery also appears to affect outcome [36, 37]. In a large randomized trial comparing systematic sampling of the mediastinum to complete mediastinal lymph node dissection in 471 patients with stages I–IIIA NSCLC, complete mediastinal dissection was associated with a median survival time of 59 months, compared to 34 months in those who underwent systematic sampling ($p = 0.0001$) [36].

Since lymph node involvement is such a powerful prognostic factor in lung cancer, early knowledge of nodal involvement may be beneficial in order to recommend adjuvant therapy. Intraoperative sentinel lymph node mapping [38] may serve as such a tool in patients with small primary tumors and clinically negative lymph nodes. Once the sentinel node is identified, it may then be thoroughly examined for the presence of micrometastases with sensitive pathologic techniques (e.g., cytokeratin staining, serial sectioning, reverse transcriptase polymerase chain reaction).

Adjuvant therapy has been recommended for surgically treated patients with adverse pathologic findings

in an effort to improve local control and survival. Lee et al. reported prognostic factors in patients treated with surgery and adjuvant thoracic irradiation [39]. High risk factors for local failure included mediastinal adenopathy, wedge resection, positive surgical margins, and multiple positive nodes. The 3-year survival rate was 54% for N0, compared with 39% for N2 disease, 44% for patients treated with pneumonectomy, compared with 31% with wedge resection, 50% with negative surgical margins, compared with 39% with positive margins, and 48% with 0-1 positive node, compared with 30% with ≥2 positive nodes. The use of adjuvant radiation therapy employing modern radiation techniques achieved 80% locoregional disease control; however, distant metastatic failure remained a significant cause of death, with an actuarial distant failure rate of 55% at 3 years and 20% survival 1 year after detection of metastatic disease.

The potential prognostic significance of blood vessel invasion (BVI) and lymphatic vessel invasion (LVI) has been evaluated with conflicting results. Maccharini et al. found BVI to be a strong predictor for both OS and disease-free survival [40]. BVI and LVI as prognostic indicators were examined in a series of 96 patients with surgically treated stage I-IV NSCLC [41]. The authors found a correlation between LVI and regional node metastasis and pathological TNM (pTNM) stage, and between venous BVI and T-factor and pTNM stage. LVI was an independent prognostic factor for both recurrence and survival. Angeletti et al. evaluated the surgical specimens of 96 patients with stage IIIA (N2) NSCLC treated by curative resection with or without adjuvant radiation therapy and/or chemotherapy [42]. Here, the presence of BVI had no prognostic significance for either recurrence or survival. On multivariate analysis, only microvessel count (MC), a measure of tumor angiogenesis, retained significance as an independent prognostic factor. The use of adjuvant treatment significantly improved survival in the subset of pIIIA (N2) patients with MC > 31.

14.3.2 Patients Treated with Primary Radiation Therapy

Technically resectable patients with early stage (I–II) NSCLC who refuse surgery or are medically inoperable may be managed with definitive radiation therapy, and 5-year survival rates of up to 30% are reported. Reviews of pertinent literature in this patient population define prognostic factors of radiation dose/fractionation, tumor size/stage, treatment volume, and the use of chemotherapy [26, 43]. Improved local control and/or survival correlate with small tumor size, careful selection of high-risk patients for elective nodal irradiation, high treatment dose in the range of 65–70 Gy [44], continuous versus split course [45], and dose/fractionation scheme [46, 47]. The authors also cite numerous conflicting reports in the literature on the potential prognostic factors of PS, patient age, histology (squamous cell versus adenocarcinoma), and tumor location (upper or superior segment lower lobes versus lower or central versus peripheral).

A dose–response relationship for NSCLC has been established for tumors ≤ 3 cm treated by conventional radiation therapy techniques [44]. Technical advances in the delivery of thoracic irradiation by three-dimensional conformal radiation therapy (3D-CRT) techniques have enabled dose escalation without increased toxicity. The RTOG dose escalation study 93-11 [48] determined the safety of 3D-CRT techniques in delivering doses of up to 83.8 Gy for stages I–III NSCLC patients with a volume of normal lung exceeding 20 Gy (V_{20}) value of $\leq 25\%$ and to 77.4 Gy for patients with V_{20} values between 25 and 36%, using fraction sizes of 2.15 Gy. The 90.3-Gy dose level was too toxic, resulting in dose-related deaths in two patients. The observed locoregional control and OS rates were each similar among the study groups within each dose level. So far there has been no convincing evidence that radiation therapy dose escalation results in improved survival in patients with NSCLC, particularly with larger tumors. In a series of 207 patients treated with primary radiation therapy, Bradley et al. identified gross tumor volume (GTV), as determined by CT and 3-D CRT, planning as the single most important prognostic variable over T, N, or overall stage [49]. Stage for stage, patients with low-volume disease had the best local control, OS, and cause-specific survival (CSS). Patients with volumes of ≤ 33 cm^3, 34–70 cm^3, 71–112 cm^3, 113–179 cm^3, and > 180 cm^3 had a 3-year OS rate of 49%, 26%, 21%, 21%, and 14%, respectively, a 3-year CSS rate of 70%, 26%, 28%, 27%, and 17%, respectively, and local control of 78%, 44%, 50%, 58%, and 30%, respectively. In addition, a total dose of > 70.0 Gy correlated with improved local control and CSS (44% vs. 26%) over all GTV groups. In a similar series of 150 patients, Etiz and associates identified CT-defined a total tumor volume of < 80 cm^3 as a strong predictor of OS, local progression-free survival, and distant failure-free survival for stage I–III patients treated with definitive irradiation [50]. Willner et al. found similar results in 135 patients in whom local control was limited to patients with tumors < 100 cm^3 (6 cm maximum diameter) treated with ≥ 70.0 Gy [51].

Werner-Wasik and associates reported a serial CT-scan-based study examining changes in tumor size and volume for patients with locally advanced NSCLC treated with radiation with or without chemotherapy [52]. Improved local control and survival correlated with smaller initial tumor size. Local control at 24 months was 79% for tumor volumes ≤ 124 cm^3 and 0% for larger volumes. Mean survival time (MST) was > 53 months for tumors ≤ 63 cm^3 and 17.3 months for larger volumes. Tumor size evaluation by largest diameter, product of perpendicular dimensions, and volume had essentially equivalent prognostic significance when measuring tumor response following chemoradiotherapy, which supported the new Response Evaluation Criteria In Solid Tumors. Maximal tumor response was not observed until 5–11 months after completion of radiation therapy, a factor with implications for follow-up and response assessment. Tumor volume is therefore emerging as the most important predictive factor for survival in patients receiving definitive radiation therapy.

Elective nodal irradiation for subclinical disease has not been proven to improve outcome, but the larger target volume does increase the potential toxicity and limits the total dose [26, 43]. In an attempt to define prognostic factors for clinically undetectable mediastinal node metastasis, Sawyer et al. examined histologic specimens from 346 patients with clinical N0 NSCLC who underwent curative resection [53]. High risk of pathologic node involvement was seen for patients with positive preoperative bronchoscopy (i.e., centrally located tumors) and high-grade histology. The authors suggest inclusion of prophylactic mediastinal irradiation in inoperable cN0 patients with large (> 3 cm) high-grade primary tumors detectable by bronchoscopy. The RTOG dose-escalation trial omits elective node irradiation and may therefore better define its role in the nonsurgical management of NSCLC.

14.4 Locally Advanced, Nonmetastatic NSCLC

14.4.1 Patients Treated with Thoracic Radiation Therapy

It is important to define subsets of patients with inoperable, locally advanced NSCLC in whom aggressive nonsurgical management is likely to be beneficial. Potential benefit must be weighed against risk of treatment-related toxicity. Recursive partitioning analysis (RPA) on a 1,592-patient RTOG database defined KPS, weight loss, and age as the most significant patient-related variables, in addition to anatomic extent of disease prognostic for survival with nonsurgical treatment [54]. KPS was the most important factor on RPA, which identified distinct favorable prognostic classes. Patients with a KPS of > 70 had a median survival of 9.9 months and a 2-year survival of 19%, compared with 5.9 months and 7%, respectively for patients with a KPS of ≤ 70. In the most favorable group of patients, with a KPS of > 70 and N0, 2-year survival was 24%, compared with 17% for patients with a KPS of > 70 and N+. Absence of malignant effusion was linked to improved outcome for patients with a KPS of ≤ 70, who had a 2-year survival of 8% without and 5% with effusion. For patients with minimal weight loss, a radiation dose of >66 Gy correlated with improved survival of 26%, compared with 16% at 2 years. In another review of stage III nonoperative patients, hyperfractionated versus conventional radiation therapy (5-year survival 16–21% vs. 4.9%, respectively; MST 13–18 months vs. 8 months, respectively), female versus male gender (5-year survival 38% vs. 0%, respectively; MST 25 months vs. 10 months, respectively), age ≥60 years vs. <60 years (5-year survival 24% vs. 0%, respectively; MST 18 months vs. 7 months, respectively), KPS ≥80 years versus <80 years (5-year survival 17% vs. 0%, respectively; MST 16 months vs. 6 months, respectively), weight loss ≤5% vs. >5% (5-year survival 31% vs. 2.8%, respectively; MST 24 months vs. 8 months, respectively), and stage IIIA versus IIIB (5-year survival 31% vs. 24%, respectively; MST 23 months vs. 7 months, respectively) were significant prognostic factors [55].

A prognostic index (PI) model has been proposed as a more relevant predictor of local control than TNM stage for patients treated with radiation therapy [23]. Important prognostic factors for local control with radiation included tumor size, earlier clinical stage, and higher total dose in shortened overall treatment time. The model identifies four patient groups with median local progression-free survival of 35.1, 26.9, 14, and 6.8 months for PI <0.8, 0.8–1.3, 1.3–1.7, and ≥1.7, respectively. Choi et al. reported findings of the first International Workshop on Prognostic and Predictive Factors in Lung Cancer [56]. Prognostic indicators fell into four groups: tumor-related (anatomic) factors, host-related (clinical) factors, technical factors related to radiation therapy delivery, and biological/radiobiological/metabolic factors. Tumor-related factors include tumor size, anatomic structures involved, and nodal status. Host-related factors include poor PS, weight loss >10% within 6 months prior to diagnosis, and comorbidity. Radiation therapy technical factors include target volume, dose/fractionation schedule, total dose, and 3D-CRT planning. The fourth major category includes relatively newer investigational factors, some of which will be discussed later, that may ultimately have clinical utility. Subcategories within this last broad group include: (1) aberrant gene expression and mutated tumor-suppressor genes, (2) tumor-cell proliferation kinetics, oxygenation, radiosensitivity, and DNA content, and (3) enzyme/hormonal factors of neuron-specific enolase, serum lactate dehydrogenase, and enhanced glucose metabolic rate.

Herbert et al. reported outcome data on 63 patients <50 years of age with stage I–III disease treated with radiation therapy alone [57]. Compared to 695 older patients, younger age correlated with poor outcome. Age <50 years correlated with advanced stage at presentation, high tumor grade, and increased distant metastatic failure, particularly brain metastasis.

Recently, PET scanning has found wide applications in the evaluation and management of NSCLC. In a large series of 153 consecutive patients with unresectable NSCLC who were considered candidates for radical radiation therapy after conventional staging, after PET scan 30% were diagnosed to have metastatic disease and 12%, more extensive locoregional disease than suspected initially [58, 59]. For radically treated patients, post-PET stage, but not pre-PET stage was strongly associated with survival. In addition, PET scanning allows the assessment of a tumor's metabolic activity (presumably correlating with its "aggressiveness") through measurement of the peak standardized uptake value (SUV). In a retrospective review of 155 patients with newly diagnosed NSCLC [60], patients with primary lesions with SUV >10 ($n=118$) had the worst prognosis, with a MST of 11.4 months, compared with 24.6 months for those with SUV <10 ($n=37$). Multivariate analysis demonstrated that an SUV >10 provided prognostic information independent of the clinical stage and lesion size. In another report, SUV >7 was correlated with a poor survival in 125 potentially operable patients with NSCLC, with a prognostic significance at least equal to those of the PS and stage [61].

There are some preliminary data to indicate that posttherapy FDG-PET may be useful in predicting long-term outcome in patients with unresectable stage III NSCLC treated with either radiation therapy alone or chemoradiation. Patients with posttreatment SUVs of 3.5 or less had a local failure rate of 17% compared with those with SUVs of greater than 3.5 who had a local failure rate of 77%. In this study, 45 patients with stage I, II, and IIIA NSCLC were treated primarily with radiation therapy alone, and the median time from completion of radiation therapy to PET imaging was 4 months (range 1–18 months) [62]. In another recent study, PET response, but not CT response predicted eventual outcome [58, 59]. The relative death rates for those with PET-based nonresponse and progressive disease were 5.71 and 13.9, respectively, when compared with those with PET-based complete response. RTOG is planning to launch a prospective study in collaboration with American College of Radiology Imaging Network to define the utility of posttherapy PET imaging in patients with unresectable stage III NSCLC.

14.4.2 Patients Treated with Radiation and Chemotherapy

Patients who fall into the category of locally advanced disease may nonetheless attain long-term survival with chemotherapy and radiation, and the use of which is recommended in practice outside of clinical trials based on a meta-analysis of prospective randomized trials [63]. Within this group, the subset of patients with good PS, no weight loss, concurrent chemoradiation, and neoadjuvant chemoradiation have been associated with improved outcome. Six of eight phase III randomized trials for patients with stage III disease showed improved MST (12–22 months vs. 9.7–14 months) and a 2-year survival rate (21–52% vs. 12–38%) with chemoradiation versus radiation alone. In the reported Southwest Oncology Group (SWOG) data, cisplatinum-based chemotherapy was a significant independent favorable prognostic indicator and showed survival benefit in all prognostic subsets defined by RPA [64].

RPA of 1,999 patients with locally advanced NSCLC treated on 9 RTOG protocols with radiation therapy with or without chemotherapy identified the use of chemotherapy as a positive prognostic factor for improved survival for patients with KPS≥90 [9]. Again, the presence of malignant pleural effusion was a strong negative prognostic indicator for all patient subsets, prompting the authors to suggest staging patients with pleural effusion as IV rather than IIIB. Five patient subgroups were identified with significantly different MSTs: (1) group I, KPS≥90, who received chemotherapy (MST 16.2 months), (2) group II, KPS≥90, who received no CT, but had no pleural effusion (11.9 months), (3) group III, KPS<90, younger than 70 years, with non-large-cell histology (9.6 months), (4) group IV, KPS≥90, but with pleural effusion, or KPS<90, younger than 70 years, and with large-cell histology, or older than 70 years, but without pleural effusion (5.6–6.4 months), and (5) group V, older than 70 years, with a pleural effusion (2.9 months). Machtay et al. evaluated survival in the subset of stage IIIB patients with supraclavicular node involvement treated with modern chemoradiation using the RTOG database [65]. The data supported the designation of N3 disease within the stage IIIB rather than stage IV category based on statistics comparable to other IIIB patients of MST 16.2 versus 15.6 months, 4-year actuarial survival 21% versus 16%, 4-year progression-free survival 19% versus 14% for patients with versus without supraclavicular node involvement, respectively. Reported data from the RTOG 94-10 trial favor concurrent cisplatin and vinblastine chemotherapy with conventional once-daily radiation therapy over sequential chemoradiation treatment schedules [66].

The use of neoadjuvant chemotherapy and radiation in patients with locally advanced disease has resulted in a subset of stage IIIA patients previously thought unresectable for cure in whom surgery may result in improved survival. Bueno et al. reported outcome in 103 patients with N2 disease treated with neoadjuvant chemoradiation and found a 35.8% 5-year survival rate in 29 patients downstaged to N0 [67]. The authors stress the importance of accurate restaging after neoadjuvant treatment by thoracoscopy, PET scan, and lymph node biopsy sampling via esophageal ultrasound and/or mediastinoscopy in order to spare patients unnecessary surgery for persistent node-positive disease. Choi et al. reported survival data on 42 patients with stage IIIA (N2) NSCLC treated with neoadjuvant cisplatinum-

based chemotherapy and concurrent hyperfractionated (1.5 Gy bid) radiation therapy followed by postoperative chemotherapy [56]. In this series, survival correlated with extent of tumor downstaging, with 5-year survival rates of 79%, 42%, and 18% for postoperative stage 0 and I, II, and III respectively. Grunenwald et al. advocate revision of the staging system for patients with advanced disease to select patients who might benefit from surgical resection, by defining subgroups for treatment by primary surgery, induction treatment followed by surgery in responders, or nonsurgical treatment [4]. In the final report of SWOG phase II trial [6], a 26% 3-year survival rate was achieved in patients with stages IIIA (N2) and IIIB NSCLC after concurrent cisplatin/etoposide chemotherapy with thoracic radiation therapy, followed by surgical resection. Of interest, there was no survival difference between stage IIIA and stage IIIB patients at 13 and 17 months, respectively, $p = 0.81$).

As treatment intensification protocols emerge, however, issues related to treatment toxicity and quality of life (QOL) assume increasing significance. Movsas et al. defined quality-adjusted survival time (QTime), "a…survival score, to serve as a metric that allows comparison of treatment regimens. QTime provides a quantitative measurement by combining duration and QOL, weighted by the factors of toxicity and tumor progression. The scores for each patient are calculated on the basis of an explicit formula that then incorporates arbitrary weights for the severity of each symptom." (Table 14.5) [68]. The authors analyzed 979 patients with stage II–IIIB inoperable NSCLC treated on 6 pro-

Table 14.5. Weighting criteria for quality-adjusted survival time calculations. Grades not listed had a weight of 1.0. In the final calculation, disease status accounts for 50% of the QTime score, lung/esophageal/upper gastrointestinal (*GI*) toxicity accounts for 30% of the QTime score, and other toxicities account for 20% of the QTime score [68]

Item	Grade	Weight
Skin toxicity	2	0.95
	3	0.75
	4	0.25
Mucous membranes	1	0.95
	2	0.75
	3	0.50
	4	0.25
Lung/esophagus/neurotoxicity/Upper GI/spine toxicity	1	0.95
	2	95
	3	0.25
	4	0.0
Hematologic toxicity	3	0.75
	4	0.25
Metastases (kidney/adrenal/liver/Subcutaneous)	Present	0.33
Metastases-brain	Present	0.20
Metastases-bone	Present	0.25
Primary/nodal progression	Present	0.33

spective trials using different regimens of radiation alone or with chemotherapy for the impact of age, histology, KPS, and toxicity on MST and QTime. Increasing age had a negative impact on outcome with treatment intensification. Improvement in MST and QTime correlated with more aggressive chemoradiation protocols in patients <60 years of age and with radiation alone in patients >71 years of age. Induction chemotherapy and concurrent chemoradiation was the optimal treatment regimen with regard to MST and QTime for squamous cell carcinoma histology. In contrast, for patients with adenocarcinoma, optimal outcome was seen with the most intensive regimen of concurrent chemotherapy and hyperfractionated radiation. Toxicity evaluation identified upper gastrointestinal and lung toxicity as having the greatest impact on QTime. KPS did not correlate with treatment to affect MST or QTime in this study.

14.5 Metastatic NSCLC

Albain et al. reported the SWOG analysis of 2,531 patients with "extensive-stage" NSCLC, identifying good PS, female sex, and age >70 years as good prognostic factors [64]. By applying the RPA method to 904 patients, 5 patient subgroups were identified that were amalgamated into 3 prognostic subsets with 1-year survivals of 27%, 16%, and 6%. Good KPS was the most important prognostic factor, followed by hemoglobin >11 g/dl and age ≥47 years. The use of cisplatinum-based chemotherapy resulted in improved survival in all patient subgroups.

14.5.1 Patients Treated with Surgery

Patients with metastatic NSCLC are generally treated with palliative intent, with the goals of maintaining maximal functional status, relieving symptoms, delaying time to progression, and prolonging QTime. Some authors have argued for aggressive surgical management of certain subsets of M1 patients. Bonnette et al. reviewed the pertinent literature and presented their own data on 103 patients treated with surgical resection of solitary cranial metastasis followed by primary tumor resection [69]. The authors indicate prognostic variables of small primary tumor size (T1), adenocarcinoma histology, and absence of mediastinal adenopathy by CT and mediastinoscopy as selection criteria for this aggressive surgical approach, with 11% calculated 5-year survival. Other authors make a similar argument for resection of solitary adrenal metastasis [70].

For patients with advanced disease receiving chemotherapy, Brundage et al. reported extent of disease by TNM stage, PS, and weight loss to be the most sig-

nificant predictors of survival time [28]. Stewart and Pignon reported a meta-analysis of 9.387 patients with NSCLC treated on 52 randomized trials with regard to the role of modern cisplatinum-based chemotherapy. The authors found modern chemotherapy to improve outcome in all patient categories, including early and advanced disease, and in all treatment categories including definitive surgery (5% improvement at 5 years), definitive radiation (4% improvement at 2 years), and best supportive care (10% improvement at 1 year) [71].

14.6 Summary

In summary, numerous prognostic indicators for NSCLC patients have been defined and continue to be evaluated for impact on local control, survival, and treatment selection. It becomes clear that tumor induction and progression are determined by multiple steps and response to treatment on numerous codependent factors that must ultimately be considered in determining optimal treatment for any given patient. The ultimate goal would be an individualized approach to each patient considering all variables of stage, tumor biology, comorbidity, and QOL.

Key Points

- Clinical prognostic factors in locally advanced non-small-cell lung cancer of major importance have been disease stage, performance status, and weight loss.
- More recently, the volume of the tumor and ^{18}fluorodeoxyglucose positron emission tomography scan findings (both on presentation and following therapy) have been reported to be highly predictive for patient survival.
- Comorbid conditions are significantly impacting on survival, especially in patients with worse performance status.
- In patients undergoing surgery, the extent of hilar and mediastinal involvement remains crucial.
- In the near future, biologic and molecular markers may add new knowledge, allowing a more accurate prediction of outcome.

References

1. Mountain CF. Revisions in the International System for Staging Lung Cancer. Chest 1997; 111(6):1710.
2. AJCC Cancer Staging Manual, 6th edn. Springer-Verlag, New York, 2002.
3. Kameyama K, Huang CL, Liu D, Okamoto T, Hiyashi E, Yamamoto Y, Yokomise H. Problems related to TNM

staging: patients with stage III non-small cell lung cancer. J Thorac Cardiovasc Surg 2002; 124(3):503.

4. Grunenwald D. Surgery for advanced stage lung cancer. Semin Surg Oncol 2000; 18:137.

5. Goldberg Z, Gaspar L, Lara P, Roberts P, Gandara D. Combined modality treatment of non-small-cell lung cancer. Lung Cancer Princ Pract Update 2001; 1(2):1.

6. Albain KS, Rusch VW, Crowley JJ, et al. Concurrent cisplatin/etoposide plus chest radiotherapy followed by surgery for Stage III (N2) and IIIB non-small cell lung cancer: Mature results of Southwest Oncology Group Phase II study 88-05. J Clin Oncol 1995, 13:1880.

7. Okada M, Tsubota N, Yoshimura M, Miyamoto Y, Nakai R. Evaluation of TNM classification for lung carcinoma with ipsilateral intrapulmonary metastasis. Ann Thorac Surg 1999; 68:326.

8. Leong S, Lima C, Sherman C, Green M. The 1997 international staging system for non-small cell lung cancer: Have all the issues been addressed? Chest 1999; 115(1):242.

9. Werner-Wasik M, Scott C, Cox J, et al. Recursive partitioning analysis of 1999 radiation therapy oncology group (RTOG) patients with locally advanced non-small-cell lung cancer (LA-NSCLC): identification of five groups with different survival. Int J Radiat Oncol Biol Phys 2000; 48(5):1475.

10. Mountain C. Staging classification of lung cancer: a critical evaluation. Lung Cancer 2002; 23(1)103.

11. Cox J, Yesher R, Mietlowski W, Petrovich Z. Influence of cell type on failure pattern after irradiation for locally advanced carcinoma of the lung. Cancer 1979; 44:94.

12. Mountain CF, Lukeman JM, Hammar S, et al. Lung cancer classification: the relationship of disease extent and cell type to survival in a clinical trials population. J Surg Oncol 1987; 35(3S):147.

13. Schleusener J, Tazelaar H, Jung S, et al. Neuroendocrine differentiation is an independent prognostic factor in chemotherapy-treated nonsmall cell lung carcinoma. Cancer 1996; 77:1284.

14. Feinstein A, Wells C. A clinical-severity staging system for patients with lung cancer. Medicine 1990; 69(1):1.

15. Wigren T, Oksanen H, Lehtinen KP. A practical prognostic index of inoperable non-small cell lung cancer. J Can Res Clin Oncol 1977; 123:259.

16. Wigren T. Confirmation of a prognostic index for patients with inoperable non-small cell lung cancer. Radiother Oncol 1997; 44:9.

17. Stanley K. Prognostic factors for survival in patients with inoperable lung cancer. J Natl Cancer Inst 1980; 65(1)25.

18. Charlson M, Pompei P, Ales K, MacKenzie R. A new method of classifying prognostic comorbidity in longitudinal studies: Development and validation. J Chron Dis 1987; 40;373.

19. Linn B, Linn M, Gurel L. Cumulative index rating scale. J Am Geriatr Soc 1968; 16:622.

20. Firat S, Bousamra M, Gore E, Byhardt R. Comorbidity and KPS are independent prognostic factors in stage I non-small-cell lung cancer. Int J Radiat Oncol Biol Phys 2002; 52(4):1047.

21. Firat S, Byhardt R, Gore E. Comorbidity and Karnofsky Performance Score are independent prognostic factors in stage III non-small-cell lung cancer: an institutional analysis of patients treated on four RTOG studies. Int. J. Radiat Oncol Biol Phys 2002; 54(2):357.

22. Langer C, Manola J, Bernardo P, Bonomi P, Kugler A, Johnson D. Advanced age alone does not compromise outcome in fit non-small cell lung cancer (NSCLC) patients (Pts) receiving platinum (DDP)-based therapy (Tx): Implications of ECOG 5592. Proceedings of ASCO 2000; Abstract 1912:489a.

23. Chen M, Jiang G, Fu X, Wang L, Qian H, Zhao S, Liu T. Prognostic factors for local control in non-small-call lung cancer treated with definitive radiation therapy. Am J Clin Oncol 2002; 25(1):76.

24. Curran W, Cox J, Azarnia N, et al. Comparison of the Radiation Therapy Oncology Group and American Joint Committee on Cancer Staging systems among patients with non-small cell lung cancer receiving hyperfractionated radiation therapy. Cancer 1991; 68:509.

25. Ball D, Smith J, Wirth A, MacManus M. Failure of T stage to predict survival in patients with non-small-cell lung cancer treated by radiotherapy with or without concomitant chemotherapy. Int J Radiat Oncol Biol Phys 2002; 54:1007.

26. Jeremic B, Classen J, Bamberg M. Radiotherapy alone in technically operable, medically inoperable, early-stage (I/II) non-small-cell lung cancer. Int J Radiat Oncol Biol Phys 2002; 54:119.

27. Paci M, Sgarbi G, Ferrari G, DeFranco S, Annessi V. Controversies over UICC-TNM classification of non-small cell lung cancer: model for a diagnostic path. (Communications to the Editor) Chest 2002; 122(2):754.

28. Brundage M, Davies, D, Mackillop W. Prognostic factors in non-small cell lung cancer: A decade of progress. Chest 2002; 122(3):1037.

29. Bernard A, Ferrand L, Hagry O, Benoit L, Cheynel N, Favre J. Identification of prognostic factors determining risk groups for lung resection. Ann Thorac Surg 2000; 70(4):1161.

30. Naruke T, Tsuchiya, R, Kondo, Hasamura H, Nakayama H. Implications of staging in lung cancer. Chest 1997; 112(4):242S.

31. Gail M, Eagan R, Feld R, et al. Prognostic factors in patients with resected stage I non-small cell lung cancer. A report from the Lung Cancer Study Group. Cancer 1984; 54:1802.

32. Komaki R, Fugi T, Perkins P, et al. Apoptosis and mitosis as prognostic factors in pathologically staged N1 nonsmall cell lung cancer. Int J Radiat Oncol Biol Phys 1996; 36(3)601.

33. Suzuki K, Nagai K, Yoshida J, Nishimura M, Takahashi K, Yokose T, Nishiwaki Y. Conventional clinicopathologic prognostic factors in surgically resected nonsmall cell lung carcinoma. A comparison of prognostic factors for each pathologic TNM stage based on multivariate analyses. Cancer 1999; 86:1976.

34. Ruckdeschel JC, Wagner H, Robinson LA. Locally Advanced Lung Cancer: Controversies in Management. ASCO Educational Book, Alexandria, 1996, p 220.

35. Andre F, Grunenwald D, Pignon JP, et al. Survival of patients with resected N2 non-small-cell lung cancer: evidence for a subclassification and implications. J Clin Oncol 2000; 18(16):2981.

36. Wu YL, Huang ZF, Wang SY, Yang XN, W Ou. A randomized trial of systematic nodal dissection in resectable non-small cell lung cancer. Lung Cancer 2002; 36(1):1.

37. Keller SM, Adak S, Wagner H, Johnson DH. Mediastinal lymph node dissection improves survival in patients with stages II and IIIA non-small cell lung cancer. Eastern Cooperative Oncology Group. Ann Thorac Surg 2000; 70:358.

38. Liptay MJ, Grondin SC, Fry WA, et al. Intraoperative sentinel lymph node mapping in non-small cell lung cancer improves detection of micrometastases. J Clin Oncol 2002; 20:1984.

39. Lee J, Machtay M, Kaiser L, Friedberg J, Hahn S, McKenna M, McKenna W. Non-small cell lung cancer: prognostic factors in patients treated with surgery and postoperative radiation therapy. Radiology 1999; 213(3):845.

40. Macchiarini P, Fontanini G, Hardin M, et al. Blood vessel invasion by tumor cells predicts recurrence in completely

resected T1N0M0 non-small-cell lung cancer. J Thorac Cardiovasc Surg 1993; 106:80.

41. Brechot J, Chevret S, Charpentier M, et al. Blood vessel and lymphatic vessel invasion in resected nonsmall cell lung carcinoma. Correlation with TNM stage and disease free and overall survival. Cancer 1996; 78:2111.

42. Angeletti C, Lucchi M, Fontanini G, et al. Prognostic significance of tumoral angiogenesis in completely resected late stage lung carcinoma (stage IIIA-N2). Impact of adjuvant therapies in a subset of patients at high risk of recurrence. Cancer 1996; 78:409.

43. Sause W. Nonsurgical management of non-small-cell lung cancer. Hematol Oncol Clin North Am 2001; 5(2):277.

44. Dosoretz D, Katin M, Blitzer P, et al. Radiation therapy in the management of medically inoperable carcinoma of the lung: results and implications for future treatment strategies. Int J Radiat Oncol Biol Phys 1992; 24:3.

45. Haffty B, Goldberg N, Gerstley J, Fischer D, Peschel R. Results of radical radiation therapy in clinical Stage I, technically operable non-small cell lung cancer. Int J Radiat Oncol Biol Phys 1988; 15:69.

46. Graham P, Gebski V, Langlands A. Radical radiotherapy for early nonsmall cell lung cancer. Int J Radiat Oncol Biol Phys 1995; 31:261.

47. Saunders M, Dische S, Barrett A, Harvey A, Griffiths G, Parmar M (on behalf of the CHART Steering committee). Continuous hyperfractionated accelerated radiotherapy (CHART) versus conventional radiotherapy in non-small cell lung cancer: mature data from the randomized multicenter trial. Radiother Oncol 1999; 52:137.

48. Bradley J, Graham MV, Winter K, et al. Toxicity and outcome results of RTOG 9311: a phase I-II dose escalation study using three-dimensional conformal radiotherapy in patients with inoperable non-small cell lung carcinoma. Int J Radiat Oncol Biol Phys 2005; 61:318.

49. Bradley J, Ieumwananonthachai N, Purdy J, Wasserman T, Lockett M, Graham M, Perez C. Gross tumor volume, critical prognostic factor in patients treated with three-dimensional conformal radiation therapy for non-small-cell lung carcinoma. Int J Radiat Oncol Biol Phys 2002; 52(1):49.

50. Etiz D, Marks L, Zhou S, Bentel G, Clough R, Hernando M, Lind P. Influence of tumor volume on survival in patients irradiated for non-small-cell lung cancer. Int. J. Radiat Oncol Biol Phys 2002; 53(4):835.

51. Willner J, Baier K, Caragiani E, Tschammler A, Flentje M. Dose, volume, and tumor control predictions in primary radiotherapy of non-small-cell lung cancer. Int J Radiat Oncol Biol Phys 2002; 52(2):382.

52. Werner-Wasik M, Xiao Y, Pequignot E, Curran W, Hauck W. Assessment of lung cancer response after nonoperative therapy: tumor diameter, bidimensional product, and volume. A serial CT scan-based study. Int J Radiat Oncol Biol Phys 2001; 51(1):56.

53. Sawyer T, Bonner J, Gould P, Garces Y, Foote R, Lange C, Li H. Predictors of subclinical nodal involvement in clinical stages I and II non-small cell lung cancer. Int J Radiat Oncol Biol Phys 1999; 43(5):965.

54. Scott C, Sause WT, Byhardt R, Marcial V, Pajak TF, Herskovic A, Cox JD. Recursive partitioning analysis of 1592 patients on four Radiation Therapy Oncology Group studies in inoperable non-small cell lung cancer. Lung Cancer 1997; 17:59.

55. Jeremic B, Shibamoto Y. Pre-treatment prognostic factors in patients with stage III non-small cell lung cancer treated with or without concurrent chemotherapy. Lung Cancer 1995; 13:21.

56. Choi N, Corey R, Daly W, et al. Potential impact on survival of improved tumor downstaging and resection rate by preoperative twice-daily radiation and concurrent che-

motherapy in stage IIIA non-small-cell lung cancer. J Clin Oncol 1997; 15(2):712.

57. Herbert S, Curran W, Rosenthal S, Stafford P, McKenna W, Hughes E, Sandler H. Adverse influence of younger age on outcome in patients with non-small cell lung carcinoma (NSCLC) treated with radiation therapy (RT) alone. Int J Radiat Oncol Biol Phys 1992; 24:37.

58. McManus MP, Hicks R, Ball DL, et al. F-18 fluorodeoxyglucose positron emission tomography staging in radical radiotherapy candidates with nonsmall cell lung carcinoma. Cancer 2001, 92:886.

59. MacManus MP, Hicks RJ, Salminen E, et al. PET response is the most powerful predictor of survival after radical radiotherapy/chemoradiotherapy for unresectable non-small cell lung cancer. Int J Radiat Oncol Biol Phys 2001; 51(1):89.

60. Ahuja V, Coleman RE, Herndon J, Patz EF. The prognostic significance of fluorodeoxyglucose positron emission tomography imaging for patients with nonsmall cell lung carcinoma. Cancer 1998, 83:918.

61. Vansteenkiste J, Stroobants S, Dupont P, et al. Prognostic importance of the standardized uptake value on ^{18}F-Fluoro-2-deoxy-glucose-positron emission tomography scan in non-small-cell lung cancer: an analysis of 125 cases. J Clin Oncol 1999; 17:3201.

62. Rosenzweig KE, Erdi Y, Schoder H, Akhurst T, Larson SM, Leibel SA. Positron emission tomography after three-dimensional conformal radiation therapy for non-small cell lung cancer. Int J Radiat Oncol Biol Physics 2001; 51(1): 89.

63. ASCO Special Article. Clinical practice guidelines for the treatment of unresectable non-small-cell lung cancer. J Clin Oncol 1997; 15(8):2996.

64. Albain K, Crowley J, LeBlanc M, Livingston R. Survival determinants in extensive-stage non-small-cell lung cancer: The Southwest Oncology Group Experience. J Clin Oncol 1991; 9:1618.

65. Machtay M, Seiferheld W, Komaki R, Cox J, Sause W, Byhardt R. Is prolonged survival possible for patients with supraclavicular node metastases in non-small cell lung cancer treated with chemoradiotherapy? Analysis of the Radiation Therapy Oncology Group experience. Int J Radiat Oncol Biol Phys 1999; 44(4):847.

66. Curran W, Scott C, Langer C, et al. Phase III comparison of sequential vs concurrent chemoradiation for patients with unresected stage III non-small cell lung cancer (NSCLC): Initial report of Radiation Therapy Oncology Group (RTOG) 94-10. Proc Am Soc Clin Oncol 2000; 19:484a.

67. Bueno R, Richards W, Swanson S, Jaklitsch M, Lukamich J, Mentzer S, Sugarbaker D. Nodal stage after induction therapy for stage IIIA lung cancer determines patient survival. Ann Thorac Surg 2000; 70(6):1826.

68. Movsas B, Scott C, Sause W, et al. The benefit of treatment intensification is age and histology-dependent in patients with locally advanced non-small cell lung cancer (NSCLC): A quality-adjusted survival analysis of Radiation Therapy Oncology Group (RTOG) chemoradiation studies. Int J Radiat Oncol Biol Phys 1999; 45(5):1143.

69. Bonnette P, Puyo P, Gabriel C, et al. Surgical management of non-small cell lung cancer with synchronous brain metastases. Chest 2001; 119(5):1469.

70. Porte H, Sait J, Guilbert B, et al. Resection of adrenal metastases from non-small cell lung cancer: a multicenter study. Ann Thorac Surg 2001; 71:981.

71. Stewart L, Pignon J. Chemotherapy in non-small cell lung cancer: a meta-analysis using updated data on individual patients from 52 randomised clinical trials. Non-small Cell Lung Cancer Collaborative Group. BMJ 1995; 311:899.

Prognostic Factors for Small-Cell Lung Cancer

15

Chad M. DeYoung and Martin J. Edelman

Contents

15.1 Introduction

Knowledge of the factors that predict the clinical outcome of a patient with small-cell lung cancer (SCLC) is critical to guiding treatment and to determining prognosis. The benefit of defining these prognostic factors, however, goes well beyond the individual patient. In 1973 the Veterans' Administration Lung Study Group (VALSG) [1] described a staging system for SCLC that divided patients into localized disease or extensive disease based upon the ability to administer radiotherapy. With the advent of this staging system, the treatment of patients with SCLC began to become standardized across institutions. This type of classification into different prognostic groups facilitated the planning and interpretation of results of clinical trials. In turn, these trials have allowed the collection of additional data that has ultimately led to a better understanding of additional factors that predict for significant patient outcomes including response to therapy, duration of response, and survival. This better understanding further refines clinical trials and ultimately leads to improved care for all patients with SCLC. In the pages that follow, we will examine the factors that have been investigated for their prognostic significance and bring perspective to the power each factor has in determining the ultimate outcomes of patients.

15.2 Staging

Staging remains the most powerful prognostic factor for SCLC. The goal of staging is to stratify patients into risk groups in order to guide treatment decisions and ensure an appropriate balance between patient groups when designing clinical trials. The current TNM staging system for lung cancer is based upon concepts most applicable to surgical issues in non-small-cell lung cancer (NSCLC), and while roughly predictive of outcome in SCLC it is not utilized in either practice or research [2]. The system described by the VALSG in 1973 has proven to be robust, and with some modifications it continues to be used today [1]. In this system, two stages are described: limited stage, defined as disease confined to one hemithorax that can be encompassed in a "single, tolerable radiation field", and extensive stage, defined as disease that can not be encompassed in a single tolerable radiation field. The importance of accurately determining stage prior to institution of therapy cannot be underestimated. Patients with limited disease are considered to be potentially curable and will receive chemotherapy and radiation, possibly with prophylactic cranial irradiation, while those with extensive disease will (for the most part) receive chemotherapy alone with the intention of prolonging life and ameliorating symptoms, but not with curative intent.

15.2.1   Limited Stage

Roughly one-third of patients will present with limited-stage disease [3]. To date, the best outcomes reported through phase III data show that the median survival of these patients is 23 months, with a 5-year overall-survival rate of 26% [4]. Patients surviving 5 years are considered to be cured of their disease. The precise definition of what constitutes limited stage is somewhat controversial. The VALSG defines limited stage as all disease limited to one hemithorax. In 1989, the International Association for the Study of Lung Cancer published their recommendations for what should constitute limited-stage disease [5]. They recommended including patients with hilar, ipsilateral and contralateral mediastinal nodes, ipsilateral and contralateral supraclavicular nodes, and patients with isolated, ipsilateral pleural effusions whether negative or positive for malignancy by cytology. Essentially, all patients without disease beyond the chest were to be included in this category. However, it is clear that this definition is overly inclusive and is not appropriate for either daily practice or for clinical trials. We shall examine each of these subsets of limited-stage disease individually.

15.2.1.1 Very-Limited-Stage Disease
Very-limited-stage disease is an uncommon subcategory of limited-stage disease, but is likely to hold a much better prognosis. It is defined as disease limited to the lung without spread to the mediastinum or elsewhere. In the University of Toronto experience [6], patients treated with chemoradiation who had no evidence of disease in their mediastinum, by imaging or sampling, had a better median survival (17 months) and higher 5-year overall-survival (18%) than did the rest of their limited-stage patients. From their analysis, they defined a group of patients with very-limited disease who had a better prognosis (25% 5-year overall survival). These were patients with disease limited to a lung with no evidence of nodal involvement, obstructing tumors, or pleural effusions. A particularly good subgroup appears to be those patients with stage I (T1 or T2 N0M0) disease, as assessed by TNM classification, who are able to undergo surgical resection followed by chemotherapy. One of the first series to suggest a better prognosis with this subgroup evaluated 132 patients who underwent re-

section of a SCLC during the previous 15 years followed by 1 of 4 different postoperative chemotherapy regimens [7]. The 5-year overall survival rate was 60% for stage IA disease. Since this initial report, other series have demonstrated comparable results. These studies demonstrate that an improved outcome exists for stage IA, and possibly stage IB patients. Stage II patients (T1 or 2, N1M0), however, do not appear to share the same superior outcome. It remains to be demonstrated prospectively whether these outcomes are a consequence of a different natural history of disease or due to therapy (i.e., surgical resection).

15.2.1.2 Mediastinal and Hilar Lymph Nodes
Patients with involvement of their mediastinal lymph nodes represent a far more common subset of limited-stage patients. Involvement of either the ipsilateral mediastinum (N2) or the contralateral mediastinum (N3) constitutes limited-stage disease. Contralateral hilum involvement, however, remains somewhat controversial. Two phase III studies comparing once daily radiotherapy to twice daily radiotherapy excluded patients with contralateral hilar disease and contralateral supraclavicular disease [4, 8]. The results obtained in these studies represent some of the best survival data published. Although not expressly stated, these patients were excluded due to concerns regarding excessive lung toxicity from radiation. Changes in radiotherapy planning (i.e., three-dimensional conformal fields) that significantly decrease exposure of normal lung tissue should alleviate these concerns and may allow this issue to be readdressed.

15.2.1.3 Supraclavicular Lymph Nodes
Two large multicenter series, one in North America and the other in Europe, have retrospectively evaluated the outcomes of patients with involvement of the supraclavicular nodes [9, 10]. In the CALGB analysis, 1,521 patients from 5 separate studies were evaluated for prognostic factors. A total of 803 patients with limited-stage disease were identified. Seventy-nine of these had supraclavicular nodes involvement and demonstrated a trend toward poorer survival when compared to limited-stage disease without supraclavicular node involvement (11.0 months vs. 12.3 months, respectively; $p = 0.06$). However, this outcome was still substantially better than for patients with extensive disease who had a median survival of 8.6 months. The European study examined 1,370 patients with SCLC from 4 studies. Of these, 234 patients had supraclavicular nodal involvement, 65 of whom were classified as having limited-stage disease. The presence of supraclavicular node involvement at baseline was a strong predictor of distant metastases, especially to liver and bone. For patients

with limited-stage disease, the presence of supraclavicular node involvement tends toward a poorer survival; median survival 12.5 months without supraclavicular node involvement compared with 11.0 months with ($p = 0.12$). In extensive-stage disease, supraclavicular nodes do not portend to either a better or worse prognosis. The authors concluded that "[the presence of] SCLN [supraclavicular lymph node] is highly correlated with extensive forms explaining its overall prognostic value. In limited disease, SCLN is only a minor poor prognostic factor, not justifying any amendment to the staging system currently used."

15.2.1.4 Isolated Ipsilateral Pleural Effusion

Patients with isolated ipsilateral pleural effusions present a particularly difficult classification dilemma. Published case series reach differing conclusions as to the prognosis of these patients. Comparable survival to other limited-stage patients has been noted [11, 12]. Other studies describe survival closer to patients with extensive disease and one site of metastasis [9, 13]. Dearing et al., on reviewing the United States National Cancer Institute (US NCI) experience, noted that the survival of these patients was identical to that of limited-stage patients treated with chemotherapy alone, not combined modality with chemotherapy and radiation [12]. Thus this report is not applicable to limited-stage patients treated with modern approaches. A 1982 review of the Southwest Oncology Group (SWOG) experience included 56 patients with ipsilateral pleural effusion as the only evidence of metastatic spread beyond the primary tumor and regional nodes [11]. These were patients who had participated in three consecutive studies between 1974 and 1980. Effusions were cytology-positive in 24 of the 56 patients. The median survival of 54 weeks for the patients with effusions was identical to the median survival of all patients classified as having limited-stage disease. Similar to the report by Dearing et al. [12], this study occurred prior to the current era of concurrent chemoradiotherapy. Subsequently, Albain et al. evaluated the SWOG database of 2,580 patients from 10 studies performed between 1976 and 1988 [13]. This larger study with more modern data demonstrated that patients with limited-stage disease and an ipsilateral pleural effusion had a median survival time that was not significantly different from that of patients with extensive-stage disease and a single metastatic lesion (13.0 months vs. 12.0 months, respectively; $p = 0.85$) and inferior to that of those with true limited-stage disease. An additional series analyzed 1,521 patients treated by the Cancer and Leukemia Group B (CALGB) on 5 multi-institutional studies between 1972 and 1986 [9]. As with the later SWOG report, they demonstrated that patients with a pleural effusion but otherwise limited-stage disease did not have a survival that was statistically different than that for patients with extensive-stage disease with a single metastatic site ($p = 0.51$). However, only 29 of their patients fit these criteria, and after adjusting for other prognostic factors the authors acknowledge having little statistical power to detect any difference. In fact, the absolute value for median survival of this group (11.4 months) was much closer to that for patients with limited-stage disease (12.3 months) than to that for patients with extensive-stage disease with a single metastatic site (8.6 months).

Although the literature regarding the prognostic value of ipsilateral effusions remains somewhat unclear, current standards in clinical investigation have effectively altered the staging of these patients. All US-NCI-sponsored cancer cooperative groups currently exclude ipsilateral effusions from limited-stage studies.

15.2.2 Extensive Stage

Disease beyond the ipsilateral lung, ipsilateral pleura, bilateral hilar, bilateral mediastinum, or bilateral supraclavicular fossa is considered unequivocally extensive stage. As noted earlier, there is some controversy regarding the staging of patients with isolated unilateral effusions. Extensive-stage patients have a uniformly poorer prognosis than limited-stage patients. It is also clear that the prognosis for patients with extensive-stage disease is quite variable. SWOG investigators evaluated their database of 2,580 patients entered onto prospective clinical trials [13] utilizing a recursive partitioning analysis, a statistical method in which a set of factors are analyzed for significance toward a certain outcome and then reanalyzed after discarding nonsignificant factors until the most statistically significant factors are found. For extensive-stage patients the only statistically significant determinant of outcome turned out to be serum lactate dehydrogenase (LDH) level. This factor will be discussed later in this chapter. A separate analysis, also employing recursive partitioning analysis, from the Toronto group [14], determined that Eastern Cooperative Oncology Group (ECOG) performance status 2 or 3, elevated serum alkaline phosphatase level, male sex, and the presence of liver metastases were significant predictors for poorer survival. In the analysis of the CALGB database [9], poor performance status and increasing number of metastatic sites predicted for a worse outcome.

15.2.2.1 Number of Metastatic Sites

The number of metastatic sites has been described in multiple series as predictive of survival within the extensive-stage category, [9, 14–16]. In both the SWOG and CALGB publications, a single metastatic site was a strong determinant of better survival. In the SWOG study, the presence of a single metastatic lesion was a significant favorable factor when compared to multiple sites or multiple lesions. The median survival of those with a single metastatic focus was 12.0 months, compared to 6.7 months for those patients with multiple metastatic foci. In comparison, the CALGB study looked at number of sites without regard to number of lesions per site; they showed that the median survival decreased as the number of sites increased.

15.2.2.2   Site of Metastasis

There is a paucity of data concerning the relative significance of different organ sites of disease. Brain metastases appear to carry the worst prognosis. In a report from the US NCI [12], patients with brain metastases had a median survival of 7 versus 8 and 10 months for liver and bone metastases, respectively. These groups were not directly compared and they did not represent groups with metastases only to these sites. The Toronto group found that liver metastases were determined statistically to be a branch point on the prognostic tree in extensive-stage patients [14]. Patients with extensive-stage disease but no liver metastases had a survival closer to that of limited-stage patients than did patients with extensive-stage disease with liver metastases. The reported median survival of patients with brain metastases was 10.5 versus 11.0 and 10.7 months for liver and bone, respectively. Again, these groups were not directly compared. The prognostic significance of the involvement of any specific organ is also determined by the bulk of disease present. No study is needed to state that massive liver disease will carry a worse prognosis than a single metastatic lesion.

15.3   Presenting Syndromes

15.3.1   Superior Vena Cave Syndrome

Patients with SCLC can present with several clinical syndromes, which in some cases carry prognostic significance. Superior vena cava (SVC) syndrome is one of the most common presentations of SCLC. Although dramatic, patients presenting with SVC syndrome have similar outcomes to patients with comparable stage [17, 18]. Investigators at the Royal Marsden Hospital (London, UK) carried out univariate and multivariate analyses of possible prognostic factors at presentation in 333 consecutive patients [19]. They found that SVC syndrome was not a predictor of survival. A German retrospective analysis of 408 cases of limited-stage SCLC with or without SVC syndrome [20] found that patients without SVC syndrome had 5-year survival rates and a median survival time of 11% and 13.7 months, respec-

tively. In comparison, patients with SVC syndrome had 5-year survival rates of 15% and a median survival time of 16.1 months. The difference was significant in univariate analysis. In multivariate analysis, SVC syndrome was a predictor of better outcome and the authors concluded that these patients should be treated with curative intent.

15.3.2   Syndrome of Inappropriate Antidiuretic Hormone

Patients with syndrome of inappropriate antidiuretic hormone (SIADH) present with low serum sodium levels as a result of ectopic antidiuretic hormone production. Several series indicate that these patients experience worse outcomes than patients without SIADH. A report of 371 patients treated with identical chemotherapy in the context of a large, prospectively randomized clinical trial demonstrated in multiple regression analysis that plasma sodium contributed independently to survival [21]. In a series of 98 patients treated with combination chemotherapy, patients who presented with SIADH had a worse prognosis than limited-stage patients who presented without SIADH. This was true even if they had achieved a complete response [22]. In another series of 815 patients, hyponatremia had a significant negative influence on the remission duration in limited-stage disease [23].

15.3.3   Cushing's Syndrome

Cushing's syndrome resulting from ectopic corticotropin (adrenocorticotropic hormone, ACTH) production can present with edema, proximal myopathy, elevated plasma and urinary free cortisol levels, hypokalemic alkalosis, and/or hyperglycemia. Several series have demonstrated that this presentation carries adverse prognostic significance. The Toronto group in an analysis of 545 patients demonstrated that patients with Cushing's syndrome have a low response to chemotherapy, short survival, and a high rate of complication to therapy [24]. Twenty-three patients (4.5%) presented with Cushing's syndrome and ectopic ACTH production. The response rate (complete plus partial) to chemotherapy for patients who had the syndrome diagnosed at initial presentation of SCLC was only 46%, and their median survival was only 3.6 months. Complications of therapy included gastrointestinal (GI) ulceration (six patients), GI bleeding (four), perforation of a duodenal ulcer (one), pneumonia (ten), septic shock (three), and fungal infections (five). Investigators from University of Texas MD Anderson Cancer Center have attributed this poor survival to the severe opportunistic infections associated with chemotherapy, leading to clinical deterioration and death before antineoplastic benefit from chemotherapy could be achieved [25]. In their study of patients surviving less than 90 days, 82% of patients with Cushing's Syndrome (9 out of 11) died within 14 days of initiation of chemotherapy, compared with 25% of the control patients (19 out of 77). In 45% of the patients with Cushing's Syndrome (5 out of 11), death was attributed to opportunistic fungal or protozoal infection, compared with 8% of control patients (6 out of 77). The authors hypothesized that biochemical control of Cushing's Syndrome for at least 1–2 weeks before initiation of chemotherapy may ameliorate the poor prognosis.

15.4 Patient-Related Factors

Patient-related factors such as age, sex, performance status, and weight loss may be indicative of the severity of the disease at presentation as well as the underlying ability of a patient to tolerate treatment. The two largest series (from the CALGB and SWOG) of prognostic factors published [9, 13] are in agreement that older age, male sex, and poor performance status predict for worse survival outcome. In the SWOG series, age greater than 70 years, male sex in the limited-stage patients, and ECOG performance status worse than 1 were predictors of poor survival. In the CALGB series, age equal to or older than 60 years was a poor prognostic factor in the limited-stage patients, while male sex and a nonambulatory performance status were significant in both limited-stage and extensive-stage disease. The literature is replete with examples both supporting and refuting these conclusions on age [14, 26–32], sex [15, 30, 33], and performance status [15, 30, 32]. However, the statistical power of the CALGB and SWOG databases, with over 4,000 patients, make their conclusions the most definitive published to date.

15.5 Laboratory Findings

15.5.1 Serum LDH

Serum LDH is the most unequivocal laboratory marker of prognosis available. Second only to stage of disease, this parameter has been the most reliable and powerful prognostic factor. In a SWOG recursive partitioning analysis [13], the first branch point occurs at limited-stage versus extensive-stage disease. The second branch point (with a p value of < 0.00005) for both limited-stage and extensive-stage disease is LDH normal or elevated. The CALGB [14] evaluated 22 pretreatment parameters in 614 patients. The only characteristic in this multivariate analysis that is predictive of survival in the limited-stage patients was serum LDH above normal levels. In addition, the data suggested that the higher the level of LDH, the poorer the survival (55 weeks for LDH < 175 IU/l, 49 weeks for LDH = 175–275 IU/l, and 33 weeks for LDH > 275 IU/l; $p = 0.0001$). In a more modern series published from Norway [15], Bremnes et al. analyzed the pretreatment characteristics of 436 patients enrolled in a prospective, multicenter study. The investigators demonstrated serum LDH to be an independent prognostic factor in patients with extensive-stage disease. A Greek study of 516 patients showed elevated LDH to be a predictor of survival and duration of response [30], 1-year overall survival for patients with limited-stage disease has been reported to be 60.2% in patients with normal serum LDH levels and 33.1% in patients with higher serum LDH values ($p = 0.0017$) [34]. Multiple other series have described the significance of this laboratory finding on patient survival [11, 23, 35]. No other single test holds more prognostic information.

15.5.2 Serum Alkaline Phosphatase

Other laboratory findings have also been associated with poorer outcomes. In the prognostic staging system developed by the Toronto group, the worst prognostic category was defined by extent of disease, performance status, and serum alkaline phosphatase levels [14]. Levels higher than normal were associated with lower survival for patients with extensive-stage disease on both univariate and multivariate analysis. In the SWOG database, serum alkaline phosphatase levels higher than normal also had an adverse affect on survival in extensive-stage patients. This parameter was only marginally significant in the recursive partitioning analysis. In the Greek study, normal alkaline phosphatase was a favorable prognostic factor for survival, duration of response, and response [30].

15.5.3 Other Laboratory Findings

Hemoglobin levels and white blood cell count (WBC) have also been associated with survival in patients with limited-stage disease [14, 15]. In the Sagman data [14], WBC ≥ 10/dl was associated with poorer survival, while in the Bremnes data [15] both elevated WBC and low hemoglobin were predictors of poor survival.

15.6 Tumor Markers

15.6.1 Neuron-Specific Enolase

To date, no tumor marker has been definitively shown to hold significant prognostic value in patients with SCLC. Neuron-specific enolase (NSE) is the most sensitive tumor marker at initial diagnosis of SCLC, and its levels have been shown to correlate with extent of disease [36]. The value of this tumor marker as a prognostic factor, however, remains controversial; some studies have shown it to be a valuable prognostic indicator [37–39], while others have been unable to form the same conclusion [40–42]. A French study has suggested that normalization of NSE levels after 1 month of chemotherapy is a strong, independent early predictor of both complete response to therapy and survival [43]. Patients whose NSE normalized had a median survival and 2-year survival of 15.3 months and 21%, respectively, while those patients with persistent elevations had median and 2-year survivals of 8.1 months and 15%, respectively, when it was not ($p < 0.03$). Another study suggested a correlation between a decline in the NSE level at the time of remission and the duration of remission [39]. Despite encouraging results from some studies, no clear pattern has emerged in this tumor marker as a prognostic factor and it has not been widely adopted.

15.6.2   Carcinoembryonic Antigen

Similarly, carcinoembryonic antigen (CEA) has been investigated and met with mixed results [44–46]. CEA has been most extensively evaluated and is routinely utilized for the evaluation and follow-up of patients with colorectal cancer. However, a wide range of other malignancies including both SCLC and NSCLC can result in CEA elevations. In a series of 160 patients who had 619 CEA assays over 16 years, an Italian group demonstrated that CEA correlated only with treatment response, but held no other prognostic information. A Japanese group showed similar results in 66 consecutive patients, while a separate group suggested that patients with higher CEA levels had shorter survival than did patients with lower levels.

15.6.3   Pro-Gastrin Releasing Peptide

Pro-gastrin releasing peptide (Pro-GRP) has been shown to be a useful tumor marker that correlates with the presence and progression of disease in most reports, although it has not been adopted for routine clinical use [47–50]. Its value as a prognostic tool, however, has not been as consistently shown. In a report of 148 patients, Pujol et al. failed to show any relevance to survival for patients with elevated Pro-GRP levels [51]. Shibayama et al. also showed no significance to prognosis in a report of 142 patients [52]. In contrast, Sunaga et al. reported that 17 patients whose ratio of the Pro-GRP level after treatment to the level before treatment was below 50% (taking the levels before treatment as 100%) survived significantly longer than did the patients whose ratio was over 50% ($p < 0.01$) [53].

15.6.4   C-Kit Protein

The type III receptor tyrosine kinase C-kit protein (CD117) has been another target of research for its prognostic value. Several series have demonstrated that increased expression of this receptor is associated with worse survival [54–56], while others have not been able to confirm that conclusion [57, 58]. A phase II study using imatinib, a c-kit inhibitor, has been performed, but failed to show any antitumor affect of blocking the c-kit receptor [59], suggesting that if c-kit does hold prognostic value, it is not necessarily a good target for therapy. The current consensus is that the activity of imatinib requires activating mutations in c-kit, such as those found in chronic myelogenous leukemia, as opposed to simple overexpression.

15.6.5   Vascular Endothelial Growth Factor and Cyclooxygenase-2

Data regarding the potential prognostic or predictive value of vascular endothelial growth factor (VEGF) or cyclooxygenase (COX-2) levels in SCLC is scant and inconsistent. Two series have examined this, and unfortunately have arrived at differing conclusions. One study [60] examined serum taken from 68 untreated patients with SCLC at the time of diagnosis. The patients were treated with six cycles of cisplatin and etoposide, and were randomly assigned to receive recombinant interferon, leukocyte interferon, or neither. High serum levels of VEGF (> 527 pg/ml) were associated with poor survival and, in a multivariate analysis, serum VEGF and stage were the only independent prognostic factors. A separate series reviewed the clinical records from 54 cases of SCLC [61]. Immunohistochemical stains for VEGF and COX-2 were performed on all tumor specimens and no significant association was found between VEGF or COX-2 expression and survival.

15.6.6   Matrix Metalloproteinases

Matrix metalloproteinases (MMPs) are a family of zinc-containing proteolytic enzymes that are believed to facilitate tumor invasion, the establishment of metastases, and the promotion of tumor-related angiogenesis. It has been suggested that high levels of these proteins in patients with SCLC are associated with a poorer survival [62]. This study has not been replicated. A phase III study of marimastat, an MMP inhibitor, showed no improvement in survival and a worse quality of life [63].

15.6.7 Fragile Histidine Triad

The fragile histidine triad protein (FHIT) is a putative tumor suppressor and has been examined as a possible prognostic factor in patients with SCLC. In a recent report from Germany, the tumors of 225 patients were examined retrospectively for FHIT expression [64]. Lack of FHIT was significantly associated with a shorter survival time for patients, with a median of 157 ± 18 days compared with 210 ± 18 days for those patients with FHIT-positive tumors ($p = 0.0061$). Furthermore, the proportion of FHIT-positive cells within the tumor was related to survival. Patients with tumors of $< 25\%$ FHIT-positive cells had the worst survival of 155 ± 21 days, compared with 217 ± 19 days for patients with a proportion of $\geq 25\%$ of FHIT-expressing tumor cells ($p = 0.0016$). Further studies will be required to validate these results.

15.6.8 P53

The tumor-suppressor gene, *p53*, has been studied extensively in many different tumor histologies, but its prognostic significance in SCLC has not been consistently proven. Zereu et al. examined paraffin sections of 58 transbronchial biopsy specimens from patients with SCLC [65]. They found that there was a significant correlation between *p53* expression and limited-stage disease ($P < 0.001$), but expression was not correlated with disease-free survival. In a separate analysis, *p53* expression seemed to predict for survival when combined with expression of integrin beta1 [66]. Oshita et al. showed that the overall survival of patients with high expression of both integrin beta1 and *p53* was significantly worse than those of individuals whose tumors had low expressions of both ($p < 0.05$). Moreover, the overall survival of patients with a high expression of either integrin beta1 or *p53* ($n = 42$) was significantly worse than that of other patients without high expression of both integrin beta1 and *p53* ($p < 0.05$). These results suggest that p53 in isolation does not have prognostic value, but if examined as part of a gene-expression profile then some predictive value may be displayed, but this remains to be proven. In addition to *p53* expression, investigators have examined serum p53 antibodies as a simple, reproducible test for prognosis. However, this surrogate has also proven to be an ineffectual predictor of prognosis [67, 68].

15.6.9 Hu and Voltage-Gated Calcium Channel Antibodies

Other antibodies that have been studied include Hu antibody, which is associated with SCLC and paraneoplastic encephalomyelitis or sensory neuropathy, and voltage-gated calcium channel (VGCC) antibodies, which are associated with Lambert Eaton myasthenic syndrome. Hu antibodies have been shown to correlate quite significantly with response to chemotherapy [69]. However, neither Hu nor VGCC antibodies have turned out to be independent predictors of survival for patients with SCLC [69, 70]. Investigators from Norway examined the serum of 200 patients with SCLC receiving chemotherapy for the presence of Hu and VGCC antibodies. They found that the presence of Hu antibodies did not correlate with VGCC antibodies, and there was no association between Hu or VGCC antibodies and the extent of disease or survival.

Key Points

- The most important prognostic factor for small-cell lung cancer is stage: limited versus extensive. The second most important predictor for improved survival in both limited and extensive stage patients is a normal serum lactate dehydrogenase level.
- In limited-stage patients, improved survival may be seen with a TNM stage I tumor, better performance status, and female gender, while supraclavicular nodal involvement and ipsilateral pleural effusion have not consistently shown worsened survival.
- Currently, most groups have reassigned patients with ipsilateral pleural effusion or pericardial effusion to the extensive disease category. The classification of patients with supraclavicular adenopathy remains controversial.
- In extensive-stage patients, improved survival is seen with a solitary metastatic site, while worsened survival is associated with an increasing number of metastatic sites, worse performance status, male sex, and elevated serum alkaline phosphatase levels. No one site of metastasis has been consistently shown to be worse than any other site.
- Presenting with superior vena cava syndrome does not predict for worsened survival, but presenting with inappropriate antidiuretic hormone syndrome or Cushing's syndrome does.
- Tumor markers such as neuron-specific enolase and carcinoembryonic antigen, among others, have not consistently shown prognostic value.
- While numerous molecular variables have been analyzed and described as prognostic, none has yet entered routine clinical practice.

References

1. Zelen M. Keynote address on biostatistics and data retrieval. Cancer Chemother Rep 3 1973; 4(2):31.
2. Mountain CF. Revisions in the International System for Staging Lung Cancer. Chest 1997; 111(6):1710.
3. Chute CG, Greenberg ER, Baron J, et al. Presenting conditions of 1539 population-based lung cancer patients by cell type and stage in New Hampshire and Vermont. Cancer 1985; 56:2107.
4. Turrisi AT, Kim K, Blum R, et al. Twice-daily compared with once-daily thoracic radiotherapy in limited small-cell lung cancer treated concurrently with cisplatin and etoposide. N Engl J Med 1999; 340(4):265.
5. Stahel R, Aisner J, Ginsberg R, et al. Staging and prognostic factors in small cell lung cancer. Lung Cancer 1989; 5:119.
6. Shepherd FA, Ginsberg RJ, Haddad R, et al. Importance of clinical staging in limited small-cell lung cancer: a valuable system to separate prognostic subgroups. The University of Toronto Lung Oncology Group. J Clin Oncol 1993; 11:1592.
7. Shields TW, Higgins GA Jr, Matthews MJ, Keehn RJ. Surgical resection in the management of small cell carcinoma of the lung. J Thorac Cardiovasc Surg 1982; 84(4):481.
8. Bonner JA, Sloan JA, Shanahan TG, et al. Phase III comparison of twice-daily split-course irradiation versus once-daily irradiation for patients with limited stage small-cell lung carcinoma. J Clin Oncol 1999; 17(9):2681.
9. Spiegelman D, Maurer LH, Ware JH, et al. Prognostic factors in small-cell carcinoma of the lung: an analysis of 1,521 patients. J Clin Oncol 1989; 7(3):344.
10. Urban T, Chastang C, Vaylet F, et al. Prognostic significance of supraclavicular lymph nodes in small cell lung cancer: a study from four consecutive clinical trials, including 1,370 patients. "Petites Cellules" Group. Chest 1998; 114(6):1538.
11. Livingston RB, McCracken JD, Trauth CJ, Chen T. Isolated pleural effusion in small cell lung carcinoma: favorable prognosis. A review of the Southwest Oncology Group experience. Chest 1982; 81(2):208.
12. Dearing MP, Steinberg SM, Phelps R, Anderson MJ, Mulshine JL, Ihde DC, Johnson BE. Outcome of patients with small-cell lung cancer: effect of changes in staging procedures and imaging technology on prognostic factors over 14 years. J Clin Oncol 1990; 8(6):1042.
13. Albain KS, Crowley JJ, LeBlanc M, Livingston RB. Determinants of improved outcome of small-cell lung cancer: an analysis of the 2, 580-patient Southwest Oncology Group database. J Clin Oncol 1990; 8(9):1563.
14. Sagman U, Maki E, Evans WK, et al. Small-cell carcinoma of the lung: derivation of prognostic staging system. J Clin Oncol 1991; 9(9):1639.
15. Bremnes RM, Sundstrom S, Aasebo U, Kaasa S, Hatlevoll R, Aamdal S. Norwegian Lung Cancer Study Group. The value of prognostic factors in small cell lung cancer: results from a randomized multicenter study with minimum 5 year follow-up. Lung Cancer 2003; 39(3):303.
16. Tas F, Aydiner A, Topuz E, Camlica H, Saip P, Eralp Y. Factors influencing the distribution of metastases and survival in extensive disease small cell lung cancer. Acta Oncol 1999; 38(8):1011.
17. Murray N, Coy P, Pater JL, et al. Importance of timing for thoracic irradiation in the combined modality treatment of limited-stage small-cell lung cancer. The National Cancer Institute of Canada Clinical Trials Group. J Clin Oncol 1993; 11(2):336.
18. Perry MC, Eaton WL, Propert KJ, et al. Chemotherapy with or without radiation therapy in limited small-cell carcinoma of the lung. N Engl J Med 1987; 316(15):912.
19. Vincent MD, Ashley SE, Smith IE. Prognostic factors in small cell lung cancer: a simple prognostic index is better than conventional staging. Eur J Cancer Clin Oncol 1987; 23(11):1589.
20. Wurschmidt F, Bunemann H, Heilmann HP. Small cell lung cancer with and without superior vena cava syndrome: a multivariate analysis of prognostic factors in 408 cases. Int J Radiat Oncol Biol Phys 1995; 33(1):77.
21. Souhami RL, Bradbury I, Geddes DM, Spiro SG, Harper PG, Tobias JS. Prognostic significance of laboratory parameters measured at diagnosis in small cell carcinoma of the lung. Cancer Res 1985; 45(6):2878.
22. Harper PG, Souhami RL, Spiro SG, Geddes DM, Guimaraes M, Fearon F, Smyth JF. Tumor size, response rate, and prognosis in small cell carcinoma of the bronchus treated by combination chemotherapy. Cancer Treat Rep 1982; 66(3):463.
23. Osterlind K, Hansen HH, Dombernowsky P, Hansen M, Andersen PK. Determinants of complete remission induction and maintenance in chemotherapy with or without irradiation of small cell lung cancer. Cancer Res 1987; 47(10):2733.
24. Shepherd FA, Laskey J, Evans WK, Goss PE, Johansen E, Khamsi F. Cushing's syndrome associated with ectopic corticotropin production and small-cell lung cancer. J Clin Oncol 1992; 10(1):21.
25. Dimopoulos MA, Fernandez JF, Samaan NA, Holoye PE, Vassilopoulou-Sellin R. Paraneoplastic Cushing's syndrome as an adverse prognostic factor in patients who die early with small cell lung cancer. Cancer 1992; 69(1):66.
26. Gronowitz JS, Bergstrom R, Nou E, et al. Clinical and serologic markers of stage and prognosis in small cell lung cancer. A multivariate analysis. Cancer 1990; 66:722.
27. Rawson NS, Peto J. An overview of prognostic factors in small cell lung cancer. A report from the Subcommittee for the Management of Lung Cancer of the United Kingdom Coordinating Committee on the Cancer Research. [published erratum in Br J Cancer 62:550] Br J Cancer 1990; 61:597.
28. Siu LL, Shepard FA, Murray N, et al. Influence of age on treatment of limited-stage small-cell lung cancer. J Clin Oncol 1996; 14:821.
29. Osterlind K, Anderson PK. Prognostic factors in small cell lung cancer: multivariate model based on 778 patients treated with chemotherapy with or without irradiation. Cancer Res 1986; 46(8):4189.
30. Christodolou C, Pavlidis N, Samantas E, et al. Prognostic factors in Greek patients with small cell lung cancer (SCLC). A Hellenic Cooperative Oncology Group study. Anticancer Res 2002; 22(6B):3749.
31. Cerny T, Blair V, Anderson H, Bramwell V, Thatcher N. Pretreatment prognostic factors and scoring system in 407 small-cell lung cancer patients. Int J Cancer 1987; 39(2):146.
32. Pignon JP, Arriagada R, Ihde DC, et al. A meta-analysis of thoracic radiotherapy for small-cell lung cancer. N Engl J Med 1992; 327(23):1618.
33. Wolf M, Holle R, Hans K, et al. Analysis of prognostic factors in 766 patients with small cell lung cancer: the role of sex as a predictor for survival. Br J Cancer 1991; 63:986.
34. Tas F, Aydiner A, Demir C, Topuz E (2001). Serum lactate dehydrogenase levels at presentation predict outcome of patients with limited-stage small-cell lung cancer. Am J Clin Oncol 2001; 4(4):376.
35. Byhardt RW, Hartz A, Libnoch JA, Hansen R, Cox JD. Prognostic influence of TNM staging and LDH levels in small cell carcinoma of the lung (SCCL). Int J Radiat Oncol Biol Phys 1986; 2(5):771.

36. Carney DN, Marangos PJ, Ihde DC, Bunn PA Jr, Cohen MH, Minna JD, Gazdar AF. Serum neuron-specific enolase: a marker for disease extent and response to therapy of small-cell lung cancer. Lancet 1982; 1:583.

37. Jorgensen LGM, Osterlind K, Genolle J, et al. Serum neuron-specific enolase (S-NSE) and the prognosis in small-cell lung cancer (SCLC): a combined multivariate analysis on data from nine centres. Br J Cancer 1996; 74:463.

38. Harding M, McAllister J, Hulks G, et al. Neuron specific enolase (NSE) in small cell lung cancer: a tumour marker for prognostic significance? Br J Cancer 1990; 61:605.

39. Johnson PWM, Joel SP, Love S, et al. Tumour markers for prediction of survival and monitoring of remission in small cell lung cancer. Br J Cancer 1993; 67:760.

40. Gomm SA, Keevil BG, Thatcher N, Hastleton PS, Swindell RS. The value of tumour markers in lung cancer. Br J Cancer 1988; 58:797.

41. Van Der Gaast A, Van Putten WLJ, Oosterom R, Cozijnsen M, Hoekstra R, Splinter TA. Prognostic value of serum thymidine kinase, tissue polypeptide antigen and neuron specific enolase in patients with small cell lung cancer. Br J Cancer 1991; 64:369.

42. Ebert W, Muley T, Trainer C, Dienemann H, Drings P. Comparison of changes in the NSE levels with clinical assessment in the therapy monitoring of patients with SCLC. Anticancer Res 2002; 22(2B):1083.

43. Fizazi K, Cojean I, Pignon JP, et al. Normal serum neuron specific enolase (NSE) value after the first cycle of chemotherapy: an early predictor of complete response and survival in patients with small cell lung carcinoma. Cancer 1998; 82(6):1049.

44. Buccheri G, Ferrigno D. Serum biomarkers or non-neuron-endocrine origin in small-cell lung cancer: a 16-year study on carcinoembryonic antigen, tissue polypeptide antigen and lactate dehydrogenase. Lung Cancer 2000; 30(1):37.

45. Niho S, Nishiwaki Y, Goto K, et al. Significance of serum pro-gastrin-releasing peptide as a predictor of relapse of small cell lung cancer: comparative evaluation with neuron-specific enolase and carcinoembryonic antigen. Lung Cancer 2000; 27(3):159.

46. Bandoh S, Fujita J, Ueda Y, et al. Expression of carcinoembryonic antigen in peripheral-or central-located small cell lung cancer: its clinical significance. Jpn J Clin Oncol 2001; 31(7):305.

47. Schneider J, Philipp M, Salewski L, Velcovsky HG. Pro-gastrin-releasing peptide (ProGRP) and neuron specific enolase (NSE) in therapy control of patients with small-cell lung cancer. Clin Lab 2003; 49(1-2):35.

48. Oremek GM, Sapoutzis N. Pro-gastrin-releasing peptide (Pro-GRP), a tumor marker for small cell lung cancer. Anticancer Res 2003; 23(2A):895.

49. Okusaka T, Eguchi K, Kasai T, et al. Serum levels of pro-gastrin-releasing peptide for follow-up of patients with small cell lung cancer. Clin Cancer Res 1997; 3(1):123.

50. Lamy P, Grenier J, Kramer A, Pujol JL. Pro-gastrin-releasing peptide, neuron specific enolase and chromogranin A as serum markers of small cell lung cancer. Lung Cancer 2000; 29(3):197.

51. Pujol JL, Quantin X, Jacot W, Boher JM, Grenier J, Lamy PJ. Neuroendocrine and cytokeratin serum markers as prognostic determinants of small cell lung cancer. Lung Cancer 2003; 39(2):131.

52. Shibayama T, Ueoka H, Nishii K, et al. Complementary roles of pro-gastrin-releasing peptide (ProGRP) and neuron specific enolase (NSE) in diagnosis and prognosis of small-cell lung cancer (SCLC). Lung Cancer 2001; 32(1):61.

53. Sunaga N, Tsuchiya S, Minato K, et al. Serum pro-gastrin-releasing peptide is a useful marker for treatment monitoring and survival in small-cell lung cancer. Oncology 1999; 57(2):143.

54. Naeem M, Dahiya M, Clark JI, Creech SD, Alkan S. Analysis of c-kit protein expression in small-cell lung carcinoma and its implication for prognosis. Hum Pathol 2002; 33(12):1182.

55. Micke P, Basrai M, Faldum A, et al. Characterization of c-kit expression in small cell lung cancer: prognostic and therapeutic implications. Clin Cancer Res 2003; 9(1):188.

56. Rohr UP, Rehfeld N, Pflugfelder L, et al. Expression of the tyrosine kinase c-kit is an independent prognostic factor in patients with small cell lung cancer. Int J Cancer 2004; 111(2):259.

57. Potti A, Moazzam N, Ramar K, Hanekom DS, Kargas S, Koch M. CD117 (c-KIT) overexpression in patients with extensive-stage small-cell lung carcinoma. Ann Oncol 2003; 14(6):894.

58. Boldrini L, Ursino S, Gisfredi S, et al. Expression and mutational status of c-kit in small-cell lung cancer: prognostic relevance. Clin Cancer Res 2004; 10(12 Pt 1):4101.

59. Johnson BE, Fischer T, Fischer B, et al. Phase II study of imatinib in patients with small cell lung cancer. Clin Cancer Res 2003; 9(16 Pt 1):5880.

60. Salven P, Ruotsalainen T, Mattson K, Joensuu H. High pre-treatment serum level of vascular endothelial growth factor (VEGF) is associated with poor outcome in small-cell lung cancer. Int J Cancer 1998; 79(2):144.

61. Dowell JE, Amirkhan RH, Lai WS, Frawley WH, Minna JD. Survival in small cell lung cancer is independent of tumor expression of VEGF and COX-2. Anticancer Res 2004; 24(4):2367.

62. Michael M, Babic B, Khokha R, et al. Expression and prognostic significance of metalloproteinases and their tissue inhibitors in patients with small-cell lung cancer. J Clin Oncol 1999 ; 17(6):1802.

63. Shepherd FA, Giaccone G, Seymour L, et al. Prospective, randomized, double-blind, placebo-controlled trial of marimastat after response to first-line chemotherapy in patients with small-cell lung cancer: a trial of the National Cancer Institute of Canada-Clinical Trials Group and the European Organization for Research and Treatment of Cancer. J Clin Oncol 2002; 20(22):4434.

64. Rohr UP, Rehfeld N, Geddert H, et al. Prognostic relevance of fragile histidine triad protein expression in patients with small cell lung cancer. Clin Cancer Res 2005; 11(1):180.

65. Zereu M, Vinholes JJ, Zettler CG. p53 and Bcl-2 protein expression and its relationship with prognosis in small-cell lung cancer. Lung Cancer 2003; 4(5):298.

66. Oshita F, Kameda Y, Hamanaka N, Saito H, Yamada K, Noda K, Mitsuda A. High expression of integrin beta 1 and p53 is a greater poor prognostic factor than clinical stage in small-cell lung cancer. Am J Clin Oncol 2004; 27(3):215.

67. Rosenfeld MR, Malats N, Schramm L, et al. Serum anti-p53 antibodies and prognosis of patients with small-cell lung cancer. J Natl Cancer Inst 1997; 89(5):381.

68. Jassem E, Bigda J, Dziadziuszko R, et al. Serum p53 antibodies in small cell lung cancer: the lack of prognostic relevance. Lung Cancer 2001; 31(1):17.

69. Graus F, Dalmou J, Rene R, et al. Anti-Hu antibodies in patients with small-cell lung cancer: association with complete response to therapy and improved survival. J Clin Oncol 1997; 15(8):2866.

70. Monstad SE, Drivsholm L, Storstein A, et al. Hu and voltage-gated calcium channel (VGCC) antibodies related to the prognosis of small-cell lung cancer. J Clin Oncol 2004; 22(5):795.

Section IV:
Management of Localized Non-Small-Cell Lung Cancer

Surgical Management of Localized and Locally Advanced Non-Small-Cell Lung Cancer

16

George Ladas

Contents

16.1 Introduction

Lung cancer was a rare disease at the beginning of the 20th century, but now, mainly as a result of smoking, it presents a significant health problem, with 170,000 new cases being diagnosed annually in the USA alone. It is also an extremely lethal disease, responsible for more deaths than any other solid tumor, and it accounts for nearly 1,000,000 deaths worldwide every year [1]. Surgical resection still remains the best treatment option when the disease is localized, but unfortunately up to 70% of patients have advanced, inoperable disease at the time of presentation, which highlights the need for early diagnosis [2]. The reported cumulative 5-year survival for patients with primary lung cancer treated with resection has increased from 23% in 1960 to about 54% in 1990, but this improvement is largely due to better patient selection. Whilst the role of surgery is clear in early tumors, the task of identifying subsets of patients with locally advanced disease who can still benefit from extended resections represents a major challenge for the modern thoracic surgeon. Similarly, the use of parenchyma-sparing techniques allows us to perform curative resections in patients with otherwise prohibitive lung function. Unfortunately, more than 85% of lung cancer patients are expected to die ultimately from the disease, even though approximately 35% of them are surgical candidates.

16.2 Historical Note

Successful resection of lung cancer was first reported in the end of the 19th century. The first dissection lobectomy for lung cancer was performed by Hugh Moriston

Davies in 1912, but the patient unfortunately died from empyema 8 days later [3].

The development of underwater pleural cavity drainage heralded the modern era of thoracic surgery in general and lung cancer surgery in particular. The first successful one-stage lobectomy was reported by Brunn [4]. However, it was the historically successful pneumonectomy by Graham [5] that led to the popularity and standardization of the surgical treatment of lung cancer, with pneumonectomy being the procedure of choice [6]. Further milestones were the introduction of segmentectomy [7], radical pneumonectomy with en bloc mediastinal nodal resection [8], and bronchoplastic (sleeve) resection by Price-Thomas in 1947 [9].

16.3 Preoperative Assessment

The number and nature of preoperative investigations necessary for the selection of patients for surgery differs from one patient to the another, but the aim is always to answer the two fundamental questions that define suitability for surgical treatment: (1) Is the extent of the disease as defined by staging amenable to surgery? and (2) Is the patient fit enough for the planned procedure? Clearly, the answer to both of these questions must be affirmative before embarking on surgery.

16.3.1 Staging

Pretreatment staging is a logical and progressive process to obtain sufficient information to arrive at a treatment decision. Accurate staging is the mainstay of the modern multidisciplinary approach to the management of lung cancer. Since 1986 the international tumor, node, metastasis (TNM) system has been used universally for the staging of lung cancer [10]. Briefly, tumors confined within the parenchyma without regional or distal metastases are classified as stage I. Tumors that involve the peribronchial or hilar lymph nodes (level N1) or extend directly to invade the chest wall, diaphragm, or pericardium (T3) but without any nodal involvement are stage II. Locally advanced tumors with mediastinal or distal nodal involvement or invasion of noble mediastinal structures or the vertebral bodies, or presenting with a malignant pleural effusion are stage III. Finally, tumors with hematogenous metastases, either intrapulmonary or distant, are stage IV.

Clinical and surgical preoperative staging is aimed at identifying those patients who are candidates for a complete resection and are therefore likely to benefit from surgery. The 5-year survival following complete resection for lung cancer is stage dependent, whilst incomplete resection is very unlikely to result in cure.

Complete resection of stage IA tumors results in 5-year survival rates of 60–70% [11]. It has to be kept in mind that the staging system was constructed so as to reflect the worsening prognosis of increasingly advanced disease, and only a small minority of highly selected patients in advanced stages will be candidates for surgery.

Several studies have highlighted the limitations of clinical staging. Fernando reported an accuracy of clinical staging with the use of helical computed tomography (CT) scan and mediastinoscopy of 55.3% for nodal status, 81.6% for tumor status, and 46.6% for tumor and nodal status combined, as assessed by pathological staging [12]. Although positron emission tomography (PET) scanning shows some promise [13], it is crucial that the surgeon performs a thorough intraoperative staging as an integral part of every operation for lung cancer in order to optimize and finalize his treatment plan. Specifically, a systematic nodal dissection (SND) has been accepted by the International Association for the Study of Lung Cancer, to be an important component of intrathoracic staging [14, 15].

16.3.2 Fitness for Surgery

For some patients this assessment can be completed quickly during a single outpatient consultation, but for others an admission to hospital and complex investigations will be required before a decision can be reached. Often, a period of optimization with smoking cessation, intensive physiotherapy, and bronchodilator treatment together with control of hypertension or arrhythmias, as required, is used before the final assessment, and also serves to prepare the patient best for the challenges ahead.

16.3.2.1 Age

The peak incidence of lung cancer in the UK occurs in patients between the age of 75 and 80 years [16], with over half of the 500,000 patients diagnosed annually worldwide being over 70 years old [17]. Whilst the risks of surgery do increase with advancing age, clearly the biological rather than the chronological age is more important. The fit elderly person with adequate organ function should be offered similar treatment to younger patients [18].

The mortality from lesser resections does not increase in elderly patients [19], but prolonged surgery and extensive resections do result in increased morbidity and mortality [20]. There is an intolerance to pneumonectomy in elderly patients, and the combination of ischemic heart disease and need for right pneumonectomy is a relative contraindication for surgery [21].

16.3.2.2 Pulmonary Function

An operation to completely resect a lung cancer by definition results in loss of lung parenchyma. In this sense, assessment of the respiratory function and reserves is pivotal in deciding fitness for surgery. Poor respiratory function not only leads to increased perioperative morbidity and mortality, but can also herald postoperative long-term disability and poor quality of life. The risks are proportional to the correlation between preoperative lung function and the extent of planned surgery.

A major cause of morbidity and mortality postoperatively is sputum retention. Spirometry is useful to depict the ability of a patient to generate adequately high airway flow rates and produce an effective cough, so serves as the initial selection tool. Patients who have a preoperative forced expiratory volume in 1 s (FEV_1) of more than 1.5 l for a lobectomy and more than 2 l for a pneumonectomy, when optimized with bronchodilators and in the absence of interstitial lung disease or unexpected disability due to dyspnea, require no further respiratory function tests and face a mortality rate of around 5% [22–25]. All patients who are not clearly operable on the basis of spirometry alone should proceed to have: (1) full lung function studies including estimation of lung transfer for carbon monoxide (TLCO) factor, (2) measurement of arterial blood gases and oxygen saturation at rest, and (3) quantitative isotope ventilation/perfusion (V/Q) lung scan, particularly if pneumonectomy is planned.

These data are used to calculate the estimated postoperative FEV_1 and TLCO, expressed as percentage of predicted for the patient's age, height, and gender. This can be achieved using either the regional perfusion values from the V/Q scan, or an anatomical equation, taking into account whether the segments to be removed are ventilated or obstructed. One often finds that the presence of a malignancy in a certain part of the lung results in diminished blood flow in that area, so that the physiological impact of resection is much smaller than initially anticipated (Fig. 16.1). Figure 16.2 shows a detailed algorithm for the selection of patients for surgery [25]. Patients who are classified as high risk for surgery should be considered for limited resections (segmentectomy) or referred for radiotherapy/chemotherapy.

16.3.2.3 Ischemic Heart Disease

Lung cancer usually affects those age groups most susceptible to ischemic heart disease. In addition, patients are often smokers, which puts them at a high risk of developing cardiovascular disease. Preexisting coronary

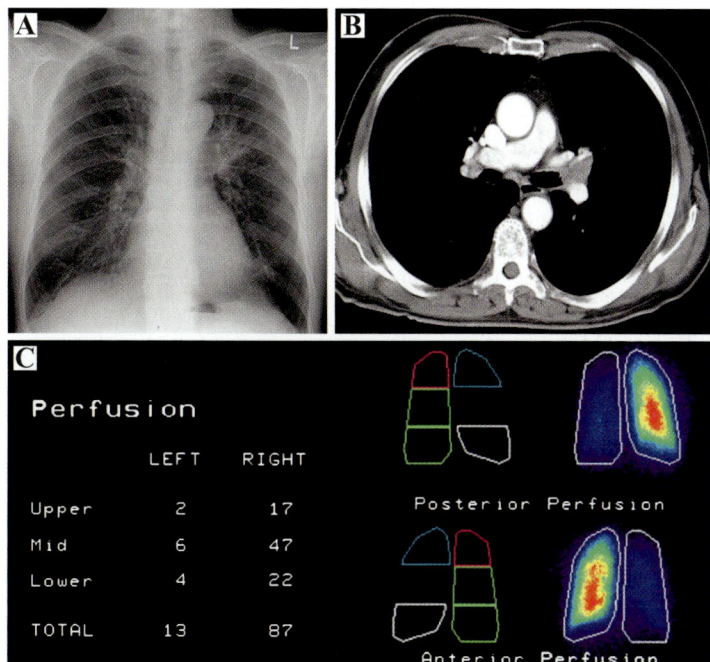

Fig. 16.1. A Chest radiograph of a patient with a left hilar opacity. **B** Computerized tomography scan (CT) of the same patient showing a left hilar mass, biopsy sampling at bronchoscopy confirmed squamous carcinoma. **C** Quantitative ventilation/perfusion scan (V/Q scan) shows that the whole of the left lung receives only 13% of the total perfusion, so the predicted post left pneumonectomy forced expiratory volume in 1 s (FEV_1) and lung transfer for carbon monoxide ($TLCO$) would be 87% of the preoperative values. *epoFEV$_1$* Estimated postoperative FEV_1, *preFEV$_1$* preoperative FEV_1, *segs.* segments, *SaO$_2$* arterial oxygen saturation, *epoTLCO* estimated postoperative TLCO, *ppoFEV$_1$* predicted postoperative FEV_1, *ppoTLCO* predicted postoperative TLCO, *VO$_2$* oxygen consumption

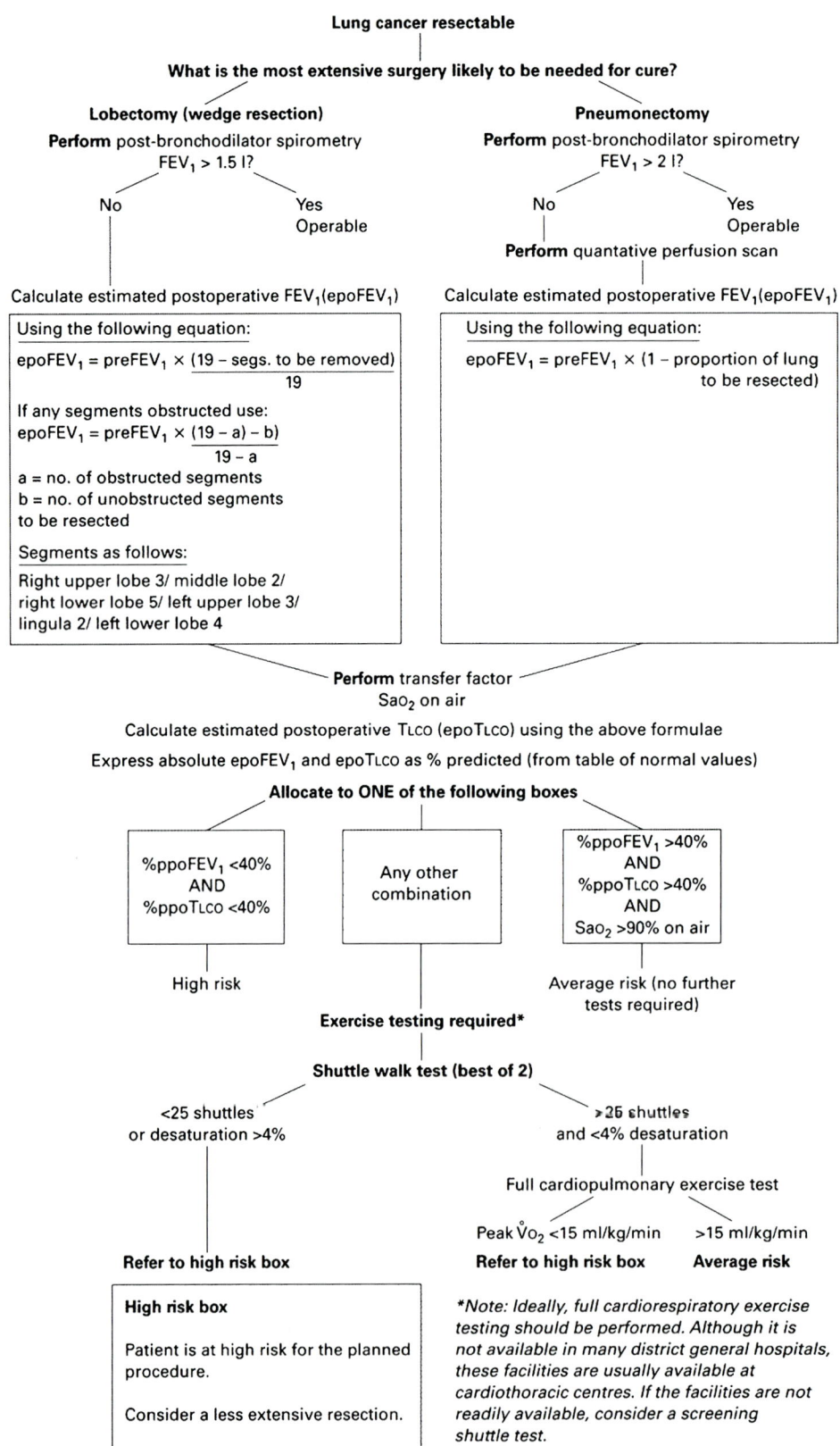

Lung cancer resectable

What is the most extensive surgery likely to be needed for cure?

Lobectomy (wedge resection)
Perform post-bronchodilator spirometry
$FEV_1 > 1.5$ l?

No   Yes
                     Operable

Calculate estimated postoperative FEV_1 (epoFEV_1)

Using the following equation:

$$epoFEV_1 = preFEV_1 \times \frac{(19 - \text{segs. to be removed})}{19}$$

If any segments obstructed use:
$$epoFEV_1 = preFEV_1 \times \frac{(19 - a) - b)}{19 - a}$$
a = no. of obstructed segments
b = no. of unobstructed segments
to be resected

Segments as follows:

Right upper lobe 3/ middle lobe 2/
right lower lobe 5/ left upper lobe 3/
lingula 2/ left lower lobe 4

Pneumonectomy
Perform post-bronchodilator spirometry
$FEV_1 > 2$ l?

No   Yes
                     Operable
Perform quantative perfusion scan

Calculate estimated postoperative FEV_1 (epoFEV_1)

Using the following equation:

$$epoFEV_1 = preFEV_1 \times (1 - \text{proportion of lung to be resected})$$

Perform transfer factor
Sao_2 on air

Calculate estimated postoperative T_{LCO} (epoT_{LCO}) using the above formulae

Express absolute epoFEV_1 and epoT_{LCO} as % predicted (from table of normal values)

Allocate to ONE of the following boxes

%ppoFEV_1 <40%
AND
%ppoT_{LCO} <40%

Any other
combination

%ppoFEV_1 >40%
AND
%ppoT_{LCO} >40%
AND
Sao_2 >90% on air

High risk

Exercise testing required*

Average risk (no further
tests required)

Shuttle walk test (best of 2)

<25 shuttles
or desaturation >4%

>25 shuttles
and <4% desaturation

Full cardiopulmonary exercise test

Peak $\overset{\circ}{V}o_2$ <15 ml/kg/min   >15 ml/kg/min

Refer to high risk box   **Refer to high risk box**   **Average risk**

High risk box

Patient is at high risk for the planned
procedure.

Consider a less extensive resection.

Consider radical radiotherapy.

*Note: Ideally, full cardiorespiratory exercise
testing should be performed. Although it is
not available in many district general hospitals,
these facilities are usually available at
cardiothoracic centres. If the facilities are not
readily available, consider a screening
shuttle test.*

Fig. 16.2. Algorithm for selection of patients suitable for resection for lung cancer [25]

artery disease increases the risk of nonfatal myocardial infarction (MI) or death within 30 days of noncardiac surgery [26, 27]. The risk of developing a second, perioperative MI steadily declines in the months following an initial MI, so when feasible, an operation should be delayed for at least 6 weeks [28]. In patients with angina, a full cardiological assessment, including exercise stress test, cardiac echocardiogram, thallium scan, and coronary angiography as required, will define whether there is scope for optimization with noninvasive or invasive means before lung surgery. Patients who undergo successful coronary artery bypass surgery are not at an increased risk from general surgical operations for at least 5 years after the procedure in the absence of new symptoms. The American College of Cardiology and the American Heart Association have published comprehensive guidelines for the clinical prediction of perioperative risk [26, 27, 29].

16.3.2.4 Performance Status

Performance status (as defined by the Karnofsky, World Health Organization – WHO – or European Cooperative Oncology Group – ECOG – scales) is correlated with prognosis in inoperable lung cancer [30]. In one surgical series of 331 patients, the Karnofsky score was not an independent predictor of complications, but only a few patients with poor performance had surgery [31]. Patients with a preoperative weight loss of 10% or more and/or a performance status of WHO 2 or worse are highly likely to have advanced disease and require a particularly thorough staging assessment and search for comorbidity [25].

16.4 Principles of Surgical Management

The goal of surgery in non-small-cell lung cancer (NSCLC) is to achieve complete resection of the primary tumor with no macroscopic tumor remaining and microscopically free margins. Only patients in whom a complete resection is anticipated are selected for surgery. These include patients with T1 to T4 and N0 to N1 tumors, and selected N2 patients. It is important to follow clear oncological principles in managing these potentially curable patients [32]:

1. Whenever possible, the tumor and all intrapulmonary lymphatic drainage should be removed completely, most frequently by lobectomy or pneumonectomy.
2. The tumor should not be disrupted during dissection to avoid spillage.
3. In case of direct invasion of extrapulmonary structures, en bloc resection is the treatment of choice rather than discontinuous resection.

4. Resection margins should be checked with frozen section analysis, including bronchial, vascular, and any other margins with close proximity to the tumor. If positive margins are encountered, wider excision should be performed when possible.
5. All accessible mediastinal lymph node stations should be removed for pathological evaluation. These should be clearly identified by the surgeon and properly labeled.

Surgical resection is the treatment of choice for early stage NSCLC and is generally offered to all patients with stage I and II disease and selected patients with stage III disease, but also the occasional, highly selected patient with solitary metastasis and completely resectable primary disease.

16.4.1 Intraoperative Strategy

At the time of thoracotomy, the surgeon should follow a clearly defined intraoperative strategy. This intrathoracic assessment should be performed in a noncommittal way, so that no structures are sacrificed until the final decision to resect is reached, and it aims to provide answers to four fundamental questions before proceeding to a resection: (1) What is the diagnosis? (2) Is the tumor resectable with a pneumonectomy? (3) If a pneumonectomy is feasible is it also justified by the extent of the disease? and (4) Can we then achieve complete resection with a lesser procedure?

16.4.1.1 What is the Diagnosis?

When a diagnosis is not available preoperatively, it is essential that confirmation of malignancy is secured at the time of thoracotomy, particularly if a pneumonectomy is anticipated. This can be achieved by either an incisional biopsy or a core needle biopsy of the tumor, and frozen-section examination. Obtaining a representative sample can be challenging when a small central tumor results in extensive distal obstructive pneumonitis and consolidation. Before any handling of the tumor takes place though, a pleural lavage is performed and the aspirate sent for cytology. We and others have found that in 4.5–9% of patients with apparently early stage NSCLC, pleural lavage cytology yields malignant cells. This micrometastatic disease has a devastating impact on survival and is an independent prognostic indicator for staging NSCLC, with a median survival of 13 months in patients with positive lavage cytology, compared with 49 months in patients with negative lavage cytology (Fig. 16.3) [33].

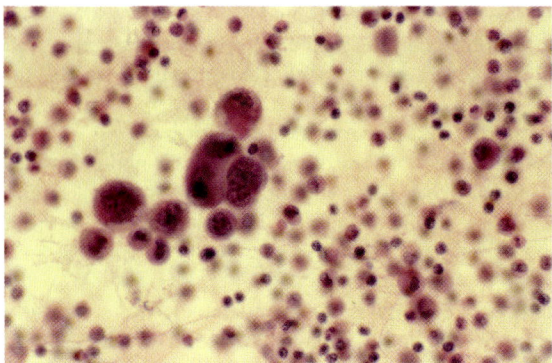

Fig. 16.3. Pleural lavage cytology. Malignant cells visible amidst normal mesothelial cells and lymphocytes

16.4.1.2 Is the Tumor Resectable with a Pneumonectomy?

Having confirmed malignancy, the surgeon must next define the T status of the tumor and confirm that it is resectable at least with a pneumonectomy in the worst-case scenario. This involves dissecting free the main pulmonary vessels and the main bronchus at the hilum, ready to be ligated and divided with tumor-free margins. When intrapericardial extension is suspected, then a limited pericardiotomy away from the phrenic nerve allows the assessment of resectability. Large T3 tumors directly extending to the chest wall will often require en bloc resection of the involved part of the chest wall, without the opportunity to first assess the hilum. This can be done with impunity, as long as a thorough preoperative staging including mediastinoscopy has demonstrated resectability and excluded N2 disease.

16.4.1.3 If a Pneumonectomy is Feasible is it also Justified by the Extent of the Disease?

A full reappraisal of the clinical staging in the light of the intrathoracic findings takes place at this point. The T status can change, for example, by the intraoperative confirmation or dismissal of clinically suspected invasion of adjacent structures, or indeed the discovery of satellite tumor nodules, altering the staging dramatically. What is extremely important is the final definition of N status, as this carries a major impact on prognosis. It is universally recognized that resection alone has no place in the management of patients with clinical N2 disease [34] and preoperative confirmation of mediastinal nodal involvement excludes the patient from primary surgery. An SND in each and every patient is now a recognized part of the intrathoracic staging and involves two separate steps.

Initially, the surgeon systematically resects lymph nodes from all accessible nodal stations of the ipsilateral mediastinum en bloc with the surrounding fat. The lymph nodes are clearly marked according to one of

the recognized nodal maps like the one proposed by Naruke (Figs. 16.4 and 16.5) [35]. These are then incised by the surgeon and appropriate samples from important stations are sent for frozen section, to define their status (Fig. 16.6). Whilst the mediastinal node specimens are processed the surgeon proceeds to systematically dissect and remove lymph nodes at the N1 level, which are then examined the same way. Efforts have been made to apply the principle of sentinel node biopsy in NSCLC patients, but the detection rate and sensitivity currently does not match the rates reported for breast cancer or melanoma, and the clinical usefulness of this method is limited [36]. At the Royal Brompton Hospital, the average number of nodal stations dissected per pneumonectomy patient is currently 9.3, rising to 12.5 for segmentectomy patients, compared to 8.5 nodal stations in exploratory (open-close) thoracotomies [37]. In our experience, this detailed assessment has led to the discovery of "unexpected" N2 disease in nearly 20% of the patients [14]. If this unexpected N2 involvement is limited to one nodal station then complete resection still results in an acceptable 5-year survival in the order of 20%, but multilevel involvement has poor prognosis and as such would not justify an extended resection such as a pneumonectomy [38]. SND is the only way to accurately define nodal status, allowing valid comparisons between patients. There is increasing evidence that SND appears to prolong relapse-free survival, with a borderline effect on overall survival in patients with limited nodal involvement [39, 40].

In the rare case where extensive unexpected mediastinal involvement is discovered intraoperatively, it is still possible to withdraw without performing a futile and possibly hazardous resection, since no structures have been sacrificed during the assessment up to this point.

16.4.1.4 Can we then Achieve Complete Resection with a Lesser Procedure?

Procedures involving removal of less than a whole lung are defined as "parenchyma sparing" and include wedge resection, segmentectomy, lobectomy, sleeve lobectomy, and bilobectomy. In order to decide whether a parenchyma-sparing operation is acceptable from the oncological point of view, the surgeon now has to assess the hilum and fissures for evidence of direct invasion by the tumor, of hilar structures supplying adjacent lobes or segments, as well as the presence and extent of N1 nodal disease. Examination of lymph nodes proceeds in a centrifugal fashion until the appropriate level of resection is defined. For example, a segmentectomy requires that the regional nodes down to level 13 (segmental) are shown to be normal on frozen section. There is no therapeutic benefit in performing a more extensive resection than that required to achieve complete resection

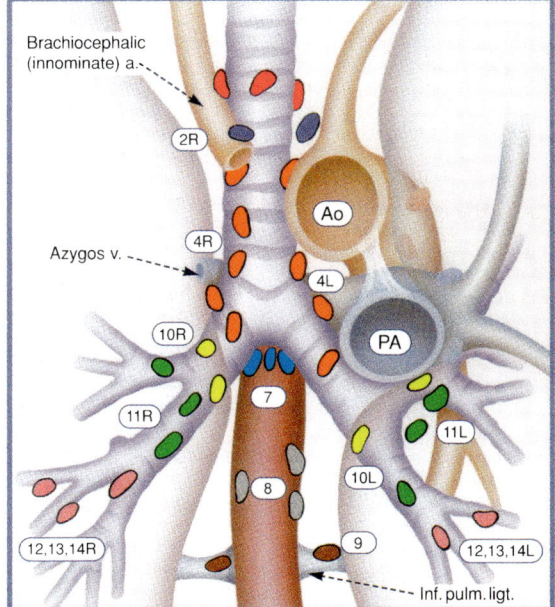

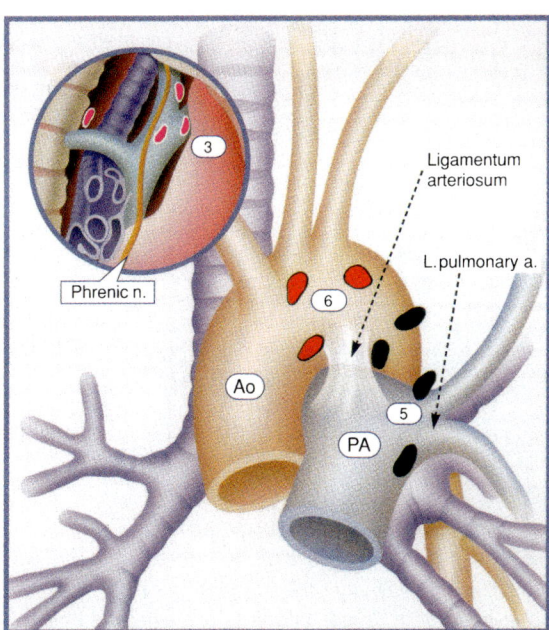

Fig. 16.4. Nodal station map

Superior Mediastinal Nodes

🔴 **1** Highest Mediastinal

🟣 **2** Upper Paratracheal

🔴 **3** Pre-vascular and Retrotracheal

🟠 **4** Lower Paratracheal
   (including Azygos Nodes)

N₂ = single digit, ipsilateral
N₃ = single digit, contralateral or supraclavicular

Aortic Nodes

⚫ **5** Subaortic (A-P window)

🔴 **6** Para-aortic (ascending
   aorta or phrenic)

Inferior Mediastinal Nodes

🔵 **7** Subcarinal

⚪ **8** Paraesophageal
   (below carina)

🟤 **9** Pulmonary Ligament

N₁ Nodes

🟡 **10** Hilar

🟢 **11** Interlobar

🔴 **12** Lobar

🔴 **13** Segmental

🔴 **14** Subsegmental

of the tumor as outlined above, although the Lung Cancer Study Group suggested that a lobectomy should be the minimum in patients with adequate pulmonary reserves [41]. Certainly, pneumonectomy does not offer any oncological advantage compared to lobectomy [42] and is actually associated with a shorter survival due to non-cancer-related mortality [43].

Bronchoplastic (sleeve) lobectomy is an excellent alternative to pneumonectomy in the appropriate circumstances, with low operative mortality and morbidity and excellent prognosis in addition to improved quality of life due to the sparing of lung parenchyma [44].

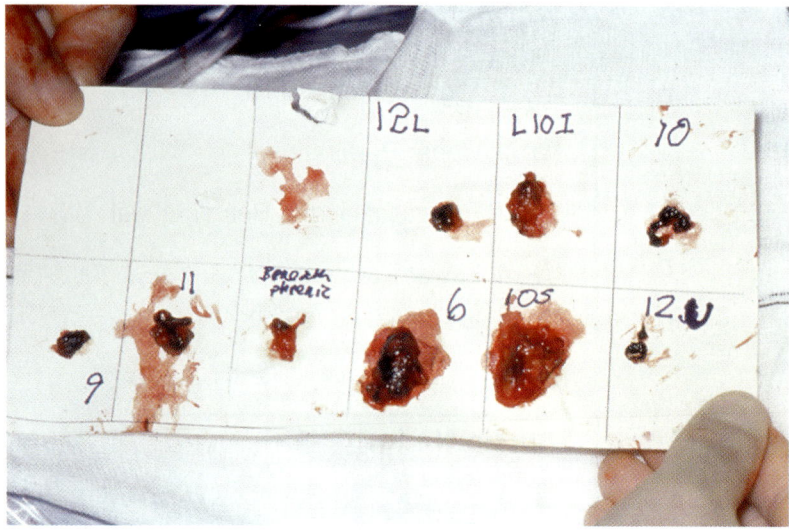

Fig. 16.5. Intrathoracic staging: lymph nodes harvested and labeled during systematic nodal dissection

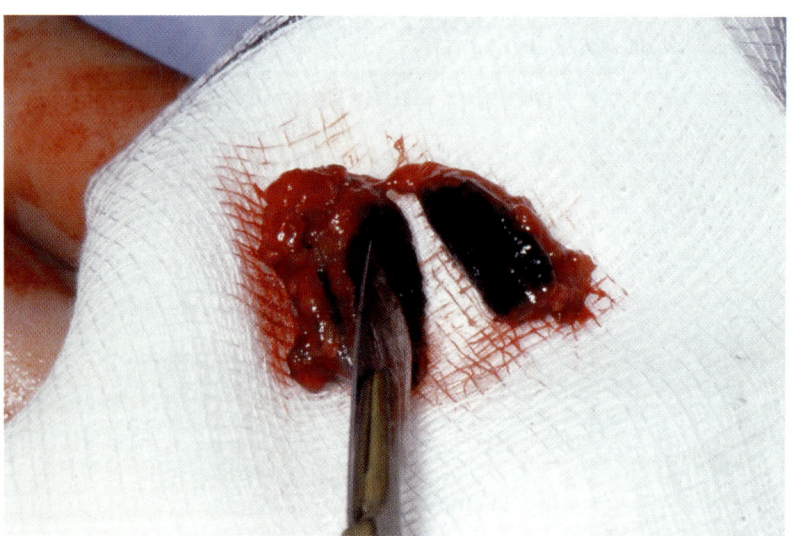

Fig. 16.6. Intrathoracic staging: nodes sectioned by the surgeon, specimens selected and sent for frozen section examination whilst the operation proceeds

16.5   Outline of Surgical Techniques

Only a brief outline is included here. A detailed description of thoracic surgical techniques is available elsewhere [45].

16.5.1   Anesthetic principles

Detailed invasive monitoring is essential in the intraoperative and early postoperative period for patients undergoing pulmonary resection for lung cancer. We would regularly perform rigid bronchoscopy right after the induction of anesthesia to confirm the endobronchial extent of the tumor and clarify the bronchial anatomy, which is particularly relevant when assessing the

need for a bronchoplastic resection. The use of one of various available designs of double-lumen endotracheal tube (Fig. 16.7) is essential in providing single-lung anesthesia. This technique allows full isolation and passive collapse of the operated lung whilst ventilation is diverted to the nonoperated side, which greatly facilitates surgical maneuvers. Accurate positioning of the double-lumen tube is critical and is often guided by the fiberoptic bronchoscope.

16.5.2   Thoracotomy

The majority of resections for lung cancer are performed via a posterolateral thoracotomy (Fig. 16.8) as it provides excellent exposure and versatility. Most surgeons use muscle-sparing techniques, where at least the

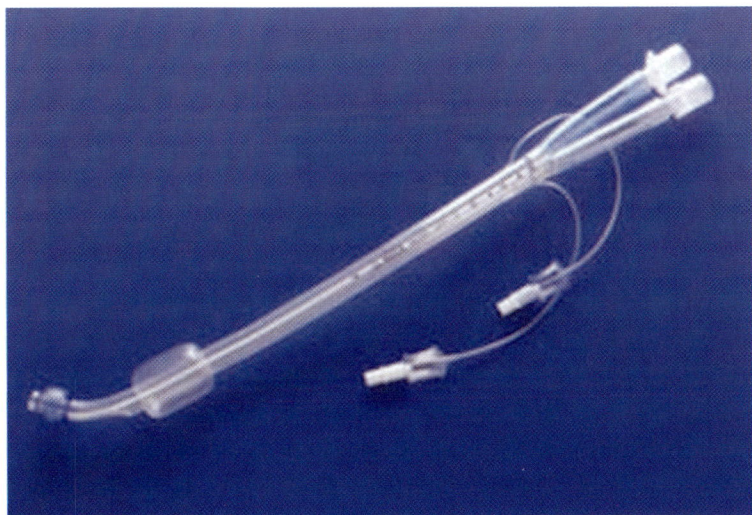

Fig. 16.7. A double-lumen endotracheal tube for single-lung anesthesia. The two lumens and the tracheal and bronchial cuffs are visible. Accurate positioning of the tube is crucial to avoid atelectasis

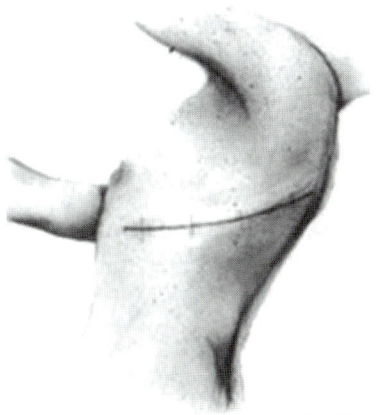

Fig. 16.8. The most commonly used incision is a posterolateral thoracotomy

serratus anterior and sometimes even the latissimus dorsi muscles are spared division.

Entry into the hemithorax is gained by dividing the intercostal muscles, usually at the level of the fifth interspace. The intercostal space is then widened with appropriate rib spreaders to obtain the necessary exposure. No ribs are removed or cut in the process, unless there is direct invasion by the tumor. At the end of the procedure, one or two interpleural drains are used and connected to underwater seal bottles. The ribs are reapproximated using pericostal sutures and the wound closed in layers.

16.5.3 Pneumonectomy and Lobectomy

Pneumonectomy means removal of a whole lung. The term "completion pneumonectomy" is used when a partial resection of this same lung (e.g., lobectomy) has taken place previously and removal of all remaining parenchyma is now performed. An anatomical resection of any part of the lung requires that the corresponding vessels and bronchi are secured and divided. In the case of pneumonectomy this involves ligation and division of the main pulmonary artery and the superior and inferior pulmonary veins, as well as the main bronchus. It has been suggested that the pulmonary veins draining the area of the tumor should be ligated first to limit shedding of cancer cells in the systemic circulation [46].

A pneumonectomy may be required even for small tumors if they directly invade the main hilar structures. Tumors arising in the apical segments of the lower lobes, or in the middle lobe in particular, can extend early to adjacent lobes across the fissures, making a more extensive resection necessary. Pneumonectomy carries an overall mortality rate of 6–8% [21, 47], but this increases significantly with advancing age, ischemic heart disease, right-sided procedure, and previous chemoradiotherapy [21, 47, 48]. Removal of one lobe is in principle much better tolerated by the patient and this is reflected in the lower reported mortality figures of 2–4% [21, 47, 48]. There seems to be no significant difference in the postoperative morbidity rates between lobectomy (28%) and pneumonectomy (31.9%) [47].

Overall survival results have changed little in 30 years and largely reflect TNM stage [42, 49], but comparison between historical [50] and modern series [51, 52] shows an improving trend, possibly due to better patient selection.

There are reports suggesting a potent adverse impact on long-term survival for stage I patients treated with pneumonectomy compared to those undergoing lesser resections, which stresses the need to preserve lung parenchyma whenever possible [43].

16.5.4   Sublobar Resections (Segmentectomy Wedge)

These techniques allow the removal of a usually small, peripheral tumor either by excising a nonanatomical wedge of lung tissue or, preferably, by resecting the relative bronchopulmonary segment. These are very useful in patients with limited pulmonary reserves who cannot tolerate a lobectomy and who are at the same time poor candidates for radical radiotherapy due to the risks of radiation pneumonitis and lung fibrosis. Anatomical segmentectomy is a superior technique from the oncological point of view but is technically much more demanding. Sublobar resections in general are ideally suited for stage I tumors. The reported operative mortality is low, ranging from 1.4 to 3.5% [53–56]. Local recurrence rates are higher than those following lobectomy, ranging between 14 and 23% [56, 57], and are much higher, reaching 59% when these techniques are used in stage III patients [55]. A recent prospective randomized study reported a 75% increase in overall and 300% in locoregional relapse rates following limited resection, compared to lobectomy [41]. There have been major criticisms of this study, however, the main one being that many nonanatomical wedge resections were included. There was no significant difference in survival in this study, but importantly, patients developing local recurrence following a wedge resection were then offered completion lobectomy. A number of reports have suggested that long-term survival is 5–10% lower with sublobar resections than following lobectomy [53, 57].

In our experience, an anatomical segmentectomy in the absence of nodal disease proximal to level 14 as confirmed by SND (see section 16.4.1.3) is an oncologically sound procedure for patients with limited reserves and stage I tumors, but meticulous surgical technique is crucial. The differential lung inflation technique after division of the segmental bronchus in order to develop the intersegmental plane is far superior to the blind application of a stapler as it helps ensure clear margins at this point.

Currently, whilst it is still generally accepted to perform a lobectomy as a minimum for patients with ample reserves even for limited lung cancer, an active effort is underway to redefine the role of sublobar resections. In a recent report by Koike and colleagues, from a series of 689 cases of cT1N0M0 tumors, 74 patients with tumors of 2 cm or less who underwent a limited resection had a survival rate of 89.1% [58].

16.5.5   Sleeve Resections

The term "sleeve resection" is used mainly to describe tracheoplastic and bronchoplastic resections, which allow the use of lobectomy and pneumonectomy procedures in circumstances where the tumor would normally lie at the resection margin. Therefore, a bronchoplastic lobectomy involves resecting a lobe en bloc with a sleeve of the main bronchus that is involved by tumor. The continuity of the remaining airways is then reestablished with a bronchial anastomosis, thus achieving a complete resection whilst avoiding a pneumonectomy. Equally, a sleeve pneumonectomy allows resection of a whole lung en bloc with the involved part of the main carina, followed by reanastomosis of the trachea to the stump of the contralateral main bronchus.

Sleeve lobectomies are technically demanding, but mortality rates range between 2.5 and 6% and are generally comparable to those for standard resections [59–62]. The somewhat increased incidence of local recurrence (17%) [62] is acceptable considering that these parenchyma-sparing procedures are used in patients who would otherwise be inoperable due to their poor lung function. There has been considerable interest in recent years in combined bronchoplastic and angioplastic or double-sleeve lobectomies. These procedures are becoming routine in major thoracic surgical centers. A large series of 52 patients was reported by Rendina in 1999, with no operative deaths and an overall 5-year survival of 38.3% [63].

Sleeve pneumonectomy is a rare, very major operation with high morbidity, and mortality in the order of 7.2–29% even in the most experienced hands [64, 65]. It is normally reserved for relatively young, fit patients with tumors directly invading the carina but with no mediastinal nodal involvement. For T4N0 tumors the 5-year survival reaches 51%, but is only 12% in T4N2 tumors [66].

16.6   Surgical Treatment by Stage

16.6.1   Occult Lung Cancer

Occult lung cancers are defined as those tumors not evident on radiological imaging but discovered by sputum cytology or incidentally at bronchoscopy. They represent less than 1% of all patients. When diagnosed on cytology it is essential to carefully inspect the upper aerodigestive tract, since one in three patients with positive sputum cytology and negative chest radiograph has a carcinoma in the head and neck region [67]. The new sophisticated techniques of in vivo fluorescent staining of mucosal malignancies during fiber-optic bronchoscopy are extremely helpful in localizing such lesions in the accessible parts of the bronchial tree, and are described elsewhere in this book.

The treatment for invasive lesions is surgical resection with the techniques described above, and in radiologically occult tumors this results in a 5-year survival approaching 100%. Whilst recurrences are rare, new lung primaries are frequent in this group of patients, with as many as 45% subsequently developing new carcinomas [67]. Regular follow-up including laserlight-induced fluorescence endoscopy bronchoscopy is therefore essential [68]. For occult in situ cancers, photodynamic therapy using transbronchoscopic laser-induced photoexcitation of porphyrins has been shown to be effective in eradicating these lesions and is widely used [69, 70].

16.6.2 Stage I Disease (T1N0M0 and T2N0M0)

The prognosis for surgically treated patients with T1N0M0 NSCLCs is generally good, with typical 5-year survival rates around 80% [11, 71]. For small, 2 cm or less in diameter tumors, 5-year survival rates of up to 89.1% have been reported even following sublobar resection [58]. Tumor size does make a difference in the survival of patients, even after complete resection. Typically, in a series reported by Martini and colleagues, the 5- and 10-year survival rates were 82% and 74%, respectively for T1N0 tumors compared to 68% and 60%, respectively, for T2N0 tumors. In a recent report on 7,620 patients with completely resected stage I tumors, Wisnivesky and colleagues found a statistically significant difference in the 12-year survival rate of 69% for tumors 5–15 mm in diameter, compared to 43% for tumors larger than 45 mm [72]. Ishida and colleagues felt that this difference may be partly due to increased incidence of occult lymph node metastasis with larger tumors not detected preoperatively or even by intraoperative nodal sampling [51].

Visceral pleura involvement may be a significant prognostic factor in stage I patients. Ichinose and colleagues found on univariate analysis a significant difference in survival between patients with tumors not extending beyond the elastic layer and not exposed on the pleural surface (P1), compared to those exposed to the pleural surface (P2) [73].

The histological type of tumor is a determinant of survival and time to recurrence in completely resected stage I patients, with worse results in nonsquamous histology tumors. Typically, in a Lung Cancer Study Group series, the 5-year survival for T1N0 patients was 83% for squamous carcinomas and 69% for adenocarcinomas, whilst for T2N0 tumors the figures were 64% and 57%, respectively [74, 75].

There is ongoing controversy regarding the optimal extent of resection in this group of patients with early cancers, and particularly the T1N0 subgroup. Video-assisted thoracoscopic lobectomy has been used by some centers in the last few years, but data regarding survival and recurrence rates to help define its role are only now starting to become available.

16.6.3 Stage II Disease (T1–2 N1 and T3N0)

16.6.3.1 T1–2N1

These are tumors confined to the lung or bronchus that involve the bronchopulmonary or hilar, but not mediastinal nodes. They represent less than 5% of all lung cancer cases and account for less than 10% of all resected lung cancers. Following resection, the overall 5-year survival rates are in the order of 55% for T1N1 tumors and 40% for T2N1 tumors [76]. In a series of 214 patients with resected T1N1 and T2N1 tumors from the Memorial Sloan-Kettering Cancer Center, the best survival was found in patients with tumors less than 3 cm in size and with only one nodal station involved. The authors insisted that these patients should be treated with primary surgery, with SND being an essential part of the procedure [77]. SND appears to offer a survival benefit in these patients compared to nodal sampling in several reports [39, 40]. In this group of patients, sleeve resections are particularly relevant and their value has been demonstrated (Fig. 16.9). If a complete resection can be achieved by a bronchoplastic lobectomy with or without a vascular sleeve resection, combined with SND, then the results are identical with those following pneumonectomy [63, 78, 79].

At this stage of disease, patients are more likely to develop distant metastases, highlighting the need for an effective systemic treatment. The data from recent reports on the use of adjuvant chemotherapy in early resected lung cancers are encouraging and are discussed elsewhere in this book.

As with stage I patients, tumor size and histology are significant prognostic factors following resection, with 5-year survival rates in T1N1 tumors of 75% for squamous cell carcinoma and 52% for adenocarcinoma, whilst for T2N1 tumors the corresponding figures were 53% for squamous cell carcinoma and 25% for adenocarcinoma [74, 75].

The location and number of involved N1 nodes have also been found to be significant indicators of prognosis, with 5-year survival rates of 45% for single, compared to 31% for multiple node involvement following resection [77]. Yano and colleagues found significantly better survival in patients with lobar N1 disease compared to those with hilar N1 disease (5-year survival 64.5% versus 39.7%, respectively) [80].

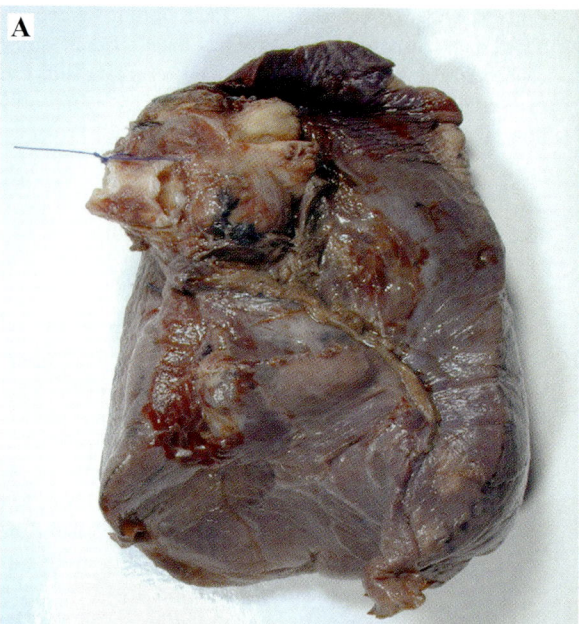
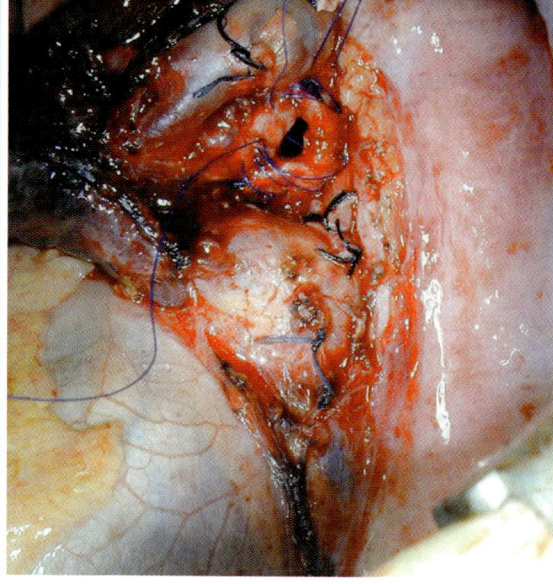

Fig. 16.9. A Specimen from a reverse, left, lower, sleeve lobectomy. The central tumor extending to the attached sleeve of the main bronchus is clearly visible. The suture marks the proximal bronchial margin for identification. Clear proximal and distal bronchial margins have been confirmed intraoperatively with frozen section examination. **B** The continuity of the airway is reestablished by a continuous suture anastomosis of the stump of the left main bronchus to the stump of the upper lobe bronchus

16.6.3.2 T3N0

Tumors that extend outside the lung parenchyma to invade the chest wall, including the superior sulcus, mediastinal pleura, pericardium or diaphragm, or endobronchial tumors within 2 cm of the main carina are classified as T3. The 5-year survival rate is around 35–40% for completely resected T3N0 tumors, but decreases to around 15–20% once N1 disease occurs. Achieving a complete resection is of paramount importance, as demonstrated in the results of a series of 61 patients with resected T3 tumors reported by Nakahashi; the 5-year survival following complete resection was 42%, compared to 10% for incomplete resection [81].

16.6.3.3 Tumors Invading the Chest Wall

Several studies have confirmed a favorable outcome when complete en-bloc resection of both lung and involved part of chest wall can be achieved in the absence of nodal involvement, to the point that T3N0 tumors were reclassified as stage IIB in the revision of the staging system in 1997. The presence of nodal involvement results in significantly worse survival and T3N1–2 tumors remain stage IIIA as before [76]. Diagnosing the presence of chest-wall invasion preoperatively is important in the planning of the operation. CT scan is helpful only when frank rib destruction is seen, but mere loss of fat planes is not diagnostic as it can be the result of simple contact or even the presence of inflammatory adhesions. The most reliable diagnostic finding is the combination of localized chest-wall pain and a positive bone scan or indeed PET scan.

The surgical technique involves division of the invaded ribs with a wide free margin of at least 5 cm either side of the tumor, and one free intercostal space above and below. The invaded part of the chest wall is then left attached to the tumor whilst the parenchyma resection is performed. Since chest-wall resection takes place before there is a chance to access the hilum or mediastinum, it is crucial that thorough preoperative staging including mediastinoscopy has eliminated the possibility of the presence of N2 disease. At the end of the operation the chest-wall defect is repaired with a variety of techniques so as to avoid paradox. For defects larger than 5 cm×5 cm and not covered by the scapula, a variety of prosthetic materials can be used. We have used a composite Marlex mesh and methylmethacrylate resin prosthesis with excellent results (Fig. 16.10).

These procedures are very well tolerated, with reported mortality rates historically ranging between 3 and 5%. Significant prognostic indicators are completeness of resection, nodal status, and depth of invasion [82, 83]. In a recent series of 104 patients with completely resected chest-wall tumors there was no operative mortality, and the overall 5-year survival was 61.4%. More specifically, the 5-year survival for T3N0 tumors was 67.3%, in contrast with 17.9% for T3N2 tu-

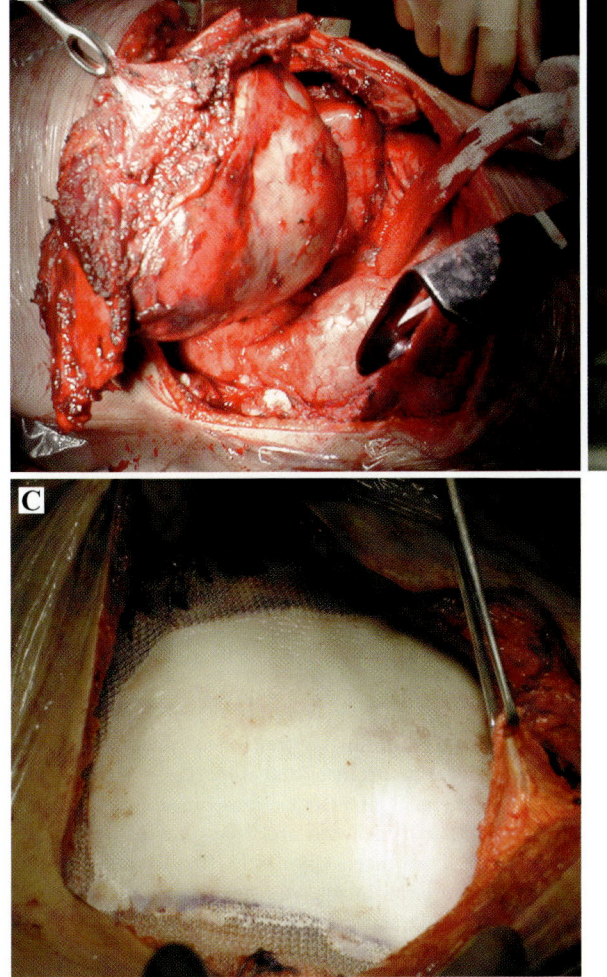

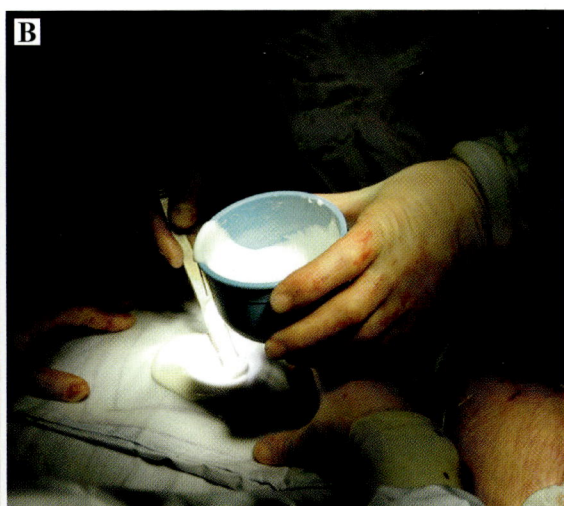

Fig. 16.10. A Large T3 tumor resected en bloc with parts of three ribs. **B** The composite chest wall prosthesis is fashioned and prepared by impregnating the polypropylene mesh with two part methyl-methacrylate resin (bone cement), which sets into a rigid but light plate. **C** The chest wall defect is repaired by securing the prosthesis in place with multiple sutures

mors. Furthermore, when invasion was limited to the parietal pleura only, the 5-year survival was 79.1%, compared to 54% when deeper invasion into muscle or bone was present [82].

There is certainly no role for adjuvant radiotherapy following complete resection of T3 tumors that invade the chest wall. Similarly, no survival benefit was found from using adjuvant radiotherapy in incompletely resected tumors [83, 84].

For tumors invading the diaphragm, the same principles of complete resection of the tumor en bloc with the invaded part of the diaphragm apply (Figs. 16.11). The prognosis, though, appears to be worse for this subgroup even after complete resection, possibly due to the high vascularity of the diaphragm with propensity for hematogenous metastases. In a series of 63 patients with tumors invading the diaphragm reported by Yokoi and colleagues, the overall 5-year survival after complete resection was 22.6%, but with no survivors beyond 4 years following incomplete resection. Furthermore, after complete resection, the 5-year survival rate

was 28.3% for T3N0 and 18.1% for T3N1–2 tumors. Depth of invasion was a significant prognostic indicator, as invasion limited to the diaphragmatic pleura or subpleural tissue resulted in a 5-year survival of 33%, compared to 14.3% when deep invasion of muscle or peritoneum was present. The authors argue that because of their poor prognosis these tumors should not be classified as T3 [85].

16.6.3.4 Superior Sulcus Tumors

Superior sulcus tumors, or Pancoast tumors, are those developing at the apex of the lung. Due to their location they extend early to invade adjacent structures, including the first two or three ribs (T3), vertebral bodies (T4), stellate ganglion, subclavian vessels and lower part of brachial plexus (T4), causing Pancoast syndrome [86, 87]. This early invasion of noble structures makes achieving complete resection difficult or impossible, a fact reflected in the significantly worse survival of the patients in this group as a whole compared to patients

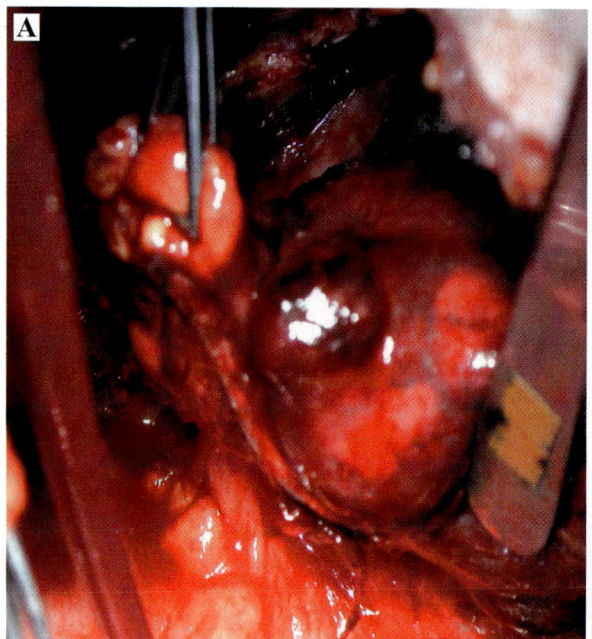
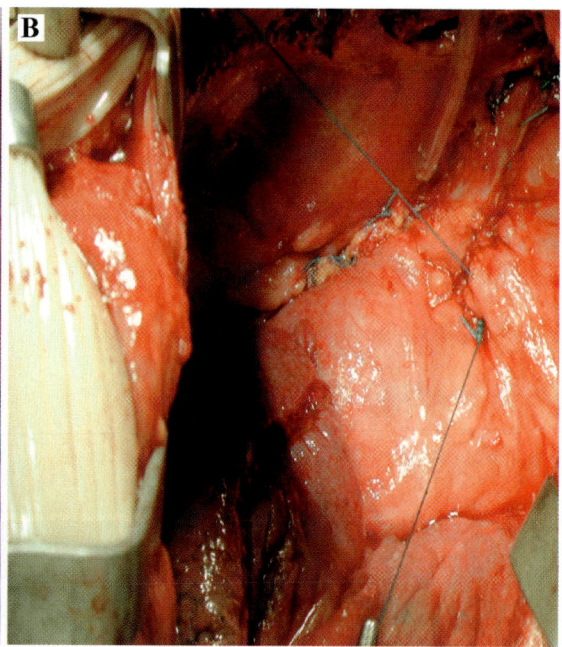
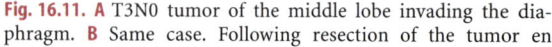

Fig. 16.11. **A** T3N0 tumor of the middle lobe invading the dia-phragm. **B** Same case. Following resection of the tumor en bloc with a wide disc of diaphragm, the diaphragm is repaired directly. If necessary a prosthesis can be used

with simple chest-wall invasion. CT and magnetic reso-nance imaging scans are helpful in clarifying the anato-my of the tumor and planning the necessary procedure.

Shaw and Paulson reported the first series of cura-tive resections for apical cancers in 1961 [87]. This se-ries included only a small number of true Pancoast tu-mors, but still their strategy of preoperative radiother-apy of 30 cGy over 3 weeks followed by resection via a high posterolateral thoracotomy remained the standard treatment until relatively recently. The reported 5-year survival for patients with completely resected superior sulcus tumors and N0 nodal status varies between 30 and 50%, but only a handful of patients with N2 disease survive in the long term, highlighting again the need to exclude N2 involvement preoperatively [88–90].

Historically, true invasion of the subclavian vessels by the tumor was considered a sign of inoperability [89]. This has changed with the introduction of the anterior cervical approach by Dartevelle in 1993 (Fig. 16.12 A) [91]. This involved resection of the medi-al half of the ipsilateral clavicle to expose the underly-ing structures of the thoracic inlet, allowing complete resection of involved parts of the subclavian vessels or the brachial plexus (Fig. 16.12 B). Vascular grafts were used to reestablish vascular continuity as required. Dar-tevelle's approach initially involved wedge resection of the lung apex, but it was subsequently modified to in-clude a full thoracotomy with nodal dissection. The sur-vival in his series of 29 patients with true Pancoast tu-mors was 50% at 2 years and 31% at 5 years, and pa-tients were offered adjuvant chemoradiotherapy. Whilst

16 patients died ultimately from their cancer, only 2 did so from local recurrence, and importantly, for the first time the presence of vascular invasion did not decrease survival [91]. Grunenwald and Spaggiari further refined this cervical approach (Fig. 16.13) by leaving the ster-noclavicular joint intact, which leads to an improved cosmetic result, much shorter recovery time, and pre-servation of the function of the shoulder girdle, and this has become the technique of choice in our practice (Figs. 16.14) [92].

Recent reports suggest that induction chemo/radio-therapy offers a significant survival benefit compared with induction radiotherapy alone in patients with Pan-coast tumors. In a retrospective study of 35 patients re-ported by Wright, complete resection was possible in 80% of patients in the radiotherapy group, with survival at 2 and 4 years of 49% and 49%, respectively, whilst in the chemo/radiotherapy group complete resection was achieved in 93% of the patients, and survival was 93% and 84% at 2 and 4 years, respectively. Local recurrence occurred in 30% and 0% of the patients in either group, respectively [93]. The phase II Southwestern Oncology Group (SWOG) 94-16 trial evaluated the role of concur-rent cisplatin at a dose of 50 mg/m^2 on days 1, 8, 29, and 36, and etoposide at a dose of 50 mg/m^2 on days 1–5 and days 29–33, with 45 Gy of thoracic radiation therapy over 5 weeks followed by two additional cycles of chemotherapy in mediastinoscopy-negative patients with superior sulcus tumors in a multi-institutional set-ting [94]. These authors demonstrated that this therapy was associated with acceptable morbidity and mortality,

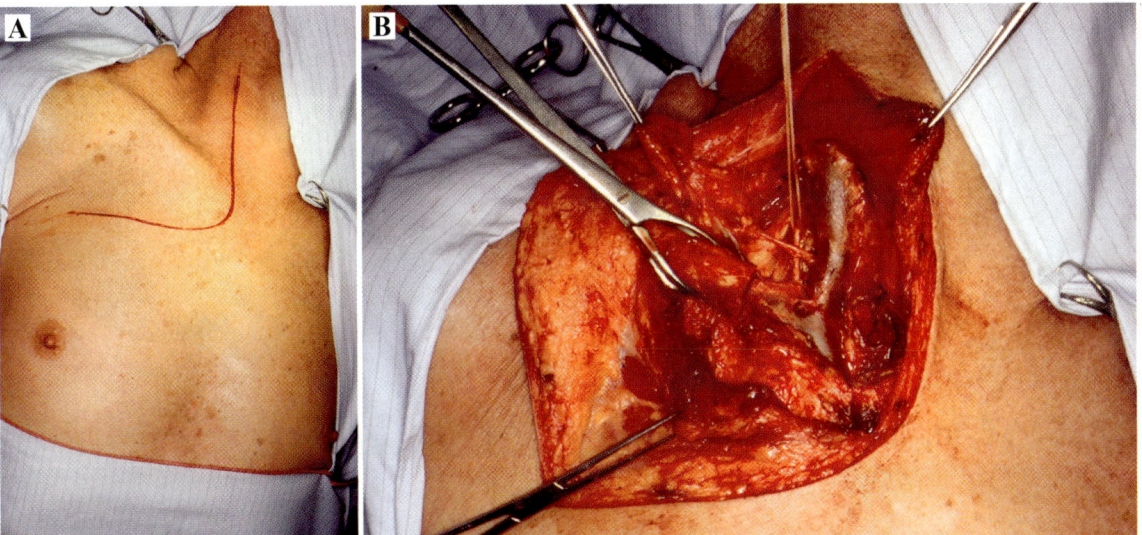

Fig. 16.12. A Anterior cervical incision circumscribing the clavicle. Dartevelle's procedure for Pancoast tumors. **B** Same patient. The medial half of the right clavicle has been resected allowing excellent exposure of the structures at the thoracic inlet. The right internal jugular, brachiocephalic, and subclavian veins are clearly visible, as well as the phrenic nerve (ensnared) on the anterior scalene muscle. Division of the scalene muscle exposes the subclavian artery underneath

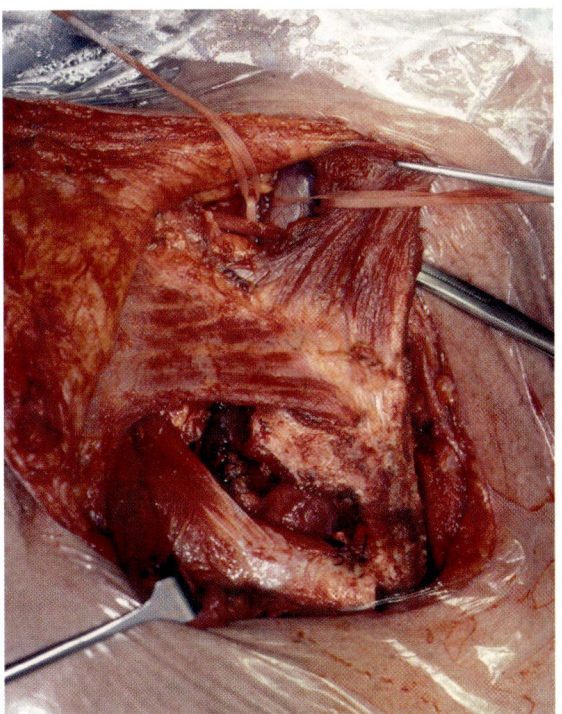

Fig. 16.13. Grunenwald technique for Pancoast tumors. The clavicle remains intact and instead the manubrium is incised at the midline, and the ipsilateral 2nd and 1st costal cartilages divided. The clavicle can then be lifted with attached manubrium, providing excellent exposure, whilst preserving the shoulder girdle integrity

and that complete resection rates of 92% where obtainable with this regimen. Of those who went on to surgery, 66% had either pathologic complete responses (36%) or minimal microscopic disease (30%) on resection. Of the patients who completed induction therapy and went on to surgery, the 2-year survival rates were 55% for all patients and 70% for those who underwent complete resection. Updated results noted a 33-month median survival and a 5-year overall survival rate of 41% for the total cohort [95].

16.6.3.5 Proximal Airway Tumors

Tumors within 2 cm of the main carina (T3) are appropriate for surgical treatment in the absence of N2 disease. Sleeve resections are particularly useful in this subgroup, in order to avoid the high mortality and long-term morbidity resulting from pneumonectomy. The long-term survival following bronchoplastic resections is equal to or better than that following pneumonectomy when adjusted for stage, to the point that they are now the procedure of choice whenever possible in all patients, and not just in those with limited respiratory reserves [96]. See also 16.5.

16.6.4   Stage III Tumors

16.6.4.1 Tumors Involving the Vertebral Bodies (T4)

True vertebral body involvement has historically been a contraindication to surgical intervention, as even isolated vertebral invasion resulted in dismal prognosis with no long-term survivors. A series of 12 patients

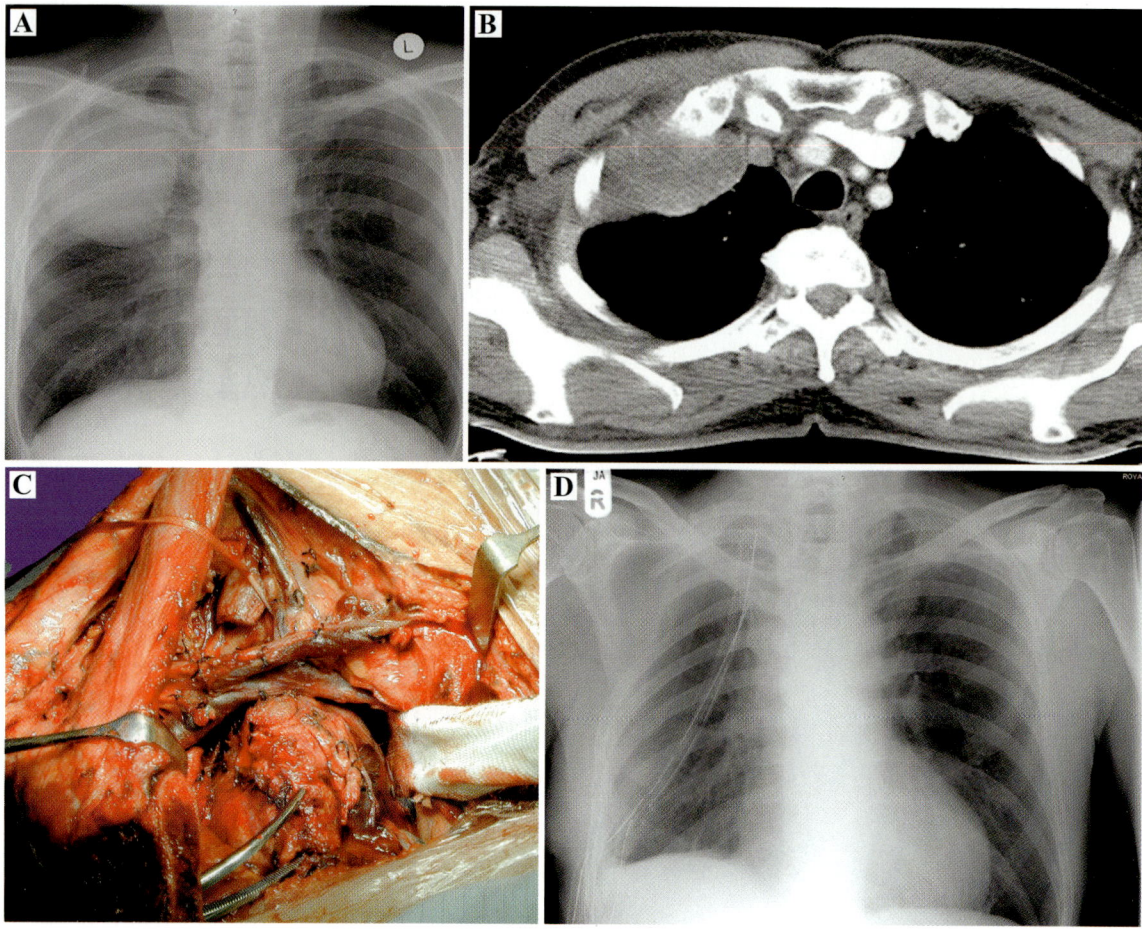

Fig. 16.14. A Chest radiograph of a patient with a large right superior sulcus tumor. **B** CT scan of same patient showing the upper pole of the tumor extending to the thoracic inlet between the first rib and the clavicle. **C** The patient was managed with Grunenwald's technique, the neck dissection is shown here. The tumor with attached parts of ribs 1, 2, and 3 was mobilized completely and allowed to fall inside the hemithorax. The neck wound was closed, and then a right thoracotomy and upper lobectomy with systematic nodal dissection followed. **D** Postoperative chest radiograph of same patient. The cut ends of upper ribs on the right are visible. The patient remains alive and disease free 3.5 years postoperatively. *L* Left, *R* right

with tumors "adherent" to the spine who underwent preoperative radiotherapy followed by en bloc resection with a wedge of vertebra reported by DeMeester and colleagues is typical of that era, with overall headline 5-year survival of 42%, but at the same time none of the patients with true bony invasion surviving more than 3 months postoperatively [97].

However, with advances in surgical techniques and better preoperative staging, tumors that were deemed unresectable may now undergo resection. Recently, Grunenwald and colleagues described a technique of radical en bloc resection for lung cancers with true invasion of the spine [98]. The procedures often lasted for more than 12 h and were performed jointly by a thoracic and a spinal surgery team. There were 19 patients, 11 of whom had induction chemo/radiotherapy. The spinal component of the operation involved hemivertebrectomy in 15 patients, and total vertebrectomy of up to 3

whole vertebral bodies in 4 patients, with spinal reconstruction using metal rods. There were no operative deaths, but there significant morbidity with complications occurred in 52% of the patients, often related to the spine. Survival was 59% at 1 year, and 14% at 5 years. There was a 47% local recurrence rate. The consensus is that although technically feasible, the utility of surgery in the subset of patients with true vertebral body invasion remains to be proven, and cannot be considered standard treatment at this point in time.

16.6.4.2 Tumors Invading the Main Carina (T4)
The majority of tumors involving the carina and lower trachea are so extensive that resection is not feasible. This is certainly the case when bulky subcarinal N2 disease (station 7) erodes through the airway. However, in selected patients, a sleeve pneumonectomy may be ap-

propriate (see 16.5). Sleeve pneumonectomy is a complex, very major operation with high morbidity, and mortality in the order of 7.2–29% even in the most experienced hands [64, 65, 99]. It is normally reserved for relatively young, fit patients with tumors directly invading the carina but with no mediastinal nodal involvement. For such T4N0 tumors, the 5-year survival following sleeve pneumonectomy reaches 51%, but is only 12% in T4N2 tumors [66].

16.6.4.3 Tumors Invading the Mediastinum (T4)

Tumors invading the mediastinal structures, including the heart, esophagus, great vessels, and mediastinal fat, are considered T4 tumors and have a dismal prognosis. They invariably represent locally very advanced, usually unresectable disease. Surgery can only be considered in highly selected patients with N0 disease and where a complete resection seems possible. In a series of 101 operated patients reported by Tsuchiya in 1994, complete resection was achieved in 66% of the cases, with an operative mortality of 13%. The 5-year survival and median survival time was 19% and 13.8 months, respectively for completely resected patients, the majority of them with N0 disease, and 0% and 6.5 months, respectively for incompletely resected patients. Only 3 out of 62 patients with T4N2 disease (4.9%) were long survivors. The 5-year survival after complete resection of tumors directly invading the left atrium was 22% (Figs. 16.15 and 16.16) [100].

There have been reports on the use of neoadjuvant chemotherapy in this challenging subgroup of patients. Macchiarini and colleagues in 1994 reported on a series of 23 patients who had induction with either chemotherapy or chemo/radiotherapy before surgery. Complete resection was achieved in 91% of the patients, with treatment-related mortality of 22% and an overall 3-year survival of 54%. Treatment-related morbidity was significantly higher in the chemo/radiotherapy group (42%) compared to chemotherapy alone (9%) [101].

16.6.4.4 Tumors with Mediastinal Nodal Involvement (N2)

Based on the collected series of 5,230 patients with NSCLC seen in the period 1975–1988 at the MD Anderson Cancer Center and reported by Clifton Mountain in the 1997 revision of lung cancer staging criteria, 30% of all patients have locally advanced disease at initial presentation. Of those, one-third (10% of the total) have stage IIIA with ipsilateral N2 lymph node metastases, with 17,000 new patients diagnosed yearly in the USA. This group possibly represents the most therapeutically challenging and controversial subset of patients with lung cancer, with a published 5-year survival of only 23% [76].

This overall poor prognosis reflects the fact that the presence of N2 disease signals an increased probability of micrometastatic disease. This is why heroic efforts to treat this subgroup of patients surgically in the 1970s and 1980s, gave such disappointing results. A large historical series of 702 operated patients with N2 disease from the Memorial Sloan-Kettering Cancer Center, illustrates this clearly. Amongst those patients who had clinical N0 or N1 disease (minimal N2), complete resection was achieved in 53%, compared to only 18% in patients with preoperatively identified, clinical (bulky) N2 disease. Furthermore, the 5-year survival was 29.8% in pa-

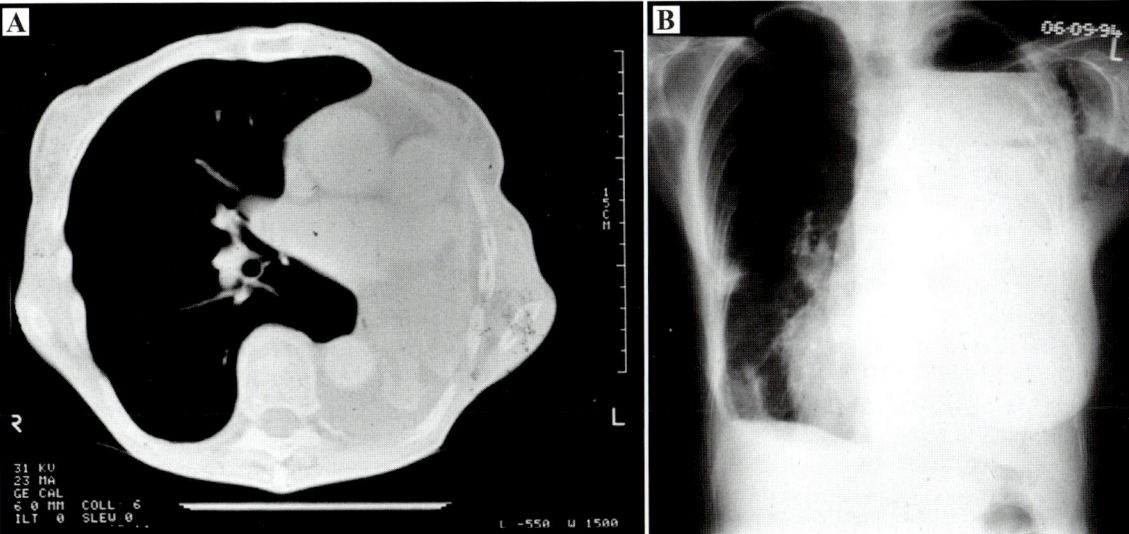

Fig. 16.15. A T4 tumor of the left lower lobe invading the left atrium and presenting with total atelectasis of the left lung. A filling defect at the atrium is visible on the left following contrast injection. **B** Same patient 6 months after left intrapericardial pneumonectomy en bloc with part of the wall of the left atrium and primary repair. Note the normal, gradual filling of the pneumonectomy space with fluid

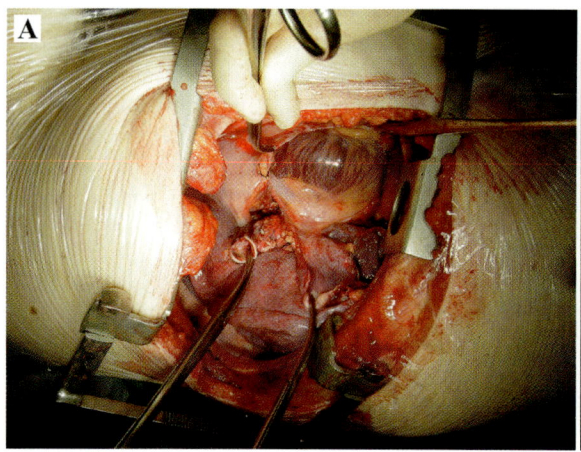
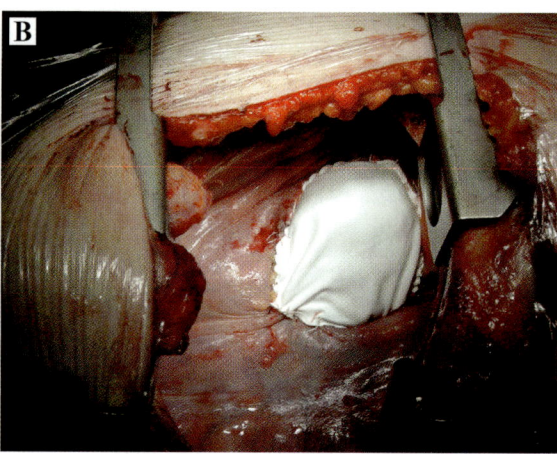
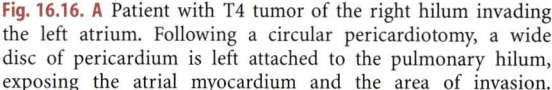

Fig. 16.16. A Patient with T4 tumor of the right hilum invading the left atrium. Following a circular pericardiotomy, a wide disc of pericardium is left attached to the pulmonary hilum, exposing the atrial myocardium and the area of invasion.

B Same patient following intrapericardial pneumonectomy en bloc with the wall of the left atrium and primary repair. A polytetrafluoroethylene prosthetic patch has been used to reconstruct the pericardial defect and prevent cardiac herniation

tients with clinical N0–1 status (minimal N2 disease) compared with 9% in those with bulky N2 disease when focusing on the completely resected subset within each group, but only 17.8% and 1.6%, respectively, when all patients in each group were included [34].

The effort to identify a favorite subset of patients with minimal N2 disease who would benefit from surgery continued. In 1982, Pearson drew attention to the fact that patients with N2 disease who underwent complete resection had a better prognosis if they had been mediastinoscopy negative before proceeding to thoracotomy, and mediastinal nodal involvement was only discovered intraoperatively (unexpected N2 disease). The 5-year survival in this case was 24%, compared to 8% in patients who had positive mediastinoscopy and still proceeded to surgery [102].

These results were confirmed by other authors. Daly and colleagues reported a 5-year survival of 31% in patients with unexpected N2 disease who had negative mediastinum on preoperative CT scan, and 45% in those with peripheral tumors [38, 103]. Important prognostic indicators were reported to include the number of involved nodal stations (one versus several), nodal involvement contained within the capsule, and squamous cell histology [38]. Patterson and colleagues pointed out that completely resected tumors of the left upper lobe with isolated N2 disease at the aortopulmonary window nodes (station 5) have a relatively good prognosis, with a 5-year survival of up to 42% [104]. The value of SND has been highlighted by several reports [37, 105]. Recent papers report a survival benefit in patients with limited N2 disease who had SND as opposed to sampling [39, 40]. Accordingly, in patients with an occult, single-station, mediastinal node metastasis that is recognized at thoracotomy following SND (unexpected minimal N2 disease), lung resection seems

appropriate as long as complete resection of the nodes and primary tumor is technically possible.

The next milestone in the management of N2 disease was the recognition of the value of chemotherapy as primary treatment. Roth's classic paper has sometimes been cited to demonstrate the value of the neoadjuvant approach to N2 disease, but the study design really only serves to prove the importance of induction chemotherapy rather than the value of the added resection [106].

The results of the RTOG 89-01 phase III trial that was designed to define whether surgery or radiotherapy represents the optimal local treatment following initial induction chemotherapy in patients with histologically proven N2 disease, were reported recently [107]. This study showed no significant difference between surgery and radiotherapy with regard to 1-year survival (70% vs. 66%) or median survival time (19.4 months vs. 17.4 months). Interestingly the median survival time in patients receiving induction chemotherapy only was 8.9 months. Whilst these results are inconclusive, this may well be due to the small number of patients enrolled in the study.

There does seem to be a specific subset of patients, however, who benefit from induction chemotherapy followed by surgery. A recent study by Bueno and associates emphasized the significance of eradicating N2 disease after induction therapy in stage IIIA tumors [108]. In their study, the long-term survival stratified by nodal status after induction therapy and lung resection found that 28% of patients downstaged to pathologic N0 had a 35.8% 5-year survival, whereas the remainder of patients with residual nodal disease at surgery had only a 9% 5-year survival. This and other studies suggest that surgical resection should be avoided in patients who, after induction therapy, have definite biopsy-proven residual tumor in the mediastinal nodes.

Clinical restaging with standard chest CT scans is not accurate enough to predict pathologic response in the lymph nodes, as recently reported by Margaritora and colleagues [109]. The use of PET scanning after induction therapy to determine response to therapy looks promising, but has limitations. In a retrospective review of the accuracy of PET scans after induction chemotherapy, radiotherapy, or both in 56 patients who underwent subsequent surgery, Akhurst and colleagues found that PET had a 98% positive predictive value for detecting residual viable disease in the primary tumor site [110]. However, PET overstaged the nodal status in 33%, understaged it in 15%, and was correct in only 52%. Therefore, until further studies are available, it is premature to routinely employ post-induction-therapy PET scans for restaging in order to make decisions about surgical resectability and nodal involvement. A more reliable approach could include histological confirmation of N2 disease at presentation using ultrasound-guided transbronchial needle biopsy of PET-positive nodes. Following the completion of induction chemotherapy, definitive assessment of the mediastinum can be performed by cervical videomediastinoscopy in order to select those patients who are downstaged to N0 to proceed to resection.

16.6.4.5 Tumors with Ipsilobar Satellite Nodules (T4)

As discussed earlier, tumors with ipsilobar satellite nodules are classified as T4 according to the most recent revision of the TNM staging system [76]. Even though their presence is an adverse prognostic indicator, it appears that in the absence of disease elsewhere and as long as they are confined to the same lobe as the primary tumor, then resection is appropriate, as it results in an acceptable 5-year survival of around 20%. This compares favorably with other subsets of T4 tumors.

16.6.4.6 Tumors with Contralateral Mediastinal Node Involvement (N3)

The presence of contralateral mediastinal lymph node involvement is an ominous prognostic sign, and patients classified into this subset of IIIB disease have an absolute contraindication to surgical resection.

16.7 Controversies

16.7.1 Video-Assisted Thoracoscopic Surgery

Video assisted thoracoscopy (VATS) represents the thoracic equivalent of laparoscopy. It allows intrathoracic pathology to be visualized by minimally invasive means, but also makes it possible to perform a wide variety of procedures. Initially, these were limited to biopsy sampling of lung and pleura, or drainage of pleural effusions.

VATS has proven very useful in the evaluation of lung cancer, particularly in the assessment of pleural dissemination. Small, peripheral, suspicious lesions can be removed and biopsied, sparing the patient the morbidity of a major thoracotomy if proven benign. Mediastinal lymph nodes not accessible by mediastinoscopy can occasionally be sampled. Furthermore, uncovering evidence of unresectability (e.g., pleural implants or tumor invasion of mediastinal structures) can avert a major thoracotomy.

Whilst the role of VATS in the diagnosis and staging of lung cancer is widely recognized, significant controversy exists regarding the suitability of this approach for the treatment of NSCLC, although there are several reports on the use of VATS for major pulmonary resections, including lobectomy and pneumonectomy [111–114].

It is generally believed that palpation plays an important role in the assessment of the tumor mass and its invasion of other structures. This "hands on" evaluation is lost with VATS. In addition, the palpation of the remaining lung for occult tumor nodules is not possible. It is technically very difficult to perform an SND as thoroughly as via an open thoracotomy. Also, even after the intended lobe or lung is separated from adjacent structures, its removal from the pleural cavity requires a much larger incision, the so-called utility thoracotomy. As a result, the potential advantage of small incisions may be lost. In addition, there is a temptation to perform less than a standard resection for small peripheral lesions. This has significant implications for local control, recurrence, and survival. There are several reports of tumor implants developing at the site of port incisions. This incidence appears to be low, less than 1%, but still represents a failure to achieve tumor eradication [115].

Lobectomies are still only rarely performed via VATS. The limited available data suggest that the perioperative morbidity and mortality are similar to open resection [113], while perioperative pain is reduced [116]. Long-term survival, as judged by 3-year results following resection of bronchogenic carcinoma, is showing a similar trend to that of open lobectomy [113, 116].

This surgical strategy is too early in its development to allow firm conclusions to be drawn regarding its effectiveness. Further evaluation should ideally take place within the context of a randomized prospective study.

16.8 Conclusion

Significant progress has been made in recent years in the strategies for managing lung cancer. The multidisciplinary lung cancer team principle has allowed more cohesive and timely treatment for the patients and better communication between specialists. New sophisticated techniques allow the modern thoracic surgeon to offer potentially curative treatment to selected patients with either locally advanced disease or very limited pulmonary reserves, who were previously denied surgery.

Key Points

- Surgical resection is the treatment of choice for early stage non-small-cell lung cancer (NSCLC) and is generally offered to all patients with stage I and II disease and selected patients with stage III disease.
- It is also occasionally offered to highly selected patient with solitary metastasis and completely resectable primary disease.
- The goal of surgery in NSCLC is to achieve complete resection of the primary tumor with no macroscopic tumor remaining and microscopically free margins. Only patients in whom a complete resection is anticipated are selected for surgery.
- Preoperative investigations are necessary to identify the extent of the disease as defined by staging and to reassure that the patient is fit enough for the planned procedure.

References

1. American Cancer Society. Lung Cancer Resource Centre online. *http://www.cancer.org*
2. McCaughan B. Recent advances in managing non small cell lung cancer. Med J Aus 1997; 166(Supp):S7.
3. Davies HM. Recent advances in the surgery of the lung and the pleura. Br J Surg 1913; 1:228.
4. Brunn HB. Surgical principles underlying one stage lobectomy. Arch Surg 1929; 18:490.
5. Graham EA, Singer JJ. Successful removal of the entire lung for carcinoma of the bronchus. JAMA 1933; 101:1371.
6. Churchill ED. The surgical treatment of carcinoma of the lung. J Thorac Surg 1933; 2:254.
7. Churchill ED, Belsey HR. Segmental pneumonectomy in bronchiectasis. Ann Surg 1939; 109:481.
8. Alison PR. Intrapericardial approach to the lung root in the treatment of bronchial carcinoma by dissection pneumonectomy. J Thorac Surg 1946; 15:991.
9. Price-Thomas C. Conservative resection of the bronchial tree. J R Coll Surg Edinb 1956; 1:169.
10. AJCC Cancer Staging Manual, Chap 19, 5th edn. Lippincott-Raven, Philadelphia, 1997.
11. Martini N, Bains MJ, Burt ME, et al. Incidence of local recurrence and second primary tumors in resected stage I lung cancer. J Thorac Cardiovasc Surg 1995; 109:120.
12. Fernando HC, Goldstraw P. The accuracy of clinical evaluative intrathoracic staging in lung cancer as assessed by post-surgical pathologic staging. Cancer 1990; 65:2503.
13. Reed CE, Harpole DH, Posther KE, et al: Results of the American College of Surgeons Oncology Group Z0050 trial: the utility of positron emission tomography in staging potentially operable non small cell lung cancer. J Thorac Cardiovasc Surg 2003, 126:1943.
14. Graham ANJ, Chan KJM, Pastorino U, et al. Systematic nodal dissection in the intrathoracic staging of patients with NSCLC. J Thorac Cardiovasc Surg 1999; 117:246.
15. Ginsberg RJ. Continuing controversies in staging NSCLC: an analysis of the revised 1997 staging system. Oncology 1998; 12(Suppl 2):51.
16. Brown JS, Eraut D, Trask C, et al. Age and the treatment of lung cancer Thorax 1996; 51:564.
17. Deppermann KM. Influence of age and comorbidities on the hemotherapeutic management of lung cancer. Lung Cancer 2001; 33(suppl 1):S115.
18. Booton R, Jones M, Thatcher N. Management of lung cancer in elderly patients. Thorax 2003; 58:711.
19. De Perrot M, Licker M, Reymond MA. Influence of age on operative mortality and long-term survival after lung resection for bronchogenic carcinoma. Eur Respir J 1999; 14(2):419.
20. Licker M, Spiliopoulos A, Frey JG, et al. Management and outcome of patients undergoing thoracic surgery in a regional chest medical centre. Eur J Anesthesiol 2001; 18:540.
21. Au J, el-Oakley R, Cameron EW. Pneumonectomy for bronchogenic carcinoma in the elderly. Eur J Cardiothorac Surg 1994; 8:247.
22. Boushy SF, Billig DM, North LB, et al. Clinical course related to preoperative and postoperative pulmonary function in patients with bronchogenic carcinoma. Chest 1971; 59:383
23. Wernly JA, DeMeester TR, Kirchner PT, et al. Clinical value of quantitative ventilation-perfusion lung scans in the surgical management of bronchogenic carcinoma. J Thorac Cardiovasc Surg 1980; 80:535.
24. Miller JI. Physiologic evaluation of pulmonary function in the candidate for lung resection. J Thorac Cardiovasc Surg 1993; 105:347.
25. British Thoracic Society. Guidelines on the selection of patients with lung cancer for surgery. Thorax 2001; 56:89.
26. Eagle KA, Rihal CS, Mickel MC, et al. Cardiac risk of noncardiac surgery. Influence of coronary disease and type of surgery in 3368 operations. Circulation 1997; 96:1882.
27. Eagle KA, Brundage BH, Chaitman BR, et al. Guidelines for perioperative cardiovascular evaluation for noncardiac surgery: an abridged version of the report of the American College of Cardiology/American Heart Association task force on practice guidelines. Mayo Clin Proc 1997; 72:524.
28. Goldman L, Caldera DL, Nussbaum SR, et al. Multifactorial index of cardiac risk in noncardiac surgical procedures. N Engl J Med 1977; 297:845.
29. Eagle KA, Brundage BH, Chaitman BR, et al. ACC/AHA Task Force Special Report. Guidelines for perioperative cardiac evaluation for noncardiac surgery. Circulation 1996; 93:1278.
30. Thatcher N, Ranson M, Anderson H, et al. In: Spiro S (ed.) Carcinoma of the Lung. European Respiratory Monograph, Sheffield, UK, 1995; p 270.
31. Kearney DJ, Lee TH, Reilly JJ, et al. Assessment of operative risk in patients undergoing lung resection. Chest 1994; 105:753.
32. Ginsberg RJ, Martini N. Non-small cell lung cancer. Surgical management In: Pearson FG (ed.) Thoracic Surgery. Churchill Livingstone, Philadelphia, 2002; p 837.
33. Lim E, Ali A, Theodorou P, et al. Intraoperative pleural lavage cytology is an independent prognostic indicator for staging non-small cell lung cancer. J Thorac Cardiovasc Surg 2004; 127:1113.
34. Martini N, Flehinger BJ. The role of surgery in N2 lung cancer. Surg Clin North Am 1987; 67:1037.
35. Naruke T, Suemasu K, Ishikawa S. Lymph node mapping and curability of various levels of metastasis in resected lung cancer. J Thorac Cardiovasc Surg 1978; 76:832.

36. Tiffet O, Nicholson AG, Khaddage A, et al. Feasibility of the detection of the sentinel lymph node in peripheral non-small cell lung cancer with radio isotopic and blue dye techniques. Chest. 2005; 127(2):443.

37. Watanabe SI, Ladas G, Goldstraw P. Inter observer variability in systematic nodal dissection: comparison of European and Japanese nodal designation. Ann Thorac Surg 2002; 73:245.

38. Goldstraw P, Mannam GC, Kaplan DK, et al. Surgical management of non small cell lung cancer with ipsilateral mediastinal node metastasis. J Thorac Cardiovasc Surg 1994; 107:1.

39. Izbicki JR, Passlick B, Pantel K, et al. Effectiveness of radical systematic mediastinal lymphadenectomy in patients with resectable NSCLC: results of a prospective randomised trial. Ann Surg 1998; 227(1):138.

40. Keller SM, Adak S, Wagner H, et al. Complete mediastinal lymph node dissection improves survival in patients with resected stages II and IIIa non small cell lung cancer. Eastern Cooperative Oncology Group. Ann Thorac Surg 2000; 70(2):358.

41. Ginsberg RJ, et al. Randomised trial of lobectomy versus limited resection for T1N0 non small cell lung cancer. Lung Cancer Study Group. Ann Thorac Surg 1995; 60:615.

42. Wilkins EW, Scannell JG, Craver JG. Four decades of experience with resection for bronchogenic carcinoma at the Massachusetts General Hospital. J Thorac Cardiovasc Surg 1978; 76:364.

43. Alexiou C, Beggs D, Onyeaka P, et al. Pneumonectomy for stage I (T1N0 and T2N0) NSCLC has potent, adverse impact on survival. Ann Thorac Surg 2003; 76:1023

44. Mehran RJ, Deslauriers J, Piraux M, at al. Survival related to nodal status after sleeve resection for lung cancer. J Thorac Cardiovasc Surg 1994; 107:578.

45. Waters P, et al. Surgical techniques. In: Pearson FG (ed.) Thoracic Surgery. Churchill Livingstone, Philadelphia, 1988; p 974.

46. Sienel W, Seen-Hibler R, Mutschler W, Pantel K, Passlick B. Tumour cells in the tumour draining vein of patients with non-small cell lung cancer: detection rate and clinical significance. Eur J Cardiothorac Surg 2003; 23(4):451.

47. Deslauriers J, Ginsberg RJ, Piantadosi S, et al. Prospective assessment of 30 day operative morbidity for surgical resections in lung cancer. Chest 1994; 106(Suppl):329.

48. Pierce RJ, Copland JM, Sharpe K, et al. Preoperative risk evaluation for lung cancer resection: predicted postoperative product as a predictor of surgical mortality. Am J Respir Crit Care Med 1994; 150:947.

49. Paulson D, Reisch JS. Long term survival after resection for bronchogenic carcinoma Ann Surg 1976; 184:324.

50. Belcher JR. Thirty years of surgery for carcinoma of the bronchus. Thorax 1983; 38:428.

51. Ishida T, Yokoyama H, Kaneko S, et al. Long term results of operation for non small cell cancer in the elderly. Ann Thorac Surg 1990; 50:919.

52. Kadri MA, Dussek JE. Survival and prognosis following resection of primary non small cell bronchogenic carcinoma. Eur J Cardiothorac Surg 1991; 5:132.

53. Jensik RJ, Faber LP, Kittle CF. Segmental resection for bronchogenic carcinoma. Ann Thorac Surg 1979; 28:475.

54. Errett LE, Wilson J, Chiu RC. Wedge resection as an alternative procedure for peripheral bronchogenic carcinoma in poor-risk patients. J Thorac Cardiovasc Surg 1985; 90:656.

55. Temeck BK, Schafer PW, Saini N. Wedge resection for bronchogenic carcinoma in high risk patients. South Med J 1992; 85:1081.

56. Weissberg D, Straehley CJ, Scully NM, et al. Less than lobar resections for bronchogenic carcinoma. Scand J Thorac Cardiovasc Surg 1993; 27:121.

57. Warren WH, Penfield Faber L. Segmentectomy versus lobectomy in patients with stage I pulmonary carcinoma. J Thorac Cardiovasc Surg 1994; 107:1087.

58. Koike T, Yamato Y, Yoshiya K, et al. Criteria for intentional limited pulmonary resection in cT1N1M0 peripheral lung cancer. Jpn J Thorac Cardiovasc Surg 2003; 51:515.

59. Frist WH, Mathieson DJ, Hilgenberg AD, et al. Bronchial sleeve resection with and without pulmonary resection. J Thorac Cardiovasc Surg 1987; 93:350.

60. Voigt-Moykopf I, Fritz T, Meyer G, et al. Bronchoplastic and angioplastic operation in bronchial carcinoma: long-term results of a retrospective analysis from 1973 to 1983. Int Surg 1986; 71:211.

61. Van Schil PE, Brutel de la Riviere A, Knaepen PJ, et al. TNM staging and long term follow up after sleeve resection for bronchogenic tumours. Ann Thorac Surg 1991; 52:1096.

62. Deslauriers J, Mehran RJ, Guimont C, et al. Staging and management of lung cancer: sleeve resection. World J Surg 1993; 17:6.

63. Rendina EA, Venuto F, De Giacomo T, et al. Sleeve resection and prosthetic reconstruction of the pulmonary artery for lung cancer. Ann Thorac Surg 1999; 68:995.

64. Deslauriers J, Beaulieu M, McClish A. Tracheal sleeve pneumonectomy. In: Shields TW (ed.) General Thoracic Surgery, 3rd edn. Lea and Febiger, Philadelphia, 1989; p 382.

65. Mathieson DJ, Grillo HC. Carinal resection for bronchogenic carcinoma. J Thorac Cardiovasc Surg 1991; 102:16.

66. Mitchell JD, Mathisen DJ, Wright CD, et al Resection for bronchogenic carcinoma involving the carina: long-term results and effect of nodal status on outcome. J Thorac Cardiovasc Surg. 2001 Mar; 121(3):465.

67. Martini N, Melamed MR. Occult carcinomas of the lung. Ann Thorac Surg 1980; 30:215.

68. Weigel TL, Kosco PJ, Dacic S. Fluorescence bronchoscopic surveillance in patients with a history of NSCLC Diagn Ther Endosc 1999; 6:1.

69. Hayata Y, Kato H, Konaca C. Photoradiation therapy with hemato-porphyrin derivative in early and stage I lung cancer. Chest 1984; 86:169.

70. Cortese DA, Edell ES, Kinsey JH. Photodynamic therapy for early stage squamous cell carcinoma of the lung. Mayo Clinic Proc 1997; 72:595.

71. Williams DE, Pairolero PC, Davis CS, et al. Survival of patients surgically treated for stage I lung cancer. Eur J Cardiothorac Surg 2004; 26:197.

72. Wisnivesky JP, Yankelevitz D, Henschke CI. The effect of tumor size on curability of stage I non-small cell lung cancers. Chest 2004 Sep; 126(3):761.

73. Ichinose Y, Yano T, Asoh H, Yokoyama H, Yoshino I, Katsuda Y. Prognostic factors obtained by a pathologic examination in completely resected non-small-cell lung cancer. An analysis in each pathologic stage. J Thorac Cardiovasc Surg 1995; 110:601.

74. Mountain CF, Lukeman JM, Hammar SP. Lung cancer classification: the relationship of disease extent and cell type to survival in a clinical trials population. J Surg Oncol 1987; 35:147.

75. Gail MH, Eagan RT, Feld R, et al. Prognostic factors in patients with resected stage I non-small cell lung cancer. A report from the Lung Cancer Study Group. Cancer 1984; 54:1802.

76. Mountain CF. Revisions in the international system for staging lung cancer. Chest 1997; 111:1710.

77. Martini N, Burt ME, Bains MS, McCormack PM, Rusch VW, Ginsberg RJ. Survival after resection of stage II non-small cell lung cancer. Ann Thorac Surg 1992; 54:460.

78. Icard P, Regnard JF, Guilbert L, et al. Survival and prognostic factors in patients undergoing parenchymal saving bronchoplastic operation for primary lung cancer. A series of 110 consecutive patients. Eur J Cardiothorac Surg 1999; 15:426.

79. Lausberg HF, Graeter TP, Wendler O, et al. Bronchial and bronchovascular sleeve resection for treatment of central lung tumors. Ann Thorac Surg 2000; 70:367.

80. Yano T, Yokohama T, Inoue T, Asoh H, Tayama K, Ichinose Y. Surgical results and prognostic factors of pathologic N1 disease in non-small-cell carcinoma of the lung. Significance of N1 level: lobar or hilar nodes. J Thorac Cardiovasc Surg 1994; 107:1398.

81. Nakahashi H, Yasumoto K, Ishida T, et al. Results of surgical treatment of patients with T3 non-small cell lung cancer. Ann Thorac Surg 1988; 46:178.

82. Facciolo F, Cardillo G, Lopergolo M, et al. Chest wall invasion in non-small cell lung carcinoma: a rationale for en bloc resection. J Thorac Cardiovasc Surg 2001; 121:649.

83. Magdeleinat P, Alifano M, Benbrahem C, et al. Surgical treatment of lung cancer invading the chest wall: results and prognostic factors. Ann Thorac Surg 2001; 71:1094.

84. Piehler JM, Pairolero PC, Weiland LH, Offord KP, Payne WS, Bernatz PE. Bronchogenic carcinoma with chest wall invasion: factors affecting survival following en bloc resection. Ann Thorac Surg 1982; 34:684.

85. Yokoi K, Tsuchiya R, Mori T. Results of surgical treatment of lung cancer involving the diaphragm. J Thorac Cardiovasc Surg 2000; 120:799.

86. Attar S, Krasna MJ, Sonett JR, et al. Superior sulcus (Pancoast) tumor: experience with 105 patients. Ann Thorac Surg 1998; 66:193.

87. Pancoast HK. Superior pulmonary sulcus tumors. JAMA 1932; 99:1391.

88. Shaw RR, Paulson DL, Kee JL. Treatment of the superior sulcus tumor by irradiation followed by resection. Ann Surg 1961; 154:29.

89. Hilaris BS, Martini N, Wong GY, Nori D. Treatment of superior sulcus tumor (Pancoast tumor). Surg Clin North Am 1987; 67:965.

90. Alifano M, D'Aiuto M, Magdeleinat P, et al. Surgical treatment of superior sulcus tumors: results and prognostic factors. Chest 2003 Sep; 124(3):996.

91. Dartevelle PH, Chapelier AR, Macchiarini P, et al. Anterior transcervical thoracic approach for radical resection of lung tumors invading the thoracic inlet. J Thorac Cardiovasc Surg 1993; 105:1025.

92. Grunenwald D, Spaggiari L. Transmanubrial osteomuscular approach for apical chest tumors. Ann Thorac Surg 1997; 63:563.

93. Wright CD, Menard MT, Wain JC, et al. Induction chemoradiation compared with induction radiation for lung cancer involving the superior sulcus. Ann Thorac Surg 2002; 73(5):1541.

94. Rusch VW, Giroux DJ, Kraut MJ, et al. Induction chemoradiation and surgical resection for non-small cell lung carcinomas of the superior sulcus: initial results of Southwest Oncology Group Trial 9416 (Intergroup Trial 0160). J Thorac Cardiovasc Surg 2001; 121:472.

95. Rusch VW, Giroux D, Kraut MJ, et al. Induction chemoradiotherapy and surgical resection for non-small cell lung carcinomas of the superior sulcus (Pancoast tumors): mature results of Southwest Oncology Group trial 9416 (Intergroup 0160). Proc Am Soc Clin Oncol 2003; 22:2548a.

96. Tronc F, Grégoire J, Rouleau J, Deslauriers J. Long-term results of sleeve lobectomy for lung cancer. Eur J Cardiothorac Surg 2000; 17:550.

97. DeMeester TR, Albertucci M, Dawson PJ, et al .Management of tumor adherent to the vertebral column. J Thorac Cardiovasc Surg 1989; 97:373.

98. Grunenwald D, et al. Radical en bloc resection for lung cancer invading the spine. J Thorac Cardiovasc Surg 2002; 123:271.

99. Dartevelle PG, Macchiarini P, Chapelier A. Tracheal sleeve pneumonectomy. Ann Thorac Surg 1995; 60:1854.

100. Tsuchiya R, Asamura H, Kondo H, et al. Extended resection of the left atrium, great vessels, or both for lung cancer Ann Thorac Surg 1994; 57:960.

101. Macchiarini P, Chapelier AR, Monnet I. Extended operations after induction therapy for stage IIIb (T4) non-small cell lung cancer. Ann Thorac Surg 1994; 57 (4):966.

102. Pearson FG, Delarue NC, Ilves R, Todd TR, Cooper JD. Significance of positive superior mediastinal nodes identified at mediastinoscopy in patients with resectable cancer of the lung. J Thorac Cardiovasc Surg 1982; 83:1.

103. Daly BD, Mueller JD, Faling LJ, et al. N2 lung cancer: outcome in patients with false-negative computed tomographic scans of the chest. J Thorac Cardiovasc Surg 1993; 105:904.

104. Patterson GA, Piazza D, Pearson FG, et al. Significance of metastatic disease in subaortic lymph nodes. Ann Thorac Surg 1987; 43:155.

105. Naruke T, Goya T, Tsuchiya R, Suemasu K. The importance of surgery in non-small cell carcinoma of lung with mediastinal lymph node metastasis. Ann Thorac Surg 1988; 46:603.

106. Roth J, Fossella F, Komaki R, et al. A randomized trial comparing perioperative chemotherapy and surgery with surgery alone in resectable stage IIIA non-small cell lung cancer. J Natl Cancer Inst 1994; 86:673.

107. Johnstone DW, Byhardt RW, Ettinger D, et al. Phase III study comparing chemotherapy and radiotherapy with preoperative chemotherapy and surgical resection in patients with non-small-cell lung cancer with spread to mediastinal lymph nodes (N2); final report of RTOG 89–101. Radiation Therapy Oncology Group. Int J Radiat Oncol Biol Phys. 2002; 54(2):365.

108. Bueno, R, Richards, W, Swanson, S, et al Nodal stage after induction therapy for stage IIIA lung cancer determines survival. Ann Thorac Surg 2000; 70:1826.

109. Margaritora, S, Cesario, A, Galetta, D, et al. Ten year experience with induction therapy in locally advanced non-small cell lung cancer (NSCLC): is clinical re-staging predictive of pathologic staging? Eur J Cardiothorac Surg 2001; 19:894.

110. Akhurst, T, Downey, RL, Ginsberg, MS, et al. An initial experience with FDG-PET in the imaging of residual disease after induction therapy in lung cancer. Ann Thorac Surg 2002; 73:259.

111. Daniels LJ, Balderson SS, Onaitis MW, et al. Thoracoscopic lobectomy: a safe and effective strategy for patients with stage I lung cancer. Ann Thorac Surg 2002; 74(3):860.

112. Lewis RJ. The role of video-assisted thoracic surgery for carcinoma of the lung: wedge resection to lobectomy by simultaneous individual stapling. Ann Thorac Surg 1993; 56:762.

113. Lewis RJ, Caccavale RJ, Sisler G, et al. One hundred video-assisted thoracic surgical simultaneously stapled lobectomies without rib spreading. Ann Thorac Surg 1997; 63:1415.

114. Lewis RJ, Caccavale RJ, Bocage JP, et al. Video-assisted thoracic surgical non-rib spreading simultaneously stapled lobectomy: a more patient-friendly oncologic resection. Chest 1999; 116(4):1119.

115. Parekh K, Rusch V, Bains M, et al. VATS port site recurrence: a technique dependent problem. Ann Surg Onc 2001; 8(2):175.

116. Walker WS. VATS lobectomy: the Edinburgh experience. Semin Thorac Cardiovasc Surg 1998; 10:291.

Radical Radiotherapy in the Management of Locally Advanced Non-Small-Cell Lung Cancer

17

Katie Newbold and Christopher M. Nutting

Contents

17.1 Introduction

The typical overall 5-year survival rate for patients diagnosed with non-small cell lung cancer (NSCLC) is 15% [1]. Historically, surgery and radiotherapy have been used independently to gain control of disease both at the local site and mediastinal lymphatic drainage areas. The role of chemotherapy has changed over the last 2 decades from being used predominantly in the metastatic setting to prolong symptom-free life, to now being employed in a multimodality setting with both surgery and radiotherapy to improve disease-free and overall survival. Surgery continues to offer the best chance of cure and should always be considered initially.

Radical radiotherapy in non-small-cell lung cancer (NSCLC) is considered in two groups of patients. Those who are technically operable but are medically unfit for surgery or who decline surgery, stages I, II (T1–3 N0, T1–2 N1) and some IIIA (T1-3 N2, T3 N1), and those who are surgically inoperable, usually stages IIIA and IIIB (T1–3 N1-2, T4 N0–2), but not stage IV, nor those stage IIIB with a cytologically malignant pleural effusion. The American Society of Clinical Oncologists (ASCO) Guidelines 2004 for candidates for definitive thoracic radiotherapy are that they should have a world health organization (WHO) performance status score of 0, 1, or possibly 2, adequate pulmonary function, and disease confined to the thorax. Patients with malignant pleural effusions or distant metastatic disease are not appropriate candidates for definitive thoracic radiotherapy [2]. Adequate pulmonary function is often stated as a forced expiratory volume in 1 s of >1.5 l, but should be variable depending upon the site and size of the target volume, and therefore rests on the radiation oncologist's clinical judgment.

Most radiotherapy for NSCLC is given as external beam radiotherapy (EBRT). Improved techniques such as three-dimensional conformal radiotherapy (3D-CRT) and intensity-modulated radiotherapy (IMRT) lead to improved accuracy of delivery of the radiation to the tumor target and minimize doses to normal tissues, allowing higher doses to the tumor itself. Brachytherapy is occasionally used in the curative setting, usually in conjunction with EBRT, or more frequently is used with palliative intent.

17.2   Results of Radical radiotherapy in NSCLC (Stages I–IIIB)

Historically, conventional radical radiotherapy has produced 3-year survival rates of 30–40% and 5-year survival rates of 10–20% [3–9]. These results presented in Table 17.1 come from studies of conventional radiotherapy administered as EBRT either from a radioactive source such as cobalt-60 or, since the 1980s, produced by a linear accelerator. The patient is usually treated in a supine position with their arms above their head. In the past the radiotherapy target volume was based on X-rays and diagnostic computed tomography (CT), but now modern-day radiotherapy planning is with a CT scan performed from the thoracic inlet to the diaphragm at 5- to 10-mm slice intervals, with a slice thickness of 3–8 mm.

Targets should be outlined according to International Commission on Radiological Units and Measurements 62 guidelines [10]. The gross tumor volume (GTV) is determined from the diagnostic CT (both lung and soft-tissue windows) with reference to clinical details and bronchoscopy reports. The clinical target volume (CTV) is the GTV with a 0.3- to 0.7-cm margin to account for microscopic spread. The CTV does not usually involve elective mediastinal nodes, as this has not been shown in retrospective studies to improve local control [11–13]. The CTV should be defined on the prechemotherapy tumor extent if induction chemotherapy has been used, and using the lung windows on the CT scan. The planning target volume (PTV) is the CTV

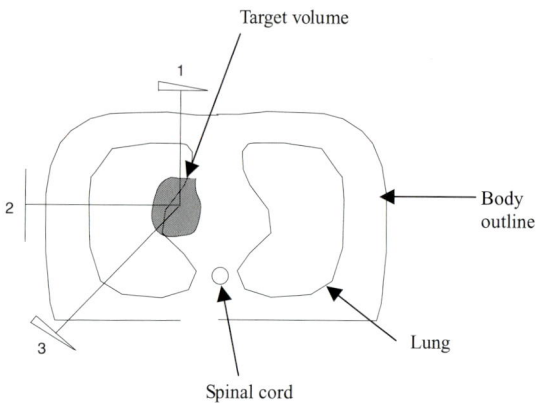

Fig. 17.1. Standard three-field arrangement viewed in the axial plane; beam 2 is weighted approximately 50% to reduce exit dose through the contralateral lung

plus 1 cm margin in the axial plane and 1.5 cm in the longitudinal plane. The extent of these margins is variable and heavily debated, particularly as recent studies on the dynamics of tumor position throughout respiration show eccentric patterns of movement in all planes [14, 15]. Typically for 3D-CRT, a single phase of treatment is used and two to four angled fields may be employed (Fig. 17.1). A second phase may be introduced to provide better overall protection of normal tissues, particularly if the spinal cord is within the phase I volume.

Doses should be calculated with inhomogeneity correction, as air-filled lungs cause little attenuation. Shielding is used to minimize the dose to normal tissues. The critical structures are the spinal cord, at risk of radiation-induced myelopathy, which should receive a dose of no greater than 46 Gy in 2-Gy fractions. The normal lung should receive as low a dose as possible. Commonly used indices are the V20 or V30 (percentage of lung volume receiving more than 20 Gy or 30 Gy), or the mean lung dose, which at our institution should be kept below 20 Gy. The heart is also at risk of late toxicity, although realistically not within the life expectancy of these patients and as such should not limit a radical target dose prescription. Dose to the myocardium should, where possible, remain below 40 Gy, with no more than one-third of the heart receiving the full, prescribed dose.

In the UK a dose of 55 Gy in 20 daily fractions over 4 weeks is often prescribed for smaller medically inoperable tumors (stage I and II). However, for larger tumors a dose of 60–70 Gy in 2-Gy fractions is given over 6.5–7 weeks. At the Royal Marsden Hospital, stage T1/2 tumors may receive 55 Gy in 20 fractions over 4 weeks, whilst T3/4 N0-3 tumors receive 64 Gy in 32 fractions over 6.5 weeks. In the USA, doses of more than 2 Gy per fraction are unusual.

Brachytherapy is only of use as a single modality in patients with very localized tumors who have too poor

Table 17.1. Results of conventional radiotherapy in non-small-cell lung cancer (NSCLC)

Study	n	Dose (Gy)	3-year Survival (%)	5-year Survival (%)
Morita et al. 1997 [3]	149	65	34	22
Jeremic et al. 1997 [4]	49	69.6	46	30
Krol et al. 1996 [5]	108	60–65	31	15
Slotman et al. 1996 [6]	31	48	42	8
Graham et al. 1995 [7]	103	60	35	14
Kaskowitz et al. 1993 [8]	53	63	19	6
Dosoretz et al. 1992 [9]	152	60–69	40	10

Table 17.2. Brachytherapy as single-modality treatment in NSCLC

Study	n	Stage	Dose	Median survival	2-year Survival	5-year Survival
Tredaniel et al. 1994 [16]	29	T1N0	7.5 Gy at 1 cm × 4–6	>23 months		23
Gollins et al. 1996 [17]	37	T1N0<2cm	15–20 Gy at 1 cm, single fraction	23	49	14

lung function to manage EBRT. This may be administered either as a fractionated dose [16] or a single fraction [17].

17.3 Prognostic Factors

Tumor-related factors of prognosis may be biological (e.g., mutation of the *p53* gene or activation of K-*ras*) predicting a poor prognosis, histopathologic (e.g., stage of disease or tumoral vessel density), or serological (e.g., cytokeratin markers). Host-related factors include clinical (e.g., performance status and weight loss) or hematological (e.g., lactate dehydrogenase, albumin, and D-Dimer levels) [18].

From the radiotherapy point of view, factors such as the delivery, fractionation, and amount of radiation dose applied, have been shown to have an impact on outcome.

17.4 Radiation Therapy Dose

Several studies have shown a dose–response of radiation in NSCLC. Perez conducted a radiation dose-escalation trial (Radiation Therapy Oncology Group, RTOG 73-01) to determine the optimal radiation dose using single daily fractions. The radiographic local control and 3-

year relapse-free survival were improved with doses of 60 Gy compared with lower doses [19]. Slawson et al. [20] and Cox et al. [21] have also shown this in the subsequent RTOG randomized studies (Table 17.3).

17.5 Complications of Conventional Radiotherapy

High-dose thoracic radiotherapy can cause significant toxicities. The type and severity of the toxicity depends on the anatomical site, the extent of the target volume, the total dose, and the fraction size of the prescribed radiation. In the thorax, the spinal cord, lung, esophagus, and heart are the organs at risk of radiation-induced damage.

17.5.1 The Lung

Radiation-induced pneumonitis can be divided into acute and late. Acute typically presents 1–4 months after the start of radiotherapy, with symptoms of shortness of breath and cough. This usually responds well to steroids. Acute pneumonitis typically resolves over 4–6 weeks. Late complications arise months to years after the radiotherapy in the form of progressive lung fibrosis. This is usually asymptomatic, but patients with

Table 17.3. Results of the Radiation Therapy Oncology Group (RTOG) series of studies investigating radiation dose for NSCLC. *Conv* Conventional 5 days per week, *Hypo* hypofractionation, *Hyper* hyperfractionation twice daily

Study	Total dose/ no./week	Fraction	n	Median survival (months)	2-year Survival (%)
RTOG 73-01	40/10/4	Split 2 week	101	9.2	
Perez et al. 1986 [19]	40/20/4	Conv	102	11.5	
	50/25/5	Conv	90	10.2	
	60/30/6	Conv	86	11.7	
RTOG 82-01	60/30/6	Conv	63	10	23
Slawson et al. 1988 [20]	60/12/12	Hypo	57	12	29
RTOG 83-11	60/50/5	Hyper	83	9.2	16
Cox et al. 1990 [21]	64.8/54/5.4		127	6.3	14
	69.6/58/5.9		220	10	20
	74.4/62/6.1		211	8.7	15
	79.2/66/6.4		207	10.5	20

poor lung function may present with increasing breathlessness. Treatment is aimed at symptom relief with steroids and oxygen, if required. Kwa et al. [22] found that the incidence of pneumonitis for which steroids were prescribed was 10% for a mean dose of 18 Gy averaged across both lungs. Hernando et al. [23] related the incidence of pneumonitis to the V_{30} (the percentage of lung volume receiving more than 30 Gy), finding 6% with a V_{30} of up to 18%, 21% with a V_{30} between 18 and 32%, and 30% with V_{30} of more than 32%.

17.5.2   The Spinal Cord

Radiation myelopathy is the most feared radiation complication of thoracic radiotherapy. Initial symptoms are nonspecific and although much quoted as a predictor of permanent myelopathy, Lhermitte's sign is rarely the harbinger of permanent myelopathy. Transient demyelination may be seen on magnetic resonance imaging. Symptoms may progress with worsening neurological function. The published safe limits of spinal cord doses have been as high as 60 Gy in 2-Gy fractions [24], but in practice levels are kept between 45 and 50 Gy in conventional fraction sizes.

17.5.3   The Esophagus

Esophageal toxicity only occurs when the mediastinum is irradiated (stage III but not stage I or II disease). The first symptoms of acute esophagitis occur in the 2nd or 3rd week of radiation, commonly at a dose of 18–20 Gy. Patients describe having difficulty in swallowing (dysphagia) and heartburn. This may lead on to pain on swallowing (odynophagia). Most patients will experience mild to moderate esophagitis (30–80%) [25]. The incidence of severe (European Organization for Research and Treatment of Cancer grade 3 or higher) acute esophagitis as a result of thoracic radiotherapy is 1.3% [26]. Symptoms of acute esophagitis usually resolve by 3–4 weeks after the last fraction of radiation. Late esophageal damage may occur at 3–8 months after completion of radiotherapy and patients may present with dysphagia to solids caused by strictures. These can usually be successfully dilated endoscopically.

17.6   Postoperative Radiotherapy

Surgery remains the treatment of choice for NSCLC, but only about 20% are suitable for curative resection [27]. For those with completely resected disease, survival is around 40% at 5 years. In an effort to improve both local control rates and survival, adjuvant or postoperative

radiotherapy (PORT) [28] has been explored. The PORT meta-analysis Trialists Group published their first review in 1998. Data from 2,128 patients from 9 randomized trials of PORT versus surgery alone were observed. The median follow-up was 3.9 years. This group reported a significant detrimental effect for those receiving radiotherapy, with a relative increase in risk of death of 21%, and an absolute detriment of 7% at 2 years. Overall survival was reduced from 55% to 48% ($p = 0.001$). It was concluded that PORT is detrimental to patients with stage I and II disease, and that there was no clear evidence that it was either detrimental or beneficial in those with stage III, N2 disease. The cause of this detrimental effect was not clear from these analyses; however, the excess mortality in those receiving PORT was thought to be due to causes other than cancer. It may be that radiation effects such as pneumonitis and cardiotoxicity on a background of lungs impaired by surgery and smoking contributed to this.

Okawara et al. [29] also reviewed available literature for PORT and concluded that it was not indicated for patients with completely resected stage I and II disease, and there was weak evidence for PORT in stage IIIA (T3 N0 and T1–3 N1/2).

In cases where there are histopathological positive margins or node-positive disease, the case for PORT is not defined and practice varies between centers and on individual cases.

17.7   Methods to Improve the Results of Radiotherapy

17.7.1   Three-Dimensional Conformal Radiotherapy

Three-dimensional CRT allows the shaping of treatment fields and dose distribution to the target volume. It aims to deliver an adequate dose to diseased tissue and minimal dose to adjacent critical normal tissues, which for lung cancer are the normal lung, spinal cord, heart, and esophagus. The GTV and critical structures are delineated on every planning CT slice upon which they are visible. The software then gives a complete picture of the disease and normal tissues that can be viewed in three dimensions.

Conformal shielding is provided by customized lead blocks or by a multileaf collimator. Beams eye views (BEVs) are images provided on the treatment planning systems allowing the radiation oncologist to visualize and check that the field positioning is appropriate to provide adequate target volume coverage and avoidance of organs at risk. The BEV is able to rotate the reconstructed patient within the computer and enable the planner to view the patient in the same orientation as the radiation beam pointed in that direction.

Studies comparing conventional techniques to 3D-CRT for NSCLC have shown the potential to deliver an increased dose to the target whilst maintaining a tolerance dose to the normal surrounding tissues by reducing the volume of tissue irradiated (Fig. 17.2) [30].

17.7.2 Conventional Dose Escalation

Evidence suggests that there is a direct correlation between dose and tumor control and that increasing the tumor dose results in an improvement of local control [19, 31]. Early phase III trials conducted by RTOG 73-01 [19] and RTOG 83-01 [20] confirmed improved local control with radiotherapy doses up to 70 Gy using conventional radiotherapy techniques. Rengan et al. [32] published a retrospective review of 72 patients with stage III disease and divided them into groups receiving greater or less than 64 Gy. They found that 2-year local failure rates were 47% and 76% for those receiving greater than 64 Gy and those receiving less than 64 Gy, respectively. Median survival was 20 months for the higher-dose group, compared to 15 months for the lower dose. Belderbos et al. [33] published preliminary data of a phase I/II dose-escalation trial. Five risk groups were defined by the relative mean lung dose, and the dose prescribed accordingly (Table 17.4). Mature data from this study are awaited.

Table 17.4. Table of escalation doses

Stage	Risk groups				
	I	II	III	IV	V
I	81 Gy	74.3 Gy	74.3 Gy	74.3 Gy	60.8 Gy
II	87.8 Gy	81 Gy	81 Gy	81 Gy	67.5 Gy
IIIa	94.5 Gy	87.8 Gy	87.8 Gy	87.8 Gy	74.3 Gy
IIIb	101.3 Gy	94.5 Gy	94.5 Gy	94.5 Gy	81 Gy

17.7.3 Altered Fractionation and Acceleration

Conventional radiotherapy regimens use once-daily fractions of 2 Gy over 6–7 weeks. This is applied to a broad spectrum of tumor sites and types. The total dose is limited by the risk of injury to normal tissues, and fractionating the dose takes advantage of the radiobiological differences in the survival curves of normal cells and malignant cells. This means that normal tissues are spared by the use of smaller fraction sizes, thus allowing repair to take place.

Newer schedules have been developed based on the principle that the therapeutic ratio could be further improved by reducing the fraction size below 2 Gy to spare the normal tissues whilst treating two to three times daily in order to give a shorter overall treatment time, therefore minimizing the possibility of repopulation of tumor cells. This approach is called accelerated hyperfractionation.

The use of twice-daily fractionation to a total dose of 69.6 Gy in 58 fractions showed improved local control and survival when compared to 60 Gy conventionally fractionated in 2-Gy fractions [21].

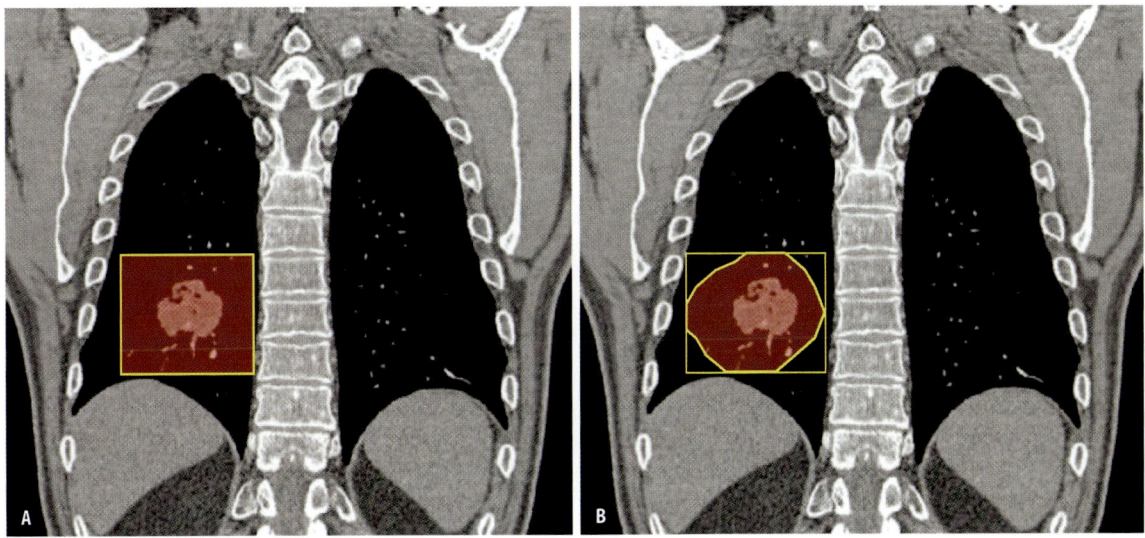

Fig. 17.2. Comparison between volumes irradiated using a conventional parallel pair, 1000 cm^3 (**A**) and three-dimensional conformal radiotherapy, 400 cm^3 (**B**)

17.7.3.1 Continuous Hyperfractionated Accelerated Radiotherapy and Continuous Hyperfractionated Accelerated Radiotherapy Weekend-less

A trial of continuous hyperfractionated accelerated radiotherapy (CHART: 54 Gy in 36 fractions twice daily over 12 days) in stages I–III NSCLC showed improved 2-year survival from 20% to 29% when compared to the conventionally fractionated 60-Gy arm [34]. In the UK the recommended standard radical treatment for inoperable, localized NSCLC is CHART. However, CHART requires radiotherapy three times a day inclusive of weekends, and due to restrictions on resources, has been difficult to implement in many centers. In response to this, a phase II study of continuous hyperfractionated accelerated radiotherapy weekend-less (CHARTWEL) delivered a higher total dose of 60 Gy in 18 days, 2-year survival was 47% [35]. This has led to a current phase III trial comparing CHARTWEL to conventional radiotherapy. Although the late treatment toxicity experienced by patients undergoing CHART is not significantly different from that seen with conventional fractionated radiotherapy, acute effects are more marked [36]. Esophagitis is more prevalent at an earlier stage and is more pronounced. Pneumonitis, however, when assessed by clinical criteria, was less significant in the CHART arm [34].

17.7.4   Methods of Boosting Radiation Dose

Intraluminal, or specifically in NSCLC, endobronchial brachytherapy is a method of applying high-dose-rate radiotherapy to the target using an iridium source. The iridium source is delivered to the target via afterloading catheters of 2–3 mm diameter contained within a designated machine (e.g., Microselectron). The proximal and distal limits of the tumor are determined by bronchoscopy. A guide wire loaded into an afterloading catheter is used to determine the tumor length and a margin of 1 cm is allowed at either end. The iridium source then replaces the guide wire and is driven along the treatment length and left to dwell there for a time calculated to deliver the prescribed dose. A concomitant endobronchial brachytherapy boost during EBRT has been shown to provide higher response rates for reexpansion of the collapsed lung compared to EBRT alone [37]. However, this beneficial effect is confined to a highly selective group of patients with obstructing tumors of the main bronchus and should be considered on a case-by-case basis only.

17.7.5   Chemoradiation

Radiotherapy alone in locally advanced NSCLC results in a 15% local control rate, a median survival of 8 months and <5% 5-year survival [1]. In an attempt to improve these statistics, combined modality treatment with chemotherapy has been explored. These two modalities can interact in four ways as described by Steel [38].

1. Spatial cooperation, where disease in a specific site is missed by one therapeutic agent, but targeted by another. For example, radiotherapy would target intrathoracic disease but chemotherapy would deal with extrathoracic disease.
2. Independent cell kill in this combination of modalities, but the chemotherapy may also kill cells targeted by radiotherapy in the chest therefore creating an additive cytotoxic effect.
3. Cytoprotective agents may be used in conjunction with radiotherapy, allowing increased radiation dose to be applied without detriment to the normal tissues.
4. One modality may have the effect of enhancing the action of the other modality; for example, chemotherapy increasing the radiation effect on a tumor. Cytoprotective agents may be used in conjunction with radiotherapy, allowing an increased radiation dose to be applied without detriment to the normal tissues.

The majority of studies have examined the impact of induction or neoadjuvant chemotherapy or concurrent chemotherapy. In their review, Shibamoto and Jeremic [39] report a survival advantage due to improvement in distant metastasis control of induction chemotherapy and improved survival due to improved locoregional control with concurrent chemoradiation.

17.7.5.1 Sequential Chemotherapy and Radiotherapy

The rationale for induction chemotherapy is to decrease intrathoracic disease bulk and the treatment of subclinical disease outside the thorax. Three large randomized studies have shown an improvement in median survival of 2 months, with a delay in development of distant metastases. Local control and long-term survival was similar to that with radiation alone (Table 17.5) [40–42]. The NSCLCCG [43] meta-analysis in 1995 reported a 13% reduction in risk of death with an absolute benefit in 2-year survival of 4% when chemotherapy was administered in patients receiving radical radiotherapy. Sequential chemotherapy and radiotherapy has been the standard of care in patients with locally advanced NSCLC and good performance status in the UK.

Table 17.5. Sequential chemoradiation

Study	n	Treatment	3-year survival (%)
LeChevalier et al. 1991 [40]	353	RT ± 4 cycles induction and adjuvant (platinum)	12 vs 4
Dillman et al. 1990 [41]	155	RT ± 2 cycles cisplatin and vinblastine	23 vs 11
Sause et al. 2000 [42]	490	RT ± 2 cycles cisplatin and vinblastine	15 vs 6

17.7.5.2 Concurrent Chemotherapy and Radiotherapy

The use of concurrent chemotherapy and radiotherapy has been introduced in an attempt firstly to utilize the spatial relationship of the two modalities, radiotherapy achieving local control and chemotherapy reducing the risk of systemic disease, and secondly to exploit the potential radiosensitizing effects of chemotherapy. There is a cost, however, with increased local toxicity.

Rowell and O'Rourke [44], in the Cochrane database review of 14 randomized trials (including 2,393 patients), demonstrated a small but significant benefit from concurrent chemoradiotherapy over radiotherapy alone (7% reduction in risk of death at 2 years) and a larger and significant benefit from concurrent over sequential chemoradiotherapy (14% reduction in death at 2 years).

Concurrent chemoradiation is the standard of care in the USA for inoperable stage III NSCLC based on the results of the RTOG 94-10 trial [45]. This three-arm study compared two cycles of neoadjuvant cisplatin and vinblastine followed by radiotherapy to 63 Gy, versus two cycles of neoadjuvant cisplatin and vinblastine followed by concomitant cisplatin and vinblastine and radiotherapy to 63 Gy, versus two cycles of neoadjuvant

cisplatin and oral etoposide followed by concomitant hyperfractionated radiotherapy to 69.6 Gy. Median survival was improved by 3 months in favor of two cycles of neoadjuvant chemotherapy followed by concomitant chemoradiation. Grade 3–4 hematological toxicity with hyperfractionated radiotherapy was in excess of 60%, with no significant improvement in median survival compared to sequential treatment. Table 17.6 [45–47].

17.7.5.3 Adjuvant Chemotherapy

There is currently a resurgence in interest in adjuvant/consolidation chemotherapy in lung cancer. The Southwest Oncology Group (SWOG) has evaluated consolidation chemotherapy following chemoradiotherapy in two phase II trials. In SWOG 9019 [48], 50 patients received concomitant chemoradiation followed by two cycles of cisplatin and etoposide. In SWOG 9504 [49], 83 patients received concomitant chemoradiation followed by two cycles of docetaxel. Better results were reported with docetaxel, resulting in a 3-year overall survival of 37% and a median survival of 26 months. Unfortunately, this was a single-arm study and so it is uncertain whether the impressive results are a real improvement, or due to patient selection.

The optimal chemotherapy regimen remains unclear, particularly with respect to the impact of taxanes, dose, and frequency of administration on outcome. The results of ongoing studies are awaited.

17.7.5.4 Toxicity

The addition of chemotherapy to radiotherapy has produced an increased risk of acute esophagitis (0–33% in those receiving radiation alone vs. 2–47% in the chemoradiotherapy group; $p = 0.001$), but adverse effects on the lung (early or late) were not seen. Concurrent and sequential regimens had similar levels of neutropenia. However, hematological toxicity is higher than with

Table 17.6. Concurrent versus sequential chemoradiation. *RT* Radiation therapy

Study	n	Treatment	Median survival (months)	Survival Concurrent vs sequential
Zatloukal et al. 2004 (Czech Lung Cancer Group) [46]	102	4 × cisplatin and vinorelbine with daily RT to 60 Gy starting at week 5 (concurrent) vs following completion of chemotherapy at week 17 (sequential)	16.6 vs 12.9	At 2 years: 34% vs 14%
Curran et al. 2003 (RTOG 94-10) [45]	402	Vinblastine and cisplatin plus daily RT (60 Gy) (concurrent) vs vinblastine and cisplatin followed by RT (sequential)	17 vs 14.6	At 4 years: 21% vs 12%
Fournel et al. 2001 [47]	216	Vinblastine and etoposide plus daily RT (66 Gy) followed by cisplatin and vinorelbine (concurrent) vs cisplatin and vinorelbine followed by RT (sequential)		At 2 years: 35% vs 23%

radiotherapy alone, with a relative risk of 1.85 for anemia ($p = 0.009$) with chemoradiotherapy [44].

17.8   Biological/Novel Agents

17.8.1   Chemotherapeutic Agents

Taxanes (paclitaxol, docetaxel), topoisomerase inhibitors (topotecan, irinotecan) and gemcitabine and vinorelbine, have all shown activity in NSCLC. It has been reasonable to incorporate these agents into combined modality trials because as many have different mechanisms of interaction with ionizing radiation and mature data from such studies is awaited.

17.8.1.1   Epidermal Growth Factor Receptor Inhibitors

Epidermal growth factor receptor (EGFR) is overexpressed in NSCLC and results in a more aggressive clinical course as it plays a role in the proliferation, invasion, angiogenesis, and development of metastases, and is antiapoptotic. Radiotherapy appears to trigger EGFR expression, resulting in accelerated repopulation. EGFR inhibition can be induced by monoclonal antibodies to EGFR such as cetuximab, small-molecule tyrosine kinase inhibitors such as Iressa, and anti-EGF vaccines, which are currently undergoing phase I trials.

17.9   Methods of Reducing Toxicity

17.9.1   Image-Guided Procedures

Advances in imaging have enabled more accurate staging of the disease, permitting improved patient selection for appropriate treatment modality. For example, positron emission tomography (PET) using ^{18}F-fluorodeoxyglucose (FDG-PET) has shown sensitivity and accuracy in NSCLC [50, 51]. The role of FDG-PET in target definition within radiotherapy planning is being evaluated. Bradley et al. [25] noted changes of up to 50% where disease was distinguished from atelectasis and previously unknown nodal disease was identified.

17.9.2   Intensity-Modulated Radiotherapy

Just as 3D-CRT made it possible to reduce toxicity to critical structures whilst increasing the radiation dose to the target by increased conformity of the beam to the target, so the emergence of intensity-modulated radiotherapy (IMRT) can further build on this by increasing conformity in more than one plane. In IMRT,

intensity modulation within the radiation beam is designed on the basis of the target prescription and a set of dose constraints for sensitive structures using inverse planning. The capability of differentiating the weight of individual rays allows sculpting of the isodose distributions for optimal conformity. However, this technique requires further evaluation to assess fully the damaging effect of greater volumes of normal lung being irradiated to a low, but possibly significant dose.

17.9.3   Overcoming Tumor Motion

One of the challenges in lung cancer irradiation is overcoming tumor motion due to respiratory movement. At present, margins of 1–2 cm are added to the clinical target volume to account for this. Consequently the PTV will always enlarge and, therefore, will the amount of normal tissue that is irradiated. Methods of minimizing error and possibly permitting smaller margins are currently under evaluation. This can be approached from two different angles, stopping the movement and irradiating at that point, for example the active breathing control (ABC) device [52] or deep inspiration breath hold (DIBH) and radiotherapy gating, or tracking the movement of either the tumor or the patient.

Use of the ABC device, where respiration is temporarily suspended for a few seconds during the planning and treatment, eliminates the PTV margin for motion because the GTV need only be defined at one point during respiration. Problems arise, however, with the compliance of the patients, who more often than not have compromised lung function and may not tolerate this technique. DIBH does not require any special apparatus; the patient is verbally coached through a modified slow vital capacity maneuver and brought to a reproducible deep inspiration breath-hold level. The goal is to immobilize the tumor and to expand the normal lung out of the high-dose region [53]. However, the results are not accurately reproducible and the technique is tiring for patients during a full course of radiotherapy treatment.

Image-guided radiotherapy techniques rely on a surrogate marker for the tumor coupled with an imaging technique to detect its position. This allows tracking of the tumor during free breathing with apparatus coupled to the patient and the linear accelerator treatment beam. Tumor position varies in all directions during respiration, and the complexity of this type of treatment delivery can in itself be subject to further errors.

With respiratory-gated radiotherapy, radiation is only delivered at a certain phase of respiration, sometimes referred to as the 'gate'. The position and width of the gate within a respiratory cycle are determined by monitoring the respiratory motion, using either an external respiratory signal (e.g., movement of the chest wall) or an internal fiducial marker. Gated therapy is an active research area and results are pending; there is a drawback of increased treatment time.

Motion-adaptive X-ray therapy has been described by Keall et al. [54], where synchronous adjustment of the treatment field shape using multileaf collimators, tracks the movement of the target during respiration. The radiation is delivered in synchrony with the target movement using respiratory-gated radiotherapy equipment.

17.10 Conclusions

Radiotherapy has played a part in the management of locally advanced NSCLC for decades. It has provided an option of radical treatment in patients who present with inoperable disease. Recent advances in radiotherapy techniques and the combined modality treatment with chemotherapy have improved the outcome for these patients. Future developments for more accurate staging of disease with both anatomical and functional imaging, improved radiotherapy conformity with IMRT and image-guided radiotherapy, and the use of novel chemotherapeutic agents and biological agents in conjunction with radiotherapy, will further improve the outcome for NSCLC.

Key Points

- Radiotherapy with chemotherapy: there is evidence of a survival benefit of concurrent chemoradiotherapy over sequential chemotherapy and radiotherapy in the treatment of locally advanced non-small-cell lung cancer (NSCLC).
- Methods of decreasing toxicity of radiotherapy: reduction of toxicity caused by radiation dose to normal tissues surrounding the target volume is being reduced by greater conformity of radiation treatments following advances in technical delivery (e.g., image-guided radiotherapy and tracking of physiological target movement, intensity-modulated radiotherapy).
- Radiation dose escalation: there is evidence of a correlation between dose and tumor control, and with increasing conformity of radiotherapy volumes, escalation of dose to the target is possible and is the subject of ongoing trials.
- Novel modalities: the impact of newer-generation cytotoxic drugs (e.g., taxanes and biological agents such as epidermal growth factor inhibitors) on radiotherapy regimens is awaited.

References

1. Jemal A, Thomas A, Murray T, et al. Cancer statistics, 2002. CA Cancer J Clin 2002; 52:23.
2. Pfister DG, Johnson DH, Azzoli CG, et al. American Society of Clinical Oncology treatment of unresectable non-small-cell lung cancer guideline: update 2003. J Clin Oncol 2004; 22:330.
3. Morita K, Fuwa N, Suzuki Y, et al. Radical radiotherapy for medically inoperable non-small cell lung cancer in clinical stage I: a retrospective analysis of 149 patients. Radiother Oncol 1997; 42:31.
4. Jeremic B, Shibamoto Y, Acimovic L, et al. Hyperfractionated radiotherapy alone for clinical stage I nonsmall cell lung cancer. Int J Radiat Oncol Biol Phys 1997; 38:521.
5. Krol AD, Aussems P, Noordijk EM, et al. Local irradiation alone for peripheral stage I lung cancer: could we omit the elective regional nodal irradiation? Int J Radiat Oncol Biol Phys 1996; 34:297.
6. Slotman BJ, Antonisse IE, Njo KH. Limited field irradiation in early stage (T1-2N0) non-small cell lung cancer. Radiother Oncol 1996; 41:41.
7. Graham PH, Gebski VJ, Langlands AO. Radical radiotherapy for early nonsmall cell lung cancer. Int J Radiat Oncol Biol Phys 1995; 31:261.
8. Kaskowitz L, Graham MV, Emami B, et al. Radiation therapy alone for stage I non-small cell lung cancer. Int J Radiat Oncol Biol Phys 1993; 27:517.
9. Dosoretz DE, Katin MJ, Blitzer PH, et al. Radiation therapy in the management of medically inoperable carcinoma of the lung: results and implications for future treatment strategies. Int J Radiat Oncol Biol Phys 1992; 24:3.
10. Landberg T, Chavaudra J, Dobbs HJ. ICRU Report 62. Prescribing, recording and reporting photon beam therapy (supplement to ICRU Report 50). International Commission on Radiotherapy Units and Measurements, Bethesda, MD, 1999.
11. Senan S, Burgers S, Samson MJ, et al. Can elective nodal irradiation be omitted in stage III non-small-cell lung cancer? Analysis of recurrences in a phase II study of induction chemotherapy and involved-field radiotherapy. Int J Radiat Oncol Biol Phys 2002; 54:999.
12. Rosenzweig KE, Sim SE, Mychalczak B, et al. Elective nodal irradiation in the treatment of non-small-cell lung cancer with three-dimensional conformal radiation therapy. Int J Radiat Oncol Biol Phys 2001; 50:681.
13. Sibley GS. Radiotherapy for patients with medically inoperable Stage I nonsmall cell lung carcinoma: smaller volumes and higher doses – a review. Cancer 1998; 82:433.
14. van Sornsen de Koste JR, Lagerwaard FJ, Nijssen-Visser MR, et al. Tumor location cannot predict the mobility of lung tumors: a 3D analysis of data generated from multiple CT scans. Int J Radiat Oncol Biol Phys 2003; 56:348.
15. Sixel KE, Ruschin M, Tirona R, et al. Digital fluoroscopy to quantify lung tumor motion: potential for patient-specific planning target volumes. Int J Radiat Oncol Biol Phys 2003; 57:717.
16. Tredaniel J, Hennequin C, Zalcman G, et al. Prolonged survival after high-dose rate endobronchial radiation for malignant airway obstruction. Chest 1994; 105:767.
17. Gollins SW, Burt PA, Barber PV, et al. Long-term survival and symptom palliation in small primary bronchial carcinomas following treatment with intraluminal radiotherapy alone. Clin Oncol (R Coll Radiol) 1996; 8:239.
18. Buccheri G, Ferrigno D. Prognostic factors. Hematol Oncol Clin North Am 2004; 18:187.

19. Perez CA, Bauer M, Edelstein S, et al. Impact of tumor control on survival in carcinoma of the lung treated with irradiation. Int J Radiat Oncol Biol Phys 1986; 12:539.

20. Slawson RG, Salazar OM, Poussin-Rosillo H, et al. Once-a-week vs conventional daily radiation treatment for lung cancer: final report. Int J Radiat Oncol Biol Phys 1988; 15:61.

21. Cox JD, Azarnia N, Byhardt RW, et al. A randomized phase I/II trial of hyperfractionated radiation therapy with total doses of 60.0 Gy to 79.2 Gy: possible survival benefit with greater than or equal to 69.6 Gy in favorable patients with Radiation Therapy Oncology Group stage III non-small-cell lung carcinoma: report of Radiation Therapy Oncology Group 83-11. J Clin Oncol 1990; 8:1543.

22. Kwa SL, Lebesque JV, Theuws JC et al. Radiation pneumonitis as a function of mean lung dose: an analysis of pooled data of 540 patients. Int J Radiat Oncol Biol Phys 1998; 42:1.

23. Hernando ML, Marks LB, Bentel GC, et al. Radiation-induced pulmonary toxicity: a dose–volume histogram analysis in 201 patients with lung cancer. Int J Radiat Oncol Biol Phys 2001; 51:650.

24. Kim YH, Fayos JV. Radiation tolerance of the cervical spinal cord. Radiology 1981; 139:473.

25. Bradley J, Thorstad WL, Mutic S, et al. Impact of FDG-PET on radiation therapy volume delineation in non-small-cell lung cancer. Int J Radiat Oncol Biol Phys 2004; 59:78.

26. Werner-Wasik M, Yu X, Marks LB, et al. Normal-tissue toxicities of thoracic radiation therapy: esophagus, lung, and spinal cord as organs at risk. Hematol Oncol Clin North Am 2004; 18:131.

27. Silverberg E, Boring CC, Squires TS. Cancer statistics, 1990. CA Cancer J Clin 1990; 40:9

28. PORT Meta-analysis Trialists Group. Postoperative radiotherapy for non-small cell lung cancer. The Cochrane Database of Systematic Reviews 2003: Art.No.:CD002142. DOI: 10.1002/14651858.CD002142.

29. Okawara G, Ung YC, Markman BR, et al. Postoperative radiotherapy in stage II or IIIA completely resected non-small cell lung cancer: a systematic review and practice guideline. Lung Cancer 2004; 44:1.

30. Emami B. Three-dimensional conformal radiation therapy in bronchogenic carcinoma. Semin Radiat Oncol 1996; 6:92.

31. Martel MK, Ten Haken RK, Hazuka MB, et al. Estimation of tumor control probability model parameters from 3-D dose distributions of non-small cell lung cancer patients. Lung Cancer 1999; 24:31.

32. Rengan R, Rosenzweig KE, Venkatraman E, et al. Improved local control with higher doses of radiation in large-volume stage III non-small-cell lung cancer. Int J Radiat Oncol Biol Phys 2004; 60:741.

33. Belderbos JS, De Jaeger K, Heemsbergen WD, et al. First results of a phase I/II dose escalation trial in non-small cell lung cancer using three-dimensional conformal radiotherapy. Radiother Oncol 2003; 66:119.

34. Saunders M, Dische S, Barrett A, et al. Continuous hyperfractionated accelerated radiotherapy (CHART) versus conventional radiotherapy in non-small-cell lung cancer: a randomised multicentre trial. CHART Steering Committee. Lancet 1997; 350:161.

35. Saunders MI, Rojas A, Lyn BE, et al. Experience with dose escalation using CHARTWEL (continuous hyperfractionated accelerated radiotherapy weekend less) in non-small-cell lung cancer. Br J Cancer 1998; 78:1323.

36. Dische S, Saunders MI. The CHART regimen and morbidity. Acta Oncol 1999; 38:147.

37. Langendijk H, de Jong J, Tjwa M, et al. External irradiation versus external irradiation plus endobronchial bra-

38. Steel G. Basic Clinical Radiobiology, 3rd edn. Hodder Arnold, London, 2002.

39. Shibamoto Y, Jeremic B. Biologic premises of combined radiation therapy and chemotherapy in lung cancer. Hematol Oncol Clin North Am 2004; 18:29.

40. LeChevalier TAR, Lacombe-Terrier M-J, et al. Radiotherapy alone versus combined chemotherapy and radiotherapy in nonresectable non-small-cell lung cancer: first analysis of a randomised trial in 353 patients. J Natl Cancer Inst 1991; 83:417.

41. Dillman RO, Herndon J, Seagren SL, et al. Improved survival in stage III non-small-cell lung cancer: seven-year follow-up of cancer and leukemia group B (CALGB) 8433 trial. J Natl Cancer Inst 1996; 88:1210.

42. Sause W, Kolesar P, Taylor S, et al. Final results of phase III trial in regionally advanced unresectable non-small cell lung cancer: Radiation Therapy Oncology Group, Eastern Cooperative Oncology Group, and Southwest Oncology Group. Chest 2000; 117:358.

43. NSCLCCG. Chemotherapy in non-small cell lung cancer: a meta-analysis using updated data on individual patients from 52 randomised clinical trials. Non-small Cell Lung Cancer Collaborative Group. BMJ 1995; 311:899.

44. Rowell N, O'Rourke N. Concurrent chemoradiotherapy in non-small cell lung cancer. Cochrane Database Syst Rev 2004:CD002140.

45. Curran WJ, Scott CB, Langer CJ, et al. Long-term benefit is observed in a phase III comparison of sequential vs concurrent chemoradiation for patients with unresected stage III NSCLC: RTOG 9410. Proc Am Soc Clin Oncol 2003:621.

46. Zatloukal P, Petruzelka L, Zemanova M, et al. Concurrent versus sequential chemoradiotherapy with cisplatin and vinorelbine in locally advanced non-small cell lung cancer: a randomized study. Lung Cancer 2004; 46:87.

47. Fournel P, Perol M, Robinet G, et al. A randomized phase III trial of sequential chemo-radiotherapy versus concurrent chemo-radiotherapy in locally advanced non small cell lung cancer (nsclc) (glot-gfpc Npc 95-01 Study). Proc Am Soc Clin Oncol 2001; 22:621.

48. Albain KS, Crowley JJ, Turrisi AT 3rd, et al. Concurrent cisplatin, etoposide, and chest radiotherapy in pathologic stage IIIB non-small-cell lung cancer: a Southwest Oncology Group phase II study, SWOG 9019. J Clin Oncol 2002; 20:3454.

49. Gandara DR, Chansky K, Albain KS, et al. Consolidation docetaxel after concurrent chemoradiotherapy in stage IIIB non-small-cell lung cancer: phase II Southwest Oncology Group Study S9504. J Clin Oncol 2003; 21:2004.

50. Kutlu CA, Pastorino U, Maisey M, et al. Early experience with PET scanning in thoracic tumours. J Cardiovasc Surg (Torino) 2001; 42:403.

51. Prauer HW, Weber WA, Romer W, et al. Controlled prospective study of positron emission tomography using the glucose analogue [18 f]fluorodeoxyglucose in the evaluation of pulmonary nodules. Br J Surg 1998; 85:1506.

52. Wong JW, Sharpe MB, Jaffray DA, et al. The use of active breathing control (ABC) to reduce margin for breathing motion. Int J Radiat Oncol Biol Phys 1999; 44:911.

53. Mah D, Hanley J, Rosenzweig KE et al. Technical aspects of the deep inspiration breath-hold technique in the treatment of thoracic cancer. Int J Radiat Oncol Biol Phys 2000; 48:1175.

54. Keall PJ, Kini VR, Vedam SS, et al. Motion adaptive x-ray therapy: a feasibility study. Phys Med Biol 2001; 46:1.

Palliative Radiotherapy in the Management of Non-Small-Cell Lung Cancer

18

Katie Newbold and Christopher M. Nutting

Contents

18.1 Introduction

Lung cancer is now the leading cause of cancer deaths in men and women in the UK. Non-small cell lung cancer (NSCLC) accounts for approximately 80% of all lung cancer and two-thirds of these patients will present with advanced disease. The 5-year survival rates for stage IIIB is 5% and for stage IV less than 1% in the UK [1].

Radiotherapy has been used to treat tumors within the chest since the 1960s. In approximately 20% of lung cancer patients, radiotherapy, usually as part of a multimodality approach with chemotherapy, can be used to provide long-term control or even cure of the disease, but more often it is used in lower doses with the aim of controlling or palliating local symptoms such as cough, hemoptysis, pain, and breathlessness. Estimates of clinical practice in the UK suggest that lung cancer constitutes 20–25% of radiation oncologists' time and 90% of these treatments are palliative [2]

Patients with advanced NSCLC are increasingly being treated with chemotherapy as the first line of treatment [3]. Palliative radiotherapy, however, continues to have an important role in this setting. Palliation should control symptoms, and with this goal the avoidance of side effects and maintaining quality of life must be the main aim of treatment.

The main groups of patients falling into the palliative management setting are those with symptomatic stage I–IIIB disease who are not suitable for radical treatment, and stage IV disease where the symptoms are principally related to thoracic disease. Patients with disseminated disease with predominantly extrathoracic symptoms are better managed with palliative chemotherapy.

18.2 Symptoms

The symptoms experienced by patients with advanced lung cancer can be divided into those due to the location of the tumor and systemic effects caused by the tumor. Local effects include dysphagia due to extrinsic pressure on the esophagus, stridor due to compression of the airway, venous distension, headaches, and edema due to superior vena caval obstruction, hemoptysis from erosion of the tumor into an airway, and chest pain. Systemic effects of the tumor include cachexia and fatigue.

18.3 Radiotherapy

Most radiotherapy used in the palliative setting will be external-beam radiotherapy (EBRT), either from a radioactive source such as cobalt-60 or, more usually now since the 1980s, a linear accelerator. Brachytherapy applied endobronchially may also be used.

18.3.1 Which Regimen?

There is little evidence that patients get better palliation of symptoms from higher radiation doses compared to low doses or longer-lasting doses. There is good evidence that higher doses give more toxicity, especially radiation-induced esophagitis. Therefore short, hypofractionated regimens make sense in keeping hospital visits to a minimum for the patient [4].

In 1991 and 1992, the British Medical Research Council (MRC) published its first two randomized trials of radiotherapy in the palliative setting (Table 18.1).

The first compared 30 Gy in ten fractions over 2 weeks with 17 Gy in two fractions over 8 days [5]. A total of 369 patients of all performance status (PS) were randomized and no significant difference was seen in terms of palliation of symptoms, acute toxicity, or survival. The second MRC trial randomized 235 patients with poor PS to either 17 Gy in two fractions or 10 Gy in one single fraction. The single-fraction arm was as effective at palliating symptoms and caused less esophagitis. There was no difference in survival [6]. In both of these trials, palliation of the main symptoms was achieved in high proportions of patients. The duration of this palliation was for 50% or more of survival, PS improved in approximately half.

The question arose as to whether in a selected group of better PS; the survival could be affected using a different fractionation regimen. The third MRC trial compared 17 Gy in 2 fractions with 39 Gy in 13 fractions in 509 patients with good PS and showed an improvement in 2-year survival, 12% vs 9%, in favor of the 13-fraction regimen [7].

Bezjak et al. 2002 carried out a phase III randomized study comparing 10-Gy single-fraction radiotherapy with 20 Gy in five fractions in the palliation of thoracic symptoms from lung cancer in 230 patients [8]. At 1 month after radiotherapy, no difference was found in symptom control between the two arms. The changes in the scores on the Lung Cancer Symptom Scale indicated that the fractionated radiotherapy (five fractions) group had greater improvement in symptoms related to lung cancer ($p = 0.009$), pain ($p = 0.0008$), ability to carry out normal activities ($p = 0.037$), and better global quality of life ($p = 0.039$). The European Organization for Research and Treatment of Cancer QLQ-C30 scores showed that patients receiving five fractions had a greater improvement in scores with respect to pain ($p = 0.04$). No significant difference was found in treatment-related toxicity. Patients who received five fractions survived on average 2 months longer ($p = 0.0305$) than patients who received one fraction.

Cross et al. irradiated 23 patients with symptomatic NSCLC with two fractions of 8.5 Gy 1 week apart [9]. The most common symptoms were dyspnea (100%), cough (96%), anorexia (65%), and chest pain (52%). Between treatment completion and 4 months after treatment, improvement was seen as follows: dyspnea (33%), cough (60%), anorexia/nausea (67%), chest pain (75%), hoarseness (25%), hemoptysis (100%), and dysphagia (100%).

18.3.2 Toxicity

Effective symptom relief is achieved with 17 Gy in two fractions or a 10-Gy single fraction, which are widely used regimens. Toxicities reported include nausea, chest pain, fever, and rigors during the first 24 h after large single fractions to the chest [10–12]. Incidence of radiation myelitis was reported in the Medical Research Council (MRC) studies 1991, 1992, and 1996 following 17 Gy in two fractions with an actuarial incidence of myelopathy of 0.6% at 1 year and 2.2% at 2 years (Table 18.1); advice from Macbeth et al. in the Cochrane database systematic review, suggests that methods to reduce the spinal cord dose when using 17 Gy in two fractions should be used [4].

18.3.3 Technique

The patient is treated in the supine position. Targets should be outlined according to International Commission on Radiological Units and Measurements 62 guide-

Table 18.1. Randomized trials comparing different regimens of radiotherapy in the palliative setting. *MRC* Medical Research Council Lung Cancer Working Party, *F* fractions, *NA* not available, *PS* performance status

Study	Regimens	Patients n, PS	Symptom control	Esophagitis	Survival
MRC 1991	30 Gy/10F 17 Gy/2F	369, any PS	No difference	No difference	No difference
MRC 1992	10 Gy/1F 17 Gy/2F	235, PS 2–4	No difference	Worse with 17 Gy	No difference
MRC 1996	36–39 Gy/12-13F 17 Gy/2F	509, PS 0–1	No difference	Worse with 39 Gy	Better for 39 Gy 9% vs. 12% at 2 years
Reinfuss 1999	50 Gy/25F 40 Gy/10F (split) 20–25 Gy/5F (delayed)	240, KPS >60 (no metastases)	NA	No difference	Better for 50 Gy; 18% vs 6% vs 0% at 2 years
Sundstrom 2004	17 Gy/2F 42 Gy/15F 50 Gy/25F	421, all PS	No difference	NA	No difference

lines [13, 14]. Gross tumor volume (GTV) is determined from chest radiographs, bronchoscopy report, and diagnostic computed tomography scan (preferably both lung and soft-tissue windows). Planning target volume (PTV) is defined as the GTV responsible for symptoms with an additional margin. Anterior and posterior fields are used to encompass the PTV with a 1- to 2-cm margin. Normal tissue shielding is used as appropriate. Care should be taken to avoid including excessive amounts of normal lung within the treatment fields. In general, palliative radiotherapy regimes fall within spinal cord tolerance. Physical factors that increase the dose to the cord (such as greater anterior-posterior separation) may exacerbate this risk. The latency of radiation myelopathy (greater than 8 months in most cases) suggests that regimes where the cord dose is close to tolerance are best used in those with a limited life expectancy. This dose is prescribed as a mid-plane dose without lung correction.

18.3.4 Superior Vena Caval Obstruction

Superior vena caval obstruction (SVCO) is an uncommon manifestation of carcinoma of the lung. It is characterized by neck swelling and distended chest veins, but is also accompanied by breathlessness, hoarseness of voice, and headache. SVCO occurs when the superior vena cava is compressed either by the primary tumor, usually arising in the right main or upper lobe bronchus, or by involved mediastinal lymphadenopathy. Treatment is either of the symptoms or of the underlying cause. Traditionally, treatment has included systemic steroids and either radiotherapy (for non-small-cell cancers) or chemotherapy (mostly for small-cell cancers). However, in those cases that do not respond to either chemotherapy or radiotherapy, or relapse rapidly after treatment, the positioning of percutaneous expandable stents within the superior vena cava can restore blood flow. Rowell and Gleeson, in the Cochrane database systematic review [15], report rates of relief of SVCO of around 60% for both chemotherapy and radiotherapy in NSCLC; 19% of those treated had a recurrence of SVCO. Insertion of an superior vena cava stent relieved SVCO in 95% of cases; 11% of those treated had further SVCO but recanalization was possible in the majority, resulting in a long-term patency rate of 92%. Chemotherapy and radiotherapy are effective in relieving SVCO in some patients, whilst stent insertion may provide relief in a higher proportion and more rapidly. The effectiveness of steroids and the optimal timing of stent insertion (whether at diagnosis or following failure of other modalities) remain uncertain.

The radiotherapy technique applied would be as described above using a parallel pair approach, prescribing 20 Gy in five fractions over 1 week to the mid-plane dose.

18.3.5 Stridor

Emergency radiotherapy is indicated for airway obstruction at the level of the trachea or carina producing stridor. High-dose dexamethasone is given prior to and during radiotherapy. A mid-plane dose of 20 Gy in five fractions over 1 week is generally appropriate.

18.3.6 Retreatment

Where possible, endobronchial laser treatment or bronchial stenting should be considered prior to reirradiation. Reirradiation may be considered in symptomatic patients who achieved a symptomatic and radiological response following a course of radiotherapy given 6 or more months previously. Where the spinal cord has been treated previously and life expectancy is greater than 6 months, anterior and posterior oblique fields are used to avoid the cord and deliver a dose of 2 0Gy at the isocenter in five fractions over 1 week. Large fields should be avoided.

18.4 Conclusion

All patients with advanced NSCLC should be considered for palliative treatment. There is reasonable evidence that palliative radiotherapy is effective in symptom control and may prolong life in some patients. There remain questions as to how best to select patients who will gain a benefit from treatment and those who will not. Where palliation aims to improve quality of life, the impact of possible side effects should be carefully considered. Palliative radiotherapy should be just part of the multimodality management of these patients.

Key Points

- For patients with poor performance status, a regimen of one or two fractions is recommended in order to minimize time spent in hospital and discomfort. The rare but serious side effect of radiation myelitis can be avoided either by shielding the cord for the second fraction or by reducing the dose to 15 Gy in two fractions.
- For good-performance patients a higher dose regimen such as 39 Gy in 13 fractions or 40 Gy in 15 fractions can be justified for the small survival benefit.
- The optimal multimodality approach with radiation, chemotherapy, or biological agents is not yet known.

References

1. Janssen-Heijnen ML, Smulders S, Lemmens VE, Smeenk FW, van Geffen HJ, Coebergh JW. Effect of comorbidity on the treatment and prognosis of elderly patients with non-small cell lung cancer. Thorax 2004; 59:602.
2. Maher EJ, Timothy A, Squire CJ, et al. Audit: the use of radiotherapy for NSCLC in the UK. Clin Oncol (R Coll Radiol) 1993; 5:72.
3. NSCLCCG. Chemotherapy in non-small cell lung cancer: a meta-analysis using updated data on individual patients from 52 randomised clinical trials. Non-small Cell Lung Cancer Collaborative Group. BMJ 1995; 311:899.
4. Macbeth F, Toy E, Coles B, Melville A, Eastwood A. Palliative radiotherapy regimens for non-small cell lung cancer. Cochrane Database Syst Rev 2001:CD002143.
5. Medical Research Council Lung Cancer Working Party. Inoperable non-small-cell lung cancer (NSCLC): a Medical Research Council randomized trial of palliative radiotherapy with two fractions or ten fractions. Report to the Medical Research Council by its Lung Cancer Working Party. Br J Cancer 1991; 63:265.
6. Medical Research Council Lung Cancer Working Party. A Medical Research Council (MRC) randomised trial of palliative radiotherapy with two fractions or a single fraction in patients with inoperable non-small-cell lung cancer (NSCLC) and poor performance status. Medical Research Council Lung Cancer Working Party. Br J Cancer 1992; 65:934.
7. Macbeth FR, Wheldon TE, Girling DJ, et al. Radiation myelopathy: estimates of risk in 1048 patients in three randomized trials of palliative radiotherapy for non-small cell lung cancer. The Medical Research Council Lung Cancer Working Party. Clin Oncol (R Coll Radiol) 1996; 8:176.
8. Bezjak A, Dixon P, Brundage M, et al. Randomized phase III trial of single versus fractionated thoracic radiation in the palliation of patients with lung cancer (NCIC CTG SC.15). Int J Radiat Oncol Biol Phys 2002; 54:719.
9. Cross CK, Berman S, Buswell L, Johnson B, Baldini EH. Prospective study of palliative hypofractionated radiotherapy (8.5 Gy × 2) for patients with symptomatic non-small-cell lung cancer. Int J Radiat Oncol Biol Phys 2004; 58:1098.
10. Devereux S, Hatton MQ, Macbeth FR. Immediate side effects of large fraction radiotherapy. Clin Oncol (R Coll Radiol) 1997; 9:96.
11. Lupattelli M, Maranzano E, Bellavita R, Chionne F, Darwish S, Piro F, Latini P. Short-course palliative radiotherapy in non-small-cell lung cancer: results of a prospective study. Am J Clin Oncol 2000; 23:89.
12. Vyas RK, Suryanarayana U, Dixit S, Singhal S, Bhavsar DC, Neema JP, Baboo HA. Inoperable non-small cell lung cancer: palliative radiotherapy with two weekly fractions. Indian J Chest Dis Allied Sci 1998; 40:171.
13. Landberg T, Chavaudra J, Dobbs HJ. ICRU Report 62. Prescribing, recording and reporting photon beam therapy (supplement to ICRU Report 50). International Commission on Radiotherapy Units and Measurements, Bethesda, MD, 1999.
14. ICRU Report 62, Prescribing, Recording and Reporting Photon Beam Therapy (Supplement to ICRU Report 50).
15. Rowell NP, Gleeson FV. Steroids, radiotherapy, chemotherapy and stents for superior vena caval obstruction in carcinoma of the bronchus. Cochrane Database Syst Rev 2001:CD001316.

Integration of Radiotherapy in the Management of Locally Advanced Non-Small-Cell Lung Cancer

19

Francesc Casas, Frank B. Zimmermann, Branislav Perin and Branislav Jeremic

Contents

19.1   Introduction

Locally advanced (LA) non-small-cell lung cancer (NSCLC) is the major target group for clinical investigation in thoracic oncology because of the number of patients falling into this category and a possibility of "cure" in such a huge population. The latter issue has been debated over decades, due to somewhat different interpretations of the "cure", when one considers the poor survival figures obtained with the available treatment modalities. With standard-fraction radiation therapy (RT) alone, these figures have been disappointingly low, with a 5-year survival rate of 5% and a median survival time of 8–10 months [1–3]. Therefore, nonbelievers were frequently asking the question: to treat or not? But nowadays this question, and even its softer variant, "should we treat immediately or not?", especially with regard to asymptomatic patients, seems to be irrelevant because all treatment modalities are becoming ever more efficient, and in the year 2006, "cure" has become imperative.

Notorious characteristics of LA NSCLC are the great local/regional tumor burden and micrometastases, which are frequently present from the outset. The poor survival figures obtained with both high-dose RT and chemotherapy (CHT), given as single-treatment modali-

ties, were probably the major factors underlying the palliative approach to this disease. The Medical Research Council (MRC) in the UK conducted two prospective randomized trials to investigate most optimal palliative fractionation RT. In these two consecutive studies, single-fraction RT (10 Gy) was shown to be equally effective as two fractions of 8.5 Gy given 1 week apart, or a more protracted regimen consisting of 39 Gy given in 13 daily fractions [4, 5] with regard to both overall survival and palliation of symptoms. The overall importance of these studies lies not just in a better understanding of particular aspects of the disease and its outcome, but to the enormous applicability of these shortened regimens, especially in countries with limited resources. It must, however, target selected patients, probably those with a poor Karnofsky performance status score (<70%), and pronounced weight loss (>5–10%), mostly falling into the stage IIIB disease category. However, this does not exclude several patients with the same stage (IIIB) from being considered suitable for curative treatment together with the vast majority of those staged as having IIIA disease, all of whom are deemed to be suitable for investigation for "curative" approaches.

Trimodality therapy has been implemented in the treatment of LA NSCLC, but no general consensus exists on its use in this disease and concern had been raised regarding the applicability of this approach [6, 7]. In order to improve the poor survival figures achievable with RT and CHT alone in this patient population, a combination of RT and CHT has also been examined. The rationale for combining RT and CHT is to achieve an improved therapeutic ratio, which should be determined as a function both of tumor response and normal tissue damage. About 25 years ago, Steel and Peckham (1979) established four basic mechanisms through which RT and CHT can interact [8].

1. Spatial cooperation describes the situation in which disease in a particular anatomical (distant) site that is missed by one therapeutic agent (RT) is dealt with

adequately by another (CHT). This combination of RT and CHT does not require interaction between the two anticancer agents. The interaction represents the situation in which treatment with one agent modifies the response of a tissue (normal or tumor) to the second agent.

2. Independent cell kill (simple addition of the antitumor effects) describes the situation that occurs when two partially effective anticancer agents are combined without having to substantially reduce their dose levels. An improvement in therapeutic result can be expected with this methodology. One would expect that two such agents are more effective than a single agent, provided that they do not interact negatively to the extent that the overall level of tumor cell kill is less than which could be produced by the best agent. In NSCLC, both RT and CHT can act on intrathoracic disease independently, leading to a cell kill that is higher than that obtained by the most effective treatment (i.e., RT) given alone. Again, this mechanism does not require an interaction between RT and CHT.

3. Protection of normal tissues is another mechanism of combined RT and CHT, whereby the combination of the two treatments allows delivery of a greater dose of radiation to be given than would be tolerated otherwise. This could happen only if tumor cells are not similarly protected. In NSCLC, this would mean that a particular CHT (or any other) agent protects normal tissue (e.g., the esophageal mucosa) without protecting an intrathoracic tumor. This mechanism does require an interaction between RT and CHT.

4. Enhancement of tumor response is the mechanism of combination of RT and CHT that produces a greater antitumor response than would be expected from the response achieved with the agents used separately. This mechanism also requires interaction between RT and CHT. These mechanisms have been discussed extensively from a clinical standpoint.

Any one of these mechanisms by itself could give an improved therapeutic strategy compared with RT and CHT used alone. A particular combination of RT and CHT may simultaneously exploit more than one mechanism. If one attempts to achieve enhancement of tumor response using anticancer agents that have no overlapping toxicity with RT, there may be a benefit from the simple addition of antitumor effects (independent cell kill), while CHT may also deal with the disease outside the RT field (spatial cooperation).

Of particular interest over the years has been the enhancement of tumor response. There are a variety of processes that may be exploited in principle in an attempt to achieve enhancement of tumor response: (1) modification of the initial radiation damage (modification of the slope of the dose–response curves), (2) decreased accumulation or inhibition of repair of radia-

tion-induced damage in tumor cells, (3) exploitation of induced cell-cycle synchrony (perturbation in cell kinetics), (4) improved drug access following irradiation, and (5) decrease of the tumor bulk by irradiation, leading to more rapid proliferation and greater chemosensitivity of the tumor cells.

There are several possible combinations of exclusive RT and CHT, and these will be detailed further in this chapter, which emphasizes the integration of RT in the management of LA NSCLC, a matter that has been debated continuously over the years [9–11].

19.2   Induction Chemotherapy and Radiotherapy

The major aim of this type of radiochemotherapy is to decrease the tumor burden and to combat micrometastatic disease. When RT follows induction CHT, the effects of CHT may permit delivery of RT to a reduced tumor volume. Increased drug delivery with less overall toxicity is also possible compared to concurrent administration. Potential disadvantages of induction treatment include a prolonged overall treatment time, excessive toxicity due to CHT preventing or delaying the delivery of RT, and CHT-induced tumor-cell resistance resulting in reduced radiation efficacy, as well as accelerated tumor clonogen repopulation, which is also expected to occur during the CHT [12, 13].

Several smaller randomized trials have failed to confirm a survival benefit for the addition of induction CHT, but these trials may have lacked the power to detect small differences in survival [14–17]. The Cancer and Leukemia Group B (CALGB) 8433 trial was the landmark positive study of sequential radiochemotherapy versus RT alone for the treatment of LA NSCLC [18]. Between 1984 and 1987, 155 patients with clinical or surgical T3 or N2 and M0 NSCLC were randomized to induction CHT followed by RT or RT alone. All patients had a good performance status and minimal weight loss. Induction CHT consisted of cisplatin (100 mg/m^2, given on days 1 and 29) and vinblastine (5 mg/m^2, given on days 1, 8, 15, 22, and 29). RT to a total dose of 60 Gy in 30 fractions was the same in both arms and began on day 50 in the combined-modality arm. The addition of CHT did not impair the ability to deliver RT, with 88% of patients in the combined-modality arm and 87% of patients on the RT alone arm completing RT as per the protocol. The addition of CHT increased the number of hospital admissions for vomiting (5% vs. 0%) and infection (7% vs. 3%), although there were no treatment-related deaths on either arm. In the initial report, induction CHT improved median survival (13.8 vs. 9.7 months, $p = 0.0066$) and doubled the number of long-term survivors, with 23% of patients treated with radiochemotherapy surviving 3 years, compared to 11% of those treated with RT alone, prompting early closure of the study. Long-term (7-year) follow-up confirmed that induction CHT improves long-term and median survival (13.7 vs. 9.6 months, $p = 0.012$) compared to RT alone [19]. Three other modern cisplatin-based trials have confirmed the CALGB experience.

The Radiation Therapy Oncology Group (RTOG)/ Eastern Cooperative Oncology Group (ECOG) trial randomized 458 eligible patients with good performance status, minimal weight loss, and LA NSCLC to receive once daily RT to 60 Gy in 2-Gy fractions with or without induction cisplatin and vinblastine [20]. Patients randomized to a third arm received RT twice daily to a total dose of 69.6 Gy. Median survival was statistically superior ($p = 0.03$) for the combined modality arm (13.8 months) versus either the standard RT arm (11.4 months), or the twice-daily RT arm (12.3 months). The final results of this study confirmed an improvement in median survival for combined-modality therapy, but 5-year survival rates remained poor at less than 10% [21].

Additional experience with induction CHT followed by RT was provided in a French trial with RT versus combined chemoradiation [22]. In this trial, 353 patients with unresectable LA squamous cell or large-cell lung carcinoma were randomized to receive either RT alone (65 Gy in 2.5-Gy fractions) or three monthly cycles of cisplatin-based CHT followed by the same RT regimen. There was a significant decrease in distant metastases for the combined-modality arm, and the median (12.0 vs. 10.0 months) and 2-year survival rates (21% vs. 14%, $p = 0.02$) were also improved [23]. Reanalysis revealed that only 8% of patients had continued local control at 5 years [24]. Five-year survival rates remained poor at 6% and 3% for the RT alone and CHT/ RT groups, respectively, secondary to the high rate of local failure on both arms.

The MRC also randomized 447 eligible patients with good performance status and localized, inoperable NSCLC to receive RT alone or cisplatin-based induction CHT followed by RT [25]. The median RT dose was 50 Gy on both arms. Median survival was improved with the addition of CHT (13.0 vs. 9.9 months, $p = 0.056$), although this difference was of borderline significance.

What was demonstrated by the aforementioned randomized trials was that the addition of platinum-based induction CHT to RT results in improved survival versus RT alone. This was particularly true for short-term survival, but modest improvements in long-term survival have also been observed. In addition, three large meta-analyses have demonstrated a small but consistent survival benefit for the addition of induction CHT to RT for LA NSCLC [26–28].

Since it was recognized that this type of combined RT and CHT may bring an increase in the locoregional failures, attempts were made to include a more intensive second part of the treatment. In such an attempt, Clamon et al. (1999) from CALGB compared induction CHT consisting of cisplatin/vinblastine followed by standard RT (60 Gy in 30 daily fractions) with or without concurrent 100 mg/m^2/week carboplatin (CALGB 9130) [29]. There was no difference regarding overall survival (the median survival time: 13.4 vs. 13.5 months; 4-year survival: 13% vs. 10%; $p = 0.74$) between the radiosensitized and nonradiosensitized groups. These results demonstrate a sobering picture regarding induction cisplatin/vinblastine followed by standard RT in that it does not necessarily obtain good and consistent results, being inferior in the study of Clamon et al. [29] to that expected from the previous two studies [18, 20]. They have shown that even when sensitized by carboplatin, standard-fraction RT can not compensate for the accelerated proliferation of surviving tumor clonogens, which occurs during the induction phase of treatment. Furthermore, the results of the CALGB 9130 study of Clamon et al. [29] are not different from those obtained by hyperfractionated RT alone in the RTOG/ECOG study [20] or the same hyperfractionated RT with 69.6 Gy using 1.2 Gy twice-daily [30].

More recently, in an attempt to further intensify the second, RT, part of this combined treatment approach, Vokes et al. [31] reported on a randomized phase II study of CALGB (9431), which used two cycles of induction CHT (cisplatin/gemcitabine or cisplatin/paclitaxel or cisplatin/vinorelbine) followed by two cycles of the same CHT concurrently with conventionally fractionated radical RT (66 Gy) in 175 patients with unresectable stage III NSCLC. Response rates were 74%, 67%, and 73% for the three arms, respectively. While the median survival time for all patients was 17 months, 3-year survival rates for the three groups were 28%, 19%, and 23%, respectively. Authors concluded that the use of concurrent radiochemotherapy could have led to the improvement in outcome when compared to previous CALGB experience with induction treatments [18, 19, 29], which was indeed true. However, the results with concurrent radiochemotherapy seemed far better than these.

19.3 Concurrent Radiochemotherapy

This combined-modality approach denotes the administration of both modalities at the same time, meaning that CHT is given during the RT course. Several variations exist, including CHT being administered on a 3-weekly basis, bi-weekly, weekly, or daily, although concurrent radiochemotherapy employing third-generation drugs (e.g., paclitaxel) also witnessed administration of the drug twice or trice weekly. Whatever the design of concurrent radiochemotherapy, its main aim is to address the issue of locoregional and distant disease at the same time, from the outset. This, unfortunately, may lead to increased toxicity (mostly acute), which may require dose reductions or treatment interruptions, both adversely influencing treatment outcome. The latter issue does not exist only for LA NSCLC [32], but was recently shown to detrimentally affect treatment outcome even in early stage NSCLC [6, 7]. On the other hand, with concurrent radiochemotherapy three of radiobiological premises, namely spatial cooperation, independent cell kill, and synergistic action, as postulated by Steel and Peckham [8], can be exploited.

The initial question regarding the effectiveness of concurrent radiochemotherapy was whether it is more effective than RT alone. In several studies, RT alone was tested against concurrent radiochemotherapy, the latter aiming mostly toward an improvement in local tumor control. Several prospective randomized phase III studies investigated this issue [30, 33–40]. Some of the negative studies may be criticized because of a relatively low total RT dose [33, 35] and CHT being given in an insufficient total dose [33], as well as use of the single agent CHT [33, 35, 39], which was probably when given concurrently with RT. All three positive studies used protracted CHT dosing. While a European Organization for Research and Treatment of Cancer study [34] tested both daily and weekly cisplatin with split-course RT, showing superior outcome for daily cisplatin/RT, Jeremic et al. first used biweekly, and weekly [37] and then daily [30] carboplatin/etoposide with hyperfractionated RT doses of 64.8 [37] and then 69.6 Gy [30] (Table 19.1). In these two consecutive studies, the best results were obtained with low-dose daily CHT given during the hyperfractionated RT course, with very encouraging 4- to 5-year survival rates being approximately 20% [30, 37]. As a rule, survival advantage in these three studies was a consequence of an advantage at local tumor level. Obviously, low-dose daily CHT acted synergistically with RT, enhancing its effects. An interesting finding was that shorter (4.5- to 5.0-h) interfraction intervals were associated with a significantly improved survival and local control than longer (5.5- to 6.0-h) interfraction intervals [41–43]. As expected, no influence on distant metastasis control was noted.

Recently, Cakir and Egehan [44] provided additional evidence that concurrent RT (64 Gy in 32 daily fractions) and cisplatin (20 mg/m^2, days 1–5, weeks 2 and 6) offers a survival advantage over the same RT alone. At 3 years, 10% of patients survived in the combined group, while only 2% survived in the RT-alone group. A combined treatment approach also offered better locoregional control ($p=0.0001$) and disease-free survival ($p=0.0006$), confirming previous observations of the superiority of combined RT and platinum CHT over RT alone.

In addition, no impact on distant metastasis control or local control was observed in those studies/arms that used high-dose CHT concurrently with RT. Another advantage of low-dose concurrent CHT over high-dose CHT and concurrent RT is that the former type of concurrent radiochemotherapy leads to less high-grade acute toxicity and, consequently, better treatment compliance and fewer treatment interruptions, which influences treatment outcome [32].

19.4 Optimal Sequencing of Radiochemotherapy

The induction CHT studies showed a survival advantage for the combined approach owing to the improvement in the distant metastasis control, a finding opposite to that of the concurrent approach studies, which unequivocally showed an improvement in survival due to the improvement in locoregional tumor control. Putting these data into the perspective of exploitable mechanisms of combined RT and CHT [8], one must identify the induction regimens as those enabling the therapeutic benefit due to spatial cooperation only. No indepen-

Table 19.1. Concurrent radiochemotherapy studies, University Hospital, Kragujevac, Serbia.

Study	Phase	Year[a]	N	Hfx RT (Gy/fx)	CHT (drugs/schedule)	MST (months)	4-year (%)	5-year (%)
I	III	1995	61	64.8/54	–	8	7	5
			56	64.8/54	CE/week 1, 3, 5	13	16	16
			52	64.8/54	CE/weeks 1–5	18	21	21
II	III	1996	66	69.6/58	–	14	9	
			65	69.6/58	CE/daily	22	23	
III	II	1998	41	69.6/58	CE/daily + week-end	25	29	29
IV	III	2001	98	69.6/58	CE/daily	20	20	20
			97	69.6/58	CE/daily + week-end	22	23	23
V	II	2005	64	67.6/52	CP/daily	28	28	26

[a] Year of publication, *Hfx RT* hyperfractionated radiation therapy, *CHT* chemotherapy, *MST* median survival time, *C* carboplatin, *E* etoposide, *P* paclitaxel

dent cell kill can be noted because there was no significant difference in locoregional tumor control, as one may expect if such independent cell kill would have happened. In addition, no enhancement of tumor response can be noted for the same reason. Contrary to these findings, in concurrent studies, spatial cooperation did not work, while both independent cell kill and enhancement of tumor response may have occurred. In the low-dose (daily) CHT arms of the concurrent studies, however, it seems unlikely that independent cell kill occurred (and if so, then to a much lesser degree), thus leaving enhancement of tumor response as the only viable alternative. Confirmation of these premises was recently provided by El Sharouni et al. [45], who investigated the influence of waiting times for RT after induction CHT by comparing computed tomography scans performed at the end of induction CHT and those performed for the purpose of RT planning. Of the potentially curable tumors, 41% turned into incurable ones, with the median potential tumor doubling time being 29 days, much less than previously thought.

Since both of these approaches proved to be feasible and effective in practice, the next step was to compare induction CHT followed by radical RT to concurrent RT and CHT. Currently, there are only two prospective randomized phase III studies evaluating concurrent versus induction CHT and RT and. Furuse et al. [46, 47] were the first to compare mitomycin, cisplatin, and vindesine CHT given as either induction followed by RT (56 Gy) or given concurrently with RT. First publication showed a superior median survival time and 5-year survival for the concurrent regimen (16.5 vs. 13.3 months and 16% vs. 9%, respectively; $p = 0.039$) [46]. Subsequent data analysis, focusing on patterns of failure, identified an improvement in local tumor control (median time, 10.6 vs. 8.0 months; 5-year, 34% vs. 20%; $p = 0.0462$) as a reason for an improvement in survival [47]. More recently, Curran et al. [48] and Komaki et al. [49] reported on an RTOG 9410 study that evaluated induction CHT followed by RT, like the CALGB 8433 [18] and RTOG 8808/ECOG 4508 studies [20] versus concurrent either standard-fraction RT (60 Gy) and cisplatin/etoposide versus hyperfractionated RT (69.6 Gy) and cisplatin/etoposide. Both the standard radiochemotherapy and hyperfractionated radiochemotherapy arms had better median survival times than the induction arm (17.0 vs. 16.0 vs. 14.6 months, respectively), although only standard radiochemotherapy was statistically significantly better than induction CHT [48]. The pattern of failure analysis showed that the best local control was in the hyperfractionated radiochemotherapy arm, confirming indirectly the observations of Jeremic et al. [30, 37] that high-dose hyperfractionated RT is an advantageous approach. Furthermore, and contrary to studies using low-dose CHT concurrent with high-dose RT, it was shown again that high-dose CHT bears a risk of exceptional acute toxicity when given with high-dose

standard or hyperfractionated RT. This finding is not just limited to RTOG 9410, but was also seen in similar studies [50–52] as well. Confirmation of more frequent high-grade toxicity recently came from preliminary results from the recent Canadian meta-analysis [53]. In that analysis, RT and concurrent low-dose, daily, CHT carried a somewhat lower risk of acute toxicity, including high-grade neutropenia, when compared to that observed with RT and concurrent high-dose CHT, another advantage of RT and concurrent low-dose, daily CHT.

Finally, the preliminary data provide during American Society of Clinical Oncology 2004 analysis of CALGB study 39801 (Vokes, personal communication) seems to confirm the ineffectiveness of induction CHT in a general treatment plan for LA NSCLC. When induction CHT consisting of carboplatin and paclitaxel followed by radical RT given concurrently with carboplatin/paclitaxel during the course of RT (66 Gy) was compared to the same exclusive concurrent RT/CHT, no difference was found in either median survival time (14 vs. 11.4 months) or 1-year survival (54% vs. 48%; $p = 0.154$). Induction CHT offered absolutely no gain when preceded by concurrent RT/CHT, but added significantly higher incidence of grade 4 toxicity (41% vs. 24%; $p = 0.001$).

19.5 Optimization of Concurrent Radiochemotherapy

These prospective randomized trials solved the question of the "standard" treatment option in LA NSCLC. Additional evidence that concurrent radiochemotherapy should be the standard of care in LA NSCLC comes also from a recent Southwest Oncology Group (SWOG) phase II study [54], which used two cycles of cisplatin/etoposide concurrently with conventionally fractionated 45 Gy in pathologic stage IIIB NSCLC. In the absence of progressive disease, an additional 16 Gy was administered with two additional cycles of cisplatin/etoposide. The median survival time was 15 months, and 5-year survival was 15%. However, grade 4 neutropenia was observed in 32% of patients, grade 3–4 anemia in 28% of patients, and grade 3–4 esophagitis in 20% of patients.

Recent attempts to refine concurrent RT and platinum-based CHT include reports of Jeremic et al. [55, 56] (Table 19.1) and Lau et al. [57], who both tried to address the issue of somewhat poorer distant metastasis control by increasing the dose of CHT. While Jeremic et al. [55] first tested the addition of weekend carboplatin/etoposide to concurrent hyperfractionated RT (69.6 Gy) and low-dose daily carboplatin/etoposide in a phase II study, which demonstrated a promising median survival time of 29 months and 5-year survival rate of 25%, the results of their subsequent prospective randomized trial showed no advantage for weekend CHT when compared to no-weekend CHT (median survival time, 22 vs. 20 months; 5-year survival, 23% vs. 20%; $p = 0.57$) [56]. Lau et al. [57] used concurrent RT (61 Gy) and CHT consisting of twice-weekly paclitaxel for 6 weeks and once-weekly carboplatin for 6 weeks. Two cycles of consolidation paclitaxel and carboplatin were offered to patients who achieved a complete response (CR), partial response (PR), or stable disease (SD). The median survival time was 17 months and the 2-year actuarial survival rate was 40%. More recently, and quite encouragingly, the SWOG reported a trial in which concurrent cisplatin/etoposide/RT was followed by three cycles of adjuvant high-dose docetaxel [58]. The median survival in this phase II study was 26 months. Most recently, Sakai et al. [59] reported on a phase II study that employed biweekly docetaxel and carboplatin with concurrent RT (60 Gy in 30 daily fractions) followed by consolidation CHT with docetaxel plus carboplatin in patients with stage III unresectable NSCLC. Among 32 evaluable patients, an impressive response rate of 91% was obtained. The median survival time was 27 months and the 2-year survival rate was 61%. High-grade toxicity was low.

These contemporary consolidations studies have two parts, a concurrent one and a consolidation one, with the same or different drugs being administered during the latter part of combined treatment. Regardless of the underlying principle for such an intervention, these studies provided a toxicity pattern divided between the concurrent and the consolidation parts. While these studies presented a very detailed pattern of failure in general, this was done for the whole time period of the study, but not which type of failure was observed when (i.e., after concurrent or after consolidation part), and in particular in which patients after the concurrent part, although some studies mandated consolidation chemotherapy in nonprogressing patients. This is important from several standpoints. First, there are several types of patient after the initial (concurrent) part of radiochemotherapy and they can easily be separated according to their response. While it is extremely unlikely that those achieving a SD would benefit from consolidation CHT, those with either a CR or a PR seem to be likely candidates (although not all of them) to benefit from consolidation CHT. Separation, therefore, of pattern of failure occurring in likely (CR and PR) and unlikely (SD) candidates could be used for further studies using similar design with respect to, for example, eligibility criteria. Second, and more importantly, among those candidates likely to benefit from consolidation CHT (CR and PR), a distinction should be made between those achieving CR and those achieving PR after concurrent radiochemotherapy because different mechanisms (more precisely, different locations) of action of consolidation CHT would be expected. In the CR patients, consolidation CHT would target microscopic disease both intrathoracically and extrathoracically, while in the PR patients it would have to deal with clinically

overt intrathoracic disease and microscopic extrathoracic disease. It is obvious that the pattern of failure of these two distinct groups of patients would then clearly show how and where consolidation CHT is actually acting and to what extent (clinical versus subclinical). Of additional importance is that with a clear pattern of failure, we would be able to begin to investigate the determinants of treatment outcome such as cross-resistance between drugs or between drugs and CHT. This would also lead to further investigation of the inherent nature of these treatment modalities, such as total dose or fractionation (for CHT) or one or more drug(s) combinations (e.g., the same or different drugs in the concurrent and the consolidation part of the treatment), as recently stressed [42].

Although identifying the pattern of failure in patients achieving different responses after concurrent radiochemotherapy may require some additional measures and may place additional burden on investigators and hospitals, this effort would eventually be rewarding. This way we would be able to discriminate between different patients and different options and to proceed (or not) with a consolidation therapy in one or more patient subsets, an approach that would ultimately lead to better patient-tailored treatment sequences, a must for a clinical research in lung cancer in the future.

One of the unsolved questions regarding the optimization of concurrent radiochemotherapy, particularly from the standpoint of RT, is the type of fractionation: conventional, once daily, or altered fractionation, employing multiple fractions per day (hyperfractionation). The RTOG 8311 study [60] showed a possible advantage only for a hyperfractionated radiation therapy dose of 69.6 Gy, 1.2-Gy twice daily. fractionation (but not beyond it) over the standard 60 Gy given in 30 daily fractions in a favorable subset of LA NSCLC, RTOG 9410, while not statistically designed to directly compare standard vs. altered fractionation, appeared to show no survival difference between conventional, once daily, and hyperfractionated RT when given with concurrent CHT. Interestingly, when compared to conventionally fractionated RT, hyperfractionated radiochemotherapy offered better local control in the RTOG 9410 trial, but this did not translate into a difference in survival. Another study came to the same conclusion, albeit with a somewhat different treatment approach. In the North Central Cancer Treatment Group/Mayo Clinic phase III study [61], conventionally fractionated RT (60 Gy) was compared to split-course hyperfractionated RT using 30 Gy given in 20 fractions in 10 treatment days over 2 weeks with a 2-week break, after which another 30 Gy was given using the same fractionation. Both conventionally fractionated and hyperfractionated RT groups received concurrent cisplatin/etoposide. No difference in toxicity was seen and no statistically significant difference in treatment outcome, although hyperfractionated RT offered numerically slightly better survival and local control.

More recently, the ECOG completed a randomized trial comparing standard fractionation RT versus hyperfractionated accelerated RT. All patients in both arms received induction chemotherapy with carboplatin/paclitaxel, although concurrent CHT was not used. Unfortunately, the study did not meet its accrual goals and was closed early; nonetheless 111 patients were analyzed and the results suggest a slight but statistically insignificant advantage to hyperfractionated accelerated RT (median survival and 2- and 3-year actuarial survival: 22.2 months, 48% and 20% vs. 13.7 months, 33% and 15%, respectively) [62].

Further attempts to optimize the treatment approach in this disease include RT given concurrently with third-generation drugs. While all third-generation drugs have been tested in this setting, prospective randomized phase III studies are lacking. Regardless, it seems that the paclitaxel/carboplatin combination has similar efficacy and probably less toxicity than either cisplatin-based or other multiagent-based chemotherapy [63, 64]. Several phase II studies tested this combination with promising results [57, 65, 66]. The very first prospective study comparing RT/paclitaxel versus RT alone showed an advantage for RT/paclitaxel (the median survival time, 15.2 vs. 12 months; $p = 0.027$) [67]. Testing the paclitaxel/carboplatin combination and standard-fraction RT (63 Gy) in three schedules, Choy et al. [68] used either pre-RT CHT followed by RT (arm 1), pre-RT and concurrent radiochemotherapy (arm 2), and concurrent radiochemotherapy and post-RT CHT (arm 3). Although this phase II randomized study was not designed to statistically compare treatment arms, nevertheless, the best results were achieved in arm 3 (median survival time, 16.1 months; 2-year survival, 33%). Also, in arm 2 there was suboptimal compliance with concurrent radiochemotherapy after induction CHT. It is expected that several ongoing or recently completed studies will bring new insight into the issue of optimization of RT and CHT in this disease.

A unique and rather innovative radiochemotherapy approach consisting of hyperfractionated RT and concurrent low-dose daily paclitaxel and carboplatin has recently been pioneered (Table 19.1). In order to increase the likelihood of successfully combating the accelerated proliferation of tumor clonogens, they have adapted their initial standard regimen (69.6 Gy in 58 fractions of 1.2 Gy given twice daily) in 6 weeks to 67.6 Gy in 52 fractions of 1.3 Gy, also given twice daily, but in a 5-week total treatment time, saving approximately 1 week. Paclitaxel was given in a daily dose of 10 mg/m^2, while carboplatin was given in a daily dose of 25 mg/m^2. In 64 patients with stage III NSCLC they have obtained very promising median survival time of 28 months and a 5-year survival rate of 26%, all accompanied with low incidence of high-grade toxicity. These results again reconfirm the effectiveness and low toxicity of concurrent hyperfractionated RT and low-dose daily CHT.

19.6 New Approaches in Combined Radiochemotherapy

A wide application of powerful computers has made a substantial impact on RT treatment planning and delivery. Three-dimensional conformal RT (3D-CRT) is now increasingly being practiced worldwide. With RT fields tailored to include only detectable tumor, more focused and escalated RT doses can be given. Phase I/II studies have shown that RT doses at the order of ≥80 Gy are being frequently used with acceptable levels of toxicity [69–71], and that the RT concepts of the necessity of elective nodal irradiation (ENI) may be challenged. It should be mentioned, however, that even with limited-field RT in 3D-CRT, some "incidental" ENI always occurs, and may reach a dose level of 45–50 Gy, the dose considered necessary for elective treatment [72, 73], a matter that must be taken into account when one defines the nature of ENI [43]. In addition to increasing target coverage and allowing escalation, the use of 3D-CRT also allows a more accurate prediction of the toxicity of a given course of RT [74, 75].

Intensity-modulated radiotherapy (IMRT) has also been used in LA NSCLC, and its potential advantages become evident when one compares 3D-CRT and IMRT plans [76]. With IMRT, in the majority of cases the prescription dose could be increased. This is coupled with a decreased lung dose and improved planning target volume uniformity, as well as a significantly reduced cumulative RT dose to the esophagus while maintaining the same or higher dose to gross disease [77]. While extracranial stereotactic radiosurgery (SRS) and stereotactic fractionated RT (SFRT) were initially used only for small (early stage) tumors [78–86], its application is slowly extending to tumors being classified as locally advanced. It is not unrealistic to expect that extracranial SRS and SFRT will play an important role in LA NSCLC, particularly in cases with favorable characteristics (e.g., response to chemotherapy, smaller lesions, more peripheral location), possibly as the boost after external beam RT. However, it should be clearly emphasized that the proper selection of patients remains a prerequisite for the use of these new technologies in LA NSCLC.

It is also expected that more new drugs will become more readily available in the future and that the process of their initial clinical testing (phase I–III) include testing for their radioenhancing potential, which would go in parallel to its testing for anticancer CHT purposes. This way, we would be able to learn earlier about the properties of novel drugs, both alone and in combination with RT, and to address the important issues of optimal sequencing radiation therapy and chemotherapy in LA disease. Some of the ongoing studies are listed in Table 19.2.

Table 19.2. Ongoing studies with radiotherapy and novel drugs

ZD 1839 and Radiotherapy in NSCLC		
ZD 1839 Regimen	Eligibility	Study group
Maintenance	Unresectable Stage III	SWOG
Concurrent	Unresectable Stage III	CALGB
Angiogenesis Inhibitors and Radiotherapy in NSCLC		
Angiogenesis Inhibitor	Eligibility	Study Group
Thalidomide	Stage III	ECOG
AE 941(Neovastat)	Stage III	MD Anderson
Celecoxib	Stage III	RTOG

NSCLC Non-small-cell lung cancer, SWOG Southwestern Oncology Group, CALGB Cancer and Leukemia Group B, ECOG Eastern Cooperative Oncology Group, RTOG Radiation Therapy Oncology Group

The use of radioprotectors has faced renewed clinical interest with respect to protection against RT-induced toxicity. Several studies have reported on the use of amifostine during RT and CHT in lung cancer. In a randomized phase III trial of RT with or without daily amifostine in patients with LA NSCLC [87], the incidence of pneumonitis ≥2 was significantly lower in the amifostine group, as was the incidence of esophagitis ≥grade 2, and the protective effect of amifostine enabled a lower incidence of late damage, with no effect on treatment outcome. Komaki et al. [88] also administered amifostine twice weekly before treatment in patients with LA NSCLC treated with concurrent radiochemotherapy to observe that morphine intake to reduce severe esophagitis was significantly lower in the amifostine arm, as was the incidence of acute pneumonitis in the treatment arm. Finally, a randomized double-blind study [89] showed a trend toward fewer patients exhibiting toxicity in the amifostine group. RTOG has just reported preliminary results on study 98-01, which randomized patients to intensive chemoradiation (induction carboplatin/paclitaxel followed by hyperfractionated RT to 69.6 Gy with concurrent weekly carboplatin/paclitaxel) with or without amifostine four times per week during RT. Although there was no difference in the rate of grade 3 esophagitis, patient-reported area-under-the-curve swallowing dysfunction scores were significantly lower in the amifostine group [90]. It is expected that more studies regarding the issue of optimal protection with amifostine will provide more data on further optimization before becoming a standard adjunct to RT or radiochemotherapy treatments in the future.

Key Points

- Concurrent radiotherapy (RT)/chemotherapy (CHT) is a treatment of choice in locally advanced NSCLC since it is superior to either RT alone or induction CHT followed by RT.
- Induction CHT offered absolutely no gain when preceded by concurrent RT/CHT, but added a significantly higher incidence of grade 4 toxicity to that observed with RT/CHT alone.
- Consolidation CHT after concurrent RT/CHT may hold promise for the future, but only after patterns of failure data and the long-term data from randomized phase III studies become available.
- Optimization of concurrent RT/CHT will include the precise definition of an optimal time–dose-fractionation regimen and the choice and optimal sequence and the dose of concurrent CHT given during the course of RT.
- Novel approaches, such as the dose escalation by better three-dimensional tumor and target volume tailoring, the use of the third-generation drugs, and the use of protectors, await additional verification in prospective randomized studies.

References

1. Choi NCH, Doucette JA. Improved survival of patients with unresectable non-small cell bronchogenic carcinoma by an innovated high-dose en bloc radiotherapeutic approach. Cancer 1981; 48:101.
2. Perez C, Stanley K, Grundy G, et al. Impact of irradiation technique and tumor extent in tumor control and survival of patients with unresectable non-oat cell carcinoma of the lung. Cancer 1982; 50:1091.
3. Petrovich Z, Stanley K, Cox JD, Paig C. Radiotherapy in the management of locally advanced lung cancer of all cell types: final report of randomized trial. Cancer 1981; 48:1335.
4. Medical Research Council Working Party. Inoperable non-small-cell lung cancer (NSCLC): a Medical Research Council randomized trial of palliative radiotherapy with two fractions or ten fractions. Br J Cancer 1991; 63:265.
5. Medical Research Council Working Party. A Medical Research Council (MRC) randomized trial of palliative radiotherapy with two fractions or a single fraction in patients with inoperable non-small-cell lung cancer (NSCLC) and poor performance status. Br J Cancer 1992; 65:934.
6. Jeremic B, Zimmermann F, Molls M. Induction chemotherapy followed by concurrent radiochemotherapy and surgery in locally advanced non-small-cell lung cancer. Ann Thorac Surg 2003; 76:979.
7. Jeremic B, Shibamoto Y, Milicic B, et al. Impact of treatment interruptions due to toxicity on outcome of patients with early stage (I/II) non-small-cell lung cancer (NSCLC) treated with hyperfractionated radiation therapy (Hfx RT) alone. Lung Cancer 2003; 40:317.
8. Steel GG, Peckham MJ. Exploitable mechanisms in combined radiotherapy-chemotherapy. Int J Radiat Oncol Biol Phys 1979; 5:85.

9. Jeremic B. Optimal integration of radiotherapy and che-motherapy in stage III non-small cell lung cancer. Eur Respir Rev 2002; 12:187.

10. Machtay M, Jeremic B. Complex and controversial issues in locally advanced non-small cell lung carcinoma. Semin Surg Oncol 2003; 21:128.

11. Jeremic B, Machtay M. Concurrent radiochemotherapy in the treatment of locally advanced non-small lung cancer. Hematol Oncol Clin N Am 2004; 18:91.

12. Byhardt RW, Scott C, Sause WT, et al. Response, toxicity, failure patterns, and survival in five Radiation Therapy Oncology Group (RTOG) trials of sequential and/or concurrent chemotherapy and radiotherapy for locally advanced non-small-cell carcinoma of the lung. Int J Radiat Oncol Biol Phys 1998; 42:469.

13. Byhardt RW. Toxicities in RTOG combined-modality trials for inoperable non-small-cell lung cancer. Oncology (Williston Park) 1999; 13(10 Suppl 5):116.

14. Mattson K, Holsti LR, Holsti P, et al. Inoperable non-small cell lung cancer: radiation with or without chemotherapy. Eur J Cancer Clin Oncol 1988; 24:477.

15. Morton RF, Jett JR, McGinnis WL, et al. Thoracic radiation therapy alone compared with combined chemoradiotherapy for locally unresectable non-small cell lung cancer. A randomized, phase III trial. Ann Intern Med 1991; 115:681.

16. Crino L, Latini P, Meacci M, et al. Induction chemotherapy plus high-dose radiotherapy versus radiotherapy alone in locally advanced unresectable non-small-cell lung cancer. Ann Oncol 1993; 4:847.

17. Planting A, Helle P, Drings P, et al. A randomized study of high-dose split course radiotherapy preceded by high-dose chemotherapy versus high-dose radiotherapy only in locally advanced non-small-cell lung cancer. An EORTC Lung Cancer Cooperative Group trial. Ann Oncol 1996; 7:139.

18. Dillman RO, Seagren SL, Propert KJ, et al. A randomized trial of induction chemotherapy plus high-dose radiation versus radiation alone in stage III non-small-cell lung cancer. N Engl J Med 1990; 323:940.

19. Dillman RO, Herndon J, Seagren SL, et al. Improved survival in stage III non-small-cell lung cancer: seven-year follow-up of Cancer and Leukemia Group B (CALGB) 8433 trial. J Natl Cancer Inst 1996; 88:1210.

20. Sause WT, Scott C, Taylor S, et al. Radiation Therapy Oncology Group 88-08 and Eastern Cooperative Oncology Group 4588: preliminary results of a phase III trial in regionally advanced, unresectable nonsmall cell lung cancer. J Natl Cancer Inst 1995; 87:198.

21. Sause W, Kolesar P, Taylor S IV, et al. Final results of phase III trial in regionally advanced unresectable non-small cell lung cancer: Radiation Therapy Oncology Group, Eastern Cooperative Oncology Group, and Southwest Oncology Group. Chest 2000; 117:358.

22. Le Chevalier T, Arriagada R, Quoix E, et al. Radiotherapy alone versus combined chemotherapy and radiotherapy in nonresectable non-small-cell lung cancer: first analysis of a randomized trial in 353 patients. J Natl Cancer Inst 1991; 83:417.

23. Le Chevalier T, Arriagada R, Tarayre M, et al. Significant effect of adjuvant chemotherapy on survival in locally advanced non-small cell lung carcinoma. J Natl Cancer Inst 1992; 84:58 (letter).

24. Arriagada R, Le Chevalier T, Rekacewicz C, et al. Cisplatin-based chemotherapy (CT) in patients with locally advanced non-small cell lung cancer (NSCLC): late analysis of a French randomized trial. Proc Am Soc Clin Oncol 1997; 16:16 (abstract).

25. Cullen MH, Billingham LJ, Woodroffe CM, et al. Mitomycin, ifosfamide and cisplatin (MIC) in non-small cell lung cancer (NSCLC): 1. Results of a randomised trial in patients with localised, inoperable disease. Lung Cancer 1997; 18(suppl 1):5 (abstract 10).

26. Non-small Cell Lung Cancer Collaborative Group. Chemotherapy in non-small cell lung cancer: a meta-analysis using updated data on individual patients from 52 randomised clinical trials. BMJ 1995; 311:899.

27. Marino P, Preatoni A, Cantoni A. Randomized trials of radiotherapy alone versus combined chemotherapy and radiotherapy in stages IIIa and IIIb nonsmall cell lung cancer. A meta-analysis. Cancer 1995; 76:593.

28. Pritchard RS, Anthony SP. Chemotherapy plus radiotherapy compared with radiotherapy alone in the treatment of locally advanced, unresectable, non-small-cell lung cancer: a meta-analysis. Ann Intern Med 1996; 125:723.

29. Clamon G, Herndon J, Cooper R, et al. Radiosensitization with carboplatin for patients with unresectable stage III non-small-cell lung cancer: a phase III trial of the cancer and Leukemia group B and the Eastern Cooperative Oncology Group. J Clin Oncol 1999; 17:4.

30. Jeremic B, Shibamoto Y, Acimovic LJ, Milisavljevic S. Hyperfractionated radiation therapy with or without concurrent low-dose daily carboplatin/etoposide for stage III non-small-cell lung cancer: a randomized study. J Clin Oncol 1996; 14:1065.

31. Vokes EE, Herndon JE, II, Crawford J, et al. Randomized phase II study of cisplatin with gemcitabine or paclitaxel or vinorelbine as induction chemotherapy followed by concomitant chemoradiotherapy for stage IIIB non-small-cell lung cancer: Cancer and Leukemia Group B Study 9431. J Clin Oncol 2002; 20:4191.

32. Cox JD, Pajak TF, Asbell S, et al. Interruptions of high-dose radiation therapy decrease long-term survival of favorable patients with unresectable non-small cell carcinoma of the lung: analysis of 1244 cases from 3 Radiation Therapy Oncology Group (RTOG) trials. Int J Radiat Oncol Biol Phys 1993; 27:493.

33. Soresi E, Borghini U, Zucali R, et al. A randomized clinical trial comparing radiation therapy versus radiation therapy plus cis-Dichlorodiamine Platinum (II) in the treatment of locally advanced non small cell lung cancer. Semin Oncol 1988; 15 (Suppl. 7):20.

34. Schaake-Koning C, van den Bogaert W, Dalesio O, et al. Effects of concomitant cisplatin and radiotherapy on inoperable non-small cell lung cancer. N Engl J Med 1992; 326:524.

35. Trovo MG, Minatel E, Franchin G, et al. Radiotherapy versus radiotherapy enhanced by cisplatin in stage III non small cell lung cancer. Int J Radiat Oncol Biol Phys 1992; 24:11.

36. Blanke C, Ansari R, Mantravadi R, et al. Phase III trial of thoracic irradiation with or without cisplatin for locally advanced unresectable non-small cell lung cancer: a Hoosier Oncology Group Protocol. J Clin Oncol 1995; 13:1425.

37. Jeremic B, Shibamoto Y, Acimovic L, Djuric L. Randomized trial of hyperfractionated radiation therapy with or without concurrent chemotherapy for stage III non-small-cell lung cancer. J Clin Oncol 1995; 13:452.

38. Bonner JA, McGinnis WL, Stella PJ, et al. The possible advantage of hyperfractionated thoracic radiotherapy in the treatment of locally advanced non small cell lung cancer. Results of a North Central Cancer Treatment Group phase III study. Cancer 1998; 82:1037.

39. Groen HJG, van de Leest AHW, Fokkema E, et al. Phase III study of continuous carboplatin over 6 weeks with radiation versus radiation alone in stage III non small cell lung cancer. Ann Oncol 2004; 15:427.

40. Ball D, Bishop J, Smith J, et al. A randomised phase III study of accelerated or standard fraction radiotherapy with or without concurrent carboplatin in inoperable

non-small cell lung cancer: final report of a multi-centre trial. Radiother Oncol 1999; 52:129.

41. Jeremic B, Shibamoto Y. Effect of interfraction interval in hyperfractionated radiotherapy with or without concurrent chemotherapy for stage III nonsmall cell lung cancer. Int J Radiat Oncol Biol Phys 1996; 34:303.

42. Jeremic B, Zimmermann F, Nieder C, Molls M. Necessity of identifying the patterns of failure after concurrent radiochemotherapy part of a combined modality approach in patients with stage III non-small cell lung cancer. Lung cancer, 2004; 46(2):263.

43. Jeremic B, Milicic M, Dagovic A, et al. Interfraction interval in patients with stage III non-small cell lung cancer treated with hyperfractionated radiation therapy with or without concurrent chemotherapy. Final results in 536 patients. Am J Clin Oncol (CCT), 2004; 27(6):616.

44. Cakir S, Egehan I. A randomized clinical trial of radiotherapy plus cisplatin versus radiotherapy alone in stage III non-small cell lung cancer. Lung Cancer 2004; 43:309.

45. El Sharouni SY, Kal HB, Battermann JJ. Accelerated regrowth of non-small-cell lung tumors after induction chemotherapy. Br J Cancer 2003; 89:2184.

46. Furuse K, Nishikawa H, Takada Y, et al. Phase III study of concurrent versus sequential thoracic radiotherapy in combination with mitomycin, vindesine and cisplatin in unresectable stage III non-small-cell lung cancer. J Clin Oncol 1999; 17:2692.

47. Furuse K, Hosoe S, Masuda N. Impact of tumor control on survival in unresectable stage III non-small cell lung cancer (NSCLC) treated with concurrent thoracic radiotherapy (TRT) and chemotherapy (CT). Proc Am Soc Clin Oncol 2000; 19:(Abstract 1893).

48. Curran WJ Jr, Scott C, Langer C. Phase III comparison of sequential Vs concurrent chemoradiation for pts with unresected stage III non-small cell lung cancer (NSCLC): initial report of Radiation Therapy Oncology Group (RTOG) 9410. Proc Am Soc Clin Oncol 2000; 19:484a (abstract 1891).

49. Komaki R, Seiferheld W, Curran Wl. Sequential vs. concurrent chemotherapy and radiation therapy for inoperable non-small cell lung cancer (NSCLC): analysis of failures in a phase III study (RTOG 9410). Proc Am Soc Ther Radiol Oncol 2000; 42:113, (abstract 5).

50. Byhardt RW, Scott CB, Ettinger DS, et al. Concurrent hyperfractionated irradiation and chemotherapy for unresectable nonsmall cell lung cancer. Results of Radiation Therapy Oncology Group 90-15. Cancer 1995; 75:2337.

51. Lee JS, Scott C, Komaki R, et al. Concurrent chemoradiation therapy with oral etoposide and cisplatin for locally advanced inoperable non-small-cell lung cancer: Radiation Therapy Oncology Group protocol 91-06. J Clin Oncol 1996; 14:1055.

52. Komaki R, Scott C, Ettinger D, et al. Randomized study of chemotherapy/radiation therapy combinations for favorable patients with locally advanced inoperable nonsmall cell lung cancer: Radiation Therapy Oncology Group (RTOG) 92-04. Int J Radiat Oncol Biol Phys 1997; 38:149.

53. Rakowitch E, Tsao M, Ung Y, et al. Comparison of the efficacy and acute toxicity of weekly versus daily chemoradiotherapy for non-small-cell lung cancer: a meta-analysis. Int J Radiat Oncol Biol 2004; 58:196.

54. Albain KS, Crowley JJ, Turrisi AT, III, et al. Concurrent cisplatin, etoposide, and chest radiotherapy in pathologic stage IIIB non-small-cell lung cancer: a Southwest Oncology Group Phase II study, SWOG 9019. J Clin Oncol 2002; 20:3454.

55. Jeremic B, Shibamoto Y, Milicic B, et al. Concurrent radiochemotherapy for patients with stage III non-small cell lung cancer (NSCLC). Long-term results of a phase II study. Int J Radiat Oncol Biol Phys 1998; 42:1091.

56. Jeremic B, Shibamoto Y, Acimovic LJ, et al. Hyperfractionated radiation therapy and concurrent low-dose, daily carboplatin/etoposide with or without week-end carboplatin/etoposide chemotherapy in stage III non-small-cell lung cancer: a randomized trial. Int J Radiat Oncol Biol Phys 2001; 50:19.

57. Lau D, Leigh B, Gandara D, et al. Twice-weekly paclitaxel and weekly carboplatin with concurrent thoracic radiation followed by carboplatin/paclitaxel consolidation for stage III non-small-cell lung cancer: a California Cancer Consortium phase II study. J Clin Oncol 2001; 19:442.

58. Gandara DR, Chansky K, Albain KS, et al. Consolidation docetaxel after concurrent chemoradiotherapy in stage IIIB non-small-cell lung cancer: phase II Southwest Oncology Group Study S9504. J Clin Oncol 2003; 21:2004.

59. Sakai H, Yoneda S, Kobayashi K et al. Phase II study of bi-weekly docetaxel and carboplatin with concurrent thoracic radiation therapy followed by consolidation chemotherapy with docetaxel plus carboplatin for stage III unresectable non-small cell lung cancer. Lung Cancer 2004; 43:195.

60. Cox JD, Azarnia N, Byhardt RW, et al. A randomized phase I/II trial of hyperfractionated radiation therapy with total doses of 60.0 Gy to 79.2 Gy: possible survival benefit with > 69.6 Gy in favorable patients with Radiation Therapy Oncology Group Stage III non-small cell lung carcinoma: report of Radiation Therapy Oncology Group 83-11. J Clin Oncol 1990; 8:1543.

61. Schild SE, Stella PJ, Geyer SM, et al. Phase III trial comparing chemotherapy plus once-daily or twice-daily radiotherapy in stage III non-small-cell lung cancer. Int J Radiat Oncol Biol Phys 2002; 54:370.

62. Belani CP, Wang W, Johnson DH, et al. Induction chemotherapy followed by standard thoracic radiotherapy (Std.TRT) vs. hyperfractionated accelerated radiotherapy (HART) for patients with unresectable stage III A & B non-small-cell lung cancer (NSCLC): phase III study of the Eastern Cooperative Oncology Group (ECOG 2597). Proc Am Soc Clin Oncol 2003; 21:622 (abstract 2500).

63. Kelly K, Crowley J, Bunn PA Jr, et al. Randomized phase III trial of paclitaxel plus carboplatin versus vinorelbine plus cisplatin in the treatment of patients with advanced NSCLC: a SWOG trial. J Clin Oncol 2001; 19:3210.

64. Schiller JH, Harrington D, Belani CP, et al. Comparison of four chemotherapy regimens for advanced NSCLC. N Engl J Med 2002; 346:92.

65. Choy H, Akerley W, Safran, Graziano S, et al. Multiinstitutional phase II trial of paclitaxel, carboplatin, and concurrent radiation therapy for locally advanced non-small-cell lung cancer. J Clin Oncol 1998; 17:3316.

66. Choy H, DeVore RF, Hande KR, et al. A Phase II study of paclitaxel, carboplatin, and hyperfractionated radiation therapy for locally advanced inoperable non-small cell lung cancer (a Vanderbilt cancer center affiliate network study). Int J Radiat Oncol Biol Phys 2000; 47:931.

67. Choy H, Curran WJ, Scott CB. Preliminary report of locally advanced multimodality protocol (LAMP):ACR 427: a randomized phase II study of three chemo-radiation regimens with paclitaxel, carboplatin, and thoracic radiation (TRT) for patients with locally advanced non small cell lung cancer (LA-NSCLC) Proc Am Soc Clin Oncol 2002; 291a (abstract 1160).

68. Ulutin HC, Pak Y. Preliminary results of radiotherapy with or without weekly paclitaxel in locally advanced non-small cell lung cancer. J Cancer Res Clin Oncol 2003; 129:52.

69. Armstrong JG, Burman C, Leibel SA, et al. Three-dimensional conformal radiation therapy may improve the therapeutic ratio of high dose radiation therapy for lung cancer. Int J Radiat Oncol Biol Phys 1993; 26:685.

70. Armstrong JG, Raben A, Zelefsky M, et al. Promising survival with three-dimensional conformal radiation therapy for non-small cell lung cancer. Radiother Oncol 1997; 44:17.
71. Robertson JM, Ten Haken RK, Hazuka MB. Dose escalation for non small cell lung cancer using conformal radiation therapy. Int J Radiat Oncol Biol Phys 199737:1079.
72. Martel MK, Sahijdak WM, Hayman JA. Incidental dose to clinically negative nodes from conformal treatment fields for nonsmall cell lung cancer. Int J Radiat Oncol Biol Phys 1999; 45:3S:244 (abstract).
73. Rosenzweig KE, Sim SE, Mychalczak B, et al. Elective nodal irradiation in the treatment of non-small-cell lung cancer with three-dimensional conformal radiation therapy. Int J Radiat Oncol Biol Phys 2001; 50:681.
74. Graham MV. Predicting radiation response. Int J Radiat Oncol Biol Phys 1997; 39:561.
75. Kwa Sl, Lebesque JV, Theuws JC, et al. Radiation pneumonitis as a function of mean lung dose: an analysis of pooled data of 540 patients. Int J Radiat Oncol Biol Phys 1998; 42:1.
76. Yorke E. Advantages of IMRT for dose escalation in radiation therapy for lung cancer. Med Phys 2001; 28:1291.
77. Giraud P, Rosenzweig KE, Yorke E. Radiotherapy for lung cancer: can IMRT decrease the risk of esophagitis? Proc. Am. Soc. Ther. Radiol. Oncol. (ASTRO). San Francisco, Int J Radiat Oncol Biol Phys 2001; 355 (abstract 2250).
78. Uematsu M, Shioda A, Tahara K, et al. Focal, high-dose, and fractionated modified stereotactic radiation therapy for lung carcinoma patients. A preliminary experience. Cancer 1998; 82:1062.
79. Hara R, Itami J, Kondo T, et al. Stereotactic single high dose irradiation of lung tumors under respiratory gating. Radiother Oncol 2002; 63:159.
80. Fukumoto S, Shirato H, Shimizu S, et al. Small-volume image-guided radiotherapy using hypofractionated coplanar and noncoplanar multiple fields with inoperable stage I nonsmall cell lung carcinomas. Cancer 2002; 95:1546.
81. Nagata Y, Negoro Y, Aoki T, et al. Clinical outcomes of 3D conformal hypofractionated single high-dose radiotherapy for one or two lung tumors using a stereotactic body frame. Int J Radiat Oncol Biol Phys 2002; 52:1041.
82. Whyte RI, Crownover R, Murphy MJ, et al. Stereotactic radiosurgery for lung tumors: preliminary report of a phase I trial. Ann Thorac Surg 2003; 75:1097.
83. Hof H, Herfarth K, Munter M, et al. Stereotactic single-dose radiotherapy of stage I non-small-cell lung cancer (NSCLC). Int J Radiat Oncol Biol Phys 2003; 56:3345.
84. Timmerman R, Papiez L, McGarry R, et al. Extracranial stereotactic radioablation. Results of a phase I study in medically inoperable stage I non-small cell lung cancer. Chest 2003; 28:1946.
85. Onimaru R, Shirato H, Shimizu S, et al. Tolerance of organs at risk in small-volume, hypofractionated, image-guided radiotherapy for primary and metastatic lung cancers. Int J Radiat Oncol Biol Phys 2003; 56:126.
86. Zimmermann FB, Schill S, Geinitz H, et al. Stereotactic hypofractionated radiation therapy for stage I non-small cell lung cancer. Lung Cancer 2005; 48(1):107.
87. Antonodou D, Coliarakis N, Synodinou M, et al. Clinical Radiation Oncology Hellenic Group. Randomized phase III trial of radiation treatment +/- amifostine in patients with advanced-stage lung cancer. Int J Radiat Oncol Biol Phys 2001; 51:915.
88. Komaki R, Lee JS, Kaplan B, et al. Randomized phase III study of chemoradiation with or without amifostine for patients with favorable performance status inoperable stage II-III non-small cell lung cancer: preliminary results. Semin Radiat Oncol 2002; 12 (1 suppl. 1):46.
89. Leong SS, Tan EH, Fong KW, et al. Randomized double-blind trial of combined modality treatment with or without amifostine in unresectable stage III non-small-cell lung cancer. J Clin Oncol 2003; 21:1767.
90. Movsas B, Scott C, Langer. Phase III study of amifostine in patients with locally advanced non-small cell lung cancer (NSCLC) receiving chemotherapy and hyperfractionated radiation (chemo/HFxRT): Radiation Therapy Oncology Group (RTOG) 98-01. Proc Am Soc Clin Oncol 2003; 21:636 (abstract 2559).

Integration of Chemotherapy in the Management of Locally Advanced Non-Small-Cell Lung Cancer

20

Cesare Gridelli and Paolo Maione

20.1   Introduction

About one-third of lung cancer patients present with stage III (locally advanced) non-small cell lung cancer (NSCLC). Locally advanced NSCLC, which accounts for more than 40,000 cases annually in the USA, represents a heterogeneous group of patients and several clinically distinct substages. Surgery is currently still considered the standard of care as initial treatment for patients with operable NSCLC, which includes stages I and II disease, and selected early subsets of IIIA disease. The existence of N2 disease (stage IIIAN2 disease) remains the most controversial area for primary surgical management of NSCLC and generally for the primary therapeutic approach to select. Minimal IIIAN2 disease is defined as single-station lymph node involvement with microscopic foci of disease not clinically apparent on clinical staging. This early-stage disease is usually dis-

covered at the time of thoracotomy or at pretreatment mediastinoscopy, and patients with minimal IIIAN2 disease may still be considered as candidates for radical surgery. Tumors with mediastinal involvement beyond that described as minimal IIIAN2 disease constitute the majority of patients presenting with stage IIIA disease; this more advanced, bulky or multistation N2 disease can usually be identified preoperatively and is termed "clinical N2 disease". Patients with clinical IIIAN2 disease have an overall 5-year survival rate of only 10–15%, although this falls to 2–5% in those with bulky mediastinal N2 involvement. Patients with clinical IIIAN2 disease or with stage IIIB disease are generally considered inoperable by primary surgery. The role of surgery following induction therapy in these advanced stage III patients is at the moment not conclusively defined.

Patients with unresectable stage IIIA or IIIB NSCLC have traditionally been treated with radiotherapy alone. Since all known macroscopic disease is confined to the chest, therapy was given in theory with curative intent. However, only 5–10% of patients survived beyond 5 years. This was frequently owing to distant disease progression (outside the radiation field), which occurred in up to 70% of patients and reflects the presence of systemic micrometastases at the time of initial therapy. Disease in a large proportion of patients also progressed within the irradiated volume, reflecting the inability of radiotherapy to eliminate all macroscopic disease. Efforts to increase cure rates have, therefore, attempted to increase both locoregional and systemic control. In practice, sequential chemoradiotherapy or concomitant chemoradiotherapy have been studied to achieve these goals. several randomized clinical trials and meta-analyses support the conclusion that combined-modality approaches using cisplatin-based chemotherapy improve survival compared with radiotherapy alone in patients with surgically unresectable stage III disease. Currently, in unresectable stage III disease, combinations of chemotherapy and radiotherapy are the standard treatment approach for patients with good performance status (PS). Depending on the strategy used, chemotherapy may play a cytotoxic role by eradi-

Table 20.1. Phase III randomized trials on concurrent versus sequential chemoradiotherapy. *MST* Median survival time, *CRT* concurrent chemoradiotherapy, *SRT* sequential chemoradiotherapy

Author	Regimens	Efficacy (MST)	Toxicity
Furuse et al. 1999 [20]	Cisplatin/vindesine/mitomycin + CRT vs. Cisplatin/vindesine/mitomycin + SRT	16.5 months 13.3 months	Myelosuppression significantly greater in the concurrent arm
Curran et al. 2003 [19]	Cisplatin/vinblastine + CRT vs. Cisplatin/vinblastine + SRT vs. Cisplatin/oral etoposide + CHRT	17.0 months 14.6 months 15.6 months	Acute grade 3–4 non-hematologic toxicity rates higher in the concurrent arms

* Statistically significant versus sequential treatments

cating distant micrometastases, a radiosensitizing role by improving local control, or both. Sequential approaches to chemoradiotherapy, in which platinum-based chemotherapy precedes thoracic radiation, have generally improved outcome by reducing distant failure rates. In contrast, in a phase III trial concurrent chemoradiotherapy using low-dose cisplatin was reported to improve survival by reducing local recurrence, without an effect on distant metastases. In view of these observations, concurrent chemoradiotherapy approaches integrating both radiosensitizing agents and dose levels of chemotherapy effective against micrometastases have been the most studied strategies. Recently, two randomized trials, one by the West Japan, Lung Cancer Group and the other by the Radiation Therapy Oncology Group (RTOG), have directly compared sequential and concurrent chemoradiotherapy regimens (Table 20.1). Each demonstrated superior survival with concurrent approach. Because distant metastases remain the major site of failure, it is likely that more effective chemotherapy or other systemic antitumor agents will be required to further improve the current level of response and survival of locally advanced NSCLC patients.

20.2 Rationale for Combined Chemoradiotherapy

Chemotherapeutic drugs can add to or modify the damage caused to tumor DNA by radiotherapy [1]. Examples of this include the effect of cisplatin on adduct formation in the presence of radiation-induced single-strand breaks and etoposide-induced double-strand breaks in addition to radiation-induced G2 blockade.

Radiosensitization linked to inhibition or alteration of radiation-induced DNA damage may also be achieved with some agents, notably the fluoropyrimidines, thymidine analogs, gemcitabine, and hydroxyurea.

Sensitizing arises most notably through the cytokinetic cooperation of drugs or radiation linked to the specific phases of the cell cycle. The S phase is the most radioresistant, and the G2/M phase is the most radiosensitive. Thus, increased radiosensitivity can be achieved by exposing proliferating cells to radiation at about the same time as drugs that kill cells in the S phase of replication. Responses to radiotherapy may also be enhanced by synchronization (or accumulation) of cells in the radiosensitive G2/M phase: this has been proposed as the mechanism underlying the in vitro radiosensitization of cells by some fluoropyrimidines.

20.3 Neoadjuvant Chemotherapy and Chemoradiotherapy

Neoadjuvant or preoperative therapy is defined as any cytoreductive treatment that is administered prior to surgery. During the past decade, several phase II trials showed that in general, it is feasible to perform pulmonary resection following chemotherapy or chemoradiation therapy. Although surgery can be more difficult after preoperative treatment, morbidity and mortality are generally acceptable.

The greater effectiveness of current chemotherapeutic regimens in settings of reduced disease bulk suggested that their use prior to surgery, either alone or in combination with radiation therapy, might increase both resectability and survival in patients with stage IIIA or IIIB NSCLC. Multiple phase II trials have shown such an approach to be feasible; however, it is not clear that such a strategy of neoadjuvant therapy and surgery improves survival over best nonsurgical chemoradiotherapy among patients who initially have clinical N2 disease.

Preoperative chemotherapy has several potential advantages over adjuvant (postoperative) chemotherapy, including delivery of chemotherapy through intact vasculature, early treatment of distant micrometastases, cytoreduction of bulky mediastinal lymph nodes and improved chemotherapy tolerance and compliance. Surgeons have a wide variety of opinions regarding the use of preoperative irradiation. A few surgeons believe that irradiation should never be given preoperatively, but most of them believe that the preoperative dose should be limited to 45–50 Gy.

Preoperative chemotherapy alone gained popularity in the mid-1990s primarily because of the encouraging results of two small randomized trials [2, 3], both of which were closed early to accrual when significant survival differences emerged favoring the chemotherapy arm over treatment with surgery alone. A French randomized trial, with 373 patients enrolled, compared preoperative chemotherapy to surgery alone in resectable stage I, II, and IIIa NSCLC [4]. Chemotherapy consisted in the MIC regimen (mitomycin 6 mg/m^2 on day 1, ifosfamide 1.5 g/m^2 on days 1–3, and cisplatin 30 mg/m^2 on days 1–3). Disease-free survival was significantly longer in the patients randomized to receive neoadjuvant chemotherapy than in those treated with surgery alone ($P=0.02$). Surprisingly, the most striking benefit of chemotherapy was seen in patients who had minimal lymphoadenopathy (either N0 or N1; $P=0.008$). Survival was superior in the preoperative chemotherapy group and was 9–10% higher in this group at years 3–5. However, the P value showed only a trend toward superiority ($P=0.09$) because the study was underpowered to show an improvement of this magnitude [4]. Survival differences were statistically significant only for the subgroup of patients with stage I and II disease. No excessive complications were seen in the chemotherapy-treated patients. Recently, the results of some phase II trials on last-generation neoadjuvant platin-containing chemotherapy have been reported. Cappuzzo et al. performed a phase II study aimed at determining the activity in terms of response rate and surgical resectability, and the tolerability of the new three-drug combination gemcitabine-cisplatin-paclitaxel in unresectable stage IIIAN2 and IIIB NSCLC [5, 6]. Complete resection of the tumor was obtained in 38% of patients, whereas a pathological complete response was achieved in 7% of patients. The regimen was globally well tolerated but the authors concluded that the activity profile, both in terms of response and surgical resection rate, is comparable to that obtained with standard doublets [5, 6]. Recently, a phase II trial evaluated the activity and safety of one of the newer platinum-based doublets, cisplatin and gemcitabine, as a neoadjuvant regimen in patients with unresectable stage IIIA-bulky N2 and stage IIIB NSCLC. This regimen proved to be a highly active and safe chemotherapy in this clinical setting. In fact, a 62% partial response rate was achieved, with 31% of patients undergoing surgery and 2% of patients achieving a pathological complete response rate [5, 6]. Another last-generation, platinum-based doublet recently tested as an induction regimen is carboplatin and paclitaxel. In a phase II study this regimen proved to be an active and very well tolerated induction chemotherapy, resulting in a response rate of 64% [7]. Some large randomized trials on neoadjuvant chemotherapy are ongoing in the USA and Europe and will elucidate the role of this approach in the general population.

At the same time, an alternative approach of preoperative treatment was explored in several phase II trials (i.e., concurrent chemoradiotherapy). The largest of these trials, Southwest Oncology Group (SWOG) 8805, administered preoperative cisplatin-etoposide with concurrent thoracic radiation to 45 Gy to 126 patients with stage IIIAN2 and selected stage IIIB NSCLC. This regimen was highly active, producing a pathologic complete response

in 21% of patients who underwent surgical resection. Another 37% of patients were left with only a few microscopic foci of disease, resulting in a major pathologic response in almost 60% of cases. Overall survival was promising, with an encouraging 26% 3-year survival rate. At a 6-year follow-up, more than 20% of patients remained alive in both the stage IIIA and IIIB subsets, documenting the potential for long-term survival with this type of combined-modality therapy [8].

The results of SWOG-8805 and a subsequent SWOG trial of definitive chemoradiotherapy (SWOG-9019) [9] provided the basis for the two arms of the recently reported Intergroup study (INT 0139) [10], designed to define the role of additional surgery in stage IIIAN2 disease. INT 0139 randomized patients with stage IIIAN2 NSCLC to either preoperative cisplatin and etoposide with concurrent thoracic radiotherapy to 45 Gy (as in SWOG 8805), or to the same chemotherapy with definitive radiotherapy to 61 Gy (as in SWOG 9019). The preliminary analysis of this trial, demonstrated superior disease-free survival in the arm that received induction chemoradiotherapy followed by surgery (3-year disease progression-free survival 29% vs. 19% in the surgical and chemoradiotherapy arms, respectively; $P=0.02$). The pathologic complete response rate on the surgical arm was 36%. More treatment-related deaths occurred on the surgical arm (7%, vs. 1.6% on the chemoradiation arm). However, to date there is no statistically significant difference in overall survival for the two groups, with the improvement in disease-free survival counterbalanced by increased mortality in the surgical arm. Specifically, the median survival for each arm was 22 months ($P=0.51$); there were more early noncancer deaths on the surgical arm, but overall survival curves crossed so that by year 3, overall survival was 15% better on the surgical arm (absolute: 38% vs. 33%). Longer follow-ups will be needed to determine whether surgery significantly prolongs survival in patients with stage IIIApN2 NSCLC. Moreover, the contribution of radiation to the preoperative regimen in INT 0139 cannot be determined. Would preoperative chemotherapy alone have been equally efficacious, and would it have been accompanied by less morbidity and treatment-related mortality? The argument for preoperative chemoradiotherapy over chemotherapy alone is predicated on the observation that the rate of complete responses in the primary tumor and mediastinal lymph nodes seems to be higher with combined-modality therapy. Indeed, trials performed to date, including SWOG 8805, have reported a positive correlation between achieving mediastinal lymph node sterilization and long-term survival after either preoperative chemoradiotherapy or chemotherapy alone [8, 11].

In conclusion, the standard treatment for initially resectable stage III NSCLC remains surgery with neoadjuvant chemotherapy, representing a promising experimental approach. In selected patients, preoperative treatment may have a favorable effect on outcome in surgically resectable stage III NSCLC. On the contrary, the standard treatment for initially unresectable stage III NSCLC is to be considered definitive chemoradiotherapy, with the role of additional surgery yet to be defined.

20.4   Definitive Combined Chemoradiotherapy

In the past, radiation therapy was considered the standard therapy for patients with stage IIIA or IIIB disease. Long-term survival was poor, in the range of 5–10%, with poor local control and early development of distant metastatic disease. The dominant pattern of failure in curatively resected or radically irradiated patients is distant metastatic failure. Thus, the rationale for chemotherapy given to potentially curative patients with NSCLC is prevention of distant relapse. Indeed, it is reported that at least 80% of patients treated with local modalities alone will have micrometastases and will, therefore, relapse [12, 13]. It has been shown that chemoradiotherapy is more efficient than either chemotherapy alone or radiation alone for the therapeutic management of localized unresectable NSCLC [14]. In the Cambridge meta-analysis, aimed at evaluating the efficacy of cytotoxic chemotherapy on survival in NSCLC patients, 9,387 patients enrolled in 52 randomized studies were distributed into 4 broad categories as a function of stage of disease. One of these categories consisted of a comparison between radiotherapy and radiotherapy plus chemotherapy. The combination of radiotherapy and cisplatin-based chemotherapy significantly reduced the risk of death by 13% (hazard ratio 0.87; $P=0.005$). The 2-year survival rate was 15% and 19% in the radiotherapy group and the radiotherapy plus chemotherapy group, respectively; the 5-year survival rate was 5% and 7% in the radiotherapy group and the radiotherapy plus chemotherapy group, respectively (Non-Small-Cell Lung Cancer Collaborative Group 1995). Several randomized trials have compared thoracic irradiation alone with chemoradiation therapy in patients with stage III NSCLC. Some of them employed sequential chemoradiation therapy and others concurrent chemoradiation therapy.

20.4.1   Sequential Chemoradiotherapy

The benefit of induction chemotherapy before radiotherapy in stage III NSCLC was established by the Cancer and Leukemia Group B (CALGB) 8433 trial [15] and subsequently verified by the RTOG 8808 [16] randomized phase III studies. In the CALGB 8433 trial, induction chemotherapy consisted of cisplatin, 100 mg/m^2 on days 1 and 29, plus vinblastine, 5 mg/m^2 weekly for 5 weeks. Standard irradiation consisted of 60 Gy given in 30 fractions beginning on day 1 in the standard radiotherapy arm and on day 50 in the chemoradiotherapy arm. After a follow-up of more than 7 years of 155 initially evaluated patients, median survival times in the chemoradiotherapy arm and the radiotherapy-only arm were 13.7 and 9.6 months, respectively ($P=0.012$). The rate of tumor response was 56% for the chemoradiotherapy arm and 43% for the radiotherapy arm ($P=0.092$). The authors concluded that although there was a 4.1-month increase in median survival favoring sequential chemoradiotherapy over radiotherapy alone, about 80–85% of the patients enrolled onto this trial died within 5 years, with treatment failure occurring both in the irradiated field and at distant sites [15]. Further improvement in both local and systemic treatment of disease was necessary. In the RTOG 8808 trial, patients were randomized to three treatment arms: sequential chemoradiotherapy, standard radiotherapy, and hyperfractionated radiotherapy. The sequential chemoradiotherapy arm and the standard radiotherapy arm comprised the same regimens used in the CALGB 8433 trial. In the third treatment arm, patients received hyperfractionated irradiation at 1.2 Gy twice daily to a total of 69.6 Gy. In that study, with 458 initially evaluable patients, overall survival was statistically superior for the patients receiving chemotherapy and radiation versus the other two radiotherapy-only arms of the study ($P=0.04$). Median survival times after 5 years were 11.4 months with standard irradiation, 13.2 months with chemoradiotherapy, and 12 months with hyperfractionated irradiation. The respective 5-years survivals were 5% for standard radiation therapy, 8% for chemotherapy followed by radiation therapy, and 6% for hyperfractionated irradiation. The twice-daily radiation therapy arm, although better, was not statistically superior in survival compared with standard radiation arm [16].

20.4.2   Concurrent Chemoradiotherapy

One of the first trials evaluating concurrent chemoradiation therapy versus radiation alone, the European Organization for Research and Treatment of Cancer (EORTC) trial 08844, compared radiotherapy alone with radiotherapy and concomitant (daily or weekly) low-dose cisplatin therapy [17]. This study demonstrated a significant survival advantage for daily cisplatin and radiotherapy compared with radiotherapy alone (3-year survival rates, 16% vs. 2%); the weekly cisplatin/radiation therapy arm produced intermediate results (3-year survival rate, 13%). Another phase III concurrent chemoradiation therapy trial showed that the combination of hyperfractionated radiation therapy and low-dose daily chemotherapy (carboplatin plus etoposide) was superior to hyperfractionated radiation therapy alone (to 69.6 Gy), with 4-year survival rates of 23% vs. 9% ($P=0.02$) [18].

After several randomized trials comparing sequential and concurrent chemoradiotherapy to radiation alone and demonstrating the superiority of the combined approaches, the superiority of concurrent administration of chemotherapy and radiotherapy over sequential therapy has been supported by two influential studies: RTOG 9410 [19] and a study from Japan [20]. The RTOG 9410 study assessed 597 patients with stage II–III NSCLC. Cisplatin 100 mg/m^2 on days 1 and 29, with vinblastine, 5 mg/m^2 weekly for 5 weeks, and with radiotherapy beginning on day 50 and administered to a total dose of 60 Gy, was compared with the same chemotherapy regimen plus radiotherapy beginning on day 1. A third group received concomitant chemoradiotherapy involving cisplatin/oral etoposide and hyperfractionated radiotherapy (total dose, 69.6 Gy). Median survival times for the three respective treatment groups were 14.6, 17.0, and 15.6 months. The 4-year survival rates with concurrent cisplatin/vinblastine and once-daily irradiation was 21%, compared with 12% with sequential treatment ($P=0.04$). The third treatment arm (concurrent cisplatin/oral etoposide and hyperfractionated irradiation) was intermediate, with a 4-year survival of 17%. These data show a strong trend favoring concurrent chemotherapy with standard radiation therapy over sequential or hyperfractionated treatment groups. The rates of acute grade 3–4 nonhematologic toxicity were reported to be higher with concurrent than with sequential therapy, but late toxicity rates were similar. Movsas et al. reported the results of a quality-adjusted time without symptoms of toxicity (QTWiST) analysis of RTOG 94-10. Despite the increase in reversible nonhematologic toxicities in the concurrent arms, the overall mean toxicity was highest in the sequential arm, which involved the longest treatment time. The concurrent once-daily arm had the optimal QTWiST, further supporting concurrent chemoradiation therapy as a new treatment paradigm [21]. Thus, delivering hyperfractionated radiation with concurrent chemotherapy produced higher toxicity rates with no increase in survival over once daily radiation concurrent with chemotherapy. The West Japan Lung Cancer Group studied 314 evaluable patients with unresectable stage III NSCLC and showed a 3.2-month median survival advantage (median survival 16.5 vs. 13.3 months, 5-year survival rates 15.8% vs. 8.9%, $P=0.04$) when irradiation was administered in what is currently considered an outdated schedule, with 28 Gy in 14 fractions at 5 fractions per week administered twice in a split-course regimen (total dose 56 Gy) concurrently with cisplatin, vindesine, and mitomycin rather than sequentially after the completion of chemotherapy at 5 fractions weekly to a total of 56 Gy. Despite the disadvantages of split-course techniques, which allow not only the repair of normal tissues but also proliferation of tumor clones during the break,

the 5-year survival rate significantly favored the concurrent approach. The authors also reported the patterns of failure, which demonstrated a benefit of concurrent chemoradiotherapy in improving the local relapse-free survival ($P=0.04$) but not the distant relapse-free survival ($P=0.6$). Myelosuppression was reported to be significantly greater among patients on the concurrent arm than on the sequential arm ($P=0.0001$).

As supported by clinical trials, the Patterns of Care Study for lung cancer, aimed at determining the national patterns of radiation therapy practice in patients treated for nonmetastatic lung cancer in 1998–1999, demonstrated that patients with clinical stage III NSCLC received chemotherapy plus radiation therapy more than radiotherapy alone ($P<0.0001$). Factors correlating with increased use of chemotherapy included lower age ($P<0.0001$), histology (SCLC more than NSCLC, $P<0.0001$), increasing clinical stage ($P<0.0001$), increasing Karnofsky PS ($P<0.0001$), and lack of comorbidities ($P=0.0002$), but not academic versus nonacademic facilities ($P=0.81$). Of all patients receiving chemotherapy, approximately three-quarters received it concurrently with radiotherapy. Only 3% of all patients were treated on Institutional-Review-Board-approved trials, demonstrating the need for improved accrual to clinical trials [22].

20.5 New Strategies of Combined Chemoradiotherapy

At present no one chemoradiotherapy regimen can be considered standard of care in surgically unresectable stage III NSCLC. Randomized trials demonstrating that concurrent chemoradiation is more effective than sequential chemoradiation were performed before the availability of newer chemotherapeutic agents with relatively higher levels of activity against NSCLC, such as paclitaxel, docetaxel, gemcitabine, and vinorelbine. Consequently, clinical research efforts have focused on incorporating newer chemotherapeutic agents, either singly or in combination with a platinum compound, into concurrent chemoradiation regimens for locally advanced NSCLC. Some phase I and II studies have been reported, many of which have shown encouraging results [23, 24, 25]. However, for many newer chemotherapeutic agents, dose-limiting toxicities require that lower doses be given during the concurrent phase. Thus the issue of how to best address the dual goals of local control and eradication of distant micrometastases while avoiding excessive toxicity remains controversial. Specifically, although delivery of full-dose chemotherapy may be required to reduce distant failure rates, toxicities such as esophagitis or pneumonitis may necessitate lowering chemotherapy doses during concurrent administration of thoracic irradiation.

Analyses of the positive randomized trials favoring chemoradiation over radiation therapy alone suggest a difference in the patterns of failure that relates to the method of combining chemotherapy with thoracic radiotherapy. In fact, in the trials employing sequential chemoradiation therapy, the improvement in survival rates over irradiation alone appeared to be linked to a decrease in the development of distant metastases. In contrast, in the positive trials employing concurrent chemoradiation therapy, the survival advantage appeared to be associated with an improvement in locoregional control. It may be that the use of high-dose induction chemotherapy combats systemic disease, whereas the simultaneous delivery of low-dose chemotherapy (cisplatin or carboplatin) with irradiation may be necessary to improve local tumor control. Based on these observations, new strategies of combined chemoradiotherapy are currently being tested to improve survival outcomes of treatment for locally advanced NSCLC.

Recently, two treatment paradigms have emerged that may optimize the delivery of chemotherapy and radiation for stage III NSCLC: induction chemotherapy followed by concurrent chemoradiation (induction-first), and concurrent chemoradiation followed by consolidation chemotherapy (concurrent-first). The rationale underlying these approaches lies in the improvements in survival seen with sequential chemoradiotherapy coupled with the apparent superiority of concurrent therapy over sequential regimens. In this field, several phase II and III studies are ongoing. Definitive data are available from the trial (9504) of the Southwest Oncology Group (SWOG) in 83 patients with stage IIIB NSCLC, in which a regimen consisting of cisplatin, 50 mg/m^2 on days 1 and 8 in weeks 1, 2, 5, and 6, with etoposide, 50 mg/m^2 on days 1–5 during weeks 1 and 5, was given in conjunction with radiotherapy to 61 Gy over 6 weeks. This combined therapy was then followed by consolidation docetaxel, $75–100 \text{ mg/m}^2$ every 21 days for three cycles [26]. The reported median survival time from this study is 26 months, median progression-free survival 16 months and 1-, 2-, and 3-year survival rates 76%, 54%, and 37%, respectively. These results are remarkably better than the median survival of 15 months and 1-, 2-, and 3-year survival rates of 58%, 34%, and 17%, respectively, reported previously in SWOG 9019, a study of 50 patients treated with cisplatin/etoposide and concurrent radiation followed by 2 consolidation cycles with cisplatin and etoposide [9]. Toxicity during consolidation consisted primarily of neutropenia (56% grade 4). In the trial S9504, brain metastasis was the most common site of failure.

Another innovative approach to be tested consists of induction chemotherapy followed by chemoradiotherapy. Vokes et al. conducted a randomized phase II study

of two cycles of induction chemotherapy followed by two additional cycles of the same drugs with concomitant radiotherapy [24]. Four cycles of gemcitabine (arm 1) or paclitaxel (arm 2) or vinorelbine (arm 3) in combination with cisplatin were administered to 175 patients. Response rates after completion of radiotherapy were 74%, 67%, and 73% for arms 1, 2, and 3, respectively. Median survival for all patients was 17 months. One-, 2-, and 3-year survival rates for the patients on the three arms were 68%/37%/28%, 62%/29%/19%, and 65%/40%/23%, respectively. The observed survival rates exceeded those of previous trials performed by the same group (CALGB). Induction chemotherapy added to concomitant chemoradiotherapy is being evaluated in a phase III randomized trial.

Choy et al. performed a randomized phase II study in 276 patients of 3 chemoradiation therapy regimens with paclitaxel, carboplatin, and thoracic irradiation in their locally advanced multimodality protocol (LAMP). Arm 1 (sequential) gave two cycles of carboplatin (AUC 6)/paclitaxel (200 mg/m^2) followed by daily radiotherapy; arm 2 (induction-first) gave induction chemotherapy with carboplatin/paclitaxel followed by weekly carboplatin (AUC 2)/paclitaxel (45 mg/m^2) plus concurrent radiotherapy; arm 3 gave concurrent carboplatin/paclitaxel followed by carboplatin/paclitaxel. They found that concurrent chemoradiation therapy followed by adjuvant chemotherapy appeared to have the best therapeutic outcome, with a median survival of 16.1 months, compared with either induction chemotherapy followed by concurrent chemoradiation therapy (median survival of 11 months and reduced delivery of concurrent chemoradiation) or sequential chemotherapy followed by irradiation (median survival, 12 months; Table 20.2) [27].

Table 20.2. Main phase II trials on new combination regimens of chemoradiotherapy. *W* Weekly, *C/P* carboplatin/paclitaxel, *CRT* concurrent chemoradiotherapy

Author	Strategy	Regimen
Lau et al. 2001 [23]	Concurrent-first	W C/P + CRT followed by C/P
Choy et al. 2002 [27]	Concurrent-first vs. Induction-first	C/P + CRT followed by C/P
		C/P followed by W C/P + CRT
Vokes 2002 et al. [24]	Induction-first	Cisplatin/gemcitabine or paclitaxel or vinorelbine followed by the same regimen + CRT
Albain 2002 et al. [9]	Concurrent-first	Cisplatin/etoposide + CRT followed by cisplatin/etoposide
Gandara 2003 et al. [26]	Concurrent-first	Cisplatin/etoposide + CRT followed by docetaxel

20.6 Integration of Targeted Therapies in the Management of Locally Advanced NSCLC

Although some progress has been made in the treatment of locally advanced NSCLC by combining chemotherapy with radiotherapy, treatment outcomes in this clinical setting are still disappointing. Thus, clinical research of new treatment strategies is warranted. Advances in the knowledge of tumor biology and mechanisms of oncogenesis have granted the singling out of several molecular targets for NSCLC treatment. Targeted therapies are designed to interfere with specific aberrant biologic pathways involved in tumorigenesis. A large amount of preclinical in vivo and in vitro data have been gathered on the antitumor properties of several new biological agents, both as single agents and combined with other conventional treatment modalities such as chemotherapy and radiotherapy. Consequently, several targeted agents have been introduced into clinical trials in NSCLC, with many phase I and II studies already completed and the first phase III study results being recently made available. To date, only few of these new agents can offer hope of a substantial impact on the natural history of the disease, and negative results are more commonly reported than positive ones. Nevertheless, clinically meaningful advances have already been achieved in chemotherapy-refractory advanced NSCLC patients, with erlotinib, an epidermal growth factor receptor (EGFR) tyrosine kinase inhibitor, representing a further chance after chemotherapy of tumor control and/or symptom palliation. To date, targeted therapies with the major implications in locally advanced NSCLC treatment are epidermal growth factor receptor family inhibitors and angiogenesis inhibitors.

20.6.1 Epidermal Growth Factor Receptor Inhibitors

Molecular pathways that regulate tumor growth, invasion, and metastases include the ErbB family of receptor tyrosine kinases. The pathways associated with activation of the EGFR have been identified as pivotal for the unregulated growth of many epithelial cancers including lung cancer. EGFR overexpression occurs in 50–80% of NSCLCs, and 81–93% of NSCLCs express the EGFR ligand, transforming growth factor-alpha (TGF-α) [28]. The EGFR pathway can be upregulated by radiation, resulting in radioresistance [29, 30], and interference of this pathway has been to shown to amplify radiation cytotoxicity in a variety of human tumor models [31, 32]. Clinically, agents that target the extracellular binding domain of the EGFR, such as cetuximab (IMC-C225, Erbitux), or the intracellular tyrosine kinase domain, such as gefitinib (ZD1839, Iressa) or erlotinib

(OSI-774, Tarceva), are well tolerated with chronic administration. Monotherapy trials of these agents demonstrated toxicity profiles that differ from those of conventional chemotherapy drugs, primarily acneiform rashes and diarrhea [33]. A palliative role in the treatment of chemotherapy-refractory NSCLC has been already established for gefitinib and erlotinib [34–36]. Encouraging preclinical data employing anti-EGFR agents alone or in combination with radiation has led to the incorporation of anti-EGFR compounds with radiation in human clinical trials. For example, the CALGB is currently conducting a clinical trial in patients with locally advanced NSCLC (CALGB 30106). Patients are treated with induction chemotherapy and gefitinib followed by concurrent gefitinib and radiation. Patients go on to receive maintenance gefitinib. Specifically, in patients with PS 0–1, gefitinib is being added to carboplatin/paclitaxel induction chemotherapy followed by concomitant chemoradiotherapy, while in patients with PS 2 or 0–1 with weight loss ≥5% to induction chemotherapy followed by single-modality radiotherapy. In fact, the investigators hypothesize that the addition of gefitinib as a single agent to radiotherapy will result in more tolerable toxicities than those associated with traditional concomitant chemoradiotherapy, and thus, might define a feasible approach to the treatment of patients with a PS of 2 or pretreatment weight loss exceeding 5%. At the University of Colorado, a regimen combining fixed-dose gefitinib (250 mg) with conformal three-dimensional radiation and concurrent chemotherapy in patients with locally advanced, inoperable NSCLC is being evaluated. This phase I trial is a radiation dose-escalation trial with a dose range of 63–70.2 Gy. Rischin et al. have reported the preliminary toxicity and response data in patients with stage III NSCLC. Patients with an Eastern Cooperative Oncology Group (ECOG) PS of 0–1 and no prior radiation were eligible for this phase I trial. Patients received fixed-dose radiation to 60 Gy/30 fractions/6 weeks to the primary site and involved regional nodes. Concurrent oral gefitinib 250 mg/day and weekly carboplatin AUC 2 were administered with radiation on dose level 1, and weekly paclitaxel was added at 25, 35, and 45 mg/m^2 at dose levels 2, 3, and 4, respectively. Initially patients continued on maintenance gefitinib; however, this was stopped after the first six patients due to concerns regarding the development of interstitial pneumonitis. Dose escalation up to dose level 4 has been completed with 15 patients enrolled. No dose-limiting toxicities were observed. Treatment was well tolerated, with three patients experiencing grade three esophagitis and no reported grade three pneumonitis (grade 2, $n=5$; 4 of which occurred in patients who continued gefitinib after chemoradiation). Interestingly, positron emission tomography analysis indicated a complete response rate in 11 evaluable patients of 55%. The chemotherapy complete response rate was 27% and the partial response rate was 64%, for an over-

Table 20.3. Possible strategies of integration of targeted therapies in the treatment of locally advanced non-small-cell lung cancer. *PS* Performance status

PS 0/1 patients	PS 2 patients
Added to chemotherapy and to concurrent chemoradiotherapy in induction-first and concurrent-first experimental regimens	Concurrently with radiotherapy in sequential chemoradiotherapy regimens
As consolidation after concurrent chemoradiotherapy	As consolidation after sequential chemoradiotherapy
Added to and as consolidation after concurrent chemoradiotherapy	Concurrently with radiotherapy and as consolidation after sequential chemoradiotherapy

all response rate of 91% [37]. Another trial, a phase I study, is currently investigating the addition of erlotinib to chemoradiotherapy in stage III NSCLC. Erlotinib is added in increasing doses to alternating cohorts of patients receiving either an induction-first or a concurrent-first regimen (Table 20.3).

20.6.2 Angiogenesis Inhibitors

In exploring novel approaches to treating NSCLC it is known that irradiation upregulates vascular endothelial factor (VEGF) and cyclooxygenase-2 (COX-2) production in tumor cells, which in turn stimulates tumor angiogenesis [38]. Teicher's work in the 1990s was instrumental in demonstrating that inhibiting angiogenesis enhances radiation cytotoxicity [39]. To this end, it has been shown recently that COX-2 inhibition on tumors improved the response to radiotherapy in an animal model, possibly through an antiangiogenic mechanism [40]. The RTOG is currently conducting a phase I/II trial of a COX-2 inhibitor, Celebrex (Celecoxib), with limited field radiation for intermediate-prognosis patients with locally advanced NSCLC (RTOG 0213). Altorki et al. recently reported a phase II trial that showed enhancement of antitumor activity of neoadjuvant chemotherapy with carboplatin and paclitaxel in 29 patients with stages IB–IIIA NSCLC with the addition of celecoxib 400 mg twice daily. In fact, the response rate of 65% compared favorably with historical controls, and moreover, the addition of celecoxib abrogated the marked increase in prostaglandin E2 detected in primary tumors after treatment with paclitaxel and carboplatin alone [41]. In the near future, Celecoxib may also prove to be useful in the treatment of locally advanced NSCLC, combined with chemoradiation.

Interfering with BEGF receptor (VEGFR) signaling is under investigation in preclinical studies alone and with radiation. A randomized phase II study of bevacizumab (7.5 or 15 mg/kg), a recombinant humanized monoclonal antibody to VEGF, in combination with carboplatin and paclitaxel or carboplatin plus paclitaxel (control) in 99 patients with stage IIIB or IV NSCLC has been carried out [42]. Response rates with the antibody were about 10% higher, and the time to tumor progression was prolonged by approximately 3 months (from 4.5 to 7.5 months) in the high-dose antibody group. However, a development warranting concern was that six patients developed severe hemoptysis (four episodes were fatal). In an evaluation of potential risk factors, it was found that the squamous histologic subtype and bevacizumab treatment were the only factors associated with hemoptysis. Patients with nonsquamous cell histology appeared to be a subpopulation with improved outcome and acceptable safety risks. The ECOG is currently evaluating the effect of adding 15 mg/kg bevacizumab to carboplatin and paclitaxel in patients with advanced nonsquamous NSCLC. The very promising results achieved in the advanced disease suggest that the approach of combining bevacizumab with chemotherapy is also worth testing in the treatment of locally advanced NSCLC.

In lung cancer models, promising preclinical data have been reported using orally bioavailable small-molecule VEGFR-tyrosine kinase inhibitors. ZD6474 is an example of this class of molecules currently under investigation in human clinical trials in patients with advanced NSCLC. ZD6474 appears to have dual inhibitory action against both VEGFR and EGFR signaling. In preclinical studies using an orthotopic lung cancer model, combinations of ZD6474 and radiation were superior to paclitaxel and radiation in preventing pleural effusions due to the tumor, as well as reducing tumor burden and preventing metastasis. Enhanced apoptosis and decreased microvessel density were observed in the animals treated with ZD6474 and radiation [43]. ZD6474 is considered to be a promising agent to test in combination with chemoradiotherapy in the treatment of locally advanced NSCLC.

20.7 Treatment of Locally Advanced NSCLC in the Elderly

NSCLC may be considered typical of advanced age. More than 50% of cases are diagnosed in patients over the age of 65 years, and about 30% of cases are diagnosed in patients over the age of 70 years [44, 45]. Specific approaches for elderly patients are needed. In fact, elderly patients may tolerate chemotherapy poorly because of comorbidity and physiological organ failure. The prevalence of these comorbid conditions is about twice as high as in the general population [46]. The most important coexisting pathologies in lung cancer patients are cardiovascular and pulmonary diseases, which are common among cigarette smokers. Moreover, it is common to find a geriatric syndrome among the elderly, in which most of their functional reserve is exhausted. Decreased hepatic, renal, and bone-marrow functions have a negative impact on the degree of toxicity, in particular on cisplatin toxicity. In order to plan the treatment of elderly NSCLC patients, a multidimensional geriatric evaluation including not only assessment of comorbidities, but also functional, mental, and nutritional status is needed.

Thus in clinical practice, combined chemoradiotherapy, even if sequential, can be contraindicated in elderly patients. In fact, this patient population often presents at diagnosis with cardiovascular and/or pulmonary comorbidities that increase the risk of severe side-effects from chemoradiotherapy. The issue is rendered more complicated by the paucity of prospective, specifically designed clinical trials on the treatment of locally advanced NSCLC of elderly patients.

20.7.1 Prospective Studies on Combined Chemoradiotherapy in the Elderly

Very few prospective studies on combined chemoradiotherapy in elderly patients with locally advanced NSCLC have been performed [47]. Although with limited samples, the phase II trials that have been performed are interesting because they investigated alternative schedules of treatment, potentially more suitable for elderly patients; mainly the administration of low-dose chemotherapy. These regimens were found to be both feasible and effective in the elderly population.

Atagi et al. reported on a phase II study during which radiotherapy and concurrent low-dose daily carboplatin (as a radiosensitizing agent), were given in patients with unresectable NSCLC. A response rate of 50% was reported with 1- and 2-year survival rates of 52.6% and 20.5%, respectively. The main toxicities were hematological toxicities, with grade 3–4 leukopenia, neutropenia, thrombocytopenia, and anemia occurring in 71%, 55%, 29%, and 34% of patients, respectively. The authors suggested that this chemoradiotherapy regimen is effective and feasible in elderly patients with NSCLC [48]. Nakano et al. conducted a pilot study to assess the tolerance and efficacy of concurrent cisplatin and thoracic radiation in elderly patients with locally advanced, unresectable NSCLC [49]. The most common grade 3 toxicities included leukopenia (20%) and thrombocytopenia (9%). The overall confirmed response rate was 82%, and the median overall survival was 23 months. The authors concluded that this chemoradiotherapy regimen is well tolerated, with promising responses and survival in elderly patients with unresectable NSCLC [49]. Very recently, D'Angellilo et al. have reported on the feasibility of a neoadjuvant chemoradiotherapy in elderly patients with locally advanced NSCLC. Involved

field radiotherapy was combined with low-dose carboplatin or gemcitabine. The incidences of hematological and nonhematological grade 3 toxicity were 7.9% and 2.6%, respectively, and an objective response rate of 72.6% was reported. Thus, this approach was considered effective and feasible in this patient population [50].

20.7.2 Retrospective Studies on Combined Chemoradiotherapy

Some retrospective analyses on randomized trials of chemoradiotherapy compared treatment outcomes between elderly patients and their younger counterpart. Results are overall ambiguous, with some analyses showing an excess of toxicity and lack of survival benefit in the elderly subgroup, others concluding for both feasibility and efficacy of combined treatment in this population, also with a concurrent schedule, and others concluding for increased toxicity but survival rates equivalent to those achieved for younger individuals. The RTOG performed a retrospective analysis of patients included in phase II–III trials. A quality-adjusted survival analysis of 979 cases treated with radiotherapy alone or combined chemoradiotherapy showed a critical relationship between age and ability to tolerate combined treatment. In fact, elderly patients aged more than 70 years achieved the best quality-adjusted survival with standard radiotherapy only [51]. Moreover, a large analysis of survival data from 1999 patients from different RTOG trials treated with or without chemotherapy found a negative influence of older age on survival [52]. These results have been confirmed in another RTOG retrospective analysis of 749 locally advanced NSCLC patients enrolled in three separate trials and randomized to radiotherapy alone versus combined sequential or concurrent chemoradiotherapy. As therapy intensified, the incidence of grade 3–5 toxicities increased in the elderly group (>70 years). Unlike the overall patient population, elderly patients did not benefit from combined treatment and the authors concluded that specific trials are indicated [53]. The same authors, 2 years later, retrospectively evaluating treatment outcomes in elderly versus younger patients enrolled on a randomized RTOG trial of concurrent versus sequential chemoradiotherapy, concluded not only for the feasibility of combined treatment, but also for the superiority of the concurrent compared to the sequential approach, also in the elderly population. In fact, the median survival of elderly patients favored concurrent chemoradiotherapy over sequential chemoradiotherapy (22.4 months versus 10.8 months, respectively; $P = 0.069$). Long-term toxicities were similar between patients aged less and more than 70 years, but short-term toxicities (grade ≥ 3 neutropenia and grade ≥ 3 esophagitis) were more pronounced in the elderly compared with patients aged less than 70 years [54]. Very recently, the North Central Cancer Treatment Group performed a secondary analysis of a phase III trial on two different schedules of radiation therapy (twice daily versus daily) combined to chemotherapy in stage III NSCLC to examine the relationship between patient age and outcome. This retrospective analysis compared the outcomes of patients aged ≥70 years with those of younger individuals. Of the 244 assessable patients, 63 (26%) were elderly, and 181 (74%) were younger. The 2- and 5-year survival rates were 39% and 18%, respectively, in patients younger than 70 years, compared with 36% and 13%, respectively, in elderly patients ($P = 0.4$). Toxicity ≥grade 4 occurred in 62% of patients younger than 70 years, compared with 81% of elderly patients ($P = 0.007$). Hematologic toxicity ≥grade 4 occurred in 56% of patients younger than 70 years, compared with 78% of elderly patients ($P = 0.003$). Pneumonitis ≥grade 4 occurred in 1% of those younger than 70 years, compared with 6% of elderly patients ($P = 0.02$). In conclusion, despite increased toxicity, elderly patients treated with combined chemoradiotherapy had survival rates equivalent to those of younger individuals. Therefore, the authors concluded that fit, elderly patients with locally advanced NSCLC should be encouraged to receive combined-modality therapy, but preferably on clinical trials with cautious, judicious monitoring [55].

Only specifically designed prospective studies will elucidate the real role and feasibility of combined chemoradiotherapy in the treatment of locally advanced NSCLC of elderly patients because evidence from retrospective analyses could suffer from selection bias. In fact, elderly patients enrolled in this sort of trial are unlikely to be representative of the whole elderly population, but rather of only of a small subgroup thought to be eligible for aggressive treatments by investigators. As a consequence the generalizability of these results is poor because of possible selection bias and they could potentially put at risk many elderly patients until large prospective trials will have been performed on this issue [56].

Different options could be considered of interest in the elderly with locally advanced disease: single-agent chemotherapy and sequential radiotherapy; attenuated-dose platin-based chemotherapy and sequential radiotherapy; single-agent chemotherapy and concurrent radiotherapy; attenuated-dose platin-based chemotherapy and concurrent radiotherapy. However, while awaiting specific trials of combined chemoradiotherapy in the elderly, the aggressive concurrent approach should be considered for selected patients only.

Key Points

- Although promising, it has not yet been demonstrated that neoadjuvant chemotherapy or chemoradiotherapy improve survival over combined chemoradiotherapy among patients who initially have more than minimal IIIAN2 non-small-cell lung cancer (NSCLC).
- In unresectable stage III disease, combinations of chemotherapy and radiotherapy are the standard treatment approach for patients with good performance status. The superiority of concurrent administration of chemotherapy and radiotherapy over sequential therapy has been supported by two influential studies by Radiation Therapy Oncology Group and West Japan Lung Cancer Group.
- New strategies of combined chemoradiotherapy, as consolidation chemotherapy after chemoradiotherapy or induction chemotherapy followed by chemoradiotherapy, are currently being tested to improve survival outcomes in locally advanced NSCLC treatment.
- Targeted therapies may be integrated into the treatment paradigms either concurrently with chemoradiotherapy or as maintenance.
- Only specifically designed prospective studies will elucidate the real role and feasibility of combined chemoradiotherapy in the treatment of locally advanced NSCLC of elderly patients.

References

1. Hennequin C, Favaudon V. Biological basis for chemoradiotherapy interactions. Eur J Cancer 2002; 38:223.
2. Roth JA, Fossella F, Komaki R, et al. A randomized trial comparing perioperative chemotherapy and surgery with surgery alone in resectable stage IIIA non-small-cell lung cancer. J Natl Cancer Inst 1994; 86:673.
3. Rosell R, Gomez-Codina J, Camps C, et al. A randomized trial comparing preoperative chemotherapy plus surgery with surgery alone in patients with non-small-cell lung cancer. N Engl J Med 1994; 330:153.
4. Depierre A, Milleron B, Moro-Sibilot D, et al. Preoperative chemotherapy followed by surgery compared with primary surgery in resectable stage I (except T1N0), II, and IIIa non-small-cell lung cancer. J Clin Oncol 2002; 20:247.
5. Cappuzzo F, De Marinis F, Nelli F, et al. Phase II study of gemcitabine-cisplatin-paclitaxel triplet as induction chemotherapy in inoperable, locally advanced non-small cell lung cancer. Lung Cancer 2003; 42:355.
6. Cappuzzo F, Selvaggi G, Gregorc V, et al. Gemcitabine and cisplatin as induction chemotherapy for patients with unresectable stage IIIA-bulky N2 and stage IIIB non small cell lung carcinoma. Cancer 2003; 98:128.
7. O'Brien MER, Splinter T, Smit EF, et al. Carboplatin and paclitaxel (Taxol) as an induction regimen for patients with biopsy-proven stage IIIA N2 non-small cell lung can-

cer: an EORTC phase II study (EORTC 08958). Eur J Cancer 2003; 39:1416.

8. Albain KS, Rusch VW, Crowley JJ, et al. Concurrent cisplatin/etoposide plus chest radiotherapy followed by surgery for stages IIIAN2 and IIIB non-small-cell lung cancer:mature results of Southwest Oncology Group phase II study 8805. J Clin Oncol 2001; 13:1880.

9. Albain KS, Crowley JJ, Turrisi AT 3rd, et al. Concurrent cisplatin, etoposide, and chest radiotherapy in pathologic stage IIIB non-small-cell lung cancer: a Southwest Oncology Group phase II study, SWOG 9019. J Clin Oncol 2002; 20:3454.

10. Albain KS, Scott CB, Rusch VR, et al. Phase III comparison of concurrent chemotherapy plus radiotherapy (CT/RT) and CT/RT followed by surgical resection for stage IIIA (pN2) non-small cell lung cancer: initial results from intergroup trial 0139 (RTOG 93-09). Proc Am Soc Clin Oncol 2003; 22:621.

11. Betticher DC, Hsu Schmitz S-F, Totsch M, et al. Mediastinal lymph node clearance after docetaxel-cisplatin neoadjuvant chemotherapy is prognostic of survival in patients with stage IIIA pN2 non-small-cell lung cancer: a multicenter phase II trial. J Clin Oncol 2003; 21:1752.

12. Rosell R. The integration of newer agents into neoadjuvant therapy. Semin Oncol 1998; 25(suppl 8):24.

13. Gandara DR, Lara PN Jr, Goldberg Z, Roberts P, Lau DH. Neoadjuvant therapy for non-small cell lung cancer. Anticancer Drugs 2001; 12 (suppl 1):S5.

14. Non-Small Cell Lung Cancer Collaborative Group. Chemotherapy in non small cell lung cancer: a meta-analysis using updated data on individual patients from 52 randomised clinical trials. Br Med J 1995; 311:899.

15. Dillman RO, Herndon J, Seagren SL, Eaton WL, Green MR. Improved survival in stage III non-small-cell lung cancer: seven-year follow-up of Cancer and Leukemia Group B (CALGB) 8433 trial. J Natl Cancer Inst 1996; 88:1210.

16. Sause W, Kolesar P, Taylor S IV, et al. Final results of phase III trial in regionally advanced unresectable non-small cell lung cancer. Radiation Therapy Oncology, Eastern Cooperative Oncology Group, and Southwest Oncology Group. Chest 2000; 117:358.

17. Schaake-Koning C, van den Bogaert W, Dalesio O, et al. Effects of concomitant cisplatin and radiotherapy on inoperable non-small cell lung cancer. N Engl J Med 1992; 326:524.

18. Jeremic B, Shibamoto Y, Acimovic L, Milisavljevic S. Hyperfractionated radiation therapy with or without concurrent low-dose daily carboplatin/etoposide for stage III non-small-cell lung cancer: a randomized study. J Clin Oncol 1996; 14:1065.

19. Curran WJ Jr, Scott CB, Langer CJ, et al. Long-term benefit is observed in a phase III comparison of sequential vs concurrent chemo-radiation for patients with unresected stage III NSCLC: rTOG 9410. Proc Am Soc Clin Oncol 2003; 22:621.

20. Furuse K, Fukuoka M, Kawahara M, et al. Phase III study of concurrent versus sequential thoracic radiotherapy in combination with mitomycin, vindesine, and cisplatin in unresectable stage III non-small cell lung cancer. J Clin Oncol 1999; 17:2692.

21. Movsas B, Scott C, Curran W, Byhardt R, Langer C. A quality-adjusted time without symptoms or toxicity (QTWiST) analysis of Radiation Therapy Oncology Group (RTOG) 94-10. Proc Am Soc Clin Oncol 2001; 20:313a.

22. Movsas V, Moughan J, Komaki R, et al. Radiotherapy (RT) patterns of care study (PCS) in lung carcinoma. J Clin Oncol 2003; 21:4553.

23. Lau D, Leigh B, Gandara DR, et al. Twice weekly paclitaxel and weekly carboplatin with concurrent thoracic irradiation followed by carboplatin/paclitaxel consolidation

for stage III non-small cell lung cancer: a California Cancer Consortium phase II trial. J Clin Oncol 2001; 19:442.

24. Vokes EE, Herndon II JE, Crawford J, Leopold KA, Perry MC, Miller AA, Green MR. Randomized phase II study of cisplatin with gemcitabine or paclitaxel or vinorelbine as induction chemotherapy followed by concomitant chemoradiotherapy for stage IIIB non-small-cell lung cancer: Cancer and Leukemia Group B study 9431. J Clin Oncol 2002; 20:4191.

25. Gridelli C, Guida C, Barletta E, et al. Thoracic radiotherapy and daily vinorelbine as radiosensitizer in locally advanced non small cell lung cancer: a phase I study. Lung Cancer 2000; 29:131.

26. Gandara DR, Chansky K, Albain KS, et al. Consolidation docetaxel after concurrent chemoradiotherapy in stage IIIB non-small-cell lung cancer: phase II Southwest Oncology Group (S9504). J Clin Oncol 2003; 21:2004.

27. Choy H, Curran WJ, Scott CB, et al. Preliminary report of locally advanced multimodality protocol (LAMP): aCR 427: a randomized phase II study of three chemo-radiation regimens with paclitaxel, carboplatin, and thoracic radiation (TRT) for patients with locally advanced non small cell lung cancer (LA- NSCLC). Proc Am Soc Clin Oncol 2002; 21:291a.

28. Raymond R, Faivre S, Armand J. Epidermal growth factor receptor tyrosine kinase as a target for anticancer therapy. Drugs 2000; 60 (suppl 1):15.

29. Dent P, Reardon D, Park J, Bowers G, Logsdon C, Valerie K, Schmidt-Ullrich R. Radiation-induced release of transforming growth factor alpha activates the epidermal growth factor receptor and mitogen-activated protein kinase pathway in carcinoma cells, leading to increased proliferation and protection from radiation-induced cell death. Mol Biol Cell 1999; 10:2493.

30. Akimoto T, Hunter NR, Buchmiller L, Masou K, Ang KK, Milas L. Inverse relationship between epidermal growth factor receptor expression and radiocurability of murine carcinomas. Clin Cancer Res 1999; 5:437.

31. Huang SM, Bock JM, Harari PM. Epidermal growth factor receptor blockade with C225 modulates proliferation, apoptosis, and radiosensitivity in squamous cell carcinomas of the head and neck. Cancer Res 1999; 59:1935.

32. Bianco C, Tortora G, Bianco R, et al. Enhancement of antitumor activity of ionizing radiation by combined treatment with the selective epidermal growth factor receptor-tyrosine kinase inhibitor ZD1839 (Iressa). Clin Cancer Res 2002; 8:3250.

33. Baselga J, Herbst R, LoRusso P, et al. Continuous administration of ZD1839 (Iressa), a novel oral epidermal growth factor tyrosine kinase inhibitor (EGFR-TKI), in patients with five selected tumor types:evidence of activity and good tolerability. Proc Am Soc Clin Oncol 2000; 19:177a.

34. Kris MG, Natale RB, Herbst RS, et al. Efficacy of gefitinib, an inhibitor of the epidermal growth factor receptor tyrosine kinase, in symptomatic patients with non-small cell lung cancer: a randomized trial. JAMA 2003; 290:2149.

35. Fukuoka M, Yano S, Giaccone G, et al. Multi-institutional randomized phase II trial of gefitinib for previously treated patients with advanced non-small-cell lung cancer. J Clin Oncol 2003; 21:2237.

36. Shepherd FA, Pereira J, Ciuleanu TE, et al. A randomized placebo-controlled trial of erlotinib in patients with advanced non-small cell lung cancer (NSCLC) following failure of 1st line or 2nd line chemotherapy. A National Cancer Institute of Canada Clinical Trials Group (NCIC CTG) trial. ASCO Annual Meeting Proceedings (Post-Meeting Edition). J Clin Oncol 2004; 22(14S):7022.

37. Rischin D, Burmeister B, Mitchell P, et al. Phase I trial of gefitinib (ZD1839) in combination with concurrent carboplatin, paclitaxel and radiation therapy in patients with

stage III non-small cell lung cancer. ASCO Annual Meeting Proceedings (Post-Meeting Edition). J Clin Oncol 2004; 22(14S):7077.

38. Steinauer KK, Gibbs I, Ning S, French JN, Armstrong J, Knox SJ. Radiation induces upregulation of cyclooxygenase-2 (COX-2) protein in PC-3 cells. Int J Rad Oncol Biol Phys 2000; 48:325.

39. Teicher BA, Depuis NP, Kusumoto T, et al. Anti-angiogenic agents can increase tumor oxygenation and response to radiation therapy. Radiat Oncol Invest 1995; 2:269.

40. Kishi K, Petersen C, Hunter N, et al. Preferential enhancement of tumor radioresponse by a cyclooxygenase-2 inhibitor. Cancer Res 2000; 60:1326.

41. Altorki NK, Keresztes RS, Port JL, et al. Celecoxib, a selective cyclo-oxygenase-2 inhibitor, enhances the response to preoperative paclitaxel and carboplatin in early-stage non-small-cell lung cancer. J Clin Oncol 2003;21:2631.

42. Johnson DH, Fehrenbacher L, Novotny WF, et al. Randomized phase II trial comparing bevacizumab plus carboplatin and paclitaxel with carboplatin and paclitaxel alone in previously untreated locally advanced or metastatic non-small-cell lung cancer. J Clin Oncol 2004; 22:2184.

43. Keiko S, Komaki R, Wenjuan W, et al. Targeted therapy against VEGF and EGF signaling with ZD6474 enhances the therapeutic efficacy of irradiation in an orthotopic mouse model of human non-small cell lung cancer. Proceedings of the 46th Annual Meeting of American Society of Therapeutic Radiology and Oncology, October 3–7, 2004, abstract 35.

44. Gridelli C, Perrone F, Monfardini S. Lung cancer in the elderly. Eur J Cancer 1997; 33:2313.

45. Havlik RJ, Yancik R, Long S, Ries L, Edwards B. The National Cancer Institute on Aging and the National Cancer Institute SEER. Collaborative study on comorbidity and early diagnosis of cancer in the elderly. Cancer 1994; 74 (suppl 7):2101.

46. Janssen-Heijnen MLG, Schipper RM, Razenberg PPA, Crommelin MA, Coebergh JW. Prevalence of co-morbidity in lung cancer patients and its relationship with treatment: a population-based study. Lung Cancer 1998; 21:105.

47. Zimmermann FB, Molls M, Jeremic B. Treatment of locally advanced and metastatic non-small cell lung cancer in the elderly. Hematol Oncol Clin North Am 2004; 18:203.

48. Atagi S, Kawahara M, Ogawara M, et al. Phase II trial of daily low-dose carboplatin and thoracic radiotherapy in elderly patients with locally advanced non-small cell lung cancer. Jpn J Clin Oncol 2000; 30:59.

49. Nakano K, Yamamoto M, Iwamoto H, Hiramoto T. Daily low-dose cisplatin plus concurrent high-dose thoracic radiotherapy in elderly patients with locally advanced unresectable non-small-cell lung cancer. Gan To Kagaku Ryoho 2003; 30:1283.

50. D'Angelillo RM, Trodella L, Ramella S, et al. Neoadjuvant chemoradiotherapy followed by surgery in elderly patients with locally advanced non-small cell lung cancer: analysis of feasibility, toxicity and factors predicting surgical resection and survival. Proc Am Soc Clin Oncol 2004; 23:654.

51. Movsas B, Scott C, Sause W, et al. The benefit of treatment intensification is age and histology-dependent in patients with locally advanced non-small cell lung cancer (NSCLC): a quality-adjusted survival analysis of radiation therapy oncology group (RTOG) chemoradiation studies. Int J Radiat Oncol Biol Phys 1999; 45:1143.

52. Werner-Wasik M, Scott C, Cox JD, et al. Recursive partitioning analysis of 1999 Radiation Therapy Oncology Group (RTOG) patients with locally-advanced non-small-cell lung cancer (LA-NSCLC): identification of five groups with different survival. Int J Radiat Oncol Biol Phys 2000; 48:1475.

53. Langer C, Scott C, Byhardt R, et al. Effect of advanced age on outcome in Radiation Therapy Oncology Group studies of locally advanced NSCLC. Lung Cancer 2000; 29 (suppl 1):119.

54. Langer CJ, Hsu C, Curran WJ, et al. Elderly patients with locally advanced non-small cell lung cancer benefit from combined modality therapy:secondary analysis of Radiation Therapy Oncology Group (RTOG) 94-10. Proc Am Soc Clin Oncol 2002; 21:299a.

55. Schild SE, Stella PJ, Geyer SM, et al; North Central Cancer Treatment Group. The outcome of combined-modality therapy for stage III non-small-cell lung cancer in the elderly. J Clin Oncol 2003; 21:3201.

56. Perrone F, Gallo C, Gridelli C. Re: Cisplatin-based therapy for elderly patients with advanced non-small cell lung cancer:implications of Eastern Cooperative Oncology Group 5592, a randomized trial. J Natl Cancer Inst 2002; 94:1029.

Integration of Biological Therapies in Locally Advanced Non-Small-Cell Lung Cancer

21

Thomas E. Stinchcombe and Mark A. Socinski

Contents

21.1 Introduction

Lung cancer remains a leading cause of cancer death throughout the world, and it is estimated that 1.2 million new cases will be diagnosed worldwide each year [1]. Within the USA, lung cancer is the leading cause of cancer deaths in both men and women [2]. It is estimated that in 2005 in the USA that there will be approximately 174,000 new diagnosis of lung cancer with an estimate 160,000 deaths resulting from this disease [2]. Non-small-cell lung cancer (NSCLC) accounts for approximately 80–85% of all cases of lung cancer, and it is estimated that 35% of patients will present with stage IIIA or stage IIIB disease [3]. There is significant heterogeneity in this patient population, and the treatment strategies employed include surgical resection, surgical resection and adjuvant chemotherapy, preoperative chemotherapy, preoperative chemotherapy and radiation therapy, or chemoradiotherapy as the primary treatment. The role of surgical resection in stage III disease, the role of adjuvant chemotherapy, and the role of adjuvant radiotherapy are beyond the scope of this chapter. A significant percentage of patients will be technically unresectable or have significant cardiopulmonary co-

morbidities that will make the risks associated with surgery prohibitive. For patients who have a good functional status and who are appropriate candidates, the combination of chemotherapy and radiation therapy has become a standard of care [4]. There are several different treatment paradigms that are used to treat this group of patients. Most of these treatment paradigms, often referred to as combined modality therapy (CMT) or definitive chemoradiotherapy, involve systemic-dose chemotherapy to reduce the chances of developing distant disease and to assist in the control of local disease, and concurrent chemoradiotherapy to improve the chances of obtaining local control. Three commonly used treatment paradigms are: the use of systemic-dose chemotherapy with concurrent thoracic radiation therapy (TRT), the use of systemic-dose chemotherapy alone or induction chemotherapy followed by concurrent chemoradiotherapy, and the use concurrent chemoradiotherapy followed by systemic chemotherapy or "consolidation" chemotherapy.

The use of induction chemotherapy in stage III disease has been developed through a series of clinical trials that compared treatment with induction chemotherapy followed by TRT to TRT alone, which revealed an improved median survival and a higher rate of long-term survival [5–8]. The use of concurrent chemoradiotherapy to improve local control has been developed through trials that have revealed an improvement in local control with concurrent chemoradiotherapy over TRT [9–11]. These trials have used low-dose chemotherapy on a weekly or daily basis to acts as a radiation sensitizer to improve the efficacy of the TRT.

The integration and timing of TRT with systemic-dose chemotherapy has been explored in several phase III trials that compared the practice of sequential radiotherapy, where the radiation therapy is performed after the completion of the systemic-dose chemotherapy, to the concurrent administration of systemic-dose chemotherapy with TRT. In general these trials have indicated an improvement in the median survival and long-term survival to the approach on concurrent chemoradiotherapy [12–14]. A fourth, randomized, controlled trial revealed a trend toward improved survival; how-

Table 21.1. Selected biologic agents being studied in the treatment of non-small-cell lung cancer (NSCLC)

Agent	Target	Mechanism	Clinical setting	Phase trial
Gefitinib	EGFR	Oral TKI	Advanced	III
			Second-line therapy	III
Erlotinib	EGFR	Oral TKI	Advanced	III
			Second-line therapy	III
Cetuximab	EGFR	Monoclonal Ab	Advanced	II
			Second-line therapy	II
ABX-EGF	EGFR	Monoclonal Ab	Advanced	II
EMD 72000	EGFR	Monoclonal Ab	Advanced	I
Bevacizumab	Angiogenesis	Monoclonal Ab	Advanced	III
Thalomide	Angiogenesis	Antiangiogenesis	Advanced	II
Celecoxib	COX-2	COX-2 inhibitor	Locally advanced	II
Velcade	Proteasome	Proteasome inhibitor	Advanced	II
Bexarotene	Retinoic acid receptor	Differentiation	Advanced	III

Ab Antibody, *COX-2* cyclooxygenase inhibitor-2, *EGFR* epidermal growth factor, *TKI* tyrosine kinase inhibitor

Table 21.2. Treatment paradigms and issues in treatment of stage III NSCLC

Issue	Options	Goal of therapy
Chemotherapy dose	Low dose (radiosensitizing)	Local control
	High dose (cytotoxic)	Systemic and local control
Chemotherapy control schedule	Cyclic	Systemic and local
	Weekly	Local control
	Daily	Local control
Sequence with radiation	Sequential (Chemo → TRT)	Local and systemic
	Concurrent (Chemo/TRT)	Local and systemic
	Combinations: (Chemo/TRT → Chemo)	Local and systemic
	(Chemo → Chemo/TRT)	Local and systemic
Radiation dose and schedule	Daily vs. ≥ Twice daily	Local Control
	Dose (60 Gy vs. >60 Gy)	Local Control

Chemo Chemotherapy, *TRT* thoracic radiation therapy

ever, the trend did not reach statistically significance [15].

A recent cooperative group phase II trial evaluated the approach of combining systemic-dose chemotherapy with concurrent TRT as the initial treatment, and then following that treatment with further systemic chemotherapy, or "consolidation" therapy [16]. This phase II trial revealed a very promising median survival of 26 months with the additional systemic therapy; however, these results will have to be confirmed in the phase III setting prior to considering consolidation chemotherapy as a part of standard therapy.

Traditional cytotoxic chemotherapy agents have targeted DNA metabolism and synthesis as well as cell mitosis. Recently, several agents have been developed that attack malignant cells in different methods than traditional chemotherapy agents. These agents often take advantage of recent advances in molecular biology to target a specific target within the malignant cell or process that is responsible for cell proliferation, development or metastasis, or growth of the blood vessels that are necessary for the continued growth of the tumor. These agents have been studied largely in the advanced stage setting or in the setting of progression after standard chemotherapy in phase I, phase II, and phase III trials (Table 21.1). Many of these agents have demonstrated activity and a tolerable toxicity profile in advanced disease; however, the integration of these new agents into current treatment paradigms for stage III disease is currently being explored in phase I and phase II studies. These new agents have several potential roles in the treatment of stage III disease (Table 21.2). One potential role would be to improve the initial systemic therapy for stage III disease or to be used as a consolidation or maintenance therapy to reduce the chances of late relapse. These agents could also be incorporated into the radiotherapy portion of treatment paradigms to enhance the effectiveness of radiotherapy and to improve the rate of local control. Obviously, some agents may have both a systemic and a locoregional effect.

21.2 Oral Tyrosine Kinase Inhibitors as Systemic Therapy

Recently, a new class of biological agents has been developed in the treatment of NSCLC targeting the tyrosine kinase portion of the extracellular growth factor receptor (EGFR), also known as HER-1. These agents are administered orally and are often referred to as oral tyrosine kinase inhibitors (TKI). This class of biological agents targets malignant cells by binding to the adenosine triphosphate (ATP) pocket intracellular domain of EGFR [17]. This reduces the autophosphorylation and signal activation of this pathway and inhibits epidermal-growth-factor-dependent cell proliferation, reduces angiogenic signals, and blocks cell cycle progression [18]. There are currently two agents in this class of drugs that are available for use outside a clinical trial, erlotinib (Tarceva) and gefitinib (Iressa). These two agents have been evaluated in phase II and phase III trials in the advanced first-line setting with chemotherapy and in the treatment of progression following first-line chemotherapy (Table 21.3).

Gefitinib was evaluated in two randomized phase II trials, Iressa Dose Evaluation in Advanced Lung Cancer (IDEAL)-1 and IDEAL-2, which revealed a response rate of 10% and 19%, respectively, in patients with advanced disease who had been previously treated with chemotherapy [19–21]. The treatment was tolerated and at 250 mg daily doses; only 2% and 1% of patients on IDEAL-1 and IDEAL-2, respectively, had to discontinue the drug because of adverse events. These trials also revealed an improvement in patients' symptoms [21, 22]. Based on these trials demonstrating activity as a single agent and an acceptable toxicity profile, the combination of gefitinib with standard chemotherapy was evaluated in two randomized phase III studies, INTACT-1 and INTACT-2. These trials compared standard platinum-based chemotherapy and gefitinib to the same chemotherapy alone [23, 24[. Unfortunately, neither of these trials revealed an improvement in response, time to progression, and overall survival between the two arms.

Recently the preliminary results have been released of a randomized phase III trial, the Iressa Survival Evaluation in Lung Cancer (ISEL) trial, which compared gefitinib to best supportive care in advanced NSCLC after progression on standard chemotherapy. This trial revealed a response rate of approximately 9%; however, the treatment with gefitinib did not result in statistically significant differences in median survival and 1-year survival [25]. This trial has raised some concerns about the efficacy of gefitinib at the dose evaluated in this clinical setting.

Another oral TKI, erlotinib, has been evaluated in a phase II trial in patients with advanced disease who had progressed on standard chemotherapy, which revealed a response rate of approximately 12% and a median survival of 8.4 months. No National Cancer Institute (NCI) Common Toxicity Criteria (CTC) grade 4 events were experienced on this trial [26]. A recent phase III trial, BR.21, compared erlotinib to best supportive care in patients who had progressed on at least one line of chemotherapy, and found an improved median survival and 1-year survival with treatment on the erlotinib arm [27]. The single-agent activity of erlotinib led to the development of two randomized phase III trials, the Tarceva Assessed in Lung Cancer trial, which compared erlotinib with gemcitabine and cisplatin to gemcitabine and cisplatin and the Tarceva Response trial, which compared paclitaxel and carboplatin with erlotinib to carboplatin and paclitaxel [28, 29]. These trials are frequently known as the TALENT and TRIBUTE trials, respectively. Similar to the INTACT-1 and INTACT-2 trials, the addition of erlotinib to standard chemotherapy had little effect on median survival and time to progression in either trial.

Table 21.3. Select trials of oral TKIs

Trial	Comparison	Result
Second-line setting:		
BR 21	Erlotinib vs. BSC	Survival advantage to erlotinib
ISEL	Gefitinib vs. BSC	No survival advantage to gefitinib
First-line setting:		
TALENT	Chemotherapy vs. Chemo + Erlotinib	No survival advantage
TRIBUTE	Chemotherapy vs. Chemo + Erlotinib	No survival advantage
INTACT-1	Chemotherapy vs. Chemo + Gefitinib	No survival advantage
INTACT-2	Chemotherapy vs. Chemo + Gefitinib	No survival advantage

BSC Best supportive care

21.3 Chemotherapy in Combination and TKI Therapy

The results of the INTACT1, INTACT2, TALENT, and TRIBUTE trials [23, 24, 28, 29] have tempered enthusiasm for the combination of chemotherapy and oral TKIs, and it is unlikely that erlotinib and gefitinib will have a significant role in combination with chemotherapy in the systemic treatment of stage III NSCLC in an unselected population. However, on reviewing the accumulating data from phase II and phase III trials, it appears that certain subgroups are more likely to respond to oral TKIs. The most common clinical and pathological factors that are associated with response to this class of drugs are adenocarcinoma histology, nonsmoking history, Asian ethnicity, and female sex [30–33]. Recently, several research groups have identified genetic mutations in the ATP-binding region of the intracellular domain that are associated with response [31–33]. These mutations occur at a higher frequency in groups with the clinical and pathologic factors associated with response. This better understanding of the subgroups of patients who are most likely to respond to this type of therapy may allow for the development of clinical trials with an enhanced patient population that will have a greater potential of benefiting from TKI therapy. For instance, a subgroup analysis of the TRIBUTE trial has revealed that patients who were never smokers who and were treated with the combination of carboplatin/paclitaxel and erlotinib had a significantly longer median survival than patients treated with carboplatin/paclitaxel alone (23 months versus 10 months, hazard ratio 0.49, 95% confidence interval, CI = 0.28–0.85) [34]. These results are provocative and should be thought of as hypothesis generating about a potential role for simultaneous treatment with the combination of chemotherapy and TKI therapy in select groups of patients with stage III or stage IV disease.

The INTACT-1, INTACT-2, TRIBUTE, and TALENT trials all explored the simultaneous administration of chemotherapy and TKI therapy. It is possible that the negative results seen in these trials were due to the fact that the chemotherapy and oral TKI therapy were targeting the same susceptible population of malignant cells. The question that has been raised is whether the sequential administration of these therapies may result in better efficacy. Interestingly, the INTACT-2 trial revealed a trend toward improved survival in a subgroup of patients with adenocarcinoma who received ≥90 days chemotherapy and gefitinib 250 mg daily [24]. A survival analysis performed on patients from the TRIBUTE trial 6 months after completing therapy found a statistically significant ($p = 0.007$) improvement in survival for the patients receiving erlotinib [29]. This finding would suggest a potential benefit to continued therapy of erlotinib or gefitinib in a subset of patients with stage IV disease.

21.4   Clinical Trials with Oral TKIs for Stage III NSCLC

21.4.1   Maintenance Therapy

There has been increasing interest in incorporating the oral TKIs into stage III therapies based on data from trials performed in patients with advanced NSCLC and in patients who have progressed after one line of chemotherapy. These agents may potentially be used as additional systemic treatment in the form of maintenance therapy once definitive therapy has been completed.

Two cooperative group trials have explored the incorporation of gefitinib in CMT. The Southwest Oncology Group (SWOG) initiated a phase III trial, SWOG 0023 (Fig. 21.1), which evaluated the potential role of gefitinib maintenance therapy. All patients received systemic-dose cisplatin and etoposide with concurrent TRT. Patients with stable or responding disease received consolidation therapy with docetaxel every 21 days for three cycles, and then 1–4 weeks after completion of consolidation therapy patients were randomized to either maintenance therapy with gefitinib or observation. The accrual goal for this study was estimated to be 840 patients. However, on April 15, 2005, the Data and Safety Monitoring Committee (DSMC) of SWOG performed an interim analysis, which revealed that "the hypothesis of an improvement in survival with ZD1839 (gefitinib) was untenable" (personal communication). As a result of this finding, the DSMC recommended closure of this trial. The preliminary analysis of this trial was presented at the American Society of Clinical Oncology (ASCO) meeting in 2005 (K. Kelly, oral presentation of abstract 7058, available at *www.asco.org* [35]). This analysis revealed that 620 patients had been enrolled and 575 were determined to be eligible. The median survival for all patients enrolled on the trial was 19 months. If the median survival is determined from the time of randomization to gefitinib or placebo (i.e. patients who had progressive disease during chemoradiotherapy and consolidation therapy are excluded) the median survival on the gefitinib arm was 19 months, in comparison to the median survival on the placebo arm of 29 months ($p = 0.09$). At this time the reasons for a lack of benefit of gefitinib and the trend toward a lower median survival are unknown and are currently being evaluated. The primary cause of death was disease progression, and there was no detectable difference between the causes of death between the two arms.

The Cancer and Leukemia Group B (CALGB) had been performing a phase II trial, CALGB 30106, exploring the role of gefitinib in poor-performance-status patient with concurrent TRT, the role of gefitinib in addition to chemoradiotherapy and as maintenance therapy (Fig. 21.1). Following the announcement of the closure of the SWOG 0023 trial, the CALGB Respiratory Committee reviewed the safety and efficacy data of their trial and decided to permanently close this trial to new patient accrual (personal communication). The data regarding the toxicity and efficacy of gefitinib on this trial is currently not available.

Another clinical trial that was exploring the potential role of gefitinib in the chemoradiotherapy portion of CMT as well as maintenance gefitinib is a single-institution phase II trial at the Lineberger Comprehensive Cancer Center at the University of North Carolina. The treatment comprises two cycles of induction chemotherapy with systemic doses of carboplatin, paclitaxel, and irinotecan every 21 days followed by weekly carboplatin

1. SWOG-0023: Phase III Trial in patients with unresectable stage IIIA/B NSCLC.

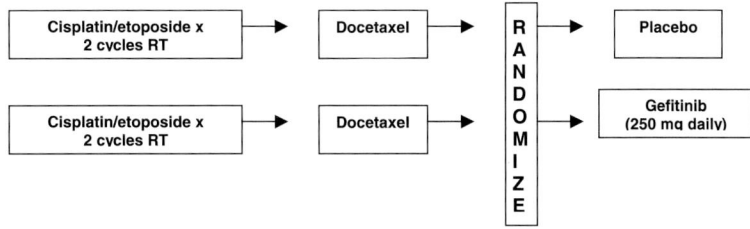

2. CALGB 30106: A phase II trial in patients with unresectable stage IIIA/B NSCLC.

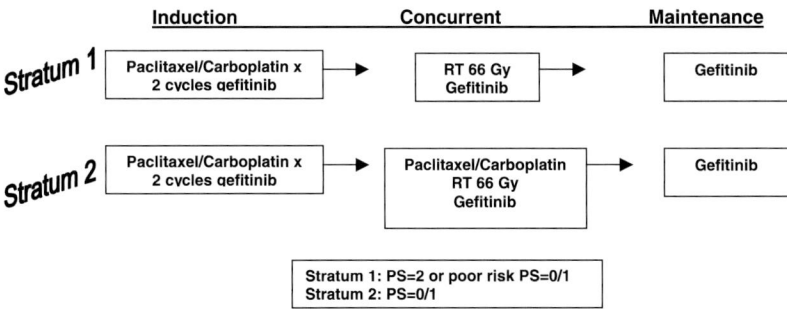

3. LCCC 0215: A phase II trial in patients with unresectable stage IIIA/B NSCLC.

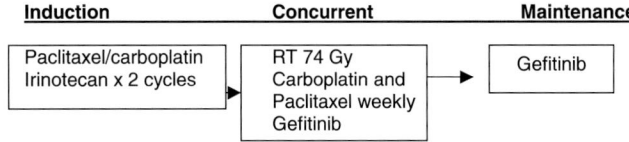

Fig. 21.1. Stage III trials with oral tyrosine kinase inhibitors. *RT* Radiotherapy, *PS* performance status, *SWOG* Southwest Oncol- ogy Group, *CALGB* Cancer and Leukemia Group B, *LCCC* Lineberger Comprehensive Cancer Center

and paclitaxel during TRT in combination with gefitinib 250 mg daily, starting with TRT [36]. The initial treatment plan was for patients to receive 2 years of maintenance gefitinib; however, after the data and the subsequent decisions of the CALGB and SWOG cooperative groups, the decision by the principal investigators was to discontinue the maintenance gefitinib portion of the trial. Patients will continue to receive gefitinib during the chemoradiotherapy portion of the trial.

The reasons for the lack of benefit and an evaluation of the potential toxicity of gefitinib treatment will be explored further when more of the data from these trials are available. However, based on the data currently available it is highly unlikely that gefitinib will have a significant role as maintenance therapy in stage III disease.

21.5 Oral TKI Therapy with Chemoradiotherapy

The potential role of oral TKI therapy in the concurrent chemoradiotherapy portion of stage III disease is currently being explored. Preclinical data indicate potential additive or synergistic interactions between radiation and oral TKIs [37–39]. Clinical trials investigating the tolerability and potential efficacy of combining oral TKIs with TRT in lung cancer have been initiated. A phase I trial explored the toxicity of combining gefitinib at 250 mg daily with weekly carboplatin (area under the plasma concentration–time curve, AUC 2 using the Calvert equation [40]) and escalating doses of weekly paclitaxel starting at a dose of 25 mg/m^2 [41]. The gefitinib was discontinued after completion of TRT. The treatment was well tolerated and dose escalation of the paclitaxel was completed up to 45 mg/m^2 without any dose-limiting toxicities (DLT). Preliminary efficacy data with limited follow-up revealed a positron emission test (PET) response rate of 55% ($n=11$), and a computed tomography (CT) compete response rate of 27% ($n=5$) and partial response rate of 64% ($n=9$). A two-arm phase I trial using the alternating, or "ping pong," trial design exploring erlotinib in combination with TRT is currently ongoing [42]. On arm A of this study, erlotinib is given daily for 7 weeks in combination with the SWOG treatment strategy of cisplatin (50 mg/m^2) on days 1 and 8, etoposide 50 mg/m^2 daily on days 1–5 and 29–33, and TRT to 66 Gy. Arm B of this study consist of the CALGB treatment strategy of induction chemotherapy with carboplatin (AUC 6) and paclitaxel (200 mg/m^2) every 21 days for two cycles followed by weekly carboplatin (AUC 2), paclitaxel (50 mg/m^2), and erlotinib daily for 7 weeks with TRT to 66 Gy. In both arms the dose of erlotinib was initiated at 50 mg daily and was escalated to 150 mg daily in 50-mg increments. This study is currently ongoing and will determine the optimal dose of erlotinib that can be used with these two commonly used treatment strategies.

A multi-institutional phase I/II study exploring the role of preoperative treatment with gefitinib 250 mg daily, cisplatin/etoposide (doses to be determined), and TRT to 45 Gy in patients with stage IIIA disease will soon be opening [39]. Patients will undergo surgical resection, and will then receive gefitinib postoperatively. The phase I portion of this trial will consist of an evaluation of the toxicity of the initial six patients after 90 days follow-up, and if there are no unexpected toxicities an additional 20 patients will be enrolled. Tissue samples will be taken at the time of diagnosis as well as at the time of surgical resection, and a molecular analysis with clinical outcome evaluation will be performed to test for any molecular correlation with response or clinical outcome.

21.6   EGFR Antibody Therapy in Stage III Disease

There are currently several monoclonal antibodies, cetuximab, EMD 72000 [43, 44], and ABX-EGF [45], that target EGFR that are being explored in clinical trials. Of these monoclonal antibodies cetuximab is currently the one that is most developed in the treatment of NSCLC. Cetuximab is a chimeric human-mouse monoclonal antibody that binds to the extracellular domain of EGFR, and blocks ligand binding. The monoclonal antibody binding inhibits the ligand induced-induced tyrosine-kinase-dependent phosphorylation and downstream signaling of the EGFR pathway. In the USA this agent is currently approved for use in the treatment of metastatic colorectal cancer. In the setting of metastatic colorectal cancer, cetuximab has demonstrated activity

as a single agent, but the response rate of combination chemotherapy and cetuximab was higher than that of cetuximab as single agent [46]. Preclinical data indicates that the combination of cetuximab and chemotherapy and radiation therapy has additive effects on tumor growth in EGFR-expressing NSCLC cell lines [47].

Cetuximab is currently being explored in phase II trials in combination with chemotherapy as initial therapy for advanced NSCLC as well as in the second-line setting. The single-agent activity of cetuximab was evaluated in a phase II study in patients who had received one or more prior treatments and who had received platinum-based therapy. The response rate was 3.3%, and 28% of patients had stable disease [48]. The median survival and 1-year survival rate were 8.1 months and 43%, respectively. This agent has successfully been combined with docetaxel in the second-line setting in another phase II study. Patients were required to have progressed on or within 3 months of completing platinum-based therapy in order to be eligible for enrollment. This phase II study found a response rate to the combination cetuximab and docetaxel of 28% [49].

Cetuximab has also been evaluated in combination with chemotherapy in the first-line setting in several phase II trials. Cetuximab given in combination with carboplatin (AUC 6) and paclitaxel (225 mg/m^2) demonstrated an impressive median survival of 15.7 months and a median time to disease progression of 4.5 months [35]. Another phase II trial in which cetuximab and carboplatin (AUC 5) and gemcitabine (1000 mg/m^2) were given in combination on days 1 and 8 found a partial response rate of 29%, and 60% of patients had stable disease [50]. A recent preliminary analysis of a randomized phase II trial that compared cisplatin (80 mg/m^2) on day 1, and vinorelbine 25 mg/m^2 on days 1 and 8 to the same chemotherapy with cetuximab found that the addition of cetuximab appeared to increase the efficacy of cisplatin/vinorelbine, particularly in patients younger than 60 years, patients with adenocarcinomas, and those with a normal lactate dehydrogenase level [51].

It appears that cetuximab can be combined with many of the commonly used doublet chemotherapy combinations, and is associated with the most commonly reported additional toxicities such as acne-like rash and hypersensitivity reactions. A phase III trial comparing a standard chemotherapy regimen to the same chemotherapy treatment with the addition of cetuximab would be required to definitively determine any increase in efficacy related to this agent. The single-agent activity and nonoverlapping toxicity profiles of cetuximab make it an attractive agent to be integrated into systemic therapy for stage III disease.

Cetuximab may also have a potential role in improving the local therapy for stage III disease. The combination of cetuximab and radiation therapy appears to be synergistic in preclinical models. Given the encouraging preclinical data, a phase III trial in patients with locally advanced squamous cell cancer of the head and neck compared the combination of cetuximab and radiation therapy to radiation therapy alone. This trial found that the combination of cetuximab and radiation therapy had a superior median survival (54 months vs. 28 months $p = 0.02$), with a relatively minimal increase in toxicity [52]. This synergy between radiation therapy and cetuximab has lead to interest in using this agent in the chemoradiotherapy portion of CMT in NSCLC. This is currently being explored in a phase II RTOG trial (0324) for unresectable stage IIIA or stage IIIB patients (www.ClinicalTrials.gov). Patients on this protocol will be treated with weekly cetuximab, carboplatin, and paclitaxel concurrent with TRT. Patients will then receive consolidation chemotherapy with two cycles of carboplatin and paclitaxel as well as weekly cetuximab for 9 weeks. This study is designed to determine the safety and feasibility of cetuximab in combination with weekly carboplatin and paclitaxel and radiotherapy.

21.7 Antiangiogenesis Therapy

Vascular endothelial growth factor (VEGF) is a glycoprotein that is considered essential for the normal development of vasculogenesis and angiogenesis [53]. Continued development of new tumor vasculature mediated through VEGF is required to maintain tumor growth. Therefore, inhibition of VEGF is promising target for antineoplastic therapy. Preclinical data indicates that an antibody to VEGF alone or in combination with chemotherapy can successfully inhibit tumor growth [54, 55]. Bevacizumab (Avastin) is a recombinant monoclonal antibody raised against VEGF that inhibits tumor growth by reducing angiogenesis. In a phase I study, bevacizumab was combined with cytotoxic chemotherapy and no exacerbation of expected chemotherapy toxicities were detected [56].

Based on the preclinical data and the favorable toxicity profile seen in the phase I study, the activity and toxicity of the combination of bevacizumab and carboplatin and paclitaxel chemotherapy for NSCLC was explored in a phase II trial [57]. This trial was a randomized phase II trial with three separate treatment arms. The control arm was given carboplatin and paclitaxel, and the two experimental arms were given carboplatin and paclitaxel with either low-dose bevacizumab (7.5 mg/kg every 3 weeks) or a higher dose of bevacizumab (15 mg/kg every 3 weeks). The patients on the higher-dose bevacizumab arm had a higher response rate than those in the control arm (31.5% vs. 18.8%, respectively), as well as a longer median time to progression (7.4 months vs. 4.2 months, respectively) and median survival time (17.7 months vs. 14.9 months, respectively). The main additional toxicity seen in this

trial was an increased risk of bleeding. The adverse bleeding events consisted of two distinct clinical events: mucocutaneous bleeding and episodes of major hemoptysis. There were six episodes of life-threatening pulmonary hemorrhage in patients receiving bevacizumab. These episodes were more frequently associated with squamous histology (4 out of 13 patients) than in adenocarcinomas (2 out of 54 patients), and in patients with centrally located tumors in close proximity to major blood vessels. In five of the six cases patients had, either at baseline or developed during the study period, cavitations or necrosis of tumors during bevacizumab therapy. These events occurred early (≤ 60 days) as well as late in the treatment course (≥ 180 days). Given the small number of episodes observed, and the tendency of squamous cell lung cancers to have a central location and to cavitate, it is difficult to determine the clinical factor that is most predictive for this complication.

Given the promising results seen in this phase II trial, a phase III trial, ECOG 4599, comparing the combination of carboplatin and paclitaxel to carboplatin, paclitaxel, and bevacizumab (15 mg/kg every 3 weeks) in patients with advanced NSCLC was initiated. The eligibility criteria were restricted to patients with adenocarcinoma, and no evidence of central nervous metastases. Patients could not be on any anticoagulation or have any history of coagulopathy or thrombosis. This study revealed an improvement in response (10% vs. 27% $p < 0.0001$), median survival time (10.2 months vs. 12.5 months $p = 0.0075$) [58]. The toxicity profile was similar between the bevacizumab arm and the standard arm. There were 11 treatment-related deaths, 2 on the chemotherapy arm and 9 on the chemotherapy and bevacizumab arm, but the difference was not statistically significant. Of the nine deaths on the bevacizumab arm, five were due to hemoptysis.

In addition to this promising phase III data, a recent phase II trial explored the combination of bevacizumab and erlotinib in patients who had progressed after one or more treatments with platinum-based chemotherapy [59]. Patients were required to have a nonsquamous histology, no evidence of central nervous system metastases, no significant bleeding history, or history of coagulopathy or thrombosis. The response rate for this combination was 20% (CI = 7.6–32.4%), and the median survival and 1-year survival were 12.6 months and 54%, respectively, which is impressive in the second-line setting. The main toxicities seen in this trial were rash and diarrhea. The incidence of epistaxis in this study was 6%. Both of these studies excluded patients with squamous histology; therefore, the toxicity and efficacy of bevacizumab in the squamous histology subtype cannot be determined.

These exciting results in the advanced setting are promising; bevacizumab may be beneficial as a systemic treatment for stage III disease. The integration of bevacizumab into therapy may be complicated by concerns about pulmonary hemorrhage related to squamous cell histology or central lesions. The restriction of bevacizumab to patients with adenocarcinoma would significantly reduce the number of patients who could potentially benefit from this therapy. Thus, a better understanding of the etiology of pulmonary hemorrhage and the clinical risk factors associated with increased risk of hemoptysis will be critical in the future. One potential method of addressing this issue may be to initiate treatment with TRT, which is the primary and most effective therapy for pulmonary hemorrhage, prior to or concurrent with bevacizumab therapy. This approach most likely would have to be investigated in the setting of a clinical trial.

Preclinical data indicates that the antiangiogenesis therapy may increase the cytotoxicity of radiation therapy [60, 61], and a phase I trial of bevacizumab and radiation in rectal cancer is currently ongoing [62]. There is potential to integrate bevacizumab therapy with TRT, which may led to reduced risks of pulmonary hemorrhage and perhaps an improvement in the efficacy of TRT. This treatment approach would have to be explored in the setting of a clinical trial designed to assess for any potential increase in toxicity.

21.8   Conclusion

The current biological agents available have demonstrated significant efficacy and an acceptable toxicity profile in the metastatic setting as well as in the second-line setting. It is unlikely that oral TKI therapy will be instigated as maintenance therapy given the recent results of two cooperative group trials. Preclinical data have indicated that oral TKI therapy also appears to have the potential to act as a radiation sensitizer, and may have a role in the chemoradiotherapy portion of stage III treatment. The use of monoclonal antibodies to target the EGFR is also an area of active interest. The fact that preliminary evidence indicates that these monoclonal antibodies can be combined with chemotherapy without a significant increase in toxicity is promising and these agents may have a role in treatment of systemic disease. The synergy between radiation therapy and monoclonal antibodies directed at EGFR may improve local-regional therapy in stage III disease. The activity of bevacizumab in combination with standard chemotherapy and in the second-line setting in a select group of patients is also quite promising. The integration of these agents into current treatment paradigms for locally advanced disease is currently being explored in many cooperative group and institutional phase II trials, and the results of these trials are eagerly awaited.

Key Points

- Several biological agents have demonstrated efficacy and an acceptable toxicity profile in non-small-cell lung cancer (NSCLC) either in the metastatic setting or as in the second-line setting.
- Preclinical data have shown that oral tyrosine kinase inhibitor therapy also appears to have the potential to act as a "radiation sensitizer" and may have a role in the chemoradiotherapy portion of stage III treatment.
- The activity of bevacizumab in combination with standard chemotherapy and in the second-line setting in a select group of patients is quite promising
- The integration of biological agents into the current treatment for locally advanced NSCLC is currently being explored in many cooperative group and institutional phase II trials, and the results of these trials are eagerly awaited.

References

1. Parkin DM. Global cancer statistics in the year 2000. Lancet Oncol 2001; 2(9):533.
2. Jemal A, Murray T, et al. Cancer statistics, 2005. CA Cancer J Clin 2005; 55(1):10.
3. Jett JR. Current treatment of unresectable lung cancer. Mayo Clin Proc 1993; 68(6):603.
4. Pfister DG, Johnson DH, et al. American Society of Clinical Oncology treatment of unresectable non-small-cell lung cancer guideline: update 2003. J Clin Oncol 2004; 22(2):330.
5. Le Chevalier T, Arriagada R, et al. Radiotherapy alone versus combined chemotherapy and radiotherapy in non-resectable non-small cell lung cancer: first analysis of randomized trial in 353 patients. J Natl Cancer Inst 1991; 83: 417.
6. Le Chevalier T, Arriagada R, et al. Significant effect of adjuvant chemotherapy on survival in locally advanced non-small cell lung carcinoma. J Natl Cancer Inst 1992; 84:58.
7. Dillman R, Herndon J, et al. Improved survival in stage III non-small cell lung cancer: seven-year follow-up of Cancer and Leukemia Group B (CALGB) 8433 trial. J Natl Cancer Inst 1996; 88:1210.
8. Sause W, Kolesar P, et al. Final results of phase III trial in regionally advanced unresectable non-small cell lung cancer: Radiation Therapy Oncology Group, Eastern Cooperative Oncology Group, and Southwest Oncology Group. Chest 2000; 117(2):358.
9. Schaake-Koning C, van den Bogaert W, et al. Effects of concomitant cisplatin and radiotherapy on inoperable non-small cell lung cancer. N Engl J Med 1992; 326:524.
10. Jeremic B, Shibamoto Y, et al. Randomized trial of hyperfractionated radiation therapy with or without concurrent chemotherapy for stage III non-small cell lung cancer. J Clin Oncol 1995; 15:452.
11. Jeremic B, Shibamoto Y, et al. Hyperfractionated radiation therapy with or without concurrent low-dose daily carboplatin/etoposide for stage III non-small cell lung cancer: a randomized study. J Clin Oncol 1996; 14:1065.

12. Furuse K, for the West Japan Lung Cancer Group. Phase III study of concurrent versus sequential thoracic radiotherapy in combination with mitomycin, vindesine, and cisplatin in unresectable stage III non-small cell lung cancer. J Clin Oncol 1999; 17:2692.

13. Curran WJ, Scott C, et al. Phase III comparison of sequential vs concurrent chemoradiation for PTS with unresected stage III non-small cell lung cancer (NSCLC): initial report of Radiation Therapy Oncology Group (RTOG) 9410. Proc Am Soc Clin Oncol 2000; 19:484a.

14. Zatloukal P, Petruzelka L, et al. Concurrent versus sequential chemoradiotherapy with cisplatin and vinorelbine in locally advanced non-small cell lung cancer: a randomized study. Lung Cancer 2004; 46(1):87.

15. Pierre F, Maurice P, et al. A randomized phase III trial of sequential chemo-radiotherapy versus concurrent chemoradiotherapy in locally advanced non-small cell lung cancer (NSCLC) (GLOT-GFPC NPC 95-01 study). Proc Am Soc Clin Oncol 2001; 20:312.

16. Gandara DR, Chansky K, et al. Consolidation docetaxel after concurrent chemoradiotherapy in stage IIIB non-small-cell lung cancer: phase II Southwest Oncology Group Study S9504.
J Clin Oncol 2003; 21(10):2004.

17. Rowinsky EK. The erbB family: targets for therapeutic development against cancer and therapeutic strategies using monoclonal antibodies and tyrosine kinase inhibitors. Annu Rev Med 2004; 55:433.

18. Moyer JD, Barbacci EG, et al. Induction of apoptosis and cell cycle arrest by CP-358,774, an inhibitor of epidermal growth factor receptor tyrosine kinase. Cancer Res 1997; 57(21):4838.

19. Kris M, Natale R, et al. A phase II trial of ZD1839 ('Iressa') in advanced non-small cell lung cancer (NSCLC) patients who had failed platinum- and docetaxel-based regimens (IDEAL-2). Proc Am Soc Clin Oncol 2001; 21: 292a.

20. Fukuoka M, Yano S, et al. Multi-institutional randomized phase II trial of gefitinib for previously treated patients with advanced non-small-cell lung cancer. J Clin Oncol 2003; 21(12):2237.

21. Kris MG, Natale RB, et al. Efficacy of gefitinib, an inhibitor of the epidermal growth factor receptor tyrosine kinase, in symptomatic patients with non-small cell lung cancer: a randomized trial. JAMA 2003; 290(16):2149.

22. Douillard J-Y, Giaccone G, et al. Improvement in disease-related symptoms and quality of life in patients with advanced non-small cell lung cancer (NSCLC) treated with ZD1839 (Iressa) (IDEAL 1). Proc Am Soc Clin Oncol 2002; 21:299a.

23. Giaccone G, Herbst RS, et al. Gefitinib in combination with gemcitabine and cisplatin in advanced non-small-cell lung cancer: a phase III trial – INTACT 1. J Clin Oncol 2004; 22(5):777.

24. Herbst RS, Giaccone G, et al. Gefitinib in combination with paclitaxel and carboplatin in advanced non-small-cell lung cancer: a phase III trial INTACT 2. J Clin Oncol 2004; 22(5):785.

25. Thatcher N, Chang A, Purvish P, Pemberton K, Archer V. Results of A Phase III placebo controlled study (ISEL) of gefitinib (IRESSA) plus best supportive care (BSC) in patients with advanced non-small cell lung cancer (NSCLC) who had received 1 or 2 prior chemotherapy regimens. Proc Am Assoc Cancer Res 2005; 46:6.

26. Perez-Soler R, Chachona A, et al. A phase II trial of the epidermal growth factor receptor (EGFR) tyrosine kinase inhibitor OSI-774, following platinum-based chemotherapy in patients (pts) with advanced, EGFR-expressing, non-small cell lung cancer (NSCLC). Proc Am Soc Clin Oncol 2001; 20:310a.

27. Shepherd FA, Pereira J, Ciuleanu TE, et al. A randomized placebo-controlled trail of erlotinib in patients with advanced non-small cell lung cancer (NSCLC) following failure of 1st or 2nd line chemotherapy. A National Institute of Canada Clinical Trials (NCIC CTG) trial. Proc Am Soc Clin Oncol 2004; 40:7023a.

28. Gatzemeier U, Pluzanska A, Szczesna A, Kaukel E, Roubec J, Brennscheidt U, DeRosa F, Mueller B, Von Pawel J. Results of a phase III trial of erlotinib HCl (OSI-744) combined with cisplatin and gemcitabine (GC) chemotherapy in advanced non-small cell lung cancer (NSCLC). J Clin Oncol 2004; 22(14S):7010a.

29. Herbst RS, Prage D, et al. TRIBUTE – A phase III Trial of erlotinib (OSI-744) combined with carboplatin and paclitaxel chemotherapy in advanced non-small cell lung cancer. J Clin Oncol 2005; 23(14S):5892.

30. Kosaka T, Yatabe Y, et al. Mutations of the epidermal growth factor receptor gene in lung cancer: biological and clinical implications. Cancer Res 2004; 64(24):8919.

31. Lynch TJ, Bell DW, et al. Activating mutations in the epidermal growth factor receptor underlying responsiveness of non-small-cell lung cancer to gefitinib. N Engl J Med 2004; 350(21):2129.

32. Paez JG, Janne PA, et al. EGFR mutations in lung cancer: correlation with clinical response to gefitinib therapy. Science 2004; 304(5676):1497.

33. Pao W, Miller V, et al. EGF receptor gene mutations are common in lung cancers from "never smokers" and are associated with sensitivity of tumors to gefitinib and erlotinib. Proc Natl Acad Sci U S A 2004; 101(36):13306.

34. Miller V, Herbst A, Prager D, et al. Long survival of never smoking non-small cell lung cancer (NSCLC) patients treated with erlotinib HCl (OSI-774) and chemotherapy: Sub-group analysis of TRIBUTE. J Clin Oncol 2004; 22(14S):7061a.

35. Kelly K, Hanna N, Rosenberg A, Bunn PA, Needle MN. Multicenter Phase I/II study of cetuximab in combination with paclitaxel and carboplatin in untreated patients with stage IV non-small cell lung cancer. Pro Am Soc Clin Oncol 2003; 22:644a.

36. Morris DE, Halle JS, Stinchcombe TE, Rosenman JG, Mears A, Tynan M, Socinski MA. Induction chemotherapy using Carboplatin (C), Irintecan (I), and Paclitaxel (P) with pegfligrastim support followed by concurrent thoracic conformal radiation therapy (TCRT) with weekly CP and daily gefitinib. J Clin Oncol 2005; 23(16S):7311a.

37. Bianco C, Tortora G, et al. Enhancement of antitumor activity of ionizing radiation by combined treatment with the selective epidermal growth factor receptor-tyrosine kinase inhibitor ZD1839 (Iressa). Clin Cancer Res 2002; 8(10):3250.

38. Solomon B, Hagekyriakou J, et al. EGFR blockade with ZD1839 ("Iressa") potentiates the antitumor effects of single and multiple fractions of ionizing radiation in human A431 squamous cell carcinoma. Epidermal growth factor receptor. Int J Radiat Oncol Biol Phys 2003; 55(3):713.

39. Kim DW, Choy H. Potential role for epidermal growth factor receptor inhibitors in combined-modality therapy for non-small-cell lung cancer. Int J Radiat Oncol Biol Phys 2004; 59(2 Suppl):11.

40. Calvert A, Newell D, et al. Carboplatin dosage: Prospective evaluation of a simple formula based on renal function. J Clin Oncol 1989; 7:1748.

41. Rischin B, Burmeister P, Mitchell P, Boyer, M, Mcmanus, M, Walpole E, Feigen, M, Tin MM, Ball D. Phase I Trial of gefitinib (ZD1839) in combination with concurrent carboplatin, paclitaxel, and radiation therapy in patients with stage III non-small cell lung cancer. J Clin Oncol 2004; 14S:7077a.

42. Mauer A, Haraf D, Hoffman PC, Rudin CM, Szeto L, Vokes EE. A Phase I study of OSI-774 in combination with chemoradiation (CRT) for unresectable, locally advanced non-small cell lung cancer (NSCLC). Proc Am Soc Clin Oncol 2003; 22:2617a.

43. Kollmannsberger C, Schittenhelm M, et al. Epidermal growth factor receptor (EGFR) antibody EMD 72000 in combination with paclitaxel (P) in patients with EGFR-positive advanced non-small cell lung cancer (NSCLC): A phase I study. Proc Am Soc Clin Oncol 2004; 22:627 2520a.

44. Vanhoefer U, Tewes M, et al. Phase I study of the humanized antiepidermal growth factor receptor monoclonal antibody EMD72000 in patients with advanced solid tumors that express the epidermal growth factor receptor. J Clin Oncol 2004; 22(1):175.

45. Crawford J, Sandler AB, et al. ABX-EGF in combination with paclitaxel and carboplatin for advanced non-small cell lung cancer (NSCLC). J Clin Oncol 2004; 22(14S):7083a.

46. Cunningham D, Humblet Y, et al. Cetuximab monotherapy and cetuximab plus irinotecan in irinotecan-refractory metastatic colorectal cancer. N Engl J Med 2004; 351(4):337.

47. Raben D, Helfrich B, et al. The effects of cetuximab alone and in combination with radiation and/or chemotherapy in lung cancer. Clin Cancer Res 2005; 11(2 Pt 1):795.

48. Lilenbaum R, Bonomi P, et al. A phase II Trial of cetuximab as therapy for recurrent non-small cell lung cancer (NSCLC): Final Results. J Clin Oncol 2005; 23(16S):7036a.

49. Kim ES, Mauer AM, et al. A Phase II study of cetuximab, an epidermal growth factor receptor (EGFR) blocking antibody in combination with docetaxel in chemotherapy refractory/resistant patients with advanced non-small cell lung cancer: Final report. Proc Am Soc Clin Oncol 2003; 22:642a.

50. Robert F, Blumenschein K, Dicke T, et al. Phase Ib/IIa study of anti-epidermal growth factor receptor (EGFR) antibody, cetuximab, in combination with gemcitabine/carboplatin in patients with advanced non-small cell lung cancer. Proc Am Soc Clin Oncol 2003; 22:643a.

51. Rossell R, Daniel C, et al. Randomized phase II study of cetuximab in combination with cisplatin (C) and vinorelbine (V) vs CV alone in the first line treatment of patients with epidermal growth factor expressing advanced non-small cell lung cancer. J Clin Oncol 2004; 22(No 14S):7012a.

52. Bonner JA, Giralt J, Harai PM, Cohen R, Jones C, Sur RK, Rabin D, Azarnia N, Needle MN, Ang KK. Cetuximab prolongs survival in patients with locoregionally advanced squamous cell carcinoma of head and neck: A phase III study of high dose radiation therapy with and without cetuximab. J Clin Oncol 2004; 22(14S):5507a.

53. Ferrara N, Gerber HP, LeCouter J. The biology of VEGF and its receptors. Nat Med 2003; 9(6):669.

54. Kim KJ, Li B, et al. Inhibition of vascular endothelial growth factor-induced angiogenesis suppresses tumour growth in vivo. Nature 1993; 362(6423):841.

55. Borgstrom P, Gold DP, Hillan KJ, Ferrara N. Importance of VEGF for breast cancer angiogenesis in vivo: implications from intravital microscopy of combination treatments with an anti-VEGF neutralizing monoclonal antibody and doxorubicin. Anticancer Res 1999; 19(5B):4203.

56. Margolin K, Gordon MS, et al. Phase Ib trial of intravenous recombinant humanized monoclonal antibody to vascular endothelial growth factor in combination with chemotherapy in patients with advanced cancer: pharmacologic and long-term safety data. J Clin Oncol 2001; 19(3):851.

57. Johnson DH, Fehrenbacher L, et al. Randomized phase II trial comparing bevacizumab plus carboplatin and paclitaxel with carboplatin and paclitaxel alone in previously untreated locally advanced or metastatic non-small-cell lung cancer. J Clin Oncol 2004; 22(11):2184.

58. Sandler AB, Gray R, Brahmer J, Dowlati A, Schiller JH, Perry MC, Johnson DH Randomized Phase II/III Trial of paclitaxel (P) plus carboplatin (C) with or without bevacizumab in patients with advanced non-squamous cell lung cancer (NSCLC): An Eastern Cooperative Oncology Group (ECOG) Trial-E4599. J Clin Oncol 2005; 23(16S):4a.

59. Herbst RS, Johnson DH, et al. Phase I/II trial evaluating the anti-vascular endothelial growth factor monoclonal antibody bevacizumab in combination with the HER-1/epidermal growth factor receptor tyrosine kinase inhibitor erlotinib for patients with recurrent non-small-cell lung cancer. J Clin Oncol 2005; 23(11):2544.

60. Mauceri HJ, Hanna NN, et al. Combined effects of angiostatin and ionizing radiation in antitumour therapy. Nature 1998; 394(6690):287.

61. Lee CG, Heijn M, et al. Anti-vascular endothelial growth factor treatment augments tumor radiation response under normoxic or hypoxic conditions. Cancer Res 2000; 60(19):5565.

62. Willett CG, Boucher Y, et al. Direct evidence that the VEGF-specific antibody bevacizumab has antivascular effects in human rectal cancer. Nat Med 2004; 10(2):145.

Section V:
Management
of Advanced Non-Small-Cell Lung Cancer

Platinum-Based Chemotherapy for Advanced Non-Small-Cell Lung Cancer

22

Anne M. Traynor and Joan H. Schiller

Contents

22.1 Cisplatin-Based Chemotherapy Versus Best Supportive Care

Lung cancer clinical practice guidelines from the American Society of Clinic Oncology (ASCO) recommend that a two-drug chemotherapy doublet be given to pa-tients with stage IV non-small-cell lung cancer (NSCLC) and a good performance status in an effort to prolong survival [1]. Platinum-based regimens have formed the backbone of systemic treatment in metastatic NSCLC since the 1980s, with cisplatin demonstrating a single-agent response rate activity of 10–17% [2]. However, the impact on patient survival using platinum-based doublets in combination with older agents such as mitomycin and vindesine remained in doubt, as multiple trials comparing cisplatin-based chemotherapy with best supportive care (BSC) drew conflicting conclusions [3–10]. For example, a Canadian study of two different types of chemotherapy detected treatment response rates of 15–25% and a statistically significant prolongation in survival, compared to BSC (28.7 weeks versus 17 weeks), whereas a British trial found a response rate of 28% with cisplatin and vindesine, but failed to confirm a significant improvement in survival [3, 5]. Preliminary results from a multicenter trial of over 700 patients with advanced NSCLC compared outcomes with the use of cisplatin-based chemotherapy versus BSC [10]. A statistically significant survival advantage resulted from the use of chemotherapy (hazard ratio of death 0.77, $P = 0.0015$), with an improvement of 2 months in median survival, from 5.7 to 7.7 months.

Although conclusive prolongations in survival were not consistently seen with the use of chemotherapy in the advanced disease setting in the eight studies [3–10] compared to BSC, its use was frequently associated with symptom relief and improvements in quality of life [8, 9]. For example, investigators in the Big Lung Trial found that the use of cisplatin-based chemotherapy was associated with less grade 3 and 4 breathlessness and less pain, but worsened peripheral neuropathy, compared to patients receiving supportive care only [11]. In addition, quality of life as assessed by the European Organization for Research and Treatment of Cancer (EORTC) QLC-LC13 questionnaire after 6 weeks of therapy confirmed an improvement for patients receiving cisplatin-based chemotherapy [12].

Due to discrepant survival results in BSC trials, meta-analyses of chemotherapy versus BSC trials have been helpful in determining the role of systemic treatment in these patients. A 1993 analysis of six randomized trials concluded that the use of chemotherapy in this setting was associated with a statistically significant 24% reduction in the risk of death at 1 year, and that treatment was associated with a lengthening of overall survival from 16.7 weeks to 27.4 weeks [13]. A 1994 meta-analysis of published literature results and individual patient data confirmed the benefit of treatment, determining an odds ratio of death of 0.44 and an increase in estimated median survival from 3.9 months for BSC to 6.7 months for patients with advanced disease receiving chemotherapy [14]. The largest meta-analysis of individual patient data was compiled from 11 studies from 1965 to 1991, and was reported in 1995 [15]. Findings from this analysis of over 1,100 patients reveal that the use of cisplatin-based regimens was associated with a 27% reduction in the risk of death for patients with advanced NSCLC, translating into an absolute improvement in survival at 1 year of 10% (from 5% to 15%). The use of non-platinum-containing regimens was not beneficial in the setting of advanced disease.

22.2 Cisplatin-Based Doublets Using Newer Agents: Improved Survival Compared to Cisplatin Alone

The clinical development of newer, so called third-generation, chemotherapeutic agents in the treatment of NSCLC, such as the taxanes, gemcitabine, and vinorelbine, was active in the 1990s, with resultant improvements in the therapeutic index [16–20]. These agents demonstrated single-agent antitumor response rates in the range of 13–19%, leading to improved survival and/ or quality of life when compared to BSC in advanced disease [21–24].

Table 22.1 demonstrates that the combination of these newer agents with cisplatin often resulted in a doubling of the antitumor response rate and increased the 1-year survival rate more than 10% [25–28]. For example, cisplatin/vinorelbine was compared to cisplatin alone in a 1998 SWOG trial of 432 chemonaive patients [25]. The increased antitumor activity seen in this study with the combination, at 26% compared to 12% with single-agent cisplatin, was associated with a significant prolongation in 1-year overall survival for patients receiving the combination, at 36%, versus 20% for patients in the cisplatin-alone arm. This improved length of survival did come at the cost of higher rates of grade 3 and 4 neutropenia, although frequencies of nonhematologic toxicities were similar between the two treatment arms. A prospective trial randomizing 522 patients with advanced disease to either cisplatin alone or combined with gemcitabine confirmed the superiority of the combination in terms of treatment activity and survival, whereas an international trial of 446 patients, likewise, detected significant improvements in antitumor response and overall survival when tirapazamine, a cytotoxic drug that works best under hypoxic conditions, was combined with cisplatin, compared to cisplatin alone [27, 28]. Combination therapy in these two studies was well tolerated, with no significant worsening of side effects, compared to single agent treatment.

However, not all cisplatin-based combination trials have proved beneficial in terms of survival when combined with a newer agent. Gatzemeier et al. published an EORTC trial of 414 patients randomized to receive either single-agent cisplatin or combination therapy with cisplatin and paclitaxel [26]. Although the response rate of the combination exceeded that for the single agent, at 26% versus 17%, and time to progression was statistically lengthened with use of the combination, overall survival was not prolonged, at 8.6 months for the control arm and 8.1 months in the combination arm. However, more patients receiving single-agent cisplatin received second-line chemotherapy, compared to those agents receiving initial combination treatment, possibly confounding the survival comparison. In addition, patients receiving the cisplatin/paclitaxel upfront treatment did experience slightly better outcomes of quality of life measurements, with respect to nausea and vomiting, appetite loss, and constipation [26].

Table 22.1. Randomized trials of cisplatin alone versus newer cisplatin-based combinations. *NS* Not significant

Study	N	Therapy	Overall response rate (%)	Median survival (months)	One-year overall survival (%)	P value
Wozniak et al. 1998 [25]	432	Cisplatin	12	6	20	
		Cisplatin/vinorelbine	26	8	36	0.0018
Sandler et al. 2000 [27]	522	Cisplatin	11.1	7.6	28	
		Cisplatin/gemcitabine	30.4	9.1	39	0.004
von Pawel et al. 2000 [28]	446	Cisplatin	13.7	6.9	22.5	
		Cisplatin/tirapazamine	27.5	8.7	45	0.0078
Gatzemeier et al. 2000 [26]	414	Cisplatin	17	8.6	36	
		Cisplatin/paclitaxel	26	8.1	30	NS

In summary, Table 22.1 provides evidence that doublet, platinum-based chemotherapy combined with a newer active, third-generation agent impacts positively on survival in most studies, without significantly worsening toxicity. Large cooperative groups, therefore, selected one of these doublets as their reference arm for treatment in subsequent comparative trials.

22.3   Cisplatin Versus Carboplatin

Cisplatin has been associated with a significant number of side effects, most notably nausea and vomiting. Although this toxicity has become much more manageable with the advent of the HT3 antiemetics, concerns remain regarding renal toxicity, neuropathy, ototoxicity, and generalized fatigue and asthenia. To alleviate some of these side effects, clinicians have turned toward the platin analogue carboplatin. Although carboplatin has a relatively low single-agent response rate, data from most, but not all, randomized trials supports equivalent clinical benefit between cisplatin and carboplatin [29–32]. For example, in the Eastern Cooperative Oncology Group (ECOG) 1594 trial, four different chemotherapy doublets were compared to each other; the comparator arm involved cisplatin and paclitaxel, while one of the experimental arms included carboplatin and paclitaxel [33]. Although the dose and infusion rate of paclitaxel differed between the two arms (135 mg/m^2 over 24 h in the cisplatin arm, and 225 mg/m^2 over 3 h in the carboplatin arm), the overall response and median survival did not differ significantly (22% and 7.8 months, respectively, in the cisplatin/paclitaxel arm, and 17% and 8.1 months in the carboplatin/paclitaxel arm, respectively). Three European trials

compared platinum doublets head-to-head using either cisplatin or carboplatin [29, 31, 32]. All three studies found more frequent and severe nausea, vomiting, and diarrhea with cisplatin, and two found either worsened renal or neurotoxicity. Paccagnella et al. used quality of life and symptom control as their primary endpoint when comparing mitomycin and vinblastine with either cisplatin or carboplatin; in this study, use of carboplatin was associated with better quality of life outcomes, although either platinum led to similar control of lung-cancer-associated symptoms [32]. In contrast, when comparing platinums combined with the same dose and schedule of paclitaxel, (as contrasted to the ECOG study, where the dose and schedule of paclitaxel varied), Rosell et al. found no difference in global quality of life or functional status outcomes [29]. Rosell et al. also were the only group to determine a statistically significant improvement in median survival; 9.8 months in the cisplatin arm, compared to 8.5 months in the carboplatin arm [29, 34].

Two recent meta-analyses comparing cisplatin and carboplatin in advanced NSCLC suggest improved antitumor efficacy with use of cisplatin [35, 36]. However, Hotta et al. incorporated only abstracted data, rather than individual patient data, into their meta-analyses, while the report of Zojwalla et al. is preliminary. As such, these meta-analyses at this point represent only hypothesis-generating findings, rather than definitive conclusive comparisons of the clinical experience with these two agents. Therefore, although it could be debated as to whether carboplatin produces exactly the same efficacy outcomes as cisplatin in advanced NSCLC, results appear to be roughly similar, and with improved tolerability seen with the use of carboplatin. Given the paramount importance of limiting toxicity and optimizing quality of life in the advanced disease setting, it certainly seems reasonable

Table 22.2. Randomized trials of platinum-base doublets versus newer single agents

Study	N	Therapy	Overall response rate (%)	Median survival (months)	One-year overall survival (%)	P value
Le Chevalier et al. 1994 [37]	612	Cisplatin/vindesine	19	8.3	29	
		Vinorelbine	4	9.0	34	
		Cisplatin/vinorelbine	30	10.8	34	0.001*
ten Bokkel Huinink et al. 1999 [38]	147	Gemcitabine	17.9	6.6	26	
		Cisplatin/etoposide	15.3	7.6	24	NS
Vansteenkiste et al. 2003 [41]	169	Gemcitabine	20.2	6.7	22	
		Cisplatin/vindesine	20	5.5	19	NS
Lilenbaum et al. 2005 [43]	584	Paclitaxel	17	6.7	32	
		Carboplatin/paclitaxel	30	8.8	37	< 0.05**
Sederholm 2002 [39]	332	Gemcitabine	12	9	32	
		Carboplatin/gemicitabine	30	11	44	0.0024
Georgoulias et al. 2004 [42]	307	Docetaxel	21.7	8	43	
		Cisplatin/docetaxel	36.5	10.5	44	NS
Negoro et al. 2003 [40]	398	Irinotecan	20.5	11.5	41.8	
		Cisplatin/vindesine	31.7	11.4	38.3	
		Cisplatin/irinotecan	43.7	12.5	46.5	NS

* When adjusted for treatment center. ** Wilcoxon analysis

to incorporate carboplatin as the platinating agent of choice in first-line doublet therapy. However, in earlier-stage disease, such as in the postoperative setting where curability is defined as the treatment goal, the results of Rosell et al. raise the important question of whether or not cisplatin is superior to carboplatin in terms of disease activity [29, 30]. Randomized trials comparing cisplatin and carboplatin in earlier-stage NSCLC are needed to address this question.

22.4 New Single Agents Versus a Platinum Combined with New Agents

Table 22.2 shows randomized trials comparing a newer single agent versus a newer platinum-based combination [37–43].

22.4.1 Vinorelbine

The combination of cisplatin and vinorelbine was compared to vinorelbine alone as part of a French trial of 612 patients [37]. The objective response rate was significantly higher in the combination arm, at 30%, compared to 14% in the single-agent arm, with this increased activity translating into a significant survival advantage at 1 year of 38% versus 34%, respectively. Toxicity was manageable on the cisplatin/vinorelbine arm, although neutropenia was more common.

22.4.2 Gemcitabine

Single-agent gemcitabine yielded similar efficacy outcomes but improved quality of life parameters and less toxicity compared to cisplatin-based treatment, in randomized studies out of Europe [38, 41]. A Swedish Lung Cancer Group study compared combination treatment with gemcitabine and carboplatin versus treatment with gemcitabine alone in 332 patients with advanced NSCLC. The antitumor response and overall survival at 1 year were improved with combination treatment in this study (30% and 44% for the combination and 12% and 32% for single agent gemcitabine, respectively), while the rates of grade 3 and 4 toxicity were similar between the two arms (26% for gemcitabine/carboplatin versus 28% for gemcitabine alone) [39].

22.4.3 The Taxanes

The Cancer and Leukemia Group B (CALGB) 9730 study found an improved antitumor response rate, and failure-free, median, and overall survival for patients with advanced disease receiving the combination of carboplatin and paclitaxel, compared to paclitaxel alone. Although treatment with the combination arm yielded more hematologic toxicity and nausea, febrile neutropenia and treatment-related deaths were equally low in the two arms. No significant differences were seen between the two treatments with respect to quality of life analyses [43]. As seen in Table 22.2, in a Greek trial of 339 patients, combination treatment with docetaxel and cisplatin did not yield a survival advantage compared to docetaxel alone, a result that was possibly impacted by the fact that 5 patients experienced septic death on the combination arm, compared to only 1 receiving single-agent treatment [42].

22.4.4 Irinotecan

Finally, Negoro et al. recently published the results of their comparison of irinotecan alone versus irinotecan combined with cisplatin. Although these two arms were not meant to be compared directly per the statistical design of this study, the response rate and survival at 1 year are numerically superior for the combination (43.7% and 46.5%, respectively), compared to single-agent irinotecan use (20.5% and 41.8%, respectively). The primary endpoint of this trial was satisfied in that single-agent irinotecan use was not inferior to combination therapy with the older doublet of cisplatin and vindesine [40].

On the whole, these trials show that antitumor response is improved with platinum-based doublet treatment, and that combination therapy potentially improves median survival by 2 months, although at higher rates of toxicity. Furthermore, Hotta el al. recently performed a meta-analysis (again, using abstracted data rather than individual patient data) of 8 trials comparing a newer single agent to platinum-based doublets incorporating that same newer agent; they found that doublet treatment was associated with a 13% prolongation of survival [44]. Platinum-based doublet therapy incorporating a newer cytotoxic agent has thus become the standard in the USA for first-line therapy of advanced NSCLC for patients with a good performance status.

Table 22.3. Randomized trials of older cisplatin-based doublets versus newer platinum-based doublets

Study	N	Therapy	Overall response rate (%)	Median survival (months)	One-year overall survival (%)	P value
Le Chevalier et al. 1994 [37]	612	Cisplatin/vindesine	19	8.3	29	
		Cisplatin/venorelbine	30	10.8	38	0.04*
Giaccone et al. 1998 [46]	332	Cisplatin/teniposide	28	9.9	41	
		Cisplatin/paclitaxel	41	9.7	43	NS
Belani et al. 1998 [45]	369	Cisplatin/etoposide	14	8.2	37	
		Carboplatin/paclitaxel	23	7.7	32	NS
Cardenal et al. 1999 [47]	135	Cisplatin/etoposide	21.9	7.2	26	
		Cisplatin/gemcitabine	40.6	8.7	32	NS
Bonomi et al. 2000 [48]	599	Cisplatin/etoposide	12.4	7.6	31.8	
		Cisplatin/paclitaxel (low dose)	25.3	9.5	37.4	
		Cisplatin/paclitaxel (high dose)	27.7	10	40.3	0.048**
Takiguchi et al. 2000 [49]	210	Cisplatin/vindesine	22	11.6	48	
		Cisplatin/irinotecan	29	10.5	43	NS
Grigorescu et al. 2002 [50]	198	Cisplatin/vinblastine	15	7.9	12	
		Carboplatin/gemcitabine	27	11.6	36	<0.05
Kubota et al. 2004 [51]	302	Cisplatin/vindesine	21	9.6	41	
		Cisplatin/docetaxel	37	11.3	48	0.014
Negoro et al. 2003 [40]	398	Cisplatin/vindesine	31.7	11.4	38.3	
		Cisplatin/irinotecan	43.7	12.5	46.5	NS

 * When adjusted for treatment centers.
** When survival is combined for the low- and high-dose paclitaxel arms

22.5 New Platinum Combinations Versus Older Platinum Combinations

Table 22.3 displays the results of nine randomized trials that compared an older cisplatin-based doublet with a platinum-based combination using a newer second agent [37, 45–51]. In these trials, the newer agents, including paclitaxel, gemcitabine, docetaxel, and irinotecan, are associated with the toxicities of myalgias/arthralgias/sensory neuropathy, non-clinically-significant thrombocytopenia, edema, and diarrhea, respectively, without consistently exacerbating neutropenia. Statistically significant prolongations in overall survival were seen in nearly half of the trials [37, 48, 50, 51]. For example, in the TAX-JP-301 trial, cisplatin and docetaxel were compared to cisplatin and vindesine [51]. Antitumor response and survival were statistically superior with the cisplatin/docetaxel combination, with survival at 1 year approaching 50% for patients receiving the newer regimen. Anorexia and diarrhea were worse in the docetaxel arm, but hematologic toxicity was improved in these patients, as were quality of life measures [51].

Quality of life measures were also improved for patients receiving the combinations with the newer cytotoxic agents, despite the absence of a corresponding survival benefit, in the trials of Belani et al. and Giaccone et al., revealing a clinically meaningful effect from

the third-generation agents [45, 46]. In the ECOG 5592 trial, cisplatin combined with the lower dose of paclitaxel (135 mg/m^2 over a 24-h continuous infusion) was selected as the reference arm for this cooperative group, based upon its optimal benefit/toxicity ratio, compared to the other two arms in that trial [48].

A meta-analysis of 8 trials (3,296 patients) found an improvement in response rate (absolute increase of 13%) and survival (absolute increase of 4%, risk ratio of 1.14, 95% confidence intervals: 0.00–0.08) with third-generation regimens compared to second-generation regimens. No increase in toxic deaths was found [52]. A second meta-analysis evaluated 2,425 patients in 8 studies, and concluded that newer regimen reduced the risk for response by 46% ($P=0.001$). It also reduced the risk for death by 19% ($P=0.012$) at 1 year [53].

Thus, although marked improvements in overall survival were not seen in all of these trials, the bulk of evidence pointed to the fact that the newer combinations resulted in 1-year overall survival rates consistently exceeding 30–35%, and that an efficacious platinum-based doublet could be individualized to match a patient's comorbidities contingent upon the newer agent's toxicities. As such, practice has progressed from the "one size fits all" recipe for a platinum-based doublet for patients with advanced NSCLC, therefore expanding the number of patients eligible to receive therapy.

Table 22.4. Randomized trials of newer platinum-based doublets. *NR* Not reported

Study	N	Therapy	Overall response rate (%)	Median survival (months)	One-year overall survival (%)	P value
Kosmidis et al. 2000 [54]	198	Carboplatin/paclitaxel (low dose)	25.6	9.5	37	
		Carboplatin/paclitaxel (high dose)	31.8	11.4	44	NS
Kelly et al. 2001 [55]	408	Cisplatin/vinorelbine	28	8.1	36	
		Carboplatin/paclitaxel	25	8.6	38	NS
Fossella et al. 2003 [30]	1,220	Cisplatin/vinorelbine	25	10.1	41	
		Cisplatin/docetaxel	32	11.3	46	
		Carboplatin/docetaxel	24	9.4	38	0.044*
Schiller et al. 2002 [33]	1,207	Cisplatin/paclitaxel	21	7.8	31	
		Cisplatin/gemcitabine	22	8.1	36	
		Cisplatin/docetaxel	17	7.4	31	
		Carboplatin/paclitaxel	17	8.1	34	NS
Huang et al. 2002 [56]	99	Carboplatin/paclitaxel	31	NR	NR	
		Carboplatin/docetaxel	22	NR	NR	NR
Scagliotti et al. 2002 [57]	612	Cisplatin/gemcitabine	30	9.8	37	
		Carboplatin/paclitaxel	32	9.9	43	
		Cisplatin/vinorelbine	30	9.5	37	NS
Gebbia et al. 2003 [58]	400	Cisplatin/vinorelbine	44	9.0	24	
		Cisplatin/gemcitabine	34	8.2	20	NS
Martoni et al. 2005 [61]	285	Cisplatin/vinorelbine	32.6	11.0	39.7	
		Cisplatin/gemcitabine	25.9	11.0	44.4	NS
Kubota et al. 2004 [51]	602	Cisplatin/irinotecan	31	14.2	59.2	
		Carboplatin/paclitaxel	32.4	12.3	51	
		Cisplatin/gemcitabine	30.1	14.8	60	
		Cisplatin/vinorelbine	33.1	11.4	48.3	NR
Belani 2004 [59]	444	Carboplatin/paclitaxel every 3 weeks	18	10.2	43	
		Carboplatin/paclitaxel every week	20	8.9	39.5	NR

* Cisplatin/docetaxel versus cisplatin/vinorelbine.
** Intention-to-treat analysis, as of the survival update, September 2001

22.6   Comparisons of Newer Platinum Doublets

Comparisons of platinum-based doublets incorporating third-generation agents have demonstrated improvements in treatment activity and overall survival in patients with a good performance status, but have yet to identify one clinically superior regimen [30, 33, 54–61]. Table 22.4 demonstrates that treatment with these combinations yields antitumor response rates of at least 30%, median survival times of 8–12 months, 1-year overall survival rates exceeding 30%, and for the first time, 2-year survival rates exceeding 10%. These advances are measured against median survivals of 5.3–5.8 months and 1-year survival of <20% seen with platinum-based doublets combined with older, second-generation agents [62, 63]. In terms of scheduling a particular doublet, Belani et al. recently demonstrated no difference in antitumor response or survival when comparing carboplatin administered with paclitaxel given weekly or every 3 weeks [59]. Toxicity profiles did dif-

fer, however, with more anemia with the weekly regimen and more arthralgia with the 3-weekly paclitaxel.

As noted in Tables 22.3 and 22.4, no single platinum-based doublet has proved superior in terms of efficacy outcomes; as such, there is flexibility in selecting a regimen in terms of an individual patient's comorbidities, treatment schedule, and cost. However, in an effort to identify a superior combination, Le Chevalier et al. performed a meta-analysis comparing gemcitabine-containing platinum regimens to those without gemcitabine [64]. These authors found that a small but statistically significant survival advantage of almost 4% at 1 year as a result of incorporation of gemcitabine, even when comparing only those platinum-based doublets that contained a newer, third-generation agent. In terms of making general recommendations, then, doublet treatment containing gemcitabine may offer a patient a slight survival advantage. However, these data are not sufficiently persuasive to alter our recommendation that selection of a platinum-based doublet must be made contingent upon each individual patient's unique circumstances.

Quality of life analyses were conducted in four of the trials listed in Table 22.4, with consistent, significant differences seen most strongly with the use of docetaxel in the Fossella trial [29, 30, 55, 57]. Using the EuroQoL global health scale and the Lung Cancer Symptom Scale (LCSS), these investigators showed that treatment with docetaxel/cisplatin (DC) or docetaxel/carboplatin (DCb) was associated with significant improvements in quality of life, compared to treatment with vinorelbine/cisplatin (VC): (for DC versus VC: LCSS $P = 0.064$ and EuroQoL $P = 0.016$; for DCb versus VC: LCSS $P = 0.016$ and EuroQoL $P < 0.001$). Declines in performance status and weight were mitigated with docetaxel therapy [30]. It has been noted in a discussion of these results that the cisplatin dose administered to patients in the vinorelbine arm was higher per treatment (at 100 mg/m^2, compared to 75 mg/m^2 in the docetaxel arms). In addition, a higher dose of corticosteroids was given to patients receiving docetaxel. Both of these factors may have contributed to an improvement in symptoms in patients in the docetaxel arms [65]. Regardless, in light of the efficacy plateau reached with the platinum-based doublets shown in Table 22.4, it remains paramount to incorporate quality of life and symptom management outcomes into the decision-making of selecting treatments for patients in this palliative setting. Furthermore, the therapeutic efficacy plateau achieved with the use of these newer doublets also clearly speaks to the need to incorporate newer treatments, most notably the use of targeted agents, into clinical trials of new treatment combinations.

22.7 Platinum-Based Doublets Versus Triplets

Table 22.5 shows the results of 14 trials randomizing patients with advanced NSCLC to treatment with 2 or 3 cytotoxic agents [66–79]. However, in 9 of the 14 trials, the comparison 3-agent arm contains at least 1 single agent that is older and would not be used presently as a single agent for treatment (i.e., mitomycin C or ifosfamide) [66, 69–71, 73, 74, 76, 78, 79]. The remaining five studies utilized newer, third-generation agents into their triplets; however, the final results for three of the remaining five trials have yet to be published [67, 68, 72]. Although the three-agent combination of cisplatin/gemcitabine/navelbine was found by the Southern Italian Cooperative Oncology Group (SICOG) investigators to be superior to treatment with cisplatin/navelbine, the doublet arm in this study was surprisingly toxic, and was associated with two toxic deaths, higher rates of chemotherapy discontinuation, severe neutropenia, and vomiting compared to the other arms. This unexpected rate of toxicity with this doublet may have been related to the treatment schema of administering 120 mg/m^2 of cisplatin on day 1 of each 4- to 6-week cycle [67]. The

Spanish Lung Cancer Group 98-02 study detected higher rates of hematologic toxicity with no corresponding improvement in efficacy outcomes for treatment with their 3-drug combination [75]. In contrast, preliminary results from a second SICOG study yielded improved survival with only a modest increase in toxicity with the use of either of two three-drug regimens [68]. The final results from this SICOG trial are anticipated. Finally, it should be noted that doublet therapy is not always less toxic than triplet therapy, as recently demonstrated by investigators on behalf of the British Thoracic Oncology Group trial [78]. Their preliminary findings indicate that both hematologic and nonhematologic toxicity was more severe with the use of carboplatin and docetaxel compared to their triplet standard mitomycin/ifosfamide/cisplatin or mitomycin/vinblastine/cisplatin regimens.

In summary, the consensus of evidence and opinion, including the recent publication of two meta-analyses, conclude that treatment of good-performance-status patients with advanced NSCLC with two cytotoxic agents is better than with one (see Tables 22.1 and 22.2), while the addition of a third agent is only likely to exacerbate toxicity [80, 81]. However, the majority of these findings result from studies incorporating rather inactive, older agents into the three-agent arm. Favorable results with the use of three-drug regimens from the SICOG investigators and Paccagnella et al. require confirmation before their findings would impact upon practice patterns [68, 72]. Nonetheless, incorporation of agents with novel, targeted mechanisms of action into new treatment regimens, administered to patients who are preselected based upon the molecular characteristics of their tumors, will likely bear better outcomes, rather than continuing to explore combinations of cytotoxic agents administered to patients without genomic preselection. The recently released results of SWOG 0003, revealing no improvement in efficacy outcomes for patients with advanced NSCLC receiving the three-drug regimen carboplatin, paclitaxel, and tirapazamine, confirms the need to consider molecular preselection criteria into study designs [77].

22.8 Treatment with a Nonplatinum Regimen

ASOC guidelines state that a non-platinum-containing regimen may be used as an alternative to a platinum-containing regimen in the first-line setting [1]. The use of non-platinum-containing regimens will be discussed in a subsequent chapter.

Table 22.5. Randomized trials of platinum-based doublets versus triplets

Study	N	Therapy	Overall response rate (%)	Median survival (months)	One-year overall survival (%)	P value
Crino et al. 1999 [66]	307	Mitomycin/ifosfamide/cisplatin	26	9.6	34	
		Cisplatin/gemcitabine	38	8.6	33	
		Cisplatin/vinorelbine	25	8.8	34	NS
Comella et al. 2000 [67]	180	Cisplatin/vinorelbine	30	10.5	40	
		Cisplatin/gemcitabine/vinorelbine	47	12.8	45	<0.01*
		Cisplatin/gemcitabine	42	9.3	38	
Alberola et al. 2003 [75]	557	Cisplatin/gemcitabine/vinorelbine	41	8.2	33	
		Gemcitabinevinorelbine → ifosfamide/vinorelbine	27	8.1	34	NS
		Cisplatin/gemcitabine	28	9.5	39	
Comella 2001 [68]	343	Cisplatin/gemcitabine/vinorelbine	44	12.8	47	
					46	
		Cisplatin/gemcitabine paclitaxel	48	12.8		<0.05**
Rudd et al. 2005 [79]	422	Mitomycin/ifosfamide/cisplatin	40	6.5	28	
		Carboplatin/gemcitabine	37	10	38	0.028
Melo et al. 2002 [71]	248	Mitomycin/vinblastine/cisplatin	27	6.4	NR	
		Cisplatin/vinorelbine	37.1	9.0	NR	
		Cisplatin/gemcitabine (early)	48.4	9.4	NR	
		Cisplatin/gemcitabine (late)	48.4	9.7	NR	0.05***
Paccagnella et al 2002 [72]	60	Carboplatin/paclitaxel/gemcitabine	33	NR	NR	NR
		Carboplatin/paclitaxel	15	NR	NR	
Gebbia et al. 2002 [69]	247	Mitomycin/vindesine/cisplatin	42	8	14.7	
		Cisplatin/vinorelbine	39	7	15.2	NS
Kodani et al. 2002 [70]	132	Vindesine/ifosfamide/cisplatin	49.3	12.4	49.3	
		Cisplatin/vindesine	44.6	9.3	35.3	
		Cisplatin/carboplatin/ifosfamide	25	6.0	23	NS
Sculier et al. 2002 [73]	284	Cisplatin/carboplatin/gemcitabine	31	8.5	33	
		Ifosfamide/gemcitabine	26	7.5	35	NS
Souquet et al. 2002 [74]	259	Cisplatin/ifosfamide/vinorelbine	35.7	8.2	33.7	
		Cisplatin/vinorelbine	34.6	10	38.4	NS
Danson et al. 2003 [76]	372	Mitomycin/ifosfamide/cisplatin or Mitomycin/vinblastine/cisplatin	33	8.3	32.5	
		Carboplatin/gemcitabine	30	7.9	33.2	NS
Williamson et al. 2003 [77]	396	Carboplatin/paclitaxel/tirapazamine	18	7	NR	
				9	NR	0.74
		Carboplatin/paclitaxel	27			
Lorigan 2004 [78]	432	Mitomycin/ifosfamide/cisplatin or Mitomycin/vinblastine/cisplatin	33	NR	37	
		Carboplatin/docetaxel	33	NR	32	NR

22.9   Duration of Therapy with a Platinum Doublet

The updated ASCO guidelines state that first-line therapy for stage IV NSCLC should be stopped at four cycles in patients who are not responding to treatment, with the consensus that even in responding patients, no more than six cycles should be administered in this setting [1]. These statements are supported by the results of five trials that examined the question of duration of first-line therapy in advanced NSCLC [82–86]. Socinski et al. randomized 230 patients to continuous treatment every 21 days with carboplatin and paclitaxel, versus 4 cycles of the same regimen [84]. The median number of cycles received by both groups was four, with over one-third of patients on the continuous arm stopping treatment due to disease progression and another third halting therapy due to physician and patient discretion. No difference was found between the treatment groups in terms of response activity, survival, quality of life, and toxicity, except for an increased rate of grade 2–4 neuropathy in patients receiving continuous therapy. These results, suggesting that a shorter, finite number of treatment doses is equivalent to administering additional cycles, confirm the findings of Smith et al., who detected no improvement in antitumor activity, survival, or symptom relief between patients who received either three or six cycles of mitomycin C, vinblastine, and cisplatin chemotherapy [83]. Indeed, quality of life parameters for patients receiving only three courses of treatment were better, including less fatigue and a strong trend toward reduced nausea and vomiting ($P=0.06$). In a trial using newer agents, Andresen et al. detected identical antitumor response and survival in patients who received either three or six cycles of carboplatin and vinorelbine [85]. Depierre et al. found that there was no survival benefit to adding weekly vinorelbine to patients who had responded to treatment with mitomycin, ifosfamide, and cisplatin [82]. In contrast, Krazkowski et al. recently found an improved time to progression for patients randomized to receive maintenance gemcitabine after completing four cycles of cisplatin and gemcitabine; median survival was not prolonged by maintenance therapy [86]. Although additional studies are underway examining the addition of maintenance cytotoxic therapy, the findings from Socinski et al., Smith et al., Depierre et al., and Andresen et al. have guided practitioners in limiting the number of front-line cycles of chemotherapy, as nearly all patients who respond to treatment do so within the first 3–4 cycles (all in the Socinski trial and 48/58 patients in the Smith study), and administering additional cycles only serves to expose patients to additional toxicities [82–85].

22.10 Platinum-Based Chemotherapy in Elderly Patients with Advanced NSCLC

Patients over the age of 65 years comprise a large fraction of patients with advanced NSCLC. Their treatment tends to be complicated by increased frequency of medical comorbidities and multiple concurrent medications. Moreover, therapeutic treatment decisions in the elderly are complicated by their significant underrepresentation in clinical oncology trials [87]. However, a recent review from the National Cancer Institute in Naples found that elderly patients with lung cancer do not appear to have different characteristics at disease presentation, especially related to disease stage, performance status, and histology, compared to younger patients [88]. Moreover, when asked, elderly patients are as likely as their younger counterparts to accept chemotherapy for both curative and palliative purposes [89]. Despite this,

two recent population-based analyses in the USA confirmed that elderly patients with advanced NSCLC were less likely to receive chemotherapy for their disease compared to younger patients [90, 91].

Although randomized clinical trials of single, nonplatin agents have been conducted in elderly patients with advanced NSCLC, no randomized, prospective trials have incorporated platinum-based chemotherapy [21, 92–94]. However, multiple retrospective reviews of cooperative groups and other large trials that examined subsets of elderly patients (usually defined as ≥ 65 or ≥ 70 years of age) have shown that the "fit" elderly are as likely to benefit with platin-based regimens in terms of improvements in survival and quality of life as are younger patients, albeit at the expense of a slightly higher rate of the most severe toxicities [80, 92–98]. For example, findings from CALGB 9730 suggest that patients over 70 years of age receiving the combination of carboplatin and paclitaxel benefited from doublet therapy as much as younger patients, compared to monotherapy with paclitaxel [43]. In addition, treatment with cisplatin/docetaxel appears to confer the same survival advantage over treatment with cisplatin/vinorelbine in the elderly subset of patients in the TAX326 trial as that seen with the study population as a whole [99]. In this preliminary report, moderately higher rates of grade 3–4 asthenia, infection, and pulmonary toxicities, as well as diarrhea and sensory neuropathy, were seen in the elderly cohort of patients in this trial. Likewise, investigators from ECOG showed that elderly patients benefited from cisplatin combined with paclitaxel or etoposide to the same extent as did younger patients, although at the cost of slightly higher rates of leukopenia and neuropsychiatric toxicities [96]. Treatment cessation due to toxicity occurred more frequently in elderly patients enrolled in two SWOG trials, but again, overall comparisons of toxicity and efficacy were similar to those in younger patients [95]. Finally, Hensing et al. found no differences between elderly and nonelderly patients receiving carboplatin and paclitaxel with respect to toxicity, efficacy, or quality of life outcomes [100].

Prospective data with platinating agents in the treatment of elderly patients with advanced NSCLC are lacking, in contrast to prospective data available with single-agent, nonplatinum compounds [94]. Nonetheless, robust retrospective data emphasize that age alone should not disqualify an elderly patient from consideration for platinum-based treatment in advanced NSCLC, and that elderly patients with a good performance status may experience similar rates of antitumor response, prolonged survival, improvements in quality of life, and treatment-related toxicity as do their younger counterparts [101, 102]. Further investigation of the pharmacokinetics and pharmacodynamics of chemotherapies in the elderly are needed to clarify the impact on chemotherapy-related toxicities of reduced renal function and hematopoietic reserve of the elderly [103, 104].

22.11   New Directions in the Platinum-Based Treatment of NSCLC

22.11.1   Genetic Variations in DNA Repair and Platinum-Based Chemotherapy

Platinating compounds covalently bind to DNA, forming intrastrand adducts. Variations in DNA repair capabilities have been shown to correlate inversely with sensitivity to cisplatin in cancer cell lines [105]. As such, it has been postulated that suboptimal DNA repair may predict a better clinical response to platinum therapy [106]. Lord et al. examined mRNA levels of the nucleotide excision repair gene *ERCC1* in tumors from patients with stage IIB/IV NSCLC who received treatment with cisplatin and gemcitabine [107]. Low *ERCC1* expression correlated with a prolonged median survival (61.6 weeks), compared to patients with high *ERCC1* expression (20.4 weeks; $P = 0.009$ log rank test). In addition, the presence of a single nucleotide polymorphism (SNP) at codon 118 of *ERRC1* has been associated with shortened survival (281 days for patients with the variant genotype, compared to 486 days for patients with the wild-type codon) in a study of 109 NSCLC patients who received at least two cycles of cisplatin-based chemotherapy [108].

Genetic variations in the expression of a second gene involved in DNA repair, *XPD*, have also been examined. In contrast to *ERRC1*, which must be tested in tumor tissue, *XPD* can be analyzed using constitutional DNA, such as that isolated from peripheral blood lymphocytes. Patients with *XPD* variants are seen in about half of lung cancer patients, and have been associated with impaired DNA repair capacity [109]. Gurubhagavatula et al. found that the presence of the Asp312Asn polymorphism was associated with decreased survival in a review of 103 NSCLC patients treated with platinum-based regimens: median survival of 16.3 weeks for patients with the wild-type genotype (Asp/Asp), 15.2 months for heterozygotes (Asp/Asn), and 6.6 months for those with the homozygous variant (Asn/Asn; $P = 0.003$) [106].

Recent studies have attempted to examine multiple genotypic variants in DNA repair enzymes, in order to identify patients most sensitive to platinum-based treatment. For example, Sarries et al. recently examined polymorphisms in the following DNA repair genes: *XPD*, *ERCC1*, *XRCC1*, *TP53*, and *RRM1* [110]. They found in their population of NSCLC patients treated with cisplatin and gemcitabine that shortened time to progression and overall survival correlated with the presence of both the *XPD*/751 (Gln/Gln) and *XPD*/312 Asn/Asn. Furthermore, when these two polymorphisms were combined with a third, *ERCC1*/N118N (C/C), time to progression and survival were, again, shortened [110].

These studies highlight the idea that variations in DNA repair may affect clinical outcomes in patients treated with platinums, and that detection of these polymorphisms may help to select patients with an improved chance of benefiting from platinum-based treatments. Examination of these genetic variants is now included in multiple treatment trials around the world, and should continue to shed light on the interplay between pharmacogenomic and clinical outcomes.

22.11.2   Emerging Platinum Compounds

22.11.2.1   Oxaliplatin

The platinum analogue oxaliplatin (1,2-diaminocyclohexanoeoxalato platinum II), has been studied in the treatment of NSCLC. Treatment-related toxicities include sensory neuropathy, including laryngeal spasm and cold dysesthesias, and nausea and vomiting; myelosuppression is usually mild. Single-agent activity is 15% when administered at 130 mg/m^2 intravenously very 3 weeks [111]. Phase II combinations with gemcitabine, paclitaxel, and vinorelbine have yielded response rates of 16–35%, median survivals ranging from 8–9.8 months, and 1-year survival rates of 37% [112–114]. Combination studies of oxaliplatin with newer cytotoxic agents in the treatment of advanced NSCLC continue.

22.11.2.2   Satraplatin

Satraplatin (*bis*-aceto-ammine-dichloro-cyclohexylamine platinum IV) can be administered orally; myelosuppression is its dose-limiting toxicity. Other treatment-related toxicities include nausea, vomiting, and diarrhea [115]. Multiple treatment schedules have been developed, including daily treatment for 5 or 14 days [116]. When combined in patients with NSCLC and esophageal cancer with thoracic radiotherapy at 2 Gy per day administered five times weekly, the maximum tolerated dose of concurrent satraplatin was 30 mg/m^2/day for 5 days [117]. No objective responses were seen when Judson et al. administered satraplatin at 120 mg/m^2 daily for 5 days every 3 weeks in a phase II trial of 17 patients with advanced NSCLC [118]. Further phase I studies, including in combination with docetaxel, are underway.

22.11.2.3   Nedaplatin

Nedaplatin (*cis*-diammine-glycolato-0,0′ platinum II) is an analogue of cisplatin that is currently approved for use in Japan for several cancers, including small cell lung cancer. The dose-limiting toxicity of nedaplatin in myelosuppression (thrombocytopenia and leukopenia); its use is also associated with minor abnormalities in renal function. Hirose et al. [119] and Kurata et al. [120] combined nedaplatin with gemcitabine in two recent phase I studies of patients with advanced NSCLC. They found that the combination was well tolerated and that antitumor response rates ranged from 16.7% to 35%. The recommended phase II dose of nedaplatin to be combined with 1000 mg/m^2 of gemcitabine every 3 weeks was 80–100 mg/m^2. Oshita et al. detected an antitumor response rate of 31% when nedaplatin was combined in a phase I/II study with irinotecan [121]. Takigawa et al. published a phase II study of nedaplatin with vindesine in 48 patients with relapsed NSCLC; the objective response rate was 7.5% in this second-line setting. The authors concluded that use of this combination was unsatisfactory, even though it was well tolerated [122].

22.12　Summary

Platinum compounds provide the foundation for the treatment of patients with advanced NSCLC. Treatments with such regimens offer patients with an improvement in good performance status, in quality of life and prolonged survival, compared to BSC. Carboplatin very likely offers similar efficacy outcomes compared to cisplatin in this setting, and with less toxicity. Treatment with a platinum-based doublet incorporating a newer, third-generation cytotoxic agent is the recommended therapy for good-performance-status patients with advanced NSCLC, yielding an approximate response rate of 30%, median survival of 8–12 months, 1-year survival of 30%, and 2-year survival of 10%. No single regimen is recommended as superior; selection of the regimen can be flexible, contingent upon the patient's comorbidities, treatment cost, and administration schedule. Adding a third cytotoxic agent is only likely to exacerbate toxicity, without improving efficacy. Treatment should be limited to four cycles in patients with stable disease, and possibly a maximum of six cycles, as tolerated, in responding patients. Age alone should not preclude consideration for treatment with a platinum doublet, although prospective data using platinum agents in studies restricted to elderly patients are lacking. Finally, research continues into the identification of platinum-sensitive patients based upon pharmacogenomic parameters, and the development of newer platinum compounds.

Key Points

- Treatment of good-performance-status patients with advanced non-small-cell lung cancer (NSCLC) with platinum-based chemotherapy offers prolongation of survival and improvement of quality of life, compared to best supportive care.
- Treatment of good-performance-status patients with advanced NSCLC using a platinum-based doublet incorporating a newer, second agent can be expected to result in an antitumor response rate of approximately 30%, a median survival of 8–12 months, a 1-year overall survival of 30%, and a 2-year survival of 10%, with acceptable toxicity.
- No single platinum-based doublet is recommended as the superior regimen; selection of a doublet can be made contingent upon a patient's comorbidities.
- The recommended duration of treatment is four cycles for patients with stable disease and up to six cycles in responding patients.
- Although prospective data are lacking, use of a platinum-based doublet for elderly NSCLC patients with a good performance status is supported by retrospective data from multiple, large clinical trials.

References

1. Pfister DG, Johnson DH, Azzoli CG, Sause W, Smith TJ, Baker S Jr, Olak J, Stover D, Strawn JR, Turrisi AT, Somerfield MR. American Society of Clinical Oncology treatment of unresectable non-small-cell lung cancer guideline: update 2003. J Clin Oncol 2004; 22:330.
2. Johnson D. Evolution of cisplatin-based chemotherapy in non-small cell lung cancer: a historical perspective and the Eastern Cooperative Oncology Group Experience. Chest 2000; 117:133S.
3. Rapp E, Pater J, Willan A, Cormier Y, Murray N, Evans W, Hodson D, Clark D, Feld R, Arnold A, Ayoub J, Wilson K, Lateille J, Wierzbicki R, Hill D. Chemotherapy can prolong survival in patients with advanced non-small-cell lung cancer – report of a Canadian multicenter randomized trial. J Clin Oncol 1988; 6:633.
4. Ganz PA, Figlin RA, Haskell CM, La Soto N, Siau J. Supportive care versus supportive care and combination chemotherapy in metastatic non-small cell lung cancer. Does chemotherapy make a difference? Cancer 1989; 63:1271.
5. Woods RL, Williams CJ, Levi J, Page J, Bell D, Byrne M, Kerestes ZL. A randomised trial of cisplatin and vindesine versus supportive care only in advanced non-small cell lung cancer. Br J Cancer 1990; 61:608.
6. Cellerino R, Tummarello D, Guidi F, Isidori P, Raspugli M, Biscottini B, Fatati G. A randomized trial of alternating chemotherapy versus best supportive care in advanced non-small-cell lung cancer. J Clin Oncol 1991; 9:1453.
7. Cartei G, Cartie F, Cantone A, Cousarano D, Genco G, Tobaldin A, Interlandi G, Giraldi T. Cisplatin-cyclophosphamide-mitomycin combination chemotherapy with suppor-

tive care versus supportive care alone for treatment of metastatic non-small-cell lung cancer. J Natl Cancer Inst 1993; 85:794.

8. Cullen M, Billingham J, Woodroffe C, Chetiyawardana A, Gower N, Joshi R, Ferry D, Rudd R, Spiro S, Cook J, Trask C, Bessell E, Connolly C, Tobias J, Souhami R. Mitomycin, ifosfamide, and cisplatin in unresectable non-small-cell lung cancer: effects on survival and quality of life. J Clin Oncol 1999; 17:3188.

9. Thongprasert S, Sanguanmitra P, Juthapan W, Clinch J. Relationship between quality of life and clinical outcomes in advanced non-small cell lung cancer: best supportive care (BSC) versus BSC plus chemotherapy. Lung Cancer 1999; 24:17.

10. Stephens RJ, Fairlamb D, Gower N, Maslove L, Milroy R, Napp V, Peake MD, Rudd RM, Spiro S, Thorpe H, Waller D. The big lung trial (BLT): Determining the value of cisplatin-based chemotherapy for all patients with non-small cell lung cancer (NSCLC). Preliminary results in the supportive care setting. Proc Am Soc Clin Oncol 2002; 21:291a.

11. Brown J, Thorpe H, Napp V, Stephens R, Fairlamb D, Gower N, Milroy R, Rudd R, Spiro S, Waller D, Peake M. The Big Lung Trial Quality of Life Study: Determining the effect of cisplatin-based chemotherapy for supportive care in patients with non-small cell lung cancer (NSCLC). In: 10th World Conference on Lung Cancer. Vancouver: Canada, 2003;41; 20a.

12. Billingham LJ, Cullen MH. The benefits of chemotherapy in patient subgroups with unresectable non-small-cell lung cancer. Ann Oncol 2001; 12:1671.

13. Grilli R, Oxman AD, Julian JA. Chemotherapy for advanced non-small-cell lung cancer: how much benefit is enough? J Clin Oncol 1993; 11:1866.

14. Marino P, Pampallona S, Preatoni A, Cantoni A, Inveinezzi F. Chemotherapy vs. supportive care in advanced non-small cell lung cancer: results of a meta-analysis of the literature. Chest 1994; 106:861.

15. Anonymous. Chemotherapy in non-small cell lung cancer: a meta-analysis using updated data on individual patients from 52 randomized clinical trials. Non-small Cell Lung Cancer Collaborative Group. BMJ 1995; 311:899.

16. Depierre A, Lemarie E, Dabouis G, Garnier G, Jacoulet P, Dalphin J. A phase II study of Navelbine (Vinorelbine) in the treatment of non-small-cell lung cancer. Am J Clin Oncol 1991; 14:115.

17. Fukuoka M, Niitani H, Suzuki A, Motomiya M, Hasegawa K, Nishiwaki Y, Kuriyama T, Ariyoshi Y, Negoro S, Masuda N, Nakajima S, Taguchi T. A phase II study of CPT-11, a new derivative of camptothecin, for previously untreated non-small-cell lung cancer. J Clin Oncol 1992; 10:16.

18. Murphy W, Fossella F, Winn R, Shin D, Hynes H, Gross H, Davilla E, Leimert J, Dhingra H, Raber M, Krakoff I, Hong W. Phase II study of taxol in patients with untreated advanced non-small-cell lung cancer. J Natl Cancer Inst 1993; 85:384.

19. Francis PA, Rigas JR, Kris MG, Pisters KM, Orazem JP, Woolley KJ, Heelan RT. Phase II trial of docetaxel in patients with stage III and IV non-small-cell lung cancer. J Clin Oncol 1994; 12:1232.

20. Fossella FV, Lippman SM, Shin DM, Tarassoff P, Calayag-Jung M, Perez-Soler R, Lee JS, Murphy WK, Glisson B, Rivera E, Hong WK. Maximum-tolerated dose defined for single-agent gemcitabine: a phase I dose-escalation study in chemotherapy-naive patients with advanced non-small-cell lung cancer. J Clin Oncol 1997; 15:310.

21. Anonymous. Effects of vinorelbine on quality of life and survival of elderly patients with advanced non-small cell lung cancer. The Elderly Lung Cancer Vinorelbine Italian Study Group. J Natl Cancer Inst 1999; 91:66.

22. Anderson H, Hopwood P, Stephens R, Thatcher N, Cottier B, Nicholson M, Milroy R, Maughan T, Falk S, Bond M, Burt P, Connolly C, McIllmurray M, Carmichael J. Gemcitabine plus best supportive care (BSC) vs BSC in inoperable non-small cell lung cancer–a randomized trial with quality of life as the primary outcome. UK NSCLC Gemcitabine Group. Non-Small Cell Lung Cancer. Br J Cancer 2000; 83:447.

23. Ranson M, Davidson N, Nicolson M, Falk S, Carmichael J, Lopez P, Anderson H, Gustafson N, Jeynes A, Gallant G, Washington T, Thatcher N. Randomized trial of paclitaxel plus supportive care versus supportive care for patients with advanced non-small-cell lung cancer. J Natl Cancer Inst 2000; 92:1074.

24. Roszkowski K, Pluzanska A, Krzakowski M, Smith A, Saigi E, Aasebo U, Parisi A, Tran N, Olivares R, Berille J. A multicenter, randomized, phase III study of docetaxel plus best supportive care versus best supportive care in chemotherapy-naive patients with metastatic or non-resectable localized non-small cell lung cancer (NSCLC). Lung Cancer 2000; 27:145.

25. Wozniak AJ, Crowley JJ, Balcerzak SP, Weiss GR, Spiridonidis CH, Baker LH, Albain KS, Kelly K, Taylor SA, Gandara DR, Livingston RB. Randomized trial comparing cisplatin with cisplatin plus vinorelbine in the treatment of advanced non-small-cell lung cancer: a Southwest Oncology Group study. J Clin Oncol 1998; 16:2459.

26. Gatzemeier U, von Pawel J, Gottfried M, Velde G, Mattson K, DeMarinis F, Harper P, Salvati F, Robinet G, Lucenti A, Bogaerts J, Gallant G. Phase III comparative study of high-dose cisplatin versus a combination of paclitaxel and cisplatin in patients with advanced non-small-cell lung cancer. J Clin Oncol 2000; 18:3390.

27. Sandler A, Nemunaitis J, Denham C, Von Pawel J, Cormier Y, Gatzemeier U, Mattson K, Manegold C, Palmer M, Gregor A, Nguyen B, Niyikiza C, Einhorn L. Phase III trial of gemcitabine plus cisplatin versus cisplatin alone in patients with locally advanced or metastatic non-small cell lung cancer. J Clin Oncol 2000; 18:122.

28. von Pawel J, von Roemeling R, Gatzemeier U, Boyer M, Elisson L, Clark P, Talbot D, Rey A, Butler T, Hirsh V, Olver I, Bergman B, Ayoub J, Richardson G, Dunlop D, Arcenas A, Vescio R, Viallet J, Treat J. Tirapazamine plus cisplatin versus cisplatin in advanced non-small-cell lung cancer: A report of the international CATAPULT I study group. Cisplatin and tirapazamine in subjects with advanced previously untreated non-small-cell lung tumors. J Clin Oncol 2000; 18:1351.

29. Rosell R, Gatzemeier U, Betticher D, Keppler U, Macha H, Pirker R, Berthet P, Breau J, Lianes P, Nicholson M, Ardizzoni A, Chemaissani A, Bogaerts J, Gallant G. Phase III randomized trial comparing paclitaxel/carboplatin with paclitaxel/cisplatin in patients with advance non-small cell lung cancer: a cooperative multinational trial. Ann Oncol 2000; 13:1539.

30. Fossella F, Pereira JR, von Pawel J, Pluzanska A, Gorbounova V, Kaukel E, Mattson KV, Ramlau R, Szczesna A, Fidias P, Millward M, Belani CP. Randomized, multinational, phase III study of docetaxel plus platinum combinations versus vinorelbine plus cisplatin for advanced non-small-cell lung cancer: the TAX 326 study group. J Clin Oncol 2003; 21:3016.

31. Zatloukal P, Petruzelka L, Zemanova M, Kolek V, Skrickova J, Pesek M, Fojtu H, Grygarkova II, Sixtova D, Roubec J, Horenkova E, Havel L, Prusa P, Novakova L, Skacel T, Kuta M. Gemcitabine plus cisplatin vs. gemcitabine plus carboplatin in stage IIIb and IV non-small cell lung cancer: a phase III randomized trial. Lung Cancer 2003; 41:321.

32. Paccagnella A, Favaretto A, Oniga F, Barbieri F, Ceresoli G, Torri W, Villa E, Verusio C, Cetto GL, Santo A, De Pan-

gher V, Artioli F, Cacciani GC, Parodi G, Soresi F, Ghi MG, Morabito A, Biason R, Giusto M, Mosconi P, Chiarion Sileni V. Cisplatin versus carboplatin in combination with mitomycin and vinblastine in advanced non small cell lung cancer. A multicenter, randomized phase III trial. Lung Cancer 2004; 43:83.

33. Schiller JH, Harrington D, Belani CP, Langer C, Sandler A, Krook J, Zhu J, Johnson DH. Comparison of four chemotherapy regimens for advanced non-small-cell lung cancer. N Engl J Med 2002; 346:92.

34. Jelic S, Mitrovic L, Radosavljevic D, Elezar E, Babovic N, Kovcin V, Tomasevic Z, Kovacevic S, Gavrilovic D, Radulovic S. Survival advantage for carboplatin substituting cisplatin in combination with vindesine and mitomycin C for stage IIIB and IV squamous-cell bronchogenic carcinoma: a randomized phase III study. Lung Cancer 2001; 34:1.

35. Hotta K, Matsuo K, Ueoka H, Kiura K, Tabata M, Tanimoto M. Meta-analysis of randomized clinical trials comparing Cisplatin to Carboplatin in patients with advanced non-small-cell lung cancer. J Clin Oncol 2004; 22:3852.

36. Zojwalla N, Raftopoulos H, Gralla RJ. Are cisplatin and carboplatin equivalent in the treatment of non-small cell lung carcinoma (NSCLC)? Results of a comprehensive review of randomized studies in over 2300 patients. Am Soc Clin Oncol 2004; 22:633a.

37. Le Chevalier T, Brisgand D, Douillard J, Pujol J, Alberola V, Monnier A, Riviere A, Lianes P, Chomy P, Cigolari S, Gottfried P, Ruffie P, Panizo A, Gaspard M, Ravaioli A, Beserval M, Besson F, Martinez A, Berthaud P, Tursz T. Randomized study of vinorelbine and cisplatin versus vindesine and cisplatin versus vinorelbine alone in advanced non-small-cell lung cancer: results of a European multicenter trial including 612 patients. J Clin Oncol 1994; 12:360.

38. ten Bokkel Huinink WW, Bergman B, Chemaissani A, Dornoff W, Drings P, Kellokumpu-Lehtinen PL, Liippo K, Mattson K, von Pawel J, Ricci S, Sederholm C, Stahel RA, Wagenius G, Walree NV, Manegold C. Single-agent gemcitabine: an active and better tolerated alternative to standard cisplatin-based chemotherapy in locally advanced or metastatic non small cell lung cancer. Lung Cancer 1999; 26:85.

39. Sederholm S. Gemcitabine (G) compared with gemcitabine plus carboplatin (GC) in advanced non small cell lung cancer (NSCLC): a phase III study by the Swedish Lung Cancer Study Group (SLUSG). Proc Am Soc Clin Oncol 2002; 21:291a.

40. Negoro S, Masuda N, Takada Y, Sugiura T, Kudoh S, Katakami N, Ariyoshi Y, Ohashi Y, Niitani H, Fukuoka M. Randomised phase III trial of irinotecan combined with cisplatin for advanced non-small-cell lung cancer. Br J Cancer 2003; 88:335.

41. Vansteenkiste J, Vandebroek J, Nackaerts K, Dooms C, Galdermans D, Bosquee L, Delobbe A, Deschepper K, Van Kerckhoven W, Vandeurzen K, Deman R, D'Odemont JP, Siemons L, Van den Brande P, Dams N. Influence of cisplatin-use, age, performance status and duration of chemotherapy on symptom control in advanced non-small cell lung cancer: detailed symptom analysis of a randomised study comparing cisplatin-vindesine to gemcitabine. Lung Cancer 2003; 40:191.

42. Georgoulias V, Ardavanis A, Agelidou A, Agelidou M, Chandrinos V, Tsaroucha E, Toumbis M, Kouroussis C, Syrigos K, Polyzos A, Samaras N, Papakotoulas P, Christofilakis C, Ziras N, Alegakis A. Docetaxel versus docetaxel plus cisplatin as front-line treatment of patients with advanced non-small-cell lung cancer: a randomized, multicenter phase III trial. J Clin Oncol 2004; 22:2602.

43. Lilenbaum RC, Herndon JE 2nd, List MA, Desch C, Watson DM, Miller AA, Graziano SL, Perry MC, Saville W, Chahinian P, Weeks JC, Holland JC, Green MR. Single-

agent versus combination chemotherapy in advanced non-small-cell lung cancer: the cancer and leukemia group B (study 9730). J Clin Oncol 2005; 23:190.

44. Hotta K, Matsuo K, Ueoka H, Kiura K, Tabata M, Tanimoto M. Addition of platinum compounds to a new agent in patients with advanced non-small-cell lung cancer: a literature based meta-analysis of randomised trials. Ann Oncol 2004; 15:1782.

45. Belani C, Natale R, Lee J, Socinski M, Robert F, Waterhouse D, Rowland K, Ansari R, Lilenbaum R, Sridhar K. Randomized phase III trial comparing cisplatin/etoposide versus carboplatin/paclitaxel in advanced and metastatic non-small cell lung cancer (NSCLC). Proc Am Soc Clin Oncol 1998; 17:455a.

46. Giaccone G, Splinter TA, Debruyne C, Kho GS, Lianes P, van Zandwijk N, Pennucci MC, Scagliotti G, van Meerbeeck J, van Hoesel Q, Curran D, Sahmoud T, Postmus PE. Randomized study of paclitaxel-cisplatin versus cisplatin-teniposide in patients with advanced non-small-cell lung cancer. The European Organization for Research and Treatment of Cancer Lung Cancer Cooperative Group. J Clin Oncol 1998; 16:2133.

47. Cardenal F, Lopez-Cabrerizo M, Anton A, Alberola V, Massuti B, Carrato A, Barneto I, Lomas M, Garcia M, Lianes P, Montalar J, Vadell C, Gonzalez-Larriba J, Nguyen B, Artal A, Rosell R. Randomized phase III study of gemcitabine-cisplatin versus etoposide- cisplatin in the treatment of locally advanced or metastatic non-small-cell lung cancer. J Clin Oncol 1999; 17:12.

48. Bonomi P, Kim K, Fairclough D, Cella D, Kugler J, Rowinsky E, Hiroutek M, Johnson D. Comparison of survival and quality of life in advanced non-small cell lung cancer patients treated with two dose levels of paclitaxel combined with cisplatin versus etoposide with cisplatin: results of an Eastern Cooperative Oncology Group trial. J Clin Oncol 2000; 18:623.

49. Takiguchi Y, Nagao K, Nishiwaki A. The final results of a randomized phase III trial comparing irinotecan (CPT-11) and cisplatin (CDDP) with vindesine (VDS) and CDDP in advanced non-small cell lung cancer (NSCLC). Proceedings of the Ninth World Conference on Lung Cancer. Tokyo 2000; 29:28a.

50. Grigorescu AC, Draghici IN, Nitipir C, Gutulescu N, Corlan E. Gemcitabine (GEM) and carboplatin (CBDCA) versus cisplatin (CDDP) and vinblastine (VLB) in advanced non-small-cell lung cancer (NSCLC) stages III and IV: a phase III randomised trial. Lung Cancer 2002; 37:9.

51. Kubota K, Watanabe K, Kunitoh H, Noda K, Ichinose Y, Katakami N, Sugiura T, Kawahara M, Yokoyama A, Yokota S, Yoneda S, Matsui K, Kudo S, Shibuya M, Isobe T, Segawa Y, Nishiwaki Y, Ohashi Y, Niitani H. Phase III randomized trial of docetaxel plus cisplatin versus vindesine plus cisplatin in patients with stage IV non-small-cell lung cancer: the Japanese Taxotere Lung Cancer Study Group. J Clin Oncol 2004; 22:254.

52. Baggstrom M, Socinski M, Hensing T, Poole C. Third generation chemotherapy regimens (3GR) improve survival over second generation regimens (2GR) in stage IIIB/IV non-small cell lung cancer (NSCLC): A meta-analysis of the published literature. Proc Am Soc Clin Oncol 2002; 21:306a.

53. Yana T. New chemotherapy agent plus platinum for advanced non-small cell lung cancer: a meta-analysis. Am Soc Clin Oncol, 2002; 21:328a.

54. Kosmidis P, Mylonakis N, Skarlos D, Samantas E, Dimopoulos M, Papadimitriou C, Kalophonos C, Pavlidis N, Nikolaidis C, Papaconstantinou C, Fountzilas G. Paclitaxel (175 mg/m^2) plus carboplatin (6 AUC) versus paclitaxel (225 mg/m^2) plus carboplatin (6 AUC) in advanced non-small-cell lung cancer (NSCLC): a multicenter randomized

trial. Hellenic Cooperative Oncology Group (HeCOG). Ann Oncol 2000; 11:799.

55. Kelly K, Crowley J, Bunn P, Present C, Grevstad P, Moinpour C, Ramsey S, Wozniak A, Weiss G, Moore D, Israel V, Livingston R, Gandara D. Randomized phase III trial of paclitaxel plus carboplatin versus vinorelbine plus cisplatin in the treatment of patients with advanced non-small-cell lung cancer: a Southwest Oncology Group trial. J Clin Oncol 2001; 19:3210.

56. Huang C, Langer C, Minniti C, Nahum K, Seldomridge J, Hutter B, Mintzer D. Phase III toxicity trial of carboplatin (Cb) plus either docetaxel (D) or paclitaxel (P) in advanced non-small cell lung cancer (NSCLC): Preliminary findings of OPN-001. Proc Am Soc Clin Oncol 2002; 21:337a.

57. Scagliotti G, De Marinis F, Rinaldi M, Crino L, Gridelli C, Ricci S, Matano E, Boni C, Marangolo M, Failla G, Altavilla G, Adamo V, Ceribelli A, Clerici M, Di Costanzo F, Frontini L, Tonato M. Phase III randomized trial comparing three platinum-based doublets in advanced non-small-cell lung cancer. J Clin Oncol 2002; 20:4285.

58. Gebbia V, Galetta D, Caruso M, Verderame F, Pezzella G, Valdesi M, Borsellino N, Pandolfo G, Durini E, Rinaldi M, Loizzi M, Gebbia N, Valenza R, Tirrito M, Varvara F, Colucci G. Gemcitabine and cisplatin versus vinorelbine and cisplatin versus ifosfamide+gemcitabine followed by vinorelbine and cisplatin versus vinorelbine and cisplatin followed by ifosfamide and gemcitabine in stage IIIB-IV non small cell lung carcinoma: a prospective randomized phase III trial of the Gruppo Oncologico Italia Meridionale. Lung Cancer 2003; 39:179.

59. Belani C. A multicenter, phase III randomized trial for stage IIIB/IV NSCLC of weekly paclitaxel and carboplatin vs. standard paclitaxel and carboplatin given every three weeks, followed by weekly paclitaxel. Proc Am Soc Clin Oncol, 2004; 22(14S):621a.

60. Kubota K. The Four-Arm Cooperative Study (FACS) for advanced non-small-cell lung cancer (NSCLC). Proc Am Soc Clin Oncol 2004; 22(14s):618s.

61. Martoni A, Marino A, Sperandi F, Giaquinta S, Di Fabio F, Melotti B, Guaraldi M, Palomba G, Preti P, Petralia A, Artioli F, Picece V, Farris A, Mantovani L. Multicentre randomised phase III study comparing the same dose and schedule of cisplatin plus the same schedule of vinorelbine or gemcitabine in advanced non-small cell lung cancer. Eur J Cancer 2005; 41:81.

62. Ruckdeschel J, Finkelstein D, Ettinger D, Creech R, Mason B, Joss R, Vogl S. A randomized trial of the four most active regimens for metastatic non small cell lung cancer. J Clin Oncol 1986; 4:14.

63. Weick J, Crowley J, Natale R, Hom B, Rivkin S, Coltman C, Taylor S, Livingston R. A randomized trial of five cisplatin-containing treatments in patients with metastatic non-small cell lung cancer: A Southwest Oncology Group Study. J Clin Oncol 1991; 9:1157.

64. Le Chevalier T, Scagliotti G, Natale R, Danson S, Rosell R, Stahel R, Thomas P, Rudd RM, Vansteenkiste J, Thatcher N, Manegold C, Pujol JL, van Zandwijk N, Gridelli C, van Meerbeeck JP, Crino L, Brown A, Fitzgerald P, Aristides M, Schiller JH. Efficacy of gemcitabine plus platinum chemotherapy compared with other platinum containing regimens in advanced non-small-cell lung cancer: a meta-analysis of survival outcomes. Lung Cancer 2005; 47:69.

65. Harper P, Plunkett T, Khayat D. Quality trials and quality of life in non-small-cell lung cancer. J Clin Oncol 2003; 21:3007.

66. Crino L, Scagliotti G, Ricci S, De Marinis F, Rinaldi M, Gridelli C, Ceribelli A, Bianco R, Marangolo M, Di Costanzo F, Sassi M, Barni S, Ravaioli A, Adamo V, Portalone L, Cruciani G, Masotti A, Ferrara G, Gozzelino F, Tonato M. Gemcitabine and cisplatin versus mitomycin, ifosfa-

mide, and cisplatin in advanced non-small-cell lung cancer: a randomized phase III study of the Italian Lung Cancer Project. J Clin Oncol 1999; 17:3522.

67. Comella P, Frasci G, Panza N, Manzione L, De Cataldis G, Cioffi R, Maiorino L, Micillo E, Lorusso V, Di Rienzo G, Filippelli G, Lamberti A, Natale M, Bilancia D, Nicolella G, Di Nota A, Comella G. Randomized trial comparing cisplatin, gemcitabine, and vinorelbine with either cisplatin and gemcitabine or cisplatin and vinorelbine in advanced non-small-cell lung cancer: interim analysis of a phase III trial of the Southern Italy Cooperative Oncology Group. J Clin Oncol 2000; 18:1451.

68. Comella P. Phase III trial of cisplatin/gemcitabine with or without vinorelbine or paclitaxel in advanced non-small cell lung cancer. Semin Oncol 2001; 28:7.

69. Gebbia V, Galetta D, Riccardi F, Gridelli C, Durini E, Borsellino N, Gebbia N, Valdesi M, Caruso M, Valenza R, Pezzella G, Colucci G. Vinorelbine plus cisplatin versus cisplatin plus vindesine and mitomycin C in stage IIIB-IV non-small cell lung carcinoma: a prospective randomized study. Lung Cancer 2002; 37:179.

70. Kodani T, Ueoka H, Kiura K, Tabata M, Takigawa N, Segawa Y, Moritaka T, Hiraki S, Harada M, Tanimoto M. A phase III randomized trial comparing vindesine and cisplatin with or without ifosfamide in patients with advanced non-small-cell lung cancer: long-term follow-up results and analysis of prognostic factors. Lung Cancer 2002; 36:313.

71. Melo M, Barradas P, Costa A, Cristovao M, Alves P. Results of a randomized phase III trial comparing 4 cisplatin (P)-based regimens in the treatment of locally advanced and metastatic non-small cell lung cancer (NSCLC): mitomycin/vinblastine/cisplatin (MVP) is no longer a therapeutic option. Proc Am Soc Clin Oncol 2002; 21:302a.

72. Paccagnella A. Carboplatin/paclitaxel (CP) vs carboplatin/paclitaxel/gemcitabine (CPG) in advanced NSCLC: a phase II-III multicentric study. Proc Am Soc Clin Oncol, 2002; 21:338a.

73. Sculier J, Lafitte J, Lecomte J, Berghmans T, Thiriaux J, Florin M, Efremidis A, Alexopoulos C, Recloux P, Ninane V, Mommen P, Paesmans M, Klastersky J. A three-arm phase III randomised trial comparing combinations of platinum derivatives, ifosfamide and/or gemcitabine in stage IV non-small-cell lung cancer. Ann Oncol 2002; 13:874.

74. Souquet P, Tan E, Rodrigues Pereira J, Van Klaveren R, Price A, Gatzemeier U, Jaworski M, Burillon J, Aubert D. GLOB-1: a prospective randomised clinical phase III trial comparing vinorelbine-cisplatin with vinorelbine-ifosfamide-cisplatin in metastatic non-small-cell lung cancer patients. Ann Oncol 2002; 13:1853.

75. Alberola V, Camps C, Provencio M, Isla D, Rosell R, Vadell C, Bover I, Ruiz-Casado A, Azagra P, Jimenez U, Gonzalez-Larriba JL, Diz P, Cardenal F, Artal A, Carrato A, Morales S, Sanchez JJ, de las Penas R, Felip E, Lopez-Vivanco G. Cisplatin plus gemcitabine versus a cisplatin-based triplet versus nonplatinum sequential doublets in advanced non-small-cell lung cancer: a Spanish Lung Cancer Group phase III randomized trial. J Clin Oncol 2003; 21:3207.

76. Danson S, Middleton MR, O'Byrne KJ, Clemons M, Ranson M, Hassan J, Anderson H, Burt PA, Fairve-Finn C, Stout R, Dowd I, Ashcroft L, Beresford C, Thatcher N. Phase III trial of gemcitabine and carboplatin versus mitomycin, ifosfamide, and cisplatin or mitomycin, vinblastine, and cisplatin in patients with advanced nonsmall cell lung carcinoma. Cancer 2003; 98:542.

77. Williamson S, Crowley J, Lara P, Tucker R, McCoy J, Lau D, Gandara D. S0003: paclitaxel/carboplatin (PC) v PC + tirapazamine (PCT) in advanced non-small cell lung can-

cer (NSCLC). A Southwest Oncology Group (SWOG) trial. Proc Am Soc Clin Oncol 2003; 22:622.

78. Lorigan P. Randomised phase III trial of docetaxel/carboplatin vs MIC/MVP chemotherapy in advanced non-small cell lung cancer (NSCLC) – final results of a British Thoracic Oncology Group (BTOG) trial. Proc Am Soc Clin Oncol 2004; 22(14s):632s.

79. Rudd RM, Gower NH, Spiro SG, Eisen TG, Harper PG, Littler JA, Hatton M, Johnson PW, Martin WM, Rankin EM, James LE, Gregory WM, Qian W, Lee SM. Gemcitabine plus carboplatin versus mitomycin, ifosfamide, and cisplatin in patients with stage IIIB or IV non-small-cell lung cancer: a phase III randomized study of the London Lung Cancer Group. J Clin Oncol 2005; 23:142.

80. Baggstrom MQ, Socinski MA, Hensing TA, Poole C. Addressing the optimal number of cytotoxic agents in stage IIIB/IV non-small cell lung cancer (NSCLC): A meta-analysis of the published literature. Proc Am Soc Clin Oncol 2003; 22:624.

81. Delbaldo C, Michiels S, Syz N, Soria JC, Le Chevalier T, Pignon JP. Benefits of adding a drug to a single-agent or a 2-agent chemotherapy regimen in advanced non-small-cell lung cancer: a meta-analysis. JAMA 2004; 292:470.

82. Depierre A, Quoix E, Mercier M. Maintenance chemotherapy in advanced non-small cell lung cancer (NSCLC): a randomized study of vinorelbine (V) versus observation (OB) in patients (Pts) responding to induction therapy (French Cooperative Oncology Group). Proc Am Soc Clin Oncol 2001; 20:309a.

83. Smith I, O'Brien M, Talbot D, Nicolson M, Mansi J, Hickish T, Norton A, Ashley S. Duration of chemotherapy in advanced non-small-cell lung cancer: a randomized trial of three versus six courses of mitomycin, vinblastine, and cisplatin. J Clin Oncol 2001; 19:1336.

84. Socinski M, Schell M, Peterman A, Bakri K, Yates S, Gitten R, Unger P, Lee J, Lee J, Tynan M, Moore M, Kies M. Phase III trial comparing a defined duration of therapy versus continuous therapy followed by second-line therapy in advanced-stage IIIB/IV non-small cell lung cancer. J Clin Oncol 2002; 20:1335.

85. Andresen O. Duration of chemotherapy and survival in advanced non-small cell lung cancer (NSCLC). A multicenter prospective randomized study. Tenth World Conference on Lung Cancer 2003; 41(S2):S28.

86. Krzakowski M. Gemcitabine and cisplatin (GC) +/– subsequent maintenance therapy with single-agent gemcitabine in advanced non-small cell lung cancer (NSCLC): preliminary results of a randomized trial of the Central European Cooperative Oncology Group (CECOG). Proc Am Soc Clin Oncol 2004; 22(14s):633s.

87. Hutchins LF, Unger JM, Crowley JJ, Coltman CA, Jr., Albain KS. Underrepresentation of patients 65 years of age or older in cancer-treatment trials. N Engl J Med 1999; 341:2061.

88. Montella M, Gridelli C, Crispo A, Scognamiglio F, Ruffolo P, Gatani T, Boccia V, Maione P, Fabbrocini G. Has lung cancer in the elderly different characteristics at presentation? Oncol Rep 2002; 9:1093.

89. Yellen SB, Cella DF, Leslie WT. Age and clinical decision making in oncology patients. J Natl Cancer Inst 1994; 86:1766.

90. Potosky AL, Saxman S, Wallace RB, Lynch CF. Population variations in the initial treatment of non-small-cell lung cancer. J Clin Oncol 2004; 22:3261.

91. Ramsey SD, Howlader N, Etzioni RD, Donato B. Chemotherapy use, outcomes, and costs for older persons with advanced non-small-cell lung cancer: evidence from surveillance, epidemiology and end results-Medicare. J Clin Oncol 2004; 22:4971.

92. Frasci G, Lorusso V, Panza N, Comella P, Nicolella G, Bianco A, De Cataldis G, Iannelli A, Bilancia D, Belli M, Massidda B, Piantedosi F, Comella G, De Lena M. Gemcitabine plus vinorelbine versus vinorelbine alone in elderly patients with advanced non-small-cell lung cancer. J Clin Oncol 2000; 18:2529.

93. Comella G, Comella P, De Cataldis G, Del Gaizo F, Lorusso V, Panza N, Gambardella A, Buzzi F, Muci D, Frasci G. Gemcitabine plus vinorelbine (GV) or paclitaxel (GT) vs gemcitabine (G) or paclitaxel (T) alone in elderly or unfit non-small cell lung cancer (NSCLC) patients. SICOG 9909 phase III trial. Proc Am Soc Clin Oncol 2003; 22:629.

94. Gridelli C, Perrone F, Gallo C, Cigolari S, Rossi A, Piantedosi F, Barbera S, Ferrau F, Piazza E, Rosetti F, Clerici M, Bertetto O, Robbiati S, Frontini L, Sacco C, Castiglione F, Favaretto A, Novello S, Migliorino M, Gasparini G, Galetta D, Iaffaioli R, Gebbia V. Chemotherapy for elderly patients with advanced non-small-cell lung cancer: the Multicenter Italian Lung Cancer in the Elderly Study (MILES) phase III randomized trial. J Natl Cancer Inst 2003; 95:362.

95. Kelly K, Giarritta S, Hayes S, Akerley W, Hesketh P, Wozniak A, Albain KS, Crowley J, Gandara DR. Should older patients (pts) receive combination chemotherapy for advanced stage non-small cell lung cancer (NSCLC)? An analysis of Southwest Oncology Trials 9509 and 9308. Proc Am Soc Clin Oncol 2001; 20:329a.

96. Langer C, Manola J, Bernardo P, Kugler J, Bonomi P, Cella D, Johnson D. Cisplatin-based therapy for elderly patients with advanced non-small-cell lung cancer: implications of Eastern Cooperative Oncology Group 5592, a randomized trial. J Natl Cancer Inst 2002; 94:173.

97. Rocha Lima CM, Herndon JE 2nd, Kosty M, Clamon G, Green MR. Therapy choices among older patients with lung carcinoma: an evaluation of two trials of the Cancer and Leukemia Group B. Cancer 2002; 94:181.

98. Fossella F, Belani C. Phase III study (TAX 326) of docetaxel-cisplatin (DC) and docetaxel-carboplatin (DCb) versus vinorelbine-cisplatin (VC) for the first-line treatment of advanced/metastatic non-small-cell lung cancer (NSCLC): analyses in elderly patients. Proc Am Soc Clin Oncol 2003; 22:629.

99. Langer CJ, Vangel MG, Schiller J, Harrington DP, Sandler A, Belani CP, Johnson D. Age-specific subanalysis of ECOG 1594: fit elderly patients (70-80 YRS) with NSCLC do as well as younger patients (<70). In: Grunberg SM (ed) Am Soc Clin Oncol, Chicago: ASCO, 2003; 22:639.

100. Hensing TA, Peterman AH, Schell MJ, Lee JH, Socinski MA. The impact of age on toxicity, response rate, quality of life, and survival in patients with advanced, stage IIIB or IV nonsmall cell lung carcinoma treated with carboplatin and paclitaxel. Cancer 2003; 98:779.

101. Earle CC, Tsai JS, Gelber RD, Weinstein MC, Neumann PJ, Weeks JC. Effectiveness of chemotherapy for advanced lung cancer in the elderly: instrumental variable and propensity analysis. J Clin Oncol 2001; 19:1064.

102. Peake MD, Thompson S, Lowe D, Pearson MG. Ageism in the management of lung cancer. Age Ageing 2003; 32:171.

103. Gridelli C, Maione P, Barletta E. Individualized chemotherapy for elderly patients with nonsmall cell lung cancer. Curr Opin Oncol 2002; 14:199.

104. Minami H, Ohe Y, Niho S, Goto K, Ohmatsu H, Kubota K, Kakinuma R, Nishiwaki Y, Nokihara H, Sekine I, Saijo N, Hanada K, Ogata H. Comparison of pharmacokinetics and pharmacodynamics of docetaxel and Cisplatin in elderly and non-elderly patients: why is toxicity increased in elderly patients? J Clin Oncol 2004; 22:2901.

105. Rosell R, Lord RV, Taron M, Reguart N. DNA repair and cisplatin resistance in non-small-cell lung cancer. Lung Cancer 2002b; 38:217.

106. Gurubhagavatula S, Liu G, Park S, Zhou W, Su L, Wain JC, Lynch TJ, Neuberg DS, Christiani DC. XPD and XRCC1 genetic polymorphisms are prognostic factors in advanced non-small-cell lung cancer patients treated with platinum chemotherapy. J Clin Oncol 2004; 22:2594.

107. Lord RV, Brabender J, Gandara D, Alberola V, Camps C, Domine M, Cardenal F, Sanchez JM, Gumerlock PH, Taron M, Sanchez JJ, Danenberg KD, Danenberg PV, Rosell R. Low ERCC1 expression correlates with prolonged survival after cisplatin plus gemcitabine chemotherapy in non-small cell lung cancer. Clin Cancer Res 2002; 8:2286.

108. Ryu JS, Hong YC, Han HS, Lee JE, Kim S, Park YM, Kim YC, Hwang TS. Association between polymorphisms of ERCC1 and XPD and survival in non-small-cell lung cancer patients treated with cisplatin combination chemotherapy. Lung Cancer 2004; 44:311.

109. Rosell R, Taron M, Alberola V, Massuti B, Felip E. Genetic testing for chemotherapy in non-small cell lung cancer. Lung Cancer 2003; 41 (Suppl 1): S97.

110. Sarries C. Combined DNA repair gene single nucleotide polymorphisms (SNPs) in gemcitabine (gem)/cisplatin (cis)-treated non-small-cell lung cancer (NSCLC) patients (p). Proc Am Soc Clin Oncol 2004; 22(14s):624s.

111. Monnet I, Brienza S, Hugret F, Voisin S, Gastiaburu J, Saltiel JC, Soulie P, Armand JP, Cvitkovic E, de Cremoux H. Phase II study of oxaliplatin in poor-prognosis non-small cell lung cancer (NSCLC). ATTIT. Association pour le Traitement des Tumeurs Intra Thoraciques. Eur J Cancer 1998; 34:1124.

112. Monnet I, de CH, Soulie P, Saltiel-Voisin S, Bekradda M, Saltiel JC, Brain E, Rixe O, Yataghene Y, Misset JL, Cvitkovic E. Oxaliplatin plus vinorelbine in advanced non-small-cell lung cancer: final results of a multicenter phase II study. Ann Oncol 2002; 13:103.

113. Franciosi V, Barbieri R, Aitini E, Vasini G, Cacciani GC, Capra R, Camisa R, Cascinu S. Gemcitabine and oxaliplatin: a safe and active regimen in poor prognosis advanced non-small cell lung cancer patients. Lung Cancer 2003; 41:101.

114. Winegarden JD, Mauer AM, Otterson GA, Rudin CM, Villalona-Calero MA, Lanzotti VJ, Szeto L, Kasza K, Hoffman PC, Vokes EE. A phase II study of oxaliplatin and paclitaxel in patients with advanced non-small-cell lung cancer. Ann Oncol 2004; 15:915.

115. Schiller JH. Small cell lung cancer: defining a role for emerging platinum drugs. Oncology 2002; 63:105.

116. Sessa C, Minoia C, Ronchi A, Zucchetti M, Bauer J, Borner M, de Jong J, Pagani O, Renard J, Weil C, D'Incalci M. Phase I clinical and pharmacokinetic study of the oral platinum analogue JM216 given daily for 14 days. Ann Oncol 1998; 9:1315.

117. George CM, Haraf DJ, Mauer AM, Krauss SA, Hoffman PC, Rudin CM, Szeto L, Vokes EE. A phase I trial of the oral platinum analogue JM216 with concomitant radiotherapy in advanced malignancies of the chest. Invest New Drugs 2001; 19:303.

118. Judson I, Cerny T, Epelbaum R, Dunlop D, Smyth J, Schaefer B, Roelvink M, Kaplan S, Hanauske A. Phase II trial of the oral platinum complex JM216 in non-small-cell lung cancer: an EORTC early clinical studies group investigation. Ann Oncol 1997; 8:604.

119. Hirose T, Horichi N, Ohmori T, Shirai T, Sohma S, Yamaoka T, Ohnishi T, Adachi M. Phase I study of the combination of gemcitabine and nedaplatin for treatment of previously untreated advanced non small cell lung cancer. Lung Cancer 2003; 39:91.

120. Kurata T, Tamura K, Yamamoto N, Nogami T, Satoh T, Kaneda H, Nakagawa K, Fukuoka M. Combination phase I study of nedaplatin and gemcitabine for advanced non-small-cell lung cancer. Br J Cancer 2004; 90:2092.

121. Oshita F, Yamada K, Kato Y, Ikehara M, Noda K, Tanaka G, Nomura I, Suzuki R, Saito H. Phase I/II study of escalating doses of nedaplatin in combination with irinotecan for advanced non-small-cell lung cancer. Cancer Chemother Pharmacol 2003; 52:73.

122. Takigawa N, Segawa Y, Ueoka H, Kiura K, Tabata M, Shibayama T, Takata I, Miyamoto H, Eguchi K, Harada M. Combination of nedaplatin and vindesine for treatment of relapsed or refractory non-small-cell lung cancer. Cancer Chemother Pharmacol 2000; 46:272.

Non-Platinum-Based Chemotherapy for Advanced Non-Small-Cell Lung Cancer

23

Giorgio V. Scagliotti and Giovanni Selvaggi

Contents

23.1 Introduction

Although it has been considered as a therapeutic alternative by the 2004 American Society of Clinical Oncology (ASCO) clinical guideline update [1], the value of non-platinum-based chemotherapy in the treatment of advanced non-small-cell lung cancer (NSCLC) remains a matter of debate. For patients with good Eastern Cooperative Oncology Group (ECOG) performance status (PS=0 and 1) and without significant weight loss (>5% in the 6-month period before diagnosis), cisplatin-based chemotherapy remains the cornerstone of treatment for unresectable, locally advanced and metastatic NSCLC. This information was generated by several meta-analyses [2–4]. In the largest one, based on individual patient data [4], patients with metastatic NSCLC receiving cisplatin-based chemotherapy showed in the 1st year after diagnosis a 27% reduction in the risk of death when compared to those treated with best supportive care alone; this translated into a 10% absolute improvement in the 1-year survival rate, which means a 1.5-month increment in median survival time. This meta-analysis evaluated the first- and second-generation platinum-based regimens (developed in the 1980s) before the third generation of cytotoxic agents (developed in the 1990s) including vinorelbine, docetaxel, paclitaxel, and gemcitabine established their efficacy in advanced NSCLC when combined with cisplatin and carboplatin. When compared with each other in specifically designed randomized trials, these platinum doublets including third-generation agents showed a comparable level of efficacy: the median survival time of treated patients ranged between 8.0 and 10 months, with a 1-year survival rate ranging from 31 to 43% (depending upon the proportion of stage IV patients enrolled into the individual trials) [5, 6]. Although some data seem to favor gemcitabine-based chemotherapy [7], there is clear evidence that in advanced NSCLC, standard platinum-based chemotherapy has reached a therapeutic plateau [5, 6, 8, 9]. Further improvement in efficacy with new analogues and new cytotoxic agents are quite unlikely. Therefore, the issues regarding toxicity profiles of each combination and quality of life of the patients have become priorities in the choice of the treatment.

In addition to the disappointing overall patient survival, the many toxicities associated with cisplatin, including nausea and vomiting, renal toxicity often requiring hospitalization for appropriate treatment, and long-lasting ototoxicity and cumulative peripheral neuropathy, are all of great concern for the quality of life of treated patients. Platinum-based regimens may be particularly poorly tolerated in elderly patients and patients with poor PS. Furthermore, because cisplatin needs to be routinely infused along a hydration program, its administration is extremely time-consuming. The limited efficacy associated with occasional cumbersome toxicities and the long-lasting administration schedule have led several physicians to avoid the routine use of cisplatin-based chemotherapy in the medical management of advanced NSCLC. Furthermore, cellular resistance to cisplatin has been found to be associated with elevated mRNA levels of excision repair cross-complement group 1 (*ERCC1*), a DNA-repair gene, in tumor tissues [10, 11]. High ERCC1 levels have also been associated with shorter survival in NSCLC patients treated with cisplatin/gemcitabine [12]. Therefore, NSCLC patients with high levels of ERCC1 could potentially benefit more from effective non-platinum-based cytotoxic therapy. Ongoing randomized trials are currently prospectively testing this hypothesis (e.g., the GILT trial).

To avoid the use of cisplatin, different strategies have been investigated, including the substitution of cisplatin with its analogue carboplatin and the use of nonplatinum combinations. Although it is arguable whether cisplatin produces a better survival outcome than carboplatin in advanced NSCLC [13, 14], the available results confer a marginal superiority for cisplatin, but toxicity is definitely more manageable with carboplatin. A recently published meta-analysis of 8 randomized clinical trials in patients with advanced NSCLC comparing cisplatin to carboplatin in 2,948 patients with advanced NSCLC [15, 16] found that combination chemotherapy consisting of cisplatin plus a third-generation agent (gemcitabine, taxanes) yields a substantial survival advantage compared with carboplatin plus a new agent, although it failed to find any survival difference in an analysis that included both new and old agents (etoposide, mitomycin C, vindesine, vinblastine). However, the strength of the conclusion of this specific meta-analysis is limited because only abstracted data were used, and careful interpretation is thus required.

Another strategy to avoid cisplatin side effects is to shift toward nonplatinum combination regimens. This therapeutic possibility relies on the consideration that most of the third-generation agents (vinorelbine, gemcitabine, and the taxanes) have shown a response rate of around 20% as single agents in chemotherapy-nave patients. The equivalence in efficacy of gemcitabine to the older combination of cisplatin/etoposide and to cisplatin/vindesine [17, 18] has emerged from randomized trials. In addition, a Japanese trial showed the equivalence of single-agent irinotecan when compared with the combination of cisplatin/irinotecan [19]. However, as clearly demonstrated in a huge meta-analysis summarizing the clinical experience of more than 20 years and including more than 13,600 patients from randomized clinical trials, when doublet regimens were compared to single-agent regimens, a significant increase in tumor response and 1-year and median survival time was observed in favor of the doublet regimens. When a third agent was added to a doublet, a further improvement in response rate but no additional benefits in 1-year and median survival were observed [20].

Most of the new nonplatinum agents have a markedly decreased toxicity profile, and when combined with each other in doublets, they usually lack of overlapping toxicities. This rationale was the driving force behind the exploratory phase II programs that aimed to investigate the activity of several nonplatinum doublets. Based on promising phase II data for some of these nonplatinum doublets showing an improved tolerability without losing ground on efficacy, the same combinations have been subsequently challenged against platinum-based combinations in the phase III setting.

23.2   Gemcitabine and the Taxanes

23.2.1   Gemcitabine/Paclitaxel

Gemcitabine and the taxanes (e.g., paclitaxel and docetaxel) are characterized by different mechanisms of action. Gemcitabine is a nucleoside analogue that is structurally related to cytarabine [21], while paclitaxel enhances microtubular assembly and stabilizes microtubules. In NSCLC cell lines, paclitaxel enhances the antitumor activity of gemcitabine and the combination has an additive effect [22]. Both sequences have been examined: gemcitabine before paclitaxel, and paclitaxel before gemcitabine. The administration of paclitaxel before gemcitabine induced a higher apoptotic index in NSCLC cells [23].

Gemcitabine and paclitaxel are easy to administer, and administration may occur every 3 weeks or weekly on an outpatient basis. Potentially, weekly administration offers frequent exposure of tumor cells and multiple targeting of clones with different growth kinetics. Single-agent gemcitabine, administered three times per week every 4 weeks, was investigated extensively in patients with chemotherapy-naive advanced NSCLC and showed response rates of approximately 20% [24, 25]. Gemcitabine has also demonstrated preclinical and clinical evidence of synergism with cisplatin, with remission rates of 52–54% for the combination in phase II trials [26, 27].

Paclitaxel has produced overall response rates ranging from 20 to 42% in previously untreated patients with advanced NSCLC, with a 1-year survival rate of approximately 40% [28–30]. The combination of paclitaxel and cisplatin has produced good responses in both chemotherapy-naive and previously treated patients with NSCLC, with neurotoxicity found to be the dose-limiting factor [31, 32].

These agents are characterized by at least partially nonoverlapping toxicities: both can cause myelosuppression, which does not usually require the use of hematopoietic growth factor support or significant dose reduction, which would compromise efficacy. Paclitaxel can cause peripheral neuropathy and alopecia, whereas gemcitabine can produce a flu-like syndrome, fever, rash, and elevation of liver enzymes.

Several phase I and II studies have tested the combination of gemcitabine and paclitaxel in chemonaive patients with NSCLC (Table 23.1) and they have shown response rates ranging from 24 to 47%, and reporting generally mild toxicities [33–37]. Pulmonary damage such as interstitial pneumonitis has been described, although at a very low incidence (3%). When a 3-week schedule was used, paclitaxel at 200 mg/m^2 or 175 mg/m^2) on day 1 and gemcitabine at 1,000 mg/m^2 on days 1 and 8 were the preferred doses. Alternative schedules

Table 23.1. Gemcitabine/paclitaxel: phase II trials. *Pts* Patients, *RR* response rates, *MST* median survival time, *d* days, *Q 3-wk every 3 weeks*, *GEM* gemcitabine, *PAC* paclitaxel, *NR* not reported

Author, year	GEM (mg/m^2)	PAC (mg/m^2)	Schedule	Pts n	RR (%)	MST (months)
Auerbach, 2000	1,000; d 1, 8	175 d 1	Q 3-wk	20	46	7
Giaccone, 2000	1,000; d 1, 8	150–200 d 1	Q 3-wk	49	24	NR
Douillard, 2001	1,000; d 1, 8	200 d 1	Q 3-wk	54	35	13
Isla, 2001	2,000; d 1, 15	150 d 1, 15	Q 4-wk	89	32	9.9
Bhatia, 2002	1,000; d 1, 8, 15	110 d 1, 8, 15	Q 4-wk	40	38	5
Chen, 2002	1,000; d 1, 8	175 d 1	Q 3-wk	90	40	12.6
Hirsch, 2003	1,000; d 1, 8	100 d 1, 8	Q 3-wk	40	55	9.8

Table 23.2. Gemcitabine/paclitaxel: phase III clinical trials. *CIS* Cisplatin, *CARBO* carboplatin, *AUC* area under the plasma concentration–time curve

Author, year	Regimen (Q 3-wk)	Pts n	RR (%)	MST (months)	One-year survival (%)
Kosmidis, 2002	GEM 1,000 mg/m^2; d 1, 8	257	35	9.8	41
	PAC 200 mg/m^2; d 1	252	28	10.4	41
	PAC 200 mg/m^2; d 1				
	CARBO AUC 6; d 1				
Smit, 2003	GEM 1,250 mg/m^2; d 1, 8	161	27	6.7	26
	PAC 175 mg/m^2; d 1	160	36	8.9	33
	GEM 1,250 mg/m^2; d 1, 8	159	32	8.1	35
	CIS 80 mg/m^2; d 1				
	PAC 175 mg/m^2; d 1				
	CIS 80 mg/m^2; d 1				

were also investigated: Spanish investigators assessed a biweekly regimen with gemcitabine 2,000 mg/m^2 plus paclitaxel 150 mg/m^2, reporting in 89 patients with advanced stage NSCLC a response rate of 32% and a median survival of 9.9 months, in the absence of grade 3 and 4 myelotoxicity. Another study conducted in 40 patients [38] administered gemcitabine 1,000 mg/m^2 plus paclitaxel 100 mg/m^2, on days 1 and 8 every 3 weeks, reporting a 55% response rate and a median survival of 9.8 months, with low incidence of myelosuppression. Therefore, the fractionated administration of paclitaxel and gemcitabine on the same days apparently increased the therapeutic index of the combination, supporting its use especially in elderly or unfit patients.

In a phase III randomized trial [39], gemcitabine/paclitaxel as first-line therapy was compared to carboplatin/paclitaxel. In both arms, paclitaxel was administered at 200 mg/m^2 on day 1 as a 3-h intravenous infusion, followed by either carboplatin at an area under the time–concentration curve (AUC) of 6 or gemcitabine 1,000 mg/m^2 on days 1 and 8, according to a 3-week schedule (Table 23.2). A total of 509 patients were evaluable, and an overall response rate of 28% and 35%, respectively, was achieved ($P = 0.12$). Hematologic toxicity was mild. Grade 3/4 neutropenia appeared in 15% of patients in both groups, although it was transient and of short duration, and no neutropenic sepsis

was reported. Grade 3/4 thrombocytopenia was seen in 1–2% of patients. Nonhematologic toxicity was also mild in both groups: grade 3 neurotoxicity was reported in 6–8% of patients, while grade 3–4 alopecia occurred almost universally, affecting more than 50% of patients in both arms. The overall survival time was similar: 9.8 months for gemcitabine/paclitaxel and 10.4 months for paclitaxel/carboplatin. Chemotherapy drug and outpatient clinic costs did not significantly differ between the two arms.

The European Organization for Research and Treatment of Cancer (EORTC) performed a randomized phase III trial in 480 patients with advanced NSCLC to compare two cisplatin-based chemotherapy regimens versus a nonplatinum doublet [40]. Patients were randomly assigned to receive either paclitaxel 175 mg/m^2 (3-h infusion, day 1) or gemcitabine 1,250 mg/m^2 (days 1 and 8) both combined with cisplatin 80 mg/m^2 (day 1) or paclitaxel 175 mg/m^2 (3-h infusion, day 1) combined with gemcitabine 1,250 mg/m^2 (days 1 and 8). The primary end point was comparison of the overall survival of the reference arm (cisplatin/paclitaxel) versus the two experimental arms (Table 23.2). Secondary end points included response rate and duration, progression-free survival, toxicities, quality of life, and cost of treatments. Seventy-nine percent of these patients had stage IV disease and 21% had stage IIIB disease. A nonsignificant trend toward lower overall survival (6.7, 8.1, and 8.9 months for the paclitaxel/gemcitabine, paclitaxel/cisplatin, and gemcitabine/cisplatin arms, respectively) and progression-free survival (3.5, 4.2 vs. 5.1 months for the paclitaxel/gemcitabine, paclitaxel/cisplatin, and gemcitabine/cisplatin arms, respectively) was observed in the nonplatinum arm. The paclitaxel/gemcitabine arm had a lower 1-year survival rate (26%, compared with 35% and 32% for the paclitaxel/cisplatin and gemcitabine/cisplatin arms, respectively), and response rate (27%, compared with 31% and 36% for the paclitaxel/cisplatin and gemcitabine/cisplatin arms, respectively) than the two cisplatin-based regimens. The median survival time obtained in the reference arm was comparable to that observed with the same doublet in a large four-arm phase III study reported by the ECOG. Treatment was well tolerated, and most quality of life parameters were similar, but the costs associated with the nonplatinum arm were 25% higher as compared with platinum regimens.

The gemcitabine/paclitaxel and gemcitabine/vinorelbine nonplatinum doublets were also tested in elderly patients as compared to either single agents, with overall survival as primary endpoint. Both doublets produced a longer survival than single agents. In particular, median survival time and 1-year survival were 9.2 months and 44%, respectively, with gemcitabine/paclitaxel versus 6.4 months and 25% , respectively, with paclitaxel alone. Toxicity was manageable. If carefully selected on the basis of comorbidities and performance status, elderly patients could be treated with a nonplatinum doublet.

23.2.2   Gemcitabine/Docetaxel

The combination of docetaxel and gemcitabine showed an additive effect in NSCLC cell lines [41], with a se-quence-dependent schedule, and with docetaxel to be administered 24–48 h before gemcitabine.

Docetaxel, a semisynthetic taxoid, promotes the assembly of stable microtubules and blocks mitosis in proliferating cells. Objective response rates ranging from 26 to 54% have been achieved with docetaxel in chemotherapy-nave patients with advanced NSCLC [42–47]. Docetaxel and gemcitabine have a different mechanism of action, both are active as single agent and display nonoverlapping toxicities in phase I studies in patients with NSCLC [48, 49]. Several phase II trials, using doses of docetaxel and gemcitabine of 65–100 mg/m^2 and 900–1,000 mg/m^2, respectively, according to different schedules, tested the efficacy of the combination [50–64]. The most common 3-week schedule delivered gemcitabine on days 1 and 8, with docetaxel on day 8 rather than day 1 to avoid omission of gemcitabine on day 8 (nonoverlapping myelotoxicity). The results of all these studies are summarized in Table 23.3. Response rates in studies employing the 3-week schedule ranged from 2 to 50% and median survival times from 11 to 13 months. Side effects were mild and acceptable, with neutropenia being the dose-limiting toxicity. Weekly or biweekly schedules have been associated with a reduction in the incidence of grade 3–4 and febrile neutropenia [60].

In contrast to studies using concurrent administration, a phase II randomized study from Germany tested an alternative approach of administering the drugs sequentially with one drug (gemcitabine or docetaxel) for up to six cycles, according to a 3- or 4-week schedule, and in case of disease progression switching to the other drug for up to six cycles. Docetaxel 35 mg/m^2 followed at progression by gemcitabine 1,000 mg/m^2 on a 4-week schedule was proven to be relatively ineffective (median survival time: 5 months; 1-year survival: 19%). The other schedules studied (gemcitabine 1,000 mg/m^2 followed by docetaxel 35 mg/m^2 every 4 weeks; and gemcitabine 1,250 mg/m^2 and docetaxel 100 mg/m^2 in

Table 23.3. Gemcitabine/docetaxel: phase II trials. *DOC* Docetaxel

Author, year	GEM (mg/m^2)	DOC (mg/m^2)	Schedule	Pts *n*	RR (%)	MST (months)
Ventriglia, 1998	1,000; d 1, 15	65; d 1	Q 3-wk	43	38	11
Georgoulias, 1999	900; d 1, 8	100; d 8	Q 3-wk	51	38	13
Rubio, 1999	1,000; d 1, 8	75; d 8	Q 3-wk	18	31	NR
Hejna, 2000	1,000; d 1, 10	80; d 1	Q 3-wk	34	50	13
Syrigos, 2001	1,000; d 1, 15	80; d 1, 15	Q 2-wk	25	28	NR
Rebattu, 2001	1,000; d 1, 8	85; d 8	Q 3-wk	35	29	11
Lizon, 2001	1,000; d 1, 8	75; d 8	Q 3-wk	28	25	NR
Miyazaki, 2001	800; d 1, 8	60; d 8	Q 3-wk	30	50	NR
Amenedo, 2001	1,000; d 1, 8	85; d 8	Q 3-wk	40	36	1-year 30%
Menendez, 2001	1,000; d 1, 8, 15, 29	36	weekly	21	60	NR
McKay, 2001	800; d 1, 8, 15, 29	30	Weekly/Q 8-wk	59	27	7.5
Popa, 2002	1,000; d 1, 8	40; d 1, 8	Q 3-wk	27	30	7.9
Patel, 2002	1,200; d 1, 8	40; d 1, 8	Q 3-wk	64	44	NR
Hirsch, 2004	1,000; d 1, 8	36; d 1, 8	Q 3-wk	40	10	7.7
Neubauer, 2005	900; d 1, 8, 22, 29	36	weekly	50	20	6.9

either sequence every 3 weeks) achieved a median survival of 6.5–9.5 months, and 1-year survival rates of 27–30%. Globally, the survival outcomes did not reach those observed with concomitant administration, and this approach may be considered for unfit patients.

A randomized phase II trial [62] compared two different taxane/gemcitabine regimens: in one arm patients received docetaxel at 40 mg/m^2 plus gemcitabine at 1,200 mg/m^2 and, in the other, paclitaxel at 120 mg/m^2 plus gemcitabine at 1,200 mg/m^2 (all drugs given on days 1 and 8 every 3 weeks). The response rate in 64 randomized patients was 44% with docetaxel/gemcitabine and 37% with paclitaxel/gemcitabine. The incidence of grade 3/4 neutropenia was 19% in the docetaxel arm and 13% in the paclitaxel arm. There were no cases of grade 3/4 thrombocytopenia. Asthenia and neurotoxicity occurred in 13% or fewer patients in both arms.

The phase II results were confirmed by large randomized phase III trials (Table 23.4). Georgoulias et al. [65, 66] performed a phase III study in 441 patients with stage IIIB or IV disease. Patients were randomized to receive either docetaxel 100 mg/m^2 on day 1 and cisplatin 80 mg/m^2 on day 3, every 3 weeks, or gemcitabine 1,100 mg/m^2 on days 1 and 8 and docetaxel 100 mg/m^2 on day 8 of a 3-week cycle. Colony-stimulating factor support was permitted. Both arms had similar activity (response rate, 32% vs. 30%) and survival benefit (median survival, 10 vs. 9.5 months; 1-year survival rate, 42% vs. 38%). The median duration of response and time to progression were also similar. Subset analysis revealed a significantly higher response rate in patients with adenocarcinoma in the docetaxel/gemcitabine arm, with response rates of 43 and 23%, respectively ($P=0.011$). In those patients with tumor types other than adenocarcinoma, there was a significant difference in response favoring the docetaxel/cisplatin arm. As might have been predicted, the regimen without cisplatin showed less toxicity. Grade 3/4 neutropenia (34% vs. 22%), nausea and vomiting (10% vs. 2%), and diarrhea (10% vs. 3%) were significantly worse in the docetaxel/cisplatin arm. The effect of treatment on quality of life was not evaluated in this study.

In a phase III trial, the Greek Cooperative Group for Lung Cancer compared docetaxel plus gemcitabine to vinorelbine plus cisplatin in 219 patients with stage IIIB/IV NSCLC [67, 68]. Response rates were similar (29% and 36%). The median survival was 9 months for gemcitabine/docetaxel and 11.5 months for the cisplatin doublet; the difference was not statistically significant. Toxicity, however, was lower in the gemcitabine/docetaxel arm. Thus, the nonplatinum regimen maintained efficacy and resulted in an improved toxicity profile.

Substitution of cisplatin with carboplatin could improve the tolerability of such a platinum-based combination. A phase III trial planning to include over 900 patients is ongoing, comparing carboplatin (AUC 6) and docetaxel (75 mg/m^2) to gemcitabine 1,000 mg/m^2 plus docetaxel 40 mg/m^2 on days 1 and 8 of a 3-week cycle. A recently presented interim analysis showed equivalence of efficacy between the two regimens [69].

23.2.3   Gemcitabine/Vinorelbine

The combination of gemcitabine/vinorelbine exerted additive effects when it was tested in experimental models [70, 71]. This nonplatinum regimen was tested in several phase II clinical trials in untreated advanced NSCLC and showed good tolerability and enough clinical activity to bring the combination into the phase III testing [72–83]. Doses of gemcitabine of 800–1,200 mg/m^2 and vinorelbine of 20–30 mg/m^2, have been used. Various schedules have been tested, including 3-, 4-, and 2-week schedules. The combination is generally well tolerated, with reported response rates of 19–72% and median survival times in the range of 7–13.9 months, with a 1-year survival rate of 30–55%. Grade 3/4 toxicities were mainly hematological. Neutropenia (grade 3/4) was seen in 6–38% of patients, while thrombocytopenia and anemia were seen in 2–12.5% and 1–20%, respectively. The wide range of response rates seen in these trials reflects the small sample sizes and potential differences in patient selection (Table 23.5).

A randomized phase II trial from Japan [84] compared gemcitabine/vinorelbine with carboplatin/gemcitabine. A total of 128 patients were included and randomized to gemcitabine 1,000 mg/m^2 plus vinorelbine 25 mg/m^2 on days 1 and 8 or gemcitabine 1,000 mg/m^2

Table 23.4. Gemcitabine/docetaxel: phase III trials. *VIN* Vinorelbine

Author, year	Regimen (Q 3-wk)	Pts *n*	RR (%)	MST (months)	One-year survival (%)
Georgoulias, 2001	GEM 1,100 mg/m^2; d 1, 8 DOC 100 mg/m^2; d 8 DOC 100 mg/m^2; d 1 CIS 80 mg/m^2 ; d 2	201 205	30 32	9.5 10	38 42
Kakolyris, 2002	GEM 1,000 mg/m^2; d 1, 8 DOC 100 mg/m^2; d 8 VIN 30 mg/m^2; d 1, 8 CIS 80 mg/m^2; d 8	117 102	29 36	9 11.5	NR NR

Table 23.5. Gemcitabine/vinorelbine: phase II clinical trials

Author, year	GEM (mg/m^2)	VIN (mg/m^2)	Schedule	Pts n	RR (%)	MST (months)
Isokangas, 1999	1,200; d 1, 15	35; d 1, 15	Q 4-wk	28	46	8
Lilenbaum, 2000	1,250; d 1, 8	25; d 1, 8	Q 3-wk	32	25	8.3
Krajnik, 2000	1,200; d 1, 8, 15	25; d 1, 8, 15	Q 4-wk	78	19	7
Chen, 2000	800; d 1, 8, 15	20; d 1, 8, 15	Q 4-wk	40	70	11
Lorusso, 2000	1,200; d 1, 8	30; d 1, 8	Q 3-wk	52	36	12.5
Bajetta, 2000	1,250; d 1, 8	25; d 1, 8	Q 3-wk	51	30	12
Laack, 2001	1,000; d 1, 8, 15	30; d 1, 8, 15	Q 4-wk	70	41	8.3
Palmeri, 2001	1,000; d 1, 8, 15	30; d 1, 8, 15	Q 4-wk	45	40	>8
Hirsch, 2001	1,000; d 1, 8, 15	30; d 1, 8, 15	Q 4-wk	34	53	11
Herbst, 2002	900; d 1, 8, 15	25; d 1, 8, 15	Q 4-wk	42	36	10
Hosoe, 2003	1,000; d 1, 8	25; d 1, 8	Q 3-wk*×3	44	47	15
Katakami, 2004	1,000; d 1, 8	25; d 1, 8	Q 3-wk	50	18	13.9
Kashii, 2004	1,000; d 1, 8	25; d 1, 8	Q 3-wk	65	21	10.6
Lilenbaum, 2005	1,000; d 1, 8	25; d 1, 8	Q 3-wk	82	14	7.8

* Followed by docetaxel 60 mg/m^2 Q 3-wk – three cycles

on days 1 and 8 plus carboplatin AUC 6 on day 1, every 3 weeks. Median survival time favored the platinum arm (16 vs. 10.6 months), with 1-year survival rates of 64% and 48% for the platinum and nonplatinum arms, respectively. Hematological toxicity was higher in the carboplatin arm.

Conversely, the most recent randomized phase II trial [85] showed a comparable efficacy in 165 patients with advanced NSCLC randomized between gemcitabine/vinorelbine (82 patients) and carboplatin/paclitaxel (83 patients). Treatment doses and schedules were: gemcitabine 1,000 mg/m^2 plus vinorelbine 25 mg/m^2 on days 1 and 8 or paclitaxel 200 mg/m^2 plus carboplatin AUC 6 on day 1, both arms every 3 weeks. Response rates were 14.6 and 16.9%, median survival times were 7.8 and 8.6 months, and 1-year survival rates were 38.4 and 31.9%, respectively (Table 23.5). Quality of life parameters were also similar between the two arms, although there was a lower overall incidence of toxicities in the nonplatinum arm.

To better define the potential role of this combination in the treatment of advanced NSCLC, phase III randomized trials have been conducted. A Swiss group [86] reported the results of a phase III randomized trial of gemcitabine/vinorelbine versus cisplatin/gemcitabine/vinorelbine. Three hundred patients with advanced NSCLC (stage IIIB with malignant pleural effusion or stage IV disease) were included and randomly assigned to receive gemcitabine 1,000 mg/m^2 + vinorelbine 25 mg/m^2 on days 1 and 8 or gemcitabine 1,000 mg/m^2 + vinorelbine 25 mg/m^2 on days 1 and 8 + cisplatin 75 mg/m^2 on day 2, both regimens administered every 3 weeks (Table 23.6). No statistically significant difference was observed for overall survival between the two arms, with a median survival of 35.9 versus 32.4 weeks and a 1-year survival of 33.6% versus 27.5%. The overall response rates were 13.0% for gemcitabine/vinorelbine versus 28.3% for the platinum combination ($P=0.004$;

complete responses 0% versus 3.8%; partial responses 13.0% versus 24.5%, respectively). Hematological and nonhematological toxicities were significantly lower in the nonplatinum regimen. No statistically significant differences in quality of life parameters were observed. In conclusion, the addition of cisplatin to gemcitabine/vinorelbine brought a significant increase in the response rate but no survival benefit as first-line chemotherapy in advanced NSCLC, while the nonplatinum doublet was substantially better tolerated.

A randomized phase III trial from a Spanish group [87] compared three regimens: cisplatin/gemcitabine, cisplatin/gemcitabine/vinorelbine, and gemcitabine/vinorelbine followed by ifosfamide/vinorelbine (Table 23.6). They included 562 patients with stage IIIB disease with malignant pleural effusion (21%) or stage IV disease (79%). The sequential nonplatinum doublet induced a lower response rate than the cisplatin-based regimens (24% vs. 41% and 40% for the gemcitabine/vinorelbine, cisplatin/gemcitabine, and cisplatin/gemcitabine/vinorelbine arms, respectively); however, the median survival time was not significantly different among the three arms (9.3 vs. 8.2 vs. 8.1 months, respectively). As expected, the nonplatinum arm was associated with less frequent and less severe hematological toxicity.

Another randomized phase III trial [88, 89] compared gemcitabine/vinorelbine with cisplatin/vinorelbine or cisplatin/gemcitabine (Table 23.6). Patients were randomized in a 2:1:1 manner. Doses were: gemcitabine 1,000 mg/m^2 plus vinorelbine 25 mg/m^2 on days 1 and 8, while in the control arm either gemcitabine 1,200 mg/m^2 on days 1 and 8 plus cisplatin 80 mg/m^2 on day 1, or vinorelbine 30 mg/m^2 on days 1 and 8 plus cisplatin 80 mg/m^2 on day 1. The primary end point of this study was quality of life. Patients with stage IIIB disease with pleural effusion or involved supraclavicular nodes (20%) or stage IV disease (80%) < 70 years were eligible for the study. Over 400 of the 501 patients were

Table 23.6. Gemcitabine/vinorelbine: phase III clinical trials.

Author, year	Regimen (Q 3-wk)	Pts n	RR (%)	MST (months)	One-year survival (%)
Gridelli, 2003	GEM 1,000 mg/m^2; d 1, 8	256	25	8	31
	VIN 25 mg/m^2; d 1, 8	126	30	9.2	37
	VIN 30 mg/m^2; d 1, 8	+ *			
	CIS 80 mg/m^2; d 1	126			
	GEM 1,200 mg/m^2; d 1, 8				
	CIS 80 mg/m^2; d 1				
Alberola, 2003	GEM 1,000 mg/m^2; d 1, 8 × 3 courses**	187	27	8.1	34
	VIN 30 mg/m^2; d 1, 8	188	41	8.2	33
	VIN 25 mg/m^2; d 1, 8	182	42	9.3	38
	GEM 1,000 mg/m^2; d 1, 8				
	CIS 100 mg/m^2; d 1				
	GEM 1,250 mg/m^2; d 1, 8				
	CIS 100 mg/m^2; d 1				
Laack, 2004	GEM 1,000 mg/m^2; d 1, 8	143	13	9	33
	VIN 25 mg/m^2; d 1, 8	144	28	8	27
	GEM 1,000 mg/m^2; d 1, 8				
	VIN 25 mg/m^2; d 1, 8				
	CIS 75 mg/m^2; d 2				
Abratt, 2004	GEM 1,000 mg/m^2; d 1, 8	157	28	11.5	48
	VIN 25 mg/m^2; d 1, 8	159	20	8.6	34
	VIN 30 mg/m^2; d 1, 8				
	CARBO AUC 5; d 1				

* Statistical analysis carried out on both platinum arms versus the nonplatinum arm
** Followed by ifosfamide 3 g/m^2 + vinorelbine 30 mg/m^2 Q 3-wk – three courses

assessable for quality of life analyses (statistical analysis evaluated the two platinum-based arms taken together versus the non-platinum-based regimen). After 2 months of treatment there was no significant difference in the general quality of life between the two arms. Cisplatin-based chemotherapy improved disease-related symptoms (not significantly in the multivariate analysis), but patients treated with a cisplatin-based regimen had significantly more grade 3/4 neutropenia, vomiting, alopecia, and ototoxicity. In contrast to previously described trials, no significant difference was observed in response rates (25 vs. 30%). Median survival was also similar in the two arms (32 vs. 38 weeks), whereas the cisplatin-based arms produced a significantly longer progression-free survival time (17 vs. 23 weeks). Although the extent of this advantage is below the threshold that was considered to be clinically relevant when the study was planned (9 weeks in median survival), it should be noted that survival differences of this magnitude, or even less, have been statistically significant in other trials and have led to changes in treatment strategies.

Another phase III comparison between a platinum-based doublet versus a nonplatinum regimen in advanced NSCLC was recently presented by Abratt et al. [90]. Patients were randomly assigned to receive vinorelbine 30 mg/m^2 on days 1 and 8 plus carboplatin AUC 5 on day 1 or vinorelbine 25 mg/m^2 plus gemcitabine 1,000 mg/m^2, days 1 and 8, both treatments adminis-

tered every 3 weeks (Table 23.6). A total of 316 patients were included, with response rates as the primary endpoint. The response rate was higher in the nonplatinum arm (28% vs. 20.8%) as were the median survival time (11.5 vs. 8.6 months) and 1-year survival rate (48% vs. 34%). The platinum doublet was associated with a higher incidence of hematological toxicity (neutropenia in 44% vs. 23%) and significantly more febrile neutropenia (17 patients vs. 1 patient). Gemcitabine/vinorelbine also showed an advantage in nonhematological toxicities and in terms of improvement in clinical benefit, fatigue, appetite, cough, and dyspnea. The authors concluded that the nonplatinum doublet demonstrated efficacy, tolerability, and clinical benefit comparable to their choice of platinum-based regimen. It should be noted that there was some unbalance among the major prognostic factors (gender, performance status, metastatic burden), thus favoring gemcitabine/vinorelbine; 20% of the patients in this arm received cisplatin as second-line treatment.

A different approach has been proposed by an Italian group [91]. Gemcitabine 1,000 mg/m^2 on day 1 and 1,000 or 800 mg/m^2 on day 4, ifosfamide 3 g/m^2 on day 1 (with mesna), vinorelbine 25 mg/m^2 on day 1, and 25 or 20 mg/m^2 on day 4 were administered on an outpatient basis every 3 weeks for a maximum of 6 courses to 50 chemonaive patients. Myelosuppression was the most frequent toxicity: grade 3/4 neutropenia was seen in 47% of the courses. Nonhematological toxicity was mild to moderate. A response rate of 52% was reported, with a 1-year survival rate of 46%. The combination showed promising activity with neutropenia as the dose-limiting toxicity.

A few phase II studies with the gemcitabine/vinorelbine regimen were conducted in NSCLC patients aged 70 years or older or patients who were unfit to receive cisplatin. Both elderly patients and poor-performance-status patients (Karnofsky Performance Status ≥2) are traditionally considered poor candidates for a platinum-based chemotherapy.

A phase II trial [37] was conducted to evaluate the efficacy and toxicity of gemcitabine/vinorelbine in 20 patients with a median age of 83 years and with stage IIIB or IV NSCLC. The schedule consisted in vinorelbine 20 mg/m^2 plus gemcitabine 800 mg/m^2 on days 1, 8, and 15, every 4 weeks. The overall response rate was 65%, with a median survival of 10 months. The most significant, although manageable toxicity was grade 3/4 myelosuppression.

In another study [92] vinorelbine 25 mg/m^2 plus gemcitabine 1,000 mg/m^2 were both administered on days 1, 8, and 15 every 4 weeks. Forty-nine patients were included, either older than 70 years or unfit to receive cisplatin. The overall response rate was 26%, and the 1-year survival rate was 33%. Authors concluded that the gemcitabine/vinorelbine combination was moderately active and well tolerated except in patients aged 75 years or older.

Recently two randomized studies from Italian investigators comparing a gemcitabine/vinorelbine combination to single-agent gemcitabine or vinorelbine has been reported in an elderly population with NSCLC. An improved survival with gemcitabine/vinorelbine regimen over vinorelbine alone and improvement in some tumor-related symptoms was reported in one phase II randomized study [93]. However, these results were not confirmed by the other larger randomized phase III study, which demonstrated that single-agent therapy is at least as good as combination therapy in terms of survival [88, 89].

23.3 Gemcitabine and Other Nonplatinum Agents

23.3.1 Gemcitabine/Pemetrexed

Pemetrexed is a novel antifolate that inhibits three enzymes (thymidylate synthase, dihydrofolate reductase, and glycinamide ribonucleotide transferase) that are involved in folate metabolism and DNA synthesis. The cytotoxicity of pemetrexed is caused by the inhibition of both the pyrimidine and purine pathways. The maximum tolerated dose established in phase I studies of pemetrexed was 600 mg/m^2 every 3 weeks [94]. This dose was later reduced to 500 mg/m^2 every 3 weeks in several phase II trials, particularly when used in combination with other cytotoxic agents [95]. Folic acid and vitamin B$_{12}$ supplementation became a requirement for pemetrexed-based therapy when analysis of safety data from multiple pemetrexed trials suggested that supplementation decreases toxicity [96]. Single-agent pemetrexed in two phase II trials in advanced NSCLC [95, 97] yielded response rates of 15.8% and 23.3% and median survivals of 7.2 and 9.2 months, respectively.

Both pemetrexed and gemcitabine have shown single-agent activity in NSCLC, and these two agents in combination showed cytotoxic synergy when gemcitabine was administered before pemetrexed [98, 99]. The recommended dose was gemcitabine (1,250 mg/m^2) on days 1 and 8, followed by pemetrexed (500 mg/m^2) on day 8 of a 3-week cycle. The most common dose-limiting toxicity was neutropenia. Other toxicities included nausea, fatigue, rash, and elevated hepatic transaminases.

These doses of gemcitabine/pemetrexed were tested in a recent phase II study on 60 chemonaive patients with advanced NSCLC (87% in stage IV). After the inclusion of the first 13 patients, folic acid and vitamin B$_{12}$ supplementation was added to lower pemetrexed-induced toxicity. The overall response rate was 15%, and median survival time was 10 months with a 1- and 2-year overall survival of 42% and 18%, respectively. Median progression-free survival was 5.0 months, with a median response duration of 3.3 months (Table 23.7).

Table 23.7. Gemcitabine and miscellaneous agents: phase II and phase III clinical trials. *IRI* Irinotecan, *PEM* pemetrexed

Author, year	GEM (mg/m^2)	PEM (mg/m^2)	Schedule	Pts n	RR (%)	MST (months)
Adjei, 2004	1, 250; d 1, 8	500; d 1	Q 3-wk	54	29	NR
Monnerat, 2004	1, 250; d 1, 8	500; d 8	Q 3-wk	60	15	10

Author, year	GEM (mg/m^2)	IRI (mg/m^2)	Schedule	Pts n	RR (%)	MST (months)
Georgoulias, 2004	1, 000; d 1, 8	300; d 8	Q 3-wk	76	18	9
	–	300; d 1		71	4	8
Rocha Lima, 2004	1, 000; d 1, 8	100; d 1, 8	Q 3-wk	40	12	8

The only significant grade 3/4 toxicities were fatigue and febrile neutropenia; cumulative myelosuppression was not observed.

A phase II study tested three different sequences of the gemcitabine/pemetrexed doublet at the fixed doses of 1,250 mg/m^2 and 500 mg/m^2, respectively [100]. Overall, 148 patients with advanced NSCLC were included in the three arms, and 74% experienced at least grade 3 hematological toxicity and 62% experienced grade 3 or more nonhematological toxicity, of which fatigue (17.6%), dyspnea (11.5%), and rash (8.1%) were the most common. The sequence and schedule of administration is a critical determinant of the efficacy and toxicity of this doublet. Preliminary efficacy and toxicity data indicate that pemetrexed followed by gemcitabine on day 1 with gemcitabine on day 8 is the optimal sequence, with a response rate of 29% in 54 patients and the lowest incidence of febrile neutropenia (5%).

23.3.2 Gemcitabine/Irinotecan

Irinotecan (CPT-11), which is a semisynthetic derivative of camptothecin that acts as a topoisomerase I inhibitor, was proved to be active as a single agent in NSCLC, with response rates ranging from 15% to over 30% with either weekly, 3-weekly or 4-weekly schedules. Preclinical studies documented a dose-dependent synergic interaction between gemcitabine and irinotecan [101]. In phase I trials in previously treated NSCLC, both gemcitabine and irinotecan were administered on days 1 and 15 every 4 weeks [67, 68, 102]. The maximum tolerated dose was 1,000 mg/m^2 for gemcitabine and 150 mg/m^2 for irinotecan. Diarrhea and neutropenia were the dose-limiting toxicities.

In a randomized phase II trial (Table 23.7), 147 pretreated patients with advanced NSCLC [103, 104] received either gemcitabine 1,000 mg/m^2 on days 1 and 8 and irinotecan 300 mg/m^2 on day 8 every 3 weeks (76 patients), or single-agent irinotecan 300 mg/m^2 once every 3 weeks (71 patients). Despite a higher response rate with the doublet (18%) versus single-agent irinotecan (4%), the overall survival was similar in both groups (9 and 8 months, respectively). Quality of life scores were significantly better for patients treated with the combination, resulting in better control of disease-related symptoms.

In another randomized phase II comparison of non-platinum doublets, gemcitabine with either irinotecan or docetaxel, was tested in 80 chemonaive patients with advanced NSCLC [105]. The response rates for gemcitabine/irinotecan and gemcitabine/docetaxel were relatively modest (12% and 23%, respectively), with a corresponding 1-year survival of 23% and 51% and median survival of 8 and 12.8 months, respectively. The most common hematological toxicity was neutropenia, which occurred in one-quarter of the patients in each treatment arm. Survival data, in particular with the combination gemcitabine/docetaxel, are promising.

23.4 Vinorelbine and the Taxanes

23.4.1 Paclitaxel/Vinorelbine

The regimen of paclitaxel/vinorelbine is one of the non-platinum combinations that have been tested in only a few studies [106]. Both agents have a mechanism of action that is related to the polymerization of microtubules: in vitro studies showed the synergistic cytotoxicity of this combination [107]. As mentioned previously, each agent is considered to be effective in NSCLC either alone or in combination with other cytotoxic drugs. A phase II trial of paclitaxel/vinorelbine in 58 patients with advanced NSCLC achieved a response rate of 50% with acceptable toxicity (Table 23.8) [108]. The same investigators completed a randomized phase III trial in advanced NSCLC [109], comparing a standard platinum-based regimen such as carboplatin/paclitaxel with the nonplatinum combination of paclitaxel/vinorelbine (Table 23.8). The study included 360 patients randomized to either carboplatin AUC 6 plus paclitaxel 175 mg/m^2 every 3 weeks for 6 cycles, or to paclitaxel 135 mg/m^2 plus vinorelbine 25 mg/m^2 every 2 weeks for up to 9 cycles. Overall response rates were similar, at 45% and 42%, respectively. Median survival was 11 and 10 months, respectively, 1-year survival was 42% and 37%, respectively, and 2-year survival 10% and 19%, respectively. However, neutropenia occurred significantly more frequently in the vinorelbine arm, while no major differences in the rest of the toxicity profile were seen between the two arms, thus favoring the platinum-based regimen.

23.4.2 Docetaxel/Vinorelbine

Preclinical models have indicated a synergistic effect for these two drugs. Such interaction seems to be schedule-dependent, with optimal activity being observed when docetaxel is administered immediately after vinorelbine.

In phase I studies febrile neutropenia was the dose-limiting toxicity. A 2-week schedule was considered the safest [110], but 3-week schedules with docetaxel administered on either day 1 or day 8 with weekly vinorelbine also revealed acceptable toxicity. Moreover, a weekly schedule of both docetaxel and vinorelbine proved effective in a phase I study. A 2-week schedule of vinorelbine 45 mg/m^2 and docetaxel 60 mg/m^2 with granulocyte colony-stimulating factor (G-CSF) support

Table 23.8. Vinorelbine and taxanes: phase II and phase III clinical trials

Author, year	Drugs and doses		Schedule	Pts n	RR (%)	MST (months)
	PAC (mg/m^2)	VIN (mg/m^2)				
Phase II Stathopoulos, 2003	d 1, 8	30; d 8 30; d 1	Q 3-wk	58	50	10
Phase III Stathopoulos, 2004	135; d 1, 8	25; d 1, 8	Q 3-wk	180	42	10
	175; d 1	CARBO AUC 6; d 1	Q 3-wk	180	45	11

Author, year	Drugs and doses		Schedule	Pts n	RR (%)	MST (months)
	DOC (mg/m^2)	VIN (mg/m^2)				
Phase II Trillet-Lenoir, 1996	75; d 2	25; d 1	Q 3-wk	39	23	9.4
Kourousis, 1998	60; d 1	40; d 1, 5	Q 3-wk	46	37	5
Walls, 2000	60; d 1	15; d 1, 8, 15	Q 3-wk	71	21	1-year 35%
Miller, 2000	60; d 1	45; d 1	Q 2-wk	35	51	14
Page, 2004	60; d 1	45; d 1	Q 2-wk	61	42	14

was administered to 35 and 61 advanced NSCLC patients in 2 phase II studies [110, 111]. Febrile neutropenia occurred in 8% and 14% of these patients, respectively. Response rates were 51% and 42%, respectively, with a median survival of 14 months and a 1-year survival of nearly 60% in both studies (Table 23.8).

Other phase II studies used a 3-week schedule with G-CSF support [112, 113]. The dose intensity of docetaxel was the same in all trials, but that of vinorelbine varied largely. Results were quite inferior to the aforementioned studies with a bi-weekly schedule, and the degree of hematological toxicity was higher (Table 23.8).

Despite the fact that survival data from these studies remain comparable to data from standard cisplatin-based doublets, toxicity, in terms of grade 3/4 neutropenia and neutropenic fever, remains a big concern.

23.5   Taxanes and Irinotecan

23.5.1   Docetaxel/Irinotecan

A phase I study has determined that the recommended phase II doses for irinotecan followed by docetaxel are 160 and 65 mg/m^2, respectively, administered according to a 3-week schedule [98]. Neutropenia is the dose-limiting toxicity. A more recent phase I study from Japan confirmed these results: recommended doses for phase II trials were irinotecan 150 and docetaxel 50–60 mg/m^2, respectively, administered in a 3-week schedule

[98]. In 18 patients the response rate was 33%, with a median survival of 13.6 months. Exploring weekly schedules, Murren et al. [114] found that the appropriate doses were 50 and 35 mg/m^2 for irinotecan and docetaxel, respectively, weekly for 4 weeks, or 60 and 35 mg/m^2, respectively, weekly for 2 weeks with a 1-week interval. Weekly or 3-weekly schedules were brought into phase II studies. Neutropenia and diarrhea emerged as the main toxicities.

A phase II trial in patients with locally advanced or metastatic NSCLC was prematurely closed due to the low response rates observed [115]. The treatment scheme consisted of docetaxel 50 mg/m^2 on day 2, and irinotecan 50 mg/m^2 on days 1, 8, and 15 of a 4-week cycle. The preliminary analysis among the first 14 patients showed only 1 partial response. The median survival time was 11 months and the 1-year survival was 43%. This combination chemotherapy was well tolerated with no case of severe diarrhea.

Two recent phase II studies tested either a 3-week [116] or a weekly schedule [117] of docetaxel/irinotecan in advanced NSCLC. The doublet showed an encouraging 10 months of median survival time, but the number of treated patients was limited (39 and 36 patients, respectively). Myelosuppression was moderate in both studies, but the weekly regimen showed a high incidence of grade 3–4 diarrhea (29%).

A phase II randomized study was conducted by the West Japan Thoracic Oncology Group comparing docetaxel/irinotecan to docetaxel/cisplatin [118]. Patients with advanced NSCLC were randomized to receive either docetaxel 60 mg/m^2 on day 8 plus irinotecan

60 mg/m^2 on days 1 and 8 (57 patients), or cisplatin 80 mg/m^2 plus docetaxel 60 mg/m^2, both on day 1 (51 patients), both according to a 3-week schedule. The activity of the two combinations was similar (response rates 32% vs. 37%, median survival of 46 weeks vs. 50 weeks, 1-year survival 40% vs. 47%, respectively). The toxicity profile was quite different, with a significantly higher incidence of neutropenia and diarrhea in the nonplatinum combination and more nausea and vomiting in the cisplatin arm.

23.5.2   Paclitaxel/Irinotecan

Also for paclitaxel and irinotecan, an additive or synergistic interaction has been demonstrated when the combination was tested in preclinical studies [119]. So far there have been few reports evaluating a combination of these two drugs in patients with NSCLC. In a phase I study, paclitaxel was administered on day 1 and irinotecan on days 1, 8, and 15 [120]. The starting doses of paclitaxel and irinotecan were 120 and 40 mg/m^2, respectively. This regimen produced a response rate of 31% and well-tolerated toxicities. However, the administration of irinotecan on days 8 and 15 was omitted in over 40% of cycles because of myelotoxicity, even at the recommended dose level. Another phase I study [121] evaluated paclitaxel 135 mg/m^2 on day 2 and irinotecan 50 mg/m^2 on days 1, 8, and 15, respectively. All patients at the initial dose level had dose-limiting myelotoxicity. Rosen et al. [122] also reported that dose escalation of the two drugs above the starting dose (irinotecan 225 mg/m^2 and paclitaxel 100 mg/m^2, once every 3 weeks) was not feasible because of neutropenic fever or severe diarrhea. In addition, the optimal sequence of administration using a combination of these drugs has not been definitively determined by phase I trials. The most recent phase I study [15, 16] demonstrated that the combination of irinotecan/paclitaxel on days 1 and 8 every 3 weeks at doses of 40 mg/m^2 and 50 mg/m^2, respectively, produced considerable toxicities and no promising activity for advanced NSCLC.

In conclusion, these phase I studies could show neither feasibility nor effectiveness of a two-drug combination consisting of irinotecan and paclitaxel for patients with advanced NSCLC.

23.6   Conclusion

The development of nonplatinum combinations for advanced NSCLC has aimed at equalizing or improving the survival gain already proved for cisplatin-based chemotherapy, while reducing toxicity and enhancing quality of life. This consideration is judged to be clinically relevant in the palliative setting, which still remains the main goal of chemotherapy for the management of the majority of patients with metastatic NSCLC. An additional sought-after advantage is to broaden the range of patients for whom treatment is judged suitable and practical, particularly in an outpatient setting.

Clinical trials have demonstrated that even though the cisplatin-free regimens were significantly less toxic than cisplatin-based ones, they did not always translate into an improvement in global quality of life [88, 89]. The choice of optimal regimen should be determined primarily by its expected efficacy, namely improved survival. Based on higher single-agent response rates, the initial hope was that newer nonplatinum regimens would have higher or similar levels of activity compared with platinum-containing combinations, but sparing some of the toxic effects. To date such survival improvement has not yet been demonstrated but, in the case of some nonplatinum doublets, it is quite close. Further trials of different combinations and doses of these agents are unlikely to produce better results. To date, these nonplatinum doublets may be the preferred choice for unfit patients.

In conclusion, it is very difficult to compare the data from the various studies for a variety of reasons, including different patient characteristics, different selection criteria, different primary endpoints and sample sizes, and different combination chemotherapies with different schedules. Finally, the outcome of patients with metastatic NSCLC – regardless of chemotherapy regimens – remains dismal. We need to keep focusing our efforts on understanding cancer biology to create individualized therapies aimed at specific targets on tumor cells. In this perspective, nonplatinum doublets may become a reasonable therapeutic alternative in the presence of predictive molecular factors indicating a resistance to platinum agents.

Key Points

- Cisplatin-based chemotherapy is still the cornerstone of treatment for unresectable, locally advanced, and metastatic (stage IIIB and IV) non-small-cell lung cancer (NSCLC), mainly in patients with good performance status (PS = 0–1) and without significant weight loss.
- There is clinical evidence that in advanced NSCLC, standard platinum-based chemotherapy has reached a therapeutic plateau.
- Non-platinum-based chemotherapy with doublets of newer cytotoxic agents shows a better toxicity profile than platinum-containing regimens and, in some clinical trials, comparable efficacy. As yet, no standard nonplatinum regimen has emerged as better than others.

- Platinum-based regimens may be particularly poorly tolerated in elderly patients or patients with poor performance status (PS = 2). In this subset of patients with advanced NSCLC, nonplatinum chemotherapy represents a potential therapeutic option.
- Although prospective data are lacking, use of a platinum-based doublet for elderly NSCLC patients with a good performance status is supported by retrospective data from multiple, large clinical trials.

References

1. Pfister DG, Johnson DH, Azzoli CG, et al. American Society of Clinical Oncology treatment of unresectable non-small cell lung cancer guideline: update 2003. J Clin Oncol 2004; 22:254.
2. Soquet PJ, Chauvin F, Boissel JP, et al. Polychemotherapy in advanced non-small cell lung cancer: a meta-analysis. Lancet 1993; 342:19.
3. Marino P, Pampallona S, Preatoni A, et al. Chemotherapy vs. supportive care in advanced non-small cell lung cancer: results of a meta-analysis of the literature. Chest 1994; 106:861.
4. Non-Small Cell Lung Cancer Collaborative Group. Chemotherapy in non-small cell lung cancer: a meta-analysis using updated data on individual patients from 52 randomized clinical trials. BMJ 1995; 311:899.
5. Scagliotti G, De Marinis F, Rinaldi M, et al. Phase III randomized trial comparing three platinum-based doublets in advanced non-small cell lung cancer. J Clin Oncol 2002; 20:4285.
6. Schiller JH, Harrington D, Belani CP, et al. Comparison of four chemotherapy regimens for advanced non-small-cell lung cancer. N Engl J Med 2002; 346:92.
7. Le Chevalier T, Scagliotti GV, Natale R, et al. Efficacy of gemcitabine plus platinum chemotherapy compared with other platinum containing regimens in advanced non-small-cell lung cancer: a meta-analysis of survival outcomes. Lung Cancer 2005; 47:69.
8. Kelly K, Crowley J, Bunn PA Jr, et al. Randomized phase III trial of paclitaxel plus carboplatin versus vinorelbine plus cisplatin in the treatment of patients with advanced non-small-cell lung cancer: a Southwest Oncology Group trial. J Clin Oncol 2001; 19:3210.
9. Fossella F, Pereira JR, von Pawel J, et al. Randomized, multinational, phase III study of docetaxel plus platinum combinations versus vinorelbine plus cisplatin for advanced non-small-cell lung cancer: the TAX 326 study group. J Clin Oncol 2000; 21:3016.
10. Dabholkar M, Vionnet J, Bostick-Bruton F, Yu JJ, Reed E. Messenger RNA levels of XPAC and ERCC1 in ovarian cancer tissue correlate with response to platinum-based chemotherapy. J Clin Invest 1994; 94:703.
11. Metzger R, Leichman CG, Danenberg KD, et al. ERCC1 mRNA levels complement thymidylate synthase mRNA levels in predicting response and survival for gastric cancer patients receiving combination cisplatin and fluorouracil chemotherapy. J Clin Oncol 1998; 16:309.
12. Lord RV, Brabender J, Gandara D, et al. Low ERCC1 expression correlates with prolonged survival after cisplatin plus gemcitabine chemotherapy in non-small cell lung cancer. Clin Cancer Res 2002; 1:2286.
13. Rosell R, Gatzemeier U, Betticher H, et al. Phase III randomised trial comparing paclitaxel/carboplatin with paclitaxel/cisplatin in patients with advanced non-small-cell lung cancer: a cooperative multinational trial. Ann Oncol 2002; 13:1539.
14. Zojwalla NJ, Raftopoulos H, Gralla RJ. Are cisplatin and carboplatin equivalent in the treatment of non-small cell lung cancer? Result of a comprehensive review of randomized studies in over 2300 patients. Proc Am Soc Clin Oncol 2004; 23:630 (Abstract 7068).
15. Hotta K, Ueoka H, Kiura K, et al. A phase I and pharmacokinetic study of irinotecan (CPT-11) and paclitaxel in patients with advanced non-small cell lung cancer. Lung Cancer 2004; 45:77.
16. Hotta K, Matsuo K, Ueoka H, Kiura K, Tabata M, Tanimoto M. Addition of platinum compounds to a new agent in patients with advanced non-small cell lung cancer: a literature based meta-analysis of randomized trials. Ann Oncol 2004; 15:1782.
17. Perng RP, Chen YM, Ming-Liu J, et al. Gemcitabine versus the combination of cisplatin and etoposide in patients with inoperable non-small cell lung cancer in a phase II randomized study. J Clin Oncol 1997; 15:2097.
18. Vansteenkiste JF, Vandebroek JE, Nackaerts KL, et al. Clinical-benefit response in advanced non-small cell lung cancer: a multicentre prospective randomised phase III study of single agent gemcitabine versus cisplatin-vindesine. Ann Oncol 2001; 12:1221.
19. Negoro S, Masuda N, Takada Y, et al. Randomised phase III trial of irinotecan combined with cisplatin for advanced non-small-cell lung cancer. Br J Cancer 2003; 88:335.
20. Delbaldo C, Michiels S, Syz N, Soria JC, Le Chevalier T, Pignon JP. Benefits of adding a drug to a single-agent or a 2-agent chemotherapy regimen in advanced non-small cell lung cancer: a meta-analysis. JAMA 2004; 292:470.
21. Hertel LW, Kroin JS, Misner JW, et al. Synthesis of 2-deoxy-2′,2′-difluoro-D-ribose and 2-deoxy-2′,2′-difluoro-D-ribofuranosyl nucleosides. J Org Chem 1998; 53:2406.
22. Kroep JR, Giaccone G, Voon DA, et al. Gemcitabine and paclitaxel: pharmacokinetic and pharmacodynamic interactions in patients with non-small cell lung cancer. J Clin Oncol 1999; 17:2190.
23. Kroep JR, Giaccone G, Tolis C, et al. Sequence dependent effect of paclitaxel on gemcitabine metabolism in relation to cell cycle and cytotoxicity in non-small-cell lung cancer cell lines. Br J Cancer 2000; 83:1069.
24. Shepherd FA. Phase II trials of single-agent activity of gemcitabine in patients with advanced non-small cell lung cancer: an overview. Anticancer Drugs 1995; 6:19.
25. Gatzemeier U, Shepherd FA, Le Chevalier T, et al. Activity of gemcitabine in patients with non-small cell lung cancer: a multicenter, extended phase II study. Eur J Cancer 1996; 32A:243.
26. Crino L, Scagliotti G, Marangolo M, et al. Cisplatin-gemcitabine combination in advanced non-small-cell lung cancer: a phase II study. J Clin Oncol 1997; 15:297.
27. Abratt RP, Bezwoda WR, Goedhals L, et al. Weekly gemcitabine and monthly cisplatin: effective chemotherapy for advanced non-small-cell lung cancer. J Clin Oncol 1997; 15:744.
28. Murphy WK, Fossella FV, Winn RJ, et al. A phase II study of taxol in patients with untreated advanced non-small-cell lung cancer. J Natl Cancer Inst 1993; 85:384.
29. Gatzemeier U, Heckmayer M, Neuhauss R, et al. Chemotherapy of advanced inoperable non-small cell lung cancer with paclitaxel: a phase II trial. Semin Oncol 1995; 22:24.

30. Hainsworth JD, Thompson DS, Greco FA. Paclitaxel by 1-hour infusion: an active drug in metastatic non-small-cell lung cancer. J Clin Oncol 1995; 13:1609.

31. Giaccone G, Splinter TAW, DeBruyne C, et al. Randomized study of paclitaxel-cisplatin versus cisplatin-teniposide in patients with advanced non-small-cell lung cancer. J Clin Oncol 1998; 16:2133.

32. Bonomi P, Kim K, Fairclough D, et al. Comparison of survival and quality of life in advanced non-small-cell lung cancer patients treated with two dose levels of paclitaxel combined with cisplatin versus etoposide with cisplatin: results of an Eastern Cooperative Oncology Group trial. J Clin Oncol 2000; 18:623.

33. Auerbach M, Chaudhry M, Richards P, et al. Phase II study of gemcitabine and paclitaxel in metastatic non-small cell lung cancer. Proc Am Soc Clin Oncol 2000; 19:522a (Abstract 2052).

34. Giaccone G, Smith EF, van Meerbeeck JP, et al. A phase I-II study of gemcitabine and paclitaxel in advanced non-small-cell lung cancer patients. Ann Oncol 2000; 11:109.

35. Douillard J, Lerouge D, Monnier A, et al. Combined paclitaxel and gemcitabine as first-line treatment in metastatic non-small cell lung cancer: a multicentre phase II study. Br J Cancer 2001; 84:1179.

36. Bhatia S, Hanna N, Ansari R, et al. A phase II study of weekly gemcitabine and paclitaxel in patients with previously untreated stage IIIB and IV non-small cell lung cancer. Lung Cancer 2002; 38:73.

37. Chen YM, Perng RP, Lee YC, et al. Paclitaxel plus carboplatin, compared with paclitaxel plus gemcitabine, shows similar efficacy while more cost-effective: a randomized phase II study of combination chemotherapy against inoperable non-small-cell lung cancer previously untreated. Ann Oncol 2002; 13:108.

38. Hirsh V, Whittom R, Ofiara L, et al. Weekly paclitaxel and gemcitabine chemotherapy for metastatic non-small cell lung carcinoma (NSCLC): a dose-optimizing phase II trial. Cancer 2003; 97:2242.

39. Kosmidis P, Mylonakis N, Nicolaides C, et al. Paclitaxel plus carboplatin versus gemcitabine plus paclitaxel in advanced non-small-cell lung cancer: a phase III randomized trial. J Clin Oncol 2002; 20:3578.

40. Smit EF, van Meerbeeck JP, Lianes P, et al. Three-arm randomized study of two cisplatin-based regimens and paclitaxel plus gemcitabine in advanced non-small-cell lung cancer: a phase III trial of the European Organization for Research and Treatment of Cancer Lung Cancer Group–EORTC 08975. J Clin Oncol 2003; 21:3909.

41. Zoli W, Ricotti L, Dal Susino M, et al. Docetaxel and gemcitabine activity in NSCLC cell lines and in primary cultures from human lung cancer. Br J Cancer 1999; 81:609.

42. Cerny T, Kaplan S, Pavlidis N, et al. Docetaxel (Taxotere) is active in non-small cell lung cancer: a phase II trial of the EORTC Early Clinical Trials Group (ECTG). Br J Cancer 1994; 70:384.

43. Fossella FV, DeVore R, Kerr R, et al. Randomized phase II trial of docetaxel versus vinorelbine or ifosfamide in patients with advanced non-small-cell lung cancer previously treated with platinum-containing regimens: the TAX 320 Non-Small Cell Lung Cancer Study Group. J Clin Oncol 2000; 18:2354.

44. Francis PA, Rigas JR, Kris MG, et al. Phase II trial of docetaxel in patients with stage III and IV non-small-cell lung cancer. J Clin Oncol 1994; 12:1232.

45. Miller VA, Rigas JR, Francis PA, et al. Phase II trial of a 75 mg/m² dose of docetaxel with prednisone premedication for patients with advanced non-small cell lung cancer. Cancer 1995; 75:968.

46. Roszkowski K, Pluzanska A, Krzakowski M, et al. A multicenter, randomized, phase III study of docetaxel plus best supportive care versus supportive care in chemotherapy-naïve patients with metastatic or non-resectable localized non-small-cell lung cancer (NSCLC). Lung Cancer 2000; 27:145.

47. Shepherd FA, Dancey J, Ramlau R, et al. Prospective randomized trial of docetaxel versus best supportive in patients with non-small-cell lung cancer previously treated with platinum-based chemotherapy. J Clin Oncol 2000; 18:2095.

48. Bhargava P, Marshall JL, Fried K, et al. Phase I and pharmacokinetic study of two sequences of gemcitabine and docetaxel administered weekly to patients with advanced cancer. Cancer Chemother Pharmacol 2001; 48:95.

49. Ganjoo KN, Gordon MS, Sandler AB, et al. A phase I study of weekly gemcitabine and docetaxel in patients with advanced cancer: a Hoosier Oncology Group Study. Oncology 2002; 62:299.

50. Ventriglia M, Estevez R, Alume H, et al. Docetaxel plus gemcitabine: a new combination in the treatment of patients with advanced non-small-cell lung cancer: a preliminary analysis. Ann Oncol 1998; 9(S2):96 (Abstract 365).

51. Georgoulias V, Kouroussis C, Androulakis N, et al. Frontline treatment of advanced non-small cell lung cancer with docetaxel and gemcitabine: a multicenter phase II trial. J Clin Oncol 1999; 17:914.

52. Rubio G, Blajman C, Capo A, et al. Docetaxel and gemcitabine in metastatic non-small cell lung cancer: a phase II study. Proc Am Soc Clin Oncol 1999; 18:522 (Abstract 2012).

53. Hejna M, Kornek GV, Raderer M, et al. Treatment of patients with advanced non small cell lung carcinoma using docetaxel and gemcitabine plus granulocyte-colony stimulating factor. Cancer 2000; 89:516.

54. Rebattu P, Quantin X, Ardiet C, Morere JF, Azarian MR, Schuller-Lebeau MP, Pujol JL. Dose-finding, pharmacokinetic and phase II study of docetaxel in combination with gemcitabine in patients with inoperable non-small cell lung cancer. Lung Cancer 2001; 33:277.

55. Lizon J, Feliu J, Morales S, et al. A phase II study gemcitabine plus docetaxel as a first line treatment in non-small-cell lung cancer (NSCLC). Proc Am Soc Clin Oncol 2001; 20:270b (Abstract 2833).

56. Miyazaki M, Takeda T, Ichimaru Y, et al. A phase I/II study of docetaxel and gemcitabine combination chemotherapy for advanced non-small-cell lung cancer (NSCLC). Proc Am Soc Clin Oncol 2001; 20:265b (Abstract 2812).

57. Amenedo M, Mel JR, Huidobro G, et al. Phase II multicenter clinical trial of gemcitabine and docetaxel in advanced non-small-cell lung cancer (NSCLC): final results. Proc Am Soc Clin Oncol 2001; 20:265b (Abstract 2813).

58. Menendez P, Gomez PG, Mendez M, et al. A phase II study of a combination of docetaxel and gemcitabine in a weekly schedule as a first line treatment in stages IIIB/IV non-small-cell lung cancer. GOTY STUDY GROUP. Proc Am Soc Clin Oncol 2001; 20:256b (Abstract 2777).

59. Syrigos KN, Dionellis G, Alevyzaki F, et al. Biweekly administration of gemcitabine and docetaxel in patients with advanced non-small-cell lung cancer: a phase II study. Proc Am Soc Clin Oncol 2001; 20:260b (Abstract 2791).

60. McKay CE, Hainsworth JD, Burris HA, et al. Weekly docetaxel/gemcitabine in the treatment of elderly patients (pts) with advanced non-small cell lung cancer (NSCLC): a Minnie Pearl Cancer Research Network phase II trial. Proc Am Soc Clin Oncol 2001; 20:260b (Abstract 2793).

61. Popa IE, Stewart K, Smith FP, et al. A phase II trial of gemcitabine and docetaxel in patients with chemotherapy-naive, advanced non-small cell lung carcinoma. Cancer 2002; 95:1714.

62. Patel R, Keiser LW, Justice GR, et al. ACORN 9901: a multicenter randomized trial of weekly docetaxel+gemcitabine versus weekly paclitaxel+gemcitabine in patients (pts) with non-small cell lung cancer (NSCLC). Proc Am Soc Clin Oncol 2002; 21:320a (Abstract 1276).

63. Hirsch V, Whittom R, Desjardins P, et al. Docetaxel and gemcitabine administered on day 1 and 8 for metastatic non-small cell carcinoma (NSCLC): a phase II multicenter trial. Lung Cancer 2004; 46:113.

64. Neubauer MA, Garfield DH, Kurfler PR, et al. Results of a phase II multicenter trial of weekly docetaxel and gemcitabine as first-line therapy for patients with advanced non-small cell lung cancer. Lung Cancer 2005; 47:121.

65. Georgoulias V, Papadakis E, Alexopoulos A, et al. Platinum-based and non-platinum-based chemotherapy in advanced non-small-cell lung cancer: a randomized multicenter trial. Lancet 2001; 357:1478.

66. Georgoulias V, Samonis G, Papadakis E, et al. Comparison of docetaxel/gemcitabine to docetaxel/cisplatin as first-line treatment of advanced non-small cell lung cancer: early results of a randomized trial. Lung Cancer 2001; 34 (S4):S47.

67. Kakolyris S, Tsiafaki X, Agelidou A, et al. Preliminary results of a multicenter randomized phase III trial of docetaxel plus gemcitabine (DG) versus vinorelbine plus cisplatin (VC) in patients with advanced non-small cell lung cancer. Proc Am Soc Clin Oncol 2002; 21:296a (Abstract 1182).

68. Kakolyris SS, Kouroussis C, Koukourakis M, et al. A dose-escalation study of irinotecan (CPT-11) in combination with gemcitabine in patients with advanced non-small cell lung cancer previously treated with a cisplatin-based front line chemotherapy. Anticancer Res 2002; 22:1891.

69. Rigas JR, Carey M, Cole B, et al. Multicenter Web-based phase III study to test the survival equivalence of non-platinum-based (NPB) vs. platinum-based (PB) therapy for advanced non-small cell lung cancer (NSCLC): the Dartmouth NPB Chemotherapy Trial (D0112). Proc Am Soc Clin Oncol 2004; 23:631 (Abstract 7071).

70. Herbst RS, Lynch C, Vasconcelles M, et al. Gemcitabine and vinorelbine in patients with advanced lung cancer: preclinical studies and report of a phase I trial. Cancer Chemother Pharmacol 2001; 48:151.

71. De Luca A, Grassi M, Maiello MR, et al. Does the sequence of gemcitabine and vinorelbine affect their efficacy in non-small cell lung cancer in vitro? Anticancer Res 2004; 24:2985.

72. Isokangas OP, Knuuttila A, Halme M, et al. Phase II study of vinorelbine and gemcitabine for inoperable stage IIIB–IV non small-cell lung cancer. Ann Oncol 1999; 10:1059-1063.

73. Krajnik G, Mohn-Staudner A, Thaler J, et al. Vinorelbine-gemcitabine in advanced non-small cell lung cancer (NSCLC):An AASLC phase II trial. Austrian Association for the Study of Lung Cancer. Ann Oncol 2000; 11:993.

74. Chen YM, Perng RP, Yang KY, et al. A multicenter phase II trial of vinorelbine plus gemcitabine in previously untreated inoperable (stage IIIB/IV) non-small cell lung cancer. Chest 2000; 117:1583.

75. Lorusso V, Carpagnano F, Frasci G, et al. Phase I/II study of gemcitabine plus vinorelbine as first-line chemotherapy of non-small-cell lung cancer. J Clin Oncol 2000; 18:405.

76. Lilenbaum RC, Cano R, Schwartz M, et al. Gemcitabine and vinorelbine in advanced non small cell lung carcinoma: a phase II study. Cancer 2000; 88:557.

77. Bajetta E, Chiara Stani S, De Candis D, et al. Gemcitabine plus vinorelbine as first-line chemotherapy in advanced non-small cell lung carcinoma: a phase II trial. Cancer 2000; 89:763.

78. Laack E, Mende T, Benk J, et al. Gemcitabine and vinorelbine as first-line chemotherapy for advanced non-small cell lung cancer: a phase II trial. Eur J Cancer 2001; 37:583.

79. Palmeri S, Leonardi V, Gebbia V, et al. Gemcitabine plus vinorelbine in stage IIIB or IV non-small cell lung cancer (NSCLC): a multicentre phase II clinical trial. Lung Cancer 2001; 34:115.

80. Hirsh V, Langleben A, Ayoub J, et al. Flexible chemotherapy regimen with gemcitabine and vinorelbine for metastatic non-small cell lung carcinoma: a phase II multicenter trial. Cancer 2001; 92:830.

81. Herbst RS, Khuri FR, Lu C, et al. The novel and effective nonplatinum, nontaxane combination of gemcitabine and vinorelbine in advanced non-small cell lung carcinoma: potential for decreased toxicity and combination with biological therapy. Cancer 2002; 95:340.

82. Hosoe S, Komuta K, Shibata K, et al. Gemcitabine and vinorelbine followed by docetaxel in patients with advanced non-small-cell lung cancer: a multi-institutional phase II trial of nonplatinum sequential triplet combination chemotherapy (JMTO LC00-02). Br J Cancer 2003; 88:342.

83. Katakami N, Sugiura T, Nogami T, et al. Combination chemotherapy of gemcitabine and vinorelbine for patients in stage IIIB-IV non-small cell lung cancer: a phase II study of the West Japan Thoracic Oncology Group (WJTOG) 9908, Lung Cancer 2004; 43:93.

84. Kashii T, Yamamoto N, Takada Y, et al. A randomized phase II study of carboplatin/gemcitabine (CG) versus vinorelbine/gemcitabine (VG) in patients with advanced non-small cell lung cancer (NSCLC); mature results of West Japan Thoracic Oncology Group (WJTOG) 0104. Proc Am Soc Clin Oncol 2004; 23:644 (Abstract 7124).

85. Lilenbaum RC, Chen CS, Chidiac T, Schwarzenberger PO, Thant M, Versola M, Lane SR. Phase II randomized trial of vinorelbine and gemcitabine versus carboplatin and paclitaxel in advanced non-small-cell lung cancer. Ann Oncol 2005; 16:97.

86. Laack E, Dickgreber N, Müller T, et al. Randomized phase III study of gemcitabine and vinorelbine versus gemcitabine, vinorelbine, and cisplatin in the treatment of advanced non-small-cell lung cancer: from the German and Swiss Lung Cancer Study Group. J Clin Oncol 2004; 22:2348.

87. Alberola V, Camps C, Provencio M, et al. Cisplatin plus gemcitabine versus a cisplatin-based triplet versus non-platinum sequential doublets in advanced non-small-cell lung cancer: a Spanish lung cancer group phase III randomized trial. J Clin Oncol 2003; 21:3207.

88. Gridelli C, Gallo C, Shepherd FA, et al. Gemcitabine plus vinorelbine compared with cisplatin plus vinorelbine or cisplatin plus gemcitabine for advanced non-small cell lung cancer: a phase III trial of the Italian GEMVIN investigators and the National Cancer Institute of Canada Clinical Trials Group. J Clin Oncol 2003; 21:3025.

89. Gridelli C, Perrone F, Gallo C, et al. Chemotherapy for elderly patients with advanced non-small cell lung cancer: the Multicenter Italian Lung Cancer in the Elderly Study (MILES) phase III randomized trial. J Natl Cancer Inst 2003; 95:362.

90. Abratt RP, Szczesna A, Mattson K, et al. Vinorelbine (NVB)-carboplatin (CBDCA) vs. non-platinum doublets in inoperable non-small cell lung cancer (NSCLC) patients (pts) – final results of the Glob 2 phase III with patient benefit analysis. Proc Am Soc Clin Oncol 2004; 23:619 (Abstract 7016).

91. Baldini E, Ardizzoni A, Prochilo T, Cafferata MA, Boni L, Tibaldi C. Gemcitabine, ifosfamide and Navelbine (GIN): a platinum-free combination in advanced non-small-cell

lung cancer (NSCLC). Cancer Chemother Pharmacol 2000; 49 (S1):S25.

92. Feliu J, Lopez Gomez L, Madronal C, et al. Gemcitabine plus vinorelbine in nonsmall cell lung carcinoma patients age 70 year or older or patients who cannot receive cisplatin. Oncopaz Cooperative Group. Cancer 1999; 86:1463.

93. Frasci G, Lorusso V, Panza N, et al. Gemcitabine plus vinorelbine versus vinorelbine alone in elderly patients with advanced non-small-cell lung cancer. J Clin Oncol 2000; 18:2529.

94. Adjei AA. Pemetrexed (Alimta): a novel multitargeted antifolate agent. Expert Rev Anticancer Ther 2003; 3:145.

95. Rusthoven JJ, Eisenhauer E, Butts C, et al. Multitargeted antifolate LY231514 as first-line chemotherapy for patients with advanced non-small-cell lung cancer: a phase II study. National Cancer Institute of Canada Clinical Trials Group. J Clin Oncol 1999; 17:1194.

96. Niyikiza C, Baker SD, Seitz DE, et al. Homocysteine and methylmalonic acid: markers to predict and avoid toxicity from pemetrexed therapy. Mol Cancer Ther 2002; 1:545.

97. Clarke SJ, Abratt R, Goedhals L, et al. Phase II trial of pemetrexed disodium (ALIMTA, LY231514) in chemotherapy-naive patients with advanced non-small-cell lung cancer. Ann Oncol 2002; 13:737.

98. Adjei AA, Erlichman C, Sloan JA, et al. Phase I and pharmacologic study of sequences of gemcitabine and the multitargeted antifolate agent in patients with advanced solid tumors. J Clin Oncol 2000; 18:1748.

99. Adjei AA, Klein CE, Kastrissios H, et al. Phase I and pharmacokinetic study of irinotecan and docetaxel in patients with advanced solid tumors: preliminary evidence of clinical activity. J Clin Oncol 2000; 18:1116.

100. Adjei AA, Nair S, Reuter N, et al. Pemetrexed (Pem)/gemcitabine (Gem) as front-line therapy for advanced NSCLC: a randomized, phase II trial of three schedules. Proc Am Soc Clin Oncol 2004; 23:630 (Abstract 7070).

101. Bahadori HR, Rocha Lima CMS, Green MR, Safa AR. Synergistic effect of gemcitabine and irinotecan (CPT-11) on breast and small cell lung cancer cell lines. Anticancer Res 1999; 19:5423.

102. Nishio M, Oyanagi F, Karato A, et al. Phase I study of biweekly chemotherapy with gemcitabine (GEM) and irinotecan (CPT-11) in previously treated patients (pts) with non-small-cell lung cancer (NSCLC). Proc Am Soc Clin Oncol 2002; 21:219b (Abstract 2693).

103. Georgoulias V, Ardavanis A, Agelidou A, et al. Docetaxel versus docetaxel plus cisplatin as front-line treatment of patients with advanced non-small-cell lung cancer: a randomized, multicenter phase III trial. J Clin Oncol 2004; 22:2602.

104. Georgoulias V, Kouroussis C, Agelidou A, et al. Irinotecan plus gemcitabine vs. irinotecan for the second-line treatment of patients with advanced NSCLC pretreated with docetaxel and cisplatin: a multicenter, randomized, phase II study. Br J Cancer 2004; 91:482.

105. Rocha Lima CM, Rizvi NA, Zhang C, et al. Randomized phase II trial of gemcitabine plus irinotecan or docetaxel in stage IIIB or stage IV NSCLC. Ann Oncol 2004; 15:410.

106. Breton JL, Westeel V, Jacoulet P, et al. Phase I study of paclitaxel (taxol) plus vinorelbine (navelbine) in patients with untreated stage IIIB and IV non-small-cell lung cancer. Lung Cancer 2001; 31:295.

107. Kano Y, Akutsu M, Suzuki K, et al. Schedule-dependent interactions between vinorelbine and paclitaxel in human carcinoma cell lines in vitro. Breast Cancer Res Treat 1999; 56:79.

108. Stathopoulos GP, Veslemes M, Georgatou N, et al. Paclitaxel and vinorelbine combination in advanced inoperable

adenocarcinoma of the lung. A phase II study. Anticancer Res 2003; 23:3479.

109. Stathopoulos GP, Veslemes M, Georgatou N, Antoniou D. Front-line paclitaxel-vinorelbine versus paclitaxel-carboplatin in patients with advanced non-small-cell lung cancer: a randomized phase III trial. Ann Oncol 2004; 5:1048.

110. Miller VA, Krug LM, Ng KK, Pizzo B, Perez W, Heelan RT, Kris MG. Phase II trial of docetaxel and vinorelbine in patients with advanced non-small-cell lung cancer. J Clin Oncol 2000; 18:1346.

111. Page RD, Smith FP, Geils GF, et al. Prospective multi-center phase II trial of docetaxel and vinorelbine with filgrastim support in subjects with advanced non-small cell lung cancer (NSCLC). Proc Am Soc Clin Oncol 2004; 23:647 (Abstract 7138).

112. Kouroussis C, Androulakis N, Kakolyris S, et al. First-line treatment of advanced non-small cell lung carcinoma with docetaxel and vinorelbine. Cancer 1998; 83:2083.

113. Walls JA, O'Rourke M, Garfield D, Asmar L. First-line therapy of Taxotere and Navelbine in patients with advanced non-small cell lung cancer (NSCLC). Proc Am Soc Clin Oncol 2000; 19:547a (Abstract 2158).

114. Murren JR, Davies M. Irinotecan and taxane combination for non-small cell lung cancer. Clin Lung Cancer 2002; 3 (S1):S5.

115. Raez LE, Rosado MF, Santos ES, Reis IM. Irinotecan and docetaxel as first-line chemotherapy in patients with stage IIIB/IV non-small cell lung cancer: experience from a prematurely closed phase II study. Lung Cancer 2004; 45:131.

116. Ziotopoulos P, Chandrinos V, Samaras N, et al. A phase II study of docetaxel plus irinotecan (DOCIRI) in chemo-naïve patients with non small cell lung cancer (NSCLC). Proc Am Soc Clin Oncol 2004; 23:679 (Abstract 7267).

117. Ramalingam S, Dobbs TW, Coke DE, Wojtowicz-Praga S, Belani CP. Weekly docetaxel and irinotecan for patients with advanced non-small cell lung cancer (NSCLC): results of a multi-center, phase II study. Proc Am Soc Clin Oncol 2004; 23:687 (Abstract 7298).

118. Yamamoto N, Fukuoka M, Negoro S, et al. Randomized phase II study of docetaxel/cisplatin versus docetaxel/irinotecan in advanced non-small cell lung cancer (NSCLC): a West Japan Thoracic Oncology Group study (WJTOG9803). Br J Cancer 2004; 90:87.

119. Pei XH, Nakanishi Y, Takayama K, et al. Effect of CPT-11 in combination with other anticancer agents in lung cancer cells. Anticancer Drugs 1997; 8:231.

120. Kasai T, Oka M, Soda H, et al. Phase I and pharmacokinetic study of irinotecan and paclitaxel for patients with advanced non-small cell lung cancer. Eur J Cancer 2002; 38:1871.

121. Yamamoto N, Negoro S, Chikazawa H, Shimizu T, Fukuoka M. Pharmacokinetic interaction of the combination paclitaxel and irinotecan in vivo and clinical study. Proc Am Soc Clin Oncol 1999; 18:187a (Abstract 718).

122. Rosen P, Schaaf LJ, Knuth DW, et al. Phase I and pharmacokinetic trial of CPT-11 and paclitaxel in patients with advanced cancers. Proc Am Soc Clin Oncol 1999; 18:177a (Abstract 679).

123. Isla D, Rosell R, Sanchez JJ, et al. Phase II trial of paclitaxel plus gemcitabine in patients with locally advanced or metastatic non-small-cell lung cancer. J Clin Oncol 2001; 19(4):1071.

124. Monnerat C, Le Chevalier T, Kelly K, et al. Phase II study of pemetrexed-gemcitabine combination in patients with advanced-stage non-small-cell lung cancer. Clin Cancer Res 2004; 10(16):5439.

Second-Line Chemotherapy for Non-Small-Cell Lung Cancer

24

Eleni Karapanagiotou and Konstantinos N. Syrigos

Contents

24.1 Background

Chemotherapy for non-small-cell lung cancer (NSCLC) patients with stage IIIB or IV has only a palliation role, since their disease is incurable and the 5-year survival is less than 2% [1, 2]. Best supportive care (BSC) offers to this group of patients only 3.6 months (range 2.4–4.9 months), while platinum-based chemotherapy offers an improvement in the median overall survival time of 6–8 weeks. It has also doubled the 1-year survival rate and demonstrated important gains in secondary end points of clinical trials, such as the time to disease progression and the quality of life [3–5]. Based on the results of several randomized clinical trials and meta-analyses, the American College of Chest Physician Lung Cancer Guidelines Committee approved the administration of chemotherapy to fit patients with advanced-unresectable or metastatic disease, with grade of recommendation A. Currently, the platinum-based regimens comprise the gold standard as first-line treatment for advanced and metastatic.

Despite the undoubted gains from chemotherapy for stage IIIB or IV NSCLC patients, a proportion of approximately 50% of those who have received first-line platinum-based regimens will relapse during treatment or soon after completing it. These patients might be young, with good performance status, and their disease is expressed with only minor symptoms. In addition, clinical oncologists often come across patients with refractory disease who are willing to accept considerable toxicity in order to achieve a small prolongation in survival. Once the disease progresses the median survival time is approximately 3 months. It is clear that there is strong motivation for these patients to receive second-line chemotherapy [3, 6–10].

24.2 Docetaxel

Until recently the role of second-line chemotherapy was undefined. Fossella and colleagues tried to review the data surrounding this field of chemotherapy, with disappointing results. The majority of studies were small single-institute studies in which drug dosages and schedules were totally different and response rates were not reported. Moreover, no phase III clinical trials had been conducted. However, the agent demonstrating the most consistent responses in the second-line setting was docetaxel, which was evaluated in refractory platinum-based patients in seven phase-II clinical trials. A total of 312 participants received 100 mg/m^2 docetaxel every 3 weeks, resulting in response rates ranging from 14 to 24%, median overall survival time greater than 7 months, and 1-year survival rates ranging from 25 to 44% [11].

Docetaxel is a second-generation taxane that is derived from the needles of the European yew tree. It has a large spectrum of antitumor activity that is expressed basically by inhibiting microtubule dynamics. The principal mechanism of action for both taxanes (docetaxel and paclitaxel) is to promote microtubulin assembly and stabilize the polymers against depolymerization. Docetaxel has exhibited documented cytotoxicity in murine tumor models and human tumor xenografts, and this preclinical promise has successfully translated into clinical practice. Several clinical trials have proved the efficacy of docetaxel in NSCLC patients in front-line treatment as combination therapy or monotherapy.

A large randomized phase-III clinical trial (TAX317) has been conducted to determine whether docetaxel as a single agent is effective in the second-line treatment of NSCLC patients. The primary outcome measure was survival and secondary end points were response rate, time to progression, toxicity, and quality of life. Eligible participants were those who had documented progressive disease after receiving a platinum-containing (cisplatin or carboplatin) regimen, but not a taxane. Forty-nine patients received 100 mg/m² docetaxel and 55 received 75 mg/m² docetaxel once every 21 days, while the control group of 100 patients received only BSC. The docetaxel dosage changed from 100 mg/m² to 75 mg/m² during the study due to an unacceptably high toxic death rate in the experimental arm. The results of this trial were really encouraging. The median overall survival was 7.0 months for the chemotherapy arm and 4.6 months for the BSC arm, while the 1-year survival rates for the chemotherapy and BSC arm were 29 and 19%, respectively, and the overall response rate was 7%. The key point of this clinical trial was the docetaxel dosage. Prolongation of median overall survival was seen with both doses of docetaxel, but the most marked improvement was associated with the lower dose, for which the 1-year survival rate was significantly higher, at 37%. Moreover, the prolongation of patients' life was in line with the improvement of patient quality of life (well-being). The quality-of-life analysis demonstrated less worsening of performance status and less common use of tumor-related medications for docetaxel patients. Only 32% of docetaxel patients versus 49% of the BSC arm required morphine-equivalent medication for the pain, and 39% versus 55% patients, respectively, required nonmorphine analgesics. Palliation radiotherapy was required for fewer docetaxel patients (26%) than BSC patients (37%). The safety profile of docetaxel administration was satisfactory. Grade 3 or 4 neutropenia occurred in 67% of those patients administered 75 mg/m² docetaxel, and only one patient (1.8%) developed febrile neutropenia. Grade 3 or 4 anemia occurred in three (5.5%) patients at the lower dose. Severe thrombocytopenia was observed in less than 1% of the patients, without any reported bleeding episodes. Nonhematological toxicities were similar, although sometimes worse for the BSC patients in terms of more asthenia and neurotoxicity. This trial concluded that good-performance NSCLC patients who have progressed after receiving a platinum-based regimen should be offered the chance of a second-line docetaxel-based chemotherapy with the aim of prolongation of survival as well as

a significant improvement in disease-related symptoms [11, 12].

In another phase III trial (TAX320) that examined the efficacy of docetaxel as second-line chemotherapy in NSCLC patients, 373 patients who had received 1 or more platinum-based regimens with no exclusion of prior exposure to paclitaxel were randomized to 3 arms: the first received 100 mg/m² docetaxel, the second 75 mg/m² docetaxel (both arms in a cycle of 21 days), and the control arm was represented by 123 patients who received either vinorelbine (n = 89) or ifosfamide (n = 34). The 1-year survival rate was significantly greater in docetaxel-treated patients (32% at 75 mg/m² and 21% at 100 mg/m²) compared to the vinorelbine/ifosfamide-treated patients (19%). There was only a trend toward improved overall survival for the docetaxel group, although 26-week progression-free survival was significantly favored for the docetaxel-treated patients. Both docetaxel arms presented a slight increased hematological toxicity, the incidence of febrile neutropenia being 8% for those receiving the lower docetaxel dose, compared to 1% for the control arm. The nonhematological side effects were similar across treatment groups [13].

A finding from this trial that was of important clinical significance was that prior paclitaxel therapy did not predict the likelihood of a patient's response to docetaxel. This was proved by the partial response rates between patients with prior paclitaxel therapy (n = 91) and those without paclitaxel exposure (n = 157), which were rather equivalent at 10.5% and 8.5%, respectively [13].

In an attempt to minimize docetaxel toxicity, three clinical trials were conducted whereby the standard dose of 75 mg/m² every 3 weeks was compared to one weekly dose of 33 mg/m². In a landmark analysis of a total of 524 patients, no significant differences were found for either response rates or toxicity. The median time to progression and the overall survival were rather similar between arms, while the weekly administration of docetaxel was associated with less hematological toxicity, the rate of severe neutropenia being particularly lower. In conclusion, weekly docetaxel represents another option for patients at risk for severe neutropenia and its consequences [14–16].

Although the recent advances in chemotherapy are welcome, the outcome expectations from chemotherapy administration remain slim. In economical terms, is it cost-effective to administer docetaxel as palliation therapy? A retrospective economic evaluation of docetaxel clinical trial (TAX 317) was undertaken using data from the 63 patients using the Canadian health-care system in 1999. This analysis concluded that the cost per life-year gained by using docetaxel at the recommended dose of 75 mg/m² was approximately US$20,000, which is similar to the care expenditures for palliative chemotherapy of other solid tumors [17].

There is an increasing body of evidence suggesting that the administration of second-line treatment in fit patients who are experiencing progressive disease after receiving platinum-containing regimens is recommended. In this context, the USA Food and Drug Administration (FDA) and the European Agency for the Evaluation of Medical Products approved Docetaxel as standard treatment in the second-line setting.

24.3 Pemetrexed

Patients who are candidates for second-line chemotherapy expect only a modest prolongation of life and a better quality of life with minimal disease symptoms. They are eager to receive chemotherapy, but at the same time are reluctant to spend a considerable part of their limited life in hospital due to treatment-related complications. Due to its toxicity profile, docetaxel is still greeted with a degree of unease and there have been attempts to identify new compounds with the same efficacy but reduced toxicity. One such compound, a novel chemotherapeutic agent, is pemetrexed (Alimta). It is the first multitargeted antifolate with minimal pyrimidine nucleus differences from the common antifolates. Pemetrexed inhibits more than one enzyme in the cell cycle, including thymidylate synthase, dihydrofolate reductase, glycinamide ribonucleotide formyl transferase, aminoimidazole carboxamide ribonucleotide formyltransferase, and is implicated in the inhibition of pyrimidine and purine synthesis. The fact that a tumor is composed of a heterogeneous group of cells with varying predominant enzymes may provide an explanation regarding the multitargeted cytotoxid mechanisms of action of pemetrexed [18].

Several trials on the efficacy and toxicity of pemetrexed in malignant mesothelioma and NSCLC patients have been conducted; these have found an increase in the response rates of accrued patients, but also increased side effects of the treatment. A retrospective analysis of serious adverse events was performed consecutively. Plasma levels of homocysteine, which represent a surrogate for folate nutritional status, and plasma levels of methylmelonic acid, which is an indicator of B12 vitamin status, were markedly elevated in patients with neutropenia, thrombocytopenia, and nonhematologic toxicities such as infection, mucositis, and diarrhea. There was also an increased death rate related to this new agent. After treatment with pemetrexed, patients were prescribed a daily dose of 350–1,000 µg acid folic and 1,000 µg vitamin B12, given intramuscularly every 9 weeks, resulting in a considerable improvement in drug toxicity [19–21].

Based on the results of several phase II clinical trials, Hanna and coworkers conducted a large phase III clinical trial in an attempt to examine the superiority of pemetrexed compared to docetaxel, the standard second-line chemotherapy. In the largest phase III clinical

Table 24.1. Phase III clinical trial: Pemetrexed vs. Taxotere. *G-CSF* Granulocyte colony-stimulating factor

Toxicity	Docetaxel	Pemetrexed
Grade 3/4 neutropenia	40.2%	5.3%
Febrile neutropenia	12.7%	1.9%
Infections with grade 3/4 neutropenia	3.3%	0%
Requirements for G-CSF[a]	19.2%	2.6%
Hospitalizations related to drug	13.4%	1.5%
Alopecia	37.7%	6.4%

[a] Requirements for G-CSF: % of cycles

trial of second-line therapy, 571 NSCLC patients were accrued who had documented disease progression after receiving only 1 front-line regimen. Of these, 283 patients received 500 mg/m^2 of pemetrexed once every 21 days with acid folic and vitamin B12 supplementation, and 288 patients received 75 mg/m^2 docetaxel in the same cycle. Both arms received dexamethasone premedication. From the randomized patients, 90% had previously been treated with platinum regimens and 28% with taxanes regimens. This study met the primary and secondary endpoints. The overall response rates were 9.1% for the pemetrexed-treated group and 8.8% for docetaxel-treated group; both groups had the same 1-year survival rate. With regard to toxicity, pemetrexed presented a more safety profile with less episodes of hospitalization related to drug administration and febrile neutropenia (Table 24.1). The requirements for granulocyte colony-stimulating factor were increased in the docetaxel arm. Notably, due to vitamin B12 and acid folic supplementation, pemetrexed-related myelotoxicity, diarrhea, and mucositis were limited. The prophylactic use of dexamethasone lessened the occurrences and intensity of skin rash [22].

Based on data obtained from this clinical trial, in the summer of 2004 the USA FDA approved pemetrexed as a single-agent chemotherapy agent as an alternative to docetaxel in the second-line setting for NSCLC patients.

24.4 Other Agents on Trial

New agents have been tested in several clinical trials in the treatment of NSCLC patients, as monotherapy or in combination regimens. They can be divided into the following classes: mitotic spindle inhibitors (vinorelbine), antimetabolites (gemcitabine), inhibitors of topoisomerase I (irinotecan and topotecan), and taxanes (paclitaxel and docetaxel). If we exclude docetaxel and pemetrexed, which have been approved for use by the FDA as second-line chemotherapy agents, the new agents represent some options as salvage therapy in different combinations.

24.4.1 Vinorelbine

Vinorelbine is a semisynthetic derivative of vinca rosea, the Madagascar periwinkle, which is used as an antimitotic agent through its property of affecting the dynamics of spindle microtubules. Vinca alkaloids interact with tubulin subunits to prevent microtubule assembly, and consecutively induce chromosome segregation in dividing cells and cause aneuploidy. Vinorelbine has shown interesting results with respect to response rates, time to progression, and median overall survival when was tested as single, first-line treatment; its basic treatment-related toxity is neutropenia. It has been involved in few clinical trials as second-line treatment, and with moderate results. There were no responses in two studies of patients who had previously failed to respond to platinum-based regimens, and in a third study a response rate of 20% was reported but with no other information [23–25].

Patient preference and the need for fewer visits in hospital, as well as concerns and difficulties with intravenous access have driven the development of oral vinorelbine. Several clinical trials have tried to evaluate the feasibility and safety profile of oral vinorelbine in treatment of recurrent NSCLC patients [26].

The feasibility of vinorelbine as an active agent in the salvage therapy of NSCLC patients has been explored in clinical trials in combination with other active agents such as platinol, carboplatin, docetaxel, and irinotecan. Ongoing studies are evaluating the tolerability and activity of these combinations. Those studies evaluating the efficacy of vinorelbine in combination with either platinol or carboplatin are based on small numbers (range 17–44) of pretreated patients and use different regimens and schedules, although encouraging results regarding to objective responses and 1-year survival rate with acceptable toxicity have been presented [27–30].

24.4.2 Gemcitabine

Gemcitabine is a novel deoxycytidine analogue that has been implicated in the inhibition of DNA and cellular apoptosis. It is a prodrug that, once transported into the cell, is phosphorylated by deoxycytidine kinase into an active form. This active form can be incorporated into the terminal part of elongating DNA strands, inhibiting the activity of DNA polymerases. Gemcitabine is indicated in combination with cisplatin in the front-line treatment of inoperable NSCLC patients. Response rates of 20% have been demonstrated in several phase II trials, and so gemcitabine has been evaluated in previously treated NSCLC patients at a dosage of 1,000 mg every 3–4 weeks. The published response rates range from 0 to 21% and the median overall survival was between 5.5 and 9 months. The 1-year survival was scarcely reported. In conclusion, these results are not encouraging for the use of gemcitabine as monotherapy in salvage therapy [31–35].

However, better responses were obtained when gemcitabine and vinorelbine were combined in several phase II clinical trials. The number of patients enrolled in these was small and larger studies should therefore be performed. Excluding the Camps study, which enrolled 16 patients and presented disappointing results with only 1 complete responder, no partial responders, and a median survival of 25 weeks [36], the following studies present a hint of success, which translates into a median survival ranging from 6.5 to 8.5 months and a 1-year survival rate reaching 35%. Further evaluation of this combination is needed and may represent another option for relapsing patients after receiving a platinum–taxane combination in the front-line setting (Table 24.2) [37–42].

Table 24.2. Clinical trials phase II of combination gemcitabine plus navelbine in second-line setting

	Hainsworth [37]	Kosmas [38]	Pectasides [39]	Herbst [40]	Chen [41]	Park [42]
Dose and schedule	V 20 mg/m^2 G 1,000 mg/m^2 days 1, 8, 15, q28d	V 25 mg/m^2 G 1,000 mg/m^2 days 1, 8, q21d	V 25 mg/m^2 G 800 mg/m^2 days 1, 8, q21d	V 25 mg/m^2 G 900 mg/m^2 days 1, 8, 15, q21d	V 20mg/m^2 G 800 mg/m^2 days 1, 8, 15, q28d	V 30 mg/m^2 G 1,000 mg/m^2 days 1, 8, q21d
Pts (n)	55	40	39	78 (36)	17	38
Prior CHT (%)	85	100	100	46	100	100
PR (%)	18	22.5	2.6	17	31.3	21
SD (%)	48	32.5	35.9	50	N/R	55
TTP (months)	5	4.5	4.7	N/R	4.6	3.9
Median survival (months)	6.5	7	7.3	8.5	8.3	8.1
One-year survival (%)	20	17	35	30	34	N/R
Grade 3–4 neutropenia (%)	36	33	5.2	67	52.9	28
Grade 3–4 thrombocytopenia (%)	22	0	0	13.9	17.64	N/R

V Vinolrebine, *G* gemcitabine, *Pts* patients, *CHT* chemotherapy, *PR* partial response, *SD* stable disease, *TTP* time to progression, *q28d* every 28 days, *q21d* every 21 days, *N/R* not reported

24.4.3 Inhibitors of Topoisomerase I

The topoisomerases (I and II) are nuclear enzymes that play a role in DNA synthesis and transcription. The role of both enzymes in the cell cycle is to relieve DNA torsional strain by forming a reversible complex with it and by introducing transient enzyme-bridged strand breaks. When the transcription is finished, the enzymes reseal the break and dissociate from the DNA. Topoisomerase inhibitors play a role in the stabilization of topoisomerase in a complex with DNA, resulting in double- stranded DNA break and subsequent programmed cell death. Examples of topoisomerase I inhibitors are irinotecan and topotecan, and these represent an interesting class of agents for the treatment of NSCLC.

24.4.3.1 Irinotecan

Preclinical studies suggest that irinotecan has a substantial activity either alone or in combination with other agents in palliation therapy of NSCLC. There are several small studies exploring the efficacy of irinotecan in the second-line setting, reporting response rates between 0 and 29% [43–45]. Unfortunately, when this novel agent was added to docetaxel in a combination regimen and compared to standard second-line chemotherapy docetaxel at 75 mg/m^2 in a 3-weekly schedule in two large phase II clinical studies, not only was there no improvement in response rates and 1-year survival rates, there was also increased gastrointestinal toxicity [46, 47]. Moreover, irinotecan has been studied in phase II clinical trials as a second-line treatment, in more than one combination with docetaxel, vinorelbine, cisplatin, capecitabine, or gemcitabine. The reported results showed response rates ranging between 29 and 48% and median survival ranging between 25 and 32 weeks, while the reported hematologic and nonhematologic toxicities were acceptable (Table 24.3) [48–52]. In a phase II study, Georgoulias and coworkers compared the combination of irinotecan and gemcitabine

versus irinotecan in docetaxel- and cisplatin-pretreated patients ($n = 147$). The response rates were 18.4% and 4.2%, respectively in the two arms. The combined schedule resulted in a higher response rate but without any improvement in the overall survival [53].

24.4.3.2 Topotecan

Topotecan is a semisynthetic derivative of camptothecin, which has been approved for the second-line treatment of small-cell lung cancer and ovarian cancer. In several phase II clinical trials in previously untreated patients with advanced NSCLC, the intravenous administration of topotecan at a dose of 1.5–2 mg/m^2/day for 5 consecutively days resulted in moderate response rates of 15–16%, and another study reported stable disease in half of the enrolled patients [54–56].

In the second-line setting, topotecan was evaluated in combination with gemcitabine in a small trial. Thirty-five previously treated patients received 0.75 mg/m^2 topotecan and gemcitabine 400 mg/m^2 for 5 days in a 3-week cycle. A partial response was experienced by 11% of the participants, and another 23% experienced stable disease. The median survival time was 7 months and the 1-year survival rate was 20%. Modest hematologic toxicity was observed [57].

An oral formulation of topotecan has been tested in a large, 800-patient study as second-line treatment in NSCLC patients. Topotecan at a dose of 2.3 mg/m^2 (given orally) for 5 consecutive days in a 21-day cycle has been compared to standard-therapy docetaxel 75 mg/m^2; the trial results are pending.

24.4.4 Taxanes

Paclitaxel, like docetaxel, is a microtubule stabilizer that results in cell cycle arrest and impairment of mitotic progression. Paclitaxel has been investigated extensively in several solid tumors including NSCLC. It has gained a position in the front-line treatment of NSCLC patients

Table 24.3. Irinotecan in several combinations as second-line treatment

	Font [48]	Gonzalez [49]	Kakolyris [50]	Nakanishi [51]	Han [52]
Schedule	I 70 mg/m^2, D 25 mg/m^2 days 1, 8, 15, q28 d	I 300 mg/m^2 day 1 V 30 mg/m^2 days 1, 14, q28d	I 100 mg/m^2 days 1, 8 P 80 mg/m^2 day 8, q21d	I 60 mg/m^2 P 30 mg/m^2 days 1, 8, 15, q28d	I 90–100 mg/m^2 days 1, 8 C 2,000 mg/m^2 days 1–14 q21d
Pts (n)	51	33	44	21	37
RR%	43	48	42	29	45.7
Median survival	8 months	25 weeks	8 months	32 weeks	7.4 months (6-month follow up)
One-year survival (%)	30	N/A	N/A	43	N/A
Toxicity	Mild	Mild	Increased	Increased	Acceptable

I Irinotecan, *D* docetaxel, *P* cisplatin, *C* capecitabine, *RR* response rate, *N/A* not assessed

in combination with other active agents. Paclitaxel has also been investigated as a single agent in the second-line setting of this target group. The results from several clinical trials using paclitaxel at very different doses and schedules show a clinical benefit rate ranging from 0 to 42% and median overall survival ranging from 16 to 52 weeks with acceptable toxicities. In summary, paclitaxel represents a favorable chemotherapeutic approach in this setting (Table 24.4) [58–70].

In an effort to maximize the efficacy of paclitaxel, it was combined with other active agents such as gemcitabine, cisplatin, and irinotecan in small phase II studies. These combinations resulted in active schemes with acceptable levels of toxicity, but future trials will clarify the role of paclitaxel-based combinations in the salvage therapy of NSCLC patients. In a randomized study including 71 patients, weekly administration of docetaxel at a dose of 36 mg/m^2 was compared to weekly administration of paclitaxel at a dose of 80 mg/m^2 for 6 weeks followed by a 2-week rest. Partial response was experienced by one and five patients, median time to progression was 74 and 68 days, and the median overall survival was 184 and 105 days with docetaxel and paclitaxel, respectively. Both taxanes showed a discrete efficacy in this population [71].

An oral formulation of taxane under the code name BMS-275183 has been approved for participation in combination with pemetrexed in a clinical phase I–II study in patients with recurrent pretreated NSCLC [72].

24.5 Targeted Therapy

Even with the introduction of new antineoplastic agents and more effective chemotherapeutic combinations, the prognosis for refractory NSCLC patients receiving second-line chemotherapy remains dismal. Recently, our knowledge of molecular oncology has significantly increased, endorsing recognition of the main signaling pathways that promotes malignant cell transformation. This in turn has raised hopes for the development of a novel therapeutic strategy that would target neoplastic cells, whilst minimizing both damage to noncancerous cells and any side effect resulting from the given therapy.

Two main representatives of targeted therapy have been explored in this subpopulation of patients, the epidermal growth factor receptor (EGFR) pathway inhibitors and the neoangiogenesis inhibitors.

24.5.1 EGFR Inhibitors

The EGFR family autocrine pathway plays a critical role in the malignant and metastatic development potential of NSCLC. Ligands binding to their extracellular domain initiate a molecular cascade that promotes cellular proliferation and differentiation. EGFR targeting can be achieved through two principal mechanisms: (1) through monoclonal antibodies that prevent ligand binding, or (2) by means of small-molecule tyrosine-kinase inhibitors (TKIs) that inhibit the adenosine triphosphate binding site of the growth factor receptor.

Table 24.4. Paclitaxel as a single agent in phase II clinical trials in the second-line setting

	Tan [58]	Murphy [59]	Ruchdeschel [60]	Hainsworth [61]	Nauman [62]	Socinski [63]	Chang [64]	Juan [65]	Socinski [66]	Sculier [67]	Buccheri [68]	Ceresoli [69]	Yasuda [70]
Schedule	135–400 mg/m^2, 24-h 175 mg/m^2, 3-h	175–200 mg/m^2, 24-h	250 mg/m^2, 24-h	200 mg/m^2 135 mg/m^2, 1-h	130–175 mg/m^2, 1-h	140 mg/m^2, 96-h	50–100 mg/m^2, weekly	80 mg/m^2, weekly	80 mg/m^2, weekly	225 mg/m^2, 1-h	100 mg/m^2, weekly	80 mg/m^2, weekly	80 mg/m^2, weekly
Pts (n)	11	40	14	16 10	16	13	13	40	62	67	38	55	39
Clinical benefit (%)	9	22.5	28.5	38/0	N/R	31	N/R	37.5	8	27	42	36	31
Median survival	N/R	N/R	4 months	N/R	10 months	N/R	N/R	9.7 months	5.2 months	4.5 months	58 weeks	N/R	43 weeks
One-year survival (%)	N/R	N/R	N/R	N/R	45	N/R	N/R	N/R	20	19	N/R	N/R	N/R
Toxicity	N/R	Mild	Mild	N/R	N/R	Mild	N/R	Mild	Mild	Acceptable	Mild	Mild	Acceptable

-h Hourly

Gefitinib and erlotinib act as TKIs, while cetuximab is a monoclonal antibody that targets the extracellular domain of the human EGFR.

24.5.1.1 Gefitinib

Gefitinib has been approved for NSCLC patients as third-line treatment after receiving platinum- and docetaxel-based regimens. Its approval by the FDA was based on the Iressa Dose Evaluation in Advanced Lung Cancer (IDEAL 2) study, which showed a response rate of 10.6% and a symptom improvement rate of 40% without the existence of any randomized trial demonstrating superior survival rates for patients treating with this drug [73]. The data obtained in two clinical studies suggesting the administration of gefitinib as monotherapy and not in combination with chemotherapy is of great clinical importance [74]. Gefitinib treatment appears to be more efficacious in nonsmoking women with bronchoalveolar carcinoma. Preliminary results of the SWONG 0126 trial showed a response rate of 12% in previously treated patients [75]. Gefitinib toxicity is limited to diarrhea and skin rash and is generally well-tolerated.

A large phase III clinical trial involving gefitinib is ongoing, with the purpose of comparing a dose of 250 mg/day (taken orally) to the standard second-line chemotherapy of docetaxel at 75 mg/m^2 every 3 weeks. The results are pending [76].

24.5.1.2 Erlotinib

Erlotinib, the other orally available EGFR TKI that demonstrated a response rate of 26% in a trial involving patients with bronchoalveolar carcinoma, was evaluated in a large phase III clinical trial compared to placebo. All 731 of the participants, had received 1 or 2 chemotherapeutic regimens and they were randomized in two arms. The results were encouraging. The median survival was 6.7 and 4.7 months, the 1-year survival rate was 31% and 22%, and the time to progression was 2.23 and 1.84 months for the erlotinib- and placebo-treated arms, respectively. Moreover, disease-related symptoms were better controlled in the erlotinib-treated group. Toxicity was limited to rash and diarrhea [77].

24.5.1.3 Cetuximab

Cetuximab is a recombinant human/mouse chimeric IgG1 monoclonal antibody that targets the extracellular domain of the human EGFR. Its efficacy has been demonstrated in solid tumors. A multicenter, open-label, randomized, phase III clinical trial is currently open to recruitment for patients with relapsed NSCLC after failure of initial platinum-based chemotherapy. Four experimental arms are presented: cetuximab plus docetax-el, cetuximab plus pemetrexed, docetaxel alone, or pemetrexed alone [78].

24.5.1.4 Neoangiogenesis Inhibitors – Bevacizumab

Bevacizumab is a humanized anti-vascular endothelial growth factor antibody that is currently under investigation in a variety of solid tumors. Several ongoing studies are under way in NSCLC in front-line treatment as well as in salvage therapy. Phase II studies explore the efficacy of bevacizumab combinations with erlotinib and/or cetuximab in previously treated NSCLC patients.

24.6 Conclusions

The role of second-line chemotherapy is the subject of a longstanding debate. In 1997, the American Society of Clinical Oncology (ASCO) guidelines stated that it could be neither confirmed nor refuted that second-line chemotherapy improves survival in patients with advanced NSCLC [79]. One year later, the ASCO guidelines stated that second-line treatment may be appropriate for good-performance-status patients for whom an investigational protocol is not available or desired, or for patients who respond to initial chemotherapy and then experienced a long progression-free interval off treatment [80]. Some years later, two large randomized phase III clinical trials with realistic and appropriate objectives were conducted. These trials showed a superiority for docetaxel regarding survival prolongation and quality of life when it was compared either to BSC or chemotherapy. In addition, these studies presented an acceptable toxicity profile. As a result, some questions have been answered. Chemotherapy in the second-line setting is of value in fit patients, offering a survival and clinical benefit. The American College of Chest Physicians Lung Cancer Guidelines Committee approved the administration of second-line chemotherapy in platinum-refractory NSCLC patients with grade of recommendation B [3]. An alternative to docetaxel chemotherapy is presented by pemetrexed, which achieves the same goals in treatment targets with minor toxicities. Moreover, several drug combinations are under investigation in an attempt to be determine the best regimen with the least toxic profile.

Although current data offer a hint of victory in this war, the research efforts have been driven to molecular oncology. Targeted therapies gain new ground in the second- line treatment of NSCLC patients. New anti-EGFR and antiangiogenesis agents are being widely investigated in phase II and III clinical trials in combination with chemotherapeutic agents or alone. Research advances are orientated toward the adoption of drugs tailored to the tumor's molecular profile, with the aim of greater efficacy and less toxicity.

Key Points

- Second-line treatment of non-small-cell lung cancer patients offers a survival and clinical benefit.
- It is appropriate for good-performance-status patients for whom an investigational protocol is not available or desired, or for patients who respond to initial chemotherapy and then experience a long progression-free interval off treatment.
- Several drug combinations are currently under investigation in an attempt to obtained the best regimen with the least toxic profile.

References

1. Parker SL, Tong T, Bolden S, et al. Cancer statistics, 1996. CA Cancer J Clin 1997; 47:5.
2. Ginsberg JK, Kris MG, Armstrong JG. Cancer of the lung: non-small cell lung cancer. In: De Vita VT, Hellman S, Rosenberg SA (eds.) Cancer: Principles and Practice of Oncology, 4th edn. Lippincott, Philadelphia, 1993; p 673.
3. Socinski MA, Morris DE, Masters GA, et al. Chemotherapeutic management of stage IV non-small cell lung cancer. Chest 2003; 123:226S.
4. Johnson DH. Locally advanced, unresectable non-small cell lung cancer: new treatment strategies. Chest 2000; 117(2):123S.
5. Non-Small Cell Lung Cancer Collaborative Group. Chemotherapy in non-small cell lung cancer: a meta-analysis using updated data on individual patients from 52 randomized clinical trials. Br Med J 1995; 311:899.
6. Buccheri G, Vola F, Ferrigno D. Aspects of quality of life in patients with lung cancer: a three observer evaluation study. Int J Oncol 1993; 2:537.
7. Slevin ML, Stubbs L, Plant HJ. Attitudes to chemotherapy: comparing views of patients with cancer and those of doctors, nurses, and general public. Br Med J 1990; 300:1458.
8. Faller H, Lang H, Schilling S, et al. Emotional distress and hope in lung cancer patients as perceived by patients, relatives, physicians and interviewers. Psychol Oncol 1995; 4:21.
9. Le Chevalier T, Brisgand D, Douillard J-Y, et al. Randomized study of vinorelbine and cisplatin vs vindesine and cisplatin in advanced non-small cell lung cancer: results of a European multicenter trial including 612 patients. J Clin Oncol 1994; 12:360.
10. Sandler AT, Nemunaitis J, Denham C, et al. Phase III trial of gemcitabine plus cisplatin VS cisplatin alone in patients with locally advanced or metastatic non-small cell lung cancer. J Clin Oncol 2000; 18:122.
11. Shepherd FA, Dancey J, Ramalau R, et al. Prospective randomized trial of docetaxel versus best supportive care in patients with non-small- cell lung cancer previously treated with platinum-based chemotherapy. J Clin Oncol 2000; 18:2095.
12. Dancey J, Shepherd FA, Gralla RJ, et al. Quality of life assessment of second-line docetaxel versus best supportive care in patients with non-small-cell lung cancer previously treated with platinum-based chemotherapy: results of a prospective, randomized phase III trial. Lung Cancer 2004; 43:183.
13. Fossella FV, DeVore R, Kerr RN, et al. Randomized phase III trial of docetaxel versus vinorelbine or ifosfamide in patients with advanced non-small-cell lung cancer previously treated with platinum-containing regimens. J Clin Oncol 2000; 18:2354.
14. Gridelli C, Gallo C, Di Maio M, et al. A randomized clinical trial of two docetaxel regimens (weekly vs 3 week) in the second-line treatment of non-small-cell lung cancer. The DISTAL 01 study. Br J Cancer 2004; 91(12):1996.
15. Gervais R, Ducolone A, Breton JL, et al. Phase II randomized trial comparing docetaxel given every 3 weeks with weekly schedule as second-line therapy in patients with advanced non-small-cell lung cancer (NSCLC). Ann Oncol 2005; 16(1):90.
16. Camps C, Massuti B, Jimenez AM, et al. Second-line docetaxel administered every 3 weeks versus weekly in advanced NSCLC: a Spanish Lung Cancer Group (SLCG) phase III trial. Proc Am Soc Clin Oncol 2003; 22:625.
17. Leighl NB, Shepherd FA, Kwong R, et al. Economic analysis of the TAX 317 trial: docetaxel versus best supportive care as second-line therapy of advanced non-small-cell lung cancer. J Clin Oncol 2002; 20(5):1344.
18. Shih C, Chen VJ, Gossett LS, et al. LY 231514, a pyrolo (2, 3-d) pyromidine-based antifolate that inhibits multiple folate requiring enzymes. Cancer Res 1997; 57:1116.
19. Hammond L, Baker SD, Villalona-Calero SG, et al. A phase I and pharmacokinetic study of the multitargeted antifol (MTA) LY 231514 with folic acid (abstract). Ann Oncol 1998; 9:620.
20. Niyikiza C, Baker SD, Switz DE, et al. Homocysteine and methylmalonic acid: markers to predict and avoid toxicity from pemetrexed therapy. Mol Cancer Ther 2002; 1:545.
21. Vogelzang NJ, Rusthoven JJ, Symanowski J, et al. Phase III study of pemetrexed in combination with cisplatin versus cisplatin alone in patients with malignant pleural mesothelioma. J Clin Oncol 2003; 21:2636.
22. Hanna N, Shepherd FA, Fossella FV, et al. Randomized phase III trial of pemetrexed versus docetaxel in patients with non-small-cell lung cancer previously treated with chemotherapy. J Clin Oncol 2004; 22:1589.
23. Pronzato P, Landucci M, Vaira F. Failure of vinorelbine to produce responses in pre-treated non-small-cell lung cancer. Anticancer Res 1994; 14:1413.
24. Rinaldi M, Della Giulia M, Venturo I. Vinorelbine as single agent in the treatment of advanced non-small-cell lung cancer. Proc Am Soc Clin Oncol 1994; 13:360A.
25. Santoro A, Maiorino L, Santoro M. Second-line with vinorelbine in the weekly monochemotherapy for the treatment of advanced non-small-cell lung cancer. Lung Cancer 1994; 11(130):1.
26. Depierre A, Freyer G, Jassem J, et al. Oral vinorelbine: feasibility and safety profile. Ann Oncol 2001; 12(12):1677.
27. De Pas T, De Braud F, Mandala M, et al. Cisplatin and vinorelbine as second-line chemotherapy in patients with advanced non-small-cell lung cancer (NSCLC) resistant to taxol plus gemcitabine. Lung Cancer 2001; 31(2-3):267.
28. Chen YM, Lee CS, Lin WC, et al. Phase II study with vinorelbine and cisplatin in advanced non-small-cell lung cancer after failure of previous chemotherapy. J Chin Med Assoc 2003; 66(4):241.
29. Agelaki S, Bania H, Kouroussis C, et al. Second-line treatment with vinorelbine and carboplatin in patients with advanced non-small-cell lung cancer. A multicenter phase II study. Lung Cancer 2001; 34(4):S77.
30. Seo-Young S, Won SK, Kihyun K, et al. Vinorelbine, Ifosfamide, and Cisplatin combination in advanced non-small-cell lung cancer. Jpn J Clin Oncol 2003; 33(10):509.
31. Rosvold E, Langer CJ, Scholder R, et al. Salvage therapy with gemcitabine in advanced non-small-cell lung cancer progressing after prior carboplatin-paclitaxel. Proc Am Soc Clin Oncol 1998; 17:463a.

32. Crino L, Mosconi AM, Scagliotti G, et al. Gemcitabine as second-line treatment for advanced non-small-cell lung cancer: a phase II trial. J Clin Oncol 1999; 17:2081.

33. Rossi A, Perrone F, Barletta E, et al. Activity of gemcitabine in cisplatin pretreated patients with non-small-cell lung cancer: a phase II trial. Proc Am Soc Clin Oncol 1999; 18:484a.

34. Reddy GR, Gandara DR, Edelman MJ, et al. Gemcitabine in platinum treated non-small-cell lung cancer. Proc Am Soc Clin Oncol 1999; 18:521a.

35. Garfield DH, Dakhil SR, Whittaker TL, et al. Phase II randomized multicenter trial of two dose schedules of gemcitabine as second-line therapy in patients with advanced non-small-cell lung cancer. Proc Am Soc Clin Oncol 1998; 17:484a.

36. Camps C, Martinez EN, Jaime AB. Second-line treatment with gemcitabine and vinorelbine in non-small-cell lung cancer (NSCLC) cisplatin failures: a pilot study. Lung Cancer 2000; 27(1):47.

37. Hainsworth JD, Burris HA 3rd, Litchy S, et al. Gemcitabine and vinorelbine in the second-line treatment of non small cell lung carcinoma patients: a Minnie Pearl cancer research network phase II trial. Cancer 2000; 88(6):1353.

38. Kosmas C, Tsavaris N, Panopoulos C, et al. Gemcitabine and vinorelbine as second-line therapy in non-small-cell lung cancer after prior treatment with taxane+platinum-based regimens. Eur J Cancer 2001; 37(8):972.

39. Pectasides D, Kalofonos HP, Samantas E, et al. An out-patient second-line chemotherapy with gemcitabine and vinorelbine in patients with non-small cell lung cancer previously treated with cisplatin-based chemotherapy. A phase II study of the Hellenic Co-operative Oncology Group. Anticancer Res 2001; 21(4B):3005.

40. Herbst RS, Khuri FR, Lu C, et al. The novel and effective nonplatinum, nontaxane combination of gemcitabine and vinorelbine in advanced non small cell lung carcinoma: potential for decreased toxicity and combination with biological therapy. Cancer 2002; 95(2):340.

41. Chen YM, Perng RP, Lee CS, et al. Phase II study of gemcitabine and vinorelbine combination chemotherapy in patients with non-small cell lung cancer not responding to previous chemotherapy. Am J Clin Oncol 2003; 26(6):567.

42. Park YH, Lee JC, Kim CH, et al. Gemcitabine and vinorelbine as second-line therapy for non-small cell lung cancer after treatment with paclitaxel plus platinum. Jpn J Oncol 2004; 34(5):245.

43. Negoro S, Fukuoka M, Niitani H, et al. A phase II study of CPT-11, An camptothecin derivative, in patients with primary lung cancer. CPT-11 co-operative group. Jpn J Cancer Chemother 1991; 18:1013.

44. Nakai H, Fukuoka M, Furuse K, et al. An early phase II study of CPT-11 for primary lung cancer. Jpn J Cancer Chemother 1991; 18:607.

45. Nakanishi Y, Takayama K, Takano K, et al. Second-line chemotherapy with weekly cisplatin and irinotecan in patients with refractory lung cancer. Am J Clin Oncol 1999; 22:399.

46. Watchers FM, Groen HJ, Biesma B, et al. A randomized phase II trial of docetaxel vs docetaxel and irinotecan in patients with stage IIIb-IV non small cell lung cancer who failed first-line treatment. Br J Cancer 2005; 92(1):15.

47. Pectasides D, Pectasides M, Farmakis D, et al. Comparison of docetaxel and docetaxel-irinotecan combination as second-line chemotherapy in advanced non-small-cell lung cancer: a randomized phase II trial. Ann Oncol 2005; 16(2):294.

48. Font A, Sanchez JM, Taron M, et al. Weekly regimen of irinotecan/docetaxel in previously treated non-small cell lung cancer patients and correlation with uridine diphos-

49. phate glucuornosyltransferase 1A1 (UGT1A1) polymorphism. Invest New Drugs 2003; 21(4):435.

49. Gonzalez Cao M, Aramendia JM, Salgado E, et al. Second-line chemotherapy with irinotecan and vinorelbine in stage IIIB and IV non-small cell lung cancer: a phase II study. Am J Clin Oncol 2002; 25(5):480.

50. Kakolyris S, Kourousis C, Souglakos J, et al. Cisplatin and irinotecan (CPT-11) as second-line treatment with advanced non-small cell lung cancer. Lung Cancer 2001; 34(4):S71.

51. Nakanishi Y, Takayama K, Takano K, et al. Second-line chemotherapy with weekly cisplatin and irinotecan in patients with refractory lung cancer. Am J Clin Oncol 1999; 22(4):399.

52. Han JY, Lee DH, Kim HY, et al. A phase II study of weekly irinotecan and capecitabine in patients with previously treated non-small cell lung cancer. Clin Cancer Res 2003; 9(16):5909.

53. Georgoulias V, Kouroussis C, Agelidou A, et al. Irinotecan plus gemcitabine vs irinotecan for the second-line treatment of patients with advanced non-small-cell lung cancer pretreated with docetaxel and cisplatin: a multicentre, randomized, phase II study. Br J Cancer. 2004; 9:482.

54. Lynch TJ Jr, Kalish L, Strauss G, et al. Phase II study of topotecan in metastatic non-small-cell lung cancer. J Clin Oncol 1994; 12:347.

55. Perez-Soler R, Fossella FV, Glisson BS, et al. Phase II study of topotecan in patients with advanced non-small-cell lung cancer previously untreated with chemotherapy. J Clin Oncol 1996; 14:503.

56. Weitz JJ, Marschke RF Jr, Sloan JA, et al. A randomized phase II trial of two schedules of topotecan for the treatment of advanced stage non-small-cell lung cancer. Lung Cancer 2000; 28:157.

57. Rinaldi DA, Lormand NA, Brierre JE, et al. A phase II trial of topotecan and gemcitabine in patients with previously treated, advanced non small cell lung carcinoma. Cancer 2002; 95(6):1274.

58. Tan V, Herrera C, Einzig AJ, et al. Taxol is active as a 3- or 24-h infusion in non-small cell lung cancer. Proc Am Soc Clin Oncol 1995; 14:366A.

59. Murphy WK, Winn RJ, Huber M, et al. Phase II study of Taxol in patients with non-small cell lung cancer who have failed platinum-containing chemotherapy. Proc Am Soc Clin Oncol 1994; 13:363A.

60. Ruckdeschel J, Wagner H, Williams C, et al. Second-line therapy for resistant metastatic non-small cell lung cancer: the role of Taxol. Proc Am Soc Clin Oncol 1994; 13:357A.

61. Hainsworth JD, Thompson DS, Greco FA, et al. Paclitaxel by 1-h infusion: an active drug in metastatic non-small cell lung cancer. J Clin Oncol 1995; 13:1609

62. Nauman C, DeLaney TF, Park J, et al. Paclitaxel (Taxol) as a single agent salvage therapy in non-small cell lung cancer (NSCLC). Proc Am Soc Clin Oncol 1997; 16:476A.

63. Socinski MA, Steagal A, Gillenwater H, et al. Second-line chemotherapy with 96-h infusional paclitaxel in refractory non-small cell lung cancer: report of a phase II study. Cancer Invest 1999; 17:181.

64. Chang AY, Boros L, Garrow A, et al. Paclitaxel by 3-hour infusion followed by 96-hour infusion on failure in patients with refractory malignant disease. Semin Oncol 1995; 22(6):124.

65. Juan O, Albert A, Ordono F, et al. Low-dose paclitaxel as second-line treatment for advanced non-small cell lung cancer: a phase II study. Jpn J Clin Oncol 2002; 32(11):449.

66. Socinski MA, Schell MJ, Bakri K, et al. Second-line, low-dose, weekly paclitaxel in patients with stage IIIB/IV non-small cell lung carcinoma who failed first-line chemother-

apy with carboplatin plus paclitaxel. Cancer 2002; 95(6):1265.

67. Sculier JP, Berghmans T, Lafitte JJ, et al. A phase II study testing paclitaxel as second-line single agent treatment for patients with advanced non-small cell lung cancer failing after a first-line chemotherapy. Lung Cancer 2002; 37(1):73.

68. Buccheri G, Ferrigno D, Cuneo Lung Cancer Study Group. Second-line weekly paclitaxel in patients with inoperable non-small cell lung cancer who fail combination chemotherapy with cisplatin. Lung Cancer 2004; 45(2):227.

69. Ceresoli GL, Gregore V, Cordio S, et al. Phase II of weekly paclitaxel as second-line therapy in patients with advanced non-small cell lung cancer. Lung Cancer 2004; 44(2):231.

70. Yasuda K, Igishi T, Kawasaki Y, et al. Phase II study of weekly paclitaxel in patients with non-small cell lung cancer who have failed previous treatments. Oncology 2004; 66(5):347.

71. Esteban E, Gonzalez de Sande L, Fernandez Y, et al. Prospective randomized phase II study of docetaxel versus paclitaxel administered weekly in patients with non-small cell lung cancer previously treated with platinum-based chemotherapy. Ann Oncol 2003; 14(11):1640.

72. Clinical trial phase I-II: Oral taxane in combination with Pemetrexed (Alimta) in patients with recurrent non-small cell lung cancer. *www.cancer.gov.*

73. Kris MG, Natale RB, Herbst RS, et al. A phase II trial of ZD 1839 ('Iressa') in advanced non-small cell lung cancer

(NSCLC) patients who had failed platinum- and docetaxel-based regimens (IDEAL-2). Proc Am Soc Clin Oncol 2002; 21:292a.

74. Giaccone G, Johnson D, Scagliotti GV, et al. Results of a multivariate analysis of prognostic factors of overall survival of patients with advanced non-small cell lung cancer (NSCLC) treated with gefitinib (ZD 1839) in combination with platinum-based chemotherapy (CT) in two large phase III trials (INTACT 1 and 2). Proc Am Soc Clin Oncol 2003; 22:627a.

75. West HL, Franklin WA, Gurnerlock P, et al. ZD1839 (Iressa) in advanced bronchioalveolar carcinoma (BAC): a preliminary report of SWOG S0126. 10th World Conference on Lung Cancer, Vancouver, Canada, Lung Cancer 2003; 30; 81A.

76. Clinical trial phase III. Oral ZD1839 (Iressa) versus intravenous Docetaxel in patients with non-small cell lung cancer. *www.cancer.gov.*

77. Erlotinib (Tarceva) extends survival in advanced lung cancer. ASCO annual meeting, New Orleans, June 5, 2004. *www.cancer.gov.*

78. Docetaxel or Pemetrexed with or without Cetuximab in patients with recurrent or progressive non-small cell lung cancer. *www.cancer.gov.*

79. American Society of Clinical Oncology Treatment Guidelines for Unresectable NSCLC. J Clin Oncol 1997; 15:2996.

80. American Society of Clinical Oncology. Clinical practice guidelines for treatment of unresectable non-small-cell lung cancer. J Clin Oncol 1998; 15(8):2996.

Management of Patients with Advanced Non-Small-Cell Lung Cancer and Performance Status 2

Rogerio Lilenbaum

25

Contents

25.1 Introduction

Patients with a performance status (PS) of 2 represent a substantial percentage of advanced non-small-cell lung cancer (NSCLC) patients seen in clinical practice, yet these patients have been largely excluded from clinical research in the last two decades. As a result, the management of PS 2 patients remains inconsistent. Recent efforts have led to a greater awareness of the unique challenges presented in the management of PS 2 patients. However, there is still considerable debate as to how these patients should be treated. In contrast to widely adopted evidence-based guidelines for PS 0–1 patients, those with PS 2 can be offered, at random, supportive care, single-agent therapy, or combination chemotherapy [1].

25.2 Identification of PS 2 Patients

Two PS scales are used in clinical practice: the Karnofsky Performance Scale (KPS) and the Eastern Cooperative Oncology Group (ECOG) scale (Table 25.1). Other US cooperative groups, such as the Cancer and Leukemia Group B (CALGB) and the Southwest Oncology Group (SWOG), use scales that are adaptations of the ECOG scale. Although they do not share precisely the same definition, there is a strong correlation between the two scales [2]. In both, PS 2 patients are described

as patients whose symptoms are severe enough to impact upon their lifestyle and impair their ability to work, but are not severe enough to lead to a state of permanent disability. From a functional standpoint, PS 2 patients differ from those with milder symptoms who maintain an active lifestyle and retain their ability to work (PS 1), and from those with more severe disability who spend the majority of their time in bed and require constant assistance for personal needs (PS 3 and lower).

Despite efforts to reach a uniform definition, studies have shown great variability in the assessment provided by physicians compared to nurses and patients [3]. A study by Ando et al. demonstrated a significant difference in the PS assignments by the three groups, with physicians giving the healthiest scores and patients the poorest [4]. However, there was a better correlation between the PS provided by the physicians and survival, whereas the patients' assessment failed to distinguish between patients with PS 1 and PS 2 with respect to survival. Furthermore, correlation between PS and overall functional status can be challenging. Comorbidity is a diverse and complex variable. While a low PS in patients with advanced NSCLC is often a reflection of cancer-related symptoms, some patients present with a variety of comorbid conditions that are primarily re-

Table 25.1. Performance status (*PS*) scales

ECOG PS scale		Karnofsky scale
0	Asymptomatic and fully active	100%
1	Symptomatic; fully ambulatory; restricted in physically strenuous activity	80–90%
2	Symptomatic; ambulatory; capable of self-care; more than 50% of waking hours are spent out of bed	60–70%
3	Symptomatic; limited self-care; spends more than 50% of time in bed, but not bedridden	40–50%
4	Completely disabled; no self-care; bedridden	20–30%

ECOG Eastern Cooperative Oncology Group

sponsible for their low functional status. Indeed, a recent study investigated the relationship between PS and functional status in patients with stage III and IV NSCLC and found significant differences between the ECOG PS and other objective measures of functional capacity [5].

Although there are no data indicating that these two subgroups of PS 2 patients have distinct outcomes, or can be even identified accurately, there are reasons to believe that they should be managed differently in clinical practice. Patients who are previously healthy and present with rapidly progressive symptoms and declining PS may benefit from more aggressive chemotherapy. On the other hand, patients whose low PS preceded the diagnosis of NSCLC are not likely to tolerate aggressive therapy. This hypothesis, while plausible, has not been tested prospectively.

25.3 Prevalence of PS 2 Patients

The true prevalence of PS 2 patients in clinical practice is not known. Few studies have attempted to estimate the percentage of PS 2 patients. A population-based study of over 20,000 women with lung cancer in Poland estimated that 30% of the patients who had advanced disease presented with a PS of 2 [6]. The idiosyncrasies of this particular population may preclude generalizations to North America or Western Europe, but it represents a rough estimate.

A more recent study from Chicago attempted to estimate the percentage of PS 2 patients with various types of cancer, as assessed by health care practitioners and by the patients themselves (D. Cella, personal communication). In a population of 493 patients with lung cancer, the estimate of PS 2 patients was approximately 25%, ranging from 20% (according to health care providers) to slightly higher than 30% (as assessed by the patients themselves). Moreover, the diagnosis of advanced lung cancer conferred a 5.0 higher relative risk of presenting with PS 2 as opposed to patients with localized breast cancer (relative risk = 1.0).

Another estimate of the prevalence of PS 2 patients comes from large multicenter clinical trials. In the CALGB 9730 trial, which compared combination chemotherapy with single-agent therapy, 18% of the eligible patients had a PS of 2 [7]. In the European trial led by Le Chevalier, which compared cisplatin/vinorelbine to cisplatin/vindesine and single-agent vinorelbine, approximately 20% of the eligible patients had PS 2 [8]. A similar percentage of PS 2 patients was enrolled in the combined mitomycin, ifosfamide, cisplatin (MIC) trials in the UK [9], including both locally advanced (MIC 1) and advanced NSCLC (MIC 2). However, enrollment figures probably underestimate the actual number of PS 2 patients in clinical practice, since only those patients

who are judged by their physicians to be fit enough for chemotherapy are actually enrolled. Furthermore, physicians are more likely to enroll PS 2 patients in trials that include single-agent therapy than trials that are limited to combination chemotherapy.

25.4 Prognostic Significance of PS 2

The classical report by Stanley and colleagues established the prognostic significance of PS [10]. In a sample of approximately 5,000 patients with inoperable NSCLC treated in different protocols sponsored by the Veterans Administration between 1968 and 1978, the most important prognostic factors were the initial KPS, extent of disease, and prior weight loss, with KPS retaining the strongest prognostic power. Albain and colleagues published another landmark analysis of prognostic factors in advanced NSCLC. It included 2,531 patients who were entered in 14 phase II and III trials conducted by the SWOG between 1974 and 1988 [11]. Performance status was the most powerful predictor of outcome, with 1-year survival rates of 20% for patients with PS 0–1 and 9% for PS 2 patients. In a subset of 904 patients treated with modern cisplatin-based chemotherapy, the median survival time (MST) for PS 0–1 patients was 6.7 months, compared with 3.8 months for patients with PS 2, a highly statistically significant difference. Other prognostic factors in this subset included age, hemoglobin level, and lactate dehydrogenase level.

In a similar experience form Europe, Paesmans analyzed 1,052 patients with unresectable NSCLC entered in 7 separate clinical trials performed by the European Lung Cancer Working Party between 1980 and 1991 [12]. All trials employed platinum-based chemotherapy. After disease extent, PS was the most important determinant of outcome.

A more recent report by ECOG investigators analyzed 1,960 patients with advanced NSCLC treated with cisplatin-based chemotherapy between 1981 and 1992 [13]. Most patients were male (68%) and had a PS of 0–1 (86%). Median age was 60.7 years (range, 19–82 years). MST was correlated with PS at presentation: 9.0 months, 6.4 months, and 3.9 months, for patients with PS 0, 1, and 2, respectively. Gender and weight loss were also important determinants of outcome.

25.5 Treatment Data

25.5.1 First-Line Chemotherapy

A trial published by ECOG investigators in the 1980s was one of the first to illustrate the poor prognosis of PS 2 patients with advanced NSCLC [14]. A total of 486 patients, of whom 92 (19%) had PS 2, were randomized to 4 platinum-based combination regimens. The MST for PS 0 and PS 1 patients was 36 and 26 weeks, respectively, whereas it was 10 weeks for PS 2 patients ($p = 0.001$). Furthermore, there was a 10% incidence of treatment-related deaths in PS 2 patients, which was significantly higher than that observed in PS 0–1 patients. The investigators concluded that patients with advanced NSCLC and a PS of 2 did not benefit form chemotherapy and should be excluded from future phase III clinical trials. A subsequent meta-analysis performed by the Non-Small-Cell Lung Cancer Collaborative Group evaluated the benefit of chemotherapy in 1,190 patients with advanced disease, and described a survival advantage for cisplatin-based chemotherapy compared to supportive care [15]. A subset analysis showed that this benefit was seen through all the cohorts including PS 2 patients. The meta-analysis did not include the newer chemotherapeutic agents, nor did it compare single-agent with combination chemotherapy. However, the encouraging observation that PS 2 patients also seem to benefit from chemotherapy led investigators to restart, including these patients in large clinical trials.

In the phase III study by Le Chevalier and colleagues [8], the combination of cisplatin and vinorelbine was found to be superior to cisplatin-vindesine and to single-agent vinorelbine. A subsequent analysis showed no significant interaction between treatment and various prognostic factors, except for low PS, which was of borderline significance ($p = 0.056$). In the PS 2 subset, there was no benefit of cisplatin-vinorelbine over the other two regimens, and single-agent vinorelbine was suggested as a reasonable treatment approach [16].

Billingham and Cullen from the UK reported two phase III trials of MIC chemotherapy versus no chemotherapy in patients with locally advanced disease and metastatic disease, respectively [9]. Chemotherapy significantly improved survival in the combined analysis, with an overall 16% reduction in the risk of death compared to supportive care. In subgroups defined by age, gender, and histology, the overall treatment effect was similar [17]. However, there was a trend toward decreasing effectiveness of chemotherapy with worsening PS, with no apparent benefit seen in PS 2 patients.

In the US, ECOG investigators reported an influential analysis of PS 2 patients treated with modern chemotherapy. ECOG trial 1594 randomized over 1,200 patients to 4 frequently used platinum-based regimens [18]. After 68 PS 2 patients were enrolled, accrual was stopped due to a high incidence of adverse events, including 5 deaths. However, a more in-depth analysis showed that the overall toxicity experienced by PS 2 patients was not significantly different from that experienced by the PS 0–1 population [19]. In fact, only two of the five deaths were directly attributed to toxicity, while the others were felt to be secondary to disease progression. The outcome of PS 2 patients was significantly inferior to that reported for PS 0–1 patients, with a medial survival time of 4.1 months and a 1-year survival rate of 19%. Based on this subset analysis, the ECOG investigators reinforced their initial recommendation, made 15 years before, that patients with advanced NSCLC and a PS of 2 should not be treated with platinum-based combinations.

The CALGB 9730 trial was a phase III study that randomized patients with advanced NSCLC to single-agent paclitaxel or the combination of carboplatin-paclitaxel [7]. As stated above, out of a total of 581 eligible patients, 99 PS 2 patients were enrolled (18%). When compared to PS 0–1 patients, who had an MST of 8.8 months and a 1-year survival of 38%, the corresponding figures for PS 2 patients were 3.0 months and 14%, respectively. Furthermore, when PS 2 patients were analyzed by treatment arm, those who received combination chemotherapy had a higher response rate (24% vs. 10%), a longer MST (4.7 vs. 2.4 months), and superior 1-year survival (18% vs. 10%) compared to those treated with single-agent paclitaxel (Table 25.2).

Table 25.2. Combination chemotherapy in PS 2 patients

Study	Number of PS 2 patients	Objective response	Median survival time (months)	One-year survival
ECOG 1594				
All four arms combined	68	14%	4.1	19%
CALGB 9730				
Paclitaxel	50	10%	2.4	10%
Paclitaxel + carboplatin	49	24%	4.7	18%
ECOG 1599				
Cisplatin + gemcitabine	49	22%	6.7	25%
Carboplatin + paclitaxel	53	13%	6.1	19%
Kosmidis				
Gemcitabine	47	4%	4.8	17.8%
Carboplatin + gemcitabine	43	14%	6.7	20%

More recently, two prospective trials dedicated to PS 2 patients have been completed. The first, by Langer and colleagues (ECOG 1599), was a phase II randomized trial of attenuated doses of cisplatin-gemcitabine (CG) and carboplatin-paclitaxel (CP) in the first-line treatment of advanced NSCLC and PS 2 [20]. CG yielded a higher response rate (21% vs. 10%), but timer to disease progression and MST were similar between the two arms. The MST of approximately 6 months in both arms was longer than expected based on historical controls (Table 25.2). Myelosuppression, particularly thrombocytopenia, was more common with CG, whereas peripheral neuropathy was more frequent with CP.

The second trial was conducted by Kosmidis and colleagues from Greece [211]. A total of 102 patients were randomized to gemcitabine with or without carboplatin. The MST for those treated with a single agent was 4.8 months, compared to 6.7 months for those who received the combination. One-year survival rates were comparable (17.8% and 20%, respectively). Hematologic toxicity was higher in the combination arm. A separate analysis of symptom improvement showed no difference between the two arms.

25.5.2 Second-Line Chemotherapy

A recent phase III study compared pemetrexed to docetaxel as second-line therapy in 571 eligible patients [22]. Efficacy was comparable between the two arms, but toxicity was more favorable in the pemetrexed arm. In that study, 12% of the patients had PS 2, and their MST was significantly inferior to patients with PS 0–1: 2.2 and 3.6 months for docetaxel and pemetrexed, respectively, compared to 9.1 and 9.4 months, respectively, for PS 0-1 patients.

Other studies have investigated the role of molecular targeted agents, such as gefitinib and erlotinib, in this patient population. In the IDEAL-2 trial, conducted in the USA, 216 patients (20% with PS 2) who had previously failed at least two prior regimens were randomized to receive gefitinib at a dose of 250 mg or 500 mg per day [23]. The rates of radiographic response and symptom improvement did not differ significantly in

patients with PS 0,1, or 2, and the benefit of gefitinib seemed to be similar among the three PS subgroups. The most convincing data with respect to the benefits of second- or third -line treatment of PS 2 patients with NSCLC come from the BR-21 trial. This phase III study enrolled 731 patients who failed at least 1 prior regimen, who were randomized to receive erlotinib or placebo [24]. Of the 488 patients treated with erlotinib, 26% had PS 2 and 9% had PS 3. The results showed a significant improvement in survival for patients who received erlotinib (MST: 6.7 months; 1-year survival: 31%) compared to placebo (MST: 4.7 months; 1-year survival: 21%). This effect persisted across PS 0, 1, 2, and 3 patients (Table 25.3).

Key Points

- Patients with performance status (PS) 2 represent a sizable percentage of our practice, yet they have been excluded from clinical research in the last 10–15 years. More recently, dedicated trials and prospective subset analyses have contributed greatly to our understanding and management of this patient population.
- There is now randomized evidence that chemotherapy improves disease-related symptoms and prolongs survival compared to no treatment in PS 2 patients. However, their overall prognosis remains poor compared to PS 0–1 patients.
- No firm statement can be made about single-agent versus combination chemotherapy in PS 2 patients. Combination chemotherapy should be considered in those PS 2 patients who are ill primarily from the cancer and have no major comorbidities. Better methods of assessing PS are urgently needed.
- Dedicated studies in PS 2 patients are ongoing and will hopefully clarify further the role of chemotherapy molecular-targeted agents in these patients.

Table 25.3. IDEAL 2 tBR-21 results

Study	No. of patients	Response rate	Median survival (months)	One-year survival
Gefitinib IDEAL 2				
250 mg	102	12%	7.0	27%
500 mg	114	9%	6.0	24%
Erlotinib BR-21				
150 mg	488	9%	6.7	31%
Placebo	243	1%	4.7	22%

References

1. Pfister DG, Johnson DH, Azzoli CG, et al. American Society of Clinical Oncology treatment of unresectable non-small-cell lung cancer guideline: Update 2003. J Clin Oncol 2003; 22:330.
2. Buccheri G, Ferrigno D, Tamburini M. Karnofsky and ECOG performance status scoring in lung cancer: a prospective, longitudinal study of 536 patients from a single institution. Eur J Cancer 1996; 32A:1135.
3. Taylor AE, Olver IN, Sivanthan T, Chi M, Purnell C. Observer error in grading performance status in cancer patients. Support Care Cancer 1999; 7(5):332.

4. Ando M, Ando Y, Hasegawa Y. Prognostic value of performance status assessed by patients themselves, nurses, and oncologists in advanced non-small cell lung cancer. Br J Cancer 2001; 85(11):1634.

5. Dalzell M-A, Kreisman H, Small D, et al. Is performance status related to functional capacity in patients with non-small cell lung cancer (NSCLC)? Proc Am Soc Clin Oncol 2204; 23:669.

6. Radzikowska E, Glatz P, Roszkowski, et al. Lung cancer in women: age, smoking, histology, performance status, stage, initial treatment and survival. Population-based case study of 20,561 cases. Ann Oncol 2002; 13:1087.

7. Lilenbaum RC, Herndon J, List M, et al. Single-agent versus combination chemotherapy in advanced non-small cell lung cancer: The Cancer and Leukemia Group B (study 9730). J Clin Oncol 2005; 23:190.

8. Le Chevalier T, Brisgand D, Douillard JY, et al. Randomized study of vinorelbine and cisplatin versus vindesine and cisplatin versus vinorelbine alone in advanced non-small-cell lung cancer: results of a European multicenter trial including 612 patients. J Clin Oncol 1994; 12:360.

9. Cullen MH, Billingham LJ, Woodroffe CM, et al. Mitomycin, ifosfamide, and cisplatin in unresectable non-small-cell lung cancer: effects on survival and quality of life. J Clin Oncol 1999; 17(10):3188.

10. Stanley KE. Prognostic factors for survival in patients with inoperable lung cancer. J Natl Cancer Inst 1980; 65:25.

11. Albain K, Crowley J, LeBlanc M, et al. Survival determinants in extensive-stage non-small lung cancer: The Southwest Oncology Group Experience. J Clin Oncol 1991; 9:1618.

12. Paesmans M, Sculier JP, Libert P, et al. Prognostic Factors for survival in advanced non-small cell lung cancer: univariate and multivariate analyses including recursive partitioning and amalgamation algorithms in 1,052 patients. J Clin Oncol 1995; 13:1221.

13. Jiroutek M, Jahnsosn D, Blum R, et al. prognostic factors in advanced non-small cell lung cancer: Analysis of the Eastern cooperative group trials from 1981–1992. Proc Am Soc Clin Oncol 1998; 17:461 (abstract).

14. Ruckdeschel J, Finkelstein D, Ettinger D, et al. A randomized trial of the four most active regimens for metastatic non-small cell lung cancer. J Clin Oncol 1986; 4:14.

15. Non-small Cell Lung Cancer Collaborative Group. Chemotherapy in non-small cell lung cancer: a meta-analysis using updated data on individual patients from 52 randomised clinical trials. BMJ 1995; 311:899.

16. Le Chevalier T, Brisgand D, Soria JC, et al. Long term analysis of survival in the European randomized trial comparing vinorelbine/cisplatin to vindesine/cisplatin and vinorelbine alone in advanced non-small cell lung cancer. Oncologist 2001; 6:8.

18. Billingham L, Cullen M. The benefits of chemotherapy in patient subgroups with unresectable non-small-cell lung cancer. Ann Oncol 2001; 12(12):1671.

19. Schiller, JH, Harrington D, Belani CP, et al. Comparison of four chemotherapy regimens for advanced non-small-cell lung cancer. N Engl J Med 2002; 346:92.

20. Sweeney CJ, Zhu J, Sandler AB. Outcome of patients with a performance status of 2 in Eastern Cooperative Oncology Group Study E1594: a phase II trial in patients with metastatic nonsmall cell lung carcinoma. Cancer 2001; 92:2639.

21. Tester WJ, Stephenson P, et al. ECOG 1599: randomized phase II study of paclitaxel/carboplatin or gemcitabine/cisplatin in performance status (PS) 2 patients with advanced non-small cell lung cancer (NSCLC). Annual Meeting of the American Society of Clinical Oncology 2004; 23:7023a

22. Kosimidis, PA, Kimopoulos MA, Syrigos C, et al. Gemcitabine (G) vs gemcitabine-carboplatin (GCB) for patients with advanced non-small cell lung cancer (NSCLC) and PS:2. A prospective randomized phase II study of the Hellenic Co-operative Oncology Group. Proc Am Soc of Clin Oncol 2004; 23:7058a.

23. Hanna N, Shepherd FA, Fossella FV, et al. Randomized phase III trial of pemetrexed versus docetaxel in patients with non-small cell lung cancer previously treated with chemotherapy. J Clin Oncol 2004; 22:1589.

24. Kris MG, Natale RB, Herbst RS, et al. Efficacy of gefitinib, an inhibitor of the epidermal growth factor receptor tyrosine kinase, in symptomatic patients with non-small cell lung cancer. JAMA 2003; 290:2149.

25. Shepherd FA, Pereira J, Ciuleanu TE, et al. A randomized placebo-controlled trial of erlotinib in patients with advanced non-small cell lung cancer following failure of first- or second-line chemotherapy. A National Cancer Institute of Canada Clinical Trials Group (NCIC-CTG). Proc Am Soc Clin Oncol 2004; 23:12.

Targeted Therapy of Non-Small-Cell Lung Cancer

26

Kristin L. Hennenfent and Ramaswamy Govindan

Contents

26.1 Introduction

In the USA, lung cancer will claim the lives of an estimated 163,000 people in 2005. Non-small cell lung cancer (NSCLC) accounts for more than 80% of all cases of lung cancer [1]. Nearly 40% of patients diagnosed with NSCLC present with metastatic disease at the time of initial diagnosis, a stage at which long-term survival is rarely achieved with conventional systemic chemotherapy [2]. Systemic chemotherapy produces a modest survival benefit compared to best supportive care in this setting [3]. During the 1990s, several new chemotherapeutic agents were identified to have single-agent activity in lung cancer, including paclitaxel, docetaxel, vinorelbine, gemcitabine, and irinotecan. When utilized in combination with a platinum analogue, randomized trials have not demonstrated a survival advantage with any particular regimen. Nonplatinum doublets have not been found to offer an advantage over a platinum doublet. Thus, four to six cycles of platinum-based combination chemotherapy remains the standard treatment option for the majority of patients. Unfortunately, the 1-year survival has reached a plateau of approximately 40% following administration of conventional cytotoxic agents in advanced NSCLC [4]. Both the toxicities and drug resistance that ensue following administration limit the curative potential of systemic chemotherapy. Thus, in an effort to improve survival, several molecular targets of potential importance have been identified in NSCLC and targeted for therapeutic intervention.

Our understanding of several specific tumorigenic processes has evolved recently and several new agents that target these processes are under clinical development. Lung cancer cells obtain growth advantages through numerous genetic changes of normal cell physiology, including self-sufficiency in growth signaling, evasion of apoptosis, insensitivity to growth-inhibitory signaling, uninhibited replicative potential, defects in DNA repair, sustained angiogenesis, and the ability to invade and metastasize. Four primary therapeutic approaches have been employed, including immunotherapy approaches (e.g., monoclonal antibodies, vaccines), antisense oligonucleotides, small-molecule inhibitors, and gene therapy [5]. The discussion that follows reviews the targets of molecular therapy and summarizes the current clinical evidence of these agents.

26.2 Definition of Targeted Therapy

Targeted therapies, unlike conventional cytotoxic chemotherapy, focus on cell signaling and other biologic pathways that are involved in tumorigenesis. In most cases, the molecular aberrations involved in malignant transformation include, among others, growth-factor receptors on cell surfaces, proteins or enzymes in signal-transduction pathways, enzymes involved in cell replication, apoptosis, migration, and infiltration, or alterations in deoxyribonucleic acid [6]. Targeted therapies interfere with specific critical steps associated with the initiation and maintenance of the malignant phenotype. Due to their specific targeted mechanisms of action, these novel therapies generally demonstrate improved tolerability profiles compared to their conventional cytotoxic chemotherapeutic counterparts. Targeted therapies can be offered to heavily pretreated patients or to those patients with a performance status that renders them unsuitable for other treatment options [6].

26.3 Targets for Therapeutic Intervention in Lung Cancer

Major agents that are involved in cell signal transduction pathways, such as protein tyrosine kinases (PTKs), ras/mitogen-activated protein kinase (MAPK), and protein kinase C (PKC), are emerging as potential targets for therapeutic intervention in lung cancer. The protein kinases regulate most of the cell signal transduction processes in eukaryotic cells and can become potent oncogenes upon genetic mutation. These important pathways appear to be altered within lung cancer cells, leading to dysregulation of cell signaling and aberrant cell proliferation, and represent potential selective targets for lung cancer therapies. Compounds that target tyrosine kinases, their ligands, and signal transducers have been studied recently in NSCLC. In addition, antagonism of ligands at growth factor binding sites has been investigated as a therapeutic mechanism through antibodies aimed at both growth factors and their receptor sites [5].

26.4 Epidermal Growth Factor Receptor-Targeted Agents

The epidermal growth factor (EGF) receptor (EGFR) is a transmembrane receptor tyrosine kinase of the ErbB (HER) family that appears to be abnormally activated in many epithelial malignancies. Four tyrosine kinases, ErbB1/HER1, ErbB2-HER-2/neu, ErbB3-HER3, and ErbB4-HER4, make up the ErbB family [7]. Receptors may be activated by numerous mechanisms, including receptor overexpression, gene amplification, activating mutations, overexpression of receptor ligands, and loss of negative regulatory mechanisms [8]. Mendelsohn and colleagues first proposed the EGFR as a target for cancer therapy several decades ago, but only recently has EGFR inhibition been associated with improved survival in patients with advanced cancer. There are monoclonal

antibodies directed at the extracellular domain of EGFR and small-molecule tyrosine-kinase inhibitors targeting signal transduction through the EGFR pathway. In preclinical models, EGFR inhibition by monoclonal antibodies or by the use of tyrosine kinase inhibitors has been associated with decreased cell proliferation, increased apoptosis, and decreased angiogenesis [9–11].

EGFR is commonly overexpressed in NSCLC, the incidence ranging from 43% to 89% [12]. The difference in reported rates of EGFR expression is probably due to nonstandard assessment methods, differences in definition of overexpression, and variation in the study population [13]. Overexpression is most likely to be observed with squamous cell carcinoma (70%), followed by adenocarcinoma (50%) and large-cell carcinoma. There is increasing evidence that bronchioalveolar carcinomas express an extraordinarily high amount of EGFR [14]. The mechanism responsible for EGFR activation in lung cancer cells is largely unknown [13, 15]. Overexpression has been associated with a poor prognosis [16–18]. The prognostic significance of EGFR expression and ability to predict response to EGFR-targeted pharmacologic agents is the subject of current research.

26.4.1
Monoclonal antibodies

26.4.1.1 Cetuximab
Cetuximab (C-225, Erbitux) is a recombinant chimeric IgG1 monoclonal antibody directed against the extracellular domain of EGFR to inhibit receptor-ligand binding and subsequent autophosphorylation of EGFR [19]. This leads to cell cycle arrest, increased expression of proapoptoic proteins, and decreased expression of antiapoptotic proteins [19]. In preclinical models, cetuximab has demonstrated synergism with chemotherapeutic agents, including cisplatin and paclitaxel, as well as with radiation therapy [20]. In phase I testing, cetuximab was well tolerated, producing most notably a hypersensitivity reaction (1%) and grade 3 or 4 acneiform rash (11%) [21]. A nonlinear dose-dependent pharmacokinetic profile has been observed, with drug elimination saturation occurring at dose levels between 200 and 400 mg/m^2. The dosing regimen recommended for further clinical testing was a loading dose of 400 mg/m^2, followed by a weekly maintenance dose of 250 mg/m^2.

Lilenbaum and colleagues recently reported the final results of a phase II trial of cetuximab monotherapy in patients with recurrent stage IIIB or IV NSCLC [22]. Patients previously failing a platinum-based chemotherapeutic regimen initially received cetuximab 400 mg/m^2 on day 1, followed by 250 mg/m^2 weekly until disease progression ($n = 66$). Of the sixty patients evaluable for response, partial response was observed in two (3.3%,

95% confidence interval, 95% CI = 0.41–11.53). Median time to progression and overall survival were 2.3 and 8.1 months, respectively. Single-agent cetuximab was well tolerated in this population, with rash being the most frequently reported adverse event (77%; grade 3, 6.1%).

In a small phase I/II trial ($n = 31$), cetuximab was administered in combination therapy with paclitaxel and carboplatin in previously untreated cases of metastatic NSCLC [23]. In this trial, paclitaxel was administered at a dose of 225 mg/m^2, intravenously, in combination with carboplatin (area under the time–plasma concentration curve, AUC 5) every 3 weeks for a maximum of six cycles. Cetuximab was given as a loading dose of 400 mg/m^2 intravenously, followed by a weekly dose of 250 mg/m^2. This regimen produced predictable toxicities of myalgia/arthralgia, neutropenia, and rash. Cetuximab was administered for a median of 19 weeks, and produced a promising median survival of 15.7 months (95% CI = 10.2–17.5 months). The median time to disease progression was 4.5 months (95% CI = 2.8–5.8 months). A similarly designed phase II study evaluated cetuximab in combination with gemcitabine and carboplatin for the first-line treatment of metastatic NSCLC [24]. This combination regimen produced a similar time to disease progression (165 days, 95% CI = 144–188 days) and toxicity profile; rash (20%) and fatigue (14%) were the most commonly reported grade 3 adverse effects. Furthermore, partial response was observed in 29%, and the 1-year overall survival was 43%.

Gatzemeier and colleagues conducted a randomized phase II study of cetuximab in combination with cisplatin and vinorelbine versus cisplatin and vinorelbine alone for the treatment of previously untreated NSCLC [25]. Those patients randomized to receive cetuximab in combination with chemotherapy had a higher overall response rate (53%, 95% CI = 36.1–69.8% vs. 26%, 95% CI = 18.6–49.9%). The time to progression and overall survival data are not yet available. Although these findings are promising, large, prospective, randomized studies are needed to determine whether the addition of cetuximab to platinum-based combination chemotherapy improves the survival of patients with metastatic NSCLC.

Investigators at the MD Anderson Cancer Center have also evaluated cetuximab in patients with relapsed NSCLC resistant or refractory to platinum-based chemotherapy [26]. In this trial, cetuximab (loading dose 400 mg/m^2, followed by 250 mg/m^2 weekly dose) was administered concurrently with docetaxel (75 mg/m^2, administered intravenously every 3 weeks). The overall response rate observed was 28%, with nearly 66% achieving stable disease. These results are encouraging given the disease-refractory patient population.

Several questions regarding the role of cetuximab in patients with NSCLC remain outstanding, including the role of cetuximab in combination with radiation therapy, cytotoxic agents, and other biological agents.

26.4.1.2 ABX-EGF

ABX-EGF is a fully humanized IgG2 monoclonal antibody that binds with a higher affinity to EGFR than does cetuximab [7]. In a dose-dependent manner, ABX-EGF blocks the EGF binding site on its receptor, and subsequent cell signal transduction. In a preclinical study, ABX-EGF completely eradicated human tumor xenograft models with high EGFR expression and demonstrated some synergy with conventional chemotherapy agents [27]. In a phase I clinical study of ABX-EGF in 43 patients with NSCLC, Figlin and colleagues demonstrated a dose-dependent transient acneiform rash as well as tumor response and/or stabilization, even at low doses [28]. In a phase II trial of ABX-EGF in combination with cytotoxic chemotherapy, 19 patients with stage IIIB or IV NSCLC and EGFR overexpression received ABX-EGF intravenously (dosing cohorts: 1 mg/kg, 2 mg/kg, and 2.5 mg/kg) weekly in combination with 6 cycles of paclitaxel/carboplatin in a 3-weekly manner [29]. One patient (5%) achieved an objective response at ABX-EGF 1 mg/kg and four patients (two at the 2 mg/kg dose and two at the 2.5 mg/kg dose) achieved partial response. Skin rash was the most commonly reported adverse event. In contrast to the phase I data, skin rash did not appear to be related to the dose in this trial. There was no pharmacokinetic interaction between ABX-EGF and standard chemotherapy.

26.4.2 Small-Molecule Tyrosine Kinase Inhibitors

The small-molecule tyrosine kinase inhibitors compete with ATP binding to the intracellular tyrosine kinase domain of the EGFR receptor, which inhibits tyrosine kinase activation and subsequently blocks cell signaling through the EGFR pathway. These agents cause decreased cellular proliferation and tumor regression by increasing apoptosis and inhibiting angiogenesis. Gefitinib (ZD1839, Iressa) and erlotinib (OSI 774, Tarceva), anilinoquinazoline derivatives that specifically target the HER-1 protein, are the two most developed small-molecule tyrosine kinase inhibitors used to treat advanced NSCLC.

26.4.2.1 Gefitinib

In preclinical studies, gefitinib demonstrated its ability to inhibit and perhaps induce complete response of xenografts models, and possibly sensitize tumor cells to the effects of ionizing radiation [9, 30, 31]. In a phase I trial conducted by Herbst and colleagues, nausea and vomiting, acneiform rash, and diarrhea were the most common adverse effects. At the maximum tolerated dose of 800 mg/day, the acneiform rash and diarrhea were dose limiting [32]. Daily doses of 250–500 mg were chosen for further phase II/III clinical evaluation.

The results of IDEAL-1 and -2, two large randomized phase II trials evaluating gefitinib in pretreated patients with NSCLC, have now been reported [33]. The IDEAL-1 trial recruited patients from Australia, Europe, South Africa, and Japan, whereas the IDEAL-2 trial enrolled patients from the USA. Preclinical models revealed no clear correlation between EGFR overexpression and response to gefitinib; patient selection was thus not performed in these trials. In each of the IDEAL trials, patients with advanced NSCLC (stage III/IV) who had failed at least one platinum-based chemotherapeutic regimen were randomized to receive either gefitinib 250 or 500 mg/day until disease progression. In both studies, there were no differences between the two dosing groups with respect to overall survival, response rate, or time to progression. The median survival in these two studies ranged from 6 to 8 months, similar to that seen with docetaxel in the second-line setting [34]. Four factors, including female gender, adenocarcinoma histology, Asian origin, and never-smokers, were most likely to respond to gefitinib therapy [35]. The frequency of rash and diarrhea were greater in the higher-dose arm, thus given the similar response rates of the two dose levels, 250 mg/day gefitinib has emerged as the standard dose in this setting. Notably, rapid symptomatic improvement was observed in a significant proportion of patients (40.3%). Mean time to improvement was 8–10 days after beginning therapy [36]. Based on the results of these two phase II studies, gefitinib was approved for clinical use in Japan and the USA [37].

Thatcher and colleagues recently reported the results of a phase III placebo-controlled study (ISEL) comparing gefitinib to best supportive care in recurrent advanced NSCLC [38]. A total of 1,692 patients who had received 1 or 2 prior chemotherapy regimens were randomized to gefitinib 250 mg daily ($n = 1129$) or placebo ($n - 563$). At a median follow-up of approximately 7 months, an improvement in median survival for the gefitinib arm was observed compared to placebo-treated patients, but this did not reach statistical significance (5.6 and 5.1 months, respectively; hazard ratio, HR = 0.89; 95% CI = 0.77–1.02; $p = 0.089$). Planned subgroup analyses did reveal survival advantages for gefitinib-treated patients of Asian origin (9.5 vs. 5.5 months; HR = 0.66, 95% CI = 0.48–0.91; $p = 0.01$) and those that had never smoked (8.9 vs. 6.1 months; HR = 0.67; 95% CI = 0.49–0.92; $p = 0.012$).

Two further trials, INTACT 1 (USA) and INTACT 2 (Europe), which are randomized, multicenter phase III evaluations of gefitinib in combination with standard chemotherapeutic regimens in treatment-nave patients with unresectable stage IIIB or INSCLC, have been completed [39, 40]. Gefitinib improved the efficacy of cyto-

toxic chemotherapy against several human tumor xenografts, including lung cancer, regardless of EGFR expression [9, 41]. In these trials, patients were randomized to receive gefitinib (250 or 500 mg/day) or placebo in combination with cisplatin plus gemcitabine (INTACT 1, $n = 1093$) or paclitaxel plus carboplatin (INTACT 2, $n = 1037$). The addition of gefitinib did not extend the median overall survival in either trial, nor did it improve the secondary endpoints, including time to progression and treatment response rate. In INTACT 2, Herbst and colleagues showed a trend toward improved survival in the subgroup of patients with adenocarcinoma receiving at least 90 days of chemotherapy and gefitinib 250 mg/day, perhaps suggesting a benefit to gefitinib monotherapy for maintenance after chemotherapy. There did not appear to be any differences in adverse events between all treatment arms except for acneiform rash and diarrhea, which occurred at a higher incidence in both gefitinib groups compared to the placebo group. Rare interstitial-lung-disease-type events were observed in each of the trials, but were generally similar across all treatment groups. Gefitinib 250 mg/day was associated with fewer adverse events, dose reductions, and treatment interruptions.

The reasons for the disappointing efficacy results observed in the INTACT 1 and INTACT 2 trials are still not clear. It was speculated that recurrent NSCLC (IDEAL 1 and IDEAL 2) perhaps depends upon EGFR ligands as survival factors after platinum-based chemotherapy [42, 43]. It may be possible that each agent targets the susceptible subpopulation of tumor cells, resulting in lack of additive activity, or that concomitant administration impairs the function of one of the agents, resulting in antagonism [39, 44]. Notably, patients were not included in the study based upon EGFR their expression, but whether patient selection impacts gefitinib sensitivity is subject to further evaluation.

26.4.2.2 Erlotinib

Phase I studies of erlotinib showed that diarrhea, rash, nausea, headache, emesis, and fatigue were the most commonly reported side effects [45]. At 200 mg/day, diarrhea was dose limiting but easily managed with loperamide or dose reduction to 150 mg/day. This prompted the selection of 150 mg/day as the dose for phase II investigations. In contrast, the doses chosen for clinical investigation of gefitinib (250 and 500 mg/day) were much lower than the 800 mg maximum tolerated dose (MTD) observed in early clinical studies, raising the question of the appropriateness of dosing of anti-EGFR agents. Interestingly, erlotinib results in a plasma AUC that is one order higher than that achieved with gefitinib [46].

Two phase II trials of erlotinib have been completed, one in patients with advanced NSCLC and one in patients with bronchioalveolar carcinoma [47, 48]. Single-agent erlotinib induced an objective response in 12 and 26% of patients with advanced NSCLC and bronchioalveolar carcinoma, respectively. Subsequent to these results, researchers at the National Cancer Institute of Canada conducted a randomized phase III trial in which erlotinib was administered to patients with stage IIIB or IV NSCLC after failure of first- or second-line chemotherapy ($n=731$) [49]. Of the enrolees, 50% had received two prior chemotherapy regimens, the majority (93%) of which had included a platinum analogue. In this study, the overall response was 8.9% and erlotinib significantly prolonged overall survival compared to placebo (6.7 months vs. 4.7 months, $p=0.001$). The results of the study led to the approval of erlotinib in the second-line therapy of advanced NSCLC. Not surprisingly, rash and diarrhea were the most frequently reported adverse effects.

The TALENT and TRIBUTE trials, two randomized phase III trials, have evaluated the role of erlotinib in combination with chemotherapy for the first-line treatment of advanced NSCLC [49, 50]. In the TALENT trial, previously untreated patients with advanced NSCLC were randomized to receive erlotinib 150 mg daily plus gemcitabine and cisplatin combination chemotherapy or chemotherapy alone ($n=1172$) [51]. Chemotherapy was administered for a maximum of six cycles and erlotinib was continued until disease progression. Unfortunately, the addition of erlotinib to platinum-based chemotherapy did not significantly prolong overall survival or time to progression and, as expected, was associated with an increased incidence of grade 3/4 diarrhea and skin rash. In the parallel trial, TRIBUTE, the role of erlotinib in combination with carboplatin and paclitaxel was explored ($n=1059$) [50]. Similar to the results of the TALENT trial, erlotinib did not confer a survival advantage over carboplatin/paclitaxel chemotherapy (overall survival, 10.8 versus 10.6 months, $p=0.95$) and the overall toxicity profiles were equivalent except for diarrhea and skin rash. Interestingly, a subgroup analysis of never-smokers enrolled in the TRIBUTE trial revealed that the addition of erlotinib did in fact markedly extend survival (23 vs.10 months, 95% CI = 0.28–0.85) in this subpopulation [52]. Confirmation of this finding in a randomized trial is warranted.

26.5 Vascular Endothelial Growth Factor (VEGF)-Targeted Agents

26.5.1 Antibody-Directed Therapy

Angiogenesis plays a key role in tumor cell growth and the metastatic process associated with many malignancies [53]. Regulation of angiogenesis is accomplished by a multitude of stimulatory and inhibitor regulators, the balance of which determines whether angiogenesis occurs in a particular setting [53, 54]. It appears to be required both in tumorigenesis and some normal tissue processes including wound healing and ovulation [55]. In the early 1970s, Folkman first described the theory of the "angiogenic switch," a process postulated to be required for tumor growth and metastasis. It is merely the change from an avascular state accompanied by the acquisition of angiogenic properties, and is considered a hallmark of the malignant process [55, 56].

Advances in the understanding of angiogenesis over the past several decades are the foundation for the emergence of antiangiogenesis as a therapeutic approach for NSCLC. VEGF is thought to be the most potent endogenous positive regulator of angiogenesis, and expression of VEGF has been associated with advanced tumor stage and poor prognosis in a variety of human malignancies [56]. Moreover, microvessel density, an indicator of angiogenic activity, is an independent poor prognostic factor for patients with NSCLC [57]. Thus, identifying therapeutic strategies to inhibit VEGF signaling have gained intense interest. The best-studied strategies under clinical investigation in NSCLC include antibody-based therapies to target the ligand, and inhibition of receptor signaling by small-molecule inhibitors [58].

According to the manufacturer, Bevacizumab (Avastin; Genentech, South San Francisco, CA, USA) is a recombinant humanized (93% human IgG1; 7% murine) monoclonal antibody that competitively blocks the binding of all VEGF isoforms to their receptors and inhibits the biologic activities of VEGF. The VEGF receptors most closely linked with angiogenesis include VEGFR-1 and VEGFR-2 [53]. Bevacizumab is currently being evaluated in several human tumor types, including NSCLC. Administration of bevacizumab has proved promising thus far in breast cancer, renal cell carcinoma, and colorectal cancer. Positive results were recently demonstrated in a phase III trial of bevacizumab in combination with irinotecan/5-flourouracil/leucovorin chemotherapy for metastatic colorectal cancer and provide the first clinical validation of the antiangiogenic treatment approach [59].

In preclinical models, bevacizumab has exhibited inhibitory effects against human tumor cell lines in murine xenograft models, including the CALU-6 NSCLC model [60–63]. Bevacizumab may act synergistically with conventional chemotherapy and radiation therapy, as it demonstrated the ability to enhance the activity of both modalities by inhibiting the activity of VEGF produced during hypoxic conditions [60, 63]. In addition, administration of bevacizumab was able to reverse the protective effects of endogenous VEGF against the antiangiogenic effects of docetaxel in endothelial cells both in vitro and in vivo [64].

Johnson and colleagues evaluated the addition of bevacizumab to paclitaxel/carboplatin combination chemotherapy versus paclitaxel/carboplatin alone in patients with stage IIIB (with pleural effusion), stage IV, or recurrent NSCLC ($n = 99$). In this randomized, phase II study, patients received carboplatin (target AUC = 6 mg/ml/min) and paclitaxel (200 mg/m^2) plus or minus bevacizumab at 7.5 mg/kg (low-dose group) or 15 mg/kg (high-dose group). All agents were administered every 21 days. The addition of bevacizumab (15 mg/kg) resulted in a greater response rate (31.5% vs. 18.8%) and significantly extended time to disease progression (7.4 months vs. 4.2 months, $p = 0.02$) compared to conventional chemotherapy alone. A small improvement in median overall survival (17.7 vs. 14.9 months) was also observed. Nineteen patients randomized to receive platinum-based combination chemotherapy alone were allowed to crossover to single-agent bevacizumab (15 mg/kg) upon disease progression; no objective responses were observed, but 5 patients did demonstrate disease stabilization.

Bevacizumab was well tolerated, both in a phase I clinical study in patients with advanced solid tumors and in this phase II trial of NSCLC [65]. No dose-limiting toxicities were reported in the phase I study and the most common adverse events reported included hypertension, thrombosis, transient epistaxis, and proteinuria. In combination with cytotoxic chemotherapy, bevacizumab did not appear to increase the incidence or severity of nausea/vomiting, nephropathies, or neuropathies. Although a dose-related increase in leukopenia was observed, the main tolerability concern was the occurrence of bleeding events; hemoptysis or hematemesis was reported in six patients, four of which were fatal events.

Recently, Herbst and colleagues reported the results of a phase I/II clinical study evaluating the use of bevacizumab in combination with the HER-1/EGFR tyrosine kinase inhibitor erlotinib in patients with recurrent stage IIIB/IV NSCLC [66]. The MTD utilized for the phase II portion of this study was that determined previously during single-agent evaluations of each respective agent [45, 67]. Bevacizumab 15 mg/kg was administered intravenously every 3 weeks and 150 mg/day erlotinib was administered orally. Thirty-four patients were enrolled at the phase II dose (40 patients enrolled overall), the majority of who were diagnosed with adenocarcinoma. Eight patients (20%) achieved a partial response with this combination, but most (65%) had disease stabilization as their best response. Interestingly, all patients who demonstrated a partial response had adenocarcinoma. The median overall survival for those patients treated both at the phase II dose and the overall study population was 12.6 months. Mild to moderate rash, diarrhea, and proteinuria were the most commonly reported adverse events and all were easily managed. Bleeding events were not observed in this trial.

When given in combination, a pharmacokinetic interaction was not apparent, which suggests that it is feasible to administer these two agents together.

26.5.2
Small-Molecule Tyrosine Kinase Inhibitors

26.5.2.1 ZD6474

ZD6474 is a novel small-molecule tyrosine kinase inhibitor of VEGFR-2 whose activity limits the cell signaling necessary for endothelial cell proliferation and growth [68]. This agent also possesses modest inhibitory activity against EGFR tyrosine kinase cell signal transduction as well. Based upon its promising antitumor activity in preclinical in vivo models, Minami and colleagues initiated a phase I clinical investigation in Japan [69]. Eighteen Japanese patients with refractory solid tumors, 9 of whom had a diagnosis of NSCLC, received a single oral dose of ZD6474 at a dose ranging from 100 to 400 mg/day, followed by a 7-day washout period and then received daily ZD6474 for a total of 28 days. The remainder of the treatment cycles was administered continuously. Overall, the agent was well tolerated at doses less than 300 mg/day, with the most common adverse events being rash, asymptomatic QTc prolongation, diarrhea, proteinuria, and hypertension. Evidence of corrected QT interval prolongation necessitated routine electrocardiogram monitoring throughout the study. At a dose level of 400 mg/day, dose-limiting toxicities of liver transaminase elevation and hypertension were observed. Tumor regression was noted in four patients (44%) with NSCLC and was maintained despite dose modification in two patients. Based on these results, ZD6474 at doses ranging from 100 to 300 mg/day was determined to be appropriate for further phase II clinical investigation.

A randomized phase II clinical study of ZD6474 in combination with docetaxel chemotherapy was conducted in patients with locally advanced or metastatic NSCLC after failure of platinum-based chemotherapy [70]. Initially, patients received docetaxel intravenously at a dose of 75 mg/m^2 every 3 weeks and ZD6474 100 mg/day orally. If no dose-limiting toxicities occurred within 4 weeks of treatment initiation, the dose of ZD6474 was escalated to 400 mg/day for the next patient cohort. At the time of study presentation, 15 patients were enrolled, 11 of who received ZD6474 at a dose of 400 mg/day. Patients received a median 4 four cycles of docetaxel and 12 cycles of ZD6474. Of the nine patients who received at least three cycles of combination therapy, six reported grade 3 acneiform or desquamating rash with associated photosensitivity. The rash was reversible with dose interruption and subsequent modification. Mild nausea and vomiting as well as grade 3/4 myelosuppression was reported; myelosuppression was most likely related to docetaxel administration. A pharmacokinetic analysis of the combination did not reveal any significant changes in drug exposure with either agent when administered concomitantly, and the overall toxicity profile was manageable.

26.5.2.2 CP-547, 632

CP-547, 632 is another selective VEGFR-2 small-molecule tyrosine kinase inhibitor that is under ongoing clinical investigation [71]. In a phase I trial, Cohen and colleagues evaluated the antitumor activity of CP-547, 632 at doses ranging from 100 to 250 mg/day in combination with conventional chemotherapeutic agents, paclitaxel (225 mg/m^2) and carboplatin (AUC = 6 mg/ml/min), on a 3-weekly schedule as first-line therapy for patients with stage IIIB or IV NSCLC. Twenty-nine patients received a median of at least 2 cycles of therapy. The most commonly reported adverse events were diarrhea and rash. The MTD of CP-547, 632 for phase II investigation was determined to be 200 mg/day when given in combination with paclitaxel and carboplatin. Of the 24 patients evaluable for tumor response, 20% achieved an objective response. A pharmacokinetic analysis of this combination is ongoing. Based on the antitumor activity and minimal toxicity profile, phase II studies evaluating this combination are being planned.

26.6 Eicosanoid Pathway Inhibitors

Targeting the cyclooxygenase (COX) pathway may have a role in slowing lung cancer growth and thereby decrease the lethality of this disease. The COX pathway is made up of two COX enzymes, COX1 and COX2 enzymes. The COX1 enzymes play a role in most normal tissues and are responsible for the physiologic functioning of the gastrointestinal tract. Recent evidence suggests that the COX-2 isoform is stimulated by interleukin-1, tumor necrosis factor alpha, platelet-derived growth factor, and EGFR, among others, and may play a role in epithelial tumorigenesis [72, 73]. COX-2 appears to be upregulated in NSCLC regardless of the stage of development [74–79]. The correlation between COX-2 expression and lung cancer prognosis has been reported in numerous multiple-patient groups, ranging from early stage to advanced disease [80, 81]. Overexpression of COX-2 results in inhibition of apoptosis, modulation of cell immunity, increased angiogenesis, and enhanced tissue invasion [72].

A phase II clinical trial of docetaxel (75 mg/m^2 given intravenously every 3 weeks) and celecoxib (400 mg given orally, twice daily) combination therapy was conducted in patients with recurrent NSCLC based on preclinical evidence of additive cytotoxic activity with

these two agents in this disease [82]. Of the 34 patients evaluable for response, partial response was observed in 4 (12%), and disease stabilization was seen in 8 patients. Time to progression and overall survival were not reported in this investigation. Nugent and colleagues conducted a similar phase II study that produced a slightly lower objective response rate (4.5%), a higher rate of disease stabilization (82%), and promising time to progression (19.6 weeks) [83]. Both of these early trials suggest that celecoxib enhances the efficacy of single-agent docetaxel in the second-line setting.

Takahashi and colleagues evaluated the activity of meloxicam, a selective COX-2 inhibitor, in combination with paclitaxel and carboplatin in treatment-nave patients with advanced NSCLC based on the inhibition of COX-2-positive lung cancer cells by meloxicam in vitro [84]. In addition, paclitaxel is known to upregulate COX-2, which may contribute to decreased paclitaxel antitumor activity. COX2 may also play a role in mediating neuropathic pain after paclitaxel-induced nerve damage [85]. In this trial, 25 patients received paclitaxel (200 mg/m^2) plus carboplatin (AUC 6) every 21 days in combination with meloxicam 10 mg/day, given orally. Eleven patients (44%) achieved treatment response and 12 achieved disease stabilization. A majority of the study subjects (88%) experienced grade 3 or 4 neutropenia, but neutropenic fever was observed in only two patients. Grade 3 or 4 peripheral neuropathy was observed in only one patient after repeated administration of platinum-based chemotherapy. Compared to a historical overall response rate of 33% in Japanese patients, meloxicam may improve the antitumor activity of paclitaxel/carboplatin combination chemotherapy [86]. Cancer and Leukemia Group B (CALGB) has recently completed a phase II study (30203) evaluating the activity of eicosanoid pathway modulators (celecoxib or zileuton, a 5-lipoxygenase inhibitor, or combination of celecoxib and zileuton) in combination with gemcitabine and carboplatin in advanced NSCLC.

26.7 Bcl-2-Targeted Agents

Regulation of apoptosis is critical to the maintenance of normal cell growth and proliferation. Bcl-2 is one of the key antiapoptotic proteins that have emerged as a strategy for therapeutic intervention in lung cancer [87]. Bcl-2 is located on the inner membrane of the mitochondria and maintains mitochondrial structure by inhibiting cytochrome c release [88]. By inhibiting programmed cell death, bcl-2 expression confers resistance to treatment with traditional cytotoxic chemotherapy, radiation, and monoclonal antibodies [89, 90]. In fact, overexpression of the bcl-2 protein correlates with a poor treatment response to standard chemotherapy or hormonal therapy in both solid and hematologic malignancies, including non-Hodgkin's lymphoma, acute myelogenous leukemia, multiple myeloma, and prostate cancer [91–96]. In addition, nontumorigenic cell lines in xenograft models can be made malignant by transfection of the *bcl-2* gene [92, 97, 98].

The role of *bcl-2* expression in NSCLC remains under investigation. Early studies suggested that in NSCLC, *bcl-2* overexpression is associated with a decreased risk of metastases and potentially enhanced overall survival. However, in a small study of patients with advanced NSCLC, *bcl-2* expression did not correlate with treatment response [99]. Whether expression of *bcl-2* is a clinical prognostic factor has not been clearly identified.

Oblimersen sodium (G3139, Genasense) is an antisense phosphorothioate oligonucleotide compound that was designed to bind to the first six codons of the human bcl-2 mRNA and subsequently decrease bcl-2 protein translation and intracellular concentration [87]. Data from preclinical models suggest that this compound enhances the therapeutic activity of cytotoxic chemotherapy and biologic agents. In a xenograft model of NSCLC, oblimersen improved the cytotoxic effects of single-agent docetaxel compared to either agent alone [100]. Similar results were achieved in xenograft models of aggressive human breast cancer cells [101]. In addition, oblimersen is the first oligonucleotide to demonstrate downregulation of the bcl-2 protein in human cell lines [102].

Early phase I/II studies in patients with refractory small-cell lung cancer (SCLC) and malignant melanoma indicated that oblimersen achieves biologically relevant plasma levels and downregulates the bcl-2 protein within 5 days of initiating therapy [103, 104]. In the study of patients with platinum-refractory SCLC ($n = 12$), oblimersen (3 mg/kg on days 1–8) was administered in combination with paclitaxel (150 mg/m^2 on day 6) on a thrice-weekly basis [104]. Although no patients achieved an objective response, four patients (33%) achieved disease stabilization after two treatment cycles and one patient remained free of progression for over 1 year; this patient demonstrated consistently high plasma oblimersen levels. These results were promising enough to prompt a phase I evaluation of oblimersen in combination with platinum-based chemotherapy in treatment-nave patients with SCLC [105]. In NSCLC, a randomized, multicenter trial of docetaxel (75 mg/m^2 on day 5) with or without oblimersen (7 mg/kg on days 1–8), administered every 21 days, as second-line therapy in relapsed or refractory stage IIIB-IV disease is underway [87]. The primary endpoint of this trial is overall survival.

26.8 Proteasome Inhibitors

Bortezomib is a small-molecule inhibitor of the 26S proteasome, often called the "cellular housekeeper" because it functions to ubiquinate and eliminate cellular proteins slated for degradation. Proteins regulated by the proteasome include those involved in cell cycle regulation (e.g., cyclins, cyclin-dependent kinases, and cyclin-dependent kinase inhibitors) and those inhibitors of apoptosis (e.g., nuclear factor κB, NF-κB) [106].

Several preclinical models have evaluated the in vitro and in vivo activity of bortezomib. Ling and colleagues evaluated the efficacy of bortezomib, again in human NSCLC cell lines, including those with p53 mutations [107]. In this trial, a concentration- and time-dependent cell cycle blockade in the G$_2$-M phase was observed. Sunwoo et al. examined the in vitro effects of bortezomib on human squamous carcinoma cell lines and found that bortezomib slowed cell growth and was associated with inhibition of NF-κB and increased caspase-induced apoptosis. In vivo, doses of 1–2 mg/kg administered three times per week inhibited the growth of squamous cell carcinoma xenografts in athymic mice [108]. Finally, Mack and colleagues demonstrated that bortezomib exposures stimulated an increase in p21, cell cycle accumulation in the G$_2$-M phases, activation of caspase, and increased apoptosis in lung cancer cells [109].

The sequence of drug administration, specifically with docetaxel, has been shown to influence treatment response in preclinical models [110]. In that study, the administration of docetaxel prior to bortezomib produced a greater cytotoxicity when compared with the reverse sequence of administration of these two agents. Similar studies have been performed with bortezomib in combination with gemcitabine and carboplatin against the A549 NSCLC cell line. Sequential administration of gemcitabine/carboplatin followed by bortezomib induced the greatest degree of apoptosis.

Bortezomib does not appear to exhibit traditional mechanisms of resistance to chemotherapy or radiation. It has demonstrated the ability to circumvent multicellular drug resistance and is not a substrate for the multidrug resistance p-glycoprotein MDR1 [111]. In addition, as demonstrated by Ling and colleagues, bortezomib-induced cytotoxicity does not seem to be affected by mutation of the p53 gene.

In a phase I clinical trial conducted by Orlowski et al. in patients with refractory hematologic malignancies, a MTD of 1.4 mg/m^2 on days 1, 4, 8, and 11 administered intravenously every 3 weeks was established [112]. Dose-limiting toxicities at this dose level included thrombocytopenia, fatigue, hypokalemia, and hyponatremia. Pharmacodynamic studies demonstrated that bortezomib induced time- and dose-dependent inhibition of the 26S proteasome. Responses were observed in patients with multiple myeloma, follicular lymphoma, and mantle cell lymphoma. A phase II evaluation has now been conducted in patients with multiple myeloma and shown to induce major responses in this malignancy [113].

Currently there are no published trials of bortezomib in patients with lung cancer, although several clinical studies in this patient population have just been completed or are still ongoing. These include a randomized phase II study evaluating bortezomib alone versus in combination with docetaxel that has demonstrated a manageable toxicity profile in both treatment arms. Patients receiving bortezomib in combination with conventional chemotherapy did experience fatigue and neutropenia more frequently than those in the single-agent arm. Efficacy results have not yet been presented [114]. In addition, bortezomib is currently being evaluated in phase I clinical studies in combination with conventional chemotherapeutic agents, including gemcitabine, etoposide plus cisplatin, paclitaxel plus carboplatin, and gemcitabine plus carboplatin [109]. Assuming that bortezomib displays activity against NSCLC as a single agent, the results of these combination regimens in early clinical trials should lead to advanced clinical testing [106]. As these trials unfold, several important clinical issues including the optimal dose schedule, optimal sequence with conventional chemotherapeutic regimens, duration of treatment, risk of cumulative toxicity with long-term administration, and potentially dose-limiting neurotoxicity must be considered [109].

26.9 Cyclin-Dependent Kinase Inhibitors

The cyclin-dependent kinases (cdks) make up a family of enzymes that play a critical part in the regulation of the cell cycle and RNA transcription [115]. The cdks facilitate orderly progression through the cell cycle. Overexpression of cyclins or absence of their inhibitors is thought to promote selective growth of human cancer cells [116, 117]. Production of cdk inhibitors by tumor cell lines restores command of the cell cycle, usually causing cells to stop in the G_1 or resting phase [118]. Based upon these observations, targeting these enzymes has emerged as a possibility for therapeutic intervention in clinical human cancer.

Flavopiridol is the first pan-cdk inhibitor to undergo clinical investigation. It is a flavone that directly competes with the ATP substrate for binding of multiple cyclins, including cdk1, cdk2, cdk4, cdk6, cdk7, and cdk9, resulting in cell cycle arrest in the G_1-S and G_2-M phase of the cell cycle and impairment of RNA elongation of antiapoptotic proteins. In preclinical models, 200–300 nM of flavopiridol induced cell cycle arrest in most solid tumors, indicating inhibition of cdks 1, 2, 4, and 6 [119, 120]. Apoptosis does occur; however, maximal effects do not appear to be reached for at least 72 h after

therapy initiation and requires flavopiridol concentrations higher than that necessary for cdk inhibition [121, 122]. Thus, the antitumor activity derived from the administration of flavopiridol monotherapy in many solid tumors is probably cytostatic rather than cytotoxic [115]. Consistent with this finding, 4 of the 20 patients with previously untreated NSCLC enrolled in a phase II trial of single-agent flavopiridol achieved disease stabilization as a best response [123]. No objective responses were seen in this trial.

Evidence of synergistic activity between chemotherapeutic agents with the ability to cause S-phase recruitment (e.g., gemcitabine, and cisplatin) and flavopiridol has been shown in preclinical evaluations in a sequence-dependent fashion [124, 125]. Therefore, the schedule of administration may play a significant role in achieving antitumor activity. In a phase I trial of gemcitabine followed by flavopiridol (24-h continuous infusion), three of the nine treated patients with NSCLC achieved a partial response [126].

As mentioned previously, flavopiridol monotherapy stops cell cycle progression from the G_2 phase through mitosis. Thus, when administered before or concomitantly with taxane chemotherapy, it is antagonistic [124, 127]. By contrast, if flavopiridol is administered after taxane, then the cytotoxic effects are synergistic. Gries and colleagues completed a phase I trial in patients with treatment-nave NSCLC, exploring the activity of carboplatin (AUC 5), paclitaxel (175 mg/m^2), and flavopiridol combination therapy [128]. Carboplatin and paclitaxel were administered on day 1 on a 3-weekly basis and flavopiridol was administered intravenously over 24 h on day 2 in this trial ($n=18$). Partial responses were observed in 36% of enrollees. Dose-limiting toxicities observed included neutropenia and thromboembolic events. Docetaxel and flavopiridol combination therapy in patients with NSCLC after platinum-based chemotherapy failure has been evaluated in a phase I clinical study [129]. In this trial, 15 patients received flavopiridol as a 1-hour infusion, starting 24 h after docetaxel administration, on a weekly basis in combination with docetaxel (75 mg/m^2), intravenously every 21 days. Seven of the treated patients achieved stabilization of disease; partial response was observed in one patient. A randomized phase II trial evaluating two schedules of this combination (interval between agents either 3–4 h or 16–24 h) versus docetaxel monotherapy is ongoing [115].

26.10 Farnesyl Transferase Inhibitors

The Kirsten ras (K-ras) gene was initially discovered as a retrovirus-encoded gene that initiated sarcomas in rats [130, 131]. The ras family of genes has been identified as a potential target for therapeutic treatment of lung cancer, as *K-ras* is mutated in approximately 20% of NSCLCs, most commonly in adenocarcinomas [132]. After translation of mRNA to the ras protein, farnesyl transferase covalently links a farnesyl group to the ras protein, enabling the protein to move from the cytoplasm to the cell membrane and participate in cell signaling and ultimately cell proliferation. Farnesyl transferase inhibitors (FTIs) have been developed to prevent the linkage of the farnesyl group to the ras protein, thereby blocking cell signal transduction, inhibiting cell proliferation, and promoting apoptosis.

FTI's have shown promising results, in both in vitro and in vivo studies of a broad spectrum of human cancer cells lines, including NSCLC [133–135]. Contrary to the proposed mechanism of action, tumor cell lines bearing the wild-type *ras* or mutated *H-ras* genes appear to be most sensitive to the FTIs, rather than those bearing *K-ras* mutations [133, 136]. Based on the FTIs ability to retard the growth NSCLC tumor cell lines, clinical testing was initiated.

Two agents of the FTI class, R115777 (tipifarnib) and L-778, 123 (lonafarnib) have undergone phase I testing in patients with advanced malignancies, and demonstrated a relatively tolerable toxicity profile [137–139]. The dose-limiting toxicities observed were fatigue, myelosuppression, and neurotoxicity. The doses recommended for further clinical investigation were 300–400 mg/m^2 given orally twice daily for 14–21 days, and 560 mg/m^2 intravenously, daily for 14 days for R115777 and L-778, 123, respectively. To determine the role of this pharmacologic class in NSCLC, phase II studies with each agent were initiated in patients with previously untreated advanced disease [140, 141]. Although both of these agents exhibited tolerable toxicities in the front-line phase II trials, no antitumor activity has been observed with either trial. Moreover, the observed time to progression was relatively short (approximately 6–8 weeks), which is less than the 4–6 cycles of platinum-based chemotherapy routinely administered to patients at this advanced stage of NSCLC. Interestingly, the study employing R115777 did demonstrate at least partial inhibition of farnesyl transferase activity in the majority of patients (80%), indicating that the biologic effects were achieved in the surrogate tissues. Based on this finding, a means of identifying patients more likely to respond or biomarkers correlated to improve clinical benefit might be sought. Another phase II trial of lonafarnib plus paclitaxel in taxane-refractory/resistant NSCLC did show a modest treatment response (15% partial response rate) that has prompted a phase III randomized study to investigate the combination of an FTI and standard chemotherapy (lonafarnib plus paclitaxel/carboplatin). The report of this trial is not yet available [132]. The role of the FTIs in the treatment of NSCLC is unclear at the present time.

Key Points

- Targeted therapies, unlike conventional cytotoxic chemotherapy, focus on cell signaling and other biologic pathways that are involved in tumorigenesis.
- Targeted therapies interfere with specific critical steps associated with the initiation and maintenance of the malignant phenotype.
- Due to their specific targeted mechanisms of action, targeted therapies generally demonstrate improved tolerability profiles compared to their conventional cytotoxic chemotherapeutic counterparts. They can be offered to heavily pretreated patients or to those patients with a performance status that renders them unsuitable for other treatment options.

References

1. Socinski MA, Morris DE, Masters GA, Lilenbaum R. Chemotherapeutic management of stage IV non-small cell lung cancer. Chest 2003; 123:226S.
2. Ginsberg RJ, Vokes EE, Rosenzweig K. Non-small cell lung cancer. In: DeVita VT, Hellman S, Rosenberg (eds), Cancer: Principles and Practice of Oncology, 6th edn., volume 1. Lippincott, New York, 2001; p 925.
3. Non-Small Cell Lung Cancer Collaborative Group. Chemotherapy in non-small cell lung cancer: a meta-analysis using updated data on individual patients from 52 randomised clinical trials. Br Med J 1995; 311:899
4. Schiller JH, Harrington D, Belani CP, et al. Comparison of four chemotherapy regimens for advanced non-small cell lung cancer. N Engl J Med 2002; 346:92.
5. Dy GK, Adjei AA. Novel targets for lung cancer therapy: part I. J Clin Oncol 2002; 20(12):2881.
6. Korfee S, Gauler T, Hepp R, Pottgen C, Eberhardt W. New targeted treatments in lung cancer – overview of clinical trials. Lung Cancer 2004; 45:S199.
7. Sridhar SS, Seymour L, Shepherd FA. Inhibitors of epidermal-growth-factor receptors: a review of clinical research with a focus on non-small cell lung cancer. Lancet Oncol 2003; 4:397
8. Balsega J, Arteaga CL. Critical update and emerging trends in epidermal growth factor receptor targeting in cancer. J Clin Oncol 2005; 23(11):1.
9. Sirotnak FM, Zakowski MF, Miller VA, Scher HI, Kris MG. Efficacy of cytotoxic agents against human tumor xenografts is markedly enhanced by coadministration of ZD1839 (Iressa), an inhibitor of EGFR tyrosine kinase. Clin Cancer Res 2000; 6: 4885.
10. Yarden Y. The EGFR family and its ligands in human cancer: signaling mechanisms and therapeutic opportunities. Eur J Cancer 2001; 37(Suppl 4):S3.
11. Lei W, Mayotte JE, Levitt ML. Enhancement of chemosensitivity and programmed cell death by tyrosine kinase inhibitors correlates with EGFR expression in non-small cell lung cancer cells. Anticancer Res 1999; 19:221
12. Hirsch F, Scagliotti GV, Langer CJ, Varella-Garcia M, Franklin WM. Epidermal growth factor family of receptors in preneoplasia and lung cancer: perspectives for targeted therapies. Lung Cancer 2003; 41:S29.

13. Scagliotti GV, Selvaggi GV, Novello S, Hirsch FR. The biology of epidermal growth factor receptor in lung cancer. Clin Cancer Res 2004; 10:4227s.

14. Hirsch FR, Verella-Garcia M, Bunn PA Jr, et al. Epidermal growth factor receptor in non-small cell lung carcinomas: correlation between gene copy number and protein expression and impact on prognosis. J Clin Oncol 2003; 21:3798.

15. Reinmuth N, Brandt B, Kunze WP, et al. Ploidy, expression of erbB1, erbB2, P53 and amplification of erbB1, erbB2, erbB3 in non-small cell lung cancer. Eur Respir J 2000; 16:991.

16. Woodburn JR. The epidermal growth factor receptor and its inhibition in cancer therapy. Pharmacol 1999; 82:241.

17. Brabender J, Danenberg KD, Metzger R, et al. Epidermal growth factor receptor and HER2-neu mRNA expression in non-small cell lung cancer is correlated with survival. Clin Cancer Res 2000; 7:1850.

18. Nicholson RI, Gee JM, Harper ME. EGFR and cancer prognosis. Eur J Cancer 2001; 37(Suppl 4):S9.

19. Kies MS, Harari PM. Cetuximab (Imclone/Merck/Bristol-Myers Squibb). Curr Opin Invest Drugs 2002; 3:1092.

20. Govindan R. Cetuximab in advanced non-small cell lung cancer. Clin Cancer Res 2004; 10:4241s.

21. Robert F, Ezekiel MP, Spencer SA, et al. Phase I study of anti-epidermal growth factor receptor antibody cetuximab in combination with radiation therapy in patients with advanced head and neck cancer. J Clin Oncol 2001; 19:3234.

22. Lilenbaum R, Bonomi P, Ansari R, Lynch T, Govindan R, Janne P, Hanna N. A phase II trial of cetuximab as therapy for recurrent non-small cell lung cancer: final results. Proc Am Soc Clin Oncol 2005; 23:7036.

23. Kelly K, Hanna N, Rosenberg A, Bunn PA, Needle MN. Mutlicentered Phase I/II study of cetuximab in combination with paclitaxel and carboplatin in untreated patients with stage IV non-small cell lung cancer. Proc Am Soc Clin Oncol 2003; 22:644.

24. Robert F, Blumenschien G, Dicke K, Tseng J, Saleh MN, Needle M. Phase Ib/IIa study of anti-epidermal growth factor receptor (EGFR) antibody, cetuximab, in combination with gemcitabine/carboplatin in patients with advanced non-small cell lung cancer (NSCLC). Proc Am Soc Clin Oncol 2003; 22:643.

25. Gatzemeier U, Rosell R, Ramlau R, et al. Cetuximab (C225) in combination with cisplatin/vinorelbine vs. cisplatin/vinorelbine alone in the first-line treatment of patients (pts) with epidermal growth factor receptor (EGFR) positive advanced non-small cell lung cancer (NSCLC). Proc Am Soc Clin Oncol 2003; 22:643.

26. Kim ES, Mauer AM, Tran HT, et al. A phase II study of cetuximab, an epidermal growth factor receptor (EGFR) blocking antibody, in combination with docetaxel in chemotherapy refractory/resistant patients with advanced non-small cell lung cancer: final report: Proc Am Soc Clin Oncol 2003; 22:642.

27. Lynch DH, Yang XD. Therapeutic potential of ABX-EGF: a fully human anti-epidermal growth factor receptor monoclonal antibody for cancer treatment. Semin Oncol 2002; 29(1 suppl 4):47-50.

28. Figlin RA, Belldegrun AS, Crawford J, et al. ABX-EGF, a fully human anti-epidermal growth factor receptor monoclonal antibody in patients with advanced cancer: phase I clinical results. Proc Am Soc Clin Oncol 2002; 21:35.

29. Crawford J, Sandler AB, Hammond LA, et al. ABX-EGF in combination with paclitaxel and carboplatin for advanced non-small cell lung cancer. Proc Am Soc Clin Oncol 2004; 22:7083.

30. Wakeling AE, Guy SP, Woodburn JR, Ashton SE, Curry BJ, Barker AJ, Gibson KH. ZD1839 (Iressa): an orally active inhibitor of epidermal growth factor signaling with potential for cancer therapy. Cancer Res 2002; 62:5749.

31. Bianco C, Tortora G, Bianco R, et al. Enhancement of antitumor activity of ionizing radiation by combined treatment with the selective epidermal growth factor receptor-tyrosine kinase inhibitor ZD1839 (Iressa). Clin Cancer Res 2002; 8:3250.

32. Herbst RS, Maddox AM, Rothenberg ML, et al. Selective oral epidermal growth factor receptor tyrosine kinase inhibitor ZD1839 is generally well-tolerated and has activity in non-small cell lung cancer and other solid tumors: result of a phase I trial. J Clin Oncol 2002; 20:3815.

33. Kris MG, Natale RB, Herbst RS, et al. A phase II trial of ZD1839 (Iressa) in advanced non-small-cell lung cancer (NSCLC) patients who had failed platinum- and docetaxel-based regimens (IDEAL 2). Proc Am Soc Clin Oncol 2002; 21:1166.

34. Shepherd FA, Dancey J, Ramlau R, et al. Prospective randomized trial of docetaxel versus best supportive care in patients with non-small-cell lung cancer previously treated with platinum-based chemotherapy. J Clin Oncol 2000; 18:2095.

35. Fukuoka M, Yano S, Giaccone G, et al. A multi-institutional randomized phase II trial of ZD1839 ('Iressa') for previously treated patients with advanced non-small cell lung cancer (the IDEAL 1 trial). J Clin Oncol 2003; 21:2237.

36. Vansteenkiste J, Natale R, Giaccone G, et al. Two randomized, double-blind studies of ZD1839 ('Iressa') in 425 patients with pretreated advanced non-small cell lung cancer (IDEAL1 and IDEAL2). Eur Respir J 2002; 20(Suppl 38):399S.

37. Cohen MH, Williams GA, Sridhara R, Chen G, Pazdur R. FDA drug approval summary: Gefitinib (ZD1839) (Iressa) tablets. Oncologist 2003; 8:203.

38. Thatcher N, Chang A, Parikh P, Pemberton K, Archer V, on behalf of the ISEL Investigators. Results of a phase III placebo-controlled study of gefitinib plus best supportive care in patients with advanced non-small cell lung cancer who had received 1 or 2 prior chemotherapy regimens. Proc Am Assoc Cancer Res 2005; 46:LB-6.

39. Gianccone G, Herbst RS, Manegold C, et al. Gefitinib in combination with gemcitabine and cisplatin in advanced non-small-cell lung cancer: a phase III trial – INTACT 1. J Clin Oncol 2004; 22(5):777.

40. Herbst RS, Giaccone G, Schiller JH, et al. Gefitinib in combination with paclitaxel and carboplatin in advanced non-small-cell lung cancer: a phase III trial – INTACT 2. J Clin Oncol 2004; 22(5):785.

41. Ciardiello F, Caputo R, Bianco R, et al. Antitumor effect and potentiation of cytotoxic drugs activity in human cancer cells by ZD-1839 (Iressa), an epidermal growth factor receptor-selective tyrosine kinase inhibitor. Clin Cancer Res 2000; 6:2053.

42. Goldman CK, Kim J, Wong WL, King V, Brock T, Gillespie GY. Epidermal growth factor stimulates vascular endothelial growth factor production by human malignant glioma cells: A model of glioblastoma multiforme pathophysiology. Mol Biol Cell 1993; 4:121.

43. Ravindranath N, Wion D, Brachet P, Djakiew D. Epidermal growth factor modulates the expression of vascular endothelial growth factor in the human prostate. J Androl 2001; 22:432.

44. Giaccone G. The role of gefitinib in lung cancer treatment. Clin Cancer Res 2004; 10:4233s.

45. Hildago M, Siu LL, Nemunaitis J, et al. Phase I and pharmacologic study of OSI-774, an epidermal growth factor receptor tyrosine kinase inhibitor, in patients with advanced solid malignancies. J Clin Oncol 2001; 19:3267.

46. Perez-Soler R. The role of erlotinib (tarceva, OSI 774) in the treatment of non-small cell lung cancer. Clin Cancer Res 2004; 10: 4238s.

47. Perez-Soler R, Chachoua A, Huberman M, et al. Final results of a phase II study of erlotinib monotherapy in patients with advanced non-small cell lung cancer following failure of platinum-based chemotherapy. Lung Cancer 2003; 41:S56.

48. Patel JD, Miller VA, Kris MG, et al. Encouraging activity and durable responses demonstrated by the EGFR tyrosine kinase inhibitor erlotinib in patients with advanced bronchioalveolar cell carcinoma. Lung Cancer 2003; 41:S56.

49. Shepherd FA, Pereira J, Ciuleanu TE, et al. A randomized placebo-controlled trial of erlotinib in patients with advanced non-small cell lung cancer following failure of 1st line or 2nd line chemotherapy: a National Cancer Institute of Canada Trials Group (NCIC CTG) trial. Proc Am Soc Clin Oncol 2004; 22:7022.

50. Herbst RS, Prager D, Hermann V, et al. TRIBUTE – a phase III trial of erlotinib HCl combined with carboplatin and paclitaxel chemotherapy in advanced non-small cell lung cancer. Proc Am Soc Clin Oncol 2004; 22:7011.

51. Gatzemeier U, Pluzanska A, Szczesna A, et al. Results of a phase III trial of erlotinib combined with cisplatin and gemcitabine chemotherapy in advanced non-small cell lung cancer. Proc Am Soc Clin Oncol 2004; 22:7010.

52. Miller VA, Herbst R, Prager D, et al. Long survival of never smoking non-small cell lung cancer patients treated with erlotinib HCl and chemotherapy: sub-group analysis of TRIBUTE. Proc Am Soc Clin Oncol 2004; 22:7061.

53. Bergsland EK. Vascular endothelial growth factor as a therapeutic target in cancer. Am J Health-Syst Pharm 2004; 61:S4.

54. Fernando NH, Hurwitz HI. Inhibition of vascular endothelial growth factor in the treatment of colorectal cancer Semin Oncol 2003; 30(3):39.

55. Folkman J. Role of angiogenesis in tumor growth and metastasis. Semin Oncol 2002; 29(6):15.

56. Hicklin DJ, Ellis LM. Role of vascular endothelial growth factor pathway in tumor growth and angiogenesis. J Clin Oncol 2005; 23(5):1011.

57. Fontanini G, Lucchi M, Vignati S, et al. Angiogenesis as a prognostic indicator of survival in non-small-cell lung carcinoma: a prospective study. J Natl Cancer Inst 1997; 89:881.

58. Bergsland EK. Update on clinical trials targeting vascular endothelial growth factor in cancer. Am J Health-Syst Pharm 2004; 61:S12.

59. Hurwitz H, Fehrenbacher L, Novotny W, et al. Bevacizumab plus irinotecan, 5-flourouracil, and leucovorin for metastatic colorectal cancer. N Engl J Med 2004; 350(23):2335

60. Lee CG, Heijn M, di Tomaso E, et al. Anti-vascular endothelial growth factor treatment augments tumor radiation response under normoxic or hypoxic conditions. Cancer Res 2000; 60:5565.

61. Phan CD, Roberts TP, van Bruggen N, et al. Magnetic resonance imaging detects suppression of tumor vascular endothelial growth factor. Cancer Invest 1998; 16:225.

62. Kim KJ, Li B, Winer J, Armanini M, Gillett N, Phillips HS, Ferrara N. Inhibition of vascular endothelial growth factor-induced angiogenesis suppresses tumour growth in vivo. Nature 1993; 362:841.

63. Kabbinavar FF, Wong JT, Ayala RE, et al. The effect of antibody to vascular endothelial growth factor and cisplatin on the growth of lung tumors in nude mice. Proc Am Cancer Res 1995; 36:488.

64. Sweeney CJ, Miller KD, Sissons SE, et al. The antiangiogenic property of docetaxel is synergistic with a recombi-

nant humanized monoclonal antibody against vascular endothelial growth factor or 2-methoxyestradiol but antagonized by endothelial growth factors. Cancer Res 2001; 61:3369.

65. Gordon MS, Margolin K, Talpaz M, et al. Phase I safety and pharmacokinetic study of recombinant human anti-vascular endothelial growth factor in patients with advanced cancer. J Clin Oncol 2001; 19:843.

66. Herbst RS, Johson DH, Mininberg E, et al. Phase I/II trial evaluating the anti-vascular endothelial growth factor monoclonal antibody bevacizumab in combination with the HER-1/epidermal growth factor receptor tyrosine kinase inhibitor erlotinib for patients with recurrent non-small cell lung cancer. J Clin Oncol 2005; 23(14):2544.

67. Johnson DH, Kabbinavar F, Fehrenbacher L, et al. Randomized phase II trial comparing bevacizumab plus carboplatin and paclitaxel with carboplatin and paclitaxel alone in previously untreated locally advanced or metastatic non-small cell lung cancer. J Clin Oncol 2004; 22:2184.

68. Basser R, Hurwitz H, Barge A, et al. Phase 1 pharmacokinetic and biological study of angiogenesis inhibitor, ZD6474, in patients with solid tumors. Proc Am Soc Clin Oncol 2001; 22:396.

69. Minami H, Ebi H, Tahara Y, et al. A phase I study of an oral VEGF receptor tyrosine kinase inhibitor ZD6474, in Japanese patients with solid tumors. Proc Am Soc Clin Oncol 2003; 22:778.

70. Heymach JV, Dong RP, Dimery I, et al. ZD6474, a novel antiangiogenic agent, in combination with docetaxel in patients with NSCLC: results of the run-in phase of a two-part, randomized phase II study. Proc Am Soc Clin Oncol 2004; 22:3051.

71. Cohen RB, Simon G, Langer CJ, et al. Phase I trial of oral CP-547, 632 (VEGFR2) in combination with paclitaxel and carboplatin in advanced non-small cell lung cancer. Proc Am Soc Clin Oncol 2004; 22:3014.

72. Brown JR, DuBois RN. Cyclooxygenase as a target in lung cancer. Clin Cancer Res 2004; 10:4266s.

73. Gupta RA, DuBois RN. Colorectal cancer and the cyclooxygenase pathway. Nat Rev Cancer 2001; 1:11-21.

74. Hida T, Yatabe Y, Achiwa H, et al. Increased cyclooxygenase 2 occurs frequently in human lung cancers, specifically adenocarcinomas. Cancer Res 1998; 58:3761.

75. Hosomi Y, Yokose T, Hirose Y, Nakajima R, Nagai K, Nishiwaki Y, Ochiai A. Increased cyclooxygenase 2 (COX-2) expression occurs frequently in precursor lesions of human adenocarcinoma of the lung. Lung Cancer 2000; 30:73.

76. Anderson WF, Umar A, Viner JL, Hawk ET. The role of cyclooxygenase inhibitors in cancer prevention. Curr Pharm Des 2002; 8:1035.

77. Wolff H, Saukkonen K, Anttila S, Karjalainen A, Vainio H, Ristimaki A. Expression of cyclooxygenase-2 in human lung carcinoma. Cancer Res 1998; 58:4997.

78. Huang M, Stolina M, Sharma S, et al. Non-small cell lung cancer cyclooxygenase-2-dependent regulation of cytokine balance in lymphocytes and macrophages: up-regulation of interleukin 10 and down-regulation of interleukin 12 production. Cancer Res 1998; 58:1208.

79. Fang HY, Lin TS, Lin JP, Wu YC, Chow KC, Wang LS. Cyclooxygenase-2 in human non-small cell lung cancer. Eur J Surg Oncol 2003; 29:171.

80. Achiwa H, Yatabe Y, Hida T, et al. Prognostic significance of elevated cyclooxygenase 2 expression in primary, resected lung adenocarcinomas. Clin Cancer Res 1999; 5:1001.

81. Brabender J, Park J, Metzger R, et al. Prognostic significance of cyclooxygenase 2 mRNA expression in non-small cell lung cancer. Ann Surg 2002; 235:440.

82. Hida T, Kozaki K, Muramatsu H, et al. Cyclooxygenase-2 inhibitor induces apoptosis and enhances cytotoxicity of various anticancer agents in non-small cell lung cancer cell lines. Clin Cancer Res 2000; 6:2006.

83. Nugent FW, Graziano S, Levitan N, et al. Docetaxel and COX-2 inhibition with celecoxib in relapsed/refractory non-small cell lung cancer (NSCLC): promising progression-free survival in a phase II study. Proc Am Soc Clin Oncol 2003; 22:2697.

84. Tsubouchi Y, Mukai S, Kawahito Y, Yamada R, Kohno M, Inque KI, Sano H. Meloxicam inhibits the growth of non-small cell lung cancer. Anticancer Res 2000; 20(5A):2867.

85. Ma W, Eisenach JC. Cyclooxygenase 2 in infiltrating inflammatory cells in injured nerve is universally up-regulated following various types of peripheral nerve injury. Neuroscience 2003; 121:691.

86. Ohe Y, Saijo N, Ohashi Y, et al. Preliminary results of the four-arm cooperative study (FACS) for advanced non-small cell lung cancer in Japan. Proc Am Soc Clin Oncol 2003; 22:2509.

87. Herbst RS, Franke SR. Oblimersen sodium (genasense bcl-2 antisense oligonucleotide): a rational therapeutic to enhance apoptosis in therapy of lung cancer. Clin Cancer Res 2004; 10: 4245s.

88. Reed JC. Dysregulation of apoptosis in cancer. J Clin Oncol 1999; 17:2941.

89. Kitada S, Takayama S, De Riel K, Tanaka S, Reed JC. Reversal of chemoresistance of lymphoma cells by antisense-mediated reduction of bcl-2 gene expression. Antisense Res Dev 1994; 4:71.

90. Schmitt CA, Rosentahl CT, Lowe SW. Genetic analysis of chemoresistance in primary murine lymphomas. Nat Med 2000; 6:1029.

91. Reed JC. Bcl-2 and the regulation of programmed cell death. J Cell Biol 1994; 124:1.

92. Miyashita T, Reed JC. Bcl-2 oncoprotein blocks chemotherapy-induced apoptosis in a human leukemia cell line. Blood 1993; 81:151.

93. Gazit Y, Fey V, Thomas C, Alvarez R. Bcl-2 overexpression is associated with resistance to dexamethasone, but not melphalan, in multiple myeloma cells. Int J Oncol 1998; 13:397.

94. Feinman R, Koury J, Thames M, Barlogie B, Epstein J, Siegel DS. Role of NF-kappaB in the rescue of multiple myeloma cells from glucocorticoid-induced apoptosis by bcl-2. Blood 1999; 93:3044.

95. Furuya Y, Krajewski S, Epstein JI, Reed JC, Isaacs JT. Expression of bcl-2 and the progression of human and rodent prostatic cancers. Clin Cancer Res 1996; 2:389.

96. Lipponen P, Vesalainen S. Expression of the apoptosis suppressing protein bcl-2 in prostatic adenocarcinoma is related to tumor malignancy. Prostate 1998; 32:9.

97. Ben-Ezra JM, Kornstein MJ, Grimes MM, Krystal G. Small cell carcinomas of the lung express the Bcl-2 protein. Am J Pathol 1994; 145:1036.

98. Koty PP, Zhang H, Levitt ML. Antisense bcl-2 treatment increases programmed cell death in non-small cell lung cancer cell lines. Lung Cancer 1999; 23:115.

99. Krug LM, Miller VA, Filippa DA. Bax, Bcl-2 and drugs affecting tubulin. J Int Assoc Study Lung Cancer 2000; 29:S1.

100. Klasa RJ, Gillum AM, Klem RE, Frankel SR. Oblimersen bcl-2 antisense: facilitating apoptosis in anticancer treatment. Antisense Nucleic Acid Drug Dev 2002; 12:193.

101. Yang D, Ling Y, Almazan M, et al. Tumor regression in human breast carcinomas by combination therapy of anti-bcl-2 antisense oligonucleotide and chemotherapeutic drugs. Proc Am Assoc Cancer Res 1999; 40:729.

102. Lebedeva I, Stein CA. Antisense oligonucleotides: promise and reality. Annu Rev Pharmacol Toxicol 2001; 41:403.

103. Jansen B, Wacheck V, Heere-Ress E, et al. Clinical, pharmacologic, and pharmacodynamic study of Genasense (G3139, Bcl-2 antisense oligonucleotide) and dacarbazine (DTIC) in patients with malignant melanoma. Proc Am Soc Clin Oncol 2001; 1429.

104. Rudin CM, Otterson GA, Mauer AM, et al. A pilot trial of G3139, a bcl-2 antisense oligonucleotide, and paclitaxel in patients with chemorefractory small-cell lung cancer. Ann Oncol 2002; 13:539.

105. Rudin CM, Kosloff M, Hoffman PC, Edelman MJ, Vokes EE. Phase I study of G3139, a bcl-2 antisense oligonucleotide, combined with carboplatin and etoposide in patients with small cell lung cancer. J Clin Oncol 2004; 22:1110.

106. Bunn PA. The potential role of proteasome inhibitors in the treatment of lung cancer. Clin Cancer Res 2004; 10:4263s.

107. Ling YH, Liebes L, Jiang JD, et al. Mechanisms of proteasome inhibitor PS-341-induced G(2)-M-phase arrest and apoptosis in human non-small cell lung cancer cell lines. Clin Cancer Res 2003; 9:1145.

108. Sunwoo JB, Chen Z, Dong G, et al. Novel proteasome inhibitor PS-341 inhibits activation of nuclear factor-B, cell survival, tumor growth, and angiogenesis in squamous cell carcinoma. Clin Cancer Res 2001; 7:1419.

109. Mack PC, Davies AM, Lara PN, Gumerlock PH, Gandara DR. Integration of the proteasome inhibitor PS-341 (Velcade) into the therapeutic approach to lung cancer. Lung Cancer 2003; 41:S89-96.

110. Gumerlock PH, Kawaguchi T, Moisan LP, Lau AH, Mack PC, Lara PN, Gandara DR. Mechanisms of enhanced cytotoxicity from docetaxel plus PS-341 combination in non-small cell lung carcinoma. Proc Am Soc Clin Oncol 2002; 21:1214.

111. Frankel A, Man S, Elliott P, Adams J, Kerbel RS. Lack of multicellular drug resistance observed in human ovarian and prostate carcinoma treated with the proteasome inhibitor PS-341. Clin Cancer Res 2000; 6:3719.

112. Orlowski RZ, Stinchcombe TE, Mitchell BS, et al. Phase I trial of the proteasome inhibitor PS-341 in patients with refractory hematologic malignancies. J Clin Oncol 2002; 20:4420.

113. Richardson PG, Barlogie B, Berenson J, et al. Phase 2 study of bortezomib in relapsed, refractory myeloma. N Engl J Med 2003; 348(26):2609.

114. Fannuci MP, Belt RJ, Fossella FV, et al. Phase 2 study of bortezomib ± docetaxel in previously treated patients with advanced non-small cell lung cancer (NSCLC): preliminary results. Proc Am Soc Clin Oncol 2004; 22(14S):7107.

115. Shapiro GI. Preclinical and clinical development of the cyclin-dependent kinase inhibitor flavopiridol. Clin Cancer Res 2004; 10: 4270s.

116. Sherr CJ. Cancer cell cycles. Science 1996; 13:1501.

117. Hall M, Peters G. Genetic alterations of cyclins, cyclin-dependent kinases, and cdk inhibitors in human cancer. Adv Cancer Res 1996; 68:67.

118. Shapiro GI, Harper JW. Anticancer drug targets: cell cycle and checkpoint control. J Clin Invest 1999; 104:1645.

119. Shapiro GI. Small molecule inhibitors of cyclin-dependent kinases. In: Blagosklonny M (ed), Cell Cycle Checkpoints and Cancer. Landes Bioscience, Georgetown, TX, 2003; p 208.

120. Sedlacek HH. Mechanisms of action of flavopiridol. Crit Rev Oncol Hematol 2001; 38:139.

121. Bible KC, Kaufmann SH. Flavopiridol: a cytotoxic flavone that induces cell death in noncycling A549 human lung carcinoma cells. Cancer Res 1996; 56:4856.

122. Shapiro GI, Koestner DA, Matranga CB, Rollins BJ. Flavopiridol induces cell cycle arrest and p-53 independent apoptosis in non-small cell lung cancer cell lines. Clin Cancer Res 1999; 5:2925.

123. Shapiro GI, Supko JG, Patterson A, et al. A phase II trial of the cyclin-dependent kinase inhibitor flavopiridol in patients with previously untreated stage IV non-small cell lung cancer. Clin Cancer Res 2001; 7:1500.

124. Bible KC, Kaufmann SH. Cytotoxic synergy between flavopiridol and various antineoplastic agents: the importance of sequence of administration. Cancer Res 1997; 57:3375.

125. Jung CP, Motwani MV, Schwartz GK. Flavopiridol increases sensitization to gemcitabine in human gastrointestinal cancer cell lines and correlates with down-regulation of the ribonucleotide reductase M2 subunit. Clin Cancer Res 2001; 7:2527.

126. Goffin J, Appleman L, Ryan D, et al. A phase I trial of gemcitabine followed by flavopiridol in patients with solid tumors. Lung Cancer 2003; 41:S179.

127. Motwani M, Delohery TM, Schwartz GK. Sequential dependent enhancement of caspase activation and apoptosis by flavopiridol on paclitaxel-treated human gastric and breast cancer cells. Clin Cancer Res 1999; 5:1876.

128. Gries JM, Kasimis B, Schwartzenberger P, et al. Phase I study of HMR1275 (flavopiridol) in non-small cell lung cancer patients after 24 hr IV administration in combination with paclitaxel and carboplatin. Proc Am Soc Clin Oncol 2002; 22:94a.

129. Kasimis B, Rocha-Lima C, Cogswell J, Mahany JJ, Rodriguez L, Gries JM. Phase I study evaluating 1-hr flavopiridol (HMR1275) in combination with docetaxel in previously treated non-small cell lung cancer patients. Proc Am Soc Clin Oncol 2003; 22:669.

130. Crul M, de Klerk GJ, Beijnen JH, Schellens JH. Ras biochemistry and farnesyl transferase inhibitors: a literature survey. Anticancer Drugs 2001; 12(3):163.

131. Ghobrial IM, Adjei AA. Inhibitors of the ras oncogene as therapeutic targets. Hematol Oncol Clin N Am 2001; 16(5):1065.

132. Johnson BE, Heymach JV (2004). Farnesyl transferase inhibitors for patients with lung cancer. Clin Cancer Res 2004; 10: 4254s.

133. End DW, Smets G, Todd AV, et al. Characterization of the antitumor effects of the selective farnesyl protein transferase inhibitor R115777 in vivo and in vitro. Cancer Res 2001; 61(1):131.

134. Sepp-Lorenzino L, Ma Z, Rands E, Kohl NE, Gibbs JB, Oliff A, Rosen N. A peptidomimetic inhibitor of farnesyl:protein transferase blocks the anchorage-dependent and independent growth of human tumor cell lines. Cancer Res 1995; 55(22):5302.

135. Liu M, Bryant MS, Chen J, et al. Antitumor activity of SCH 66336, an orally bioavailable tricyclic inhibitor of farnesyl protein transferase, in human tumor xenograft models and wap-ras transgenic mice. Cancer Res 1998; 58(21):4947.

136. Nagasu T, Yoshimatsu K, Rowell C, Lewis MD, Garcia AM. Inhibition of human tumor xenograft growth by treatment with the farnesyl transferase inhibitor B956. Cancer Res 1995; 55(22):5310.

137. Britten CD, Rowinsky EK, Soignet S, et al. A phase I and pharmacologic study of the farnesyl protein transferase inhibitor with solid malignancies. Clin Cancer Res 2001; 7(12):3894.

138. Crul M, de Klerk GJ, Swart M, et al. Phase I clinical and pharmacologic study of chronic oral administration of the farnesyl transferase inhibitor R115777 in advanced cancer. J Clin Oncol 2002; 20(11):2726.

139. Zujewski J, Horak ID, Bol CJ, et al. Phase I and pharmacokinetic study of farnesyl protein transferase inhibitor R115777 in advanced cancer. J Clin Oncol 2000; 18(4):927.

140. Adjei AA, Mauer A, Bruzek L, et al. Phase II study of the farnesyl transferase inhibitor R115777 in patients with advanced non-small cell lung cancer. J Clin Oncol 2003; 18(4):927.

141. Evans TL, Fidias P, Skarin A, et al. A Phase II study of the farnesyl-protein transferase inhibitor L-778, 123 as first-line therapy I patients with advanced non-small cell lung cancer (NSCLC). Proc Am Soc Clin Oncol 2002; 2:13.

Management of Cerebral Metastasis in Patients with Non-Small-Cell Lung Cancer

27

Kevin J. Harrington, Konstantinos N. Syrigos and
Christopher M. Nutting

Contents

27.1 Introduction

Cerebral metastasis is a frequent occurrence in patients with non-small-cell lung cancer (NSCLC) and represents a highly significant cause of both morbidity and mortality. Commonly cited rates for cerebral metastases from lung cancer are in the range of 20–40%. Such considerations have guided the current wave of studies that seek to assess the role of prophylactic cranial irradiation for patients with NSCLC [1, 2]. As yet, the potential value of such an approach has not received the same attention that has been given to small-cell lung cancer (SCLC), as reviewed elsewhere in this volume.

A large population-based estimate of the incidence of brain metastases in patients diagnosed with cancer in a large metropolitan district between the years 1973 and 2001 reported that of all cancers, the rate was highest in patients with lung cancer (19.9%) and that this was more than thrice the rate of the next three commonest tumors (melanoma, 6.9%; renal cell cancer,

6.5%; breast cancer, 5.1%). Interestingly, the rates of cerebral metastases from lung cancer were higher in black patients, in females, and in patients aged between 40 and 49 years.

Cerebral metastases from NSCLC can present at any phase of a patient's malignant illness. Patients may experience neurological symptoms as the presenting feature of an occult primary tumor, or may be found to have cerebral metastases during the initial staging investigations (synchronous disease). Cerebral metastasis frequently represents a manifestation of disease relapse (metachronous disease). Bajard et al. [3] have conducted a multivariate analysis of factors predictive of relapse with cerebral metastasis in patients with localized NSCLC. They analyzed the records of 305 patients and showed that factors that were predictive of the development of brain metastases were age (62 years or lower), T4 primary tumor, N2 or N3 nodal disease, and adenocarcinomatous histology.

No matter what the clinical scenario, the development of cerebral metastases represents a life-threatening event, and one that patients seldom survive long-term. Therefore, the aims of treatment are to alleviate the immediate symptoms of raised intracranial pressure and neurological dysfunction and to attempt to secure local control of the disease in the brain to prevent progressive neurological deterioration. A small number of patients should be considered for aggressive local management with the aim of curing the disease, and the others should receive either best supportive care or short-course palliative radiotherapy.

27.2 Therapeutic Options

The available modalities for treatment of cerebral metastases are summarized in Table 27.1. As can be seen, these treatment options range from aggressive therapy with curative intent to short-term best supportive care in patients with very poor prognosis disease. Careful selection of patients for the most appropriate treatment approach is an essential component of the management of cerebral

Table 27.1. Treatment modalities for cerebral metastasis from lung cancer

Surgery
Radiotherapy (RT)
● Whole brain RT
● Stereotactic RT (radiosurgery)
Chemotherapy
Epidermal growth factor receptor inhibitors
Symptom control (best supportive care)

Table 27.2. Selection criteria for surgical management of cerebral metastases from lung cancer

1. Solitary deposit
2. NSCLC
3. Operable lesion in an area with predicted good functional outcome
4. Good performance status
5. Local site controlled or synchronous tumors with no evidence of other systemic metastasis
6. Long disease-free interval (in patients with metachronous disease)

NSCLC Non-small-cell lung cancer

metastases. In general terms, the initial decision should select patients for either palliative or radical treatment. Most patients will be candidates for palliative treatment alone by virtue of the fact that they have multiple lesions, poor performance status, or uncontrolled extracranial disease. However, there are several situations in which the intent is to achieve long-term local control, even with the goal of curing a small minority of cases.

As a means of predicting the utility of palliative radiotherapy, the Radiation Therapy Oncology Group (RTOG) has devised a recursive partitioning analysis (RPA) system to divide patients in to different prognostic groups [4]. This classification is based on the following factors: age, the presence or absence of extracranial metastasis, and the Karnofsky Performance Status (KPS) [5]. RPA class 1 is assigned to those with KPS ≥70%, age less than 65 years, and controlled primary and no extracranial metastasis. RPA class 3 is assigned to those with KPS <70%, and RPA class 2 to all others (i.e., KPS ≥70%, age ≥65 years, uncontrolled primary or evidence of extracranial metastases). This classification has been shown to be a reliable means of predicting outcome following palliative whole-brain radiation therapy (WBRT) in several tumor types including lung and breast cancers and melanoma [5, 6]. Patients in RPA class 1 have a relatively good prognosis and should be seen as candidates for aggressive local management, whereas patients in class 3 have a very poor prognosis and are seldom suitable for anything more than best supportive care. Patients in class 2 have a more variable prognosis and careful consideration is required to select the most appropriate approach to their disease. Lock et al. [7] have also reported that performance status and the number of metastatic sites is a useful predictor of early death and can be used to select poor-prognosis patients for best supportive care.

27.3 Surgical Management of Cerebral Metastases

The potential value of a surgical approach should be considered for all patients who present with cerebral metastases from lung cancer. In the vast majority of patients, this will result in a clear decision against such treatment.

However, it is becoming clear that there are certain situations in which surgical intervention can result in a significant palliation of symptoms, durable local control, and even, on rare occasions, long-term survival [8].

There is no clear-cut agreement on the selection criteria that should be used in deciding whether or not a patient with cerebral metastases from lung cancer should undergo a surgical procedure, but Table 27.2 shows several factors that may be taken in to account. In general terms, surgery should be considered in patients with solitary accessible metastases from NSCLC in whom there is a reasonable expectation that surgical excision will not cause serious functional morbidity. For example, a patient presenting with a lesion in the nondominant cerebral hemisphere may be expected to have a better functional outcome than a patient with a lesion adjacent to the speech area in the dominant cortex. Ideally, patients should present either with an isolated cerebral relapse or with synchronous pulmonary and cerebral disease (but no evidence of other extracranial metastasis). Following surgical resection (or ultrasonic aspiration), most patients would be considered for "adjuvant" radiotherapy, usually to the whole brain (see below). The different clinical situations in which patients may undergo surgical excision are considered in more detail below.

27.3.1 Synchronous Pulmonary and Cerebral Disease

The presence of cerebral metastases at the time of diagnosis of the primary lung cancer is not uncommon, but usually occurs in the setting of widely disseminated disease. In the rare situation in which a patient presents with a primary lung cancer and a synchronous isolated cerebral metastasis, the option of radical treatment should be considered very carefully. If the primary tumor is potentially curable, patients should be evaluated for their suitability for surgical excision of the cerebral metastasis.

Several studies have demonstrated that in this situation, surgery can play an important role. Magilligan et al. [9] reported on 25 years experience in which they treated 41 patients (37 NSCLC, 4 SCLC). In all cases, the primary lung tumor was treated surgically: wedge resection in 4, lobectomy in 23, and pneumonectomy in 14. Following resection of the cerebral disease, 25 patients received postoperative cranial radiotherapy. The survival rates at 1 and 2 years were 55% and 31%, respectively. A further series was reported by Hankins et al. [10], who treated 20 patients (19 NSCLC, 1 carcinoid) over a period of 22 years. The survival rates at 1 and 5 years were 65% and 45%, respectively. Granone et al. [11] reported a group of 30 patients with NSCLC who were treated over a 10-year period. Twenty of the patients had synchronous disease and 10 had metachronous cerebral metastasis. The patterns of survival were significantly better for patients who presented with synchronous disease, with 1- and 2-year survival rates of 95% and 47%, respectively, compared with 50% and 30%, respectively, for patients with metachronous disease. Koutras et al. [12] have reported survival rates of 53% at 1-year and a median survival of 13.5 months in a group of 32 patients with single cerebral metastasis from NSCLC. Thirteen patients developed relapse in the brain, and 6 of these underwent re-operation.

27.3.2 Metachronous Cerebral Metastases

As has been described briefly above, the survival rates for patients who undergo surgical treatment of metachronous cerebral metastasis are less favorable than for those treated for synchronous disease [11]. However, this does not necessarily mean that patients with disease relapse in the brain will not benefit from a more radical approach. Moazami et al. [13] have assessed the factors associated with a better outcome in 91 patients who presented with cerebral metastases as a sign of relapse of stage III NSCLC. The median survival for the whole group of patients was 5.2 months, and the 1- and 2-year survival rates were 22% and 10%, respectively. The factors that were associated with improved survival were isolated cerebral relapse, previous resection of the primary lung tumor, young age, maintained performance status, stage IIIA disease, and aggressive management of the cerebral disease with either resection or radiosurgery. Therefore, it would appear that patients who meet these criteria should be considered for intensive management of the cerebral relapse.

27.4 Palliative WBRT

Patients who are considered unsuitable for surgical resection of cerebral disease are generally considered for palliative WBRT. Patients are treated in a supine position in a simple immobilization device, such as a thermoplastic or Perspex shell. Treatment is delivered using two parallel-opposed lateral fields that aim to treat all of the cerebral tissue above the skull base. This can be accomplished either by simulating the treatment field or as a clinical mark-up, treating all of the tissues above a line joining the mastoid process to the lateral aspect of the supraorbital ridge. Treatment is normally given using a ^{60}Co source or a linear accelerator generating 6–10 MV photons. It is routine practice to give steroid cover during palliative WBRT because of the risk of increasing cerebral edema during this treatment.

Several factors can be considered when judging the efficacy of WBRT, including radiation dose and fractionation, the use of WBRT after surgical resection, and the use of radiosensitizing agents during WBRT. Each of these areas will be reviewed briefly below.

27.4.1 Radiation Fractionation in WBRT

Several studies have sought to define the optimal fractionation schedule for WBRT for cerebral metastases. There have been interesting differences in the emphasis of the research approaches adopted in the USA and in the UK, with the former assessing the potential value of radiation dose escalation and hyperfractionation (delivering more than one fraction per day) and the latter evaluating the effect of shortening the treatment course by delivering a small number of large radiation fractions. Of course, the underlying hypotheses for these studies had different bases: in the USA there was a belief that more aggressive therapy would yield improved survival rates, while in the UK it was felt that studies should focus on achieving the same (dismal) results with the least impact on the patients' quality of life and with minimal outlay of health resources.

The RTOG conducted an initial phase I/II dose-escalation study in which patients received WBRT to a dose of 32 Gy in twice-daily, 1.6-Gy fractions with successive cohorts receiving tumor boosts to achieve total doses of 48, 54.4, 64, and 70.4 Gy [14]. The results of this trial, which are shown in Table 27.3, suggest that there is a benefit to escalating the dose of radiation to the tumor in patients with cerebral metastases. Although there seemed to be additional neurological benefits from increasing the radiation dose from 54.4 to 70.4 Gy, there was no real difference in the 1-year survival rates between these two treatment doses, and so the lower dose was selected for subsequent randomized study. The follow-up randomized phase III study (RTOG 9104) evaluated the effect of twice-daily hyperfractionated radiotherapy to a dose of 54.4 Gy against once-daily standard radiotherapy to a dose of 30 Gy in 10 fractions in a group of 445 patients (65% of whom had lung cancer) [15]. The median survival for each group of patients was 4.5 months, and the 1-year survival rates were not significantly different (16% for the standard arm and 19% for the hyperfractionated arm).

Table 27.3. Survival data from the Radiation Therapy Oncology Group 85-28 trial of dose escalation with hyperfractionated radiotherapy

Dose (Gy)	Median survival (months)	One-year survival (%)	Neurological improvement (%)
48	4.9	20	25
54.4	5.4	33	38
64	7.2	28	50
70.4	8.2	37	63

In the UK, the emphasis has been toward reducing the number of treatment fractions, with the obvious goals of reducing the impact of treatment on the patients' quality of life and limiting the usage of machine time. The Royal College of Radiologist's randomized phase III study of two different fractionation schedules compared the standard arm of 30 Gy in 10 fractions with 12 Gy in 2 fractions in 533 patients, the majority of who had lung cancer [16]. The median survivals for the two groups of patients were statistically significantly different (84 days for 30 Gy in 10 fractions versus 77 days for 12 Gy in 2 fractions), although this is clearly not a result that represents a clinically significant benefit. The incidence of side effects in the two treatment groups was similar: 8% for 30 Gy in 10 fractions versus 12% for 12 Gy in 2 fractions. Interestingly, the majority of centers in the UK currently use neither of the above regimens as their standard of care, rather preferring to use an intermediate schedule of 20 Gy in five fractions over 1 week.

A nonrandomized study has examined the effect of three different fractionation schedules in 125 patients treated with WBRT [17]. Patients received 50 Gy in 25 fractions (21%), 30 Gy in 10 fractions (38%), or 20 Gy in 5 fractions (33%). The 6- and 12-month survival rates were equivalent between the different groups, with no evidence of a benefit from a more extended treatment course.

When viewed together, the results of these various studies suggest that for patients with cerebral metastases and poor prognosis features, the use of an abbreviated fractionation schedule is preferable to a more protracted course of treatment. Therefore, the use of a schedule of 20 Gy in five fractions or 30 Gy in ten fractions should be viewed as standard. However, for patients with poor performance status or in whom a limited number of journeys to the hospital is preferable, a treatment regimen of 12 Gy in two fractions may be justifiable.

27.4.2 Postoperative WBRT Following Resection of Cerebral Metastases

The role of postoperative radiotherapy after resection of brain metastases has not been examined formally in a randomized clinical trial. Smalley et al. [18] reported a series of 85 patients who were treated in a nonrandomized study. Thirty-four patients received postoperative radiotherapy and 51 patients were entered on to an observation policy. The median survivals of the two treatment groups were 21 months and 11.5 months, respectively. At the time of analysis, 29% of patients treated with surgery and postoperative radiotherapy were free of disease, compared with 4% of patients in the observation policy. In multivariate analysis, the delivery of WBRT showed the strongest association with local control in the brain ($p < 0.0001$).

Of course, in this setting it is difficult to attribute the beneficial effect of the postoperative WBRT either to its activity in improving local control of an incompletely excised brain metastasis or its effect against other subclinical deposits in the brain. Nonetheless, in most patients who undergo excision of cerebral metastases from NSCLC, postoperative WBRT would be considered as routine practice in most centers.

27.4.3 WBRT and Radiosensitizing Agents

An interesting approach to enhancing the radiation response of cerebral metastases is the use of the radiosensitizing agents. One such agent that has received recent attention is motexafin gadolinium (gadolinium III texaphyrin). This agent has been shown to be selectively cytotoxic in hematological malignancies by localizing in areas of metabolic activity, where it inhibits cellular respiration. This agent has been subjected to a randomized phase III trial in patients with cerebral metastases from NSCLC (251 patients), breast (75 patients), and other cancers (75 patients) [19, 20]. Patients received WBRT to a dose of 30 Gy in ten fractions either with or without motexafin gadolinium. There was no significant difference in median survival rates (5.2 months for WBRT plus motexafin gadolinium versus 4.9 months for WBRT alone) for the whole group of patients, although there was a significant improvement in time to neurological progression in the patients with cerebral metastasis from lung cancer. In a subsequent study, patient outcome was measured in terms of neurocognitive function, and this demonstrated a trend toward improved memory and executive function in patients with NSCLC (but not the other tumor types) who received motexafin gadolinium [20].

Recently, a randomized phase III trial has evaluated the potential benefit of adding carboplatin chemotherapy to WBRT in patients with cerebral metastases from

NSCLC [21. In what was a very small study, 42 patients received WBRT to a dose of 20 Gy in 5 fractions either with or without concomitant carboplatin at a dose of 70 mg/m^2 with each of the radiotherapy fractions. There was no difference in the median survivals of the two treatment arms, although the concomitant chemotherapy group had a poorer outcome. Maraveyas et al. [22] have recently reported a phase I study of gemcitabine concomitant with WBRT of 30 Gy in ten fractions. These authors have defined a dose of gemcitabine for phase II study and these data will be awaited with interest. Similarly, further studies with agents such as temozolomide may yield interesting data.

27.5 Radiosurgery

An alternative or adjunctive approach to WBRT is the delivery of localized radical radiotherapy to tumor deposits. This approach has been called radiosurgery in an attempt to highlight the precise ablative nature of this treatment. This field of treatment has certainly received a great deal of attention in recent years, not least because it represents the development of powerful techniques in the delivery of high-precision radiation therapy. However, its use is not yet strongly supported by data from randomized clinical trials and conducting these studies should be seen as a major goal of trials in patients with cerebral metastases in the next decade.

Radiosurgery can be performed by using two main techniques: stereotactic radiotherapy using a linear accelerator, and the gamma knife. In the former approach, linear-accelerator-based conformal radiotherapy is used, and in the latter, multiple ^{60}Co sources are used to produce a highly focused radiation beam in the targeted area. Many (but not all) nonrandomized studies involving radiosurgery appear to demonstrate a potential advantage in terms of securing local control in the brain. Nieder et al. [23] reported a series of 25 patients with 31 lesions in the brain between them. Fifteen of the patients were suffering from NSCLC. The patients received WBRT to a dose of 30 Gy in ten fractions and then received a stereotactic radiosurgery boost to a dose of 10 Gy at the isocenter, with the tumor volume enclosed by the 90% isodose. The median survival of this group of patients was only 2.3 months, with 10 patients dying of progressive brain metastases and 13 patients dying from extracranial disease progression. In a further study, 29 patients received WBRT (30–40 Gy) combined with fractionated stereotactic radiosurgery (12–40 Gy) [24]. The actuarial 1- and 2-year local control rates were 78% and 71%, respectively. The median survival for the group of patients was 13 months. Noel et al. [25] reported their experience of treating 145 metastases in 92 patients: 34 patients were treated with stereotactic radiosurgery alone, 36 with radiosurgery for re-

current disease after previous WBRT, and 22 for with radiosurgery in association with WBRT. The median survival for all 92 patients was 9 months, but the number of patients in each group was not sufficient to allow conclusions to be drawn about the differences between the three treatment approaches. However, analysis of prognostic factors revealed that controlled extracranial disease, good performance status, and a low number of cerebral metastases were associated with a better outcome.

The use of gamma knife radiosurgery has been reported in a large series (273 patients with 627 NSCLC metastases) spanning a period of 14 years [26]. There was evidence of tumor reduction or stabilization in 84% of cases. The median survival time was 15 months from the time of diagnosis of cerebral metastasis. Factors predictive of survival were female gender, performance status, adenocarcinomatous histology, active systemic disease, and interval between lung cancer diagnosis and the development of brain disease. Prior surgical resection or WBRT were not associated with improved patient outcome. In another large series (458 patients, 1305 lesions), 21% of the patients had lung cancer. This report showed that performance status, activity of systemic disease, histology, and volume of intracranial disease were factors that influenced survival.

Flannery et al. [27] reported their experience of gamma knife radiosurgery in a group of 72 patients with solitary cerebral metastasis from NSCLC in the absence of extracranial disease. Patients were treated to a median dose of 18 Gy, with 45 patients receiving additional WBRT. The median survival for the whole group was 15.7 months and the 5-year actuarial survival was 10%. Interestingly, patients who were treated for metachronous tumors had a significantly better survival (33 months versus 9 months) than those treated for synchronous tumors (in contrast to the data on surgical excision described above). This translated in to 5-year actuarial survival rates of 13.2% and 8.1%, respectively. In this series of patients, there was no additional benefit from the use of additional WBRT. Jawahar et al. [28] treated 44 patients with the Leksell gamma knife: 50% of patients had a single metastasis and the rest had between 2 and 6 deposits. Local control of disease in the brain was achieved in 32 patients, and only 10 patients were considered to have died from local recurrence in the brain or the development of new cerebral metastases. The median duration of overall survival was 7 months, with a median time of freedom from new brain metastases of 17 months. Varlotto et al. [29] have analyzed the results of gamma knife radiosurgery in 208 lesions in 137 patients, 37% of whom had NSCLC: 96 patients received WBRT, although 27 of these were treated in the context of failure after WBRT. At 1 and 5 years follow-up, the local tumor control rates were 90% and 63%, respectively, and the complication rates were 3% and 11%, respectively. Factors that were shown to be associated with loss of local control were increased tumor volume, failure to deliver WBRT, and extensive cerebral edema. The incidence of posttreatment complications was directly related to the volume of brain tissue irradiated.

Jawahar et al. [30] have attempted to determine the potential benefit of delivering gamma knife radiosurgery and WBRT. In their series of 61 patients (27 solitary tumors, 34 multiple tumors) with 103 lesions, 43 patients were treated with only radiosurgery and 18 had received prior WBRT. The additional use of WBRT was not associated with improved outcome.

When viewed in their entirety, these data suggest that radiosurgery represents a powerful technique for the treatment of cerebral metastases; it certainly delivers high rates of local control in the individual treated lesions. However, for many of the series that have been reported in the literature, the median survival rates are similar to those reported in trials of palliative WBRT and this reflects the fact that many patients with metastatic lung cancer will succumb to further extracranial or intracranial disease.

Andrews et al. [31] have recently published data from a phase III randomized trial of WBRT with or without stereotactic radiosurgery boost in patients with between one and three brain metastases. Approximately two-thirds of the patients in the study had lung cancer. Patients were eligible for inclusion if the largest lesion was no greater than 4 cm in diameter and, in the case of multiple brain metastases, if the other lesion(s) were no greater than 3 cm in diameter. Patients were stratified for the study on the basis of the number of cerebral metastases and the status of their extracranial disease. A total of 331 patients were analyzed (164 WBRT alone, 167 WBRT plus stereotactic boost). Analysis of overall survival for the entire group showed no significant difference between the two groups (6.5 months for WBRT plus boost versus 5.7 months for WBRT). The univariate analysis demonstrated a median survival advantage (6.5 months versus 4.9 months) in patients with single brain metastases treated with WBRT plus stereotactic boost, but this effect was absent in multivariate analysis. There was also a greater likelihood of stable or improved performance status at 6 months in those patients who received the boost. In the multivariate analysis, only RTOG RPA class 1 and a lung primary tumor were associated with a favorable outcome, with treatment modality failing to reach statistical significance. Interestingly, there was absolutely no difference between outcomes for patients treated with linear-accelerator-based stereotaxy and gamma knife. Further research in this area must focus on randomized trials to assess the effect of treatment parameters (dose, number of lesions, tumor volume), prognostic factors and the integration of radiosurgery alongside palliative WBRT.

27.6 Cytotoxic Chemotherapy for Cerebral Metastases

The use of chemotherapy as a therapeutic option for patients with cerebral metastases from lung cancer has been rather limited because of a presumed lack of efficacy due to the presence of the blood-brain barrier [32]. However, it is likely that in the region of a metastatic deposit the blood-brain barrier is nonfunctional, and this leakiness may be further augmented by prior radiotherapy. As a result, there is reason to believe that cerebral metastases may respond to conventional cytotoxic drugs. Several recent small trials have demonstrated the efficacy of chemotherapy in the context of both NSCLC and SCLC [33–35]. It is likely that this will represent an area of increased interest in the coming years and it is hoped that randomized trials will address appropriate questions in the near future.

27.7 Epidermal Growth Factor Receptor Inhibitors

Epidermal growth factor receptor (EGFR) is overexpressed in many cancers including lung cancer [36, 37], where it has been shown to correlate with an aggressive course and, when activated, with poor prognosis. Higher levels of EGFR expression are found in more advanced disease and in the squamous cell carcinoma subtype (reviewed in [38]). Various approaches to EGFR inhibition have confirmed antiproliferative effects and validated it as a target for cancer therapeutics. Several studies have demonstrated that this class of drugs may be beneficial in patients with lung cancer (reviewed by Rogers et al. [38]). However, the initial enthusiasm for this class of drugs has been tempered by the results of randomized trials in patients with NSCLC (reviewed in [37]). Nonetheless, several studies have suggested that EGFR tyrosine kinase inhibitors (EGFR-TKIs) have activity against brain metastases from NSCLC.

Ceresoli et al. [39] reported the results of treating 41 consecutive patients with cerebral metastases from NSCLC with the EGFR-TKI gefitinib (ZD1839, Iressa) at a dose of 250 mg/day by mouth. The majority of patients had been treated previously: 37 patients had received prior chemotherapy and 18 patients had received WBRT. A partial response was observed in four patients (10%) and stable disease in 7 (17%). The median duration of the partial response was 13.5 months, although the median progression-free survival for all 41 patients was only 3 months. Previous WBRT and adenocarcinoma histological subtype were predictors of a better outcome. Hotta et al. [40] reported the results of gefitinib in a group of 57 Japanese patients with advanced

NSCLC, 14 of who had cerebral metastases. Of the patients with cerebral metastases, six had an objective response to gefitinib (one complete response, five partial responses) and eight had stable disease. It is of interest that six of the patients who had objective responses to the disease in the brain also had a response in extracranial disease. For the entire group of 57 patients, the response rate to gefitinib was only 27%. Female gender, age of 70 years or more, and the presence of cerebral metastases were shown to predict a response to gefitinib on multivariate analysis. The median duration of response and median survival were 7.7 months and 9.1 months, respectively. A further study from Taiwan has reported on the outcome of 76 patients with cerebral metastases from NSCLC who were treated with single-agent gefitinib. The objective response rate was 33% in the 57 patients with measurable disease, and for all patients the disease control rate was 63%. The median progression-free survival and overall survival rates were 5 months and 9.9 months, respectively.

On the basis of these studies, it would appear that the EGFR-TKIs represent an interesting class of drugs for further study in patients with brain metastasis from NSCLC. These drugs are generally well tolerated, with common side effects including folliculitic skin rash, diarrhoea, and lethargy. A rare side effect of this treatment is the occurrence of an interstitial lung disease, which affects < 1% of patients.

Key Points

- Cerebral metastasis is a frequent occurrence in patients with non-small-cell lung cancer (NSCLC) and represents a highly significant cause of both morbidity and mortality.
- The available modalities for the treatment of cerebral metastases range from aggressive therapy with curative intent to short-term best supportive care in patients with very poor prognosis disease.
- Surgery, whole-brain radiation therapy, and radiosurgery may all have a role in the treatment of NSCLC cerebral metastases.
- Careful selection of patients for the most appropriate treatment approach is essential. The Radiation Therapy Oncology Group recursive partitioning analysis classification, which is based on age, the presence or absence of extracranial disease, and the Karnofsky performance status, functions as a useful means of dividing patients in to groups with different possible outcomes.
- Most patients will be candidates for palliative treatment alone by virtue of the fact that they have multiple lesions, poor performance status, or uncontrolled extracranial disease. However, there are several situations in which the intent is to achieve long-term local control, even with the goal of curing a small minority of cases.

27.8　Conclusions

The development of cerebral metastases represents a life-threatening condition in patients with NSCLC. The approach to management should be guided initially by consideration of the relevant prognostic factors. The RTOG RPA classification, which is based on age, the presence or absence of extracranial disease, and the Karnofsky performance status, functions as a useful means of dividing patients into groups with different outcomes. The RPA can be used to select patients for either aggressive management with potentially curative intent (for patients in RPA class 1), more palliative treatment (RPA class 2), or best supportive care (RPA class 3). Surgery, WBRT and radiosurgery may all have a role in treatment. There is a pressing need for appropriately controlled randomized trials to define more accurately the indications for each of these modalities.

References

1. Gore E, Choy H. Non-small cell lung cancer and central nervous system metastases: should we be using prophylactic cranial irradiation? Semin Radiat Oncol 2004; 14:292.
2. Lester JF, Macbeth FR, Coles B. Prophylactic cranial irradiation for preventing brain metastases in patients undergoing radical treatment for non-small-cell lung cancer. Cochrane Database Syst Rev 2005; (2):CD005221.
3. Bajard A, Westeel V, Dubiez A, et al. Multivariate analysis of factors predictive of brain metastases in localized non-small cell lung carcinoma. Lung Cancer 2004; 45:317.
4. Gaspar L, Scott C, Rotman M, et al. Recursive partitioning analysis (RPA) of prognostic factors in three Radiation Therapy Oncology Group (RTOG) brain metastases trials. Int J Radiat Oncol Biol Phys 1997; 37:745.
5. Gaspar LE, Scott C, Murray K, Curran W. Validation of the RTOG recursive partitioning analysis (RPA) classification for brain metastases. Int J Radiat Oncol Biol Phys 2000; 47:1001.
6. Morris SL, Low SH, A'Hern RP, Eisen TG, Gore ME, Nutting CM, Harrington KJ. A prognostic index that predicts outcome following palliative whole brain radiotherapy for patients with metastatic malignant melanoma. Br. J. Cancer 2004; 91:829.
7. Lock M, Chow E, Pond GR, et al. Prognostic factors in brain metastases: can we determine patients who do not benefit from whole-brain radiotherapy? Clin Oncol (R Coll Radiol) 2004; 16:332.

8. Korinth MC, Delonge C, Hutter BO, Gilsbach JM. Prognostic factors for patients with microsurgically resected brain metastases. Onkologie 2002; 25:420.

9. Magilligan DJ Jr, Duvernoy C, Malik G, Lewis JW Jr, Knighton R, Ausman JI. Surgical approach to lung cancer with solitary cerebral metastasis: twenty-five years' experience Ann Thorac Surg 1986; 42:360.

10. Hankins JR, Miller JE, Salcman M, et al. Surgical management of lung cancer with solitary cerebral metastasis. Ann Thorac Surg 1988; 46:24.

11. Granone P, Margaritora S, D'Andrilli A, Cesario A, Kawamukai K, Meacci E. Non-small cell lung cancer with single brain metastasis: the role of surgical treatment. Eur J Cardiothorac Surg 2001; 20:361.

12. Koutras AK, Marangos M, Kourelis T, et al. Surgical management of cerebral metastases from non-small cell lung cancer. Tumori 2003; 89:292.

13. Moazami N, Rice TW, Rybicki LA, et al. Stage III non-small cell lung cancer and metachronous brain metastases. J Thorac Cardiovasc Surg 2002; 124:113.

14. Epstein BE, Scott CB, Sause WT, et al. Improved survival duration in patients with unresected solitary brain metastasis using accelerated hyperfractionated radiation therapy at total doses of 54.4 gray and greater. Results of Radiation Therapy Oncology Group 85-28. Cancer 1993; 71:1362.

15. Murray KJ, Scott C, Greenberg HM, et al. A randomized phase III study of accelerated hyperfractionation versus standard in patients with unresected brain metastases: a report of the Radiation Therapy Oncology Group (RTOG) 9104. Int J Radiat Oncol Biol Phys 1997; 39:571.

16. Priestman TJ, Dunn J, Brada M, Rampling R, Baker PG. Final results of the Royal College of Radiologists' trial comparing two different radiotherapy schedules in the treatment of cerebral metastases. Clin Oncol (R Coll Radiol) 1996; 8:308.

17. Portaluri M, Bambace S, Giuliano G, et al. Fractionations in radiotherapy of brain metastases. Tumori 2004; 90:80.

18. Smalley SR, Schray MF, Laws ER Jr, O'Fallon JR. Adjuvant radiation therapy after surgical resection of solitary brain metastasis: association with pattern of failure and survival. Int J Radiat Oncol Biol Phys 1987; 13:1611.

19. Mehta MP, Rodrigus P, Terhaard CH, et al. Survival and neurologic outcomes in a randomized trial of motexafin gadolinium and whole-brain radiation therapy in brain metastases. J Clin Oncol 2003; 21:2529.

20. Meyers CA, Smith JA, Bezjak A, et al. Neurocognitive function and progression in patients with brain metastases treated with whole-brain radiation and motexafin gadolinium: results of a randomized phase III trial. J Clin Oncol 2004; 22:157.

21. Guerrieri M, Wong K, Ryan G, Millward M, Quong G, Ball DL. A randomised phase III study of palliative radiation with concomitant carboplatin for brain metastases from non-small cell carcinoma of the lung. Lung Cancer 2004; 46:107.

22. Maraveyas A, Sgouros J, Upadhyay S, et al. Gemcitabine twice weekly as a radiosensitiser for the treatment of brain metastases in patients with carcinoma: a phase I study. Br J Cancer 2005; 92:815.

23. Nieder C, Nestle U, Walter K, Niewald M, Schnabel K. Dose-response relationships for radiotherapy of brain metastases: role of intermediate-dose stereotactic radiosurgery plus whole-brain radiotherapy. Am J Clin Oncol 2000; 23:584.

24. Kim HJ, Hong S, Kim S, et al. Efficacy of whole brain radiotherapy combined with fractionated stereotactic radiotherapy in metastatic brain tumors, and prognostic factors. Radiat Med 2003; 21:155.

25. Noel G, Medioni J, Valery CA, et al. Three irradiation treatment options including radiosurgery for brain metastases from primary lung cancer. Lung Cancer 2003; 41:333.

26. Sheehan JP, Sun MH, Kondziolka D, Flickinger J, Lunsford LD. Radiosurgery for non-small cell lung carcinoma metastatic to the brain: long-term outcomes and prognostic factors influencing patient survival time and local tumor control. J Neurosurg 2002; 97:1276.

27. Flannery TW, Suntharalingam M, Kwok Y, et al. Gamma knife stereotactic radiosurgery for synchronous versus metachronous solitary brain metastases from non-small cell lung cancer. Lung Cancer 2003; 42:327.

28. Jawahar A, Matthew RE, Minagar A, et al. Gamma knife surgery in the management of brain metastases from lung carcinoma: a retrospective analysis of survival, local tumor control, and freedom from new brain metastasis. J Neurosurg 2004; 100:842.

29. Varlotto JM, Flickinger JC, Niranjan A, Bhatnagar AK, Kondziolka D, Lunsford LD. Analysis of tumor control and toxicity in patients who have survived at least one year after radiosurgery for brain metastases. Int J Radiat Oncol Biol Phys 2003; 57:452.

30. Jawahar A, Willis BK, Smith DR, Ampil F, Datta R, Nanda A. Gamma knife radiosurgery for brain metastases: do patients benefit from adjuvant external-beam radiotherapy? An 18-month comparative analysis. Stereotact Funct Neurosurg 2002; 79:262.

31. Andrews DW, Scott CB, Sperduto PW, et al. Whole brain radiation therapy with or without stereotactic radiosurgery boost for patients with one to three brain metastases: phase III results of the RTOG 9508 randomised trial. Lancet 2004; 363:1665.

32. Schuette W. Treatment of brain metastases from lung cancer: chemotherapy. Lung cancer 2004; 45 (suppl 2):S253.

33. Christodoulou C, Bafaloukos D, Linardou H, et al. Temozolomide (TMZ) combined with cisplatin (CDDP) in patients with brain metastases from solid tumours: a Hellenic Co-operative Oncology Group (HeCOG) phase II study. J Neurooncol 2005; 71:61.

34. Chou R, Chen A, Lau D. Complete response of brain metastases to irinotecan-based chemotherapy. J Clin Neurosci 2005; 12:242.

35. Kim DY, Lee KW, Yun T, et al. Efficacy of platinum-based chemotherapy after cranial radiation in patients with brain metastasis from non-small cell lung cancer. Oncol Rep 2005; 14:207.

36. Salomon DS, Brandt R, Ciardiello F, Normanno N. Epidermal growth factor-related peptides and their receptors in human malignancies. Crit Rev Oncol Hematol 1995; 19:183.

37. El-Rayes BF, LoRusso PM. Targeting the epidermal growth factor receptor. Br J Cancer 2004; 91:418.

38. Rogers SJ, Harrington KJ, Eccles SA, Nutting CM. Combination epidermal growth factor receptor inhibition and radical radiotherapy for non-small cell lung cancer. Exp Rev Anticancer Ther 2004; 4:569.

39. Ceresoli GL, Cappuzzo F, Gregorc V, Bartolini S, Crino L, Villa E. Gefitinib in patients with brain metastases from non-small-cell lung cancer: a prospective trial. Ann Oncol 2004; 15:1042.

40. Hotta K, Kiura K, Ueoka H, et al. Effect of gefitinib ('Iressa', ZD1839) on brain metastases in patients with advanced non-small-cell lung cancer. Lung Cancer 2004; 46:255.

Management of Non-Small-Cell Lung Cancer in the Elderly

28

Eleni Karapanagiotou, Kevin J. Harrington and
Konstantinos N. Syrigos

Contents

28.1 Introduction

In Western societies, the percentage of elderly people is increasing within the population as a result of increased average lifespan. Consistently, the question remains, what is the cut-off point for the definition of "elderly". Until recently, the border between middle age and old age was at 65 years of age. This borderline is no longer considered valid. The National Institute on Aging and the National Institutes of Health have redefined the term "elderly" as the age group greater or equal to 65 years, which cover three subcategories, namely: the "young old" for those aged between 65 and 74 years, the "older old" for those aged 75 years, and the "oldest old" for subjects aged 85 years old [1, 2]. Peterman et al. offered a different viewpoint to this debate through the definition for the geriatric oncology patient: "old is a patient when his health status begins to interfere with oncological decision-making guidelines" [3]. Conclusively, the biological age of each patient is the most important parameter and should be defined individually, based on comorbidities and performance status.

The definition of "elderly" is of clinical importance in oncology due to the fact that the median age of presentation of all cancers is 69 years old in males and 67 years old in females. Sixty percent of all cancers and 66% of all cancer deaths occur over the age of 65 years

[3–5]. These data hold true for lung cancer epidemiology, with more than half of the patients being over the age of 65 years; over 30% are over 70 years old at the time of diagnosis. In the UK, the peak incidence of lung cancer is between 75 and 80 years old [6]. Furthermore, two-thirds of all patients who die of lung cancer are older than 65 years old. Four out of five lung carcinoma-related deaths occur in patients over or at the age of 60 years, while this proportion changes to one out of five for subjects older than 80 years [1, 7, 8]. Bearing this statistical analysis in mind, there is no excuse for not treating the older patient.

The elderly group is characterized by age-specific problems such as depression, alterations of mental status, reduced nutritional status, and absence of social support, which interfere with the diagnosis and treatment of their cancer. Depression is a major obstacle in lung cancer as it can lead both the patient and the physician to underestimate the symptoms. Cognitive disorders interfere with decision making to seek medical help and accept treatment. Loss of weight is often attributed to social conditions rather than to cancer cachexia. Moreover, elderly patients who are diagnosed with lung cancer show a high symptomatic burden expressed mainly by fatigue and dyspnea, along with the increased prevalence of comorbidities associated with long-term smoking. Cardiovascular disease, chronic obstructive pulmonary disease (COPD), and other malignancies are present in 23%, 22%, and 15%, respectively, in such patients [9]. Moreover, combinations of these comorbidities are often present. A review study of 966 patients with lung cancer at the median age of 70 years old showed that COPD was present with cardiac disease in 7.6% and cerebrovascular disease in 26.3%, each correlating adversely with survival. Yet, the most intriguing point of this study was the fact that more than 70% of the subjects had a performance status of 0–1 according to the Eastern Cooperative Oncology Group (ECOG) [10, 11].

Most physicians are doubtful as to the potential benefits of lung cancer treatment based solely on age in elderly patients. Surgery and chemotherapy options in such patients are limited. Patients younger than 65 years receive surgery or chemotherapy for non-small-cell lung cancer (NSCLC) in a proportion of 18% and 21%, respectively, compared to patients older than 75 years which receive the same treatment options in a percentage of 2.1% and 0%, respectively [6].

28.2 Diagnosis of Lung Cancer

Histological tumor confirmation and accurate staging are needed before treatment initiation. The elderly obtain lower histological confirmation rates, less accurate staging, and less definitive treatments [6, 9, 12]. The histological type of the tumor can be obtained by fiber optic bronchoscopy, computer tomography (CT)-guided biopsy, and other less invasive techniques. Flexible bronchoscopy is recommended by the British Thoracic Society for diagnostic procedures in the elderly. Age is not a restraining factor for the application of this technique as long as there is no marked ventilatory impairment. Morbidity and mortality due to this procedure are extremely low in every age group [13, 14].

Image-guided transthoracic fine-needle biopsy is an alternative to flexible bronchoscopy, especially for peripheral pulmonary lesions or mediastinal tumors. In a prospective study, which included 500 subjects with a maximum age of 94 years, 60% had emphysema with varying severity. In general, there was a good procedural tolerance with no remarkable complications. Similar findings were noted in another retrospective analysis of patients aged 70–90 years with a suspicion of lung malignancy who underwent a transthoracic needle biopsy. The safety and procedural tolerance were similar to those reported for younger subjects [15, 16].

Besides the histological confirmation of the tumor, an accurate staging should be performed in these elderly lung cancer patients in order to initiate appropriate accurate therapeutic management. CT and ^{18}fluoro-deoxyglucose-positron emission tomography (PET) should be used for this purpose. PET scans detect distant metastasis in 7.5% and 24% of patients staged as I and III confirmed by CT scan evaluation, respectively [17]. However, PET, in comparison to CT, downstages 10% of the patients and upstages 33% of them. Patients who have received a complete and accurate evaluation follow different therapeutic approaches, such as surgery alone or surgery plus chemotherapy or irradiation.

28.3 Surgery for the Lung Cancer Patient

Surgery offers the best potential for a cure for early stage NSCLC, provided that it can be performed at an acceptable risk. Given the fact that elderly patients present with localized disease and a lower rate of metastatic disease compared to younger patients, the perspective of radical surgery should be seriously considered [18]. Two or three decades ago, age was an inhibiting factor for surgery. A questionnaire-based study of 1,652 lung cancer patients with the goal of evaluating treatment management and 6-month survival rates among 3 age groups (under 65 years, 65–74 years, and over 75 years), has demonstrated that 37% of the patients under 65 years underwent surgical resection compared to only 15% of the patients over 75 years. Similarly, the survival was longer for younger patients [2]. During the last decade, improvements in anesthetic and operative techniques in combination with the introduction of minimally invasive chest surgery, as well as the accumulated knowledge about risk factors help change the conventional attitude. Patients with palliative and nonsurgically resolved, early stage lung cancer have an average life expectancy of only 1.5 years. The average subject in the 9th decade of life has a 50% chance of living another 5–9 years. This proves that surgical interventions should be considered very seriously for every patient [19]. Generally speaking, an elderly patient who has undergone detailed preoperative evaluation including spirometry, diffusion capacity for carbon monoxide, arterial blood gasometry, exercise tolerance tests, and, if necessary, a pulmonary ventilation/perfusion test, as well as a full cardiovascular evaluation, should be safe to undergo lung surgery [20].

Moreover, a detailed assessment of comorbidities is extremely important in the subject's preoperative evaluation. In one study, 451 patients with stage I NSCLC with mild, moderate, and severe comorbidities who underwent complete resections were evaluated for postoperative recovery and long-term survival. The relative risk of death in relation to the comorbidities was 1.44, 2.28, and 1.94, respectively [21]. Right pneumonectomy, in the presence of ischemic heart disease, is associated with a high mortality rate according to one study [22]. On the contrary, comorbidities that are often are seen in the elderly, such as diabetes, hypertension, peripheral vascular disease, and cerebrovascular disease, bear no correlation to mortality [22].

Regarding different types of surgical procedures, the most frequently performed, by far, is lobectomy, although the percentage of bilobectomies and pneumonectomies performed is also increasing among the elderly. New surgical procedures have been introduced mainly for elderly patients who cannot tolerate a lobectomy. The wedge resection, a wide local resection of the primary malignancy, represents an alternative to lobectomy, and the same applies to segmentectomy, a formal anatomical resection of the building block of a lobe. Although smaller resections are associated with better lung function, they present higher percentage of local recurrence [23, 24].

Based on published data of the surgery results of octogenarians, long-term survival of these patients treated with various surgical procedures is not influenced by age. The 5-year survival varies from 16 to 55%. In addition, the mortality from pneumonectomy in the elderly is falling. A series of 385 elderly patients has been examined over the years and has showed that the mortality rate has fallen from 11.1% in 1971–82 to 2.6% in 1983–94 [25]. Lobectomy is generally better tolerated than pneumonectomy in this age group (Table 28.1) [26–32]. Moreover, some of the largest studies, which include patients over 70 years of age who had undergone surgery for NSCLC, presented 5-year survival rates ranging between 27 and 40.1% (Table 28.2) [33–37].

When surgical procedures (lobectomy and pneumonectomy) were applied to the elderly and compared to younger patients, no significant differences regarding the 5-year survival rate were observed. It should be noted that if the deaths from those who did not die from recurrence were ignored, the survival rates for the two groups became similar (Table 28.3) [38–41]. The previous results show that 5-year survival rates are really satisfactory in the elderly. One issue regarding surgical approaches is perioperative mortality. A retrospective analysis of elderly people showed a nonsignificant difference in operative mortality for patients aged < 69 years, 70–79 years, and > 80 years, with mortality rates of 1.6%, 4.2%, and 2.8, respectively. On the contrary, some existing reviews support that patients over the age of 65 years, present with an increased morbidity and mortality as well as a shorter overall survival compared to younger patients [42, 43]. However, multivariate analysis has revealed that age is not important for long-term survival [36, 37, 44].

In their guidelines, the British Thoracic Society recommends surgery for clinical stages I and II in patients older than 70 years, after a careful assessment of comorbidities. Age should be a factor in deciding suitability for pneumonectomy. For example, age over 80 years, is not a contraindication to lobectomy or wedge resection for clinical stage I [45].

Recently, an attractive surgical procedure, video-assisted thoracoscopic surgery (VATS), has been introduced. Avoiding open thoracotomy and impairment of the ipsilateral respiratory muscles, VATS represents the preferred operation for small and peripheral nodules in elderly patients with high operative risk. Retrospective analysis of VATS lobectomy for stage I–III NSCLC showed 3- and 4-year survival rates to be 90% and 70%, respectively, and shorter or equivalent hospital days to thoracotomy [46, 47, 48].

An alternative for frail, elderly patients is radiofrequency ablation. Radiofrequency ablation entails the percutaneous insertion of an internally cooled radiofrequency electrode under CT guidance, followed by passing of an alternating current through the electrode causing heat and coagulation necrosis. It is a procedure with manageable side effects but with a high rate of recurrence.

Table 28.1. Comparison of 5-year survival rates of octogenarians after surgery

Reference	Number of patients	Five-year survival (%)
Shirakusa et al. 1989 [26]	33	55
Naunheim et al. 1991 [27]	35	26
Osaki et al. 1994 [28]	33	32
Riquet et al. 1994 [29]	11	16
Harvey et al. 1995 [30]	17	42
Pagni et al. 1997 [31]	54	43
Hanagiri et al. 1999 [32]	18	42.6

Table 28.2. Largest studies on 5-year survival rates of elderly patients following surgery

Reference	Number of patients	Age (years)	Five-year survival (%)
Breyer et al. 1981 [33]	150	>70	27
Gebitekin et al. 1993 [34]	145	70	30
Massard et al. 1996 [35]	210	70	32.9
Thomas et al. 1998 [36]	500	70	34
Oliaro et al. 1999 [37]	258	70	40.1

Table 28.3. Comparison of 5-year survival rates of the elderly and nonelderly following surgery

Reference	Number of patients	Age (years)	Five-year survival (%)
Sherman and Guidot 1987 [38]	64	>70	35.9
	75	<70	47.6
Ishida et al. 1990 [39]	185	70	48
	472	<70	41
Morandi et al. 1997 [40]	85	70	28
	130	<70	35
Kamiyoshohara et al. 2000 [41]	37	70	35.1
	123	<70	50.8

28.4 Radiation Therapy for Early and Advanced-Stage NSCLC

Although surgery for early stage NSCLC treatment has gained ground even in octogenarians, a remarkable percentage of elderly subjects remain unsuitable for such an approach due to the presence of comorbidities or simply personal refusal. Radical radiotherapy represents an alternative for them, although there are no prospective randomized studies evaluating the efficacy of radiotherapy versus surgery or radiotherapy in the elderly in comparison with younger patients. In addition, the published data are based on different treatment techniques and different radiation doses. However, a large retrospective review, which included 347 patients with median age of 70 years and stage I NSCLC treated with a dose of 50 Gy in 20 fractions over 4 weeks, showed promising results for the elderly population. The 5-year survival rate was 34% for patients older than 70 years and 22% for patients younger than 70 years. The median survival was 26 months for the older age group and 22 months for younger patients [49]. Similarly, in the Noordijk et al. study, 50 patients with a mean age of 74 years were irradiated with curative intent for NSCLC staged at T1 or T2 and N0M0. The results showed a median survival of 27 months with 2- and 5-year survival rates of 56% and 16%, respectively. This was compared favorably to the results obtained from a group of 86 patients aged >70 years treated with surgery for the same stage disease in the same hospital [50]. Moreover, it is known that the toxicity of radiation therapy, which consists mainly of interstitial pneumonitis and esophagitis, is not greater in elderly patients than in younger patients [49, 51, 52]. There is no excuse for physicians to not treat early stage NSCLC with curative intent.

Radiation therapy also plays an important role, not only in early stage lung cancer, but also in advanced-stage lung cancer, as a palliative therapy. However, it is generally accepted that the optimal time to begin radiotherapy is before symptoms develop. A systematic review showed that radical radiotherapy offers better survival in comparison to palliative radiotherapy, which offers only symptomatic alleviation [53]. Clinically important are the results of a prospective analysis showing that pain, hemoptysis, and anorexia were largely controlled by radiotherapy. Contrary to that, cough, fatigue, and dyspnea relief were not obtained [54].

Until recently, several results have been published referring to the impact of radiotherapy on the elderly patients. Lonardi et al. published the results of a group of 48 patients, aged 75 years and over, with stage IIIA–B symptomatic NSCLC who received radiation therapy at a median dose of 50 Gy. Overall survival was 48% at 6 months, 23% at 12 months, and 10% at 24 months with a median survival of 5 months. Toxicity was very mild and the management of symptoms satisfactory. These results confirmed that radiation therapy might be safely delivered to patients regardless of their age [55]. Similar results were obtained in a study by Hayakawa et al. They gave radiation therapy at a dose of 60 Gy or higher in 97 patients older than 75 years with inoperable or unresectable NSCLC and compared them to 206 patients younger than 75 years who received the same treatment. There were no statistically significant differences regarding survival rates or toxicity between the two age groups [50]. The same conclusion that age does not represent an inhibiting factor for radiotherapy in patients treated for bronchogenic carcinoma was obtained by Newaishy et al. [56]. In that study, 277 patients with histologically confirmed bronchogenic carcinoma were

included. Finally, Wurschmidt, basing his opinion on a pool of 427 patients with unresectable NSCLC, stated that after univariate and multivariate analysis, indeed age does not influence survival for stage I, II, and III NSCLC [57].

Controversial are the conclusions for the combination of radiotherapy with chemotherapy for locally advanced nonresectable NSCLC in the elderly. Five clinical trials, which examined the role of chemoradiation in older and younger patients, concluded that age does not represent a negative prognostic factor in a multivariate analysis [58–62]. Contrary to these results, a large metaanalysis of "survival" data of 1,999 patients of several Radiation Therapy Oncology Group studies treated with or without chemotherapy found a negative influence on survival in older ages [63].

In summary, radiation therapy plays a pivotal role in the treatment of NSCLC in the elderly population, not only in the context of palliation, but also in the overall control of the disease. Clinical trials need to be developed to evaluate the best therapy regimens with fewer side effects for older oncology patients.

28.5 Chemotherapy Options for Advanced and Metastatic Disease

It is universally accepted that chemotherapy administered to stage IIIB and IV NSCLC patients prolongs survival and improves quality of life. The most commonly used regimens are either cisplatin- or carboplatin-based. The primary question that has to be answered is whether this therapeutic approach is as efficient for older patients as it is for younger ones, without causing serious side effects.

Insufficient randomized trials have been performed with the purpose of answering this question. In addition, elderly patients are rarely included in large-scale phase III clinical trials. A published study has shown that patients older than 65 years are underrepresented in trials involving all cancer types except lymphomas [64]. Similarly, only 5.1% of elderly patients generally receive chemotherapy, a figure climbs to 18.8% for younger patients (based on insurance records) [65]. Oshita et al. reported that only 29% of patients with advanced NSCLC over 75 years old met the inclusion criteria for treatment with cisplatin-based chemotherapy [66]. There is a general reluctance from physicians to administer chemotherapy to elderly people. This is due primarily to the reduction in hepatic drug-metabolizing enzyme activity, particularly that of the P450 microsomal system, which is approximately 30% lower in healthy elderly people than in younger ones. Secondly, the fall in the glomerular filtration rate is a concern, which is approximately 1 ml/min for every year over the age of 40 years. Finally, the existing comorbidities in this age group are also problematic [67].

Cisplatin is not usually administered to this target group because of the associated renal and neurologic side effects and the potential hydration-related problems, while the newer chemotherapeutic agents are better tolerated with favorable therapeutic indices in the elderly. Vinorelbine, gemcitabine, and irinotecan represent some of these newer agents in addition to cisplatin and the taxanes that are being evaluated in this subpopulation.

The first randomized phase III clinical trial that compared vinorelbine plus best supportive care (BSC) versus BSC alone was the Elderly 1st and the 8th day of a 21-day cycle. The results showed an objective response rate in 19.7% of 76 patients treated with vinorelbine and a longer median overall survival that translated into 28 weeks for this group compared to 21 weeks for controls. Patients receiving vinorelbine were significantly more likely to survive 1 year (32% versus 14%), while the toxicity was mild, with grade 3/4 neutropenia in 10% of the patients and grade 2/3 anemia in 16% of the patients. An important point of this study was the improvement of the quality of life of subjects receiving chemotherapy in terms of improving lung cancer symptoms and pain as well as improved social, cognitive, and physical functioning [68].

Combination therapies are also being investigated in the elderly. Two trials have directly compared a combination therapy to monotherapy. Frasci et al. evaluated the combination of vinorelbine and gemcitabine versus monotherapy with vinorelbine in 120 patients over the age of 70 years. The results showed superiority for combination therapy, which translated into a longer median survival time (29 weeks versus 18 weeks), better response rates (22% versus 15%), and an increase in 1-year survival rates (30% versus 13%) for the monotherapy arm. Combination therapy was also associated with a clear delay in symptoms and quality of life deterioration. Most notably in this study is the low response rate of the vinorelbine group compared to other studies [69].

The next step in the evaluation of chemotherapy in the elderly population was a large-scale, randomized, multicenter phase III clinical study including 698 patients over or at 70 years of age with advanced NSCLC. Subjects were randomized into three groups assigned to receive vinorelbine 30 mg/m^2, gemcitabine 1,200 mg/m^2, or vinorelbine 20 mg/m^2 plus gemcitabine 1,000 mg/m^2, on the 1st and 8th day, every 3 weeks. Statistical analysis showed that the three regimens were equivalent and the combination regimen did not show any advantage over the single-agent therapies. Median survival was 37 weeks versus 28 weeks and 1-year survival rates were 42% versus 28% for the vinorelbine alone group and the gemcitabine alone group, respectively. Values for the combination arm fell between the single-agent arms.

Toxicity was tolerable along the three arms of the study [70]. Based on these data, single-agent chemotherapy should be considered a reasonable treatment choice for unselected elderly NSCLC patients with advanced disease. The American Society of Clinical Oncology adopted this attitude in the 2003 evidence-based guidelines. Vinorelbine is now a widely used chemotherapeutic agent, while gemcitabine represents an alternative therapeutic option.

To date, there are no phase III clinical trials designed to compare platinum-based regimens with BSC in the elderly. However, a subanalysis of large clinical trials has been performed in order to evaluate platinum efficacy and toxicity in older populations.

A retrospective analysis of the ECOG, phase III randomized trial (5592) comparing cisplatin plus either etoposide or paclitaxel in chemonaive patients with advanced NSCLC, compared the study endpoints between enrollees older and younger than 70 years. Age did not influence clinical benefit, survival, and median time to progression. Although older patients had a higher incidence of cardiovascular and respiratory comorbidities, toxicities were rather similar, with the exception of leukopenia and neuropsychiatric complications [71].

Cancer and Leukemia Group B obtained similar results through a retrospective analysis of two randomized phase III clinical trials. A cohort of 515 patients was assigned to receive paclitaxel alone or in combination with carboplatin, and a retrospective evaluation of the results, showed no significant differences in response, survival, or continuation of treatment with age. Regarding toxicity, increased leukocyte toxicity was seen in the elderly [72].

The last retrospective subgroup analysis was performed by Kelly et al. and included two randomized trials. The first one was Southwestern Oncology Group (SWOG) protocol 9509, comparing carboplatin and paclitaxel to cisplatin and vinorelbine. The second trial was SWOG protocol 9308, comparing cisplatin alone to cisplatin and vinorelbine. Patients older than 70 years of age did not present with worse hematological and nonhematological toxicities than their younger counterparts. Only a trend was observed for more toxicity, mainly in the vinorelbine/cisplatin arm, and a rather shorter median overall survival in the older group. This shorter survival could be explained by more frequent comorbidities in this population [73].

Based on the previous results, we can conclude that patients aged 70 years old or older with good performance status, who receive combination chemotherapy for advanced NSCLC do just as well as younger patients. However, these elderly patients presented a rather increased toxicity when cisplatin was used.

The role of adjuvant chemotherapy in the elderly represents another dilemma for physicians. A meta-analysis published a few years ago confirmed that patients who received surgery plus cisplatin-based chemotherapy presented a survival benefit of 5% at 5 years [74]. Based on these results, several randomized trials were conducted with conflicting outcomes. The International Adjuvant Lung Cancer Trial (IALT) enrolled 1,867 patients less than 75 years of age, and showed a survival benefit for adjuvant cisplatin-containing chemotherapy [75]. This study was followed by others using different chemotherapeutic regimens, such as cisplatin plus vinorelbine [76], carboplatin plus paclitaxel [77], or uracil plus tegafur [77, 78], which reached similar results. It appears, therefore, that adjuvant chemotherapy improves survival after surgery for stage IB–IIIA NSCLC patients. The survival benefit gained in these studies is also worthwhile for elderly patients who present with higher rates of hematological toxicities and lower rates of therapy compliance. There are no randomized trials answering this question, although available data suggest that newer chemotherapeutic agents can be used in this direction.

28.6 Targeted Therapies for the Elderly

Biological therapies constitute a significant step forward in cancer treatment. As they develop along with our understanding of molecular oncology and malignant progression, they encourage us to approach neoplasms from a new perspective; that is, one where there is a patient-tailored therapy aiming to achieve the best results at a minimal cost. Gefitinib and erlotinib represent the two major inhibitors of the epidermal growth factor receptor by binding to tyrosine kinase molecules. They have been slightly evaluated in elderly populations. Results from three randomized phase II studies evaluating the administration of gefitinib in pretreated symptomatic and asymptomatic lung cancer patients showed a rather modest disease control, but a remarkable symptomatic improvement with acceptable toxicity at a dose of 250 mg daily [79–81]. These results represented the rationale for performing several studies in elderly people. Although the number of participants was small, these trials showed that gefitinib offers an acceptable degree of disease stabilization at minimal toxicities [82–85]. With regard to erlotinib, a phase III study was conducted that showed a prolongation of overall survival compared to placebo in NSCLC patients receiving this agent as first- or second-line therapy [86]. Due to the erlotinib safety profile, a prospective phase II study involving previously untreated NSCLC patients over the age of 70 years was conducted with encouraging response rates (13.3%) and mild toxicity [87].

It is interesting that these two agents in combination with standard chemotherapy, increased the toxicity profile without providing a better result [88–90]. It is generally agreed upon that this field needs further evaluation. The results of ongoing clinical trials of biological agents in combination with chemotherapy, or not, for the treatment of elderly people are pending.

28.7 Conclusions

Although the selected information from randomized clinical trials for therapeutic management of lung cancer in the elderly seems to need further evaluation, some conclusions can be drawn from the published data. First of all, treatment approaches should be tailored to individual patients and based upon the patient's biological age and not their chronological age. For early stage lung cancer patients with good performance status and satisfactory cardiopulmonary reserves, the first therapeutic option is represented by surgery. In the presence of contraindications, radiotherapy is the alternative solution. Patients with a locally advanced disease and a good performance status should benefit more from radiochemotherapy, while frail patients should receive radiotherapy alone. Systemic chemotherapy offers the best potential results for metastatic disease. Single-agent chemotherapy with vinorelbine represents the first choice for elderly patients with good performance status, with the alternative of the single agent gemcitabine. In only very selective patients may the use of combination chemotherapeutic agents be given.

Physicians should overcome their fears for possible surgical complications or unmanageable chemoradiotherapy toxicities when treating elderly people. Careful selection of individuals and detailed clinical assessment of comorbidities leads to effective management of this disease.

Key Points

- More than half of the patients diagnosed with lung cancer are over the age of 65 years, and 35% are over 70 years old at the time of diagnosis. The peak incidence of lung cancer occurs in patients between 75 and 80 years old, and two-thirds of all patients who die of lung cancer are older than 65 years old.
- The elderly patients are characterized by age-specific problems such as depression, alterations of mental status, reduced nutritional status, and absence of social support, which interfere with the diagnosis and treatment of their cancer.
- Histological confirmation of the tumor and accurate staging should be concluded in elderly lung cancer patients in order to take therapeutic decisions.

- Treatment approaches for elderly non-small-cell lung cancer (NSCLC) patients should be patient-tailored and based upon the patient's biological, not chronological age.
- Elderly NSCLC patients with limited disease who have undergone detailed preoperative evaluation should not be deprived of a potentially curative lung surgery. Radical radiotherapy represents an alternative for them, although there are no prospective randomized studies evaluating the efficacy of radiotherapy versus surgery.
- Palliative chemotherapy improves the quality of life of fit NSCLC patients with extensive disease in terms of improving lung cancer symptoms and pain as well as the social, cognitive, and physical functioning of the individuals.
- Physicians should overcome their fear of possible surgical complications or unmanageable chemoradiotherapy toxicities when treating elderly people with NSCLC. Careful selection of individuals and detailed clinical assessment of comorbidities lead to effective management of this group of patients.

References

1. Parkin DM. Global cancer statistics in the year 2000. Lancet Oncol 2001; 2:533.
2. Peake MD, Thompson S, Lowe D, Pearson MG. Ageism in the management of lung cancer. Age Ageing 2003; 32:171.
3. Extermann M. Measuring comorbidity in older cancer patients. Eur J Cancer 2000; 36:453.
4. American Cancer Society Centers for Disease Control and Prevention National Conference on Cancer and the Older Person. Proceedings. Atlanta, Georgia, February 10–12, 1994. Cancer 1994; 74:1995.
5. Yancik R, Ries LA. Aging and cancer in America. Demographic and epidemiologic perspectives. Hematol Oncol Clin North Am 2000; 14:17.
6. Brown JS, Eraut D, Trask C, Davison AG. Age and the treatment of lung cancer. Thorax 1996; 51:564.
7. Gridelli C, Perrone F, Monfardini S. Lung cancer in the elderly. Eur J Cancer 1997; 33:2313.
8. Silverberg E, Lubera JA. Cancer statistics, 1988. CA Cancer J Clin 1988; 38:5.
9. Janssen-Heijnen ML, Schipper RM, Razenberg PP, Crommelin MA, Coebergh JW. Prevalence of comorbidity in lung cancer patients and its relationship with treatment: a population-based study. Lung Cancer 1998; 21:105.
10. Kurishima K, Satoh H, Ishikawa H, Yamashita YT, Homma T, Ohtsuka M, et al. Lung cancer patients with chronic obstructive pulmonary disease. Oncol Rep 2001; 8:63.
11. Kurishima K, Satoh H, Ishikawa H, Yamashita YT, Ohtsuka M, Sekizawa K. Lung cancer patients with cardio- and cerebrovascular diseases. Oncol Rep 2001; 8:1251.
12. Connolly CK, Crawford SM, Rider PL, Smith AD, Johnston CF, Muers MF. Carcinoma of the bronchus in the Yorkshire region of England 1976–1990: trends since 1984. Eur Respir J 1997; 10:397.
13. Hehn B, Haponik EF. Flexible bronchoscopy in the elderly. Clin Chest Med 2001; 22:301.

14. Pue CA, Pacht ER. Complications of fiberoptic bronchoscopy at a university hospital. Chest 1995; 107:430.
15. Brown TS, Kanthapillai P. Transthoracic needle biopsy for suspected thoracic malignancy in elderly patients using CT guidance. Clin Radiol 1998; 53:116.
16. Dennie CJ, Matzinger FR, Marriner JR, Maziak DE. Transthoracic needle biopsy of the lung: results of early discharge in 506 outpatients. Radiology 2001; 219:247.
17. MacManus MP, Hicks RJ, Matthews JP, Hogg A, McKenzie AF, Wirth A et al. High rate of detection of unsuspected distant metastases by pet in apparent stage III non-small-cell lung cancer: implications for radical radiation therapy. Int J Radiat Oncol Biol Phys 2001; 50:287.
18. Teeter SM, Holmes FF, McFarlane MJ. Lung carcinoma in the elderly population. Influence of histology on the inverse relationship of stage to age. Cancer 1987; 60:1331.
19. Anderson RN. United States life tables, 1997. Natl Vital Stat Rep 1999; 47:1.
20. Jaklitsch MT, Mery CM, Audisio RA. The use of surgery to treat lung cancer in elderly patients. Lancet Oncol 2003; 4:463.
21. Battafarano RJ, Piccirillo JF, Meyers BF, Hsu HS, Guthrie TJ, Cooper JD, et al. Impact of comorbidity on survival after surgical resection in patients with stage I non-small cell lung cancer. J Thorac Cardiovasc Surg 2002; 123:280.
22. Au J, el-Oakley R, Cameron EW. Pneumonectomy for bronchogenic carcinoma in the elderly. Eur J Cardiothorac Surg 1994; 8:247.
23. Keenan RJ, Landreneau RJ, Maley RH Jr, Singh D, Macherey R, Bartley S, et al. Segmental resection spares pulmonary function in patients with stage I lung cancer. Ann Thorac Surg 2004; 78:228.
24. Jacklitsch M, Mery C, Bueno R. Lesser pulmonary resections are more common in elderly non-small cell lung cancer (NSCLC) patients but do not adversely affect survival . Proc Am Soc Clin Oncol 1999; 18:471a.
25. Pagni S, McKelvey A, Riordan C, Federico JA, Ponn RB. Pulmonary resection for malignancy in the elderly: is age still a risk factor? Eur J Cardiothorac Surg 1998; 14:40.
26. Shirakusa T, Tsutsui M, Iriki N, Yoshida T, Minoda S, Iwasaki T, et al. [Results of surgical treatment in patients aged 80 years and over]. Nippon Kyobu Geka Gakkai Zasshi 1989; 37:1306.
27. Naunheim KS, Kesler KA, D'Orazio SA, Fiore AC, McBride LR, Judd DR. Thoracotomy in the octogenarian. Ann Thorac Surg 1991; 51:547.
28. Osaki T, Shirakusa T, Kodate M, Nakanishi R, Mitsudomi T, Ueda H. Surgical treatment of lung cancer in the octogenarian. Ann Thorac Surg 1994; 57:188.
29. Riquet M, Manac'h D, Le Pimpec-Barthes F, Debrosse D, Dujon A, Saab M, et al. Operation for lung cancer in the elderly: what about octogenarians? Ann Thorac Surg 1994; 58:916.
30. Harvey JC, Erdman C, Pisch J, Beattie EJ. Surgical treatment of non-small cell lung cancer in patients older than seventy years. J Surg Oncol 1995; 60:247.
31. Pagni S, Federico JA, Ponn RB. Pulmonary resection for lung cancer in octogenarians. Ann Thorac Surg 1997; 63:785.
32. Hanagiri T, Muranaka H, Hashimoto M, Nagashima A, Yasumoto K. Results of surgical treatment of lung cancer in octogenarians. Lung Cancer 1999; 23:129.
33. Breyer RH, Zippe C, Pharr WF, Jensik RJ, Kittle CF, Faber LP. Thoracotomy in patients over age seventy years: ten-year experience. J Thorac Cardiovasc Surg 1981; 81:187.
34. Gebitekin C, Gupta NK, Martin PG, Saunders NR, Walker DR. Long-term results in the elderly following pulmonary resection for non-small cell lung carcinoma. Eur J Cardiothorac Surg 1993; 7:653.

35. Massard G, Moog R, Wihlm JM, Kessler R, Dabbagh A, Lesage A, et al. Bronchogenic cancer in the elderly: operative risk and long-term prognosis. Thorac Cardiovasc Surg 1996; 44:40.

36. Thomas P, Piraux M, Jacques LF, Gregoire J, Bedard P, Deslauriers J. Clinical patterns and trends of outcome of elderly patients with bronchogenic carcinoma. Eur J Cardiothorac Surg 1998; 13:266.

37. Oliaro A, Leo F, Filosso PL, Rena O, Parola A, Maggi G. Resection for bronchogenic carcinoma in the elderly. J Cardiovasc Surg (Torino) 1999; 40:715.

38. Sherman S, Guidot CE. The feasibility of thoracotomy for lung cancer in the elderly. JAMA 1987; 258:927.

39. Ishida T, Yokoyama H, Kaneko S, Sugio K, Sugimachi K. Long-term results of operation for non-small cell lung cancer in the elderly. Ann Thorac Surg 1990; 50:919.

40. Morandi U, Stefani A, Golinelli M, Ruggiero C, Brandi L, Chiapponi A, et al. Results of surgical resection in patients over the age of 70 years with non small-cell lung cancer. Eur J Cardiothorac Surg 1997; 11:432.

41. Kamiyoshihara M, Kawashima O, Ishikawa S, Morishita Y. Long-term results after pulmonary resection in elderly patients with non-small cell lung cancer. J Cardiovasc Surg (Torino) 2000; 41:483.

42. Filippetti M, Crucitti G, Andreetti C, Mastropietro T, Santoro R, Lepiane P, et al. [Experience of 10 years with the surgical treatment of lung cancer in elderly patients]. Chir Ital 2001; 53:167.

43. Riquet M, Medioni J, Manac'h D, Dujon A, Souilamas R, Le Pimpec BF, et al. [Non-small cell lung cancer: surgical trends as a function of age]. Rev Mal Respir 2001; 18:173.

44. Bouchardy C, Fioretta G, De PM, Obradovic M, Spiliopoulos A. Determinants of long term survival after surgery for cancer of the lung: a population-based study. Cancer 1999; 86:2229.

45. BTS guidelines: guidelines on the selection of patients with lung cancer for surgery. Thorax 2001; 56:89.

46. McKenna RJ Jr, Wolf RK, Brenner M, Fischel RJ, Wurnig P. Is lobectomy by video-assisted thoracic surgery an adequate cancer operation? Ann Thorac Surg 1998; 66:1903.

47. Shiraishi T, Yoshinaga Y, Yoneda S, Okabayashi H, Iwasaki A, Kawahara K, et al. [Clinical evaluation of VATS lobectomy for lung cancer]. Kyobu Geka 2000; 53:4.

48. Solaini L, Prusciano F, Bagioni P, Di FF, Basilio PD. Video-assisted thoracic surgery major pulmonary resections. Present experience. Eur J Cardiothorac Surg 2001; 20:437.

49. Gauden SJ, Tripcony L. The curative treatment by radiation therapy alone of Stage I non-small cell lung cancer in a geriatric population. Lung Cancer 2001; 32:71.

50. Noordijk EM, vd Poest CE, Hermans J, Wever AM, Leer JW. Radiotherapy as an alternative to surgery in elderly patients with resectable lung cancer. Radiother Oncol 1988; 13.03.

51. Hayakawa K, Mitsuhashi N, Katano S, Saito Y, Nakayama Y, Sakurai H, et al. High-dose radiation therapy for elderly patients with inoperable or unresectable non-small cell lung cancer. Lung Cancer 2001; 32:81.

52. Pignon T, Gregor A, Schaake KC, Roussel A, Van GM, Scalliet P. Age has no impact on acute and late toxicity of curative thoracic radiotherapy. Radiother Oncol 1998; 46:239.

53. Rowell NP, Williams CJ. Radical radiotherapy for stage I/II non-small cell lung cancer in patients not sufficiently fit for or declining surgery (medically inoperable): a systematic review. Thorax 2001; 56:628.

54. Langendijk JA, Aaronson NK, de Jong JM, ten Velde GP, Muller MJ, Lamers RJ, et al. Prospective study on quality of life before and after radical radiotherapy in non-small cell lung cancer. J Clin Oncol 2001; 19:2123.

55. Lonardi F, Coeli M, Pavanato G, Adami F, Gioga G, Campostrini F. Radiotherapy for non-small cell lung cancer in patients aged 75 and over: safety, effectiveness and possible impact on survival. Lung Cancer 2000; 28:43.

56. Newaishy GA, Kerr GR. Radical radiotherapy for bronchogenic carcinoma: five year survival rates. Clin Oncol (R Coll Radiol) 1989; 1:80.

57. Wurschmidt F, Bunemann H, Bunemann C, Beck-Bornholdt HP, Heilmann HP. [The radiotherapy of inoperable non-small-cell bronchial carcinoma. A retrospective analysis of 427 cases]. Strahlenther Onkol 1994; 170:302.

58. Clamon G, Herndon J, Cooper R, Chang AY, Rosenman J, Green MR. Radiosensitization with carboplatin for patients with unresectable stage III non-small-cell lung cancer: a phase III trial of the Cancer and Leukemia Group B and the Eastern Cooperative Oncology Group. J Clin Oncol 1999; 17:4.

59. Furuse K, Fukuoka M, Kawahara M, Nishikawa H, Takada Y, Kudoh S, et al. Phase III study of concurrent versus sequential thoracic radiotherapy in combination with mitomycin, vindesine, and cisplatin in unresectable stage III non-small-cell lung cancer. J Clin Oncol 1999; 17:2692.

60. Jeremic B, Shibamoto Y, Milicic B, Milisavljevic S, Nikolic N, Dagovic A, et al. A phase II study of concurrent accelerated hyperfractionated radiotherapy and carboplatin/oral etoposide for elderly patients with stage III non-small-cell lung cancer. Int J Radiat Oncol Biol Phys 1999; 44:343.

61. Schaake-Koning C, van den BW, Dalesio O, Festen J, Hoogenhout J, van Houtte P, et al. Effects of concomitant cisplatin and radiotherapy on inoperable non-small-cell lung cancer. N Engl J Med 1992; 326:524.

62. Langer CJ, Hsu C, Curan WJ, et al. Elderly patients with locally advanced non-small cell lung cancer benefit from combined modality therapy: secondary analysis of Radiation Therapy Oncology Group (RTOG) 94-10. Proc Am Soc Clin Oncol 2002; 94:173.

63. Werner-Wasik M, Scott C, Cox JD, Sause WT, Byhardt RW, Asbell S, et al. Recursive partitioning analysis of 1999 Radiation Therapy Oncology Group (RTOG) patients with locally-advanced non-small-cell lung cancer (LA-NSCLC): identification of five groups with different survival. Int J Radiat Oncol Biol Phys 2000; 48:1475.

64. Hutchins LF, Unger JM, Crowley JJ, Coltman CA Jr, Albain KS. Underrepresentation of patients 65 years of age or older in cancer-treatment trials. N Engl J Med 1999; 341:2061.

65. Hillner BE, McDonald MK, Desch CE, Smith TJ, Penberthy LT, Retchin SM A comparison of patterns of care of nonsmall cell lung carcinoma patients in a younger and Medigap commercially insured cohort Cancer 1998; 83:1930

66. Oshita F, Kurata T, Kasai T, Fakuda M, Yamamoto N, Ohe Y, et al. Prospective evaluation of the feasibility of cisplatin-based chemotherapy for elderly lung cancer patients with normal organ functions. Jpn J Cancer Res 1995; 86:1198.

67. Lichtman SM, Villani G. Chemotherapy in the elderly: pharmacologic considerations. Cancer Control 2000, 7:548.

68. Gridelli C. The ELVIS trial: a phase III study of single-agent vinorelbine as first-line treatment in elderly patients with advanced non-small cell lung cancer. Elderly Lung Cancer Vinorelbine Italian Study. Oncologist 2001; 6 Suppl 1:4-7.:4.

69. Frasci G, Lorusso V, Panza N, Comella P, Nicolella G, Bianco A, et al. Gemcitabine plus vinorelbine versus vinorelbine alone in elderly patients with advanced non-small-cell lung cancer. J Clin Oncol 2000; 18:2529.

70. Gridelli C, Cigolari S, Gallo C, Manzione L, Ianniello GP, Frontini L, et al. Activity and toxicity of gemcitabine and gemcitabine + vinorelbine in advanced non-small-cell lung cancer elderly patients: Phase II data from the Multi-center Italian Lung Cancer in the Elderly Study (MILES) randomized trial. Lung Cancer 2001; 31:277.

71. Langer CJ, Manola J, Bernardo P, Kugler JW, Bonomi P, Cella D, et al. Cisplatin-based therapy for elderly patients with advanced non-small-cell lung cancer: implications of Eastern Cooperative Oncology Group 5592, a randomized trial. J Natl Cancer Inst 2002; 94:173.

72. Lilenbaum RC, Herndon JE, List MA, Desch C, Watson DM, Miller AA, et al. Single-agent versus combination chemotherapy in advanced non-small-cell lung cancer: the cancer and leukemia group B (study 9730). J Clin Oncol 2005; 23:190.

73. Kelly K, Giarritta S, Hayes S, et al. Should older patients (pts) receive combination chemotherapy for advanced stage non-small-cell lung cancer (NSCLC). An analysis of Southwest Oncology Trials 9509 and 9308. Proc Am Soc Clin Oncol 2001; 20:329a.

74. Chemotherapy in non-small cell lung cancer: a meta-analysis using updated data on individual patients from 52 randomised clinical trials. Non-small Cell Lung Cancer Collaborative Group. BMJ 1995; 311:899.

75. Arriagada R, Bergman B, Dunant A, Le CT, Pignon JP, Vansteenkiste J. Cisplatin-based adjuvant chemotherapy in patients with completely resected non-small-cell lung cancer. N Engl J Med 2004; 350:351.

76. Winton TL, Livingstone R, Johnson D, et al. A prospective randomized trial of adjuvant vinorelbine (VIN) and cisplatin (CIS) in completely resected stage IB and II non small cell lung cancer (NSCLC) Intergroup JBR 10. Proc Am Soc Clin Oncol 2004; 23:621s.

77. Strauss GM, Herndon J, Maddaus MA, et al. Randomised clinical trial of adjuvant chemotherapy with paclitaxel and carboplatin following resection in stage IB and II non-small cell lung cancer (NSCLC): Report of Cancer and Leukemia Group B (CALGB) Protocol 9633. Proc Am Soc Clin Oncol 2004; 23:621s.

78. Kato H, Ichinose Y, Ohta M, Hata E, Tsubota N, Tada H, et al. A randomized trial of adjuvant chemotherapy with uracil-tegafur for adenocarcinoma of the lung. N Engl J Med 2004; 350:1713.

79. Cella D, Herbst RS, Lynch TJ, Prager D, Belani CP, Schiller JH, et al. Clinically meaningful improvement in symptoms and quality of life for patients with non-small-cell lung cancer receiving gefitinib in a randomized controlled trial. J Clin Oncol 2005; 23:2946.

80. Fukuoka M, Yano S, Giaccone G, Tamura T, Nakagawa K, Douillard JY, et al. Multi-institutional randomized phase II trial of gefitinib for previously treated patients with advanced non-small-cell lung cancer (The IDEAL 1 Trial) [corrected]. J Clin Oncol 2003; 21:2237.

81. Kris MG, Natale RB, Herbst RS, Lynch TJ Jr, Prager D, Belani CP, et al. Efficacy of gefitinib, an inhibitor of the epidermal growth factor receptor tyrosine kinase, in symptomatic patients with non-small cell lung cancer: a randomized trial. JAMA 2003; 290:2149.

82. Cappuzzo F, Bartolini S, Ceresoli GL, Tamberi S, Spreafico A, Lombardo L, et al. Efficacy and tolerability of gefitinib in pretreated elderly patients with advanced non-small-cell lung cancer (NSCLC). Br J Cancer 2004; 90:82.

83. Gridelli C, Maione P, Castaldo V, Rossi A. Gefitinib in elderly and unfit patients affected by advanced non-small-cell lung cancer. Br J Cancer 2003; 89:1827.

84. Copin M, Kommareddy A, Behnken D, et al. Gefitinib in elderly patients with non-small cell lung cancer (NSCLC). Proc Am Soc Clin Oncol 2003; 22:758.

85. Soto Parra H, Cavina R, Zucali P, et al. Gefitinib in elderly patients with progressive, pretreated, non-small cell lung cancer. Br J Cancer 2003; 89(Suppl 2):S25-S35.

86. Shepherd FA, Pereira J, Giuleanu E, et al. A randomized placebo-controlled trial of erlotinib in patients with advanced non-small cell lung cancer (NSCLC) following failure of 1st line or 2nd line chemotherapy. A national Cancer Institute of Canada Clinical Trials Group (NCIC CTG) trial. Proc Am Soc Clin Oncol 2004; 7022.

87. Johnson BE, Lucca J, Rabin MS, et al. Preliminary results from a phase II study of the epidermal growth factor receptor kinase inhibitor erlotinib in patients 70 years of age with previously untreated advanced non-small cell lung carcinoma. Proc Am Soc Clin Oncol 2004; 23:633.

88. Scagliotti G, Rossi A, Novello S. Gefitinib (ZD 1839) combined with gemcitabine or vinorelbine as single-agent in elderly patients with advanced non-small cell lung cancer (NSCLC). Proc Am Soc Clin Oncol 2004; 23:633.

89. Gatzemeier U, Pluzanka A, Szczesna A, et al. Results of a phase III of erlotinib (OSI-774) combined with cisplatin and gemcitabine in advanced non-small cell lung cancer (NSCLC). Proc Am Soc Clin Oncol 2004; 23:617.

90. Herbst RS, Prager D, Hermann R, et al. TRIBUTE-a Phase III trial of erlotinib HCl (OSI-774) combined with carboplatin and paclitaxel (CP) chemotherapy in advanced non-small cell lung cancer (NSCLC). J Clin Oncol 2005; 23:5892.

Section VI:
Management of Small-Cell Lung Cancer

Management of Limited Disease Small-Cell Lung Cancer

29

Ritesh Rathore and Alan B. Weitberg

Contents

29.1 Introduction

Small-cell lung cancer (SCLC) represents a distinct clinicopathologic entity that is biologically and clinically distinct from other lung cancers. It is distinguished by its rapid growth characteristics accompanied by the early development of widespread metastases. Though it is extremely sensitive to both chemotherapy and radiotherapy, responses are typically of a short duration and relapse usually occurs within 2 years. Overall long-term outcomes continue to be dismal with poor 5-year survival rates.

Small-cell lung cancer represents approximately 20% of lung cancer cases diagnosed annually. Cigarette smoking is the primary risk factor and accounts for more than 90% of cases [1]. In one series, only 2% of 500 SCLC patients had no smoking history [2]. SCLC is also the most common histologic subtype among uranium miners, probably due to exposure to radioactive radon, a byproduct of uranium decay [3].

29.2 Treatment Aspects

The overriding goals in the treatment of limited disease SCLC (LD-SCLC) are those of local tumor control and treatment of micrometastatic disease. With the evolution of combination chemotherapy regimens, the rates of overall and complete responses in LD-SCLC have increased to 80–90% and 50–60%, respectively. Recent analysis of LD-SCLC patients listed in the SEER database reveals a more than doubling of the 5-year survival rate to 12.1% [4]. For patients treated on North American phase III trials between 1972 and 1992, the same analysis revealed an improvement in the median survival from 12 to 17 months.

Responses in SCLC are typically short lived with the median duration being 6–8 months. Local recurrences remain a common site of failure. Local therapeutic modalities including radiotherapy and to a lesser extent surgery are therefore considered valuable in the multimodality management of LD-SCLC. The effort to eradicate micrometastatic disease, except in the case of prophylactic cranial irradiation, has concentrated on investigational schedules and intensities of chemotherapy, investigation of newer chemotherapeutic agents, and the use of immunologic approaches. The current manage-

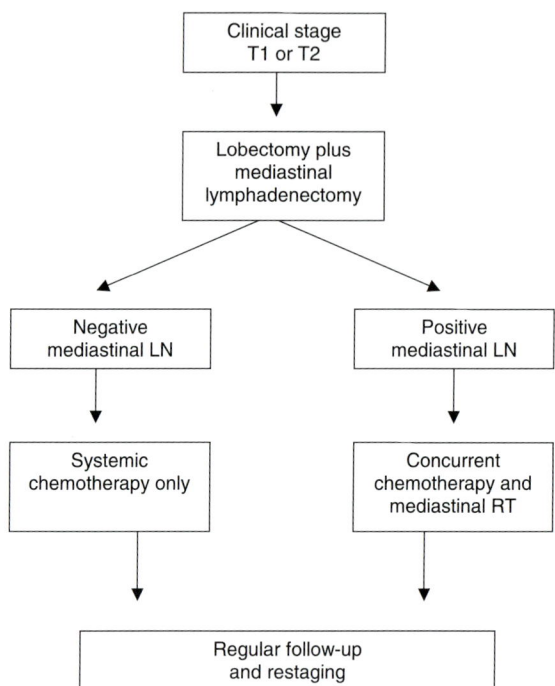

Fig. 29.1. Treatment for T1–T2 SCLC. *LN* Lymph node, *RT* radiation therapy

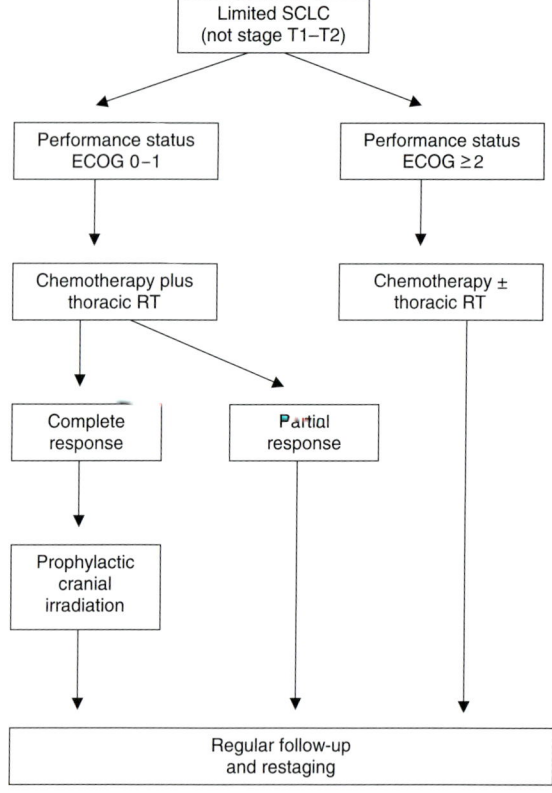

Fig. 29.2. Treatment of limited SCLC. *ECOG* Eastern Cooperative Oncology Group

ment approaches therefore rely on integrated multimodality therapy for the achievement of prolonged complete remissions (Figs. 29.1, 29.2).

29.2.1 Prognostic Factors

The presence of overt distant metastases is, by far, the worst prognostic feature. Among patients with LD-SCLC, the absence of mediastinal and supraclavicular adenopathy is considered favorable. The presence of paraneoplastic syndromes is generally believed to be associated with an adverse outcome. Elevations of lactate dehydrogenase (LDH) and alkaline phosphatase levels are considered unfavorable. Additionally, adverse determinants of prognosis include a poor performance status and weight loss. Though the effect of smoking discontinuation on prognosis is not firmly established, all patients should be encouraged to quit smoking. One recent report suggested that attainment of a complete response was a predictor for improved rates of long-term survival [5].

29.2.2 Initial Evaluation and Staging

Small-cell lung cancer typically presents as a large hilar mass with mediastinal adenopathy. A solitary peripheral nodule without central adenopathy is uncommon. As discussed below, in this situation, mediastinal staging followed by surgical resection is recommended. All SCLC patients require systemic therapy. Therefore, staging provides a therapeutic guideline for chest radiotherapy, which is indicated for limited disease but not typically indicated for extensive disease (ED-SCLC).

Staging includes a physical examination and radiologic imaging (Fig. 29.3). It should include a chest radiograph and chest and abdomen computed tomography (CT) scans that encompass the adrenal glands. Imaging of the head with gadolinium-enhanced magnetic resonance imaging (MRI) or CT is necessary. A bone scan is also required, followed by bone radiographs if necessary. Baseline complete blood cell count and a comprehensive metabolic panel including electrolytes, liver function tests, calcium, LDH, blood urea nitrogen, and serum creatinine are also required.

A unilateral bone marrow aspirate and biopsy are performed in some centers for patients believed to have LD-SCLC but not for patients with obvious ED-SCLC. Criteria for selecting patients include cytopenias, elevated LDH or alkaline phosphatase, or leukoerythroblastic features upon peripheral smear review. Marrow examination may upstage 5–10% of patients from LD-SCLC to ED-SCLC.

Thoracentesis is recommended for pleural effusion. If pleural fluid cytology is not conclusive, then thoraco-

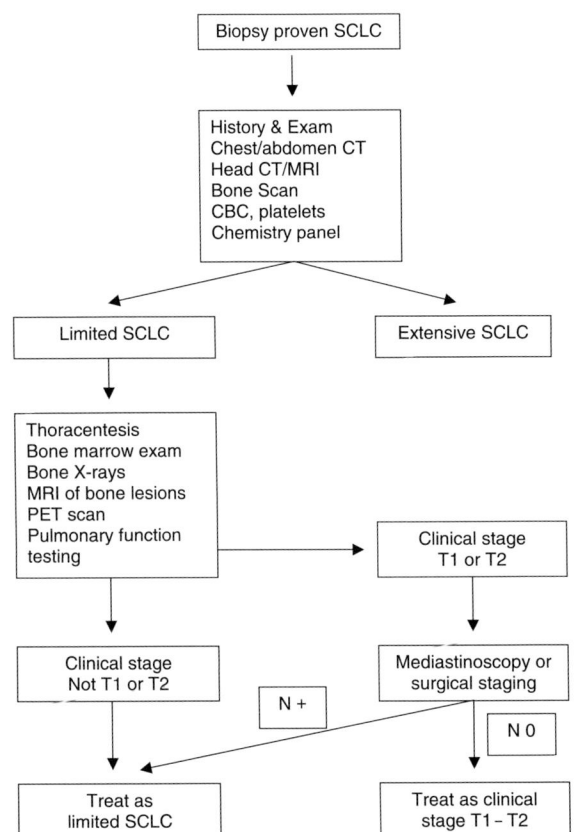

Fig. 29.3. Initial evaluation of SCLC. *CBC* Complete blood count

scopy may be attempted. However, if multiple cyto-pathologic examinations of pleural fluid are negative for cancer, then the pleural effusion should be excluded as a staging element.

29.2.3 Historical Perspectives

Small-cell lung cancer is a systemic process early on in its development. Managing this disease with locoregional modalities alone results in poor outcomes. In comparison to non-small-cell lung cancer (NSCLC), there is a much higher level of chemotherapy responsiveness in all stages of SCLC. The mainstay of therapeutic planning is around systemic chemotherapy.

In a British report from 1966, median survival for patients with unresectable, limited disease and those with extensive disease was approximately 12 and 5 weeks, respectively [6]. In another study by the Medical Research Council published in 1973, 144 patients with apparently resectable SCLC were randomized to either surgery or radiation therapy. Extremely poor survival was seen with median, 1-, and 5-year survivals of 6.5 months, 21%, and 1%, respectively, for the surgery arm and 10 months, 22%, and 4%, respectively, for the radiation arm [7].

In a single-institution report of SCLC patients seen during 1931–1971, only 7% had resectable tumors, and only 2 patients survived for 5 years [8]. Similarly, among 368 patients with SCLC who underwent surgical resection in the 1960s, the 5-year survival was less than 1% [9]. In contrast, there was a 15–25% 5-year survival for patients with the other three major histologic subtypes of lung cancer. A 1978 review of patients felt to have surgically resectable SCLC could find absolutely no advantage for the inclusion of surgery in the treatment regimen [10].

In 1969, the first report of an improvement in survival in SCLC with the use of chemotherapy was reported. The Veterans Administration Lung Cancer Study Group trial showed that three cycles of cyclophosphamide could more than double median survival when compared to supportive care in extensive SCLC [11]. Subsequently, data from many small studies showed that chemotherapy could improve survival at 2-year follow-up significantly when used in an adjuvant fashion after surgical resection. Similarly, in randomized trials, addition of chemotherapy to thoracic irradiation improved median survival. The results of these trials rapidly established combination chemotherapy as the mainstay of therapy for both limited and extensive disease SCLC by the early 1970s.

29.3 Chemotherapeutic Approaches

29.3.1 Active Agents

Numerous chemotherapeutic agents have demonstrated considerable single activity in SCLC (Table 29.1). The active single agents used in the earliest phase of the development of combination chemotherapy included cyclophosphamide, mechlorethamine, doxorubicin, methotrexate, etoposide, and vincristine. Of these, etoposide has an impressive response rate of 40–80% in previously untreated patients [12, 13] but response rates were much more modest in previously treated patients in a large report [14]. In the 1980s, cisplatin, ifosfamide, carboplatin, teniposide, epirubicin, and vindesine were documented as having significant activity. Cisplatin was evaluated as a single agent in mostly previously treated patients and has at least similar response rates as carboplatin, which produced a 60% response rate in previously treated patients in one report [15].

The 1990s have seen the introduction of a range of new chemotherapeutic agents including the topoisomerase I inhibitors topotecan and irinotecan, the taxanes paclitaxel and docetaxel, vinorelbine, and gemcitabine as active single agents in the therapy of SCLC. Topotecan has shown 39% and 25% response rates among previously untreated and treated patients, respectively [16, 17]. Irinotecan had response rates of 33–47% in pre-

Table 29.1. Chemotherapeutic agents with documented activity in SCLC

Older agents	Newer agents
Cyclophosphamide	Paclitaxel
Ifosfamide	Docetaxel
Doxorubicin	Irinotecan
Methotrexate	Topotecan
Etoposide	Gemcitabine
Vincristine	Vinorelbine
Cisplatin	Epirubicin
Carboplatin	

Table 29.2. Commonly utilized chemotherapy regimens in SCLC

Regimen	Components	Frequency
EP		
Etoposide	100 mg/m^2 IV, days 1–3	Every 3 weeks
Cisplatin	80 mg/m^2 IV, day 1; or	
	25 mg/m^2 IV, days 1–3	
EC		
Etoposide	100 mg/m^2 IV, days 1–3	Every 3 weeks
Carboplatin	300 mg/m^2 IV, day 1; or	
	AUC = 6 IV, day 1	
CAV		
Cyclophospha-mide	1,000 mg/m^2 IV, day 1	Every 3 weeks
Doxorubicin	45 mg/m^2 IV, day 1	
Vincristine	2 mg IV, day 1	
CAVE		
Cyclophospha-mide	1,000 mg/m^2 IV, day 1	Every 3 weeks
Doxorubicin	50 mg/m^2 IV, day 1	
Vincristine	1.5 mg/m^2 IV, day 1	
Etoposide	60 mg/m^2 IV, days 1–5	
CDE		
Cyclophospha-mide	1,000 mg/m^2 IV, day 1	Every 3 weeks
Doxorubicin	45 mg/m^2 IV, day 1	
Etoposide	100 mg/m^2 IV, days 1–3	
ICE		
Ifosfamide (with mesna)	5 g/m^2 CIV over 24 h, on day 1	Every 3 weeks
Carboplatin	300 mg/m^2 IV, day 1	
Etoposide	100 mg/m^2 IV, days 1–3	

viously treated patients and 50% in untreated patients [18 ,19]. Paclitaxel showed responses of 34–41% in untreated patients in cooperative group phase II trials [20, 21], while docetaxel showed a 25% response rate in previously treated patients [22]. Vinorelbine showed response rates of 13–16% in two small trials [23, 24]. Gemcitabine had a 29% response rate when evaluated in previously untreated patients [25].

29.3.2 Combination Chemotherapy

While few randomized trials have been conducted to address this point, the results with combination chemotherapy appear to have significant advantages compared to the results achievable with single-agent chemotherapy [26]. In the early 1980s, a consensus report concluded that optimal results in the treatment of SCLC could only be achieved with the use of combination chemotherapy [27]. Commonly utilized combination chemotherapy regimens (Table 29.2) include cisplatin and etoposide (EP), carboplatin and etoposide (EC), cyclophosphamide, doxorucibin, and vincristine (CAV), and cyclophosphamide, doxorubicin, and etoposide (CDE).

Among patients with limited disease, modern chemotherapy regimens are capable of producing overall response rates of 80–90%, which include complete response rates of 50–60%. Median survival times of 14–16 months have been regularly observed, and 2-year survival rates of 15–25% are possible. As will be discussed below, thoracic radiation improves local control rates from 10% to about 40–60% in patients with LD-SCLC and is associated with improved survival.

The optimal combination chemotherapy regimen remains a subject for debate. The combination of cyclophosphamide, doxorubicin, and vincristine (CAV regimen) was widely used in the late 1970s and 1980s. It repeatedly resulted in the optimal response rates and median survival duration as outlined above and was considered by many to be the "standard regimen."

In the 1980s, when etoposide became established as an active agent, trials were conducted to determine if the addition of etoposide to CAV (CAVE regimen) or the substitution of etoposide for vincristine (CDE) led to improvements in outcome. Of three trials that compared CAV with CAVE, two found greater response rates with CAVE [28–30], which did not translate into improved overall survival. Median survival in extensive-stage patients was prolonged modestly with the substitution of etoposide for either vincristine or doxorubicin, but no improvement was seen in limited-stage patients. Again, in randomized comparison of CDE to CAV, there was an improvement response duration and overall survival which was only slightly better in LD-SCLC patients [31]. These studies were thus unable to demonstrate the superiority of inclusion of etoposide in the existing regimens.

This combination of etoposide and cisplatin (EP) has been shown to be highly synergistic in preclinical studies. In previously treated patients, the EP regimen produced response rates approaching 50% in early studies [32, 33]. Subsequently, the evaluation of EP as first-line therapy led to acceptable results in both limited and extensive-stage patients. As first-line therapy, response rates as high as 90% have been reported. A pooled analysis of 294 previously treated patients with SCLC who were treated with EP produced an overall response rate of 47% [34].

The EP regimen was directly compared to the CAV regimen in two randomized studies [35, 36]. In a Japanese study including patients with limited and extensive disease, the overall survival was same in the CAV and EP arms. The Southeastern Cancer Study Group (SECSG) trial in patients with previously untreated extensive-stage disease showed no difference in response rates or overall survival for either CAV or EP. However, EP was twice as effective in relapsing patients previously treated with CAV, whereas CAV was relatively ineffective as a second-line regimen. Less neutropenia and infections were seen with EP compared to CAV in these randomized trials. While CAV appears to be comparable to EP, it has not been proven to be superior and, with its favorable toxicity profile, EP remains the choice for the treatment of limited disease in the USA. Recently, the results of a 5-year follow-up of a randomized study comparing cisplatin, epirubicin, and etoposide (CEV) to EP were published [37]. Among patients with LD-SCLC on this trial, the median survival was 14.5 and 9.7 months in the EP and CEV arms, respectively. The 2- and 5-year survival rates were better in the EP arm also. These results thus add more support to the routine use of EP as first-line therapy in LD-SCLC.

Regimens substituting carboplatin for cisplatin in combination with etoposide (EC) in SCLC appear to have similar efficacy. The Hellenic Cooperative Oncology Group randomized 143 patients (82 with LD-SCLC) to six cycles of EC or EP [38]. Complete response rates (57% and 58%) and median survival (12.5 and 11.8 months) were similar in the EP and EC groups, respectively. However, the hematologic, gastrointestinal, and neurologic toxicities were more frequent and/or severe in the EP arm. Currently, it is common practice in the USA to substitute carboplatin for cisplatin in patients with ED-SCLC but retain EP for patients with LD-SCLC.

A regimen consisting of cisplatin, ifosfamide, and etoposide (VIP) has been well studied. Phase II trials documented the activity of this regimen [39, 40]. A randomized Japanese study consisting of patients with both limited and extensive SCLC did not detect any survival or response differences with the addition of ifosfamide [41]. In a larger randomized trial, the VIP regimen was evaluated in comparison to EP in patients with previously untreated ED-SCLC [42]. Overall and median survival favored the VIP arm by a small margin, though the response rates were not markedly different. Phase II studies have incorporated carboplatin instead of cisplatin in this regimen with the resultant ICE regimen being used in patients with both limited and extensive disease [43, 44].

29.3.3 Alternating Chemotherapy

One strategy to develop clearly more effective chemotherapy regimens has been to employ alternating "non-cross-resistant" chemotherapy, which might improve tumor cell killing according to the mathematical model described by Goldie and Coldman [45]. This method can potentially overcome drug resistance by exposing tumors to an increased number of active cytotoxic agents.

Multiple randomized trials have attempted to prove this theory. A Canadian trial in 300 patients with LD-SCLC showed a non-significant improvement in complete responses (52% versus 44%, $p=0.20$), but no difference in disease-free or overall survival with alternating CAV/EP as compared with CAV followed by EP [46]. Another Canadian trial in 289 patients with ED-SCLC showed improvements in overall response rates and overall survival with alternating CAV/EP as compared with CAV alone, but it could not be definitively ascertained whether the improvements were due to alternation or due to the superiority of EP over CAV [47]. In a Japanese study of 288 patients with both limited and extensive disease, overall response rates in the EP and CAV/EP arms were superior to the CAV arm [35]. The larger SECSG trial of 437 patients with ED-SCLC demonstrated no differences in either observed responses or overall survival with CAV, EP, or alternating CAV/EP.

An EORTC randomized study evaluated CDE (cyclophosphamide, doxorubicin, and etoposide) alternating with VIMP (vincristine, ifosfamide, mesna, and carboplatin) in ED-SCLC and found no difference in median survival in comparison to standard chemotherapy [48]. Given the lack of consistent clinical benefit, alternating regimens have not gained widespread acceptance in standard practice.

29.3.4 Dose Escalation

Another approach involves increasing doses of chemotherapy in order to enhance response rates and survival. Several randomized trials have evaluated dose-response relationships in SCLC. In the late 1970s and 1980s, studies tested doxorubicin or alkylating agent-based chemotherapy of which only one study demonstrated a modest survival advantage with early dose intensification. Cisplatin-based chemotherapy has been evaluated in limited disease patients in randomized trials with conflicting results. In a French study, 105 patients received a regimen containing cisplatin, cyclophosphamide, doxorubicin, and etoposide. The treatment arms differed in cycle 1 only, with the dose-intense regimen containing cisplatin and doxorubicin at higher doses. Two-year survival rates were 43% and

26% in the dose-intense and standard arms, respectively, whereas there was no difference in toxicities between both arms [49]. A second study at the National Cancer Institute [50] randomized 90 patients to higher-dose EP or standard-dose EP. There was no reported difference in overall survival between the two arms though the dose-intense arm had higher hematologic toxicities. A 1991 meta-analysis could show no demonstrable effect on response rate or survival by increasing dose intensity [51].

29.3.5   Intensive Weekly Dosing

Another approach to dose intensification has been the rapid sequencing of a regimen incorporating several active agents over a short period. One thoroughly studied regimen, CODE, consists of weekly dosing of cisplatin, vincristine, doxorubicin, and etoposide, with the myelosuppressive and non-myelosuppressive agents being alternated. CODE was designed to increase the dose intensity of these four agents in comparison to CAV/EP. A Canadian pilot study reported a 94% overall response rate and 40% complete response rate in 48 patients with ED-SCLC [52]. The median survival was 61 weeks but grade 4 neutropenia occurred in 56% patients and 58% patients required blood transfusions. A confirmatory National Cancer Institute–Canada/Southwestern Oncology Group (SWOG) trial was prematurely closed due to an excess of toxic deaths in the CODE arm [53]. A phase III Japanese trial that randomized patients to CODE plus granulocyte colony-stimulating factor (G-CSF) versus CAV/EP failed to demonstrate any advantage in response rates or survival [54]. On the basis of these randomized trials, there is no role for dose intensification in the standard management of SCLC.

29.3.6   Dose Intensification with Cytokine Support

Dose escalation or frequent dosing when done with the concomitant use of colony-stimulating factors potentially reduces the development of excessive myelosuppression. Studies utilizing G-CSF demonstrated modest improvements in delivered dose intensity and reduction in febrile neutropenia [53, 55] without survival benefits. A randomized study of granulocyte macrophage colony-stimulating factor (GM-CSF) in LD-SCLC [56] had a significantly increased incidence and duration of life-threatening thrombocytopenia and toxic deaths. The increased toxicities were thought to be secondary to a cumulative effect of chest irradiation and GM-CSF.

A British randomized study utilizing chemotherapy consisting of vincristine, ifosfamide, carboplatin, and etoposide (V-ICE) given every 3 or 4 weeks with or without GM-CSF, revealed no difference in the incidence of myelosuppression and febrile neutropenia, though the 2-year survival rates were increased in the dose-intensified arm [57]. Another British randomized trial [58] in 403 patients (302 with LD-SCLC), utilizing doxorubicin, cyclophosphamide, and etoposide (ACE) given every 3 weeks versus every 2 weeks along with G-CSF, showed similar overall responses but higher complete responses (40% versus 28%). A modest 2-year survival benefit (13% versus 8%) was seen in the G-CSF arm and was similar in both LD- and ED-SCLC patients. G-CSF resulted in less neutropenia, but more blood and platelet transfusions were required. An EORTC study evaluated standard CDE given every 3 weeks in comparison to intensified CDE given every 2 weeks with G-CSF support. Although a 70% increase in administered dose intensity was achieved, the response rates (84% versus 79%) and median survival rates (54 weeks versus 52 weeks) were no different between the two arms.

While a few studies have suggested that dose intensification may be worthwhile, the preponderance of evidence from randomized comparisons indicate that comparisons of "high-dose" to "standard-dose" regimens employing the same agents do not produce consistent survival advantages, while toxicity, particularly myelosuppression, is greater with the dose-intense regimens.

29.3.7   Late Intensification with High-dose Chemotherapy

Small-cell lung cancer represents an appropriate disease to study in the context of late intensification with high-dose chemotherapy and autologous hematopoietic support. Multiple small studies in the 1980s demonstrated an enhanced rate of complete responses without obvious survival benefits. In the only randomized trial reported, 45 patients who had responded to induction chemotherapy were randomized to conventional or high-dose chemotherapy with marrow support [59]. Disease-free survival was enhanced, and a trend toward higher median and long-term survival was observed in the high-dose arm. A serious problem with this study was the high toxic death rate of 18%.

In a phase II study in patients with LD-SCLC who achieved complete responses or near-complete responses with conventional chemotherapy, high-dose cyclophosphamide, carmustine, and cisplatin with hematopoietic stem cell support was given, followed by thoracic and prophylactic cranial irradiation. Among 36 treated patients, the median progression-free survival (PFS) was 21 months with a toxic death rate of 8%. Overall 2-year and 5-year progression-free survival rates were 53% and 41%, respectively. In the patients who were in complete response or near-complete response prior to high-dose therapy, these rates were 57% and 53%, respectively. In a feasibility study by the European

Group for Blood and Marrow Transplantation (EBMTR), 69 patients received one to three courses of high-dose ifosfamide, carboplatin, and etoposide (ICE) with stem cell support. The rates for toxic death and febrile neutropenia were 9% and 66%, respectively. There was an 86% response rate (51% complete response). Median survival in patients with limited disease was 18 months, with 2-year survival being 32%; in extensive disease patients the corresponding rates were 11 months and 5%, respectively.

During the last decade, there has been a continual and substantial decline in the morbidity and mortality with high-dose chemotherapy and the upper age for eligible patients in many centers has increased to 65 years. SCLC patients will always have the added factor of potentially increased complications secondary to their smoking history and associated lung damage. Ongoing randomized trials will assist in determining the role of high-dose therapy in the subset of limited SCLC patients with good responses to induction chemotherapy.

29.3.8   Newer Chemotherapy Regimens

The results of the current generation of randomized trials incorporating the newer chemotherapeutic agents into combination regimens have been mixed. The most promising report is the Japanese study [60] in patients with ED-SCLC, which was prematurely closed due to improved response rates and overall survival when the cisplatin plus irinotecan regimen was compared to EP.

Among 154 patients randomized upon this study, there were significant differences in the experimental and standard arms in terms of response rates (84% versus 68%), median overall survival (12.8 months versus 9.4 months), and 2-year survival (19.5% versus 5%), respectively. The results of confirmatory larger studies with this newer regimen are awaited.

Conversely, randomized trials testing the incorporation of paclitaxel into standard regimens for LD-SCLC have failed to show a consistent benefit (Table 29.3). A Greek Lung Cancer Group study comparing paclitaxel, etoposide, and cisplatin (TEP) to standard EP was terminated due to excessive toxicity and mortality in the TEP arm after accruing 133 patients. Response rates were equal in both arms though time to progression was significantly increased in the TEP arm (11 months versus 9 months). There were eight toxic deaths in the TEP group; additionally, TEP was associated with significantly more hematologic toxicity, severe diarrhea, and febrile neutropenia.

A recent study of 614 patients (approximately 50% with LD-SCLC) evaluated paclitaxel, etoposide phosphate, and carboplatin (TEC) in comparison to carboplatin, etoposide, and vincristine (CEV). This study showed modest improvement in median survival in the TEC arm (12.7 months versus 11.7 months) though the benefit was confined to early-stage (I–IIIB) patients (17.6 months versus 16.6 months). In addition, there was less frequent hematologic toxicity with the TEC regimen. Mature results of a third study are not yet reported [61]. Thus, the current standard chemotherapeutic regimen in LD-SCLC, outside of a clinical trial, remains EP.

Table 29.3. Randomized trials of taxane-containing regimens in LD-SCLC

Study author (year)	Patients	Regimen	Stage	Survival	Comments
Reck (2003)	$n=614$ TEC: 305 pts CEV: 309 pts	T 175 mg/m^2 IV, d 4 E 125 mg/m^2 IV, d 1–3 C AUC=5 IV, d 4 vs C AUC=5 IV, d 1 Ep 159 mg/m^2 IV, d 1–3 V 2 mg IV, d 1	LD, ED	12.7 mo vs 11.7 mo ($p=0.024$)	Experimental therapy had decreased hematologic toxicity
Mavroudis (2001)	$n=133$ TEP: 62 pts EP: 71 pts	T 175 mg/m^2 IV, d 1 E 80 mg/m^2 IV, d 2–4 P 80 mg/m^2 IV, d 2 vs E 120 mg/m^2 IV, d 1–3 P 80 mg/m^2 IV, d 1	LD, ED	10.5 mo vs 11.5 mo ($p=$NS)	Experimental arm had more gastrointestinal and hematologic toxicity
Birch (2000)	$n=170$ EC: 86 pts EC+T: 84 pts	E 120 mg/m^2 IV, d 1–3 C AUC=6 IV, d 1 vs Eo 50/100 mg PO, d 1–10 C AUC=6 IV, d 1 T 200 mg/m^2 IV, d 1	LD, ED	Mature data pending	Trend for improved survival in ED (preliminary analysis)

E etoposide, *Ep* etoposide phosphate, *Eo* oral etoposide, *P* cisplatin, *I* irinotecan, *C* carboplatin, *T* paclitaxel, *V* vincristine, *LD* limited disease, *ED* extensive disease, *NS* not significant, *pts* patients, *d* day, *mo* month

29.3.9   Chemotherapy in the Elderly

In some series, age has been a poor prognostic factor in determining outcomes. When chemotherapy for elderly patients is administered, it is often administered at lower doses or for fewer cycles. Due to the infrequent inclusion of elderly patients on SCLC trials, extrapolation of results achieved with younger patients may not be accurate.

Impressive response and survival rates have been reported with the use of single-agent oral etoposide in elderly patients with extensive disease [13]. Accordingly, single-agent chemotherapy was considered as an option for elderly or poor performance status patients. However, two recent randomized trials that compared oral etoposide with intravenous multiagent chemotherapy showed that palliation of symptoms was equivalent or slightly worse with oral etoposide [62, 63]. In addition, both trials showed a small but significant survival benefit associated with multiagent chemotherapy. Thus, single-agent oral etoposide can not be considered a standard of care for elderly patients with SCLC.

29.3.10   Immunologic Approaches

Many patients experience complete responses with concurrent therapy and are thought to possess a minimal tumor burden. These patients are theoretically ideal candidates for adjuvant immunologic approaches. A number of approaches have been evaluated so far with mostly disappointing results.

In some patients with SCLC, poorer survival rates have been associated with the phenomenon of impaired response to delayed cutaneous hypersensitivity testing [64]. Similar observations by other investigators were used as the rationale for investigating biologic response modifiers and other immunologic approaches as adjunctive therapies in SCLC. Patients randomized to receive bacillus Calmette-Guérin (BCG) vaccine after chemotherapy and thoracic radiotherapy showed no improvements in responses or survival in two large studies [65, 66]. Similar disappointing results were obtained in trials evaluating addition of methanol-extractable residue of BCG to standard therapeutic approaches [67–69].

The interferons (IFNs) have been extensively evaluated in SCLC and were felt to offer promise in limited disease patients [70, 71]. Results from a Finnish study, in which responding patients were treated with maintenance IFN-α, showed an improvement in long-term survival in the IFN arm [72]. In two American cooperative group trials, further therapy with additional IFN-α [73] or IFN-γ [74] showed no improvements in responses or survival.

In a pilot study, long-term survivors were reported in SCLC patients vaccinated with the BEC2/BCG vaccine [75]. Results from an EORTC phase III study of therapy with the BEC2/BCG vaccine in responding patients with LD-SCLC were recently made available. In this large study involving 515 patients, there was no significant difference in median survival (16.3 months versus 14.3 months) or progression-free survival (6.6 months versus 5.7 months) among the standard therapy or vaccine-containing arm, respectively. Thus, there is no role for immunotherapy in the current management of SCLC outside of a clinical trial.

29.3.11   Targeted Therapies

A new class of agents, matrix metalloproteinase inhibitors (MMPIs), has been investigated in SCLC. Certain matrix metalloproteinases contribute to tumor progression and metastasis and, in one study, tumoral expression of these proteinases was associated with a negative effect on survival. In a randomized trial of 532 patients (approximately half with LD-SCLC) induction chemotherapy was followed by the MMPI marimastat versus placebo for 2 years. The use of this MMPI did not result in prolongation of survival or time to progression [76]. BAY 12-9566, another MMPI, was compared to placebo in 700 SCLC patients who had responded to chemotherapy [77]. Interim analysis revealed a significantly worse outcome and increased adverse events for patients receiving MMPI therapy, leading to early termination of the trial. Other targeted agents being investigated include bcl2 antisense drugs in combination with chemotherapy and platelet-derived growth factor (PDGF)-directed therapy with the tyrosine kinase inhibitor imatinib.

29.3.12   Summary

The introduction of combination chemotherapy as standard therapy for SCLC has contributed to significant improvements in survival in limited disease. Unfortunately, the initial enthusiasm generated by these significant therapeutic advances has waned with the realization that a plateau has been reached and no major survival increments have been gained recently. While a number of chemotherapy regimens may be equivalent to EP or EC, alternating or dose-intense regimens have not gained widespread acceptance. Four to six cycles of EP or EC without maintenance therapy appears sufficient by today's standards. If confirmed, the improvement in responses and survival with the cisplatin–irinotecan regimen would be a welcome addition to the current therapeutic armamentarium for SCLC. On the whole, it remains to be seen whether the newer chemotherapy combinations in combination with targeted therapies will move us away from this therapeutic plateau.

29.4   Surgery

Studies in the 1960s demonstrated that surgical resection alone is not a reasonable option for the management of SCLC. The role for surgery needs to be reconsidered in the context of current multimodality therapy which provides excellent response rates in LD-SCLC.

There are several theoretical advantages with the incorporation of surgery into multimodality management of LD-SCLC. Surgery conveys prognostic significance by improving staging information, may reduce local recurrences, does not limit chemotherapy intensity, and, unlike radiotherapy, there are no myelosuppressive side effects. A moderate amount of data exists on the use of surgery in the context of adjuvant and neoadjuvant chemotherapy in LD-SCLC.

29.4.1   Surgery Followed by Adjuvant Chemotherapy

Of lung cancers presenting as a solitary pulmonary nodule (SPN), 4–12% turned out to be SCLC in one report [78]. In a single-institution report, 4% (15/408) of SCLC patients were found to have presented as a SPN [79]. While there exist no controlled data, long-term survival rates of patients with SCLC-SPN who undergo surgical resection are impressive, relative to other groups of SCLC patients. Pooled data from available studies show that among SCLC-SPN patients with stage I SCLC treated with surgical resection, 40–53% survived for 5 years [78]. The role of postoperative therapy in such patients is somewhat unclear. While most resected patients received postoperative chemotherapy, some did not and still enjoy a prolonged disease-free survival. Nonetheless, in recognition of the systemic nature of most SCLC, most authorities recommend that resected SCLC-SPN patients should receive adjuvant chemotherapy with an established combination regimen. However, there exist no controlled data to definitively establish this point. Similarly, there are no data regarding the efficacy of thoracic radiation or prophylactic cranial irradiation in this setting, although it is reasonable to consider such therapy in the context of potentially curative therapy for such patients.

Impressive long-term survival rates have been reported for patients with early SCLC undergoing surgical resection. The data suggest that patients with stage I–II SCLC have a 27–42% chance of 5-year survival following resection. Long-term survival was less common among patients with more advanced disease. In a recent prospective, multicenter Japanese study utilizing postoperative adjuvant EP chemotherapy in 61 patients, impressive overall survival rates were observed with the 5-year survival being 57%. The 5-year survival rates of patients with stage I, stage II, and stage IIIA SCLC were 69%, 38%, and 40%, respectively [80]. In a follow-up

report, the same group reported a more than threefold higher rate of distant versus local recurrences in this group. A recent retrospective analysis compared outcomes of 67 LD-SCLC patients undergoing surgery and adjuvant chemotherapy to that of matched controls undergoing conventional treatment. The median survival was improved in the surgical group (22 months versus 11 months, $p<0.001$) as was the rate of local control (85% versus 45%, $p<0.001$). Local control rates thus seem to be vastly improved with the incorporation of surgery in early SCLC.

Whether the encouraging trends in resectable SCLC reflect a beneficial effect of the surgery itself or whether it reflects a reduced tumor burden among patients in whom resection is possible remains unknown. Nonetheless, such data support continued investigation of the role of surgical resection following by chemotherapy and possible radiotherapy in early-stage SCLC.

29.4.2   Chemotherapy Followed by Surgery

Most of the available data for surgical resection following neoadjuvant chemotherapy are from small phase II trials. In a review of the results of nine trials including 260 limited disease patients treated with neoadjuvant chemotherapy followed by consideration of resection among responders to initial therapy, the overall chemotherapy response rates were at least 88% in eight of the nine trials [81]. Approximately 60% of patients were taken to surgery, and about 80% of these patients underwent complete resection (approximately 50% of those entering the trials). In completely resected patients with pathologic stage I SCLC, the 5-year survival rate approached 70%. For patients with stage II–IIIA SCLC, survival was less favorable, but there were cohorts who achieved long-term disease-free survival.

In a randomized study by the Lung Cancer Study Group, the role of surgical resection was evaluated in 340 LD-SCLC patients (ISS stages I–IIIB) [82]. All patients initially received five cycles of CAV chemotherapy. Those patients who were judged to be suitable for resection were then randomized to surgery followed by thoracic radiation and prophylactic cranial irradiation, or to an identical regimen of radiation treatment without surgery. Of all patients, 66% responded to induction chemotherapy (28% complete and 38% partial responses). A total of 144 (42%) patients were randomized, 68 to the surgery arm and 76 to no surgery. No significant differences in median or overall survival were observed between the two groups. Median survival of all patients was 14 months, while it was 18 months for those patients who were randomized. Actuarial 2-year survival was 20% in both arms. Accordingly, the study failed to provide any support for the use of surgical resection in limited SCLC.

Presently, surgery can be considered an option for only certain subgroups of SCLC patients. Available evidence from non-randomized studies supports a role for resection in well-staged patients with stage I (T1–T2 lesions), and possibly some patients with stage II disease as well. Patients with involved mediastinal lymph nodes at surgery should be considered for adjuvant thoracic irradiation also. For LD-SCLC patients with stage IIIA–IIIB disease, surgery should not currently be included in their management. Unfortunately, such patients represent the vast majority and thus surgery is not indicated for most patients with LD-SCLC currently.

29.5   Thoracic Irradiation

29.5.1   Randomized Trials

In SCLC, thoracic irradiation alone produces responses in the vast majority of patients. Locoregional failure within the chest occurs in up to 80% of limited disease patients treated with chemotherapy alone [83]. This high rate of local failure provides a rationale for the use of thoracic irradiation in patients with the objectives of improving both local control and overall survival. Several randomized trials have been conducted and a review of these studies has revealed certain conclusions regarding chemotherapy and thoracic irradiation. All studies almost uniformly demonstrated that thoracic irradiation significantly decreases the rate of local failure in SCLC. Combined modality therapy also invariably increases hematologic, pulmonary, and esophageal complications.

The role of thoracic irradiation in SCLC was assessed in a comprehensive fashion in two meta-analyses [84, 85]. Thirteen randomized trials, including over 2,100 limited-stage patients, were included in the larger meta-analysis [85]. Chemotherapy regimens differed between studies as well as radiation doses and schedules. Both reports demonstrate that the addition of thoracic irradiation was associated with a 5–7% improvement in 2-year and 3-year survival rates. Local control rates were more impressively improved by 25%. Overall, local control was observed in 23% (172/737) of patients receiving chemotherapy alone compared to 48% (376/784) for patients who were treated with chemoradiation [84]. The survival benefit was greatest for patients who were less than 55 years of age and was achieved at the cost of increased toxicity among patients receiving thoracic irradiation.

29.5.2   Optimal Chemotherapy with Thoracic Irradiation

Combined modality protocols in randomized studies have evaluated alkylator-based, doxorubicin-based, or platinum-based regimens administered concurrently with thoracic irradiation. The EP regimen is more mucosa-sparing, less myelosuppressive, and has lower cardiac and pulmonary toxicity. Several pilot trials with this approach suggested an improvement in long-term outcome, compared with trials included in the meta-analyses. Results from Japanese and American randomized studies of thoracic irradiation in combination with EP showed consistent and significant improvement in survival rates in excess of 40% at 2 years. In some centers, carboplatin is utilized in place of cisplatin with a view to ease of administration and perceived lesser toxicities. Equivalent response and survival results have been obtained for both EP or EC. Currently, however, the reference arms for most clinical trials continue to utilize the EP regimen.

Building on the improvements in long-term outcome with EP and concurrent radiotherapy, the current emphasis involves evaluating the possibility of enhancing results by adding newer cytotoxic drugs to the existing regimens. This includes adding newer drugs such as the taxanes to standard chemotherapy regimens. Increased locoregional control at the cost of increased esophageal toxicity has been seen in early reports. It remains to be seen whether these results translate into improved long-term survival compared to that obtained with EP and radiation. Definite randomized trials will be needed to fully assess the impact of these newer regimens.

29.5.3   Timing of Radiation

Methods of combining thoracic irradiation with chemotherapy include:
1. Radiotherapy given with the initiation of chemotherapy
2. Induction chemotherapy followed by radiotherapy during subsequent courses
3. Chemotherapy followed sequentially by radiotherapy
4. Radiotherapy administered split between cycles of chemotherapy

Table 29.4 summarizes the randomized trials evaluating the issue of timing of thoracic irradiation in the context of delivery of chemotherapy. Previous randomized trials utilizing doxorubicin-based or alkylator-based chemotherapy, which specifically addressed this issue, have demonstrated conflicting findings. The meta-analysis by Pignon et al. [85] did not find any statistically significant differences in the timing of radiation relative to the delivery of chemotherapy. Recent trials have used

Table 29.4. Randomized trials addressing thoracic irradiation timing

Study author (year)	Chemotherapy regimen	RT timing	Number of patients	RT dose/fractions	OS at 2 years	Median survival (months)
Perry (1987)	CAVE for 18 months	Cycle 1 vs cycle 4	270	50 Gy/24	24% vs 30%	13.1 vs 14.6
Murray (1993)	CAV/EP×total 6 cycles	Cycle 2 vs cycle 6	308	40 Gy/15	40% vs 33%	21.2 vs 16
Work (1997)	EP×3 cycles plus CAV×6 cycles	Cycle 1 vs cycle 6	199	40–45 Gy/22	20% vs 19%	10.5 vs 12
Jeremic (1997)	EC with RT, plus EP×4 cycles	Cycle 1 vs cycle 3	107	54 Gy/18 BID	30% vs 15%	34 vs 26
Gregor (1997)	CDE×6 cycles	After cycle 2 vs after cycle 5	335	50 Gy/20	25.9% vs 23%	14 vs 15
Skarlos (2001)	EC×6 cycles	Cycle 1 vs cycle 4	81	45 Gy/15 BID	35.7% vs 28.2%	17.5 vs 17
Takada (2002)	EP×4 cycles	Cycle 1 vs after cycle 4	228	45 Gy/15 BID	31% vs 21%	27.2 vs 19.7

CAVE cyclophosphamide, doxorubicin, etoposide, vincristine, *CAV* cyclophosphamide, doxorubicin, vincristine, *EP* etoposide, cisplatin, *EC* etoposide, carboplatin, *CDE* cyclophosphamide, doxorubicin, etoposide, *Gy* gray (rads), *RT* radiation therapy, *BID* twice-daily radiation

EP or EC compared with radiation in the second versus sixth cycle of chemotherapy [86], in the first versus the third cycle [87], or in the first cycle versus sequential after the fourth cycle [88]. A more recent meta-analysis that included trials utilizing platinum-based chemotherapy revealed a significant improvement in 2-year overall survival for early versus delayed thoracic radiotherapy. The authors concluded that the magnitude of benefit was similar to that of adding radiation to chemotherapy or that of prophylactic cranial irradiation. Additionally, a greater benefit was seen for hyperfractionated radiation and platinum-based chemotherapy. Thus, the current weight of evidence favors concurrent thoracic irradiation initiated relatively early on with the first or second cycle of platinum-based chemotherapy.

29.5.4 Radiation Target Volume

The recommendation for standard radiation portals includes the original tumor volume with a 1.5- to 2.0-cm-free margin and is on the basis of retrospective studies. Conflicting data from these studies have suggested a twofold to threefold increase in thoracic recurrences with the use of reduced volume radiotherapy. However, a randomized trial by the South West Oncology Group addressing this issue did not reveal any differences in the intrathoracic recurrence rate with the use of wide volume radiotherapy in comparison to reduced volume radiotherapy [89]. It is not certain whether radiation portals should be designed based on the original tumor volume and uninvolved nodes, or on the shrinking volume present following a response to chemotherapy. A review of this issue [90] found no compelling evidence supporting either strategy.

29.5.5 Radiation Dose

For the past three decades, the commonly utilized dose of thoracic radiotherapy in limited SCLC has remained between 40 and 50 Gy. Presumably since SCLC is typically much more responsive to radiotherapy, the doses utilized have been lower than those used in NSCLC. However, even with current chemoradiation approaches local "in-field" recurrence rates are in the order of 30%. Most of the data addressing this issue are in the form of retrospective analyses. One retrospective study found that local failure rates for doses below 40 Gy were over 50% while those for doses between 40 and 50 Gy were 30% [91]. A study using a total radiotherapy dose of 60 Gy reported a local failure rate of only 3% [92]. In an attempt to better define the dose of thoracic radiotherapy, a cooperative group trial identified 70 Gy as the maximum tolerated dose when given in a once-daily fashion [93]. Current US cooperative group trials have started utilizing higher doses of thoracic irradiation (60–63 Gy).

29.5.6 Radiation Fractionation

Conventional radiation fractionation is administered as 1.8- to 2.0-Gy daily fractions, administered over a 5-week period. In contrast, hyperfractionation in SCLC utilizes twice-daily fractions of a lower dose of radiation, administered over a shorter 3-week period [94]. This approach results in reduction in late-effect injury and increased damage upon rapidly proliferating subpopulations of cancer cells that divide within the 24-h time interval. A number of phase II studies have suggested that hyperfractionation schedules may produce an advantage in terms of local control and possibly survival compared to standard once-daily fractionation schedules [95, 96].

Results from two large, randomized trials provide supporting data for dose-intensive radiation as a means for improving both locoregional control and long-term overall survival. In a large intergroup trial [96] involving 417 patients with LD-SCLC, overall survival was 47% at 2 years and 26% at 5 years with twice-daily accelerated radiation (45 Gy over 3 weeks) given concurrently with cycle 1 of EP. Survival rates in patients treated with standard once-daily radiation (45 Gy over 5 weeks) were 41% at 2 years and 19% at 5 years. After a median follow-up of 8 years, median survival in the twice- and once-daily groups was 23 and 19 months, respectively. The incidence of grade 3 esophagitis with accelerated radiotherapy was higher. Interestingly, survival rates in both arms were better than the 23% 2-year survival revealed in the meta-analyses.

The other randomized study examined the role of concurrent, twice-daily split-course irradiation compared to conventional once-daily irradiation in limited-stage disease patients responding after three cycles of EP [97]. A 2.5-week break after 24 Gy of hyperfractionated radiotherapy resulted in a similar dose intensity of radiation in both arms, with 48–50 Gy being delivered over 6 weeks. There were no differences with regard to locoregional control, median survival, and overall survival at 3 years. The possibility therefore arises that superior outcomes in the intergroup trial were actually a manifestation of accelerated radiation than hyperfractionation itself.

In a randomized European study comparing early versus delayed hyperfractionated radiation in limited SCLC, 30% 5-year survival was achieved with radiation given early with concurrent EC chemotherapy followed by EP chemotherapy alone [87]. However, the rates for severe esophagitis in this study were 29% and 25% in the early- and late-radiation arms, respectively, thus illustrating again the increased toxicity associated with hyperfractionated therapy.

Accelerated hyperfractionated radiotherapy is an interesting approach to management of limited SCLC. Improvement in local control and survival achieved so far are at the cost of higher acute but decreased late toxicities making it difficult to incorporate it as standard of care in the community setting.

29.5.7 Current Perspective

With the benefits of improved local control and overall survival, thoracic irradiation is firmly established as an integral component of combined modality therapy of LD-SCLC. Issues of timing, volume, and optimal chemotherapy have been largely addressed by the available data. Ongoing investigation into hyperfractionation, increased dosing, additional chemotherapy, and the use of mucoprotective agents should lead to significant refinements in the current standard delivery of thoracic irradiation.

Currently, the standard approach is to consider early integration of thoracic irradiation (first or second cycle of chemotherapy onward) with systemic platinum-based chemotherapy. Standard dosing of 45–50 Gy delivered to original tumor volume is an acceptable approach. The use of hyperfractionated radiotherapy or larger doses of radiotherapy, outside the setting of clinical trials, has currently not been adopted even though associated with promising long-term outcomes.

29.6 Summary

The use of combination chemotherapy for SCLC has contributed to significant improvements in local control and survival in limited-stage disease. The initial enthusiasm generated by these significant therapeutic advances has waned with the realization that a plateau has been reached and no additional survival increments have been gained in the last decade. While a number of chemotherapy regimens may be equivalent to EP or EC, alternating regimens or dose-intense regimens have not gained widespread acceptance. The role for thoracic irradiation and prophylactic cranial irradiation in LD-SCLC has been firmly established. What remains to be determined is whether chemotherapy combinations incorporating some of the newer "targeted" agents will move us away from this therapeutic plateau.

Key Points

- The role of chemotherapy in the management of limited disease small-cell lung cancer (LD-SCLC) is well established. Dose intensification does not improve survival.
- Late intensification with high-dose chemotherapy and autologous hematopoietic support holds promise for a therapeutic advance.
- The role of surgery as part of a treatment regimen is being reexamined and may be of benefit.
- Concurrent thoracic irradiation should be administered with the first or second cycle of platinum-based chemotherapy.
- Prophylactic cranial irradiation should be incorporated into the management of completely responding patients with LD-SCLC.

References

1. Mulshine JL, Treston AM, Brown HP, Birrer MJ, Shaw GL. Initiators and promoters of lung cancer. Chest 1993; 103(suppl 1):4S.
2. Ihde DC, Pass HI, Glatstein EJ. Small cell lung cancer. In: DeVita V, Hellman S, Rosenberg S, eds. Cancer: principles and practice of oncology. Philadelphia: Lippincott, 1993:723.
3. Janne PA, Freidlin B, Saxman S, et al. Twenty-five years of clinical research for patients with limited-stage small cell lung carcinoma in North America. Cancer 2002; 95:1528.
4. Archer VE, Saccomanno G, Jones JH. Frequency of different histologic types of bronchogenic carcinoma as related to radiation exposure. Cancer 1974; 34:2056.
5. Paesmans M, Sculier JP, Lecomte J, et al. Prognostic factors for patients with small cell lung carcinoma: analysis of a series of 763 patients included in 4 consecutive prospective trials with a minimum follow-up of 5 years. Cancer 2000; 89:523.
6. Medical Research Council of Great Britain. Working party on the evaluation of different methods of therapy in carcinoma of the bronchus: comparative trial of surgery and radiotherapy for primary treatment of small celled or oat celled carcinoma of the bronchus. Lancet 1966; 2:979.
7. Fox W, Scadding JG. Medical Research Council comparative trial of surgery and radiotherapy for primary treatment of small cell or oat cell carcinoma of the bronchus: ten-year follow-up. Lancet 1973; 2:63.
8. Martini N, Wittes RE, Hilaris BS. Oat cell carcinoma of the lung. Clin Bull 1975; 5:144.
9. Mountain CF, Carr DT, Anderson WA. A system for the clinical staging of lung cancer. AJR Am J Roentgenol 1974; 120:130.
10. Mountain CF. Clinical biology of small cell carcinoma: relationship to surgical therapy. Semin Oncol 1978; 5:272.
11. Green RA, Humphrey E, Close H, et al. Alkylating agents in bronchogenic carcinoma. Am J Med 1969; 46:515.
12. Grant SC, Gralla RJ, Kris MG, et al. Single-agent chemotherapy trials in small-cell lung cancer, 1970–1990: the case for studies in previously treated patients. J Clin Oncol 1992; 10:484.
13. Carney DN, Grogan L, Smit EF, et al. Single-agent oral etoposide for elderly small cell lung cancer patients. Semin Oncol 1990; 17(suppl 2):49.
14. Issell BF, Einhorn LH, Comis RL, et al. Multicenter phase II trial of etoposide in previously treated small cell carcinoma of the lung. Cancer Treat Rep 1985; 69:127.
15. Smith IE, Harland SJ, Robinson BA, et al. Carboplatin: a very active new cisplatin analog in the treatment of small cell lung cancer. Cancer Treat Rep 1985; 69:43.
16. Schiller JH, Kim K, Hutson P, et al. Phase II study of topotecan in patients with extensive-stage small cell carcinoma of the lung. J Clin Oncol 1996; 14:2345.
17. von Pawel J, Schiller JH, Sheperd FA, et al. Topotecan vs cyclophosphamide, doxorubicin, and vincristine for the treatment of recurrent small-cell lung cancer. J Clin Oncol 1999; 17:658.
18. Negoro S, Fukuoka M, Niitani H, et al. Phase II study of CPT-11, new campothecin derivative, in small-cell lung cancer (SCLC) (abstract). Proc Am Soc Clin Oncol 1991; 10:241.
19. Masuda N, Fukuoka M, Kusunoki Y, et al. CPT-11: a new derivative of campothecin for the treatment of refractory or relapsed small-cell lung cancer. J Clin Oncol 1992; 10:122.
20. Ettinger DS, Finkelstein DM, Sarma RP, et al. Phase II study of paclitaxel in patients with extensive-disease small-cell lung cancer: an Eastern Cooperative Oncology Group study. J Clin Oncol 1995; 13:1430.
21. Kirschling RJ, Jung Sh, Jett JT, et al. A phase II trial of taxol and G-CSF in previously untreated patients with extensive stage small-cell lung cancer (SCC) (abstract). Proc Am Soc Clin Oncol 1994; 13:326.
22. Smyth JF, Smith TB, Sessa C, et al. Activity of docetaxel (Taxotere) in small-cell lung cancer. Eur J Cancer 1994:30A:1058.
23. Jassem J, Karnicka-Mlodkowska H, van Pottelsberghe CH, et al. Phase II study of vinorelbine (Navelbine) in previously treated small-cell lung cancer patients. Eur J Cancer 1993; 29A:1720.
24. Furuse K, Kubota K, Kawahara M, et al. Phase II study of vinorelbine in heavily previously treated small-cell lung cancer. Oncology 1996; 53:169.
25. Cormier Y, Eisenhauer B, Muldal A, et al. Gemcitabine: an active new agent in previously untreated extensive stage small-cell lung cancer (SCLC). Ann Oncol 1994; 5:283.
26. Lowenbraun S, Bartolucci A, Smalley RV, et al. The superiority of combination chemotherapy over single agent chemotherapy in small cell lung carcinoma. Cancer 1979; 44:406.
27. Aisner J, Alberto P, Bitran J, et al. Role of chemotherapy in small cell lung cancer: a consensus report of the International Association for the Study of Lung Cancer workshop. Cancer Treat Rep 1983; 67:37.
28. Jett JR, Everson L, Therneau TM, et al. Treatment of limited-stage small-cell lung cancer with cyclophosphamide, doxorubicin, and vincristine with or without etoposide: a randomized trial of the North Central Cancer Treatment Group. J Clin Oncol 1990; 8:33.
29. Jackson DV Jr, Case LD, Zekan PJ, et al. Improvement of long-term survival in extensive small-cell lung cancer. J Clin Oncol 1988; 6:1161.
30. Messeih AA, Schweitzer JM, Lipton A, et al. Addition of etoposide to cyclophosphamide, doxorubicin, and vincristine for remission induction and survival in patients with small cell lung cancer. Cancer Treat Rep 1987; 71:61.
31. Bunn PA Jr, Greco FA, Einhorn L. Cyclophosphamide, doxorubicin, and etoposide as first-line therapy in the treatment of small-cell lung cancer. Semin Oncol 1986; 13(suppl 3):45.
32. Evans WK, Sheperd FA, Feld R, et al. VP-16 and cisplatin as first-line therapy for small cell lung cancer. J Clin Oncol 1985; 3:1471.

33. Porter LL, Johnson DH, Hainsworth JD, et al. Cisplatin and etoposide combination chemotherapy for refractory small cell carcinoma of the lung. Cancer Treat Rep 1985; 69:479.

34. Aisner J, Abrams J. Cisplatin for small cell lung cancer. Semin Oncol 1989; 16:2.

35. Fukuoka M, Furuse K, Saijo N, et al. Randomized trial of cyclophosphamide, doxorubicin, and vincristine versus cisplatin and etoposide versus alternation of these regimens in small-cell lung cancer. J Natl Cancer Inst 1991; 83:855.

36. Roth BJ, Johnson DH, Einhorn LH, et al. Randomized study of cyclophosphamide, doxorubicin, and vincristine versus etoposide and cisplatin versus alternation of these two regimens in extensive small-cell lung cancer: a phase III trial of the Southeastern Cancer Study Group. J Clin Oncol 1992; 10:282.

37. Sundstrom S, Bremnes RM, Kaasa S, et al. Cisplatin and etoposide regimen is superior to cyclophosphamide, epirubicin, and vincristine regimen in small-cell lung cancer: results from a randomized phase III trial with 5 years' follow-up. J Clin Oncol 2002; 20:4665.

38. Skarlos DV, Samantas E, Kosmidis P, et al. Randomized comparison of etoposide-cisplatin vs. etoposide-carboplatin and irradiation in small-cell lung cancer. A Hellenic Co-operative Oncology Group study. Ann Oncol 1994; 5:601.

39. Evans WK, Stewart DJ, Shepherd FA, et al. VP-16, ifosfamide and cisplatin (VIP) for extensive small cell lung cancer. Eur J Cancer 1994; 30A:299.

40. Loehrer PJ Sr, Rynard S, Ansari R, et al. Etoposide, ifosfamide, and cisplatin in extensive small cell lung cancer. Cancer 1992; 69:669.

41. Miyamoto H, Nakabayashi T, Isobe H, et al. A phase III comparison of etoposide/cisplatin with or without added ifosfamide in small-cell lung cancer. Oncology 1992; 49:431.

42. Loehrer PJ, Ansari R, Gonin R, et al. Cisplatin plus etoposide with and without ifosfamide in extensive small-cell lung cancer: a Hoosier Oncology Group study. J Clin Oncol 1995; 13:2594.

43. Smith IE, Perren TJ, Ashley SA, et al. Carboplatin, etoposide, and ifosfamide as intensive chemotherapy for small-cell lung cancer. J Clin Oncol 1990; 8:899.

44. Wolff AC, Ettinger DS, Neuberg D, et al. Phase II study of ifosfamide, carboplatin, and oral etoposide chemotherapy for extensive-disease small-cell lung cancer: an Eastern Cooperative Oncology Group pilot study. J Clin Oncol 1995; 13:1615.

45. Goldie JH, Coldman AJ. A mathematical model for relating sensitivity of tumors to their spontaneous mutation rate. Cancer Treat Rep 1979; 63:1727.

46. Feld R, Evans WK, Coy P, et al. Canadian multicenter randomized trial comparing sequential and alternating administration of two non-cross-resistant chemotherapy combinations in patients with limited small-cell carcinoma of the lung. J Clin Oncol 1987; 5:1401.

47. Evans WK, Feld R, Murray N, et al. Superiority of alternating non-cross-resistant chemotherapy in extensive small cell lung cancer. A multicenter, randomized clinical trial by the National Cancer Institute of Canada. Ann Intern Med 1987; 107:451.

48. Postmus PE, Scagliotti G, Groen HJ, et al. Standard versus alternating non-cross-resistant chemotherapy in extensive small cell lung cancer: an EORTC phase III trial. Eur J Cancer 1996; 32A:1498.

49. Arriagada R, Le Chevalier T, Pignon JP, et al. Initial chemotherapeutic doses and survival in patients with limited small-cell lung cancer. N Engl J Med 1993; 329:1848.

50. Ihde DC, Mulshine JL, Kramer BS, et al. Prospective randomized comparison of high-dose and standard-dose etoposide and cisplatin chemotherapy in patients with extensive-stage small-cell lung cancer. J Clin Oncol 1994; 12:2022.

51. Klasa RJ, Murray N, Coldman AJ. Dose intensity meta-analysis of chemotherapy regimens in small cell carcinoma of the lung. J Clin Oncol 1991; 9:499.

52. Murray N, Shah A, Osoba D, et al. Intensive weekly chemotherapy for the treatment of extensive-stage small-cell lung cancer. J Clin Oncol 1991; 9:1632.

53. Miles DW, Fogarty O, Ash CM, et al. Received dose-intensity: a randomized trial of weekly chemotherapy with and without granulocyte colony-stimulating factor in small-cell lung cancer. J Clin Oncol 1994; 12:77.

54. Furuse K, Fukuoka M, Nishiwaki Y, et al. Phase III study of intensive weekly chemotherapy with recombinant human granulocyte colony-stimulating factor versus standard chemotherapy in extensive-disease small-cell lung cancer. The Japan Clinical Oncology Group. J Clin Oncol 1998; 16:2126.

55. Trillet-Lenoir V, Green J, Manegold C, et al. Recombinant granulocyte colony stimulating factor reduces the infectious complications of cytotoxic chemotherapy. Eur J Cancer 1993; 29A:319.

56. Bunn PA Jr, Crowley J, Kelly K, et al. Chemoradiotherapy with or without granulocyte-macrophage colony-stimulating factor in the treatment of limited-stage small-cell lung cancer: a prospective phase III randomized study of the Southwest Oncology Group. J Clin Oncol 1995; 13:1632.

57. Steward P, von Pawel J, Gatzemeier U, et al. Effects of granulocyte-macrophage colony-stimulating factor and dose intensification of V-ICE chemotherapy in small-cell lung cancer: a prospective randomized study of 300 patients. J Clin Oncol 1998; 16:642.

58. Thatcher N, Girling DJ, Hopwood P, et al. Improving survival without reducing quality of life in small-cell lung cancer patients by increasing the dose-intensity of chemotherapy with granulocyte colony-stimulating factor support: results of a British Medical Research Council Multicenter Randomized Trial. Medical Research Council Lung Cancer Working Party. J Clin Oncol 2000; 18:395.

59. Humblet Y, Symann M, Bosly A, et al. Late intensification chemotherapy with autologous bone marrow transplantation in selected small-cell carcinoma of the lung: a randomized study. J Clin Oncol 1987; 5:1864.

60. Noda K, Nishiwaki Y, Kawahara M, et al. Irinotecan plus cisplatin compared with etoposide plus cisplatin for extensive small-cell lung cancer. N Engl J Med 2002; 346:85.

61. Birch R, Greco F, Hainsworth J, et al. Preliminary results of a randomized study comparing etoposide and carboplatin with or without paclitaxel in newly diagnosed small cell lung cancer (abstract). Proc Am Soc Clin Oncol 2000; 19:490.

62. Medical Research Council Lung Cancer Working Party. Comparison of oral etoposide and standard intravenous multidrug chemotherapy for small-cell lung cancer: a stopped multicentre randomized trial. Lancet 1996; 348:563.

63. Souhami RL, Spiro SG, Rudd RM, et al. Five-day oral etoposide treatment for advanced small-cell lung cancer: randomized comparison with intravenous chemotherapy. J Natl Cancer Inst 1997; 89:577.

64. Johnston-Early A, Cohen MH, Fossieck BE Jr, et al. Delayed hypersensitivity skin testing as a prognostic indicator in patients with small cell lung cancer. Cancer 1983; 52:1395.

65. McCracken JD, Heilbrun L, White J, et al. Combination chemotherapy, radiotherapy, and BCG immunotherapy in

extensive (metastatic) small cell carcinoma of the lung. A Southwest Oncology Group study. Cancer 1980; 46:2335.

66. McCracken JD, Chen T, White J, et al. Combination chemotherapy, radiotherapy, and BCG immunotherapy in limited small-cell carcinoma of the lung: a Southwest Oncology Group Study. Cancer 1982; 49:2252.

67. Aisner J, Wiernik PH. Chemotherapy versus chemoimmunotherapy for small-cell undifferentiated carcinoma of the lung. Cancer 1980; 46:2543.

68. Jackson DV Jr, Paschal BR, Ferree C, et al. Combination chemotherapy-radiotherapy with and without the methanol-extraction residue of bacillus Calmette-Guérin (MER) in small cell carcinoma of the lung: a prospective randomized trial of the Piedmont Oncology Association. Cancer 1982; 50:48.

69. Maurer LH, Pajak T, Eaton W, et al. Combined modality therapy with radiotherapy, chemotherapy, and immunotherapy in limited small-cell carcinoma of the lung: a phase III Cancer and Leukemia Group B Study. J Clin Oncol 1985; 3:969.

70. Olesen BK, Ernst P, Nissen MH, et al. Recombinant interferon A (IFL-rA) therapy of small cell and squamous cell carcinoma of the lung. A phase II study. Eur J Cancer Clin Oncol 1987; 23:987.

71. Newman HF, Bleehen NM, Galazka A, et al. Small cell lung carcinoma. A phase II evaluation of r-interferon-γ. Cancer 1987; 60:2938.

72. Mattson K, Niiranen A, Holsti L, et al. Low-dose of natural α-interferon as maintenance therapy for small cell lung cancer: a phase III study (abstract). Proc Am Soc Clin Oncol 1989; 8:227.

73. Kelly K, Crowley JJ, Bunn PA Jr, et al. Role of recombinant interferon alfa-2a maintenance in patients with limited-stage small-cell lung cancer responding to concurrent chemoradiation: a Southwest Oncology Group study. J Clin Oncol 1995; 13:2924.

74. Jett JR, Maksymiuk AW, Su JQ, et al. Phase III trial of recombinant interferon gamma in complete responders with small-cell lung cancer. J Clin Oncol 1994; 12:2321.

75. Grant SC, Kris MG, Houghton AN, et al. Long-term survival of patients with small cell lung cancer after adjuvant treatment with the anti-idiotypic antibody BEC2 plus bacillus Calmette-Guérin. Clin Cancer Res 1999; 5:1319.

76. Shepherd FA, Giaccone G, Seymour L, et al. Prospective, randomized, double-blind, placebo-controlled trial of marimastat after response to first-line chemotherapy in patients with small-cell lung cancer: a trial of the National Cancer Institute of Canada–Clinical Trials Group and the European Organization for Research and Treatment of Cancer. J Clin Oncol 2002; 20:4434.

77. Rigas JR, Denham CA, Rinaldi DA, et al. Randomized placebo-controlled trials of the matrix metalloproteinase inhibitor (MMPI), BAY12-9566 as adjuvant therapy for patients with small cell and non-small cell lung cancer. Proc Am Soc Clin Oncol 2003; 22:628

78. Kreisman H, Wolkove N, Quoix E. Small cell lung cancer presenting as a solitary pulmonary nodule. Chest 1992; 101:225.

79. Quoix E, Fraser R, Wolkove N, et al. Small cell lung cancer presenting as a solitary pulmonary nodule. Cancer 1990; 66:577.

80. Suzuki K, Tsuchiya R, Ichinose Y, et al. Phase II trial of postoperative adjuvant cisplatin/etoposide (PE) in patients with completely resected stage I–IIIA small cell lung cancer: the Japan Clinical Oncology Group Lung Cancer Study Group trial (JCOG9101) (abstract). Proc Am Soc Clin Oncol 2000; 19:492a.

81. Shepherd FA. Role of surgery in the management of small cell lung cancer. In: Aisner J, Arriagada R, Green MR, Martini N, Perry MC, eds. Comprehensive textbook of thoracic oncology. Baltimore: Williams and Wilkins, 1996:439.

82. Lad T, Piantadosi S, Thomas P, et al. A prospective randomized trial to determine the benefit of surgical resection of residual disease following response of small cell lung cancer to combination chemotherapy. Chest 1994; 106(suppl):320S.

83. Cohen MH, Ihde DC, Bunn PA, et al. Cyclic alternating combination chemotherapy for small cell bronchogenic carcinoma. Cancer Treat Rep 1979; 62:163.

84. Warde P, Payne D. Does thoracic radiation improve survival and local control in limited-stage small cell carcinoma of the lung? J Clin Oncol 1992; 10:890.

85. Pignon JP, Arriagada R, Ihde DC, et al. A meta-analysis of thoracic radiotherapy for small-cell lung cancer. N Engl J Med 1992; 327:1618.

86. Perry MC, Eato WL, Propert KJ, et al. Chemotherapy with or without radiation therapy in limited small-cell carcinoma of the lung. New Engl J Med 1987; 316:912.

87. Jeremic B, Shibamoto Y, Acimovic L, et al. Initial versus delayed accelerated hyperfractionated radiotherapy and concurrent chemotherapy in limited small-cell lung cancer: A randomized study. J Clin Oncol 1997; 15:893.

88. Takada M, Fukuoka M, Kawahara M, et al. Phase III study of concurrent versus sequential thoracic radiotherapy in combination with cisplatin and etoposide for limited-stage small-cell lung cancer: results of the Japan Clinical Oncology Group Study 9104. J Clin Oncol 2002; 20:3054.

89. Kies MS, Mira JC, Crowley JJ, et al. Multimodal therapy for limited small cell lung cancer. A randomized study of induction combination chemotherapy with or without thoracic radiation in complete responders; and with wide-field versus reduced volume radiation in partial responders: a Southwest Oncology Group study. J Clin Oncol 1987; 5:592.

90. Lichter AS, Turrisi AT. Small cell-lung cancer: the influence of dose and treatment volume on outcome. Semin Radiat Oncol 1995; 5:44.

91. Choi NC, Carey RR. Importance of radiation dose in achieving improved locoregional tumor control in small-cell lung carcinoma: an update. Int J Radiat Oncol Biol Phys 1989; 17:307.

92. Papac J, Son Y, Bien R, et al. Improved local control of thoracic disease in small-cell lung cancer with higher dose thoracic irradiation and cyclic chemotherapy. Int J Radiat Oncol Biol Phys 1987; 13:993.

93. Choi NC, Herndon J, Rosenman J, et al. Phase I study to determine the maximum tolerated dose (MTD) of radiation in standard daily (QD) and accelerated twice daily (BID) radiation schedules with concurrent chemotherapy (CT) for limited stage small-cell lung cancer: CALGB 8837 (abstract). Proc Am Soc Clin Oncol 1995; 14:363.

94. Turrisi AT, Glover DJ, Mason BA. A preliminary report: concurrent twice-daily radiotherapy plus platinum-etoposide chemotherapy for limited small cell lung cancer. Int J Radiat Oncol Biol Phys 1988; 15:183.

95. Johnson DH, Turrisi AT, Chand AY, et al. Alternating chemotherapy and twice-daily thoracic radiotherapy in limited-stage small-cell lung cancer: a pilot study of the Eastern Cooperative Oncology Group. J Clin Oncol 1993; 11:879.

96. Turrisi AT, Kynugmann K, Blum R, et al. Twice-daily compared with once-daily thoracic radiotherapy in limited small-cell lung cancer treated concurrently with cisplatin and etoposide. N Engl J Med 1999; 340:264.

97. Bonner JA, Sloan JA, Shanahan TG, et al. Phase III comparison of twice-daily split-course irradiation versus once-daily irradiation for patients with limited stage small-cell lung carcinoma. J Clin Oncol 1999; 17:2681.

Management of Extensive Small-Cell Lung Cancer

30

Melanie Deberne, Fabrice Andre, Benjamin Besse,
Jean-Charles Soria and Thierry Le Chevalier

Contents

30.1 Introduction

Chemotherapy is the cornerstone of the treatment of extensive small-cell lung cancer (SCLC). Some advances have been made since the association of etoposide and cisplatin has been established as the standard for treatment. The addition of anthracycline and cyclophosphamide to this treatment has been shown to improve both response rates and survival. New drugs are being tested in this setting. To date, the most interesting results have been reported with irinotecan since it has been shown that the combination of cisplatin/irinotecan was superior to the standard etoposide/cisplatin in Japan. When patients present with a poor performance status that renders at risk the administration of standard che-

motherapy, carboplatin is now a reasonable option in combination with etoposide.

30.2 Definition of Extensive Stage

The first practical staging was described by the Veteran Affairs Lung Study Group (VALG) in 1957, which defined limited-stage (LS) disease as patients with primary tumor and lymph node involvement limited to one hemithorax. The definition excluded pleural effusions and the involvement of any contralateral nodes. All other patients were classified as having extensive-stage (ES) disease.

The International Association for the Study of Lung Cancer (IASLC) [1] modified this definition, incorporating the involvement of contralateral mediastinal nodes, as well as ipsilateral non-malignant pleural effusion in LS disease, provided that all the tumor burden could be included in one radiation field. They considered all other patients to have ES disease.

The IASLC criteria are more relevant than the VALG criteria in terms of predicting patient outcome, survival, and therapeutic strategy and are therefore preferable in clinical practice.

30.3 How Etoposide/Cisplatin Regimen Became the Standard?

Early chemotherapy studies in the 1970s were based on the CAV regimen (cyclophosphamide, doxorubicin, and vincristine). The etoposide/platin (EP) regimen was introduced in the early 1980s. Etoposide is a semisynthetic podophyllotoxin alkaloid that inhibits topoisomerase II, thus preventing DNA unwinding, and DNA replication and transcription. Cisplatin is a platinum analog that covalently binds to DNA to produce DNA crosslinks, resulting in inhibition of DNA synthesis and transcription. In the late 1980s, randomized studies established the etoposide/cisplatin regimen as a standard treatment in extensive-stage small-cell lung cancer (ES-SCLC).

Fukuoka et al. [2] compared EP with CAV as front-line therapy for ES-SCLC. Patients in the EP arm had a higher response rate than those treated with CAV (78% versus 55%). Roth et al. [3] also demonstrated higher response rates with EP or an EP/CAV combination compared with only CAV (59% to 61% versus 51%). Evans et al. [4] showed that patients previously treated with CAV had a 55% response rate to EP. In addition to present a better efficacy compared to the CAV regimen, the EP regimen presents an acceptable toxicity profile. The most frequently used schedule is the administration of 80–100 mg/m^2 cisplatin on days 1 or 2, and 100 mg/m^2 of etoposide on days 1–3, repeated every 3–4 weeks.

A literature-based meta-analysis has confirmed the value of cisplatin and EP in ES-SCLC. Indeed, Pujol et al. [5] analyzed 19 trials, including 60% of ES disease, comparing cisplatin to non-cisplatin-containing regimens. This meta-analysis showed a statistically significant reduction in the risk of death at both 6 months (odds ratio=0.87, $p=0.03$) and 1 year (odds ratio=0.80, $p=0.002$) for patients treated with a cisplatin-based regimen. There were no differences in toxicity between the different chemotherapy regimens.

Since this era, several questions rise in the field of "conventional" chemotherapy: (1) Is carboplatin a reasonable alternative to cisplatin? (2) Does the addition of anthracycline and cyclophosphamide to the EP regimen increase efficacy? (3) What is the additional value of alternating regimens? (4) What is the efficacy of dose increase? (5) Are new drugs of interest in the treatment of ES-SCLC?

30.4 Is Carboplatin a Reasonable Alternative to Cisplatin-based Chemotherapy?

If platinum-based regimens have become the standard of care for ES-SCLC patients with good performance status, the question arises as to whether carboplatin is equivalent to cisplatin in regard to efficacy.

The Hellenic Oncology Group conducted a phase III trial in which patients were randomized to receive EP (platin 50 mg/m^2) or carboplatin (300 mg/m^2)/etoposide [6]. Both ES and LS were included, and there was no statistically significant difference in median survival (11.8 months for EC versus 12.5 months for EP), overall response rate (50% versus 64%), or complete response rate (16% versus 10%) in patients with disseminated SCLC. Brahmer and Ettinger reviewed all recent phase II and III data regarding the use of etoposide/carboplatin in SCLC, concluding that carboplatin is as effective as cisplatin with less toxicity (nausea, vomiting, and neuropathy).

Despite limited data to support the equivalence of carboplatin to cisplatin in SCLC, the goal of therapy in disseminated SCLC is palliative, making carboplatin a reasonable alternative to cisplatin when this latter drug is expected to be highly toxic.

30.5 Does the Addition of Anthracycline and Cyclophosphamide to the EP Regimen Increase Efficacy?

In order to decrease the probability of further drug resistance, it has been suggested to combine drugs in front-line therapy. Pujol et al. [7] have compared a standard EP regimen to a four-drug combination that included cisplatin (100 mg/m^2), etoposide (100 mg/m^2 ×3), epirubicin (40 mg/m^2), and cyclophosphamide (400 mg/m^2 ×3). This trial included 226 patients. The four-drug combination increased the overall response rate (76% versus 61%, $p=0.02$) and the overall survival (median survival 10.5 months versus 9.3 months, $p=0.006$). The documented infection rate was increased in the four-drug arm (22% versus 8%, $p=0.003$).

This trial suggested that a four-drug regimen increased endpoints for efficacy, but the magnitude of the benefit was modest, while this regimen significantly increased toxicity.

30.6 Alternating or Sequential Chemotherapy

Considering that the high response rate is associated with a short duration of response, alternating non-cross-resistant chemotherapy was an attractive concept to be tested in ES-SCLC.

Evans et al. [4] first demonstrated the superiority of this method in randomizing 279 ES-SCLC patients to either CAV or CAV alternating with EP. The CAV/EP regimen increased response rate (80% versus 63%, $p=0.002$) and survival time (9.6 months versus 8 months), but it may simply reflect the superiority of EP over CAV.

The Southeastern Cancer Study Group [4] compared EP×4 to an alternation of these two regimens (3 CAV plus 3 EP) in 437 ES-SCLC. No significant differences in treatment outcome for EP or CAV/EP were observed for response rate (61% versus 59%) or median survival (8.6 months versus 8.1 months).

Fukuoka et al. [2] compared EP to EP alternating with the CAV regimen. The response rate was similar between the two arms (78% versus 76%). No difference was observed in overall survival.

Overall, the two trials that compared the EP regimen to an alternating or sequential regimen did not report any benefit from this approach.

30.7 Does Dose Intensification Increase Efficacy?

Pujol et al. [8] investigated whether a high-dose chemotherapy regimen of cyclophosphamide 1,800 mg/m^2, 4-epidoxorubicin 60 mg/m^2, etoposide 330 mg/m^2, and cisplatin 120 mg/m^2 given monthly for 4 cycles with recombinant human granulocyte-macrophage colony-stimulating factor (rhGM-CSF) support (5 mcg/kg daily for 10 days) could improve the survival of patients with ES-SCLC compared with a standard-dose regimen (cyclophosphamide 1,200 mg/m^2, 4-epidoxorubicin 40 mg/m^2, etoposide 225 mg/m^2, and cisplatin 100 mg/m^2) given monthly for 6 cycles. A total of 125 patients were included in this randomized trial. The cumulative doses of each drug actually delivered were significantly higher in the standard-dose group. No difference in response rate was observed between the two groups. There were significantly greater hematologic toxicities, documented infections, and transfusions of RBCs and platelets in the higher-dose plus rhGM-CSF group.

Patients in this group proved to have a shorter survival duration and a shorter time to relapse than patients in the standard-dose group (median overall survival: standard dose, 10.8 months; higher dose, 8.9 months; log-rank test with adjustment for prognostic variables, $p = 0.0005$; respective probabilities of relapse at 1 year, 77 ± 0.6 and 96 ± 2.2; log-rank test, $p = 0.013$). This study showed that a dose increase was not feasible in this population of patients. In addition, this study suggests that GM-CSF could be deleterious in patients with ES-SCLC.

Another approach to increase dose density consists of reducing the treatment intervals. Several phase III studies have evaluated the efficacy of a dose-dense chemotherapy compared to a standard chemotherapy. Steward et al. [9] have compared a 3-week interval to a 4-week interval in a phase III trial that included 300 patients. Patients received chemotherapy with ifosfamide 5 g/m^2 day 1, carboplatin 300 mg/m^2 day 1, etoposide 120 mg/m^2 days 1–3, and vincristine day 15 for 6 cycles. While response rates did not differ, median survival times were improved in patients treated with a 3-week interval schedule (443 days versus 351 days). It is of note that this study included patients with both limited and extensive disease. Whether a further shortening of the interval could improve outcome was investigated in three randomized trials. Thatcher et al. [10] included 403 patients with limited or extensive disease to receive a 3-week or a 2-week interval chemotherapy (CDE protocol). Both response rates and survival were improved in the 2-week treatment arm. Ardizzoni et al. [11] also compared a 2-week versus a 3-week regimen and reported no difference in terms of survival. Finally, Sculier et al. [12] from the European Lung Cancer Working Party randomized 233 patients to either a standard regimen of epirubicin, vindesine, and ifosfamide for 6 cycles given every 3 weeks (arm A), or the same regimen given every 2 weeks with GM-CSF (arm B), or the same regimen as given in B with oral antibiotics (cotrimoxazole) (arm C). Response rates were higher in arm B compared to arm A (76% versus 59%), but there were no differences in median (264 days versus 286 days) or 2-year survival rates (6% versus 5%).

Two phase III trials have evaluated the efficacy of a weekly CODE regimen compared with a standard CAV/PE regimen. In the first trial [13], 219 patients were randomized to receive cisplatin, vincristine, doxorubicin, and etoposide (CODE) or alternating cyclophosphamide, doxorubicin, and vincristine/etoposide and cisplatin (CAV/EP). Response rates after chemotherapy were higher ($p = 0.006$) with CODE (87%) than with CAV/EP (70%). However, progression-free survival (median of 0.66 years on both arms) and overall survival (median of 0.98 years for CODE and 0.91 years for CAV/EP) were not improved. The second trial [14] included 227 patients and compared a weekly CODE regimen to a CAV/PE regimen. Overall response rates were 77% for the CAV/PE arm and 84% for the CODE arm (15% complete response in both arms). The median survival times were 10.9 months in the CAV/PE arm and 11.6 months in the CODE arm ($p = 0.10$). Overall, these two studies do not support the use of the CODE regimen in patients with ES-SCLC.

Overall, the randomized trials that evaluated a dose increase in patients with ES-SCLC failed to show a convincing significant benefit for this approach. There is therefore no place for this strategy in daily practice.

30.8 Are New Drugs Promising in the Treatment of Extensive-stage Small-Cell Lung Cancer?

30.8.1 Irinotecan

Several phase II studies, mainly performed in Japan, showed that irinotecan was active in SCLC. A recently published phase III study from Japan [15] compared standard EP to irinotecan plus cisplatin. Two hundred and thirty patients with ES-SCLC were randomized to receive either irinotecan (60 mg/m^2 on days 1, 8, and 15) + cisplatin (60 mg/m^2 on day 1) or etoposide (100 mg/m^2 on days 1–3) plus cisplatin (80 mg/m^2 on day 1).

Median survival was significantly improved in the irinotecan-treated arm (12.8 months versus 9.4 months, $p = 0.002$). The 2-year overall survivals were 19.5% and 5.2%. The toxicity profiles were different between the two arms, with more grade 3/4 myelosuppression (neutropenia 65% versus 92%) and thrombocytopenia (5% versus 18%) in the EP arm, while the irinotecan arm provided a higher rate of diarrhea. Three confirmatory phase III trials have been designed in North America and Europe to reproduce the clinical data of the Japanese trial in a larger population of western patients.

30.8.2 Topotecan

Topotecan is semisynthetic analog of the alkaloid camptothecin that is a specific inhibitor of topoisomerase I.

Topotecan in the First-line Therapy

The Eastern Cooperative Oncology Group (ECOG) conducted a randomized trial [16] that compared topotecan with observation after standard cisplatin/etoposide in 402 previously untreated patients. All patients received 4 cycles of EP. Patients with stable or responsive disease were randomized to receive either IV topotecan (1.5 mg/m^2 for 5 days for 4 cycles) or observation. There was no difference in overall survival or quality of life between the two groups.

Topotecan as a Second-line Agent

Numerous phase II trials have evaluated topotecan as single agent for second-line therapy, using the same schedule as previously described (1.5 mg/m^2 for 5 days every 3 weeks). The overall response rates ranged between 3% and 11% for refractory patients and between 19% and 37% for sensitive patients. Von Pawel [17] performed a phase III study that compared topotecan with CAV in 211 patients with recurrent LS- or ES-SCLC, whose disease had relapsed 2 months or more after completion of first-line treatment. No difference was observed in terms of response rate (24% for topotecan versus 18% for CAV, $p=0.285$) or median survival. However topotecan appeared to give patients symptomatic benefit, particularly for dyspnea ($p=0.002$).

Oral Topotecan

With an oral formulation given at 1.7 mg/m^2 daily for 5 days every 21 days, the ECOG study [18] obtained a 33% overall response rate and 37 weeks median survival. These results are comparable to IV topotecan. A randomized phase II study [19] reported results obtained with either oral or IV topotecan in 106 patients. Response rates in this phase II randomized study were 23% (12/52) in the oral topotecan arm and 15% (8/54) in the IV topotecan arm. Median survival was 32 weeks (oral) and 25 weeks (IV). No phase III study has compared these two modalities of treatment.

30.8.3 Taxanes

Paclitaxel has been combined to the standard doublet of cisplatin/etoposide in several studies [20,21]. This combination was shown to be active with response rates ranging between 83% and 90% and median survivals of 10–11 months. In another phase II study using a carboplatin/etoposide/paclitaxel regimen, 84% of ES patients had major responses including 21% complete remission. However, the median survival was above 10 months, which is similar to that achieved with the triple regimen using cisplatin.

Three phase III trials have evaluated the efficacy of paclitaxel in patients with SCLC. In the first one, Reck et al. [22] have compared the paclitaxel/etoposide/carboplatin combination to carboplatin/etoposide. Six hundred and fourteen patients have been included. The hazard ratio (HR) of death for patients receiving the standard treatment was statistically significantly higher than that for patients receiving the experimental treatment (HR=1.22, 95% confidence interval [CI]=1.03 to 1.45, $p=0.024$). There were no differences in the response rates (complete and partial combined) to the treatments (standard arm: 69.4%, 95% CI=63.9% to 74.5%; experimental arm: 72.1%, 95% CI=66.7% to 77.1%; difference=2.7%, 95% CI=4.5% to 9.9%). A second trial conducted by the CALGB [23] and comparing etoposide/cisplatin/paclitaxel to a standard did not report a survival benefit for patients treated in the paclitaxel arm. In the third trial [24], 133 chemotherapy-naive patients with histologically proven LS- or ES-SCLC were randomized to receive either paclitaxel (175 mg/m^2 IV 3-h infusion on day 1), cisplatin (80 mg/m^2 IV on day 2), and etoposide (80 mg/m^2 IV on days 2–4) with G-CSF support (5 mcg/kg SC on days 5–15) or cisplatin (80 mg/m^2 IV on day 1) and etoposide (120 mg/m^2 IV on days 1–3) in cycles every 28 days. In an intention-to-treat overall analysis both regimens were equally active with a complete and partial response rate of 50% (95% CI=37.5% to 62.4%) for TEP and 48% (95% CI=36.2% to 59.5%) for EP ($p=0.8$). The median time to disease progression was 11 months for TEP and 9 months for EP ($p=0.02$). The duration of response, 1-year survival, and overall survival were similar in the two arms.

Overall, although one randomized trial reported a benefit for patients treated with paclitaxel, it is of note that the standard arm was not optimal [22]. Since other trials did not report any survival benefit, paclitaxel should therefore not be considered as a standard chemotherapy in SCLC.

30.8.4 Gemcitabine

Gemcitabine has been reported to provide around 10% response rates in patients with SCLC who relapsed after first-line chemotherapy [25]. This drug has been evaluated in a phase III trial that compared the combination gemcitabine/carboplatin (GC) with a standard cisplatin/etoposide [26]. Two hundred and forty-one patients were included. The GC combination did not improve response rates or overall survival in this trial.

30.9 Prophylactic Cranial Irradiation (PCI)

Prophylactic cranial irradiation is recommended in localized SCLC in complete remission since it increases overall survival as shown in a recent meta-analysis [27]. It is of note that patients presenting a complete response after induction therapy for an extensive disease were also included in this meta-analysis and could therefore be considered as eligible for prophylactic cranial irradiation.

30.10 Conclusion

The treatment of patients with extensive SCLC still remains palliative. In this setting, it is highly important to include patients in clinical trials that evaluate new drugs. For patients who can not be included in trials, the treatment should be tailored according to performance status and patients' wishes. Three options can be discussed: a four-drug combination when performance status is unaltered, a standard etoposide/cisplatin regimen when there is a minimal alteration of performance status, and when the patient asks for a good quality of life. The combination of carboplatin and etoposide should be given only to patients who present an important performance status alteration or a contraindication to a standard chemotherapy.

Key Points

- The cisplatin/etoposide regimen is considered the standard treatment in extensive disease small-cell lung cancer (SCLC).
- Despite limited data to support equivalence of carboplatin to cisplatin in SCLC, the goal of therapy in disseminated SCLC is palliative, making carboplatin a reasonable alternative to cisplatin when this latter drug is expected to be highly toxic.
- Irinotecan, when combined with cisplatin, has demonstrated comparable activity, but data from the Japanese studies need further evaluation and confirmation before being universally accepted.

References

1. Stahel RA, Ginsberg R, Havemann K. Staging and prognostic features in small cell lung cancer: a consensus report. Lung Cancer 1989;59:119.
2. Fukuoka M, Furuse K, Saijo N, et al. Randomized trial of cyclophosphamide, doxorubicin, and vincristine versus cisplatin and etoposide versus alternation of these regimens in small-cell lung cancer. J Natl Cancer Inst 1991;83:855.
3. Roth BJ, Johnson DH, Einhorn LH, et al. Randomized study of cyclophosphamide, doxorubicin, and vincristine versus etoposide and cisplatin versus alternation of these two regimens in extensive small-cell lung cancer: a phase III trial of the Southeastern Cancer Study Group. J Clin Oncol 1992;10:282.
4. Evans WK, Osoba D, Feld R, et al. Etoposide and cisplatin: an effective treatment for relapse in small-cell lung cancer. J Clin Oncol 1985;3:65.
5. Pujol JL, Carestia L, Daures JP, et al. Is there a case for cisplatin in the treatment of small-cell lung cancer? A meta-analysis of randomized trials of a cisplatin-containing regimen versus a regimen without this alkylating agent. Br J Cancer 2000;83:8.
6. Skarlos DV, Samantas E, Kosmidis P, et al. Randomized comparison of etoposide-cisplatin vs etoposide-carboplatin and irradiation in small-cell lung cancer. A Hellenic Cooperative Oncology Group study. Ann Oncol 1994;5:601.
7. Pujol JL, Daures JP, Riviere A, et al. Etoposide plus cisplatin with or without the combination of 4-epidoxorubicin plus cyclophosphamide in treatment of extensive small-cell lung cancer: a French Federation of Cancer Institutes multicenter phase III randomized study. J Natl Cancer Inst 2001;93:300.
8. Pujol JL, Douillard JY, Riviere A, et al. Dose-intensity of a four-drug chemotherapy regimen with or without recombinant human granulocyte-macrophage colony-stimulating factor in extensive-stage small-cell lung cancer: a multicenter randomized phase III study. J Clin Oncol 1997;15:2082.
9. Steward WP, von Pawel J, Gatzemeier U, et al. Effects of granulocyte-macrophage colony-stimulating factor and dose intensification of V-ICE chemotherapy in small-cell lung cancer: a prospective randomized study of 300 patients. J Clin Oncol 1998;16:642.

10. Thatcher N, Girling DJ, Hopwood P, et al. Improving survival without reducing quality of life in small-cell lung cancer patients by increasing the dose-intensity of chemotherapy with granulocyte colony-stimulating factor support: results of a British Medical Research Council Multicenter Randomized Trial. Medical Research Council Lung Cancer Working Party. J Clin Oncol 2000;18:395.

11. Ardizzoni A, Tjan-Heijnen VC, Postmus PE, et al. European Organization for Research and Treatment of Cancer–Lung Cancer Group. Standard versus intensified chemotherapy with granulocyte colony-stimulating factor support in small-cell lung cancer: a prospective European Organization for Research and Treatment of Cancer–Lung Cancer Group phase III trial-08923. J Clin Oncol 2002;20:3947.

12. Sculier JP, Paesmans M, Lecomte J, et al. A three-arm phase III randomised trial assessing, in patients with extensive-disease small-cell lung cancer, accelerated chemotherapy with support of haematological growth factor or oral antibiotics. Br J Cancer 2001;85:1444.

13. Murray N, Livingston RB, Shepherd FA, et al. Randomized study of CODE versus alternating CAV/EP for extensive-stage small-cell lung cancer: an intergroup study of the National Cancer Institute of Canada Clinical Trials Group and the Southwest Oncology Group. J Clin Oncol 1999;17:2300.

14. Furuse K, Fukuoka M, Nishiwaki Y, et al. Phase III study of intensive weekly chemotherapy with recombinant human granulocyte colony-stimulating factor versus standard chemotherapy in extensive-disease small-cell lung cancer. The Japan Clinical Oncology Group. J Clin Oncol 1998;16:2126.

15. Noda K, Nishiwaki Y, Kawahara M, et al. Irinotecan plus cisplatin compared with etoposide plus cisplatin for extensive small-cell lung cancer. N Engl J Med 2002;346:85.

16. Schiller JH, Adak S, Cella D, et al. Topotecan versus observation after cisplatin plus etoposide in extensive-stage small-cell lung cancer: E7593—a phase III trial of the Eastern Cooperative Oncology Group. J Clin Oncol 2001;19:2114.

17. Von Pawel J, Schiller JH, Shepherd FA, et al. Topotecan versus cyclophosphamide, doxorubicin, and vincristine for the treatment of recurrent small-cell lung cancer. J Clin Oncol 1999;17:658.

18. Ardizzoni A. Topotecan in the treatment of recurrent small cell lung cancer: an update Oncologist 2004;9:4.

19. Von Pawel J, Gatzemeier U, Pujol JL, et al. Phase II comparator study of oral versus intravenous topotecan in patients with chemosensitive small-cell lung cancer. J Clin Oncol 2001;19:1743.

20. Glisson BS, Kurie JM, Perez-Soler R, et al. Cisplatin, etoposide and paclitaxel in the treatment of patients with extensive small-cell lung carcinoma. J Clin Oncol 1999;17:2309.

21. Hainsworth J, Gray J, Stroup S, et al. Paclitaxel, carboplatin, and extended schedule etoposide in the treatment of small cell lung cancer: comparison of sequential phase II trials using different dose-intensities. J Clin Oncol 1997;15:3464.

22. Reck M, von Pawel J, Macha HN, et al. Randomized phase III trial of paclitaxel, etoposide, and carboplatin versus carboplatin, etoposide, and vincristine in patients with small-cell lung cancer. J Natl Cancer Inst 2003;95:1118.

23. Niell HB, Herndon JE, Miller AA, et al. Randomized phase III intergroup trial of etoposide and cisplatin with or without paclitaxel and GCSF in patients with extensive stage small cell lung cancer. Proc Am Soc Clin Oncol 2002;21:1169.

24. Mavroudis D, Papadakis E, Veslemes M, et al. Lung Cancer Cooperative Group. A multicenter randomized clinical trial comparing paclitaxel-cisplatin-etoposide versus cisplatin-etoposide as first-line treatment in patients with small-cell lung cancer. Ann Oncol 2001;12:463.

25. Masters GA, Declerck L, Blanke C, et al. Eastern Cooperative Oncology Group. Phase II trial of gemcitabine in refractory or relapsed small-cell lung cancer: Eastern Cooperative Oncology Group trial 1597. J Clin Oncol 2003;21:1550.

26. James LE, Rudd R, Gower NH, et al. A phase III randomized comparison of gemcitabine/carboplatin with cisplatin/etoposide in patients with poor prognosis small cell lung cancer. Proc ASCO 2002;21:A1170.

27. Auperin A, Arriagada R, Pignon JP, et al. Prophylactic cranial irradiation for patients with small-cell lung cancer in complete remission. Prophylactic Cranial Irradiation Overview Collaborative Group. N Engl J Med 1999; 341:476.

Management of Relapsed Small-Cell Lung Cancer

31

Morten Sorensen and Heine H. Hansen

Contents

31.1 Introduction

Although first-line chemotherapy induces a high rate of response in small-cell lung cancer (SCLC), the majority of patients eventually relapse. The management of these patients constitutes a very common problem for the clinical oncologist. Evidence from numerous phase II trials indicates that selected patients may benefit by achieving clinically meaningful response rates if treated with second-line chemotherapy. As the expected life-span is short, the major purpose of treating relapsed SCLC patients is palliative, including maintaining or increasing quality of life. The number of randomized trials to elucidate the management of patients relapsing after initial treatment is scarce and no generally accepted standard for second-line treatment exists.

31.2 Selection of Patients for Second-line Treatment

In order to minimize unnecessary toxicity and maximize benefit it is crucial that the clinician selects the right patients for second-line therapy. Both retrospective and prospective studies are available which identify predictive factors for response to second-line treatment.

Retrospective studies have identified the length of the time elapsing from first-line treatment to relapse as a major predictive factor for response to salvage treatment [1]. Ardizzoni et al. designed the first phase II trial in which a prospective distinction was made between patients with a long and short treatment-free interval [2]. They confirmed that a treatment-free interval of more than 3 months increases the chances of response to subsequent therapy. Thirty-eight percent of 45 patients classified as sensitive responded to second-line therapy compared to only 6% of 47 refractory patients. Sensitive patients were defined as those responding to first-line treatment and relapsing more than 3 months after termination of first-line therapy. Patients failing first-line treatment or relapsing less than 3 months after last chemotherapy were labeled refractory patients. The choice of a cut-off point at a 3-month treatment-free interval was arbitrary and not an absolute requirement for considering salvage therapy, but the concept has been applied since then in several similar clinical trials. Furthermore, the likelihood of response increases with the length of the treatment-free interval. In the above-mentioned phase II trial response rates increased to 57% compared to 11% if the cut-off point was changed to a 6-month treatment-free interval and response rates of 56% have been reported for patients with a disease-free survival of more than 2 years [3]. Clinically meaningful response rates above 20% have also been reported by von Pawel et al. in a randomized trial treating 211 patients relapsing more than 60 days after last chemotherapy [4].

The type of response to first-line treatment, i.e., the achievement of complete response, has also been identified to be a predictive factor [1] and these patients have a high likelihood of responding to second-line treatment. Conversely, second-line therapy should be avoided in patients with poor performance status and major comorbidities.

As refractory patients do not benefit from chemotherapy, these patients should not be offered second-line treatment on a routine basis outside the setting of phase I or II trials. Instead, refractory patients should be considered for palliative measures other than chemotherapy. Patients suffering from pain due to tumor invasion, for example, superior cava syndrome, hemoptysis, and dyspnea, should receive palliative radiotherapy (e.g., 10 Gy ×1). Dyspnea caused by obstruction of a main bronchus can also be alleviated in selected cases by argon beam laser therapy, endobronchial brachytherapy, or stenting. Refractory patients in good performance status can be considered for phase I and II studies evaluating agents with new or unknown mechanisms of action.

31.3   Treatment Strategies

As mentioned, no generally accepted treatment strategy for second-line therapy exists. The scarcity of randomized trials is the main reason for our limited knowledge of this question. Accrual of 65 patients lasted 7 years in one randomized phase II study by the European Lung Cancer Working Party, illustrating that the conduction of such trials is best carried out by large cooperative groups [5]. Furthermore, our knowledge regarding the palliative effect of second-line chemotherapy stems from the assumption that responses translate into palliation. Randomized studies using best supportive care as control and quality of life as endpoint are non-existent. Only one study randomizing between two different regimens of chemotherapy actually reports quality of life data [4].

Among the randomized trials, one of the largest studies on second-line chemotherapy was performed by the Cancer Research Campaign randomizing 610 patients to four different treatment arms, including 4 versus 8 cycles of CEV (cyclophosphamide, etoposide, and vincristine) and palliative treatment versus doxorubicin and methotrexate at progression [6]. Four cycles of CEV followed by palliation was significantly inferior to the three other arms resulting in a 9-week shorter survival. Two main conclusions can be drawn. Second-line chemotherapy may compensate for inferior first-line treatment. Second-line treatment following 8 cycles of first-line chemotherapy did not extend survival as compared to palliative treatment. This study underscores the need to analyze uncontrolled phase II trials of salvage therapy in the context of the previously administered first-line treatment. The a priori chance of a high degree of benefit of second-line therapy appears to be correlated to poor first-line therapy.

Although numerous uncontrolled phase II trials of second-line therapy have been reported over the years no superior regimen has been singled out. The assessment of these trials is hampered by the differences in patient population and by the incomplete reporting of major predictive factors for response such as treatment-free interval, response to first-line therapy, and response duration. The reported response rates most probably reflect patient population rather than the second-line treatment administered. This problem is elegantly illu-

strated by trials using a design that prospectively stratifies patients into sensitive and refractory groups [2, 7]. Response rates in sensitive patients are sixfold to ninefold higher compared to refractory patients. Obviously, this difference in response rate is several orders of magnitude higher than what would be expected for a treatment effect of the tested regimens.

Different concepts of second-line treatment have been explored including re-induction with the regimen used for first-line treatment, presumably non-cross-resistant chemotherapy, and new agents including taxanes and topoisomerase I inhibitors as single agents or in combination with older drugs.

31.3.1   Re-induction

Re-induction with the regimen that induced initial response results in response rates between 46% and 67% which are among the highest response rates reported for second-line treatment in SCLC, and thus re-induction seems a justified approach in the management of relapsed SCLC patients. These data support the notion that in selected patients a subset of sensitive tumor cells remains after optimal first-line therapy. Alternatively, in patients with a very long treatment-free interval the efficacy of re-challenge with first-line drugs could be a result of the emergence of de novo sensitive tumor cells.

The use of re-induction represents a number of advantages. Both patient and healthcare workers are familiar with the regimen in question. The toxicity is manageable and predictable and in most cases costs are affordable. However, reported response rates might be biased by the fact that patients in these trials by definition have had a treatment-free interval of some length (if no treatment-free interval has elapsed treatment should be referred to as maintenance therapy). Furthermore, in order to classify salvage therapy as re-induction a response must have been induced by first-line treatment. Both these features of re-induction tend to select patients with favorable predictive factors for response to second-line treatment.

A potential limitation of re-induction is cumulative toxicity. Special attention should be drawn to cisplatin-induced renal function impairment, debilitating neuropathy, and auditory defects. Due to its favorable toxicity profile, carboplatin makes an attractive substitute for cisplatin, also with respect to its lower emetogenic potential in this palliative setting. The usefulness of carboplatin is supported by the non-significant increase in response rates from 29% to 47% and in median survivals from 4.3 to 7.6 months in a non-comparative randomized phase II trial evaluating the addition of carboplatin to second-line cisplatin and etoposide (PE) [5]. Also, the risk of inducing cardiomyopathy should be considered before re-treatment with anthracyclines.

Most of the trials on re-induction date back to the 1980s or early 1990s and since then some of the first-line drug combinations used have now been abandoned. Today, combinations of platin and epiphyllotoxin-based therapy are commonly used as first-line treatment instead of the formerly used combinations including cyclophosphamide and anthracyclines. Although reaching the same high response rates of 75%, re-induction with PE has been evaluated in only a limited number of patients [8]. Thus, the relevance of these studies in current practice could be questioned.

Despite these considerations, no trials to date have challenged the hypothesis that re-induction is at least as efficacious as other strategies, which is the reason why re-induction could be considered the relevant comparator in randomized studies testing new drug combinations in second-line treatment.

31.3.2 Non-cross-resistant Drugs

The almost inevitable relapse in SCLC patients is due to the emergence of chemotherapy-resistant cell clones. This notion has been established in both clinical tumor samples and in experimental cell line systems. Genomic instability and heterogeneity of cancer cells are major factors in the development of resistance. Extensive knowledge is available regarding mechanisms of resistance that operate in in vitro cell lines. The multidrug-resistance (MDR) tumor cells display resistance toward a number of well-defined but chemically unrelated cytotoxins. MDR cells actively extrude these drugs by an ATP-driven protein pump called the P-glycoprotein, which is overexpressed in the cellular membrane. Other mechanisms of resistance involve other protein pumps such as multidrug-resistance-associated protein (MRP) as well as alterations in the target of cytotoxins such as topoisomerase I and II. It is unknown whether resistant clones are present at the start of treatment in patients with SCLC or resistance is acquired in the course of treatment. The clinical significance of these mechanisms needs further elucidation but it has been hypothesized that the use of potentially non-cross-resistant drugs at relapse might partly overcome resistance.

A number of early trials have evaluated two potentially non-cross-resistant regimens, PE and CAV (cyclophosphamide, adriamycin, and vincristine). Second-line PE combinations following first-line CAV seem more active than the reverse sequence, i.e., second-line CAV following first-line PE. The latter-mentioned sequence resulted in response rates of 10% compared to 30% and 40% following second-line PE [9–11]. Consequently, CAV seems a suboptimal choice as second-line treatment of patients relapsing following PE. Furthermore, the data question the assumption that CAV and PE are truly non-cross-resistant regimens.

In two parallel phase II studies, the EORTC achieved responses rate above 50% when assumed non-cross-resistant second-line regimens were used in refractory patients progressing less than 3 months after cessation of first-line treatment. Twenty-five patients receiving first-line CDE (cyclophosphamide, doxorubicin, and etoposide) crossed over to VIMP (vincristine, ifosfamide, mesna, and carboplatin), and 22 patients were treated in the reverse sequence [12]. The data strongly support the concept of using truly non-cross-resistant second-line regimens as the a priori chance of response is scant in this refractory patient population. However, the implications for the practice of today are limited as both first-line CDE and VIMP increasingly have been abandoned in favor of the more commonly used PE. Unfortunately, few studies provide information on the activity of second-line treatment in PE refractory patients. One study reported a modest 11% response rate to second-line topotecan in 22 patients progressing less than 3 months after cessation of PE [13].

31.3.3 Multiagent Versus Single-agent Regimens

A vast number of uncontrolled phase II studies evaluating single agents have been published. Several newer chemotherapeutic agents have shown high response rates. One of the most extensively studied single-agent drugs in phase II trials is the topoisomerase I inhibitor topotecan reaching response rates between 14% and 38% in sensitive patients and between 2% and 11% in refractory patients. Response rates and survival are comparable in one study randomizing patients to either oral (2.3 mg/m^2) or intravenous (1.5 mg/m^2) topotecan [14]. Similarly, in a single phase II trial, another topoisomerase I inhibitor irinotecan induced responses in 35% and 4% of sensitive and refractory patients, respectively [7]. The taxanes are also highly active in SCLC. Paclitaxel resulted in an impressive 29% response rate in patients refractory to CDE [15]. Docetaxel-induced responses in 25% of patients in a population with no record of the type of first-line treatment administered. Older drugs are similarly capable of inducing high response rates. Forty percent of patients with recurrent brain metastases responded to carboplatin [16] and 46% responded to single-agent oral etoposide [17].

Phase II studies evaluating two-drug combinations seem to reach higher or at least similar response rates compared to single agents. The combination of carboplatin and paclitaxel induced a response rate of 74% (95% CI, 59% to 88%) in patients refractory to CDE [18]. Twenty-nine percent (95% CI, 19% to 42%) and 24% (95% CI, 12% to 39%) of sensitive and refractory patients responded to a combination of topotecan and cisplatin [19]. In a Japanese study, irinotecan and etoposide achieved response rates of 71% (95% CI, 53% to 89%) in a population of mainly sensitive patients [20].

Although achieving similar response rates, the two-drug combination cisplatin and etoposide (PE) resulted in a 25-week increase in survival (35 weeks versus 10 weeks, $p = 0.01$) compared to a four-drug regimen consisting of mainly alkylating drugs (BCNU, thiotepa, vincristine, and cyclophosphamide) in a SWOG trial [21]. The survival benefit only applied for a minor subset of patients ($n = 27$) classified as "good-risk patients," defined as those who were below 65 years old and tolerated first-line therapy well. Poor-risk patients had a low response rate of approximately 10% and a short survival irrespective of the received chemotherapy. The study confirms that "poor-risk patients" (i.e., age above 65 years and with low tolerance to first-line chemotherapy) do not benefit from chemotherapy. Furthermore, alkylating agents should be avoided as second-line treatment. In a subsequent retrospective analysis of four consecutive trials performed by SWOG, treatment with PE turned out as a predictor for survival in 259 patients receiving second-line therapy [22].

Recently, a large study, including 211 patients, randomized sensitive patients to single-agent topotecan or multiagent CAV. The majority of the patients relapsed after first-line PE. Response rates (24.3% versus 18.3%) and survival (25.0 weeks versus 24.7 weeks) were comparable in the two arms. However, symptom control was marginally better in the topotecan arm, indicating that patients benefited most from single-agent topotecan in this setting. The results of this study led to the FDA approval of topotecan for second-line treatment in SCLC. The study has been subject to some criticism due to the choice of the competitor regimen CAV as this regimen is regarded as suboptimal in a population relapsing after first-line PE, as mentioned previously.

In conclusion, on the basis of the available data it is not possible to determine whether single- or multiagent therapy is the superior strategy. However, two randomized studies support the use of both single-agent topotecan and PE in patients with recurrent SCLC.

31.3.4 Brain Metastases

Patients with SCLC often relapse in the brain. About 10% of patients present with brain metastases when diagnosed. At autopsy dissemination to the brain has been found in 50% of patients. With prolonged survival the likelihood of brain metastases increases dramatically reaching 50–80% after 2 years of follow-up. Brain metastases thus represent a very burdensome problem for clinicians as well as for patients and their families. Patients suffer from headache, treatment-resistant nausea, and vomiting. Changes in personality and the loss of functions are very disturbing consequences of spread

to the central nervous system (CNS) making patients dependent on the help of their carers. The mere suspicion of brain metastases should – in some cases even before final diagnostic imaging – prompt the initiation of symptomatic treatment with steroids, which can have a dramatic effect by reducing the edema surrounding the lesions. Other symptomatic treatments to be considered are anticonvulsants and antiemetics.

Whole-brain irradiation (WBI) has been used for decades as standard palliative treatment, although its benefits mostly are based on retrospective data. Few prospective trials are available, including an EORTC phase II study that accrued patients with brain-only metastases to be treated with 3 Gy ×10 [23]. They reported a 50% remission rate evaluated by CT scans. Median disease-free survival was 5.4 months. Sixty percent of patients experienced an improvement or stabilization of their neurological function score. These data confirm that WBI is an important treatment modality for the alleviation of symptoms caused by brain metastases. A decade ago, chemotherapy was seldom used in this setting because the CNS has been perceived as a pharmacological sanctuary due to the relatively low transport of cytotoxic drugs over the blood–brain barrier (BBB). The benefits of prophylactic cranial irradiation have confirmed that chemotherapy is not sufficient to eradicate subclinical micrometastases in the CNS indicating that the BBB remains intact when brain metastases are subclinical. However, in symptomatic brain metastases the BBB is probably disrupted. This notion is supported by PET studies and the clinical observation that response rates in intra- and extracerebral lesions are comparable when induced by drugs with low transport across the BBB and high activity in SCLC. Thus, the choice of chemotherapeutic agent should be based on its activity in extracranial SCLC and not on its ability to cross the BBB. The EORTC randomized 120 SCLC patients with brain metastases to either monotherapy teniposide or combined modality treatment with WBI and teniposide [24]. Almost 75% of patients suffered from relapsed SCLC and around 66% had a treatment-free interval of more than 3 months. Response rates in the combined modality arm were significantly better reaching 57% as compared to 22% in the monotherapy arm. Time to progression in the brain was significantly longer following combined therapy. The study confirms that WBI is the most effective treatment of relapses in the brain available today. Intra- and extracranial response rates were no different in the monotherapy arm confirming that chemotherapy of brain metastases is as effective as second-line therapy of extracranial disease. Thus, the decision to administer chemotherapy to patients with recurrence in the brain should follow the same guidelines that apply for second-line treatment of patients with recurrence at other sites.

Neurosurgery or stereotactic radiotherapy should be considered only in very selected cases as patients suffer from a systemic disease with multiple metastatic lesions, and have a limited remaining lifespan.

31.4 Conclusion

Patients with a treatment-free interval of less than 3 months after first-line treatment, failing first-line treatment, with poor performance status or major co-morbidities, or with low tolerance to first-line chemotherapy should in general not receive second-line chemotherapy because of very low efficacy. Instead focus should be on palliative measures such as short fractionation of radiotherapy.

Patients with a treatment-free interval exceeding 3 months have a much greater chance of benefiting from second-line treatment and should be treated if in good performance and without major comorbidities. The treatment should consist of either re-induction (i.e., PE, consider substituting cisplatin with carboplatin) or administration of a truly non-cross-resistant regimen. Single-agent topotecan is another alternative.

Brain metastases should be treated with WBI. The decision to add chemotherapy should follow the same consideration as for patients with extracranial recurrence.

Key Points

- The main purpose of treating relapsed small-cell lung cancer (SCLC) patients is palliative. Selected patients may benefit from second-line chemotherapy.
- Second-line chemotherapy should be offered to sensitive patients defined as those achieving a response to first-line treatment lasting more than 3 months after termination of first-line treatment.
- Patients refractory to first-line treatment including those failing first-line treatment or relapsing less than 3 months after end of first-line treatment do not benefit from chemotherapy and thus refractory patients should be considered for palliative measures other than chemotherapy, such as radiotherapy.
- No generally accepted treatment strategy for second-line therapy exists. The options include re-induction, the use of presumably non-cross-resistant chemotherapy, or new agents such as taxanes and topoisomerase I inhibitors.
- Patients with recurrence in the brain may benefit from whole-brain irradiation and steroids. The addition of chemotherapy should be considered for sensitive patients.

References

1. Ebi N, Kubota K, Nishiwaki Y, et al. Second-line chemotherapy for relapsed small cell lung cancer. Jpn J Clin Oncol 1997;27:166.
2. Ardizzoni A, Hansen H, Dombernowsky P, et al. Topotecan, a new active drug in the second-line treatment of small-cell lung cancer: a phase II study in patients with refractory and sensitive disease. The European Organization for Research and Treatment of Cancer Early Clinical Studies Group and New Drug Development Office, and the Lung Cancer Cooperative Group. J Clin Oncol 1997;15:2090.
3. Chute JP, Kelley MJ, Venzon D, Williams J, Roberts A, Johnson BE. Retreatment of patients surviving cancer-free 2 or more years after initial treatment of small cell lung cancer. Chest 1996;110:165.
4. von Pawel J, Schiller JH, Shepherd FA, et al. Topotecan versus cyclophosphamide, doxorubicin, and vincristine for the treatment of recurrent small-cell lung cancer. J Clin Oncol 1999;17:658.
5. Sculier JP, Lafitte JJ, Lecomte J, et al. A phase II randomised trial comparing the cisplatin-etoposide combination chemotherapy with or without carboplatin as second-line therapy for small-cell lung cancer. Ann Oncol 2002;13:1454.
6. Spiro SG, Souhami RL, Geddes DM, et al. Duration of chemotherapy in small cell lung cancer: a Cancer Research Campaign trial. Br J Cancer 1989;59:578.
7. de Vore RF, Blanke CD, Denham CA, et al. Phase II study of irinotecan (CPT-11) in patients with previously untreated small-cell lung cancer (SCLC). Proc Am Soc Clin Oncol 1998;17:A1736.
8. Masuda N, Fukuoka M, Matsui K, et al. Evaluation of high-dose etoposide combined with cisplatin for treating relapsed small cell lung cancer. Cancer 1990;65:2635.
9. Shepherd FA, Evans WK, MacCormick R, Feld R, Yau JC. Cyclophosphamide, doxorubicin, and vincristine in etoposide- and cisplatin-resistant small cell lung cancer. Cancer Treat Rep 1987;71:941.
10. Sculier JP, Klastersky J, Libert P, et al. Cyclophosphamide, doxorubicin and vincristine with amphotericin B in sonicated liposomes as salvage therapy for small cell lung cancer. Eur J Cancer 1990;26:919.
11. Roth BJ, Johnson DH, Einhorn LH, et al. Randomized study of cyclophosphamide, doxorubicin, and vincristine versus etoposide and cisplatin versus alternation of these two regimens in extensive small-cell lung cancer: a phase III trial of the Southeastern Cancer Study Group. J Clin Oncol 1992;10:282.
12. Postmus PE, Smit EF, Kirkpatrick A, Splinter TA. Testing the possible non-cross resistance of two equipotent combination chemotherapy regimens against small-cell lung cancer: a phase II study of the EORTC Lung Cancer Cooperative Group. Eur J Cancer 1993;29A:204.
13. Perez-Soler R, Glisson BS, Lee JS, Fossella FV, Murphy WK, Shin DM, Hong WK. Treatment of patients with small-cell lung cancer refractory to etoposide and cisplatin with the topoisomerase I poison topotecan. J Clin Oncol 1996;14:2785.
14. von Pawel J, Gatzemeier U, Pujol JL, et al. Phase II comparator study of oral versus intravenous topotecan in patients with chemosensitive small-cell lung cancer. J Clin Oncol 2001;19:1743.
15. Smit EF, Fokkema E, Biesma B, Groen HJ, Snoek W, Postmus PE. A phase II study of paclitaxel in heavily pretreated patients with small-cell lung cancer. Br J Cancer 1998;77:347.
16. Groen HJ, Smit EF, Haaxma-Reiche H, Postmus PE. Carboplatin as second-line treatment for recurrent or pro-

gressive brain metastases from small cell lung cancer. Eur J Cancer 1993;29A:1696.

17. Johnson DH, Greco FA, Strupp J, Hande KR, Hainsworth JD. Prolonged administration of oral etoposide in patients with relapsed or refractory small-cell lung cancer: a phase II trial. J Clin Oncol 1990; 8:1613.

18. Groen HJ, Fokkema E, Biesma B, Kwa B, van Putten JW, Postmus PE, Smit EF. Paclitaxel and carboplatin in the treatment of small-cell lung cancer patients resistant to cyclophosphamide, doxorubicin, and etoposide: a non-cross-resistant schedule. J Clin Oncol 1999;17:927.

19. Ardizzoni A, Manegold C, Debruyne C, et al. European organization for research and treatment of cancer (EORTC) 08957 phase II study of topotecan in combination with cisplatin as second-line treatment of refractory and sensitive small cell lung cancer. Clin Cancer Res 2003;9:143.

20. Masuda N, Matsui K, Negoro S, et al. Combination of irinotecan and etoposide for treatment of refractory or relapsed small-cell lung cancer. J Clin Oncol 1998;16:3329.

21. O'Bryan RM, Crowley JJ, Kim PN, et al. Comparison of etoposide and cisplatin with bis-chloro-ethylnitrosourea, thiotepa, vincristine, and cyclophosphamide for salvage treatment in small cell lung cancer. A Southwest Oncology Group Study. Cancer 1990;65:856.

22. Albain KS, Crowley JJ, Hutchins L, et al. Predictors of survival following relapse or progression of small cell lung cancer. Southwest Oncology Group Study 8605 report and analysis of recurrent disease data base. Cancer 1993;72:1184.

23. Postmus PE, Haaxma-Reiche H, Gregor A, et al. Brain-only metastases of small cell lung cancer: efficacy of whole brain radiotherapy. An EORTC phase II study. Radiother Oncol 1998;46:29.

24. Postmus PE, Haaxma-Reiche H, Smit EF, et al. Treatment of brain metastases of small-cell lung cancer: comparing teniposide and teniposide with whole-brain radiotherapy – a phase III study of the European Organization for the Research and Treatment of Cancer Lung Cancer Cooperative Group. J Clin Oncol 2000;18:3400.

Prophylactic Cranial Irradiation in Patients with Small-Cell Lung Cancer

32

Kevin J. Harrington, Christopher M. Nutting
and Konstantinos N. Syrigos

Contents

32.1 Introduction

Lung cancer demonstrates a striking propensity toward the development of cerebral metastases. Such metastases can come to medical attention at any time during the clinical course of the disease. This is especially true for small-cell lung cancer (SCLC) with some series reporting cerebral metastasis rates of 50–80% [1]. Certainly, data from autopsy series consistently show rates of intracerebral disease in the range of 50–70% [2]. Up to 10% of patients will demonstrate cerebral metastases at the time of diagnosis of the primary lung cancer [3]. However, by far the most common clinical scenario is disease relapse in the central nervous system, often in the setting of apparently controlled extracranial disease. The complete response (CR) rates for patients with limited-stage SCLC after combination chemotherapy plus thoracic radiotherapy are in the order of 50–85% [3–5]. As locoregional control rates have improved with the use of both chemotherapy and thoracic irradiation, the potential risk of cerebral relapse has assumed even greater clinical importance. Therefore, the use of prophylactic cranial irradiation (PCI) to reduce the risk of cerebral relapse of SCLC has been developed alongside improvements in systemic chemotherapy and local thoracic irradiation. In this chapter, we will review the evidence that PCI confers a benefit to disease-free and overall survival and discuss the impact of this treatment on neuropsychiatric performance in this group of patients.

32.2 Rationale for the Use of Prophylactic Cranial Irradiation

The use of fractionated courses of radiotherapy to ablate subclinical disease is of proven benefit in a range of different tumor types. For example, adjuvant radiotherapy to the tumor bed after surgery has been shown to reduce the risk of local recurrence in head and neck, breast, gastrointestinal, and gynecological cancers. Furthermore, radiotherapy to areas at high risk of harboring micrometastatic tumor deposits has also been shown to be effective, especially in the setting of the clinically and radiologically negative neck in patients with head and neck cancer [6]. Therefore, if one accepts the premise that a significant number of patients with SCLC will have subclinical disease in the brain at the time of initial diagnosis and that this disease is in a pharmacological sanctuary site that is not accessible to combination cytotoxic chemotherapy, the use of PCI represents a sound strategy for treating a potential cause of disease relapse. In the common epithelial tumors described above, radiation doses in the order of 50–60 Gy in fractions of 1.8–2.0 Gy per day are generally used to control subclinical micrometastatic disease [6–8]. However, in view of the in vitro and in vivo radiosensitivity of SCLC cell lines, such protracted treatment courses have not been used in the setting of PCI. Most current PCI regimens employ radiation doses of 24–30 Gy at 2 or 3 Gy per fraction.

32.3 Technique for Delivery of Prophylactic Cranial Irradiation

The aim of PCI is to deliver a homogeneous radiation dose to all of the cerebral tissue above the skull base. Particular attention must be paid to ensure that the most caudal structures (temporal lobes and posterior fossa) are included in the treatment fields. The techniques that are used to plan treatment can vary significantly. In a number of centers, treatment will be based on surface landmarks in which all structures cephalad of a line joining the mastoid process to the supraorbital ridge are irradiated with rectangular fields with typical dimensions of approximately 12×18 cm. In other centers, treatment planning is performed on the simulator and shaped shielding is used at the skull base. In all cases, treatment is delivered using parallel-opposed lateral fields on a linear accelerator (6–10 MV) or a ^{60}Co machine with the dose and fractionation varying in different centers. The use of steroid cover to reduce the risk of radiation-induce cerebral edema is optional.

32.4 Meta-analysis of the Effect of Prophylactic Cranial Irradiation

A number of clinical trials have been conducted in the last 25 years with the aim of determining the potential benefit of PCI in SCLC. The numbers of patients in the individual trials vary quite widely with the result that many studies were not sufficiently powered to detect differences between the treatment groups. In order to resolve this issue, the powerful statistical method of meta-analysis has been applied to these data by the Prophylactic Cranial Irradiation Overview Collaborative Group [9]. This study group identified trials in which patients with histologically proven SCLC in CR after induction chemotherapy were randomly assigned to receive PCI or no PCI. Appropriate trials were identified by means of a detailed search of electronic databases, the reference sections of published trials, review articles, and book chapters, and of the abstracts presented in the proceedings of scientific meetings. Using this search strategy, 17 trials were identified in which patients had been randomly allocated to PCI or no PCI groups. Subsequent review of these data resulted in the exclusion of 10 of the trials (929 patients) because they did not meet the strict eligibility criteria of the meta-analysis. Typical reasons for exclusion of trials included inadequate randomization methodology, randomization before the response to induction therapy was known, and delivery of mannitol (rather than no PCI) to the control group. Therefore, the data from the meta-analysis were based on 987 patients in 7 clinical trials [10–15]. Summary data for the patients included in the

Table 32.1. Summary data for the 987 patients who were included in the Prophylactic Cranial Irradiation Overview Collaborative Group study [9]

Characteristic	PCI group (n = 526)	No PCI group (n = 461)
Male	403 (77%)	352 (76%)
Median age (range)	59 (26–80%)	59 (21–29%)
Performance status		
0	212 (67%)	215 (66%)
1	96 (30%)	105 (32%)
2, 3	7 (2%)	6 (2%)
Extensive disease	62 (12%)	78 (17%)
Induction chemotherapy + thoracic radiotherapy	314 (77%)	248 (74%)
Interval between start of chemotherapy and PCI		
< 4 months	84 (27%)	77 (24%)
4–6 months	127 (41%)	152 (48%)
> 6 months	102 (33%)	91 (28%)

meta-analysis are presented in Table 32.1. As can be seen, the two groups were well matched for demographic, disease-related, and treatment-related variables.

The details of the individual studies that were included in the meta-analysis are presented in Table 32.2 and this shows that the great majority of the patients were enrolled in only 3 studies (the PCI-85 [12], PCI-88 [15], and UKCCCR/EORTC [14] trials). The criteria that were used to determine complete remission varied between the trials from a plain chest radiograph to bronchoscopy and/or chest computed tomography (CT) scan, and these differences can be seen as reflecting current practices at the time that the different trials were established. There was a wide variation in the radiation doses that were prescribed, although all of the trials initially set out to deliver a total PCI dose of 24–40 Gy and between 2 and 3 Gy per fraction. The UKCCCR/EORTC trial was initially set up to randomize patients to control and two different PCI doses (24 Gy in 12 fractions and 36 Gy in 18 fractions) but failed to accrue patients at the projected rate and so the dose recommendations were relaxed. As a consequence, patients were eventually treated to total radiation doses between 8 Gy in 1 fraction and 36 Gy in 18 fractions. It can also be seen that for many of the trials the median follow-up was extremely long, reflecting the nature of such studies in which individual patient data are gathered by the investigating collaborative group.

32.4.1 Effect of Prophylactic Cranial Irradiation on Cerebral Relapse

The pooled data from the trials included in the meta-analysis demonstrated a significant reduction in the incidence of cerebral relapse in patients in the PCI treatment group (see Table 32.2). The relative risk of cere-

Table 32.2. Details of the seven trials included in the Prophylactic Cranial Irradiation Overview Collaborative Group meta-analysis [9]

Trial	Patients	Radiotherapy dose (dose per fraction)	Percent brain metastases after PCI	Percent brain metastases after no PCI	Follow-up (years)	P value
UMCC	29	30 (3)	0	36	18.5	0.02
Okayama	46	40 (2)	22	52	11.7	<0.05
PCI-85	300	24 (3)	40	67	8.3	$<10^{-13}$
Danish-NCI	55	24 (3)	37	52	8.8	Unpublished
UKCCCR-EORTC	314	Several	38	54	3.5	0.0004
PCI-88	211	24 (3)	44	51	5.1	0.14
ECOG-RTOG	32	25 (2.5)	19	53	3.9	NS

Table 32.3. Results of Prophylactic Cranial Irradiation Overview Collaborative Group study

Endpoint	Patients in PCI group	Patients in no PCI group	Relative risk (95% CI)	P value	Rate in control group at 3 years	Absolute benefit at 3 years
OS	526	461	0.83 (0.73–0.97)	0.01	15.3%	+5.4%
DFS	526	461	0.75 (0.65–0.86)	<0.001	13.5%	+8.8%
Cumulative brain metastases	524	457	0.46 (0.38–0.57)	<0.001	58.6%	−25.3%
Cumulative other metastases	325	332	0.89 (0.69–1.15)	0.37	45.6%	−3.8%
Cumulative locoregional recurrence	323	334	0.97 (0.75–1.26)	0.84	45.1%	−1.0%

bral metastases for patients who received PCI was 0.46 with 95% confidence intervals (CI) of 0.38–0.57. Indeed, for most of the individual trials this improvement was also seen, with only the Danish-NCI and PCI-88 trials failing to show a statistically significant improvement for PCI. As regards the PCI-88 trial, this trial had originally been designed to recruit 1,100 patients but it was stopped prematurely on publication of the PCI-85 study. At that time less than 20% of the target recruitment had been enrolled and analysis of the data showed no significant differences between the two groups in terms of cerebral relapse or overall survival. A subsequent pooled analysis of the PCI-85 and PCI-88 trials demonstrated a 16% reduction in brain metastases and an 8% improvement in survival from 18% to 26% at 3 years, although this failed to reach statistical significance.

32.4.2 Effect of Prophylactic Cranial Irradiation on Survival

Analysis of the 7 trials included in the meta-analysis revealed a significant advantage to patients who received PCI. The relative risk of death for patients who received PCI was 0.84, with 95% CI of 0.73–0.97. In terms of overall survival values, there was an absolute difference of 5.4% between the two treatment groups. The 3-year survival rates for the control and PCI groups were 15.3% and 20.7%, respectively. The benefit to disease-free survival was even more impressive with a relative

risk of 0.75 with 95% CI of 0.65–0.86. As might be expected from a treatment that seeks only to attain local control in the brain, there was no impact of PCI on locoregional control in the chest or on the development of metastases at other sites (see Table 32.3).

32.4.3 Effect of Radiation Dose on Outcome of Prophylactic Cranial Irradiation

The only individual study that has attempted to evaluate the effect of radiation dose on cerebral control was the UKCCCR/EORTC trial in which patients were to have been randomized to control, 24 Gy in 12 fractions, or 36 Gy in 18 fractions. As has been described above, this trial failed to meet its recruitment targets and the design was relaxed to allow centers more freedom in the radiation dose prescription. Therefore, the authors of the meta-analysis also presented data on the effect of radiation dose on the efficacy of PCI, measured in terms of survival and cerebral metastasis. This analysis is colored by the fact that very similar doses were used in each of the trials included in the meta-analysis. Nonetheless, it was possible to group patients in to four different radiation doses (8 Gy, 24–25 Gy, 30 Gy, and 36–40 Gy). As can be seen in Table 32.4, the vast majority of patients were treated with a radiation dose between 24 and 30 Gy. The lowest radiation dose (8 Gy as a single fraction) was used in a single center in the UKCCCR/EORTC trial. The effect of the different doses

Table 32.4. Effect of radiation dose on survival and local control in the brain

Total radiation dose (Gy)	Patients in PCI group	Patients in no PCI group	Relative risk of death (95% CI)	P value	Relative risk of cerebral metastasis	P value
8	26	16	0.69 (0.35–1.37)	0.81	0.76 (0.28–2.10)	0.02
24–25	330	340	0.88 (0.75–1.04)		0.52 (0.41–0.67)	
30	119	82	0.81 (0.59–1.12)		0.34 (0.19–0.59)	
36–40	51	59	0.81 (0.54–1.20)		0.27 (0.14–0.51)	

Table 32.5. Analysis of the effect of the timing of prophylactic cranial radiotherapy relative to induction chemotherapy

Interval between chemotherapy and PCI	Patients in PCI group	Patients in no PCI group	Relative risk of death (95% CI)	P value	Relative risk of cerebral metastasis	P value
<4 months	84	77	0.92 (0.66–1.29)	0.39	0.27 (0.16–0.46)	0.01
4–6 months	127	152	0.79 (0.61–1.02)		0.50 (0.35–0.72)	
>6 months	102	91	1.01 (0.74–1.38)		0.69 (0.44–1.08)	

on survival and local control in the brain are shown in Table 32.4. Only the effect on cerebral relapse was found to be statistically significant with a trend to lower rates of brain metastases with increased radiation dose.

32.4.4 Effect of the Interval Between the Start of Induction Chemotherapy and Prophylactic Cranial Irradiation

A further subgroup analysis in the meta-analysis looked at the effect of the delay between commencement of combination chemotherapy and the first fraction of PCI (Table 32.5). This analysis confirms a significant trend for reduced cerebral metastasis with an early start to PCI. In particular, the relative risk of cerebral metastasis was only 0.27 when PCI began less than 4 months after the start of chemotherapy. This finding probably reflects the fact that prolonged courses of chemotherapy or delay in delivery of PCI leaves subclinical disease in the central nervous system untreated in a sanctuary site. Consideration of these data means that recent protocols have tended toward introduction of PCI earlier in the treatment plan.

32.4.5 Neuropsychiatric Effects of Prophylactic Cranial Irradiation

From the time of the first trials of PCI in patients with SCLC, there were concerns about the effects of treatment on brain function [16]. Early retrospective series reported clinical neurotoxicity that was thought to develop between 6 and 24 months after completion of radiotherapy. This clinical syndrome often occurred in the absence of radiological changes in the brain. Analy-

sis of the pattern of the toxicity suggested that it appeared to be related to radiotherapy fraction size, total dose, and the volume of brain tissue that was treated. It was also suggested that neuropsychiatric morbidity was associated with the delivery of combination chemotherapy during PCI, perhaps due to the effect of PCI in disrupting the blood–brain barrier and allowing access of cytotoxic drugs to what was otherwise a sanctuary site.

These early impressions of a detrimental effect of PCI resulted in the publication of a number of small retrospective studies that appeared to confirm reduced scores on a range of neuropsychometric tests for patients with SCLC. Cull et al. [17] reported a retrospective study of 64 patients who were free of relapse of SCLC more than 2 years after completion of therapy. Fifty-two patients had received PCI, of whom 50% had received concurrent chemotherapy and PCI. None of the patients had undergone pretreatment baseline neuropsychometric tests. At the time of testing, 81% of patients had impaired function in one of the four tests that were used and 54% had impaired function in more than one test.

Van Oosterhout et al. [18] published a retrospective study in 49 long-term SCLC survivors who had been evaluated with five tests. The study group included a range of clinical scenarios. Nineteen patients had received chemotherapy only, 19 had received PCI after completion of chemotherapy, and 11 had received PCI concurrent with or sandwiched between courses of chemotherapy. Once again, in this retrospective series, no baseline neuropsychometric data were available but at the time of testing the treated patients scored significantly worse than a group of healthy matched controls. Interestingly, there was no clear association between the schedule of chemotherapy and PCI and the test scores.

The same authors published a small prospective study in which 32 patients were enrolled [19]. These patients underwent pretreatment baseline neuropsychometric tests and these were significantly worse than a group of healthy matched controls. During the course of the study, 14 patients developed brain metastases and were, therefore, not evaluable for the effects of therapy on cognitive function. Only 11 patients were fully evaluable and the authors reported no deterioration in neuropsychometric scores up to 5 months after treatment. As has been discussed above, the PCI85 trial [12] involved 300 patients in complete remission after induction therapy for SCLC. As part of this study, pretreatment neuropsychometric tests were performed and 59% of patients had detectable abnormalities at baseline. The late toxicity of treatment was assessed in 229 patients (114 PCI versus 115 no PCI) and there were no significant differences between the two groups. These findings were reinforced by data from the UKCCCR/EORTC trial [14] in which prospective data were available for 136 (of 314) patients in complete remission after induction therapy. Eighty-four patients had received PCI and 52 had not. There were detectable abnormalities at baseline in both patient groups, although there were no differences at baseline between the groups. At retesting at 6 and 12 months there was no evidence of significant deterioration in either group and no emerging differences between the two groups.

More recently, another large study has reopened the question of the potential detrimental effect of delivering combination chemotherapy during PCI. Ahles et al. [20] have reported a prospective study in which they treated 347 patients who were randomised to receive intensive chemotherapy, thoracic radiotherapy, and PCI with or without warfarin. In this study, the PCI was delivered concomitant with combination chemotherapy that consisted of cisplatin, cyclophosphamide, and etoposide. A total of 295 patients were evaluated for neuropsychometric effects with evidence of a significant deterioration in function at 8 weeks after completion of PCI. Unfortunately, the late tests at 12 and 24 months that were planned by the authors were not reported because of significant patient attrition.

32.5 Conclusions

The meta-analysis performed by the Prophylactic Cranial Irradiation Overview Collaborative Group has provided clear evidence of the beneficial effects of this treatment in terms of survival and reduction of cerebral metastasis. Delivery of PCI results in a 5.4% improvement in overall survival at 3 years after the commencement of induction chemotherapy. PCI was also shown to yield a 54% proportional reduction in the incidence of cerebral metastases, from 59% to 33%, at 3 years. Subgroup analysis suggests a trend toward reduced incidence of cerebral metastasis with increased radiation dose and earlier introduction of PCI into the treatment regimen. Further studies will address the effect of different radiation doses and fractionation regimens (including twice-daily, hyperfractionated radiotherapy) and the optimal timing of PCI relative to induction chemotherapy. Evaluation of the data on the neuropsychiatric sequelae of PCI suggest that patients have significant abnormalities at baseline and that there is no demonstrable change after PCI. However, there is a suggestion that PCI delivered concomitantly with chemotherapy may be associated with a significant deterioration in cognitive function.

Key Points

- A significant number of patients with small-cell lung cancer (SCLC) have subclinical disease in the brain at the time of initial diagnosis and this disease is in a pharmacological sanctuary site that is not accessible to combination cytotoxic chemotherapy. Therefore, the use of prophylactic cranial irradiation (PCI) represents a sound strategy for treating a potential cause of disease relapse at that site.
- The aim of PCI is to deliver a homogeneous radiation dose to all of the cerebral tissue above the skull base. Particular attention must be paid to ensure that the most caudal structures (temporal lobes and posterior fossa) are included in the treatment fields.
- The meta-analysis performed by the Prophylactic Cranial Irradiation Overview Collaborative Group has provided clear evidence of the beneficial effects of this treatment in terms of survival and reduction of cerebral metastasis. Delivery of PCI results in a 5.4% improvement in overall survival at 3 years after the commencement of induction chemotherapy.
- Evaluation of the data on the neuropsychiatric sequelae of PCI suggest that patients have significant abnormalities at baseline and that there is no demonstrable change after PCI. However, there is a suggestion that PCI delivered concomitantly with chemotherapy may be associated with a significant deterioration in cognitive function.

References

1. Nugent MJ, Bunn PA, Matthews MJ, et al. CNS metastases in small cell bronchogenic carcinoma: increasing frequency and changing pattern with lengthening survival. Cancer 1979;44:1885.
2. Hirsch FR, Paulson OB, Hansen HH, et al. Intracranial metastases in small cell carcinoma of the lung: correlation of clinical and autopsy findings. Cancer 1982;50:2433.

3. Albain KS, Crowley JJ, LeBlanc M, Livingston RB. Determinants of improved in small-cell lung cancer: an analysis of the 2580-patient Southwest Oncology Group data base. J Clin Oncol 1990;8:1563.
4. Arriagada R, Kramar A, Le Chevalier T, De Cremoux H. Competing events determining relapse-free survival in limited small-cell lung carcinoma. J Clin Oncol 1992;10:447.
5. Turrisi AT III, Kim K, Blum R, et al. Twice-daily compared with once-daily thoracic radiation in limited small-cell lung cancer treated concurrently with cisplatin and etoposide. N Engl J Med 1999;340:265.
6. Fletcher GH. Subclinical disease. Cancer 1984;53:1274.
7. Withers HR, Suwinski R. Radiation dose response for subclinical metastases. Semin Radiat Oncol 1998;8:224.
8. Early Breast Cancer Trialists' Collaborative Group. Favourable and unfavourable effects on long-term survival of radiotherapy for early breast cancer: an overview of the randomized trials. Lancet 2000;355:1757.
9. Auperin A, Arriagada R, Pignon J-P, et al. Prophylactic cranial irradiation for patients with small-cell lung cancer in complete remission. N Engl J Med 1999;341:476.
10. Aroney RS, Aisner J, Wesley MN, et al. Value of prophylactic cranial irradiation given at complete remission in small cell lung carcinoma. Cancer Treat Rep 1983;67:675.
11. Ohonoshi T, Ueoka H, Kawahara S, et al. Comparative study of prophylactic cranial irradiation in patients with small cell lung cancer achieving a complete response: a long-term follow-up result. Lung Cancer 1993;10:47.
12. Arriagada R, Le Chevalier T, Borie F, et al. Prophylactic cranial irradiation for patients with small cell lung cancer in complete remission. J Natl Cancer Inst 1995;87:183.
13. Wagner H, Kim K, Turrisi A. A randomized phase III study of prophylactic cranial irradiation versus observation in patients with small cell lung cancer achieving a complete response: final report of an incomplete trial by the Eastern Cooperative Oncology Group and Radiation Therapy Oncology Group (E3589/R92-01). Proc Am Soc Clin Oncol 1996;15:376.
14. Gregor A, Cull A, Stephens RJ, et al. Prophylactic cranial irradiation is indicated following complete response to induction therapy in small cell lung cancer: results of a multicentre randomized trial. Eur J Cancer 1997;33:1752.
15. Laplanche A, Monnet I, Santos-Miranda JA, et al. Controlled clinical trial of prophylactic cranial irradiation for patients with small-cell lung cancer in complete remission. Lung Cancer 1998;21:193.
16. Vines E, Le Pechoux C, Arriagada R. Prophylactic cranial irradiation in small cell lung cancer. Semin Oncol 2003;30:38.
17. Cull A, Gregor A, Hopwood P, et al. Neurological and cognitive impairment in long-term survivors of small cell lung cancer. Eur J Cancer 1994;30A:1067.
18. Van Ousterhout AGM, Ganzevles PGJ, Wilmink JT, et al. Sequelae in long-term survivors of small cell lung cancer. Int J Radiat Oncol Biol Phys 1996;34:1037.
19. Van Ousterhout AGM, Boon PJ, Houx PJ, et al. Follow-up of cognitive functioning in patients with small cell lung cancer. Int J Radiat Oncol Biol Phys 1995;31:911.
20. Ahles TA, Silberfarb PM, Herndon J, et al. Psychologic and neuropsychologic functioning of patients with limited small-cell lung cancer treated with chemotherapy and radiation with or without warfarin: a study by the Cancer and Leukemia Group B. J Clin Oncol 1998;16:1954.

Late Effects of Small-Cell Lung Cancer Treatment

33

Daphne M. Coutroubis and Jeremy P. C. Steele

Contents

33.1 Introduction

Without treatment, small-cell lung cancer (SCLC) has an aggressive clinical course with a median survival of as little as 6–17 weeks [1]. The treatment of SCLC comprises a combination of chemotherapy and radiotherapy with the aim of controlling the tumor locally and pre-venting systemic metastases. With treatment the prognosis of SCLC greatly improves [2–4], but the overall survival at 5 years ranges from only 5% to 10% [5–7].

The amount of treatment that is beneficial varies according to prognostic factors. These include stage of cancer, gender, number of sites involved, and performance status [6, 8, 9]. Limited-stage SCLC is up to 80–90% responsive to chemotherapy with a median survival of 15–18 months [10]. In addition, chest irradiation reduces local failure rates and increases 3-year survival [11].

Administering treatment for SCLC is clearly beneficial for most patients. But treatment also has disadvantages because of both short-term side effects and long-term complications. Unfortunately the prognosis for most patients is poor so that, in most cases, long-term effects are rarely of concern. Nevertheless it is still important to be aware of them, especially as the development of improved imaging and treatments will allow more patients to survive longer.

33.2 Chemotherapy

Chemotherapy is effective, but toxic, especially when used in high doses [12]. There is no discrimination between normal and malignant cells and tissue damage occurs resulting in adverse effects that can become life-threatening [13]. There are certain factors that affect both short-term and long-term toxicity of chemotherapy. They are choice of agent, dose, schedule of administration, route of administration, predisposing factors, and comorbidities in the patient [14].

The use of high-dose chemotherapy is controversial in SCLC. On the one hand, there is evidence that it may improve prognosis because the increased dose or dose intensity can do more damage to SCLC cells [15]. Patients in or near complete response before high-dose therapy have the most favorable prognosis [16, 17]. On the other hand, high-dose chemotherapy intensification will increase the overall toxicity to the body and cause more damage to normal cells [18]. A study by Rizzo et

Table 33.1. Common acute side effects of SCLC chemotherapy

Myelosuppression (leukopenia, thrombocytopenia, anemia)
Mucous membrane ulceration
Alopecia
Nausea and vomiting

al. in 2002 showed that receiving autologous hematopoietic stem cell transplantation with high-dose chemotherapy improved the survival rate in younger patients with limited-stage SCLC [19]. Chemotherapy causes both short-term and long-term complications. This chapter deals mainly with the long-term complications but the commoner acute toxicities are summarized below in Table 33.1. These side effects result from the cytotoxic effect of chemotherapy on rapidly dividing normal cells of the epithelium and bone marrow, for example, mucous membranes, skin, and hair follicles [14].

33.2.1 General Principles of the Causation of Late Effects of Chemotherapy

Late effects to normal tissue and organs are toxicities that occur at or persist for 90 days or more from the start of therapy [20–22]. Late effects are thought to be the result of parenchymal cellular depletion of both cycling and non-cycling cells with sparing of the fibroconnective tissue stroma and microcirculation [23]. This section identifies and discusses the effects on vital organs that can cause fatalities if tolerance is exceeded.

33.2.2 Cardiac Toxicities

Damage results from chemotherapy agents such as the anthracyclines and related substances, and high-dose cyclophosphamide. Damage is seen to all cardiac structures: the pericardium, the myocardium, the peripheral vasculature, the conduction system, and the heart valves. In some settings, the heart sustains subclinical damage, and a subsequent insult triggers clinically relevant cardiac dysfunction [24]. Numerous studies on the effects of doxorubicin (Adriamycin) on the heart serve as models for anthracycline-associated and related cardiomyopathies [25–29]. A cumulative dose of doxorubicin greater than 400 mg/m^2 causes a rapid increase in cardiomyopathies [25, 27, 30]. Other anthracycline or anthracycline-derived agents, such as daunorubicin, idarubicin, epirubicin, and mitoxantrone, carry similar risks to doxorubicin [24].

A number of agents have the potential to cause myocardial ischemia, with or without overt myocardial infarction. These include vinblastine, vincristine, bleomycin, cisplatin, interleukin-2, and 5-fluorouracil [31–33].

Some agents, including paclitaxel and interleukin-2, have also been associated with hypotension and bradycardia [33, 34].

33.2.3 Pulmonary Toxicities

Chemotherapy-related pulmonary toxicities can be difficult to diagnose and have three general forms of presentation.

Chronic Pneumonitis or Fibrosis
Agents associated with fibrosis include bleomycin [35], cyclophosphamide, BCNU, busulfan, mitomycin C, and chlorambucil [23]. Type I pneumocytes degenerate and desquamate, as they are vulnerable to toxicity, and, in response, type II pneumocytes proliferate and exhibit prominent nucleoli and giant cell formation. Subsequently chronic inflammatory cell infiltration occurs, leading to further fibroblastic proliferation and fibrosis [36].

Hypersensitivity Pneumonitis and Related Conditions
Methotrexate, bleomycin, and procarbazine can cause hypersensitivity pneumonitis, acute pleuritis, or pulmonary edema [37]. Methotrexate-induced pulmonary hypersensitivity carries a mortality rate of approximately 1% and about 10% of patients will go on to develop pulmonary fibrosis [38].

Non-cardiogenic Pulmonary Edema
Agents that are associated with this complication include cytosine arabinoside, teniposide, methotrexate, bleomycin, and cyclophosphamide [37].

33.2.4 Nephrotoxicities

This is defined as a doubling in the serum creatinine estimation from normal baseline and a serum urea >40 mg/dl. Renal complications of chemotherapy include tumor-lysis syndrome, paraneoplastic glomerulonephritis, obstructive uropathy, and acute nephrotoxicity with renal failure and electrolyte disturbances [39]. It is essential to adjust the dose of different chemotherapeutic agents based on renal function and interactions with other drugs that may be delivered concomitantly, especially when high-dose chemotherapy and additional total body irradiation are used [39]. Specific types of nephrotoxicity are associated with the following SCLC drugs, and are shown in Table 33.2. Agents that have the highest risk of nephrotoxicity are cisplatin [40] and methotrexate [41]; agents associated with chronic renal

Table 33.2. Current or previously used SCLC agents associated with nephrotoxicity

Class	Drug
Alkylating agents and platins	Cisplatin
	Carboplatin
	Ifosfamide
	Nitrosoureas
Antitumor antibiotics	Mitomycin
Antimetabolites	High-dose methotrexate
Biologic agents	Interferon

failure [42] are cisplatin, carmustine, lomustine, 5-fluorouracil [43], and mitomycin C [43]; and agents associated with delayed specific tubular damage [42] are cisplatin, cyclophosphamide, lomustine [44], streptozotocin [45], carmustine, and mitomycin C [43].

Carboplatin Dosing

Carboplatin is one of the most important drugs in the treatment of SCLC. Calvert [46] derived a formula for carboplatin dosing by a retrospective analysis of 18 patients. Each patient's pretreatment glomerular filtration rate (GFR) was measured and by using the formula [dose (mg) = target AUC × (GFR + 25)] the dosage of carboplatin required to produce a clinical effect with manageable hematologic toxicity was determined. The formula accurately predicted the observed "area under the curve" (AUC) and has, hence, become applicable to combination and high-dose carboplatin as well as conventional single-agent therapy. Most other chemotherapy agents continue to be dosed by the traditional body surface area estimation method.

33.2.5 Neurotoxicities

Many cancer treatments are associated with neurotoxicity and some of the commonest are presented in Table 33.3 below. Neurologic toxicity is a dose-limiting factor and patients may suffer more from these toxicities than from the cancer itself [47, 48]. Different factors relating to continuous improvement of treatments have paradoxically resulted in an increased incidence of acute and delayed neurotoxicity. These factors include increased or intensified dosing and improved survival rates [49]. The most common consequence of intrathecal chemotherapy and cranial radiotherapy, especially when the two are combined, is the development of chronic dementia. Dementia may begin to appear 1–2 years after completion of treatment [50, 51] and is due to microvascular changes and demyelination (leukoencephalopathy) [52, 53]. Seizures of focal origin are another potential finding and are the result of focal necrosis, strokes, and ischemia [49, 54].

Table 33.3. SCLC agents causing neurotoxicities

Agent	Neurotoxicity
Methotrexate	Acute somnolence, chronic leukoencephalopathy, mineralizing microangiopathy, myelopathy from intrathecal injection
Cisplatin/carboplatin	Large fiber sensory polyneuropathy, hearing loss, tinnitus, possible optic neuropathy, retinal cone dysfunction
Vincristine	Sensorimotor polyneuropathy, autonomic neuropathy, cranial neuropathy, SIADH, possible encephalopathy, myositis
5-Fluorouracil	Cerebellar dysfunction, transient confusion and disorientation, Wernicke-Korsakoff-like syndrome, optic neuropathy, parkinsonism (rare)
Cyclophosphamide	SIADH
Ifosfamide	Reversible encephalopathy, extrapyramidal signs: athetosis, myoclonus, opisthotonic posturing
BCNU, CCNU	Necrotizing encephalopathy with intra-arterial injection, retinal toxicity with common carotid injection
Interferon	Encephalopathy, progressive vegetative state with intraventricular injection, parkinsonism with intraventricular injection, hearing loss
Paclitaxel	Peripheral neuropathy, autonomic neuropathies, seizures (rare)

33.2.6 Hematologic and Immunologic Toxicities

Most of the hematologic effects of chemotherapy toxicity are short-term, reversible, and vary according to the specific chemotherapy treatment used. Alkylating agents are examples of treatment agents that can cause cytopenias to persist [14]. Chemotherapeutic agents can predispose to the development of infections by causing long-term immunologic impairment [14]. Many agents produce severe mucositis, particularly of the gastrointestinal tract, allowing the entry of microorganisms into tissues and the bloodstream [55].

33.2.7 Secondary Malignancies

Acute myelogenous leukemia (AML), acute lymphocytic leukemia (ALL), chronic myelogenous leukemia (CML), and myelodysplastic syndrome have all been reported as second cancers following treatment with chemotherapy for solid tumors [56–58]. These chemotherapy-induced leukemias are relatively resistant to subsequent therapy and have a cure rate of only 10–20% [56–58]. Therapy with cyclophosphamide, ifosfamide, cisplatin, carboplatin, busulfan, melphalan, nitrogen mustard, and procarbazine can result in myelodysplasia or secondary leukemia. This may present in up to 20% of patients after a latency period of between 4 and 7 years and have a poor prognosis [56, 58]. Topoisomerase II inhibitors such as the epipodophyllotoxins, etoposide and teniposide, as well as anthracyclines can also cause leukemia. These leukemias occur in between 2% and 12% of patients after a short latency period of 1–3 years and have a poor prognosis [56, 58]. Secondary cancers are at even greater risk of development when leukemogenic agents are given in combination with others (e.g. doxorubicin) [57].

Data on SCLC is scanty, but the relative risk of developing a second cancer after treatment for Hodgkin's disease is between two- and fourfold, most of which are solid neoplasms [59–62]. Solid tumors reported include thyroid cancer, breast cancer, skin cancer, and secondary leukemia. As many as 25% of secondary malignancies that follow treatment of Hodgkin's disease are secondary leukemia or lymphoma [59–62].

33.2.8 Gonadal Failure and Dysfunction

In men chemotherapy treatment can lead to temporary or permanent infertility. Temporary infertility has been indicated with cyclophosphamide [63], methotrexate, vincristine, and daunorubicin. However, data are limited and effects may also vary, depending on dosages used and different combinations with other agents that may alter toxicity levels. Agents that cause permanent damage to the seminiferous epithelium include the alkylating drugs, though other agents can also cause damage [64, 65]. In widespread cancer, generalized wasting may also contribute to impaired diminished spermatogenesis.

Women receiving chemotherapy treatment develop clinical signs and symptoms of primary ovarian failure: vaginal dryness with dyspareunia, endometrial hypoplasia, decreased libido, hot flashes, oligomenorrhea evolving into amenorrhea, and low circulating levels of estrogens with compensatory elevations of FSH and LH, i.e., premature menopause [66]. The precise frequency of permanent amenorrhea and infertility depends on the drug given, the total dose, concomitant radiation exposure, and the age of the patient at the time of treatment. Agents associated with primary ovarian failure include [67] alkylating agents, cyclophosphamide [68], busulfan [69], chlorambucil [70], and etoposide [71]. In the case of breast cancer, women receiving adjuvant chemotherapy treatment become menopausal within 10 months of beginning therapy [72, 73] and those given doxorubicin and cyclophosphamide usually become anovulatory within 3 months or sooner. It is likely that similar effects would result from the use of such drugs in women with SCLC. One study from the UK found that menopause occurred, on average, 3 years earlier in women who had received chemotherapy than in those who did not [74].

33.2.9 Late Physical Effects of Specific Chemotherapy Agents Used in Small-Cell Lung Cancer

The decision as to which agent to use in treatment of SCLC varies between institutions based on particular experience. Different agents have different therapeutic potentials whether used alone or in combinations. Worldwide the commonest schedules used for the treatment of SCLC are "PE" (cisplatin and etoposide) and "CE" (carboplatin and etoposide). Older regimens containing classic alkylating drugs (such as cyclophosphamide or ifosfamide) and doxorubicin are considered obsolete, but may have a role in specific settings. Camptothecin-containing regimens may prove to be the standard of care in the next few years [75].

Late complications that are associated with specific agents used in SCLC are evident [76]. Therapy with carboplatin can exhibit peripheral neuropathy (especially in patients older than 65 years), sensorineural deafness, optic neuritis, and azotemia

Cisplatin's late complications can be bradycardia, bundle-branch block, congestive cardiac failure, nephrotoxicity, ototoxicity and tinnitus, persistent hypomagnesemia and hypokalemia, peripheral sensory neuropathy, and an altered perception to color and even cortical blindness (rare).

Treatment with cyclophosphamide can lead to cardiac necrosis, acute myopericarditis, pulmonary fibrosis, hypothyroidism, cataracts, azospermia or amenorrhea, bladder fibrosis with telangiectasis of the mucosa, and secondary cancers including acute leukemia.

Irreversible cardiomyopathy with congestive cardiac failure and muscle weakness describe doxorubicin's late effects, whereas peripheral neuropathy and secondary cancers including leukemia are characteristic for etoposide.

An array of late complications can arise with methotrexate. They are renal dysfunction, renal tubular dysfunction, pulmonary fibrosis and pneumonitis, transverse myelitis, cerebritis, leukoencephalopathy with dementia, seizures, spasticity, ataxia (all rare), liver damage, osteoporosis, dermatitis, and photosensitivity.

Hepatic and renal dysfunction are also seen in mitomycin C with or without prolonged and severe myelosuppression (particularly thrombocytopenia), hemolytic uremia-like syndrome, interstitial pneumonitis, skin erythema, and skin ulceration (months later).

Peripheral neuropathy, generalized weakness, and seizures are characteristic of paclitaxel. However, paclitaxel can also affect the heart causing atrioventricular conduction defects, ventricular tachycardia, cardiac angina, necrosis, and even myocardial infarction (rare). Paralytic ileus can also be noted.

Similarly, vincristine can cause sensorimotor polyneuropathy, autonomic neuropathy, cranial neuropathy, encephalopathy, myositis, and seizures, as well as cranial nerve palsies, optic atrophy, and cortical blindness. Paralytic ileus is a common occurrence. Tissue necrosis can also occur at the site of injection.

33.3 Radiotherapy

Radiation affects the cells of the body in two ways [23]. It can cause parenchymal cellular hypoplasia of stem cells and alteration of the fine vasculature and fibroconnective tissues.

The slowly progressive arteriolar and interstitial fibrosis that develops after irradiation contributes to delayed parenchymal hypoplasia and causes the late effects of radiation [23]. The damaging effects on the fine vasculoconnective tissue stroma (i.e., arteriocapillary fibrosis) are predominantly a late development after irradiation and are determined by a number of factors [23]. The degree of damaging effects depends upon the relationship with the parenchymal cells, the reserve vasculature, and the degree of blood flow impairment. It also depends upon the collateral circulation, the capacity of vascular regeneration, and the functional demands during pathologic and physiologic stress.

The effects of radiation depend on many factors including energy intensity, dose fraction, total dose, and the extent to which the organ is exposed to radiation (portal size and location). Radiation effects on normal tissue may occur early, even before completion of a course of radiotherapy, or they can appear years later [77].

33.3.1 General Late Physical Effects of Radiotherapy

Radiotherapy can cause damage to any normal structure of a system. The most important are listed below.

33.3.2 Cardiovascular Damage

Chronic effusive pericarditis develops over a period of months to years and eventually causes a fibrous fusion of the parietal and visceral pericardia. This then evolves into the clinical syndrome known as constrictive pericarditis. The echocardiogram usually shows thickening of the pericardium, flattening of the posterior wall during diastole, and, in some cases, pericardial calcification; pericardial effusion may be absent. Radiation injuries can also involve the myocardium, heart valves, and coronary vessels [78]. Radiation causes vascular injury by inducing thickening of the arterial wall secondary to intimal and adventitial proliferation, thus causing reduction in luminal area. This can lead to coronary occlusion, myocardial ischemia, and infarction [79]. Large

doses of radiation have also been associated with accelerated arteriosclerosis and enhance cholesterol deposition and luminal ulceration [80]. Fibrous valvular endocardial thickening presents in 80% of autopsied patients treated with high-dose radiation [79]. The mitral and tricuspid valves are most commonly affected.

33.3.3 Pulmonary Damage

Radiation pneumonitis and fibrosis are the two main manifestations of radiation injury to the lung. Acute radiation injury (pneumonitis) results from injury to vascular endothelial cells and alveolar lining cells, particularly type II pneumocytes. This usually occurs as early as 2 weeks to 3 months after treatment. It is frequently produced by total lung radiation in excess of 12 Gy delivered over a 2- to 4-day period [81]. Increased radiation toxicity and higher cumulative doses (e.g., 40–50 Gy delivered to only part of one lung over 5–6 weeks) can result in fibrosis 6–12 months following treatment. The late fibrotic phase begins 3–6 months after irradiation. The pathology evolves in a subsequent fashion [82]. First, there is a sclerosing of the alveolar wall. It is then followed by extensive endothelial damage with loss and replacement of a few capillaries. Lastly, the alveolar spaces are replaced by fibrosis rendering them functionless.

33.3.4 Cutaneous Damage

The skin is one of the most common sites of toxicity associated with radiotherapy treatment. Radiation effects can be enhanced when certain chemotherapy agents, such as bleomycin, doxorubicin, fluorouracil, and methotrexate, are given within 1 week prior to radiation therapy. This may result in desquamation, erythema, edema, bullae, erosions, ulcerations, and postinflammatory hyperpigmentation. An erythematous inflammatory reaction can appear in previously irradiated skin from as little as 8 days to years after radiation therapy [83]. This reaction is referred to as radiation recall. Docetaxel has been associated with enhancement of radiation recall [84].

33.3.5 Renal Damage

Radiation to the kidneys can result in significant renal compromise from radiation-induced nephritis. When both kidneys are irradiated, the dose tolerance is 20 Gy in adults. This decreases when only one kidney is irradiated. Glomerular filtration rate starts to decrease at 15 Gy, and is completely lost at 25–30 Gy. Some chemotherapy agents, such as cisplatin, carmustine (BCNU), and dactinomycin, tend to lower normal tissue radiation tolerance. At 6–12 months after radiotherapy, symptoms such as anemia, hypertension, edema, albuminuria, and increased creatinine are recognized indicators of treatment-induced toxicity. After 12 months the commonest finding is benign or malignant hypertension, which eventually leads to hyperreninemic hypertension. This is related to renal scarring, atrophy of cortical tubules, and glomerulosclerosis [39, 85].

33.3.6 Hepatic Damage

Large doses of radiation can cause acute inflammation of the liver, which, although silent, can then evolve into significant secondary degeneration following progressive damage to the hepatic vascular supply [82]. The onset of radiotherapy-induced liver disease usually occurs 1–2 months after irradiation, but it may present earlier or later and can persist for months [86]. Common features of radiation hepatopathy include central vein thrombosis, sinusoidal congestion, and sinusoidal fibrosis. These can eventually lead to subendothelial and adventitial fibrosis of the central veins, liver failure, and cirrhosis [87–89]. The above features most commonly occur when doses in excess of 30–35 Gy in adults are administered. Hepatic irradiation can also act synergistically with chemotherapy to cause liver toxicity.

33.3.7 Gastroenterologic Damage

Chronic radiation can cause coloproctitis or proctitis. This develops as a consequence of mucosal and bowel wall injury, including fibrosis and obliterative endarteritis with subsequent local tissue ischemia [90]. Late effects persisting 3 months postirradiation and are due to abnormalities of the colorectal mucosa, i.e., mucosal erythema, edema, mucosal telangiectasia, and extensive ulceration with necrotic material [90]. Clinical features may include abdominal or pelvic discomfort, tenesmus, and passage of loose stools and mucoid material and/or gross blood alone and mixed with feces. Bowel damage is rare in patients with SCLC because bowel spread is rare.

33.3.8 Neurologic and Ophthalmic Damage

The damaging effects of radiation therapy to the brain, spinal cord, and the peripheral nerves can present months or years after the radiation has been completed [47]. Early delayed encephalopathy occurs weeks to months after radiotherapy and symptoms may persist for days to weeks but they eventually resolve completely [91]. The most probable cause is demyelination due to radiation injury of oligodendroglia [92].

Delayed encephalopathy is the most serious complication of brain radiotherapy caused by radionecrosis developing months to years after treatment [93, 94]. The maximum radiation-dose threshold is near 60 Gy, above which radionecrosis becomes more common [95]. Radiation may also cause dementia unassociated with evidence of necrosis. This is seen on magnetic resonance imaging (MRI) as ventricular dilatation, sulcal atrophy, white-matter hyperintensity, and even ventriculoperitoneal shunting [96]. This particular finding is more prevalent in patients who have received a combination of radiotherapy and intensive systemic chemotherapy. Large doses of radiation can also cause occlusions to cervical or intracranial arteries leading to cerebral infarction [97–99]. Radiation therapy can affect endocrinologic function which may present years after treatment as hypothalamic or pituitary failure [100–102].

Progressive radiation myelopathy is a devastating complication of radiotherapy and presents months to years (median 20 months) after treatment [103]. Symptoms of radiation myelopathy usually begin with asymmetric sensory changes in the legs and progressive sensory loss, weakness, sphincter dysfunction, and pain at the level of cord damage. Brown-Séquard syndrome, plexopathies, and lower motor neuron syndrome with weakness and muscle atrophy can also occur after irradiation of the spinal cord [104].

33.3.9 Musculoskeletal Damage

Radiation has been associated with a large variety of skeletal complications [105, 106]. Osteonecrosis is a common late phenomenon that presents when doses exceeding 50–60 Gy are delivered, and increases the risk of pathologic fractures. These fractures are associated with a high rate of non-union [107]. Radiation to a joint area can cause stiffness, joint contractures, loss of motion, and eventual subcutaneous fibrosis. The most devastating and potentially fatal skeletal complication of radiation therapy is the development of a secondary tumor, in the form of sarcoma [108–110]. Radiation-induced sarcomas are highly aggressive tumors and have a high metastatic rate. Their incidence increases with increased radiation doses, i.e., 60 Gy and above. Types of radiation-induced sarcomas include osteosarcoma, malignant fibrous histiocytoma, and fibrosarcoma [111]. Secondary bone tumors are very rare in patients with SCLC because of the low overall cure rate.

33.3.10 Genitourinary Damage

Radiation therapy is associated with hemorrhagic cystitis due to its damaging effect on vascular endothelium, increased incidence of infections (preventing proper healing), and endarteritis, causing progressive ischemia, inflammation, and fibrosis. The end result is tissue necrosis. Bladder toxicity has also been associated with total body irradiation for bone marrow transplantation in 10–17% of patients [112, 113]. The risk of hemorrhagic cystitis increases when radiation is combined with specific chemotherapy agents, such as cyclophosphamide.

33.3.11 Secondary Cancers

Secondary cancers typically present within or at the margin of the irradiated field and the most common types are bone and soft tissue sarcomas. Reports of rarer presentations appear in the form of skin, brain, thyroid, and breast cancer [114–117]. The risk of a secondary malignancy increases if the radiation exposure occurs earlier in life or during periods of rapid growth of a tissue. Additional evidence suggests that radiation acts synergistically with cigarette smoking [118]. Few SCLC patients live long enough to develop secondary bone tumors.

33.3.12 Gonadal Dysfunction

In most patients with SCLC, irradiation of the testes and ovaries is unlikely to be clinically relevant, however some of the more important radiation toxicities to the reproductive organs are discussed in this section. In adults, single 4- to 6-Gy doses of testicular radiation may produce azoospermia for 5 years or longer [119]. Oligospermia/azoospermia lasting up to 24 months after as little as 2.7 Gy has been reported [120]. Total body radiation for bone marrow transplantation conditioning and cranial irradiation in conjunction with chemotherapy are treatments that have been associated with permanent azoospermia [121]. The radiation sensitivity of the ovaries has not been as precisely defined, however, similarly to men, it is dose dependent and age dependent. Single doses of 5 Gy produce menstrual irregularities in women of all ages. A dose of 6 Gy can induce menopause in women over the age of 40 years, whereas younger women aged between 20 and 30 years can tolerate up to 3 Gy if the dose is fractionated over 6 weeks [122]. All the above complications have become less frequent due to the introduction of newer techniques of radiation therapy.

33.3.13 Late Physical Effects of Radiotherapy Specific to Small-Cell Lung Cancer

Radiotherapy plays a very important role in the treatment of SCLC, both for locoregional control and as prophylactic cranial irradiation (PCI). SCLC is very responsive to radiation compared to other lung cancers. The late effects of radiation associated with SCLC can manifest in two contexts, locoregional radiation and cranial irradiation.

Locoregional Radiation

Thoracic radiotherapy has a proven role in the management of SCLC. In patients with limited-stage SCLC, thoracic radiotherapy improves the 3-year survival by 5.4%. Radiation on the SCLC tumor lying within the chest wall can be associated with complications to the local area and may impact on surrounding organs. Features that are presented are the result of radiation toxicity and are dependent on dose, frequency, and cumulative effect.

Pulmonary toxicities are known such as radiation-induced pneumonitis and chronic fibrosis. Cardiovascular toxicities are also seen and include chronic effusive pericarditis, coronary occlusion, myocardial ischemia, infarction, and fibrous valvular endocardial thickening. Secondary malignancies on the chest wall and regional area have been documented. Lastly, cutaneous manifestations on the chest wall and regional area can be seen including desquamation, erythema, edema, bullae, erosions, ulcerations, and postinflammatory hyperpigmentation.

Cranial Irradiation

Cranial irradiation is used to treat metastatic SCLC when it presents within the cranial wall and in the prophylaxis of brain metastases in patients responding well to chemotherapy. A retrospective review of many studies by Vines et al. (2003) that looked at the long-term effects of cranial irradiation in SCLC concluded that cranial irradiation improves the overall survival of patients with SCLC [123]. The late effects of radiation treatment to the area are due to the damage it can cause to all forms of tissue that are found within the cranial walls. Some of the most important neurologic complications are neurologic manifestations such as early and delayed encephalopathy, chronic dementia, and occlusions to cervical or intracranial arteries and radionecrosis. Endocrinologic manifestations comprise hypothalamic or pituitary failure (generally rare). Secondary malignancies within the cranial wall and regional area are very rare.

33.4 Effect of Continued Smoking on Survivors of Small-Cell Lung Cancer

One important issue to be considered when discussing the long-term outcomes for SCLC patients is the issue of continued smoking. Several studies have shown the importance of continued avoidance of tobacco in those successfully treated for SCLC. At the US National Cancer Institute 540 patients with SCLC were followed for a median of 6.1 years [124]. Fifty-five (10%) patients survived free of cancer for at least 2 years. Of these, 43 stopped smoking within 6 months of starting treatment, whilst 12 continued to smoke. In those who stopped smoking the relative risk of a second primary non-small-cell lung cancer was 11 (CI, 4.4–23) and in those who continued to smoke the relative risk was 32 (CI, 12–69). Smoking was also found to have a negative impact on survival if patients undergoing concurrent chemoradiotherapy for limited-stage SCLC smoked while on treatment [125].

33.5 Conclusions

In the past the prognosis of SCLC has been poor and, for most patients, long-term effects of treatment have not been a major concern. Few patients have lived long enough to develop late treatment-related effects. Newer, safer treatments are now allowing people to live longer. In the most recent series, between 10% and 20% of patients with limited-stage SCLC have been cured. The role of prophylactic cranial irradiation after chemotherapy has been more clearly defined in recent years and the long-term effects are less serious than previously thought. The most important long-term effects of current treatment include renal damage, neurotoxicities, and pulmonary fibrosis. In the future biologic agents will almost certainly have a larger role to play in the management of SCLC. As these agents are introduced, response rates and survival will improve and the long-term sequelae of therapy will become a more important issue.

Key Points

- Late effects to normal tissue are toxicities occurring 90 days or more from the start of therapy. Factors that affect long-term toxicity of chemotherapy for small-cell lung carcinoma (SCLC) include choice of agent, dose, schedule and route of administration, and comorbidities in the patient.
- Important long-term effects of chemotherapy include cardiac failure, pulmonary fibrosis and pneumonitis, renal failure, hematologic abnormalities, gonadal dysfunction, and neurologic damage. Some agents, such as etoposide, can cause secondary cancers including acute leukemia.
- High-dose chemotherapy increases the overall toxicity of SCLC therapy but has no proven role in management at present.
- Radiotherapy can affect most organ systems, but toxicities are usually confined to the irradiated field and immediately adjacent structures. Intensity modulated radiotherapy (IMRT) will reduce the risk of long-term tissue damage in future.
- Patients who smoke during or after treatment for SCLC have a higher risk of treatment failure and secondary non-small-cell lung cancers. Patients in good-prognosis groups should be encouraged to quit smoking to maximize the chances of cancer-free survival.
- Biologic anticancer agents will play a part in SCLC treatment in the next decade. These drugs will cause different long-term effects, though indications are that their overall toxicity will be less than cytotoxic drugs.

References

1. Mountain CF. Clinical biology of small cell carcinoma. Relationship to surgical therapy. Semin Oncol 1978;5:272.
2. Devita VT, Hellman S, Rosenberg SA (eds). In: Cancer: Principles and Practice of Oncology, 5th edn. Philadelphia: Lippincott Williams & Wilkins, 1999.
3. Pignon JP, Arriagada R, Ihde DC, et al. A meta-analysis of thoracic radiotherapy for small-cell lung cancer. N Engl J Med 1992;327:1618.
4. Warde P, Payne D. Does thoracic irradiation improve survival and local control in limited-stage small cell carcinoma of the lung? A meta-analysis. J Clin Oncol 1992;10:890.
5. Johnson BE, Grayson J, Makuch RW, et al. Ten-year survival of patients with small-cell lung cancer treated with combination chemotherapy with or without irradiation. J Clin Oncol 1990;8:396.
6. Lassen U, Osterlind K, Hansen M, et al. Long-term survival in small-cell lung cancer: post treatment characteristics in patients surviving 5 to 18+ years – an analysis of 1,714 consecutive patients. J Clin Oncol 1995;13:1215.

7. Fry WA, Menck HR, Winchester DP. The national cancer data base report on lung cancer. Cancer 1996;77:1947.
8. Wolf M, Holle R, Hans K, et al. Analysis of prognostic factors in 766 patients with small cell lung cancer (SCLC): the role of sex as a predictor for survival. Br J Cancer 1991;63:986.
9. Rawson NS, Peto J. An overview of prognostic factors in small cell lung cancer. A report from the subcommittee for the management of lung cancer of the United Kingdom coordinating committee on cancer research. Br J Cancer 1990;61:597.
10. McCracken JD, Janaki LM, Crowley JJ, et al. Concurrent chemotherapy/radiotherapy for limited SCLC, Southwest Oncology Group study. J Clin Oncol 1989;8:892.
11. Kumar P. The role of radiotherapy in the management of limited-stage small cell lung cancer: past, present, and future. Chest 1997;112(suppl):259.
12. Murray N, Livingston RB, Shepherd FA, et al. Randomised study of CODE versus alternating CAV/EP for extensive-stage small-cell lung cancer: an intergroup study of the National Cancer Institute of Canada clinical trials group and the Southwest Oncology Group. J Clin Oncol 1999;17:2300.
13. Devita VT, Hellman S, Rosenthal SA (eds). In: Cancer: Principles and Practice of Oncology, 6th edn. Philadelphia: Lippincott Williams & Wilkins, 2001.
14. Skeel RT (ed). Systematic assessment of patient with cancer and long term medical complications of treatment. In: Handbook of Cancer Chemotherapy, 5th edn. Philadelphia: Lippincott Williams & Wilkins, 1999:42.
15. Elias AD, Skarin AT, Richardson P, Ibrahim J, McCauley M, Frei E 3rd. Dose-intensive therapy for extensive-stage small cell lung cancer and extrapulmonary small cell carcinoma: long-term outcome. Biol Blood Marrow Transplant 2002;8:326.
16. Elias AD, Ayash L, Frei E 3rd, et al. Intensive combined modality therapy for limited-stage small-cell lung cancer. J Natl Cancer Inst 1993;85:559.
17. Arriagada R, Le Chevalier T, Pignon JP, et al. Initial chemotherapeutic doses and survival in patients with limited small-cell lung cancer. N Engl J Med 1993;329:1848.
18. Corne F, Thiberville L. The place for therapeutic intensification in small cell lung cancer. Rev Pneumol Clin 2004;60:3S104.
19. Rizzo JD, Elias AD, Stiff PJ, et al. Autologous stem cell transplantation for small cell lung cancer. Biol Blood Marrow Transplant 2002;8:273.
20. Pavy JJ, Denekamp J, Letschert J, et al. EORTC late effects working group. Late effect toxicity scoring: the SOMA scale. Radiother Oncol 1995;35:11.
21. Dische S, Warburton MF, Jones D, Lartigau E. The recording of morbidity related to radiotherapy. Radiother Oncol 1997;16:103.
22. Rubin P, Constine S, Fajardo LF, Phillips TL, Wasserman TH. RTOG late effects working group. Overview: late effects of normal tissues LENT scoring system. Int J Radiat Oncol Biol Phys 1995;31:1041.
23. Rubin P. Late effects of chemotherapy and radiotherapy: a new hypothesis. Int J Radiat Oncol Biol Phys 1984;10:5.
24. Ewer MS, Benjamin RS, Yeh ETH. Complications of cancer and its treatment: cardiac complications. In: Bast RC Jr, Kufe DW, Pollock RE, Weichselbaum RR, Holland JF, Frei E III, Gansler TS (eds) Cancer Medicine e5, 6th edn. Hamilton, Ontario: American Cancer Society, Decker, 2003;38:152.
25. Lefrak E, Pitha J, Rosenheim S, Gottlieb J. A clinicopathologic analysis of adriamycin cardiotoxicity Cancer 1973;32:302.
26. Singal P, Iliskovic N. Doxorubicin-induced cardiomyopathy. N Engl J Med 1998;339:900.
27. Ali M, Ewer M. Cardiovascular problems in the patient with cancer: effects of chemotherapy. Prim Care Cancer 1989;9:29.
28. Haq M, Legha S, Choksi J, et al. Doxorubicin-induced congestive heart failure in adults. Cancer 1985;56:1361.
29. Mackay B, Ewer M, Carrasco C, Benjamin R. Assessment of anthracycline cardiomyopathy by endomyocardial biopsy. Ultrastruct Pathol 1994;18:203.
30. Minow R, Benjamin R, Lee E, Gottlieb J. Adriamycin cardiomyopathy risk factors. Cancer 1977;39:1397.
31. Mancuso L, Bondi F, Marchi S, et al. Cardiac toxicity of 5-fluorouracil. Report of a case of spontaneous angina. Tumori 1986;72:121.
32. Ewer M, Benjamin R, Hong W, et al. Electrocardiographic changes in patients receiving chemotherapy with 5-fluorouracil and cisplatinum with and without diethyldithiocarbomate. Proc 15th Intl Cong Chemother 1987:203.
33. Ognibene F, Rosenberg S, Lotze M, et al. Interleukin-2 administration causes reversible hemodynamic changes and left ventricular dysfunction similar to those seen in septic shock. Chest 1988;94:750.
34. Rowinsky E, McGuire W, Guarnieri T, et al. Cardiac disturbances during the administration of taxol. J Clin Oncol 1991;9:1704.
35. Jules-Elysee K, White DA. Bleomycin-induced pulmonary toxicity. Clin Chest Med 1990;11:1.
36. Walker-Smith GJ. The histopathology of pulmonary reactions to drugs. Clin Chest Med 1990;11:95.
37. Cooper JAD, White DA, Matthay RA. Drug-induced pulmonary disease: part 1, cytotoxic drugs. Am Rev Respir Dis 1986;133:321.
38. Sostman HD, Matthay RA, Putman CE. Methotrexate-induced pneumonitis. Medicine 1976;55:371.
39. Logothetis CJ, Assikis V, Sarriera JE. Complications of cancer and its treatment: urologic complications. In: Bast RC Jr, Kufe DW, Pollock RE, Weichselbaum RR, Holland JF, Frei E III, Gansler TS (eds) Cancer Medicine e5, 6th ed. Hamilton, Ontario: American Cancer Society, Decker, 2003;38:151.
40. Evans B.D, Rajn KS, Calvert AH, et al. Phase II study of JM-8, a new platinum analog in advanced ovarian carcinoma. Cancer Treat Rep 1983;67:997.
41. Frei E. Methotrexate revisited. Med Pediatr Oncol 1976;2:227.
42. Weber B, Garnick MB, Rieselbach R. Nephropathies due to anti-neoplastic agents. In: Massry SG, Glassock RJ (eds) Textbook of Nephrology, 2nd edn. Baltimore: Williams & Wilkins, 1989:818.
43. Lempert KD. Haemolysis and renal impairment syndrome in patients on 5-fluorouracil and mitomycin-C. Lancet 1980;2:369.
44. Denine EP, Harrison SD, Pechkam JC. Qualitative and quantitative toxicity of sublethal doses of methyl-CCNU in BDF1 mice. Cancer Treat Rep 1977;61:409.
45. Carter SK, Broder L, Friedman M. Streptozotocin and metastatic insulinoma. Ann Intern Med 1971;74:445.
46. Calvert AH, Newell DR, Gumbrell LA, et al. Carboplatin dosage: prospective evaluation of a simple formula based on renal function. J Clin Oncol 1995;7:1748.
47. Keime-Guibert F, Napolitano M, Delattre JY. Neurological complications of radiotherapy and chemotherapy. J Neurol 1998;245:695.
48. Lowenthal RM, Eaton K. Toxicity of chemotherapy. Hematol Oncol Clin North Am 1996;10:967.
49. Gilbert MR, Yasko JM. Neurotoxicities. In: Kirkwood JM, Lotze MT, Yasko JM (eds) Current Cancer Therapeutics, 1st edn, Current Medicine. Princeton: Academic Press, 1994:284.

50. Price RA, Jamieson PA. The central nervous system in childhood, leukaemia II, subacute leukoencephalopathy. Cancer 1975;35:306.
51. Bleyer WA. Neurologic sequelae of methotrexate and ionizing radiation: a new classification. Cancer Treat Rep 1981;65(suppl 1):89.
52. Suzuki K, Takemura T, Okeda R, Hatakeyama S. Vascular changes of methotrexate-related disseminated necrotizing leukoencephalopathy. Acta Neuropathol 1984;65:145.
53. Nakazato Y, Ishida Y, Morimatsu M. Disseminated necrotizing leukoencephalopathy. Acta Pathol Jpn 1980;9:659.
54. Feinberg WM, Swenson MR. Cerebrovascular complications of L-asparaginase therapy. Neurology 1988;38:127.
55. Viscoli C, Van der Auwera P, Meunier F. Gram-positive infections in granulocytopenic patients: an important issue? J Antimicrob Chemother 1988;21(suppl C):149.
56. Tucker MA, Meadows AT, Boice JD Jr, et al. Leukemia after therapy with alkylating agents for childhood cancer. J Natl Cancer Inst 1987;78:459.
57. Felix CA. Chemotherapy-related second cancers. In: Neugut AI, Meadows AT, Robinson E (eds) Multiple Primary Cancers. Philadelphia: Lippincott, Williams & Wilkins, 1999;137.
58. Bhatia S, Davies SM, Robison LL. Leukemia. In: Neugut AI, Meadows AT, Robinson E (eds) Multiple Primary Cancers. Philadelphia: Lippincott, Williams & Wilkins, 1999;257.
59. Tucker MA, Coleman CN, Cox RS, et al. Risk of second cancers after treatment for Hodgkin's disease. N Engl J Med 1988;318:76.
60. van Leeuwen FE, Chorus AM, van den Belt-Dusebout AW, et al. Leukemia risk following Hodgkin's disease: relation to cumulative dose of alkylating agents, treatment with teniposide combinations, number of episodes of chemotherapy, and bone marrow damage. J Clin Oncol 1994;12:1063.
61. Kaldor JM, Day NE, Clarke EA, et al. Leukemia following Hodgkin's disease. N Engl J Med 1990;322:7.
62. Bhatia S, Robison LL, Oberlin O, et al. Breast cancer and other second neoplasms after childhood Hodgkin's disease. N Engl J Med 1996;334:745.
63. Buchanan JD, Fairley KF, Barrie JU. Return of spermatogenesis after stopping cyclophosphamide therapy. Lancet 1975;2:156.
64. Kreuser ED, Ziros N, Hetzel WD, Heimple H. Reproductive and endocrine gonadal capacity in patients treated with COPP chemotherapy for Hodgkin's disease. J Cancer Res Clin Oncol 1987;113:260.
65. Roeser HP, Stocks AE, Smith AJ. Testicular damage due to cytotoxic drugs and recovery after cessation of therapy. Aust N Z J Med 1978;8:250.
66. Chapman RM, Sutcliffe SB, Malpas JS. Cytotoxic-induced ovarian failure in women with Hodgkin's disease. I. Hormone function. JAMA 1979;242:1877.
67. Schilsky RL, Lewis BJ, Sherins RJ. Gonadal dysfunction in patients receiving chemotherapy for cancer. Ann Intern Med 1980;93:109.
68. Koyama H, Wada T, Nishizawa Y, et al. Cyclophosphamide-induced ovarian failure and its therapeutic significance in patients with breast cancer. Cancer 1977;39:1403.
69. Belohorsky B, Sirack J, Sandor L, Klauber E. Comments on the development of amenorrhea caused by Myleran in cases of chronic myelosis. Neoplasma 1960;7:397.
70. Freckman HA, Fry HL, Mendez ML, Maurer ER. Chlorambucil-prednisolone therapy for disseminated breast cancer. JAMA 1965;91:100.
71. Choo YC, Chan SWY, Wong LC, Ma HK. Ovarian dysfunction in patients with gestational trophoblastic neoplasm treated with short intensive courses of etoposide. Cancer 1985;55:2348.
72. Dnistrian AM, Schwartz MK, Frecchia AA. Endocrine consequences of CMF adjuvant therapy in premenopausal and postmenopausal breast cancer patients. Cancer 1983;51:803.
73. Samaan NA, de Asis DN, Buzdar AO. Pituitary-ovarian function in breast cancer patients on adjuvant chemoimmunotherapy. Cancer 1978;41:2084.
74. Bower M, Rustin GJS, Newlands ES, et al. Chemotherapy for gestational trophoblastic tumours hastens menopause by 3 years. Eur J Cancer 1998;34:1204.
75. Noda K, Nishiwaki Y, Kawahara M, et al. Irinotecan plus cisplatin compared with etoposide plus cisplatin for extensive small-cell lung cancer. N Engl J Med 2002;346:85.
76. Casciato DA, Lowitz BB. Manual of clinical oncology: cancer chemotherapeutic agents, 3rd edn. Boston: Edition Little, Brown and Co, 1995:39.
77. Fajardo Stewart L. Radiation-induced heart disease: clinical and experimental aspects. Radiol Clin North Am 1971;9:511.
78. Cohn K, Stewart J, Fajardo L, Hancock E. Heart disease following radiation. Medicine 1967;46:281.
79. Brosius F III, Waller B, Roberts W. Radiation heart disease: analysis of 16 young (aged 15–33 years) necropsy patients who received over 3,500 rads to the heart. Am J Med 1981;70:519.
80. Amromin G, Gildenhorn H, Solomon R, et al. The synergism of X-irradiation and cholesterol-fat feeding on the development of coronary artery lesions. J Atherosclerosis Res 1964;4:325.
81. Deeg HJ, Sullivan KM, Buckner CD. Marrow transplantation for acute nonlymphocytic leukemia in first remission: toxicity and long-term follow up of patients conditioned with single-dose or fractionated total body irradiation. Bone Marrow Transplant 1986;1:151.
82. Rubin P, Keys H, Poulter CA. Changing concepts in the tolerance of radioresistance and radiosensitivity of normal tissue/organs. In: McCartney D, Bolton P (eds) Biological basis and clinical importance of tumor radioresistants. New York: Masson Publishing, 1983.
83. Susser WS, Whitaker-Worth DL, Grant-Kels JM. Mucocutaneous reactions to chemotherapy. J Am Acad Dermatol 1999;40:367.
84. Yeo W, Leung S, Johnson P. Radiation-recall dermatitis with docetaxel: establishment of a requisite radiation threshold. Eur J Cancer 1997;33:698.
85. Perez C, Brady L. Principles and practice of radiation oncology, 3rd edn. Philadelphia: Lippincott-Raven, 1998:185.
86. Lawrence TS, Robertson JM, Anscher MS, et al. Hepatic toxicity resulting from cancer treatment. Int J Radiat Oncol Biol Phys 1995;31:1237.
87. Hresnchyshyn MM. Results of the Gynaecologic Oncology Group trials on ovarian cancer: preliminary report. Symposium on Ovarian Carcinoma NCI, Monograph 1975;42:155.
88. Ingold JA, Reed GB, Kaplan HS, Bagshaw MA. Radiation hepatitis. Am J Roentgenol 1965;93:200.
89. Lewin K, Millis RR. Human radiation hepatitis: a morphologic study with emphasis on the late changes. Arch Pathol 1973;96:21.
90. Babb RR. Radiation proctitis: a review. Am J Gastroenterol 1996;91:1309.
91. Armstrong C, Ruffer J, Corn B, et al. Biphasic patterns of memory deficits following moderate-dose partial-brain irradiation: neuropsychologic outcome and proposed mechanisms. J Clin Oncol 1995;13:2263.
92. Kleinschmidt-DeMasters BK. Necrotizing brainstem leukoencephalopathy six weeks following radiotherapy. Clin Neuropathol 1995;14:63.
93. Duffey P, Chari G, Cartlidge NEF, Shaw PJ. Progressive deterioration of intellect and motor function occurring several decades after cranial irradiation: a new facet in the

clinical spectrum of radiation encephalopathy. Arch Neurol 1996;53:814.

94. Fonseca R, O'Neill BP, Foote RL, et al. Cerebral toxicity in patients treated for small cell carcinoma of the lung. Mayo Clin Proc 1999;74:461.

95. Marks JE, Wong J. The risk of cerebral radionecrosis in relation to dose, time and fractionation: a follow-up study. Prog Exp Tumor Res 1985;29:210.

96. Thiessen B, DeAngelis LM. Hydrocephalus in radiation leukoencephalopathy. Results of ventriculoperitoneal shunting. Arch Neurol 1998;55:05.

97. Bitzer M, Topka H. Progressive cerebral occlusive disease after radiation therapy. Stroke 1995;26:31.

98. Brada M, Burchell L, Ashley S, Traish D. The incidence of cerebrovascular accidents in patients with pituitary adenoma. Int J Radiat Oncol Biol Phys 1999;45:693.

99. Larson JJ, Ball WS, Bove KE, et al. Formation of intracerebral cavernous malformations after radiation treatment for central nervous system neoplasia in children. J Neurosurg 1998;88:51.

100. Arlt W, Hove U, Müller B, et al. Frequent and frequently overlooked: treatment-induced endocrine dysfunction in adult long-term survivors of primary brain tumors. Neurology 1997;49:498.

101. Abrahamsen AF, Loge JH, Hannisdal E, et al. Late medical sequelae after therapy for supradiaphragmatic Hodgkin's disease. Acta Oncol 1999;38:511.

102. Nishio S, Morioka T, Inamura T, et al. Radiation-induced brain tumours: potential late complications of radiation therapy for brain tumours. Acta Neurochir (Wien) 1998;140:763.

103. Esik O, Emri M, Csornai M, et al. Radiation myelopathy with partial functional recovery: PET evidence of long-term increased metabolic activity of the spinal cord. J Neurol Sci 1999;163:39.

104. Tallaksen CME, Jetne V, Fosså S. Postradiation lower motor neuron syndrome: a case report and brief literature review. Acta Oncol 1997;36:345.

105. Blumke DA, Fishman EK, Scott WW Jr. Skeletal complications of radiation therapy. Radiographics 1994;14:111.

106. Dalinka MK, Mazzo VP. Complications of radiation therapy. Crit Rev Diagn Imaging 1985;23:235.

107. Springfield DS, Pagliarulo C. Fractures of long bones previously treated for Ewing's sarcoma. J Bone Joint Dis Surg Am 1985;67:477.

108. Laskin WB, Silverman TA, Enzinger FM. Post radiation soft tissue sarcoma: an analysis of 53 cases. Cancer 1988;62:2330.

109. Meadows AT, Strong LC, Li FP, et al. Bone sarcoma as a second malignant neoplasm in children: influence of radiation and genetic predisposition.Cancer 1980;46:2603.

110. Smith J. Postradiation sarcoma of bone in Hodgkin's disease. Skeletal Radiol 1987;16:524.

111. Huvos AB, Woodard HW, Cahan WG, et al. Post radiation osteogenic sarcoma of bone and soft tissue: a clinicopathological study of 66 patients. Cancer 1985;55:1244.

112. Kohno A, Takeyama K, Narabajashi M, et al. Hemorrhagic cystitis associated with allogeneic and autologous bone marrow transplantation for malignant neoplasm in adults. Jpn J Clin Oncol 1993;23:46.

113. Ringden Q, Remberger M, Ruutu T, et al. Increased risk of chronic graft versus host disease, obstructive bronchiolitis and alopecia with busulfan versus total body irradiation. Blood 1999;93:2196.

114. Inskip PD. Second cancers following radiotherapy. In: Neugut AI, Meadows AT, Robinson E (eds) Multiple Primary Cancers. Philadelphia: Lippincott Williams & Wilkins, 1999:91.

115. Bhatia S, Robison LL, Oberlin O, et al. Breast cancer and other second neoplasms after childhood Hodgkin's disease. N Engl J Med 1996;334:745.

116. Tucker MA, D'Angio GJ, Boice JD Jr, et al. Bone sarcomas linked to radiotherapy and chemotherapy in children. N Engl J Med 1987;317:588.

117. Ron E, Lubin JH, Shore RE, et al. Thyroid cancer after exposure to external radiation: a pooled analysis of seven studies. Radiat Res 1995;141:259.

118. Neugut AI, Murray T, Santos J, et al. Increased risk of lung cancer after breast cancer radiation therapy in cigarette smokers. Cancer 1994;73:1615.

119. Clifton DK, Bremner WJ. The effect of testicular X-irradiation on spermatogenesis in man: a comparison with the mouse. J Androl 1983;4:387.

120. Shapiro E, Kinsella TJ, Makuch RW, et al. Effects of fractionated irradiation on endocrine aspects of testicular function. J Clin Oncol 1985;3:1232.

121. Rappaport R, Brauner R, Czernichow P. Effect of hypothalamic and pituitary irradiation on pubertal development in children with cranial tumors. J Clin Endocrinol Metabol 1982;54:1164.

122. Lushbaugh C, Casarett GW. The effects of gonadal irradiation in clinical radiation therapy: a review. Cancer 1976;37:1111.

123. Vines EF, Le Pechoux C, Arriagada R. Prophylactic cranial irradiation in small cell lung cancer. Chile Semin Oncol 2003;30:38.

124. Richardson GE, Tucker MA, Venzon DJ, et al. Smoking cessation after successful treatment of small-cell lung cancer is associated with fewer smoking-related second primary cancers. Ann Intern Med 1993;119:383.

125. Videtic GM, Stitt LW, Dar AR, et al. Continued cigarette smoking by patients receiving concurrent chemoradiotherapy for limited-stage small-cell lung cancer is associated with decreased survival. J Clin Oncol 2003;21:1544.

Section VII:
Novel Therapeutic Modalities
in the Management of Lung Cancer

Novel Cytotoxic Agents in the Management of Lung Cancer

34

Ifigenia Tzannou, Kevin J. Harrington and Konstantinos N. Syrigos

Contents

34.1 Non-Small-Cell Lung Cancer

The role of chemotherapy in the treatment of non-small cell lung cancer (NSCLC) has increased greatly over recent decades. In current clinical practice, chemotherapy is used as a combined modality with radiotherapy as an adjuvant or neoadjuvant therapy. Combination chemotherapy is regarded as the standard care in the treatment of unresectable locally advanced (stage IIIB), metastatic (stage IV), or recurrent disease. In some cases of stage IIIB diseases, combined chemoradiotherapy may be administered as well [1,2]. Over recent decades, various clinical trials have demonstrated that chemotherapy was very beneficial in cases of advanced disease, despite the toxic effects of therapy and the possibility of treatment-related death. This benefit lies in objective tumor response, overall survival, time to disease progression, palliation of symptoms, and improvement of patients' quality of life [2–5].

The first generation of antineoplastic drugs used (e.g., cyclophosphamide, methotrexate, doxorubicin) had little activity against NSCLC [2]. The second generation of agents included cisplatin, carboplatin, ifosfamide, etoposide, mitomycin, and vinca alkaloids. Although these agents proved to be effective against NSCLC, single-agent platinum treatment remained the gold standard until the 1990s when a third generation of anticancer drugs emerged. Gemcitabine, vinorelbine, paclitaxel and doce-

taxel, and irinotecan were evaluated in combination with a platinum agent in several clinical trials. The combination therapy, overall, was found to offer better response rates, while toxicity was almost the same as in platinum monotherapy [6–12]. Accordingly, the guidelines of the American Society of Clinical Oncology that were published in 1996 dictated that the mainstay of treatment for advanced and metastatic NSCLC – provided that the patient has a performance status (PS) of 0 or 1 – is a platinum-based regimen [13].

In recent studies, however, it was observed that non-platinum regimens could be as effective as platinum-based ones, while causing less serious toxicity [14, 15]. The ample number of available drugs allowed the study of many combination regimens in various schedules and doses. Nevertheless, no combination seemed to be superior to others in terms of efficacy [16, 17]. A fourth generation of cytotoxic agents has recently been introduced. These new agents have unique mechanisms of action aimed at the molecular and biological targets that take part in the biological pathways of malignant cells [17, 18].

To date, it is evident that the introduction of newer antineoplastic agents over recent decades has resulted in minor improvements in survival. Even though 20–40% of patients with locally advanced or metastatic NSCLC respond to chemotherapy, long-term prognosis is not good. The median and 1-year survival for patients who received first-line therapy are only 8.5 months and 35%, respectively [17–22].

The introduction and evaluation of new agents are, therefore, of vital importance in order to improve survival rates of NSCLC patients. Agents currently under study are members of the platinum family as well as the third and fourth generations of cytostatics. The most recently approved agents that underwent this investigation are gefitinib (Iressa) and pemetrexed (Alimta).

34.1.1 Oxaliplatin

Oxaliplatin (Eloxatin) is a third generation cisplatin analog. It contains a platinum atom which is complexed with oxalate and a bulky diaminocyclohexane (DACH). Like cisplatin, it acts as an alkylating agent on DNA. It is believed to form reactive platinum complexes that appear to inhibit DNA synthesis by interstrand and intrastrand crosslinking between two adjacent guanine and/or guanine–adenine bases. This is the basis of its major cytotoxic effects [23–25]. However, DACH-Pt DNA complexes formed by Eloxatin are more bulky and hydrophobic than those formed by cisplatin and carboplatin, and are, therefore, more effective in inhibiting DNA synthesis [26].

Oxaliplatin was administered as single-agent therapy to patients with advanced cancer in two phase I studies. The first study concluded that the indicated schedule of administration was 130 mg/m^2 every 21 days and the second 85 mg/m^2 every 15 days. Neurotoxicity was the only dose-limiting toxicity (DLT). No cases of nephro- or ototoxicity were reported, and hematologic toxicity was rare and particularly mild [26, 27]. Eloxatin was then examined as a monotherapy in the treatment of NSCLC in a phase II study by Monnet et al. In this trial 130 mg/m^2 oxaliplatin were given intravenously to previously untreated patients with advanced NSCLC. The overall response rate (ORR) was 15.1% with a median survival (MS) of 8 months. The most frequently reported toxic effect was severe peripheral neuropathy [28].

The first study to evaluate oxaliplatin-based combination chemotherapy was carried out by the same group of researchers. It was a phase I/II trial, where escalating doses of vinorelbine (22–34 mg/m^2) on days 1 and 8 of 21-day cycles were administered in combination with a fixed dose of 130 mg/m^2 Eloxatin on day 1. The DLT was neutropenia. Grade 1/2 nausea and vomiting and grade 1 peripheral neuropathy were also observed. All patients were evaluated and the ORR was found to be 37%. The study concluded that the recommended dosage is 26 mg/m^2 vinorelbine on day 1 and day 8 and 130 mg/m^2 oxaliplatin on the first day of every cycle [29].

Faivre et al. later examined the combination of oxaliplatin with gemcitabine in a phase I/II study where patients with advanced NSCLC or ovarian cancer were included. Doses of gemcitabine and oxaliplatin ranged from 800 to 1,500 mg/m^2, and from 70 to 100 mg/m^2, respectively. Both agents were administered on the same day every 2 weeks. The recommended schedule consisted of 1,500 mg/m^2 gemcitabine and 85 mg/m^2 Eloxatin. No DLT was reported, even though grade 3/4 neutropenia occurred in 13 of 355 cycles and grade 3/4 thrombocytopenia was observed in two patients. Peripheral neurotoxicity and asthenia were infrequent and mild. As far as efficacy is concerned, 12 of the 44 evaluated patients achieved an objective response [30]. An Italian group recently conducted a phase I investigation of the same combination in patients with recurrent NSCLC. Patients were treated with a fixed dose of gemcitabine 1,250 mg/m^2 on day 1, followed, the next day, by oxaliplatin in doses starting from 70 up to 130 mg/m^2. Maximum tolerated dose (MTD) was not reached, since no DLT was observed. The regimen of 130 mg/m^2 oxaliplatin plus 1,250 mg/m^2 gemcitabine is already under evaluation in phase II studies [31]. In another schedule, oxaliplatin was infused into patients with advanced NSCLC and a poor prognosis at a dose of 65 mg/m^2 along with 1,000 mg/m^2 gemcitabine on days 1 and 8 every 3 weeks [32].

The combination of oxaliplatin plus docetaxel in patients with NSCLC or breast cancer was examined in a dose-escalation study. Docetaxel was administered on day 1 and oxaliplatin on day 2 every 21 days. DLTs were grade 4 neutropenia (9%), febrile neutropenia (2%; one septic death also occurred), grade 3/4 diarrhea (10%), and grade 3 fatigue (13%). The investigators recommended the dosage of 75 mg/m^2 docetaxel on day 1 and 70 mg/m^2 Eloxatin on day 2, although in the case of recombinant human granulocyte colony-stimulating factor (rhG-CSF) support the doses may be increased to 85 mg/m^2 for both agents. As far as tumor activity was concerned, 19% of NSCLC experienced a partial response (PR) [33].

Winegarden and colleagues conducted a phase II study in order to evaluate the combination of oxaliplatin 130 mg/m^2 plus paclitaxel 175 mg/m^2 administered every 3 weeks to patients with locally advanced or metastatic NSCLC. The ORR was 34.2% and MS was found to be 9.2 months. The 1- and 2-year survivals were 37% and 21%, respectively. Except for 6 of the 38 patients who presented with grade 4 neutropenia, no other significant toxicity was reported [34].

In 2004, a phase I pharmacokinetic study was published that evaluated the combination of Eloxatin plus the novel multitargeted antifolate pemetrexed (Alimta) in the treatment of patients with advanced solid tumors, including NSCLC. MTD was not reached, nevertheless, neutropenia was the most frequent toxicity. According to the trial, the indicated schedule for phase II studies is pemetrexed 500 mg/m^2 plus oxaliplatin 120 mg/m^2, both given intravenously once every 21 days [35].

34.1.2 Camptothecins

Camptothecin is a plant alkaloid, present in wood, bark, and fruit of the Asian tree *Camptotheca acuminata*. Topotecan and irinotecan are water-soluble derivatives of this five-ring structure alkaloid. Their target of antineoplastic activity is topoisomerase I, which is the key enzyme in the replication, transcription, and repair of

DNA. By binding to topoisomerase I, the camptothecins reversibly induce single-strand breaks, thereby affecting the cell's capacity to replicate [36–38].

Irinotecan

Irinotecan (Campto) has been used as a single-agent against NSCLC in several investigations. Even though the drug initially seemed active, the results were not actually as encouraging as expected [36]. The first phase I studies were carried out by Japanese researchers. DLT effects were myelosuppression, mainly neutropenia, and unpredictable diarrhea. The MTD and, therefore, the recommended dosage for phase II studies was 200 mg/m^2 every 3–4 weeks [39] or 100 mg/m^2 weekly [40].

Nakai et al. used the schedule of 200 mg/m^2 every 3 weeks in their phase II trial. The ORR was 20% for patients with NSCLC, and the most important toxicities reported were myelosuppression and gastrointestinal symptoms [41]. Baker and colleagues administered irinotecan at a dose of 350 mg/m^2 with the same interval. In this case, the response rate was also similar, i.e., 21% [42]. The majority of phase II studies, though, followed a schedule of once weekly infusion of 100 mg/m^2 irinotecan for 3 or more weeks. In one Japanese trial by Negoro et al., the response rates were 34.3% for chemonaive and 0% for previously treated non-small cell lung carcinomas [43]. In another study, where all patients enrolled were previously untreated, an objective response was demonstrated in 31.9% of treated patients and the MS was 10.5 months [44]. Baker et al., however, in a similar group of patients, observed an ORR of 15% with the MS being 6.2 months [45]. In all cases, hematologic and gastrointestinal toxicities were the chief adverse effects mentioned. In a more recent study, where irinotecan was administered as a second-line treatment to patients with refractory NSCLC that had previously received platinum and taxanes, Negoro's results [43] were not actually confirmed. In this Spanish study, the same regimen was used, but the ORR came up to 16% with an MS of 15 weeks [46].

Irinotecan as a single agent was proven to have moderate activity against NSCLC. It was encouraging, though, to observe more promising results when it was administered in combination with other cytotoxic agents. Campto was administered along with cisplatin in several doses and schedules, with quite encouraging results. In 1992 Masuda et al., in a phase I study, used a regimen of irinotecan in an escalating dose of 30–60 mg/m^2 on days 1, 8, and 15 plus 80 mg/m^2 cisplatin on day 1 every 28 days. It was indicated that the recommended dose of irinotecan was 60 mg/m^2. In terms of efficacy, the ORR was 54%, MS was found to be 10.2 months, and 1-year survival was 33% [47]. Another Japanese trial, evaluated the following schedule of administration in previously untreated patients with advanced NSCLC: continuous infusion of 20 mg/m^2 cisplatin on

days 1 and 2 plus 160 mg/m^2 irinotecan on day 1. In this trial, 58.5% of evaluated patients achieved an objective response, while the MS and 1-year survival were 44.8 weeks and 44%, respectively [48]. DeVore et al. administered Campto at a dose of 60 mg/m^2 on days 1, 8, and 15 of 4-week cycles with 80 mg/m^2 cisplatin on the first day of every cycle. Objective responses occurred in 28.8% of patients with inoperable NSCLC, and the MS was reported to be 9.9 months [49]. Ando et al. treated patients with refractory or advanced NSCLC with irinotecan in the same weekly schedule, but cisplatin, in this case, was also administered on days 1, 8, and 15 at a dose of 30 mg/m^2. The ORR in this trial was 80% and the MS 7.9 months [50]. In a Greek trial, investigators used 100 mg/m^2 irinotecan on day 1 and 110 mg/m^2 on day 8, in combination with 80 mg/m^2 cisplatin on day 8. Of all enrolled patients, 22% presented a PR, while 20% had stable disease. The MS was 8 months [51]. Another regimen that was studied as a first-line therapy, consisted of 60 mg/m^2 irinotecan and 50 mg/m^2 cisplatin both given on days 1 and 8 of four 28-day cycles. In this trial, the ORR and MS were 48% and 12.5 months, respectively [52]. Until now, only one phase III trial, using a the combination of Campto plus cisplatin, has been conducted. Patients with advanced NSCLC were randomized to receive one of the following regimens: (a) irinotecan 60 mg/m^2 on days 1, 8, and 15 and cisplatin 80 mg/m^2 on day 1; (b) cisplatin 80 mg/m^2 on day 1 and 3 mg/m^2 vindesine on days 1, 8, and 15; or (c) irinotecan 100 mg/m^2 monotherapy on days 1, 8, and 15. The response rates were 43.7% for Campto plus cisplatin, 31.7% for cisplatin plus vindesine, and 20% for the single-agent Campto. This confirms the hypothesis that the most effective and superior therapy is irinotecan plus cisplatin, compared to cisplatin plus vindesine and to irinotecan monotherapy [53]. In all of the above-mentioned studies, the major adverse effects were hematologic toxicity – mainly neutropenia – and symptoms from the gastrointestinal tract. In all cases, the investigators concluded that the combination of irinotecan and cisplatin was well-tolerated and showed good efficacy in patients with advanced, unresectable, or recurrent NSCLC.

The combination with carboplatin proved to be equally tolerated and efficient. In 2001, in a phase I study irinotecan was administered in an escalating dose starting at 30 mg/m^2 on days 1, 8, and 15 along with a fixed dose of carboplatin AUC 5 on day 1 every 4 weeks. The MTD for irinotecan was 60 mg/m^2, but the investigators recommended a dose of 50 mg/m^2 for future trials. In this study, 35.5% of the enrolled patients achieved an objective response, while the MS was 10.5 months [54]. The schedule proposed by this study (i.e., Campto 50 mg/m^2 on days 1, 8, and 15 plus carboplatin AUC 5 on day 1 every 4 weeks) was used by several study groups with similar results. Kinoshita and colleagues found an ORR of 35% with an MS of 9.3

months [55]. Takeda et al., in their own trial, observed an ORR of 25% and an MS of 10.2 months [56]. In the study of Fukuda et al., the ORR was 34% and the MS 10.0 months [57]. Once more, the predominant toxicities were myelosuppression, nausea/vomiting, and diarrhea. A group from the University of San Diego used another regimen, according to which 250 mg/m^2 irinotecan were infused along with carboplatin AUC 5 on the first day of 3-week cycles. Due to febrile neutropenia that occurred to one patient, the dose of Campto was reduced to 200 mg/m^2. With regard to efficacy, 23% of evaluated patients demonstrated a PR [58].

As far as the combination of irinotecan with taxanes is concerned, most of the information available is derived from phase I studies. Hotta et al. administered both irinotecan and paclitaxel on days 1 and 8 every 21 days. The MTD was 40 mg/m^2 for irinotecan and 50 mg/m^2 for paclitaxel. Even so, because of grade 3/4 neutropenia in 67% of the treated patients and severe non-hematologic toxicity (febrile neutropenia, supraventricular arrhythmia, and hepatic dysfunction) along with no antitumor activity whatsoever, this schedule was characterized as inappropriate for the treatment of NSCLC [59]. The schedule that Yamada and colleagues evaluated proved to be more effective while demonstrating a milder toxicity profile. In this trial, a fixed dose of 60 mg/m^2 Campto was administered to patients with advanced NSCLC in combination with an escalating dose of paclitaxel starting at 80 mg/m^2 every 2 weeks. None of the patients experienced DLT, and the recommended dose for paclitaxel was found to be 160 mg/m^2. At the same time, an objective response was attained by 58.3% of evaluated patients, and the MS was 12 months [60].

A phase I study, examined the combination of irinotecan with docetaxel, and proposed a regimen that consisted of 50 mg/m^2 Campto on days 1, 8, and 15 plus 50 mg/m^2 docetaxel on day 2 every 4 weeks. The combination showed a tolerable toxicity. An ORR of 37% was achieved and MS was 3 months [61]. In another trial that was performed by Nogami et al., irinotecan and docetaxel were both administered on the first day of 3-week cycles. The MTD was 60 mg/m^2 docetaxel plus 165 mg/m^2 irinotecan, with grade 4 neutropenia and grade 3 hepatotoxicity being the DLTs. The ORR and MS were 33.3% and 13.6 months, respectively [62]. However, phase II studies comparing the combination versus docetaxel single-agent therapy as a second-line treatment came to the conclusion that the combination was not superior to taxane monotherapy [63, 64]. For example, a group of Greek investigators used the following regimen: docetaxel 30 mg/m^2 plus Campto 60 mg/m^2 on days 1 and 8 (arm A) or docetaxel 75 mg/m^2 on day 1, every 21 days (arm B). Although the response rates were 20% for arm A versus 14% for arm B, MS was 6.5 months versus 6.4 months, while thrombocytopenia and diarrhea were more frequently observed in the combination arm [64].

Phase I studies that tested the combination of irinotecan with gemcitabine in recurrent NSCLC, recommended the following dosage: irinotecan 300 mg/m^2 on day 8 plus gemcitabine 1,200 mg/m^2 on days 1 and 8 every 21 days [65] and irinotecan 150 mg/m^2 plus gemcitabine 1,000 mg/m^2 both administered on the same day every 2 weeks [66]. Both studies revealed that the two antineoplastic agents could be combined in doses nearer to monotherapeutic levels with only mild toxicity (i.e., neutropenia, nausea/vomiting, diarrhea, asthenia). Furthermore, in the 3-week scheduled study, efficacy of the combination was evaluated and 4.5% of enrolled patients demonstrated an objective response, while 52.5% had stable disease [65]. In a Greek investigation, the administration of 150 mg/m^2 irinotecan plus 1,800 mg/m^2 gemcitabine every 15 days was evaluated in previously untreated patients. The ORR was found to be 16%, while clinical benefit was observed in 10–44% of treated patients. The MS was 8.1 months [67]. Another Greek group studied the combination of Campto at 300 mg/m^2 on day 8 plus gemcitabine at 1,000 mg/m^2 on days 1 and 8 every 3 weeks compared to monotherapy with Campto at 300 mg/m^2 every 3 weeks. Of the patients who received the combination regimen, 18.4% experienced an objective response and a significant improvement in symptoms and quality of life. However, only 4.2% of patients who received single-agent therapy with irinotecan demonstrated PR. However, the overall 1-year survivals were similar in the two groups under study [68].

The triplet combination of irinotecan with paclitaxel and carboplatin has also been evaluated for activity against NSCLC. A phase I/II study was published in 2001 by Socinski and co-workers, where the following schedule of administration was proposed: 100 mg/m^2 irinotecan on days 1 and 8, and AUC 5 carboplatin and 175 mg/m^2 paclitaxel on day 1, administered in 21-day cycles. The most frequently observed toxicities were neutropenia and diarrhea. In the phase II part of the trial, objective response was observed in 39% of evaluated patients and the MS was found to be 11 months [69, 70]. In the phase II study of the same group, the above-mentioned schedule was followed. The ORR of the triplet was 32% with the MS being 12.5 months. As far as toxicity was concerned, neutropenia (including febrile neutropenia and one death due to sepsis), anemia, gastrointestinal toxicity, and dyspnea were the most commonly observed conditions [71]. Pectasides et al. preferred a weekly infusion of carboplatin AUC 2, paclitaxel 20 mg/m^2, and irinotecan 60 mg/m^2 on days 1, 8, and 15, repeated every 5 weeks, in patients with advanced NSCLC. The regimen was well-tolerated with moderate toxicity (i.e., myelosuppression, diarrhea, vomiting, allergy, neurotoxicity, fatigue). The conclusions drawn in this trial were quite encouraging since 8% of patients achieved complete response (CR) and 48% PR (ORR 56%), and the MS was found to be 14.8 months [72].

Topotecan

Topotecan (Hycamtin) is currently approved for the treatment of recurrent small-cell lung cancer (SCLC), but it has recently shown activity against NSCLC as well [73]. Two phase I studies of single-agent topotecan determined the MTD at 1.5–2.0 mg/m^2 given intravenously daily for 5 consecutive days every 3 weeks [74] or 1.1 mg/m^2 for 3 consecutive days every 2 weeks [75]. In both studies, neutropenia was considered the DLT, while other adverse effects that occurred were anemia, thrombocytopenia, and fatigue. Lynch et al., in 1994, used 2 mg/m^2 topotecan given daily for 5 days every 3 weeks to previously untreated patients with stage IV NSCLC. The trial was preliminarily halted because of no objective response in the first 20 patients enrolled, even though 55% of them presented stable disease and the MS was 7.6 months. Toxic effects of treatment included high-grade neutropenia and rash [76]. In another phase II trial, Hycamtin was administered at a dosage of 1.5 mg/m^2 for 5 days every 3 weeks to a similar group of patients. In this case, the ORR was 15% and the MS 38 weeks. Grade 3/4 myelosuppression was the only serious toxicity, and mild nausea/vomiting and fatigue were also reported [77]. This same regimen (arm A) was examined by Weitz et al. in comparison with 1.3 mg/m^2 topotecan a day over a 72-h infusion, repeated every 4 weeks (arm B). The ORRs were 11% for arm A and 5% for arm B and the MSs were 37 and 26 weeks, respectively, thus demonstrating topotecan's limited single-agent activity [78]. Another schedule dictated administration of 0.6 mg/m^2 Hycamtin for 21 days by continuous intravenous infusion in 28-day cycles. This schedule was used by Mainwaring [79] and Kindler [80] in phase II studies in patients with advanced NSCLC. In both trials, the starting dose was decreased to 0.5 mg/m^2 in some patients, due to myelosuppression. Once more the results were disappointing. In Mainwaring's trial the ORR was 8% and in Kindler's 4%. The MS was 41 and 36 weeks, respectively.

The potential activity of oral topotecan in patients with advanced NSCLC has also been assessed. The regimen followed in a phase II study consisted of 2.3 mg/m^2 per day topotecan for the first 5 days of six 3-week cycles. The treatment was, in general, well-tolerated with only a few cases of grade 3/4 hematologic toxicity. No objective response was observed, even though 11% of treated patients had minor responses. However, the MS was 41 weeks and clinical benefit was also significant [81].

In combination with other agents, topotecan has proved to be more efficient in the treatment of NSCLC. Platinum compounds were the first agents to be studied [73]. In a phase I study, escalating doses of topotecan (starting at 0.75 mg/m^2 per day) for 5 days were combined with a fixed dose of 75 mg/m^2 cisplatin on the first day, every 3 weeks. The DLT was neutropenia, which was observed in the first level as well. Of the pa-

tients who completed therapy, 31% achieved an objective response, but the duration of response was short [82]. The combination with carboplatin was evaluated in a phase II study and proved to be significantly less toxic. Topotecan was infused at a dose of 0.5 mg/m^2 on days 1–5 and carboplatin at a dose of AUC 5 on day 1 every 21 days. In this study, the ORR was 13% and the MS was greater than 33 weeks. Toxicity was moderate and manageable, and included mainly neutro- and thrombocytopenia [83].

Rinaldi et al. administered Hycamtin plus gemcitabine as second-line chemotherapy for NSCLC in a phase I/II study. The combination was very well tolerated and the recommended schedule was 0.75 mg/m^2 topotecan on days 1–5 plus 400 mg/m^2 gemcitabine on day 5 every 2 weeks. The ORR was 18% and the MS was 10 months [84]. When this schedule was used in the treatment of both chemonaive and pretreated patients, the response rate and MS were 11% and 7 months, respectively [85]. In another phase II study of the same combination, the investigators recommended 1,250 mg/m^2 gemcitabine on days 1, 8, and 15 and topotecan 2.0 mg/m^2 on the same days every 4 weeks. Toxicity was minimal and the ORR and MS were 21% and 21 weeks, respectively [86]. Joppert et al. examined the activity of topotecan given at a dose of 1 mg/m^2 on the first 5 days of 28-day cycles along with 1,000 mg/m^2 gemcitabine on days 1 and 15. Of enrolled patients, 17% achieved an objective response and MS was 7.6 months. Hematologic toxicity, asthenia, and gastrointestinal disorders were moderate [87].

The combination with vinorelbine was also found to be effective as first- and second-line treatment of NSCLC. In the phase I/II study of Stupp et al., patients were treated with 0.5–1.0 mg/m^2 topotecan on days 1–5 and vinorelbine 20–30 mg/m^2 on days 1 and 5 every 21 days. The combination proved to be active, as the ORR was 42% and the MS 56 weeks, while demonstrating only mild toxicity [88].

In the combination with paclitaxel, topotecan was used in its oral form. In two phase I/II studies, the following regimen was given to previously untreated patients: 1.0–1.5 mg/m^2 topotecan orally on days 1–5 and 175 mg/m^2 paclitaxel on day 1 every 21 days. In both trials the MTD for topotecan was defined at 1.25 mg/m^2 because of neutropenia. Dobbs et al. observed an ORR of 28% [89], whereas in the trial by Eckart the ORR was 12% [90].

As far as triple combinations are concerned, topotecan has been evaluated along with cisplatin and gemcitabine in previously untreated patients in a phase I/II study. The patients received 0.5–2.0 mg/m^2 topotecan intravenously plus 20 mg/m^2 cisplatin plus 1,000 mg/m^2 gemcitabine on days 1, 8, and 15 of each 28-day cycle. Even though no DLT was observed, the researchers considered 1.75 mg/m^2 as the optimal dose for topotecan. Of evaluated patients, 38% showed a PR and the MS was 38 weeks [91].

34.2 Small Cell Lung Cancer

Small cell lung cancer is considered to be a systemic disease, since it tends to disseminate quickly by hematogenous spread. Combination chemotherapy, with or without concurrent radiotherapy, has become the mainstay of treatment in the management of SCLC [1, 16, 92, 93]. Cyclophosphamide was the first drug to be investigated in 1969, and was proven to be superior to supportive care with regard to survival of patients with SCLC [94]. Since then, several antineoplastic agents, including cisplatin, carboplatin, etoposide, vincristine, doxorubicin, methotrexate, lomustine, and ifosfamide, have demonstrated a response rate of 30% or greater in SCLC [1, 95].

Combination regimens were shown to be more effective than single agents in terms of symptomatic improvement, initial response, and survival prolongation [96, 97]. A number of active chemotherapy regimens have been evaluated in extensive disease (ED)-SCLC and platinum-based regimens were proven to be superior. The combination of cisplatin plus etoposide (EP) was found to be comparable with other combinations as far as response and survival were concerned, but clearly less toxic [93, 96, 98–102]. Carboplatin also shows high efficacy against SCLC, while demonstrating less toxicity than cisplatin, and its combination with etoposide (CE) became a treatment alternative [1, 93, 95, 103–105].

Patients with limited disease (LD) are usually given a platinum-based chemotherapy regimen with either concurrent or followed by radiotherapy [106, 107]. For newly diagnosed patients with ED-SCLC chemotherapy alone is the treatment of choice. A platinum agent plus etoposide is considered the most preferable regimen, since it is highly active, synergistic, and well-tolerated [93, 100, 106–110]. However, in order to decide over the optimal regimen, various factors, such as patient's age, performance status, organ function, and previous chemotherapy, should be taken into consideration. For the time being, the most frequently used combinations, apart from EP and CE, are CAV (cyclophosphamide, doxorubicin, vincristine), CAE (cyclophosphamide, doxorubicin, etoposide), (V)-ICE (vincristine, ifosfamide, carboplatin, etoposide), and CAVE (cyclophosphamide, doxorubicin, vincristine, etoposide) [93, 94, 111, 112].

These regimens have been associated with promising initial response and survival rates, as well as improved quality of life [38, 100, 111]. However, it is now known that these results are short-lived, and that for most patients cure remains elusive. For more than 90% of patients with SCLC, death from recurrent disease is inevitable [16, 38, 94, 107]. At the same time, there has only been a minimal improvement of MS over the past 25 years. Thus, it is imperative to find new agents and regimens equally active against both initially diagnosed and metastatic disease [106].

Since 1995, a number of new cytotoxic drugs, with novel non-overlapping mechanisms of action, have been introduced and evaluated in many trials, and the initial results were quite promising [108].

34.2.1 Camptothecins

Topotecan

Topotecan (Hycamtin) is probably the most extensively studied agent for the treatment of SCLC. Phase I studies, conducted by various investigators, concluded that the recommended dosage and schedule of administration is 1.5 mg/m^2 intravenously in 30 min for 5 consecutive days every 3–4 weeks. The DLT was myelosuppression [112–116].

Later, phase II and III studies demonstrated that topotecan, with or without platinum agents, was highly active against extensive stages of SCLC [117]. Previously untreated patients were treated with topotecan as a monotherapy. In this trial, the response rate was 39% and MS was 10 months [118]. When the same treatment was given to patients with refractory disease, the results were not as encouraging. This was pointed out by three studies that were carried out by Eckart et al. [119], Depierre et al. [120], and Ardizzoni et al. [121]. The overall survival in these studies was 3%, 2%, and 6%, respectively. However, better response rates were observed in patients with tumors sensitive to previous chemotherapy. In these cases, the ORRs were 19%, 17%, and 38%, respectively. In another study, topotecan was administered to patients with refractory SCLC who were previously treated with etoposide. The response rate was higher than the ones observed in the above-mentioned studies, and was found to be 12% [122]. The most important toxicity of topotecan monotherapy was grade 4 neutropenia that was observed in 47–89% of all treated patients.

Von Pawel et al. compared, in a randomized phase III study, the efficacy and cancer-related symptomatic improvement of topotecan in patients with recurrent SCLC, compared to CAV. Both regimens were equally well-tolerated, as far as non-hematologic toxicity was concerned. Patients who received topotecan more frequently developed grade 4 thrombocytopenia, but the percentage of grade 4 neutropenia was smaller in this arm compared to the CAV arm. However, myelosuppression was reversible in all cases. At least four of the eight symptoms that were evaluated demonstrated significant amelioration in patients that were treated with topotecan as opposed to those who received CAV. Dyspnea, anorexia, hoarseness, fatigue, and interference with daily activity were the main symptoms that were improved. This pivotal study led to the conclusion that topotecan is at least as effective as CAV [123].

Topotecan was later evaluated in combination with platinum agents as second-line treatment. In the EORTC study which was published in 2000, the overall response of the regimen topotecan plus cisplatin was 29% for patients with sensitive disease and 20% for patients with refractory disease [124]. In another phase II trial of the same combination, conducted by Samantas and colleagues, the ORR was 22% [125].

The Hellenic Research Oncology Group investigated the administration of cisplatin and etoposide followed by or alternating with topotecan. The alternating schedule proved to be a feasible, active, and well-tolerated regimen with an ORR of 64% and time to progression of 8 months. There were no toxic deaths reported, while non-hematologic toxicity was mild. Grade 3/4 neutropenia was observed in 13% of EP cycles and in 28% of topotecan cycles. Thrombocytopenia was 1% and 6%, respectively, and febrile neutropenia complicated 3% of EP and 1% of topotecan cycles [126]. In the sequential combination, the results were as follows: ORR to EP was 47%, and objective response was determined in 15% of the patients who received topotecan after EP. However, none of the patients with stable or progressive disease after EP, responded to topotecan. The median time to progression in this study was 6.5 months [127].

Topotecan was evaluated in combination with etoposide in a phase I study for previously untreated patients. The preliminary response rates were high (95%), and the MS was 10 months [128]. Mok and colleagues applied the sequential administration of topotecan and oral etoposide in patients with LD- and ED-SCLC. The ORRs were 5.6% and 55.6% for LD and ED, while the overall MS was 52.4 weeks [129]. It is worth mentioning, though, that two patients died due to hematologic toxicity.

A phase III study was carried out by ECOG, in order to determine the efficacy of topotecan in combination with standard chemotherapy in previously untreated patients with ED-SCLC. Four hundred and two patients were registered and treated with 4 cycles of EP. Two hundred and twenty-three of them presented stable disease or PR, and were then randomized to either receive 4 cycles of topotecan or to observation. Even though progression-free survival was highly improved for patients receiving topotecan, overall survival and quality of life were quite similar in both topotecan and observation arms [130].

The oral formulation of topotecan has improved the convenience of administration. However, it can be more easily added in combination regimens, especially multiple-day ones. A randomized phase II study, conducted by von Pawel et al. compared oral with intravenous topotecan. With regard to tumor response and overall survival, no difference was observed [131]. Many studies comparing the oral with the intravenous formation of the drug are currently under study.

Irinotecan

Irinotecan (Campto) is similar to topotecan and has been approved for the treatment of SCLC since 1994 in Japan, but not in Europe or the USA. This drug has been evaluated as a single agent in first- or second-line chemotherapy of patients with ED-SCLC [36].

Negoro and colleagues administered 100 mg/m^2 in 27 previously treated and 8 untreated patients. The response rates were 33% and 50%, respectively [132]. In another phase II study, the same treatment was given to patients with relapsed SCLC. Objective response was observed in 47% patients and MS was 6.8 months [133]. Le Chevalier et al., in their study, used another regimen: 350 mg/m^2 irinotecan were administered to chemonaive patients every 21 days. The response rate was 16% and MS was 4.5 months [134]. In both trials, the major toxicities reported were neutropenia and, most frequently, diarrhea.

Irinotecan combined with cisplatin was evaluated by Kudoh et al. in previously untreated patients with limited and extensive-stage SCLC. On days 1, 8, and 15, 60 mg/m^2 irinotecan were administered plus 60 mg/m^2 cisplatin on day 1 (every 4 weeks). ORR was reported to be 84% with 29% of patients presenting CR. MS for patients with ED was 13.2 months [135].

The same chemotherapy regimen was used by Okishio et al. as second-line chemotherapy in a phase II study. The ORR was found to be 19% and MS was 5.7 months [136]. In another Japanese study, the same dosage of irinotecan was used, but 30 mg/m^2 cisplatin was administered on days 1, 8, and 15. The overall survival in this case was 20% [137].

Irinotecan was also combined with carboplatin in patients with refractory or relapsed SCLC. In the trial of Naka and colleagues, 50 mg/m^2 irinotecan was administered on days 1, 8, and 15 plus carboplatin AUC 2 on days 1, 8, and 15 every 28 days [138]. In the trial of Hirose et al., the regimen consisted of 50 mg/m^2 irinotecan administered on days 1 and 8 and carboplatin AUC 5 on the first day of treatment every 28 days [139]. Both studies concluded that the combination was effective and with acceptable toxicity. In the first study the ORR and MS were 31% and 3.5 months, respectively, while the trial of Hirose achieved an ORR of 68.2% and an MS of 6.5 months.

The first study that actually demonstrated irinotecan's increased clinical efficacy was a phase III trial comparing 60 mg/m^2 irinotecan on days 1, 8, and 15 plus 60 mg/m^2 cisplatin on day 1 every 4 weeks (IP) to a standard regimen of 3-week cycles of 100 mg/m^2 etoposide on days 1, 2, and 3 plus 80 mg/m^2 cisplatin on day 1 (EP) in the management of ED-SCLC [107]. The response rates were 84.4% for the IP arm and 67.5% for the EP arm. However, the principle issue under investigation was overall survival. The advantage of the IP arm was evident; overall survival in the final analysis was 12.8 months, whereas in the EP arm it was 9.4

months. Moreover, 1-year survival was 58.4% for the IP group and 37.7% for the EP group and at 2 years the survival rates were 19.5% and 5.2%, respectively [140].

34.2.2 Taxanes

The taxane class of compounds shares a core ring structure called baccatin III. Their cytotoxic activity lies in the promotion of tubulin assembly into microtubules. Through this procedure, the microtubules become resistant to depolymerization. The two most important antineoplastic agents of this category are paclitaxel and docetaxel [141, 142].

Paclitaxel

The efficacy of paclitaxel in first-line treatment of SCLC was established by the phase II studies carried out by ECOG and by the North Central Cancer Treatment Group. In both trials 250 mg/m^2 paclitaxel was administered by 24-h infusion. Ettinger and colleagues, in their study, achieved a response rate of 53% and an MS of 11 months [143]. In the trial of Kirschling et al. the response rate was reported to be 68% and the MS 7.3 months [144]. The most important toxicity in both trials was neutropenia. The drug was also administered to heavily pretreated patients, relapsing within 3 months of chemotherapy. Paclitaxel was administered intravenously at a dosage of 175 mg/m^2 over 3 h every 3 weeks. Twenty-nine percent of the patients demonstrated objective PR and MS was 100 days, thus confirming that paclitaxel is an active agent against resistant SCLC [145].

Combining paclitaxel with other active antineoplastic agents improved its ORR. Nair et al. assigned patients with previously untreated ED-SCLC to receive 75 mg/m^2 cisplatin on day 1 plus paclitaxel at 135 mg/m^2 or 175 mg/m^2 infused in 3 h. In the lower dosage arm a response rate of 71% was observed, and the MS was 8.5 months, while in the higher dosage arm an objective response was obtained at a rate of 89% and the MS was 9.5 months [146]. Combined with carboplatin, 175 mg/m^2 paclitaxel was infused in 3 h and was found to be sufficiently active. Green et al. in 1999 reported a response rate of 74% in patients with SCLC resistant to CAE [147]. In a similar study by Gridelli and colleagues, the combination produced a response rate of 54.2% among patients with ED, and MS was 9.6 months [148]. The Groupe Francais de Pneumo-Cancerologie increased the dose of paclitaxel to 200 mg/m^2 and reported a response rate of 65% with an MS of 38 weeks and a 1-year survival of 22.5% [149].

In a multicenter phase II study, Kakolyris et al. tested the combination of paclitaxel 200 mg/m^2 on day 1 plus AUC 6 carboplatin on day 2 in a 4-week sched-

ule, as salvage treatment in refractory SCLC after EP or CAV first-line treatment. The regimen was relatively active. Twenty-five percent of the patients presented objective response (3% CR), while the median time to progression and survival were 5.5 and 7 months, respectively [150]. In all four of the above-mentioned trials, the regimen was, in general, well tolerated, and the most significant toxic effect was neutropenia.

Paclitaxel 130 mg/m^2 on day 5 plus topotecan 1 mg/m^2 on days 1–5 were administered to chemonaive patients with ED-SCLC, and the response rate was 92%. In the same trial, 1-year survival was 50% [151]. In a dose-escalation phase I trial, previously untreated patients received 135–175 mg/m^2 paclitaxel intravenously on day 1 and 1.25–1.5 mg/m^2 topotecan on days 1–3 every 3 weeks. Fifty-three percent of treated patients achieved PR and 18% presented stable disease [152]. Recently, in a phase II study, 135 mg/m^2 paclitaxel on day 5 plus 1 mg/m^2 topotecan on days 1–5 were administered as first-line therapy for ED-SCLC, and an ORR of 69% and an MS of 54 weeks were reported [153].

Several investigators added paclitaxel to the standard active regimen of cisplatin plus etoposide. Kelly et al. first conducted a study with escalating doses of all three antineoplastic agents (135–200 mg/m^2 for paclitaxel). Eighty-three percent of evaluated patients achieved a response, and the MS was 10.8 months [154]. In the schedule followed by Glisson and colleagues (paclitaxel 130 mg/m^2 on day 1 plus cisplatin 75 mg/m^2 and etoposide 80 mg/m^2 on days 2–4), the response rate was 96%, with 19% of patients presenting CR and an MS of 15.5 months [155].

A Greek Lung Cancer Cooperative Group phase III study compared the active (as phase I and II studies demonstrated) PET combination to PE as first-line treatment in patients with SCLC. Patients were randomized to receive either paclitaxel 175 mg/m^2 on day 1, plus cisplatin 80 mg/m^2 on day 2 and etoposide 80 mg/m^2 on days 2–4, or cisplatin 80 mg/m^2 on day 1 and etoposide 120 mg/m^2 on days 1–3. The study was terminated early due to excessive toxicity and mortality in the PET arm. In the early provisional analysis the two arms were equally active with a CR and PR rate of 50% for PET and 40% for PE. The MS and 1-year survival estimates on arms PET versus PE were 10.8 versus 9.8 months and 36.2% versus 35.7%. However, therapy-associated deaths and severe toxicity were more frequent in the PET arm [156].

In the trial of Hainsworth et al., paclitaxel 135 mg/m^2 plus AUC 5 carboplatin on day 1, and 50 mg alternating with 100 mg etoposide per os on days 1–10 were administered to patients with LD (who received concurrent radiotherapy) and patients with ED. The regimen was well tolerated and resulted in an objective response in 93% of patients with LD and 65% of patients with ED. The MS was 17 and 7 months for patients with limited and extensive SCLC, respectively [157]. A major response of 85% was also observed in the trial of Neill et al., where the regimen was paclitaxel 200 mg/m^2 plus AUC 6 carboplatin on day 1, and 80–100 mg/m^2 etoposide on days 1–3 [158].

In a Spanish study, a novel sequence of the combination was evaluated as first-line treatment. Etoposide was administered at 80 mg/m^2 on days 1–3, paclitaxel at 175 mg/m^2 on day 3, and carboplatin AUC 6 on day 3 in 3-week cycles. The ORR was similar for patients with LD and ED (73% and 74%, respectively). However, overall survival (ORS) and 1-year survival rates were 53% and 70% in LD-SCLC and 18% and 39% in ED-SCLC [159].

Many combinations of paclitaxel have been investigated. Among these are paclitaxel plus carboplatin plus topotecan [160], paclitaxel plus ifosfamide plus carboplatin [161], and etoposide plus cisplatin alternating with topotecan plus paclitaxel [162].

Docetaxel

This taxane agent has been much less investigated than paclitaxel in SCLC [163, 164]. Docetaxel was evaluated by Hesketh and colleagues as first-line therapy, using the standard dosage, i.e., 100 mg/m^2. It produced a modest response rate of 23%, while median overall survival did not exceed 36 weeks [163]. In previously treated patients, administration of the same dosage resulted in a 25% objective response, the duration of which ranged from 3.5 to 12.6 months [164].

The combination of docetaxel 75 mg/m^2 and cisplatin 75 mg/m^2 on day 1 in a 3-week schedule, as first-line chemotherapy of SCLC, showed an ORR of 71% and a median 1-year survival of 20% [165].

Docetaxel plus gemcitabine is a regimen that has been under study for the past few years. The Hellenic Cooperative Oncology Group evaluated the combination of docetaxel 50 mg/m^2 and gemcitabine 1,000 mg/m^2, both administered on days 1 and 8 every 3 weeks, in chemonaive patients with ED-SCLC. The trial was terminated early due to poor outcome with regard to response; only 6 of 20 patients under treatment obtained PR [166]. The combination proved to be inactive in second-line treatment as well. The trial that was conducted by the Hellenic Oncology Research Group demonstrated no response whatsoever. Only 5% of patients obtained stabilization, while MS was only 14 weeks [167].

34.2.3 Gemcitabine

Gemcitabine is an antimetabolite agent – a fluorine-substituted deoxycytidine analog – that inhibits DNA polymerase [168]. Gemcitabine has been evaluated as a monotherapy in a schedule of 1,000–1,250 mg/m^2 weekly in previously untreated patients, and objective response was produced at a rate of 27%. MS was 12 months and toxicity was mild with only 18% of treatment cycles leading to grade 3/4 myelosuppression [169]. These results suggested that gemcitabine could be useful in the therapy of SCLC in combination with myelosuppressive agents.

With regard to its activity response in resistant and sensitive or refractory SCLC, gemcitabine, when administered as a monotherapy, demonstrated disappointing results. In van der Lee and colleagues' trial, patients received 1,000 mg/m^2 on days 1, 8, and 15 in 3-week cycles. An ORR of 13% was confirmed in resistant SCLC with an MS of 17 weeks [170]. The results of the ECOG trial 1597, where gemcitabine's dosage was increased to 1,250 mg/m^2 weekly, were quite similar. The response rates were 5.6% for patients with refractory disease and 16.7% for patients with sensitive disease, while overall median survival (OMS) for all patients came to 7.1 months [171]. Hoang et al. also administered 1,000 mg/m^2 gemcitabine on days 1, 8, and 15 in 3-week cycles, but in this study, no responses were reported. Of 24 patients that were evaluated, 3 achieved stable disease and 21 had disease progression. MS was 8.8 months in the group with sensitive disease and 4.2 months in that of patients with refractory disease [172].

Gemcitabine combined with carboplatin (GC) was evaluated by the London Lung Cancer Group and compared to standard SCLC therapy (cisplatin plus etoposide; EP) in patients with extensive or locally advanced disease. The two regimens demonstrated similar activities with response rates of 58% versus 63%, and overall survival of 8.1 versus 8.2 months in the GC and EP arms, respectively. Toxicity, treatment-related deaths, and quality of life were quite similar in both arms [173].

Another promising combination is that of gemcitabine with etoposide. In a phase II study, chemonaive patients with ED-SCLC were treated with 1,000 mg/m^2 gemcitabine on days 1, 8, and 15 plus 80 mg/m^2 etoposide on days 8, 9, and 10 every 4 weeks. Forty-six percent demonstrated an objective response, and the MS was 10.5 months. Serious toxicities were infrequent [174].

The Hellenic Oncology Research Group (Lung Cancer Subgroup) conducted an investigation in order to evaluate efficacy and toxicity of irinotecan plus gemcitabine in pretreated patients. The schedule of treatment was 1,000 mg/m^2 gemcitabine on days 1 and 8 plus 350 mg/m^2 irinotecan on day 8 every 21 days. The combination showed modest activity. The ORR was 10% and disease stabilization was obtained in 22% of patients. The MS did not exceed 6 months. Myelosuppression was the most frequently observed toxicity (neutropenia 29%, thrombocytopenia 13%, febrile neutropenia 6%) [175].

34.2.4 Vinorelbine

Vinorelbine (Navelbine) is a newer semisynthetic vinca alkaloid. Vinca alkaloids act by binding to tubulin and inhibiting its polymerization to microtubules [168]. This agent has been evaluated as monotherapy in both first- and second-line treatments, and it has been shown to have a modest activity. In a Southwest Oncology Group study, previously untreated patients received 30 mg/m^2 vinorelbine weekly. The percentage of patients with objective response was 24% with an OMS of 32 weeks [176]. Similarly, in the phase II study of the EORTC Lung Cancer Cooperative, where the same regimen was administered as second-line treatment, the response rate was 16% [177].

However, vinorelbine when administered in combination with other cytotoxic agents produces improved response rates. Vinorelbine at 25 mg/m^2 on days 1 and 8 plus carboplatin at 300 mg/m^2 on day 1 produced an ORR of 74%. CR was documented in 23% of cases [178]. The results were equally encouraging as far as the regimen of vinorelbine, etoposide, and cisplatin was concerned. In a phase II study, patients with LD and ED-SCLC received 75 mg/m^2 cisplatin on day 1, 60 mg/m^2 etoposide on days 1–3, and 20 mg/m^2 vinorelbine on days 1 and 8 every 4 weeks. Patients with LD received concurrent radiation and achieved objective response at a rate of 78% with OMS of 13 months. For patients with ED, the response rate and MS were found to be 40% and 7 months, respectively [179].

34.2.5 Amrubicin

Amrubicin is a completely synthetic anthracycline and a potent topoisomerase II inhibitor. It has been investigated as a single-agent treatment (45 mg/m^2 every 3 weeks) in previously untreated patients with extensive SCLC. The ORR was 79%, and a CR was achieved in 15% of treated patients. The MS was 11 months [180].

34.3 Conclusion

The mainstay of treatment for both SCLC and NSCLC is chemotherapy. Platinum-based combinations remain the gold standard. Meanwhile, new antineoplastic agents and new combinations have been and are still under investigation with regard to efficacy and toxicity. Recently, platin-free combinations have proven equally as effective as platinum-based ones, and are currently used in the treatment of NSCLC. Even though tumor responses and quality of life have significantly improved, especially as far as patients with NSCLC are concerned, MS rates remain limited.

Conventional therapy has apparently reached a plateau of effectiveness. Investigators have, therefore, turned to new kinds of therapies that are based on tumor biology. Molecular targeted therapies are regarded as a promising alternative. However, only a minority of these new drugs have shown encouraging results. No definite survival benefit has been demonstrated yet. An abundant amount of research is still required in the field of lung cancer therapy.

Key Points

- The mainstay of treatment for both small cell and non-small cell lung cancer is chemotherapy.
- Although platinum-based combinations remain the gold standard, newer antineoplastic agents and combinations have been and are still under investigation with regard to efficacy and toxicity.
- Conventional chemotherapy has significantly improved tumor responses and quality of life, nevertheless median survival rates remain limited, indicating that a therapeutic plateau has been reached. Investigators have, therefore, turned to new kinds of therapies that are based on tumor biology.

References

1. Ettinger DS. Overview and state of the art in the management of lung cancer. Oncology 2004; 18:3.
2. Spigel DR, Anthony Greco F. Chemotherapy in metastatic and locally advanced non-small cell lung cancer. Semin Surg Oncol 2003; 21:98.
3. NSCLCCG. Chemotherapy in non-small cell lung cancer: a meta-analysis using updated data on individual patients from 53 randomized clinical trials. BMJ 1995; 311:899.
4. Spira A, Ettinger DS. Multidisciplinary management of lung cancer. N Engl J Med 2004; 350:379.
5. Ettinger DS. Is there a preferred combination chemotherapy regimen for metastatic in non-small cell lung cancer? Oncologist 2002; 7:226.
6. Wozniak AJ, Crowley JJ, Balcerzak, et al. Randomized trial comparing cisplatin plus vinorelbine in the treatment of advanced non-small cell lung cancer: a Southwest Oncology Group Study. J Clin Oncol 1998; 16:2459.
7. Sandler AB, Nemunaitis J, Denham C, et al. Phase III trial of gemcitabine plus cisplatin versus cosplatin alone in patients with locally advanced or metastatic non-small cell lung cancer. J Clin Oncol 2000; 18:122.
8. Gatzemeier U, von Pawel J, Gottfried M, et al. Phase III comparative study of high-dose cisplatin versus a combination of paclitaxel and cisplatin in patients with advanced non-small cell lung cancer. J Clin Oncol 2000; 18:3390.
9. Lilenbaum RC, Herndon J, List M, et al. Single-agent (SA) versus combination chemotherapy (CC) in advanced non-small cell lung cancer (NSCLC): a CALGB randomized trial of efficacy, quality of life (QOL) and cost-effectiveness. Proc Am Soc Clin Oncol 2002; 21:1a.

10. Belani CP, Langer C. First-line chemotherapy for NSCLC: an overview of relevant trials. Lung Cancer 2002; 38:S13.

11. Manegold C. Chemotherapy for advanced non-small cell lung cancer: standards. Lung Cancer 2001;34:S165.

12. Thatcher N. Chemotherapy for advanced non-small cell lung cancer. Lung Cancer 2001;34:S171.

13. ASCO. Clinical practice guidelines for the treatment of unresectable non-small cell lung cancer. J Clin Oncol 1997; 15:2996.

14. Georgoulias V, Papadakis E, Alexopoulos A, et al. Platinum-based and non-platinum-based chemotherapy in advanced non-small cell lung cancer: a randomized multicentre trial. Lancet 2001;357:1478.

15. Kosmidis PA. A randomized phase III trial of paclitaxel plus carboplatin vs paclitaxel plus gemcitabine in advanced NSCLC. A preliminary analysis. Lung Cancer 2000; 29:S147.

16. Hoffman PC, Mauer AM, Vokes EE. Lung cancer. Lancet 2000; 335:479.

17. Schiller JH, Harrington D, Belani CP, et al. Comparison of four chemotherapy regimens for advanced non-small cell lung cancer. N Engl J Med 2002; 346:92.

18. Giaccone G. Targeted therapy in non-small cell lung cancer. Lung Cancer 2002; 38:S29.

19. Gridelli C. Targeted therapy in the treatment of non-small cell lung cancer: reality and hopes. Curr Opin Oncol 2004; 16:126.

20. Fossella FV, Lynch T, Shepherd FA. Second line chemotherapy for NSCLC: establishing a gold standard. Lung Cancer 2002; 38:S5.

21. Kris MG. What does chemotherapy have to offer patients with advance-stage non-small cell lung cancer? Semin Oncol 1998; 25(suppl 8):1.

22. Rigas JR. Do newer chemotherapeutic agents improve survival in non-small cell lung cancer? Semin Oncol 1998; 25(suppl 8):5.

23. Misser JL, Bleiberg H, Sutherland W, et al. Oxaliplatin clinical activity: a review. Crit Rev Oncol Hematol 2000; 35:75.

24. Kosmidis PA, Manegold C. Advanced NSCLC: new cytostatic agents. Lung Cancer 2003; 41:S123.

25. Faivre S, Raymond E, Chapman W, et al. Lesion in cellular DNA and apoptosis induced by oxaliplatin. Proc Am Assoc Cancer Res 1997; 16:809A.

26. Extra JM, Espie M, Calvo F, et al. Phase I study of oxaliplatin in patients with advanced cancer. Cancer Chemother Pharmacol 1990; 25:299.

27. Caussanel JP, Levi F, Brienza S, et al. Phase I study of 5-day continuous venous infusion oxaliplatin at circadian rhythm modulated rate with constant rate. J Nat Cancer Inst 1990; 82:1046.

28. Monnet I, Brienza S, Hurget F, et al. Phase II study of oxaliplatin in poor prognosis non-small cell lung cancer (NSCLC). Eur J Cancer 1998; 34:1124.

29. Monnet I, Soulie P, de Cremoux H, et al. Phase I/II study of escalating doses of vinorelbine in combination with oxaliplatin in patients with advanced non-small-cell lung cancer. J Clin Oncol 2001;19:458.

30. Faivre S, Le Chevalier T, Monnerat C, et al. Phase I-II and pharmacokinetic study of gemcitabine combined with oxaliplatin in patients with advanced non-small-cell lung cancer and ovarian carcinoma. Ann Oncol 2002; 13:1479.

31. Bidoli P, Stani SC, Mariani L, et al. Phase I study of escalating doses of oxaliplatin in combination with fixed dose gemcitabine in patients with non-small cell lung cancer. Lung Cancer 2004; 43:203.

32. Franciosi V, Barbieri R, Vasini G, et al. The combination of gemcitabine and oxaliplatin (GEM-OXAL) is feasible in patients with poor prognosis advanced non-small-cell lung cancer. Results of a phase II study. Eur J Cancer 2001;37:6.

33. Kouroussis C, Agelaki S, Mavroudis D, et al. A dose escalation study of docetaxel and oxaliplatin combination in patients with metastatic breast and non-small cell lung cancer. Anticancer Res 2003; 23(1B):785.

34. Winegarden JD, Mauer AM, Otterson GA, et al. A phase II study of oxaliplatin and paclitaxel in patients with advanced non-small-cell lung cancer. Ann Oncol 2004; 15:915.

35. Misset JL, Gamelin E, Campone M, et al. Phase I and pharmacokinetic study of the multitargeted antifolate pemetrexed in combination with oxaliplatin in patients with advanced solid tumors. Ann Oncol 2004; 15:1123.

36. Pizzolato JF, Saltz LB. The camptothecins. Lancet 2003; 361:2235.

37. Chinsoo Cho L, Hak Choy MS. Topoisomerase I inhibitors in the combined-modality therapy of lung cancer. Oncology 2004; 18:S29.

38. Schiller JH. Future role of topotecan in the treatment of lung cancer. Oncology 2001;61(suppl 1):55.

39. Taguchi T, Wakui A, Hasegawa K, et al. Phase I clinical study of CPT-11. Gan To Kagaku Ryoho 1990; 17:115.

40. Negoro S, Fukuoka M, Masuda N, et al. Phase I study of weekly intravenous infusions of CPT-11, a new derivative of camptothecin, in the treatment of advanced non-small cell lung cancer. J Natl Cancer Inst 1991;21:1164.

41. Nakai H, Fukuoka M, Furuse K, et al. An early phase II study of CPT-11 in primary lung cancer. Gan To Kagaku Ryoho 1991;18:607.

42. Douillard J, Ibrahim N, Riviere A, et al. Phase II study of CPT-11 (irinotecan) in non-small cell lung cancer (NSCLC). Proc Am Soc Clin Oncol 1995; 14:365.

43. Negoro S, Fukuoka M, Niitani H, et al. A phase II study of CPT-11, a camptothecin derivative, in patients with primary lung cancer. CPT-11 Cooperative Group. Gan To Kagaku Ryoho 1991;18:1013.

44. Fukuoka M, Niitani H, Suzuki A, et al. A phase II study of CPT-11, a new derivative of camptothecin, for previously untreated non-small cell lung cancer. J Clin Oncol 1992; 10:16.

45. Baker L, Khan R, Lynch T, et al. Phase II study of irinotecan (CPT-11) in advanced non-small cell lung cancer (NSCLC). Proc Am Soc Clin Oncol 1997; 16:461a.

46. Sanchez P, Esteban E, Palacio I, et al. Activity of weekly irinotecan (CPT-11) in patients with advanced non-small cell lung cancer pretreated with platinum and taxanes. Invest New Drugs 2003; 21:459.

47. Masuda N, Fukuoka M, Takada Y, et al. CPT-11 in combination with cisplatin for advanced non-small cell lung cancer. J Clin Oncol 1992; 10:1775.

48. Mori K, Machida S, Yoshida T, et al. A phase II study of irinotecan and infusional cisplatin with recombinant human granulocyte colony-stimulating factor support for advanced non-small cell lung cancer. Cancer Chemother Pharmacol 1999; 43:467.

49. DeVore RF, Johnson DH, Crawford, et al. Phase II study of irinotecan plus cisplatin in patients with advanced non-small cell lung cancer. J Clin Oncol 1999; 17:2710.

50. Ando M, Kobayashi K, Yoshimura A, et al. Weekly administration of irinotecan (CPT-11) for refractory or relapsed non-small cell lung cancer. Lung Cancer 2004; 44:121.

51. Kakolyris S, Kouroussis C, Souglakos J, et al. Cisplatin and irinotecan (CPT-11) as second-line treatment in patients with advanced non-small cell lung cancer. Lung Cancer 2001;34(suppl 4):S71.

52. Ueoka H, Tanimoto M, Kiura K, et al. Fractionated administration of irinotecan and cisplatin for treatment of non-small cell lung cancer: a phase II study of Okayama Lung Cancer Study Group. Br J Cancer 2001;85:9.

53. Negoro S, Masuda N, Takada Y, et al. Randomized phase III trial of irinotecan combined with cisplatin for advanced non-small cell lung cancer. Br J Cancer 2003; 88:335.

54. Takeda K, Negoro S, Takifuji N, et al. Dose escalation study of irinotecan combined with carboplatin for advanced non-small cell lung cancer. Cancer Chemother Pharmacol 2001;48:104.

55. Kinoshita A, Fukuda M, et al. A phase II study of irinotecan (CPT-11) and carboplatin (CBDCA) in patients with advanced non-small cell lung cancer. Proc Am Soc Clin Oncol 2001;20:268b.

56. Takeda K, Takifuji N, Uejima H, et al. Phase II study of irinotecan and carboplatin for advanced non-small cell lung cancer. Lung Cancer 2002; 38:303.

57. Fukuda M, Oka M, Soda H, et al. Phase II study of irinotecan combined with carboplatin in previously untreated non-small cell lung cancer. Cancer Chemother Pharmacol 2004; 56:573.

58. Read W, McLeod H, Govindan R. Irinotecan and carboplatin in metastatic or recurrent NSCLC: an update. Oncology (Hunt) 2004; 18(suppl 4):15.

59. Hotta K, Ueoka H, Kiura K, et al. A phase I study and pharmacokinetics of irinotecan (CPT-11) and paclitaxel in patients with advanced non-small cell lung cancer. Lung Cancer 2004; 45:77.

60. Yamada K, Ikehara M, Tanaka G, et al. Dose escalation study of paclitaxel in combination with fixed-dose irinotecan in patients with advanced non-small cell lung cancer (JCOG 9807). Oncology 2004; 66:94.

61. Masuda N, Negoro S, Kudoh S, et al. Phase I and pharmacokinetic study of docetaxel and irinotecan in patients with advanced non-small cell lung cancer. J Clin Oncol 2000; 18:2996.

62. Nogami N, Harita S, Ueoka H, et al. Phase I study of docetaxel and irinotecan in patients with advanced non-small cell lung cancer. Lung Cancer 2004; 45:85.

63. Wachters FM, Groen HJ, Biesma B, et al. A randomized phase III trial docetaxel vs docetaxel and irinotecan in patients with stage IIIb-IV non-small cell lung cancer who failed first-line treatment. Br J Cancer 2005; 92:15.

64. Pectasides D, Pectasides M, Farmakis D, et al. Comparison of docetaxel and docetaxel and irinotecan as second-line treatment in advanced non-small cell lung cancer: a randomized phase II trial. Ann Oncol 2005; 16:294.

65. Kakolyris SS, Kouroussis C, Koukourakis M, et al. A dose-escalation study of irinotecan (CPT-11) in combination with gemcitabine in patients with advanced non-small cell lung cancer previously treated with a cisplatin-based front line chemotherapy. Anticancer Res 2002; 22:1891.

66. Nishio M, Ohyanagi F, Taguch F, et al. Phase I study of combination chemotherapy with gemcitabine and irinotecan for non-small cell lung cancer. Lung Cancer 2005; 48:115.

67. Pectasides D, Mylonakis N, Farmakis D, et al. Irinotecan and gemcitabine in patients with advanced non-small cell lung cancer previously treated with a cisplatin-based chemotherapy. A phase II study. Anticancer Res 2003; 23:4205.

68. Georgoulias V, Kouroussis C, Agelidou A, et al. Irinotecan plus gemcitabine vs irinotecan in the second-line treatment of patients with advanced non-small cell lung cancer previously treated with docetaxel and cisplatin: a multicentre, randomized, phase II study. Br J Cancer 2004; 91:482.

69. Socinski MA, Sandler AB, Miller LL, et al. Phase I study of the combination of irinotecan, paclitaxel, and carboplatin in patients with advanced non-small cell lung cancer. J Clin Oncol 2001;19:1078.

70. Socinski MA, Sandler AB, Miller LL, et al. Irinotecan (CPT-11) in triplet combinations in patients with advanced non-small cell lung cancer: a review and report of a phase I/II trial. Clin Lung Cancer 2001;2(suppl 2):S26.

71. Socinski MA, Sandler AB, Israel VK, et al. Phase II trial of irinotecan, paclitaxel, and carboplatin in patients with previously untreated stage IIIB/IV non-small cell lung carcinoma. Cancer 2002; 95:1520.

72. Pectasides D, Visvikis A, Kouloubinis A, et al. Weekly chemotherapy with carboplatin, docetaxel and irinotecan in advanced non-small cell lung cancer: a phase II study. Eur J Cancer 2002; 38:1194.

73. Stewart D. Update in the role of topotecan in the treatment of non-small cell lung cancer. Oncologist 2004; 9(Suppl 4):43.

74. Rowinski EK, Grochow LB, Hendricks CB, et al. Phase I and pharmacologic study of topotecan: a novel topoisomerase I inhibitor. J Clin Oncol 1992; 10:647.

75. Kakolyris S, Kouroussis C, Souglakos J, et al. A phase I clinical trial of topotecan given every 2 weeks in patients with refractory solid tumors. Oncology 2001;61:265.

76. Lynch TJ, Kalish L, Strauss G, et al. Phase II study of topotecan in metastatic non-small cell lung cancer. J Clin Oncol 1994; 12:347.

77. Perez-Soler R, Fossella FV, Glisson BS, et al. Phase II study of topotecan in patients with advanced non-small cell lung cancer previously untreated with chemotherapy. J Clin Oncol 1996; 14:503.

78. Weitz JJ, Marschke RF, Sloan JA, et al. A randomized phase II trial of two schedules of topotecan for the treatment of advanced non-small cell lung cancer. Lung Cancer 2000; 28:157.

79. Mainwaring PN, Nicolson MC, Hickish T, et al. Continuous infusional topotecan in advanced breast and non-small cell lung cancer: no evidence of increased efficacy. Br J Cancer 1997; 76:1636.

80. Kindler HL, Kris MG, Smith IE, et al. Phase II trial of topotecan administered as a 21-day continuous infusion in previously untreated patients with stage IIIB and IV non-small cell lung cancer. Am J Clin Oncol 1998; 21:438.

81. White SC, Cheeseman S, Thatcher N, et al. Phase II trial of oral topotecan in advanced non-small cell lung cancer. Clin Cancer Res 2000; 6:868.

82. Raymond E, Burris HA, Rowinski EK, et al. Phase I study of daily times five topotecan and single injection of cisplatin in patients with previously untreated non-small cell lung carcinoma. Ann Oncol 1997; 8:1003.

83. Pujol JL, Pawel J, Tumolo S, et al. Preliminary results of combined therapy with topotecan and carboplatin in advanced non-small cell lung cancer. Oncology 2001;61(suppl 1):47.

84. Rinaldi D, Lormand N, Brierre J, et al. A phase I-II trial of topotecan and gemcitabine in patients with previously untreated, advanced non-small cell lung cancer (LOA-3). Cancer Invest 2001;19:467.

85. Rinaldi D, Lormand N, Brierre J, et al. A phase II trial of topotecan and gemcitabine in patients with previously untreated advanced nonsmall cell lung carcinoma. Cancer 2002; 15:1274.

86. Dabrow MB, Francesco MR, Gilman PB, et al. Combined therapy with topotecan and gemcitabine in patients with inoperable or metastatic non-small cell lung cancer (LOA-3). Cancer Invest 2003; 21:517.

87. Joppert MG, Garfield DH, Gregurich MA, et al. A phase II multicenter study of combined topotecan and gemcitabine as first line chemotherapy for advanced non-small cell lung cancer. Lung Cancer 2003; 39:215.

88. Stupp R, Bodmer A, Duvoisin B, et al. Is cisplatin required for the treatment of non-small cell lung cancer? Experience and preliminary results of a phase I/II trial

with topotecan and vinorelbine. Oncology 2001;61(suppl 1):35.

89. Dobbs T, Eckart JR, Gordon NH, et al. Oral topotecan (OT) and intravenous paclitaxel (P) in patients with advanced non-small cell lung cancer (NSCLC): a phase I/II study. Proc Am Soc Clin Oncol 2000; 19:522a.

90. Eckart JR. Feasibility of oral topotecan plus intravenous paclitaxel in advanced non-small cell lung cancer. Oncology 2001;61(suppl 1):30.

91. Guarino MJ, Schneider CJ, Grubbs SS, et al. A dose-escalation study of weekly topotecan, cisplatin and gemcitabine front-line therapy in patients with inoperable non-small cell lung cancer. Oncologist 2002; 7:509.

92. Kelly K. New chemotherapy agents for small-cell lung cancer. Chest 2000; 117:156.

93. Schiller J. Current standards of care in small-cell and non-small-cell lung cancer. Oncology 2001;61(suppl 1):3.

94. Green RA, Humphrey E, Close H, et al. Alkylating agents in bronchogenic carcinoma. Am J Med 1969; 46:516.

95. Adjei AA. Management of small-cell cancer of the lung. Curr Opin Pulm Med 2000; 6:384.

96. Miklos S, Argiris A, Murren JR. Progress in the therapy of small-cell lung cancer. Crit Rev Oncol Hematol 2004; 49:119.

97. Lowenbraun S, Bartolucci A, Smalley RV, et al. The superiority of combination chemotherapy over single agent chemotherapy in small-cell carcinoma. Cancer 1979; 44:406.

98. Pujol JL, Carestia L, Daures JP. Is there a case for cisplatin in the treatment of small-cell lung cancer? A meta-analysis of randomized trials of a cisplatin containing regimen versus a regimen without this alkylating agent. Br J Cancer 2000; 83:8.

99. Chrystal K, Cheong J, Harper P. Chemotherapy of small-cell lung cancer: state of the art. Curr Opin Oncol 2004; 16:136.

100. Sudstrom S, Bremnes RM, Kaasa S, et al. Cisplatin and etoposide regimen is superior to cyclophosphamide, epirubicin and vincristine regimen in small-cell lung cancer: results from a randomized phase III trial with 5 years follow-up. J Clin Oncol 2002; 20:4665.

101. Mascaux C, Paesmans M, Berghmans T, et al. A systematic review of the role of etoposide and cisplatin in the chemotherapy of small-cell lung cancer with methodology assessment and meta-analysis. Lung Cancer 2000; 30:23.

102. Roth BJ, Johnson DH, Einhorn LH, et al. Randomized study of cyclophosphamide, doxorubicin and vincristine versus etoposide and cisplatin versus alternation of these two regimens in extensive small-cell lung cancer: a phase II trial of the Southeastern Cancer Study Group. J Clin Oncol 1992; 10:282.

103. Skarlos DV, Samantas E, Kosmidis P, et al. Randomized comparison of etoposide-cisplatin vs. etoposide-carboplatin and irradiation in small-cell lung cancer. A Hellenic Cooperative Oncology Group. Ann Oncol 1994; 5:601.

104. Kosmidis PA, Samantas E, Fountzilas F, et al. Cisplatin/etoposide versus carboplatin/etoposide chemotherapy and irradiation in small-cell lung cancer: a randomized phase III study. HECOG for lung cancer trials. Semin Oncol 1994; 21(suppl 6):23.

105. Bunn PA Jr. Review of therapeutic trials of carboplatin in lung cancer. Semin Oncol 1989; 16:27.

106. Anupama K, Hansen H. Treatment of small-cell lung cancer. Crit Rev Oncol Hematol 2004; 52:117.

107. Stupp R, Monnerat C, Turrisi AT. Small-cell lung cancer: state of the art and future perspectives. Lung Cancer 2004; 45:105.

108. Simon GR. Small-cell lung cancer. Chest 2003; 123:259S.

109. Spira A Ettinger D. Multidisciplinary management of lung cancer. N Engl J Med 2004; 350:379.

110. Thatcher N, Eckart J, Green M. Options for first and second line therapy in small-cell lung cancer: a workshop discussion. Lung Cancer 2003; 41(suppl 4):S37.

111. Okuna SH, Jett JR. Small-cell lung cancer: current therapy and promising new regimens. Oncologist 2002; 7:234.

112. Tjan-Heijnen VC, Wagener DJ, Postmus PE. An analysis of chemotherapy dose and dose intensity in small-cell lung cancer: lessons to be drawn. Ann Oncol 2002; 13:1519.

113. Schiller J. Future role of topotecan in the treatment of lung cancer. Oncology 2004; 61(suppl 1):55.

114. Rowinski EK, Grochow LD, Hendricks CB, et al. Phase I and pharmacologic study of topotecan: a novel topoisomerase I inhibitor. J Clin Oncol 1992; 10:647.

115. Saltz S, Sirott M, Young C, et al. Phase I clinical and pharmacology study of topotecan given daily for 5 consecutive days to patients with advanced solid tumours, with attempt to dose intensification using recombinant granulocyte colony stimulating factor. J Natl Cancer Inst 1993; 85:1499.

116. Verweij J, Lund B, Beijnen J, et al. Phase I and pharmacokinetics study of topotecan, a new topoisomerase I inhibitor. Ann Oncol 1993; 4:673.

117. Chinsoo Cho L, Hak Choy MS. Topoisomerase I inhibitors in the combined-modality therapy of lung cancer. Oncology 2004; 18(suppl):29.

118. Schiller JH, Kim KM, Hufson P, et al. Phase II study of topotecan in patients with extensive small-cell carcinoma of the lung: an Eastern Cooperative Oncology Group trial. J Clin Oncol 1996; 14:2345.

119. Eckart J, Gralla R, Palmer MC, et al. Topotecan (T) as second line therapy in patients with small-cell lung cancer (SCLC): a phase II study. Ann Oncol 1996; 7(suppl 5):107.

110. Depierre A, von Pawel J, Hans K, et al. Evaluation of topotecan in relapsed small cell lung cancer (SCLC): a multicentre phase II study. Lung Cancer 1997; 18(suppl 1):35.

121. Ardizzoni A, Hansen H, Dombernowsky P, et al. for the European Organization for Research and Treatment of Cancer Early Clinical Studies Group and New Drug Development Office, and the Lung Cancer Cooperative Group. Topotecan, a new active drug in the second line treatment of small-cell lung cancer: a phase II study in patients with refractory and sensitive disease. J Clin Oncol 1997; 15:2090.

122. Perez-Soler R, Glisson BS, Lee JS, et al. Phase II study of topotecan in patients with small cell lung cancer (SCLC) refractory to etoposide. Proc Am Soc Clin Oncol 1995; 14:355.

123. von Pawel J, Schiller JH, Shepherd FA, et al. Topotecan versus cyclophosphamide, doxorubicin, and vincristine for the treatment of recurrent small-cell lung cancer. J Clin Oncol 1999; 17:658.

124. Ardizzoni A, Manegold C, Debruyne C, et al. EORTC LCCG phase II study of topotecan in combination with cisplatin as second line chemotherapy of sensitive and refractory small cell lung cancer (SCLC). Lung Cancer 2000; 29:51.

125. Samantas E, Giannelou M, Onyenadum A, et al. A phase II study of cisplatin and topotecan as second line treatment in small cell lung cancer. Proc Am Soc Clin Oncol 2002; 21:218b.

126. Mavroudis D, Veslemes M, Kouroussis C, et al. Cisplatin-etoposide alternating with topotecan in patients with extensive stage small cell lung cancer (SCLC): a multicentre phase II study. Lung Cancer 2002; 38:59.

127. Mavroudis D, Pavlakou G, Blazoyiannakis G, et al. Sequential administration of cisplatin–etoposide followed by topotecan in patients with extensive stage small cell lung cancer. A multicentre phase II study. Lung Cancer 2003; 39:71.

128. O'Neill P, Clark PI, Smith D, et al. A phase I trial of a 5-day schedule of intravenous topotecan and etoposide in previously untreated patients with small-cell lung cancer. Oncology 2001;61(suppl 1):25.

129. Mok TS, Wong H, Zee B, et al. A phase I-II study of sequential administration of topotecan and oral etoposide (topoisomerase I and II inhibitors) in the treatment of patients with small cell lung carcinoma. Cancer 2002; 95:1511.

130. Schiller JH, Adak S, Cella D, et al. Topotecan versus observation after cisplatin plus etoposide in extensive-stage small-cell lung cancer: E7593 – a phase III trial of the Eastern Cooperative Oncology Group. J Clin Oncol 2001;19:2114.

131. von Pawel J, Gatzemeier U, Pujol JL, et al. Phase II comparator study of oral versus intravenous topotecan in patients with chemosensitive small-cell lung cancer. J Clin Oncol 2001;19:1743.

132. Negoro S, Fukuoka M, Niitani H, et al. A phase II study of CPT-11, a camptothecin derivative in patients with primary lung cancer. Jpn J Cancer Chemother 1991;18:1013.

133. Masuda N, Fukuoka M, Kusunoki Y, et al. CPT-11: a new derivative of camptothecin for the treatment of refractory or relapsed small-cell lung cancer. J Clin Oncol 1992; 10:1225.

134. Le Chevalier T, Ibrahim N, Chorny P, et al. A phase II study of irinotecan (CPT-11) in patients with small cell lung cancer (SCLC) progressing after initial response to first-line chemotherapy (CT). Proc Am Soc Clin Oncol 1997; 16:450A.

135. Kudoh S, Fujiwara Y, Takad Y, et al. Phase II study of irinotecan combined with cisplatin in patients with previously untreated small cell lung cancer. J Clin Oncol 1998; 16:1068.

136. Okishio K, Furuse K, Kawahara M, et al. A phase II study of irinotecan (CPT-11) and cisplatin (CDDP) in previously treated small cell lung cancer. Proc Am Soc Clin Oncol 1998; 17:497a.

137. Nakanishi Y, Takayama K, Takanoi K, et al. Second-line chemotherapy with weekly cisplatin and irinotecan in patients with refractory lung cancer. Proc Am Soc Clin Oncol 1999; 22:399.

138. Naka N, Kawahara M, Okishio K, et al. Phase II study of weekly irinotecan and carboplatin for refractory or relapsed small-cell lung cancer. Lung Cancer 2002; 37:319.

139. Hirose T, Horichi N, Ohmori T, et al. Phase II study of irinotecan and carboplatin in patients with refractory or relapsed small cell lung cancer. Lung Cancer 2003; 40:333.

140. Noda K, Nishiwaki Y, Kawahara M, et al. Irinotecan plus cisplatin compared with etoposide plus cisplatin for extensive small cell lung cancer. N Engl J Med 2002; 346:85.

141. Francis PA, Kris MG, Rigas JR, et al. Paclitaxel (Taxol) and docetaxel (Taxotere): active chemotherapeutic agents in lung cancer. Lung Cancer 1995; 12(suppl 1):S163.

142. Vaishampayan U, Parchment R, Jasti BR, et al. Taxanes: an overview of the pharmacokinetics and pharmacodynamics. Urology 1999; 54(suppl 6A):22.

143. Ettinger DS, Finkelstein DM, Sarma RP, et al. Phase II study of paclitaxel in patients with extensive disease small-cell lung cancer. An Eastern Cooperative Oncology Group study. J Clin Oncol 1995; 13:1430.

144. Kirschling RJ, Jung SH, Jett JR, et al. for the North Central Cancer Treatment Group. A phase II trial of Taxol and GCSF in previously untreated patients with extensive small cell lung cancer (SCLC). Proc Am Soc Clin Oncol 1994; 13:326.

145. Smit EF, Fokkema E, Biesma B, et al. A phase II study of paclitaxel in heavily pretreated patients with small-cell lung cancer. Br J Cancer 1998; 72:347.

146. Nair S, Marchte R, Grill J, et al. A phase II study of paclitaxel (Taxol) and cisplatin (CDDP) in the treatment of extensive stage small cell lung cancer (ESSCLC). Proc Am Soc Clin Oncol 1997; 16:454A.

147. Green HJ, Fokkema E, Biesma B, et al. Paclitaxel and carboplatin in the treatment of small cell lung cancer patients resistant to cyclophosphamide, doxorubicin and etoposide: a non-cross resistant schedule. J Clin Oncol 1999; 17:927.

148. Gridelli C, Manzione L, Perrone F, et al. Carboplatin plus paclitaxel in extensive small cell lung cancer: a multicentre phase 2 study. Br J Cancer 2001;84:38.

149. Thomas P, Castelnau O, Paillotin D, et al. Phase II trial of paclitaxel and carboplatin in metastatic small-cell lung cancer: A Groupe Francais de Pneumo-Cancerologie study. J Clin Oncol 2001;19:1320.

150. Kakolyris S, Mavroudis D, Tsavaris N, et al. Paclitaxel in combination with carboplatin as salvage treatment in refractory small-cell lung cancer (SCLC): a multicentre phase II study. Ann Oncol 2001;12:193.

151. Jett JR, Day R, Levitt M, et al. Topotecan and paclitaxel in extensive stage small cell lung cancer (ED-SCLC) patients without prior therapy. Lung Cancer 1997; 18(suppl 1):13.

152. West W, Birch R, Schnell F, et al. Phase I study of paclitaxel and topotecan for the first-line treatment of extensive-stage small cell lung cancer. Oncologist 2003; 8:76.

153. Ramalingam S, Belani CP, Day R, et al. Phase II study of topotecan and paclitaxel for patients with previously untreated extensive stage small-cell lung cancer. Ann Oncol 2004; 15:247.

154. Kelly K, Wood ME, Bun PA Jr, et al. A phase I study of cisplatin, etoposide and paclitaxel (PET) in small cell lung cancer. Lung Cancer 1997; 18(suppl 1):28.

155. Glisson BS, Kurie JM, Fox NJ, et al. Phase I-II study of cisplatin, etoposide and paclitaxel (PIT) in patients with extensive stage small cell lung cancer. Proc Am Soc Clin Oncol 1997; 16:455A.

156. Mavroudis D, Papadakis E, Veslemes M, et al. A multicentre clinical trial comparing paclitaxel-cisplatin-etoposide versus cisplatin-etoposide as first-line treatment in patients with small-cell lung cancer. Ann Oncol 2001;12:463.

157. Hainsworth JD, Gray JR, Stroup S, et al. Paclitaxel, carboplatin and extended-schedule etoposide in the treatment of small-cell lung cancer: comparison of sequential phase II trials using different dose intensities. J Clin Oncol 1997; 15:3463.

158. Neill HB, Miller AA, Clamon GH, et al. A phase II study evaluating the efficacy of carboplatin, etoposide, and paclitaxel with granulocyte colony stimulating factor in patients with stage IIIB and IV non-small-cell lung cancer and extensive disease small-cell lung cancer. Semin Oncol 1997; 24(suppl 12):S130.

159. Vietez JM, Valladares M, Gracia M, et al. Phase II study of carboplatin and 1-h intravenous etoposide and paclitaxel in a novel sequence as first-line treatment of patients with small-cell lung cancer. Lung Cancer 2003; 39:77.

160. Hainsworth JD, Morrissey L, Scullin D, et al. Paclitaxel, carboplatin, and topotecan in the treatment of patients with small cell lung carcinoma. A phase II trial of the Minnie Pearl Cancer Research Network. Cancer 2002; 94:2426.

161. Socinski M, Neubauer M, Olivares J, et al. Phase II trial of paclitaxel, ifosfamide, and carboplatin in extensive-stage small cell lung cancer. Lung Cancer 2003; 40:91.

162. Jett JR, Hatfield AK, Hilman S, et al. Alternating chemotherapy with etoposide plus cisplatin and topotecan plus paclitaxel in patients with untreated extensive-stage small cell lung cancer. Cancer 2003; 10:2498.

163. Hesketh PJ, Crowley JJ, Burris HA, et al. Evaluation of docetaxel in previously untreated extensive-stage small cell lung cancer. A Southwest Oncology Group phase II trial. Cancer J Sci Am 1999; 5:237.

164. Smyth JF, Smith IE, Sessa C, et al. Activity of docetaxel (Taxotere) in small cell lung cancer. The Early Clinical Trials Group of the EORTC. Eur J Cancer 1994; 30A:1058.

165. Lianes P, Moreno-Nogueira JA, Cardenal F, et al. Multicentre phase II clinical trial of docetaxel (D) in combination with cisplatin (P) in first line chemotherapy for small cell lung cancer extensive disease: final results. Proc Am Soc Clin Oncol 2001;20; 309.

166. Skarlos DV, Dimopoulos AM, Kosmidis P, et al. Docetaxel and gemcitabine combination, as first-line treatment in patients with extensive disease small-cell lung cancer. A phase II study of the Hellenic Cooperative Oncology Group. Lung Cancer 2003; 41:107.

167. Agelaki S, Veslemes M, Syrigos K, et al. A multicentre phase II study of the combination of gemcitabine and docetaxel in previously treated patients with small cell lung cancer. Lung Cancer 2004; 43:329.

168. Rang HP, Dale MM, et al. Drugs used in cancer chemotherapy. In: Rang HP (ed) Pharmacology. New York: Churchill Livingston, 2003:6.8.

169. Cormier Y, Eisenhauer E, Muldal E, et al. Gemcitabine is an active new agent in previously untreated extensive small cell lung cancer (SCLC). A study of the National Cancer Institute of Canada Clinical Trials Group. Ann Oncol 1994; 5:283.

170. van der Lee I, Smit EF, van Puten JW, et al. Single-agent gemcitabine in patients with resistant small-cell lung cancer. Ann Oncol 2001;12:557.

171. Masters GA, Declerck L, Blanke C, et al. Phase II trial of gemcitabine in refractory or relapsed small-cell lung cancer: Eastern Cooperative Group Trial 1597. J Clin Oncol 2003; 21:1550.

172. Hoang T, Kim T, Jaslowski A, et al. Phase II study of second-line gemcitabine in sensitive or refractory small cell lung cancer. Lung Cancer 2003; 42:97.

173. James L, Rudd R, Gower N, et al. A phase III randomized comparison of gemcitabine/carboplatin (GC) with cisplatin/etoposide (PE) in patients with poor prognosis small cell lung cancer (SCLC). Proc Am Soc Clin Oncol 2002; 21:2193.

174. Vansteenkistee J, Gatzemeier U, Manegold C, et al. Gemcitabine plus etoposide in chemonaive extensive disease small cell lung cancer: a multicentre phase II study. Ann Oncol 2001;12:835.

175. Agelaki S, Syrigos K, Christofyllakis C, et al. A multicentre phase II study of the combination of irinotecan and gemcitabine in previously treated patients with small-cell lung cancer. Oncology 2004; 66:192.

176. Higano CS, Crowley JJ, Veith RV, et al. A phase II study of intravenous vinorelbine in previously untreated patients with extensive small cell lung cancer, a Southwest Oncology Group study. Invest New Drugs 1997; 15:153.

177. Jaseem J, Karnicka-Mlodwowska H, van Pottelsberge C, et al. Phase II study of vinorelbine (Navelbine) in previously treated small cell lung cancer patients. EORTC Lung Cancer Cooperative Group. Eur J Cancer 1993; 12:1720.

178. Gridelli C, Perrone F, Iannelio GP, et al. Carboplatin plus vinorelbine, a new well-tolerated and active regimen for the treatment of extensive-stage small cell lung cancer: a phase II study. Gruppo Oncologico Centro-Sud-Isole. J Clin Oncol 1998; 16:1414.

179. Richardet E, Carranza L, Uribe A, et al. Phase II study: cisplatin (C) + etoposide (E) + Navelbine (N) in small cell lung cancer. Proc Am Soc Clin Oncol 1995; 14:373a.

180. Negoro T, Takada Y, Yokota S. Phase II study of amrubicin (SM-5887), a 9-amino-anthracycline in extensive stage small cell lung cancer (ES-SCLC): a West Japan Lung Cancer Group trial. Proc Am Soc Clin Oncol 1998; 17:704A.

Novel Targets for Lung Cancer Therapy

35

Jill M. Siegfried and Laura P. Stabile

Contents

35.1 Introduction

Lung cancer remains the number one killer from cancer of men and women in the USA, and is also a major cause of cancer deaths worldwide. The 5-year survival rate for lung cancer has barely improved in the past 20 years [1]. Since cytotoxic therapies have reached a plateau in their clinical efficacy, even in combination, new therapies that target specific cancer-related growth pathways are needed to make an impact on the course of this disease, which is still often diagnosed at late stages that do not respond well to current therapies. The recent experience with gefitinib [2] suggests that although attractive targets such as the epidermal growth factor receptor (EGFR) exist that are effectively inhibited in preclinical studies, the successful application of targeted therapies to clinical use may require different approaches, such as use in selected sensitive patients, combination therapy against several targets, sequential treatment after cytotoxic therapy, or use of drugs intermittently at high doses to induce apoptosis rather than continuously at low doses to impair cell division.

Growth factors and their receptors are attractive targets for therapy because these molecules initiate signaling pathways that control cell division and cell survival, two processes that are in imbalance in malignant cells. Data are continuing to accumulate showing that many growth factor and oncogene signaling pathways overlap and interact with each other. This suggests that not only is there redundancy in how signaling is carried out by cancer cells, but also that strategies to interrupt the cross-signaling may have additive or synergistic effects on tumor inhibition [3, 4]. This may be particularly important because, in clinical use, doses of targeted agents to the tumor that produce 50% or higher inhibition of any one target are difficult to achieve. Partially reducing two intersecting signaling components or two linear segments of the same signaling pathway may therefore improve therapeutic efficacy.

Classical steroid hormone pathways have also been successful in the treatment of breast and prostate cancer. Steroid hormone receptors are now known to be expressed in tissues outside the reproductive tract, and to have biological effects in non-reproductive tumors, including in some cases effects that are independent of steroid ligand. This suggests that the hormone receptor itself, such as the estrogen receptor, could have intrinsic biological activity in non-reproductive tissues even in the absence of its steroid ligand. This chapter will discuss three potential targets that could be clinically exploited for lung cancer therapy, based on our current understanding of the biology of these ligand-receptor signaling pathways, which have been validated in non-small cell lung cancer (NSCLC). Challenges of bringing inhibitors of these pathways to the clinic and gaps in our understanding of the biology of these pathways in both small and non-lung cancer will also be discussed.

35.2   Steroid Hormone Receptors in Lung Cancer

35.2.1   Estrogen Receptors

Several reports of sex differences in lung cancer risk and disease presentation suggest that estrogen may be involved in the etiology of this disease [5]. Estrogen receptors (ERs), members of the nuclear steroid receptor superfamily, mediate the cellular response to estrogen. Two ERs have been identified, ERα and ERβ, which are encoded by separate genes. These proteins function as sequence-specific, ligand-activated transcription factors. There have been inconsistent results reported concerning the presence of ERs in lung tumors based on antibodies and techniques used. With the identification of antibodies that distinguish between ERα and ERβ and routine immunohistochemical procedures, it is now clear that both ERα and ERβ are expressed and functional in most human NSCLC cell lines, cells derived from normal lung and lung tumor, and normal patient tissue specimens. Table 35.1 summarizes the ER expression results from our laboratory in normal and malignant cells derived from the lung. Both mRNA and protein were detected by most cell types. ERβ was almost universally present. ERα was found mainly in the cytoplasm and membrane in immunohistochemical studies and was found to be comprised of mostly alternatively spliced variants based on Western analysis and RT-PCR [6]. In contrast, ERβ was found mainly localized to the nucleus and to be comprised of mainly full-length protein in addition to some variants [6]. ER-mediated transcriptional and growth responses in lung tumors support the hypothesis that at least some forms of ER are functional [6, 7].

A population study examining lung cancer presentation and survival in pre- versus postmenopausal women revealed that the premenopausal women presented with more advanced disease including poorly differentiated tumors with less favorable histologies [8]. Interestingly, these same women had a survival advantage versus their postmenopausal counterparts (*ibid*). ER expression status was not examined in these patients. In fact, few reports relating ER status to NSCLC patient survival have been completed. Kawai et al. [9] reported that the presence of ERα and the absence of ERβ are associated with worse prognosis among NSCLC patients. Patients at higher risk at histopathologic stage I were those with no ERβ expression [9]. These results are the opposite of what has been demonstrated for ER status and prognosis of breast cancer patients [10, 11]. Whether or not this relationship is observed in other patient populations is not known at the present time.

Estrogen acts to induce cell proliferation of NSCLC cells in vitro (Fig. 35.1) and in vivo [6] and can modulate expression of genes in NSCLC cell lines that are important for control of cell proliferation [7]. Genomic estrogen signaling has been demonstrated to occur mainly through ERβ in NSCLC cells [12]. Furthermore, fulvestrant ("Faslodex"), an ER antagonist with no agonist effects, inhibits cell proliferation in vitro (Fig. 35.1) and lung tumor xenograft growth in severe combined immunodeficient (SCID) mice by approximately 40% [6]. Thus, targeting the estrogen signaling pathway may have therapeutic value to treat or prevent lung cancer.

There are currently three available strategies to target the estrogen signaling pathway in cancer cells: (a) antagonists of ER function through drugs such as tamoxifen and raloxifene; (b) downregulation of ER function through agents such as fulvestrant; and (c) reduction of estrogen levels through aromatase inhibitors, such as the reversible non-steroidal agents letrozole and anastrozole [13] and the irreversible steroidal inactivator exemestane [14]. Tamoxifen and raloxifene have partial agonist effects in certain tissues, such as endometrium. Tamoxifen has been shown to increase lung tumor xenograft growth and is not an appropriate choice of therapy for NSCLC [12]. Additionally, results from the Tamoxifen Breast Cancer Prevention Trial as part of the National Surgical Adjuvant Breast and Bowel Project did not show any decreased risk of lung cancer [15]. Seventeen tumors of the lung, trachea, and bronchus were reported among the placebo group and 20 in the women who had received tamoxifen therapy. Although not statistically significant, these results do suggest that tamoxifen may have some agonistic effects in the lung.

The aromatase enzyme catalyzes the conversion of androgens to estrogens and is expressed in the lung [16, 17]. Recent preclinical work suggests that aromatase inhibitors are also potential inhibitors for lung cancer therapy [18]. Aromatase protein was expressed in

Table 35.1. Expression of ERα and ERβ in normal lung and NSCLC cell lines and tissues

	ERα RNA	ERα protein	ERβ RNA	ERβ protein
Human bronchial epithelial cells	4/6 (66%)	5/6 (83%)	17/18 (94%)	6/6 (100%)
Normal lung fibroblast cells	6/6 (100%)	6/6 (100%)	27/28 (96%)	6/6 (100%)
NSCLC cell lines	6/7 (86%)	10/10 (100%)	7/7 (100%)	10/10 (100%)
Tumor tissue specimens	4/6 (66%)	82/110 (74%)	5/6 (83%)	107/110 (97%)

RNA was determined by RT-PCR, and protein expression was determined by Western or immunohistochemical analysis. ERα expression was considered positive even if full-length product was not present, only exon deletion variants

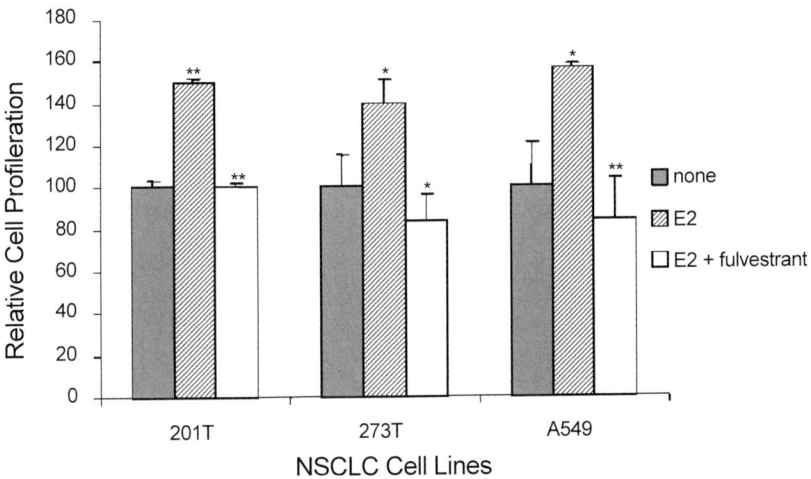

Fig. 35.1. Effect of estrogen and fulvestrant on cell proliferation. NSCLC cells were serum deprived for 48 h followed by treatments as indicated for 72 h. Cellular proliferation was measured using the CellTiter 96 Aqueous One Solution Cellular Proliferation Assay. $* P < 0.05$, $** P < 0.005$, unpaired Student's t-test, compared with no treatment (*none*) for estrogen (*E2*) treatment or compared with estrogen for fulvestrant treatment. Bars, SE

lung tumor cell lines and tumor tissue and was demonstrated to be functional. Additionally, 30% decrease in growth of lung tumor xenografts treated with anastrozole was observed. Aromatase inhibitor therapy in lung cancer is further supported by Coombes et al. [19] who reported a decreased incidence of primary lung cancer in breast cancer patients treated with exemestane after 2–3 years of tamoxifen therapy (4 cases) compared with continued tamoxifen treatment (12 cases). Because lung tumors from both male and female patients express ERs and aromatase and cell lines derived from both sexes respond to estrogens, antiestrogens, and aromatase inhibitors, these types of therapeutic treatments may be beneficial for both populations, not solely women.

In addition to the nuclear mechanisms of ER action, estrogen can also rapidly activate signaling in seconds to minutes. These rapid signaling effects are often referred to as non-genomic effects and are thought to occur via ERs located in the membrane. In human breast cancer cells, this membrane receptor was identified as a G protein-coupled receptor called GPR30 [3, 4, 20]. In NSCLC cells, extranuclear ERs have been identified in plasma membrane fractions and have been shown to promote rapid stimulation of signaling pathways [21]. These effects can be inhibited by the addition of fulvestrant. The epidermal growth factor receptor (EGFR/HER-1) is a member of the tyrosine kinase receptor family that also includes HER-2, HER-3, and HER-4 [22]. These receptors have been implicated in proliferation, cell motility, angiogenesis, cell survival, and differentiation [23]. Overexpression of EGFR correlates with poor prognosis in NSCLC patients [24]. An interaction between the ER and EGFR has been demonstrated in lung cancer cells [12]. In this regard, estrogen can rapidly activate the EGFR in lung cancer cell lines and the

combination of fulvestrant and gefitinib ("Iressa"), an EGFR tyrosine kinase inhibitor, in NSCLC can maximally inhibit cell proliferation, induce apoptosis, and affect downstream signaling pathways both in vitro and in vivo (Fig. 35.2) [12]. Furthermore, membrane ERs were found to be co-localized with EGFR in lung tumors [21]. A reciprocal control mechanism was also observed between ER and EGFR in lung cancer cells. In this respect, EGFR protein expression was downregulated in response to estrogen and upregulated in response to fulvestrant in vitro, suggesting that the EGFR pathway is activated when estrogen is depleted [12]. Conversely, ERβ protein expression was downregulated in response to EGF and upregulated in response to gefitinib providing a rationale to target these two pathways simultaneously [12].

Targeting the EGFR through small molecule tyrosine kinase inhibitors is of limited use in the absence of an EGFR mutation, which only occurs in a minority of patients. Recently, a phase I clinical trial using drugs that target these two signaling pathways was performed to assess the toxicity of combined treatment of gefitinib with fulvestrant in 22 postmenopausal women [25]. Targeting both pathways was found to be safe and have antitumor activity in stage IIIB/IV female patients. Additionally, immunohistochemical staining of nuclear ERβ was correlated with improved patient survival. Phase II trials examining the combination of erlotinib with fulvestrant are also underway. Targeting the estrogen signaling pathway via both nuclear and extranuclear receptors in conjunction with the EGFR signaling pathway should have increased beneficial antitumor effects in NSCLC as has been observed in breast cancer cells [26]. Combination therapy may increase the duration of response in patients whose tumors harbor an

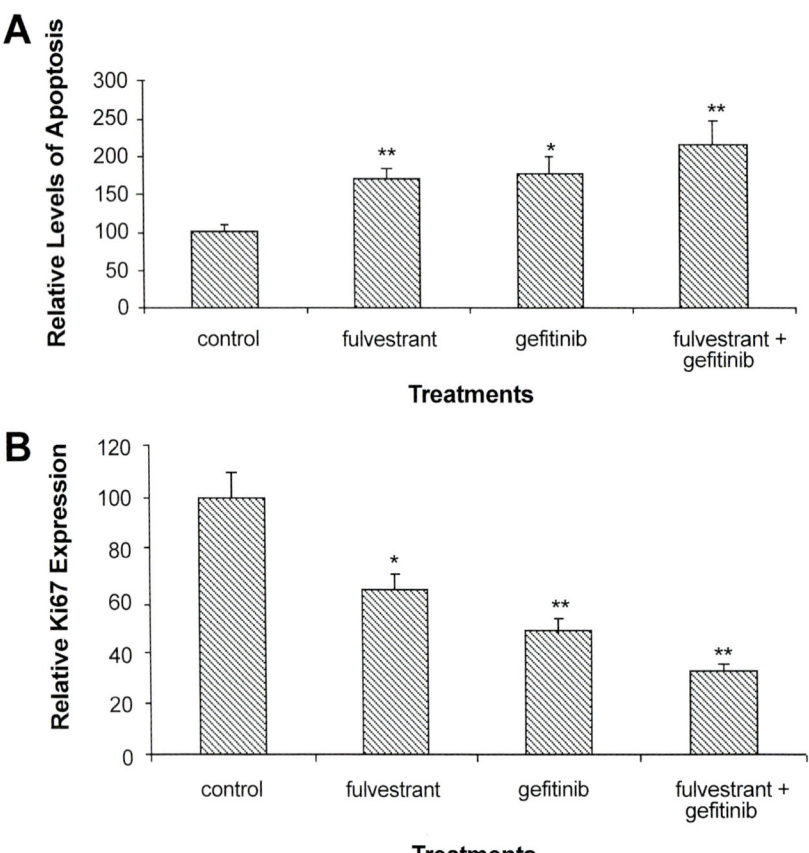

Fig. 35.2. Increased apoptosis (**a**) and decreased cell proliferation (**b**) in tumors treated with combined fulvestrant plus gefitinib versus tumors treated with individual drug treatments or controls. ** $P < 0.005$, * $P < 0.05$, unpaired Student's *t*-test, compared with control. Bars, SE. (Reprinted with permission from *Cancer Research* Stabile et al. 2005 [12])

EGFR mutation as well as improve response in patients whose tumors do not contain an EGFR mutation. Further understanding of the role of estrogen, estrogen synthesis, and ERs in lung cancer will provide the rationale for future targeting of this pathway for therapy earlier in the course of disease and possibly for lung cancer prevention. Additional understanding of the role of membrane versus nuclear ERs in lung cancer and which drugs affect which receptors will be important for designing new effective treatments.

35.2.2   Progesterone Receptors

Progesterone mediates cell differentiation through the progesterone receptor (PR). Presence of PR in breast cancer is in general an indication of a more differentiated tumor that is responsive to antiestrogen therapy, and PR is a known estrogen-responsive gene. There are several reports of expression of PR by primary NSCLC, although there is a great deal of variability in the reported frequency of expression [27, 28]. One report found no PR in NSCLC [29]. A recent report used a monoclonal antibody that recognizes both the A and B forms of PR, and found positive PR expression in 46% of cases, with a preponderance of positive PR expression in tumors from females [30]. Enzymes capable of synthesizing progesterone were also detected in many NSCLC, and a positive correlation was observed between intratumoral levels of progesterone and the presence of three enzymes that participate in progesterone synthesis (*ibid*). Exposure of NCLCs to progesterone led to growth inhibition of tumor xenografts and concomitant induction of apoptosis, in agreement with clinical data suggesting that the presence of PR was correlated with longer overall survival in NSCLC patients (*ibid*).

Progesterone derivatives have been useful in the treatment of both endometrial cancer and breast cancer [31, 32]. Agents such as medroxyprogesterone acetate, which can be given orally, have potential for treatment of lung cancer, perhaps in combination with agents that suppress either the ER pathway or act on growth factor pathways such as EGFR, c-Met, or other tyrosine kinase inhibitors. Long-term progesterone treatment might even be feasible for chemoprevention of lung cancer.

35.2.3 Androgen Receptors

Androgen receptors (ARs) have also been reported in lung cancer [28, 33, 34], and conceivably can also mediate growth-promoting signaling if androgens are present. Early studies used binding of radiolabeled ligand and/or sucrose density centrifugation to detect specific binding sites for androgens and isolation of a binding protein of the correct size for the androgen receptor in tissue from a squamous cell carcinoma of the lung [33] and in 8 of 13 small cell lung cancer (SCLC) cell lines [34]. The AR-positive cell lines were found in seven of eight men and one of three women. Growth stimulation by androgen exposure was also found in SCLC cell lines expressing the AR, as well as expression of 5a-reductase, the enzyme that produces dihydrotestosterone, the form androgenically active in the prostate gland (*ibid*). In a later study, Kaiser et al. [28] used specific antibodies directed against the AR, ligand binding, and RT-PCR to examine AR expression in lung tumor cell lines and tissues. Twelve of 17 NSCLC cell lines and 2 of 12 SCLC cell lines, as well as 17% of primary lung tumor tissues were AR positive.

As with the ER, ligand-independent signaling through AR phosphorylation has been reported in prostate cancer (reviewed by Taplin and Balk [35]). Growth factors such as insulin-like growth factor, keratinocyte growth factor, and epidermal growth factor have been shown to activate AR as evidenced by increased binding to AR response elements, in the absence of androgen. Interleukin-6 also has the ability to activate AR. A number of other proteins, such as cyclins and nuclear transcription factors, can complex with AR and might contribute to androgen-independent signaling by AR. Many of these pathways are dysregulated in lung cancer, and could allow for enhanced AR signaling in lung tumors as well, if the AR is present. Further study of AR status and signaling in lung cancer is warranted.

35.3 Hepatocyte Growth Factor (HGF)/c-Met Pathway in Lung Cancer

35.3.1 Biology and Signaling of the HGF/c-Met Pathway

Hepatocyte growth factor was first discovered as a blood-borne protein that was released immediately following liver injury; it is identical to another protein known as scatter factor and is important in the development of many organs [36, 37]. In 1991, HGF was found to be the ligand for the c-Met protein, a ubiquitously expressed tyrosine kinase receptor that is found in most epithelial cells and in endothelial cells [38]. The c-Met protein can be constitutively activated by muta-

tions [39, 40], which have been found in both SCLC and NSCLC [41, 42], and c-Met or its ligand HGF also are often overexpressed in tumors [43–45]. Both c-Met and HGF overexpression by NSCLC is associated with poor prognosis [46, 47]. High HGF content on stage I lung adenocarcinoma was strongly associated with reduced time to recurrence. The c-Met protein couples to a number of signaling systems that are initiated by the adaptor proteins Gab-1, Grb2, Shc, and c-Cbl, leading to downstream activation of the MAPK, PI-3 kinase, PLC-γ, and STAT pathways (reviewed in Christensen et al. [48]). Through these signaling pathways, HGF activation of c-Met initiates cell movement, cell growth, invasion, and angiogenesis [49–52]. High HGF content in a stage I lung cancer may increase the probability that tumor cells have migrated out of the primary tumor by the time of clinical detection. Because it is primarily involved in development, and is relatively silent in the adult except for wound healing and tissue regeneration, it may prove to be an attractive therapeutic target. Its inhibition is not expected to have severe effects on organ function unless injury is present.

Hepatocyte growth factor is involved in a number of processes that contribute to carcinogenesis. HGF induces angiogenesis, and it is known to not only locally stimulate endothelial cell migration and proliferation but also to mobilize endothelial progenitor cells from the bone marrow [53]. HGF is produced by neutrophils that infiltrate tumors, and can be detected in the bronchioalveolar lavage fluid from patients with bronchioloalveolar carcinoma, while being undetectable in healthy controls [54]. Overexpression of c-Met by squamous cell carcinoma is associated with enhanced secretion of the angiogenesis factor vascular endothelial growth factor (VEGF), a well as enhanced metastatic spread [55].

35.3.2 HGF/c-Met Inhibitors

Because of the overwhelming evidence of a role of the HGF/c-Met pathway in the pathogenesis of human cancers, therapeutic inhibitors that target this pathway are in development. Potential inhibitors of the HGF/c-Met signaling pathway include: (1) selective small molecule c-Met inhibitors (ATP-competitive kinase inhibitors such as PHA-665752 [56] and SU11274 [57]); (2) c-Met biological inhibitors (ribozymes [58, 59], c-Met antisense [60], dominant-negative receptors [61, 62], decoy receptors [63], and peptide antagonists [64, 65]); (3) HGF and c-Met neutralizing antibodies [66–68]; and (4) truncated HGF antagonists [69–72]. The following sections will focus on some of the c-Met biological inhibitors and the truncated HGF antagonists.

A recent publication demonstrated that a decoy molecule that binds to both HGF and c-Met could interfere with HGF signaling and with constitutively activated c-Met [63]. Angiogenesis, tumor growth, and tumor invasion were all inhibited by the c-Met decoy, which consists of the extracellular domain of c-Met, ending before the transmembrane domain. The decoy, when delivered by lentivirus to mice, was relatively non-toxic to normal tissues making this approach clinically useful. A c-Met antisense/U6 expression plasmid has also been shown to decrease lung tumor xenograft growth in SCID mice by 50% [60]. Apoptosis was increased in tumors treated with the c-Met antisense plasmid versus controls. Additionally, the MAPK signaling pathway and c-Met protein expression were both downregulated in the c-Met antisense treated tumors versus controls. Combined therapy to inhibit both the HGF ligand and its receptor, c-Met, may provide the most beneficial antitumor effect.

Hepatocyte growth factor has also been an attractive target for therapy; however, these inhibitors are not as well developed as the c-Met inhibitors. HGF-neutralizing antibodies demonstrate antitumor activity, however at least three monoclonal antibodies recognizing distinct epitopes are required for tumor inhibition making this approach difficult to optimize clinically [66]. Another group of potential inhibitors of HGF includes the truncated HGF molecules. Naturally occurring, alternately spliced variants of the HGF mRNA are known that produce products containing only the hairpin domain and the first kringle domain (NK1) or the first two kringle domains (NK2). These molecules appear to bind the HGF receptor, but are very inefficient at activating the receptor, as determined by autophosphorylation [73]. An antagonistic molecule called NK4 has been shown to antagonize the mitogenic, motogenic, and morphogenic activities of HGF in various cell types [69–72] and has been shown to be an angiogenesis inhibitor as well as an HGF antagonist and these activities are independent of each other [74]. In vivo NK4 gene transfer using an adenovirus vector by intratumoral or

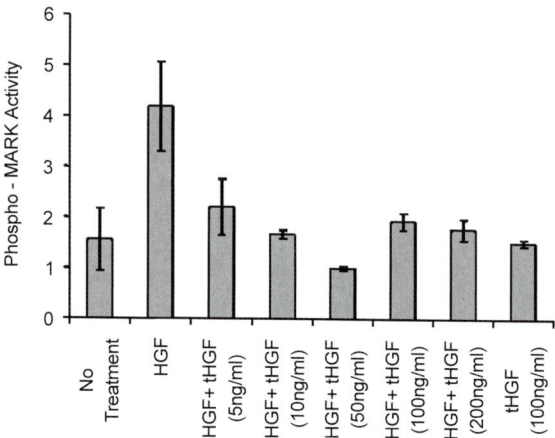

Fig. 35.3. Truncated HGF (*tHGF*) can inhibit HGF-induced MAPK activation. tHGF, 0–200 ng/ml, was added to NSCLC cells in vitro with or without exogenous HGF (10 ng/ml). Protein was isolated and equal amounts of protein from each treatment were analyzed by Western analysis for phospho-MAPK expression. Bars, SE

intraperitoneal administration significantly inhibited lung tumor xenograft growth in nude mice [75]. This variant contains the N-terminal hairpin plus the four kringle domains. A recombinant truncated HGF molecule containing the N-terminal hairpin domain, the first three kringle domains, and the first 16 amino acids of the fourth kringle domain demonstrated the ability to block HGF action in cells of liver origin [76]. It differs from the NK4 variant in that NK4 contains 42 additional amino acids of the fourth kringle domain. The ability of this molecule, which we term truncated HGF (tHGF), to inhibit HGF action in lung tumor cells shows that tHGF is able to inhibit the activation of the MAPK pathway by HGF at concentrations as low as 5 ng/ml, and showed little or no ability to activate MAPK by itself (Fig. 35.3). However, direct injection of tHGF into

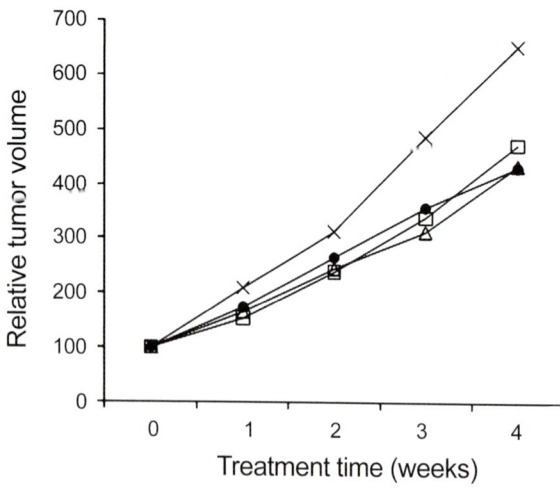

Fig. 35.4. Truncated HGF (*tHGF*) acts as an agonist at high concentrations of tHGF. In vivo lung tumor xenografts grown in SCID mice were directly injected three times per week for 4 weeks with 0–1,500 ng tHGF and measured weekly

lung tumor xenografts yielded only slight antitumor activity at low doses, and tumor growth enhancement at a high dose (Fig. 35.4). This suggests that tHGF may have partial agonist activity at high concentrations in vivo and is thus not useful for lung cancer therapy. The original NK4 molecule described above shows the most promise in this group of HGF antagonists and warrants further pursuit for lung cancer therapy, although such partial agonist properties have been reported for other HGF variants.

A recent review by Christensen et al. [48] discusses in further detail the large number of therapeutic inhibitors for this pathway. To date, there have been no clinical evaluations of an HGF/c-Met targeted therapy although there has been clinical success with other receptor tyrosine kinase inhibitors. The c-Met decoy receptor, antisense approaches, and possibly antagonists, such as NK4, offer hope for clinical evaluation in lung cancer patients, although these agents may be difficult to deliver systemically. The c-Met small molecule inhibitors developed to date demonstrate solubility problems and non-specific toxicity, and clinical development may be problematic. Further development of small molecule c-Met inhibitors is warranted. Collectively, these data show that the HGF/c-Met pathway is an attractive target for therapy because it is ubiquitously utilized by NSCLC, is important for many tumor-related phenotypes, and could be clinically useful for lung cancer treatment.

35.4 Gastrin-releasing Peptide (GRP)/GRP Receptor (GRPR) Pathways in Lung Cancer

35.4.1 Autocrine Growth Loops

Gastrin-releasing peptide is known to be secreted by many small cell lung tumors, and, via its receptor GRPR, to induce growth responses [77]. Such a self-sustaining, or autocrine, growth loop has also been found in head and neck squamous cell tumors [78] and in non-small cell tumors [79]. In fact, although GRP was once thought only to be involved in neuroendocrine tumors, it is now recognized that the GRP/GRPR pathway is expressed by many epithelial cells from different organs, such as prostate, breast, and ovary, both in the normal and malignant state [80]. Normal bronchial epithelial cells derived from airway biopsies of subjects express GRPR, and expression was linked to responsiveness to GRP and other bombesin-like peptides [46]. This implies that GRPR is involved in normal lung homeostasis, and in fact is very important in lung development [81].

35.4.2 GRPR/EGFR Cross-activation

Gastrin-releasing peptide receptor is a G protein-coupled receptor that mediates its actions mainly through the activation of Gαq subunits (Fig. 35.5). Activation of the GRPR has been linked to activation of the Src pathway, with subsequent activation of Akt, a protein important in promoting cell survival. These signal-

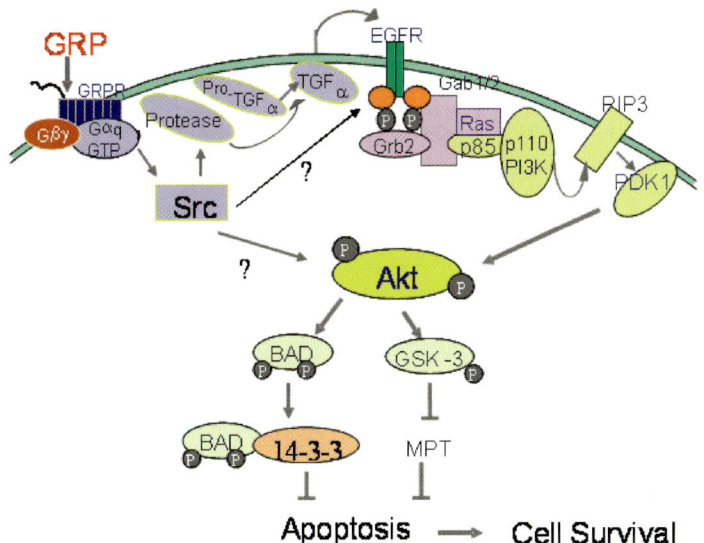

Fig. 35.5. GRPR-EGFR signaling intersections

ing events appear to be mainly dependent on EGFR activation [3, 4], although some direct Src activation may occur. This link with an important growth pathway known to be activated in lung cancer suggests GRPR activation is an important contributor to the maintenance of the malignant state. Recently GRP has also been shown to be angiogenic and GRPR is expressed by endothelial cells [82].

35.4.3   GRPR Inhibitors

There have been various attempts to develop GRPR inhibitors, but none have been developed beyond a phase II trial. A neutralizing antibody to GRP, 2A11, was developed in the 1980s that showed limited ability to treat advanced small cell carcinoma [77, 83]. Other small molecule inhibitors include RC-3094, a bombesin antagonist [84], and AN-215, which contains a doxorubicin analog covalently linked to the RC-3094 peptide antagonist [85]. AN-215 was shown to be an effective inhibitor of human ovarian cancer xenografts [86]. Because many of the peptide antagonists developed against GRPR have shown stability problems when used in vivo, even when they contain pseudopeptide bonds, a non-peptide small molecule could be very advantageous. Recently, a small molecule GRP blocker, 77427, a non-peptide amide compound, was described that substantially reduced angiogenesis and lung tumor xenograft growth, although the effect was reversible [82]. GRPR inhibition will probably be most effective in consort with other types of inhibition, perhaps of the EGFR pathway. Agents that induce apoptosis also may be effective in consort with GRPR inhibition.

35.5 Conclusions

Understanding of the steroid hormone, HGF/c-Met, and GRP/GRPR biological pathways in lung cancer is still incomplete, but these three signaling systems each have potential for exploitation in the clinic. Both steroid hormone receptors (ER and AR) that promote growth and protect against apoptosis as well as the PR pathway that promotes differentiation and apoptosis may be modulated for therapeutic benefit. Since the type of steroid receptor expressed by lung tumors may differ from that of breast or prostate cancer, simple extrapolation from the published literature on reproductive cancers may not be applicable. More in-depth understanding of steroid receptor signaling in lung cancer would be beneficial for designing therapeutic approaches and designing clinical trials using available blockers of steroid hormone action.

Hepatocyte growth factor/c-Met is an important oncogenic signaling pathway that has not yet been exploited clinically, despite the strong evidence that it participates in several important signaling pathways associated with the malignant phenotype. Although invasion, an early step in carcinogenesis that is coupled to c-Met signaling, may be a hard target for therapeutic intervention, c-Met is also important in controlling cell proliferation, cell survival, and angiogenesis. These endpoints are more amenable to clinical assessment. Truncated HGFs can inhibit the c-Met pathway, but they are large synthetically produced proteins and some have partial agonist actions. Delivery of antisense c-Met vectors is problematic, and small molecule c-Met inhibitors developed to date have solubility problems and have shown some non-specific effects in animal studies. Further drug discovery in this area is warranted. GRP/GRPR small molecule inhibitors have not yet matured to the point of therapeutic use, but they have promise.

Acknowledgements

This work was supported by National Cancer Institute grant R01 CA79882 awarded to J.M.S. and by a National Cancer Institute SPORE in Lung Cancer grant P50 CA90440 awarded to J.M.S.. L.P.S. was a Career Development Fellow supported by the SPORE in Lung Cancer grant P50 CA90440.

Key Points

- The signaling systems of the steroid hormone, hepatocyte growth factor (HGF)/c-Met, and gastrin-releasing peptide (GRP)/GRP receptor (GRPR) biological pathways have potential for exploitation in lung cancer.
- The steroid hormone receptors, estrogen and androgen receptor, that promote growth and protect against apoptosis, as well as the progesterone receptor pathway that promotes differentiation and apoptosis may be modulated for therapeutic benefit in lung cancer.
- HGF/c-Met is an important oncogenic signaling pathway that has not yet been exploited clinically, despite the strong evidence that it participates in several important signaling pathways associated with the malignant phenotype.
- GRP/GRPR small molecule inhibitors have not yet matured to the point of therapeutic use, but they have promise.

References

1. Jemel A, Murray T, Samuels A, et al. Cancer statistics, 2003 CA. Cancer J Clin 2003; 53:5.

2. Twombly R. Failing survival advantage in crucial trial, future of Iressa is in jeopardy. J Natl Cancer Inst 2005; 97:249.

3. Thomas P, Pang Y, Filardo EJ, Dong J. Identity of an estrogen membrane receptor coupled to a G protein in human breast cancer cells. Endocrinology 2005; 146:624.

4. Thomas SM, Grandis JR, Wentzel AL, Gooding WE, Lui VW, Siegfried JM. Gastrin-releasing peptide receptor mediates activation of the epidermal growth factor receptor in lung cancer cells. Neoplasia 2005; 7:426.

5. Patel J, Bach PB, Kris MG. A contemporary epidemic. JAMA 2004; 291:1763.

6. Stabile LP, Davis AL, Gubish CT, et al. Human non-small cell lung tumors and cells derived from normal lung express both estrogen receptor alpha and beta and show biological responses to estrogen. Cancer Res 2002; 62:2141.

7. Hershberger PA, Vasquez AC, Kanterewicz B, Land S, Siegfried JM, Nichols M. Regulation of endogenous gene expression in human non-small cell lung cancer cells by estrogen receptor ligands. Cancer Res 2005; 65:1598.

8. Moore KA, Mery CM, Jaklitsch MT, et al. Menopausal effects on presentation, treatment, and survival of women with non-small cell lung cancer. Ann Thorac Surg 2003; 76:1789.

9. Kawai H, Ishii A, Kiyotada W, et al. Estrogen receptor α and β are prognostic factors in non-small cell lung cancer. Clin Cancer Res 2005; 11:5084.

10. Osborne CK, Yochmowitz MG, Knight WA, McGuire WL. The value of estrogen and progesterone receptors in the treatment of breast cancer. Cancer 1980; 46:2884.

11. Thorpe SM, Rose C, Rasmussen BB, Mouridsen HT, Bayer T, Keiding N. Prognostic value of steroid hormone receptors: multivariate analysis of systemically untreated patients with node negative primary breast cancer. Cancer Res 1987; 47:6126.

12. Stabile LP, Lyker JS, Gubish CT, Zhang W, Grandis JR, Siegfried JM. Combined targeting of the estrogen receptor and the epidermal growth factor receptor in non-small cell lung cancer shows enhanced antiproliferative effects. Cancer Res 2005; 654:1459.

13. Hamilton A, Piccart M. The third-generation non-steroidal aromatase inhibitors: a review of their clinical benefits in the second-line hormonal treatment of advanced breast cancer. Ann Oncol 1999; 10:377.

14. Giudici D, Ornati G, Briatico G, Buzzetti F, Lombardi P, di Salle E. 6-Methylenandrosta-1,4-diene-3, 17-dione (FCE 24304): a new irreversible aromatase inhibitor. J Steroid Biochem 1988; 30:391.

15. Fisher B, Costantino JP, Wickerham DL, et al. Tamoxifen for prevention of breast cancer: report of the National Surgical Adjuvant Breast and Bowel Project P-1 Study. J Natl Cancer Inst 1998; 90:1371.

16. Martel C, Meiner MH, Gagne D, Simard J, Labrie F. Widespread tissue distribution of steroid sulfatase, 3 beta-hydroxysteroid dehydrogenase/delta 5-delta 4 isomerase (3 beta-HSD), 17 beta-HSD 5 alpha-reductase and aromatase activities in the rhesus monkey. Mol Cell Endocrinol 1994; 104:103.

17. Price T, Aitken J, Simpson ER. Relative expression of aromatase cytochrome P450 in human fetal tissues as determined by competitive polymerase chain reaction amplification. J Clin Endocrinol Metab 1992; 744:879.

18. Weinberg OK, Marquez-Garban DC, Chen H-W, Fishbein MC, Pietras JR. Aromatase inhibitors in human lung cancer therapy. Proc Am Assoc Cancer Res 2005; 45:4035.

19. Coombes RC, Hall E, Gibson LJ, et al. A randomized trial of exemestane after two to three years of tamoxifen therapy in postmenopausal women with primary breast cancer. N Engl J Med 2004; 350:1081.

20. Revankar CM, Cimino OF, Sklar LA, Arterburn JB, Prossnitz ER. A transmembrane intracellular estrogen receptor mediates rapid cell signaling. Science 2005; 307:1625.

21. Pietras RJ, Marquez DC, Chen HW, Tsai E, Weinberg O, Fishbein M. Estrogen and growth factor receptor interactions in human breast and non-small cell lung cancer cells. Steroids 2005; 70:372.

22. Rajkumar T, Gullick WJ. The type I growth factor receptors in human breast cancer. Breast Cancer Res Treat 1994; 29:3.

23. Yarden Y, Sliwkowski MX. Untangling the ErbB signalling network. Nat Rev Mol Cell Biol 2001; 2:127.

24. Selvaggi G, Novello S, Torri V, et al. Epidermal growth factor receptor overexpression correlates with a poor prognosis in completely resected non-small-cell lung cancer. Ann Oncol 2004; 15:28.

25. Traynor AM, Schiller JH, Stabile LP, et al. Combination therapy with gefitinib and fulvestrant (G/F) for women with non-small cell lung cancer (NSCLC). ASCO Meeting 2005; 7224.

26. Okubo S, Kurebayashi J, Otsuki T, Yamamoto Y, Tanaka K, Sonoo H. Additive antitumour effect of the epidermal growth factor receptor tyrosine kinase inhibitor gefitinib (Iressa, ZD1839) and the antioestrogen fulvestrant (Faslodex, ICI182,780) in breast cancer cells. Br J Cancer 2004; 90:236.

27. Su JM, Hsu HK, Chang H, Un SL, Chang HC, Huang MS, Tseng HH. Expression of estrogen and progesterone receptors in non-small-cell lung cancer: immunohistochemical study. Anticancer Res 1996; 16:3803.

28. Kaiser U, Hofmann J, Schilli M, et al. Steroid-hormone receptors in cell lines and tumor biopsies of human lung cancer. Int J Cancer 1996; 67:357.

29. Di Nunno L, Larsson LG, Rinehart JJ, Beissner RS. Estrogen and progesterone receptors in non-small cell lung cancer in 248 consecutive patients who underwent surgical resection. Arch Pathol Lab Med 2000; 124:1467.

30. Ishibashi H, Suzuki T, Suzuki S, et al. Progesterone receptor in non-small cell lung cancer: a potent prognostic factor and possible target for endocrine therapy. Cancer Res 2005; 65:6450.

31. Santen RJ, Manni A, Harvey H, Redmond C. Endocrine treatment of breast cancer in women. Endocr Rev 1990; 11:221.

32. Kelley RM, Baker WH. Progestational agents in the treatment of carcinoma of the endometrium. N Engl J Med 1961; 264:216.

33. Kobayashi S, Mizuno T, Tobioka N, et al. Sex steroid receptors in diverse human tumors. Jpn J Cancer Res Gann 1982; 73:439.

34. Maasberg M, Rotsch M, Jaques G, Enderle-Schmidt U, Weehle R, Havemann K. Androgen receptors, androgen-dependent proliferation, and 5 alpha-reductase activity of small-cell lung cancer cell lines. Int J Cancer 1989; 434:685.

35. Taplin ME, Balk SP. Androgen receptor: a key molecule in the progression of prostate cancer to hormone independence. J Cell Biochem 2004; 91:483.

36. Sonnenberg E, Meyer O, Weidner KM, Birchmeier C. Scatter factor/hepatocyte growth factor and its receptor, the c-met tyrosine kinase, can mediate a signal exchange between mesenchyme and epithelia during mouse development. J Cell Biol 1993; 123:223.

37. Schmidt C, Bladt F, Goedecke S, et al. Scatter factor/hepatocyte growth factor is essential for liver development. Nature 1995; 373:699.

38. Bottaro DP, Rubin JS, Faletto DL, Chan AM, Kmiecik TE, Vande Woude GF, Aaronson SA. Identification of the hepatocyte growth factor receptor as the c-met proto-oncogene product. Science 1991; 251:802.

39. Park M, Dean M, Cooper CS, Schmidt M, O'Brien SJ, Blair DG, Vande Woude GF. Mechanism of met oncogene activation. Cell 1986; 45:895.

40. Schmidt L, Duh FM, Chen F, et al. Germline and somatic mutations in the tyrosine kinase domain of the MET proto-oncogene in papillary renal carcinomas. Nat Genet 1997; 161:68.

41. Ma PC, Kijima T, Maulik G, et al. c-MET mutational analysis in small cell lung cancer: novel juxtamembrane domain mutations regulating cytoskeletal functions. Cancer Res 2003; 63:6272.

42. Ma PC, Jagdeesh S, Jagadeeswaran R, Fox EA, Christensen JG, Maulik G. c-MET expression/activation, functions, and mutations in non-small cell lung cancer. Proc Am Assoc Cancer Res 2004; 44:1875.

43. Di Renzo MF, Olivero M, Giacomini A, et al. Overexpression and amplification of the met/HGF receptor gene during the progression of colorectal cancer. Clin Cancer Res 1995; 1:147.

44. Tuck AB, Park M, Sterns EE, Boag A, Elliott BE. Coexpression of hepatocyte growth factor and receptor (Met) in human breast carcinoma. Am J Pathol 1996; 148:225.

45. Furukawa T, Duguid WP, Kobari M, Matsuno S, Tsao MS. Hepatocyte growth factor and Met receptor expression in human pancreatic carcinogenesis. Am J Pathol 1995; 1474:889.

46. Siegfried JM, Weissfeld LA, Singh-Kaw P, Weyant RJ, Testa JR, Landreneau RJ. Association of immunoreactive hepatocyte growth factor with poor survival in resectable non-small cell lung cancer. Cancer Res 1997; 57:433.

47. Ichimura E, Maeshima A, Nakajima T, Nakamura T. Expression of c-met/HGF receptor in human non-small cell lung carcinomas in vitro and in vivo and its prognostic significance. Jpn J Cancer Res 1996; 87:1063.

48. Christensen JG, Burrows J, Salgia R. c-Met as a target for human cancer and characterization of inhibitors for therapeutic intervention. Cancer Lett 2005; 225:1.

49. Furge KA, Zhang YW, Vande Woude GF. Met receptor tyrosine kinase: enhanced signaling through adapter proteins. Oncogene 2000; 1949:5582.

50. Nakanishi K, Fujimoto J, Ueki T, et al. Hepatocyte growth factor promotes migration of human hepatocellular carcinoma via phosphatidylinositol 3-kinase. Clin Exp Metastasis 1999; 17:507.

51. Royall, Lamarche-Vane N, Lamorte L, Kaibuchi K, Park M. Activation of cdc42, rae, PAK, and rho-kinase in response to hepatocyte growth factor differentially regulates epithelial cell colony spreading and dissociation. Mol Biol Cell 2000; 11:1709.

52. Kodama A, Takaishi K, Nakano K, Nishioka H, Takai Y. Involvement of Cdc42 small G protein in cell-cell adhesion, migration and morphology of MDCK cells. Oncogene 1999; 18:3996.

53. Ishizawa K, Kubo H, Yamada M, et al. Hepatocyte growth factor induces angiogenesis in injured lungs through mobilizing endothelial progenitor cells. Biochem Biophys Res Commun 2004; 324:276.

54. Wislez M, Rabbe N, Marchal J, et al. Hepatocyte growth factor production by neutrophils infiltrating bronchioloalveolar subtype pulmonary adenocarcinoma: role in tumor progression and death. Cancer Res 2003; 636:1405.

55. Dong G, Lee TL, Yeh NT, Geoghegan J, Van Waes C, Chen Z. Metastatic squamous cell carcinoma cells that overexpress c-Met exhibit enhanced angiogenesis factor expression, scattering and metastasis in response to hepatocyte growth factor. Oncogene 2004; 23:6199.

56. Christensen JG, Schreck R, Burrows J, et al. A selective small molecule inhibitor of c-Met kinase inhibits c-Met-dependent phenotypes in vitro and exhibits cytoreductive antitumor activity in vivo. Cancer Res 2003; 63:7345.

57. Ma PC, Schaefer E, Christensen JG, Salgia R. Selective small molecule c-MET inhibitor, PHA665752, cooperates with rapamycin. Clin Cancer Res 2005; 11:3212.

58. Abounader R, Ranganathan S, Lal B, Fielding K, Book A, Dietz H, Burger P, Laterra J. Reversion of human glioblastoma malignancy by U1 small nuclear RNA/ribozyme targeting of scatter factor/hepatocyte growth factor and c-met expression. J Natl Cancer Inst 1999; 91:1548.

59. Abounader R, Bachchu L, Luddy C, Koe G, Davidson B, Rosen EM, Laterra J. In vivo targeting of SF/HGF and c-met expression via U1snRNA/ribozymes inhibits glioma growth and angiogenesis and promotes apoptosis. FASEB J 2002; 16:108.

60. Kaplan O, Firon M, Vivi A, Navon G, Tsarfaty I. HGF/SF activates glycolysis and oxidative phosphorylation in DA3 murine mammary cancer cells. Neoplasia 2000; 24:365.

61. Stabile LP, Lyker JS, Huang L, Siegfried JM. Inhibition of human non-small cell lung tumors by a c-Met antisense/U6 expression plasmid strategy. Gene Ther 2004; 11:325.

62. Webb CP, Taylor GA, Jeffers M, Fiscella M, Oskarsson M, Resau JH, Vande Woude GF. Evidence for a role of Met-HGF/SF during Ras-mediated tumorigenesis/metastasis. Oncogene 1998; 17:2019.

63. Michieli P, Mazzone M, Basilico C, Cavassa S, Sottile A, Naldini L, Comoglio PM. Targeting the tumor and its microenvironment by a dual-function decoy Met receptor. Cancer Cell 2004; 6:61.

64. Bardelli A, Longati P, Gramaglia D, et al. Uncoupling signal transducers from oncogenic MET mutants abrogates cell transformation and inhibits invasive growth. Proc Natl Acad Sci U S A 1998; 95:14379.

65. Atabey N, Gao Y, Yao ZJ, et al. Potent blockade of hepatocyte growth factor-stimulated cell motility, matrix invasion and branching morphogenesis by antagonists of Grb2 Src homology 2 domain interactions. J Biol Chem 2001; 276:14308.

66. Cao B, Su Y, Oskarsson M, et al. Neutralizing monoclonal antibodies to hepatocyte growth factor/scatter factor (HGF/SF) display antitumor activity in animal models. Proc Natl Acad Sci U S A 2001; 98:7443.

67. Zheng ZAC, Moffat B, Schwall R. A chimeric Fab antibody serves as an antagonist to the HGF/SF receptor c-Met. Proc Am Assoc Cancer Res 2003; 43:5717.

68. Morton PA, Joy WD, Bobo CP, Arbuckle A, Evans ML, Huynh MS. In vitro and in vivo activity of fully human monoclonal antibody antagonists to c Met protein tyrosine kinase. Proc Am Assoc Cancer Res 2003; 43:5604.

69. Date K, Matsumoto K, Shimura H, Tanaka M, Nakamura I. HGF/NK4 is a specific antagonist for pleiotrophic actions of hepatocyte growth factor. FEBS Lett 1997; 4201:1.

70. Jiang WG, Hiscox SE, Parr C, Martin TA, Matsumoto K, Nakamura T, Mansel RE. Antagonistic effect of NK4, a novel hepatocyte growth factor variant, on in vitro angiogenesis of human vascular endothelial cells. Clin Cancer Res 1999; 5:3695.

71. Parr C, Hiscox S, Nakamura T, Matsumoto K, Jiang WG. NK4, a new HGF/SF variant, is an antagonist to the influence of HGF/SF on the motility and invasion of colon cancer cells. Int J Cancer 2000; 854:563.

72. Hiscox S, Parr C, Nakamura T, Matsumoto K, Mansel RE, Jiang WG. Inhibition of HGF/SF-induced breast cancer cell motility and invasion by the HGF/SF variant, NK4. Breast Cancer Res Treat 2000; 59:245.

73. Chan AM, Rubin JS, Bottaro DP, Hirschfield DW, Chedid M, Aaronson SA. Identification of a competitive HGF antagonist encoded by an alternative transcript. Science 1991; 254:1382.

74. Kuba K, Matsumoto K, Date K, Shimura H, Tanaka M, Nakamura T. HGF/NK4, a four-kringle antagonist of hepatocyte growth factor, is an angiogenesis inhibitor that suppresses tumor growth and metastasis in mice. Cancer Res 2000; 60:6737.

75. Maemondo M, Narumi K, Saijo Y, et al. Targeting angiogenesis and HGF function using an adenoviral vector expressing the HGF antagonist NK4 for cancer therapy. Mol Ther 2002; 52:177.

76. Yee CJ, DeFrances MC, Bell A, Bowen W, Petersen B, Michalopoulos GK, Zarnegar R. Expression and characterization of biologically active human hepatocyte growth factor (HGF) by insect cells infected with HGF-recombinant baculovirus. Biochemistry 1993; 32:7922.

77. Cuttitta F, Carney DN, Mulshine J, Moody TW, Fedorko J, Fischler A, Minna JD. Bombesin-like peptides can function as autocrine growth factors in human small-cell lung cancer. Nature 1985; 316:823.

78. Lango MN, Dyer KF, Lui VWY, Gooding WE, Gubish C, Siegfried JM, Grandis JR. Gastrin-releasing peptide receptor-mediated autocrine growth in squamous cell carcinoma of the head and neck. J Natl Cancer Inst 2002; 94:375.

79. Siegfried JM, Krishnamachary Gaither-Davis A, Gubish C, Hunt JD, Shriver SP. Evidence to autocrine actions of neuromedin B and gastrin-releasing peptide in non-small cell lung cancer. Pulm Pharmacol Ther 1999; 12:291.

80. Schally AV, Comaru-Schally AM, Nagy A, et al. Hypothalamic hormones and cancer. Front Neuroendocrinol 201; 22:248.

81. Emanuel RL, Torday JS, Mu Q, Asoknanthan N, Sikorski KA, Sunday ME. Bombesin-like peptides and receptors in normal fetal baboon lung: roles in lung growth and maturation Am J Physiol 1999; 277:L1003.

82. Martinez A, Zudaire E, Julian M, Moody TW, Cuttitta F. Gastrin-releasing peptide (GRP) induces angiogenesis and the specific GRP blocker 77427 inhibits tumor growth in vitro and in vivo. Oncogene 2005; 24:4106.

83. Chadhry A, Carrasquillo JA, Avis IL, et al. Phase I and imaging trial of a monoclonal antibody directed against gastrin-releasing peptide in patients with lung cancer. Clin Cancer Res 1999; 5:3385.

84. Radulovic S, Cai RZ, Serfozo P, et al. Biological effects and receptor binding affinities of new pseudononapeptide bombesin/GRP receptor antagonists with N-terminal D-Trp or DTpi. Int J Pept Protein Res 1991; 38:593.

85. Nagy A, Armatis P, Cai RZ, Szepeshazi K, Halmos G, Schally AV. Design, synthesis, and in vitro evaluation of cytotoxic analogs of bombesin-like peptides containing doxorubicin or its intensely potent derivative, 2-pyrrolinodoxorubicin. Proc Natl Acad Sci U S A 1997; 94:652.

86. Engel JB, Keller G, Schally AV, Halmos G, Hammann B, Nagy A. Effective inhibition of the experimental human ovarian cancers with a targeted cytotoxic bombesin analogue AN-215. Clin Cancer Res 2005; 11:2408.

Gene Therapy for Lung Cancer

36

Jack A. Roth

Contents

36.1   Introduction

Lung cancer represents a paradigm for carcinogen-induced cancers. Tobacco smoke has over 100 carcinogenic agents and the specific interactions of specific carcinogens with genes that suppress tumors and repair DNA have been identified [1]. Lung cancers show multiple genetic lesions and these can be detected even in histologically normal bronchial mucosa from individuals with a smoking history. These genetic abnormalities provide an array of targets for therapy. The p53 tumor suppressor gene appears to play a central role in lung cancer development and was the initial focus of gene therapy approaches to lung cancer.

36.2   Mechanism of p53 Tumor Suppression and Rationale for p53 Gene Therapy

Expression of some gene products, including growth factors, oncogenes, cyclins, and cyclin-dependent kinases (CDKs), drive a cell toward proliferation. Expression of tumor suppressor genes and other inhibitors of CDKs induce cell cycle arrest thus limiting the proliferation of the cell. Two interconnected pathways, the Rb (retinoblastoma gene) pathway and the p53 pathway, which are both, in turn, regulated at the protein level by oncogenes and other tumor suppressor genes, contribute to the regulation of cell proliferation. The Rb protein regulates maintenance of, and release from, the G1 phase. The p53 protein monitors cellular stress and DNA damage, either causing growth arrest to facilitate DNA repair, or inducing apoptosis if DNA damage is extensive [2]. When a cell is stressed by oncogene activation, hypoxia, or DNA damage, an intact p53 pathway may determine whether the cell will receive a signal to halt at the G1 stage of the cell cycle, whether DNA repair will be attempted, or whether the cell will self-destruct via apoptosis. The p53 gene is central in the processes of apoptosis, repair to various cell stresses, and regulation of the cell cycle and is thus referred to as the "guardian of the genome." Apoptosis plays a key role in numerous normal cellular mechanisms, from embryogenesis to self-policing of DNA damage due to random mutations, ionizing radiation, and DNA-damaging chemicals, and has more recently been implicated as a major mechanism of cell death due to DNA-damaging cancer therapies such as chemotherapy and radiation. The observation that expression of a wild-type *p53* gene in a cancer cell triggers apoptosis, sets the stage for gene therapy approaches [3]. Prior to this is was felt that gene therapy could not replace all the damaged genes in a cancer cell and thus would not have an effect. The requirement for restoring only one of the defective genes to trigger apoptosis suggests that the DNA damage present in the cancer cell may prime it for an apoptotic event which can be provided through a single pathway.

The p53 gene product acts as a transcription factor [4]. A major group of genes whose expression is in part regulated by p53 are the apoptosis genes. A precisely maintained balance between two proapoptotic versus prosurvival (antiapoptotic) signals, often compared to a rheostat, determines whether or not apoptosis will be induced. While these signals determine p53's actions, expression of many of the genes that generate these critical signals is, in turn, regulated by the activation status of *p53*, forming a complex feedback loop. p53 carries out its housekeeping duties by downregulating the "pro-survival" (or antiapoptotic) genes, including the antiapoptotic genes *bcl-2* and *bcl-XL*, and upregulating the proapoptotic genes *bax*, *bad*, *bid*, *puma*, and *noxa* [5]. Available transcripts of each of the pro- and antiapoptotic genes with *bcl2* homology-3 domains interact with one another to form heterodimers, and the relative ratio of proapoptotic to prosurvival proteins in these heterodimers determines activity of the resulting molecule, thereby determining whether the cell lives or is directed to undergo apoptosis. p53 also targets the death-receptor signaling pathway including DR5, and Fas/CD/95, the apoptosis machinery including caspase-6, Apaf-1, and PIDD, and may directly mediate cytochrome *c* release. Thus apoptosis is an important mechanism by which p53 mediates its tumor suppressor function.

The p53 pathway is regulated at the protein level by other tumor suppressor genes and by several oncogenes [2]. For example, mdm2 normally binds to the N-terminal transactivating domain of p53, prohibiting p53 activation and leading to its rapid degradation. Under normal conditions the half-life of p53 is only 20 min. In the event of genotoxic stress, resulting DNA damage causes phosphorylation of serines on p53, weakening binding to mdm2 and destabilizing the p53/mdm2 interaction and prolonging p53 half-life. The resulting increase in p53 DNA binding activity leads to an array of downstream signals that switch other genes on or off. In the normal cell, mdm2 is inhibited by expression of *p14ARF*, a tumor suppressor gene encoded by the same gene locus as *p16INK4a* but read in an alternate reading frame [6]. Deletion or mutation of the tumor suppressor gene *p14ARF*, which has been noted in some cancers, results in increased levels of mdm2 and subsequent inactivation of p53, resulting in inappropriate progression through the cell cycle. The expression of *p14ARF* is induced by hyperproliferative signals from oncogenes such as *ras* and *myc*, thus indicating an important role for p53 in protecting the cell from oncogene activation. Importantly, p53 also plays a central role in mediating cell cycle arrest. This function is significant as prolonged tumor stability has often been observed in clinical trials of p53 gene replacement suggesting that this effect is predominant in some tumors over apoptosis. p53 is involved in regulating cell cycle checkpoints and p53 expression can promote cell senescence through its control of cell cycle effectors such as p21CIP1/WAF1.

Loss of function in the p53 pathway is the most common alteration identified in human cancer to date. About 50% of common epithelial cancers have p53 mutations [7–9]. In some cancers, loss of p53 also appears to be linked to resistance to conventional DNA-damaging therapies that require functional cellular apoptosis to accomplish cell death.

36.2.1 Preclinical Studies of p53 Gene Replacement

The studies described above suggest that expressing a wild-type p53 gene in cancer cells defective in p53 function could mediate either apoptosis or cell growth arrest. Both results could be a therapeutic benefit in a cancer patient. Our initial studies showed that restoration of functional p53 suppressed the growth of some, but not all, human lung cancer cell lines [10]. Because of limitations inherent in the use of retroviruses, subsequent studies of p53 gene replacement in lung cancer made use of an adenoviral vector (*Ad-p53*) [11]. The first published study of *p53* gene therapy showed suppression of tumor growth in an orthotopic human lung cancer model using a retroviral expression vector [12]. *Ad-p53* also induced apoptosis in cancer cells with nonfunctional *p53*, without significantly affecting proliferation of normal cells [13]. Subsequent studies with *Ad-p53* demonstrated inhibition of tumor growth in a mouse model of human orthotopic lung cancer [14] and induced apoptosis and suppression of proliferation in various other cancer cell lines as well as in in vivo mouse xenograft tumor models [15–18].

Although it was first thought that the inability to transduce every cell in a tumor might limit the effectiveness of gene therapy for cancer, studies [3, 19] of three-dimensional cancer cell matrices and subcutaneous xenografts proved that therapeutic genes could potentially spread beyond the injection site to nontransduced tumor cells via a "bystander effect." Bystander killing, now known to be an important phenomenon in the success of gene therapy, appears to involve regulation of angiogenesis [20], immune upregulation [21–24], and secretion of soluble proapoptotic proteins [25].

36.2.2 Clinical Trials of p53 Gene Replacement

The first clinical trial protocol for *p53* gene replacement was carried out with a retroviral vector expressing wild-type p53 under control of the beta-actin promoter [26]. The gene/vector construct was introduced into tumors of nine patients with unresectable non-small-cell lung cancer (NSCLC) already proven resistant to other interventions. Three of the nine patients demonstrated evidence of antitumor activity with no vector-related toxicity, demonstrating the feasibility and safety of gene therapy [27, 28].

A phase I trial enrolled 28 NSCLC patients whose cancers had not responded to conventional treatments and successful gene transfer was demonstrated in 80% of evaluable patients [29]. Gene expression was detected in 46%, apoptosis was demonstrated in all but one of the patients expressing the gene, and importantly, no significant toxicity was observed. More than a 50% re-

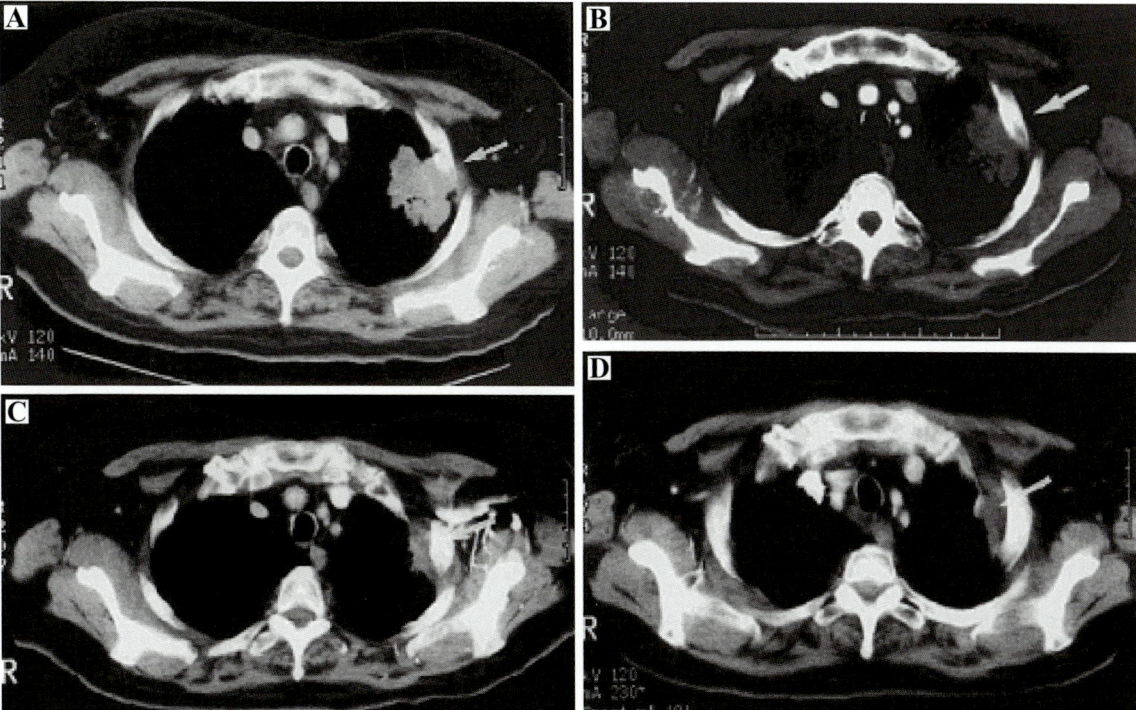

Fig. 36.1. Computed tomography (CT) scans of a patient following six courses of 109 plaque-forming units of *Ad-p53*, an adenovirus vector carrying the wild-type p53 complementary DNA. **A** Before treatment. *Arrow* shows recurrent left upper lobe adenocarcinoma, which progressed after 66 Gy of external beam radiation therapy and six courses of paclitaxel and carboplatin (CT scan volume: $3 \times 4 \times 5$ cm; 60 cm^3). **B** At 1 month after treatment. *Arrow* shows tumor regression after one course of *Ad-p53* treatment (CT scan volume: $2 \times 3 \times 5$ cm; 30 cm^3).

C At 8 months after treatment, image shows tumor regression following six courses of *Ad-p53* gene therapy (CT scan volume: $2 \times 2 \times 3$ cm; 12 cm^3). **D** Stable tumor 18 months after beginning treatment with *Ad-p53* (CT scan volume: $2 \times 2 \times 3$ cm; 12 cm^3). No viable tumor was demonstrated during the last 4 months of therapy (14 sequential percutaneous biopsies), and the patient was observed off all treatment for 12 months without evidence of tumor progression. The patient develop metastases and died 27 months after entering the study

duction in tumor size was observed in two patients, with one patient remaining free of tumor more than a year after concluding therapy and another experiencing nearly complete regression of a chemotherapy- and radiotherapy-resistant upper lobe endobronchial tumor (Fig. 36.1). Additional studies in patients with head and neck cancer helped to established *Ad-P53* gene transfer as a clinically feasible strategy resulting in successful gene transfer and gene expression, low toxicity, and strong evidence for tumor regression.

36.3 Gene Replacement in Combination with Conventional DNA-damaging Agents in Non-Small Cell Lung Cancer

Many tumors are resistant to chemotherapy and radiation therapy and, therefore, fail initial therapeutic interventions. *p53*, often missing or non-functional in radiation- and chemotherapy-resistant tumors, is known to play a key role in detecting damage to DNA and either directing repair or inducing apoptosis. Once apoptosis was

implicated as a mechanism of cell killing in response to these DNA-damaging agents, it followed that a defect in the normal apoptotic pathway might confer resistance to some tumor cells. Due to *Ad-p53*'s low toxicity (less than a 5% incidence of serious adverse events) in initial trials, therapeutic strategies combining *Ad-p53* gene replacement and conventional DNA-damaging therapies were logical extensions of earlier studies [30].

36.3.1 Preclinical Studies

The fact that overexpression of *p53* in wild-type *p53*-transfected cell lines could drive cells into apoptosis was demonstrated in several in vitro studies [31–33] and subsequent studies that examined apoptosis in tumor cells treated with radiation or chemotherapeutic agents supported a link between apoptosis induction and functional p53 expression [34–39]. Preclinical studies of *p53* gene therapy combined with cisplatin in cultured NSCLC cells and in human xenografts in nude mice demonstrated that sequential administration of cisplatin and *p53* gene therapy resulted in enhanced expression of the *p53* gene product [35,40], and similar studies of *Ad-p53* gene transfer combined with radiotherapy indicated that delivery of *Ad-p53* increase the sensitivity of *p53*-deficient tumor cells to radiation [17].

Numerous additional studies have generated additional supporting evidence for a critical link between radiation sensitivity and the ability of a cell to induce apoptosis [41–45], however, the radiosensitivity of some tumor types, for example epithelioid tumors, does not appear to be correlated with *p53* status [46–48].

36.3.2 Clinical Trials of Tumor Suppressor Gene Replacement Combined with Chemotherapy

Twenty-four NSCLC patients with tumors previously unresponsive to conventional treatment were enrolled in a phase I trial of *p53* in sequence with cisplatin [49]. Seventy-five percent of the patients had previously experienced tumor progression on cisplatin- or carboplatin-containing regimens. Up to six monthly courses of intravenous cisplatin, each followed 3 days later with intratumoral injection of *Ad-p53*, resulted in 17 patients remaining stable for at least 2 months, 2 patients achieving partial responses, 4 patients continuing to exhibit progressive disease, and 1 patient non-evaluable due to progressive disease. Seventy-nine percent of tumor biopsies showed an increase in number of apoptotic cells, 7% demonstrated a decrease in apoptosis, and 14% indicated no change.

A phase II clinical trial evaluated two comparable metastatic lesions in each NSCLC patient enrolled in the study [50]. All patients received chemotherapy, either 3 cycles of carboplatin plus paclitaxel or 3 cycles of cisplatin plus vinorelbine, and then *Ad-p53* was injected directly into one lesion. *Ad-p53* treatment resulted in minimal vector-related toxicity and no overall increase in chemotherapy-related adverse events. Detailed statistical analysis of the data indicated that patients receiving carboplatin plus paclitaxel, the combination of drugs providing the greatest benefit on its own, did not realize additional benefit from *Ad-p53* gene transfer, however, patients treated with the less-successful cisplatin and vinorelbine regimen experienced significantly greater mean local tumor regression, as measured by size, in the *Ad-p53*-injected lesion as compared to the control lesion.

36.3.3 Clinical Trials of p53 Gene Replacement Combined with Radiation Therapy

Preclinical studies suggesting that p53 gene replacement might confer radiation sensitivity to some tumors [17, 42–45] led to a phase II clinical trial of p53 gene trans-

fer in conjunction with radiation therapy [51]. Preliminary data from 19 patients with localized NSCLC revealed a complete response in 1 patient (5%), partial response in 11 patients (58%), stable disease in 3 patients (16%), and progressive disease in 2 patients (11%), while 2 patients (11%) were non-evaluable due to tumor progression or early death (Fig. 36.2). Three months following completion of therapy, biopsies revealed no viable tumor in 12 patients (63%) and viable tumor in 3 (16%). Tumors of 4 patients (21%) were not biopsied because of tumor progression, early death, or weakness. The 1-year progression-free survival rate was 45.5%. Among 13 evaluable patients after 1 year, 5 (39%) had a complete response and 3 (23%) had a partial response or disease stabilization. Most treatment failures were caused by metastatic disease but not by local progression.

In this study pre- and posttreatment biopsies of the tumor were performed so detailed studies of gene expression were possible. *Ad-p53* vector-specific DNA was detected in biopsies from 9 of 12 patients with paired biopsies (day 18 and day 19). The ratio of copies of *Ad-p53* vector DNA to copies of actin DNA was 0.15 or higher in 8 of 9 patients (range, 0.05–3.85) with 4 patients having a ratio >0.5. For 11 patients with ade-

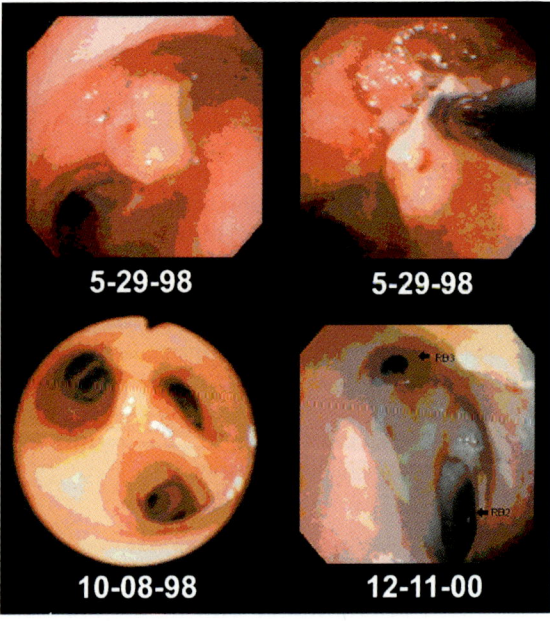

5-29-98   **5-29-98**

10-08-98   **12-11-00**

Fig. 36.2. Right upper lobe tumor in a patient unable to be treated with surgery because of poor pulmonary function and ineligible for chemotherapy because of cardiac disease and obstructed bronchus (29 May 1998). Patient was treated with three injections of *Ad-p53* (3×10^{11} virus particles) and radiation therapy (60 Gy) by bronchoscopy (29 May 1998) with a complete response 3 months after completion of therapy (10 August 1998) and no pathologic evidence of tumor 29 months after therapy (12 November 2000). The patient died from a non-cancer-related cause 2 years later

quate samples for both vector DNA and mRNA analysis, 8 showed a postinjection increase in mRNA expression associated with detectable vector DNA. Postinjection increases in *p53* mRNA were detected in 11 of 12 paired biopsies obtained 24 h after *Ad-p53* injection, with 10 of 11 increasing 3 times or greater. Preinjection biopsies that were negative for *p53* protein expression by immunohistochemistry were stained for *p53* protein expression after *Ad-p53* injection. Staining results confirmed that the *p53* protein was expressed in the posttreatment samples in the nuclei of cancer cells. Previous in vitro experiments in human NSCLC cell lines identified four genes [*p21* (*CDKN1A*), *MDM2*, *FAS*, and *BAK*] that showed the greatest increase in mRNA expression after induction of *p53* overexpression with *Ad-p53*. Therefore, in the current study, changes in mRNA levels for these four markers were determined at various time points before and during treatment using reverse transcriptase real-time PCR. The study was controlled by obtaining a pretreatment biopsy under the same conditions as the posttreatment biopsy. The inclusion of a time point during the radiation treatment allowed for a biopsy to be performed immediately before and 24 h after *Ad-p53* injection, thus allowing determination of the effects of the *Ad-p53* on mRNA expression during treatment. For *p21* (*CDKN1A*) mRNA, increases of statistical significance were noted 24 h after *Ad-P53* injection and during treatment, as compared with the pretreatment biopsy. In the case of *MDM2* mRNA, increases were noted during treatment compared with the pretreatment biopsy. Levels of *FAS* mRNA did not show statistically significant changes during treatment. *BAK* mRNA expression increased significantly 24 h after injection of *Ad-p53* and thus appeared to be the marker most acutely upregulated by *Ad-p53* injection.

Recently the first randomized clinical trial of *p53* gene therapy was reported. Ninety patients with squamous cell carcinoma of the head and neck were randomly allocated to receive intratumoral injection of *Ad-p53* (10^{12} virus particles per dose per week for a total of 8 weeks) in combination with radiation therapy (70 Gy/8 weeks) or radiation therapy alone. Complete remission was seen in 64.7% of patients receiving *Ad-p53* combined with radiation therapy compared to 20% of patients receiving radiation therapy alone, which was highly significant statistically [52].

36.4 Systemic Gene Therapy for Metastases

Local control of cancers is important, but most patients with lung cancer die from systemic metastases. Thus gene delivery to distant sites of cancer is an essential element for successful cancer gene therapy. Recently, the development of nanoscale synthetic particles that can encapsulate plasmid DNA and deliver it to cells after in-

travenous injections has been reported. This has been studied in mouse xenograft models of disseminated human lung cancer. In addition to p53, other tumor suppressor genes have been delivered using this technique. Multiple 3p21.3 genes show different degrees of tumor suppression activities in various human cancers in vitro and in preclinical animal models. One of the tumor suppressor genes at this locus is FUS1 which is not expressed in most lung cancers. When wild-type FUS1 is expressed in a lung cancer cell, apoptosis occurs. To translate these findings to clinical applications for molecular cancer therapy, we recently developed a systemic treatment strategy by using a novel FUS1-expressing plasmid vector complexed with DOTAP:cholesterol (DOTAP:Chol) liposome, termed FUS1 nanoparticle, for treating lung cancer and lung metastases [53, 54]. In a preclinical trial, we have shown that intratumoral administration of FUS1 nanoparticles to subcutaneous NSCLC H1299 and A549 tumor xenograft resulted in significant inhibition of tumor growth, and intravenous injections of FUS1 nanoparticles into mice bearing experimental A549 lung metastasis demonstrated significant decrease in the number of metastatic tumor nodules. Lung tumor bearing animals when treated with DOTAP:Chol-FUS1 complex demonstrate prolonged survival (median survival time: 80 days) compared to control animals. These results demonstrate the potent tumor suppressive activity of the FUS1 gene and is a promising therapeutic agent for the treatment of primary and disseminated human lung cancer [53, 54]. Based on these studies, a phase I clinical trial with FUS1-mediated molecular therapy by systemic administration of FUS1-nanoparticles is now underway in stage IV lung cancer patients at the University of Texas M. D. Anderson Cancer Center in Houston, Texas.

36.5 Summary and Conclusions

Current therapy such as radiation and chemotherapy controls less than 50% of lung cancers and overall 5-year survival is 15%. Combining existing treatments has reached a plateau of efficacy and the addition of conventional cytotoxic agents is limited because of toxicity. The clinical trials summarized in this article clearly demonstrate that, contrary to initial predictions that gene therapy would not be suitable for cancer, gene replacement therapy targeted to a tumor suppressor gene can cause cancer regression by activation of known pathways with minimal toxicity.

Gene expression has been documented and occurs even in the presence of an anti-adenovirus immune response, clinical trials have demonstrated that direct intratumor injection can cause tumor regression or prolonged stabilization of local disease, and the low toxicity associated with gene transfer indicates that tumor suppressor gene replacement can be readily combined with existing and future treatments. Initial concerns that the wide diversity of genetic lesions in cancer cells would prevent the application of gene therapy to cancer appear unfounded; on the contrary, correction of a single genetic lesion has resulted in significant tumor regression.

Studies combining transfer of tumor suppressor genes in combination with conventional DNA-damaging treatments indicate that correction of a defect in apoptosis induction can restore sensitivity to radiation and chemotherapy in some resistant tumors, and indications that sensitivity to killing might be enhanced in already sensitive tumors may eventually lead to reduced toxicity from chemotherapy and radiation therapy. The most recent data from the laboratory demonstrating damage to tumor suppressor genes in normal tissue and premalignant lesions even suggest that these genes may someday be useful in early intervention, diagnosis, and even prevention of cancer. Preclinical studies have shown that systemic delivery for treatment of metastases can be achieved. The ready availability of gene libraries, the ability to administer the genes without the extensive reformulation required of small molecules, and their specificity makes this an attractive therapeutic approach. In spite of the obvious promise evident in the results of these studies, it is critical to recognize that there are still gaps in knowledge and technology to address. The major issues for the future development of gene therapy include:

1. Development of more efficient and less toxic gene delivery vectors for systemic gene delivery
2. Identification of the optimal genes for various tumor types
3. Optimizing combination therapy
4. Monitoring gene uptake and expression by cancer cells
5. Overcoming resistance pathways

However, given the rapid progress in the field, it is likely that many of these technological problems will be solved in the near future.

Key Points

- Gene replacement therapy targeted to a tumor suppressor gene can cause cancer regression by activation of known pathways with minimal toxicity.
- Damage to tumor suppressor genes in normal tissue and premalignant lesions may someday be useful in early intervention, diagnosis, and even prevention of cancer.
- Correction of a defect in apoptosis induction can restore sensitivity to radiation and chemotherapy in some resistant tumors, and sensitivity to killing might be enhanced in already sensitive tumors and may eventually lead to reduced toxicity from chemotherapy and radiation therapy.
- The ready availability of gene libraries, the ability to administer the genes without the extensive reformulation required of small molecules, and their specificity makes this an attractive therapeutic approach.

References

1. Denissenko MF, Pao A, Tang M, Pfeifer GP. Preferential formation of benzo[a]pyrene adducts at lung cancer mutational hotspots in p53. Science 1996;274:430.
2. Burns T, El-Deiry W. The p53 pathway and apoptosis. J Cell Physiol 1999;181:231.
3. Fujiwaa T, Grimm EA, Mukhopadhyay T, Cai DW, Owen-Schaub LB, Roth JA. A retroviral wild-type p53 expression vector penetrates human lung cancer spheroids and inhibits growth by inducing apoptosis. Cancer Res 1993;53:4129.
4. Raycroft L, Wu H, Lozano G. Transcriptional activation by wild-type but not transforming mutants of the p53 anti-oncogene. Science 1990;249:1049.
5. Adams JM, Cory S. The Bcl-2 protein family: arbiters of cell survival. Science 1998;281:1322.
6. Kamijo T, Zindy F, Roussel MF, Quelle DE, Downing JR, Ashmun RA, et al. Tumor suppression at the mouse INK4a locus mediated by the alternative reading frame product p19ARF. Cell 1997;91:649.
7. Isobe T, Hiyama K, Yoshida Y, Fujiwara Y, Yamakido M. Prognostic significance of p53 and ras gene abnormalities in lung adenocarcinoma patients with stage I disease after curative resection. Jpn J Cancer Res 1994;85:1240.
8. Martin HM, Filipe MI, Morris RW, Lane DP, Silvestre F. p53 expression and prognosis in gastric carcinoma. Int J Cancer 1992;50:859.
9. Quinlan DC, Davidson AG, Summers CL, Warden HE, Doshi HM. Accumulation of p53 protein correlates with a poor prognosis in human lung cancer. Cancer Res 1992;52:4828.
10. Cai DW, Mukhopadhyay T, Roth JA. A novel ribozyme for modification of mutated p53 pre-mRNA in non-small cell lung cancer cell lines. Proc 3rd Antisense Workshop 1993;11–13.
11. Zhang WW, Fang X, Mazur W, French BA, Georges RN, Roth JA. High-efficiency gene transfer and high-level expression of wild-type p53 in human lung cancer cells

mediated by recombinant adenovirus. Cancer Gene Ther 1994;1:5.

12. Fujiwara T, Cai DW, Georges RN, Mukhopadhyay T, Grimm EA, Roth JA. Therapeutic effect of a retroviral wild-type p53 expression vector in an orthotopic lung cancer model [commentary]. J Natl Cancer Inst 1994;86:1437.

13. Wang JX, Bucana CD, Roth JA, Zhang WW. Apoptosis induced in human osteosarcoma cells is one of the mechanisms for the cytocidal effect of Ad5CMV-p53. Cancer Gene Ther 1995;2:9.

14. Georges RN, Mukhopadhyay T, Zhang Y, Yen N, Roth JA. Prevention of orthotopic human lung cancer growth by intratracheal instillation of a retroviral antisense K-ras construct. Cancer Res 1993;53:1743.

15. Bouvet M, Fang B, Ekmekcioglu S, Ji L, Bucana CD, Hamada K, et al. Suppression of the immune response to an adenovirus vector and enhancement of intratumoral transgene expression by low-dose etoposide. Gene Ther 1998;5:189.

16. Nielsen LL, Dell J, Maxwell E, Armstrong L, Maneval D, Catino JJ. Efficacy of p53 adenovirus-mediated gene therapy against human breast cancer xenografts. Cancer Gene Ther 1997;4:129.

17. Spitz FR, Nguyen D, Skibber J, Meyn R, Cristiano RJ, Roth JA. Adenoviral mediated p53 gene therapy enhances radiation sensitivity of colorectal cancer cell lines. Proc Am Assoc Cancer Res 1996;37:347.

18. Xu M, Kumar D, Srinivas S, Detolla LJ, Yu SF, Stass Sa, et al. Parenteral gene therapy with p53 inhibits human breast tumors in vivo through a bystander mechanism without evidence of toxicity. Hum Gene Ther 1997;8:177.

19. Cusack JC, Spitz FR, Nguyen D, Zhang WW, Cristiano RJ, Roth JA. High levels of gene transduction in human lung tumors following intralesional injection of recombinant adenovirus. Cancer Gene Ther 1996;3:245.

20. Dameron KM, Volpert OV, Tainsky MA, Bouck N. Control of angiogenesis in fibroblasts by p53 regulation of thrombospondin-1. Science 1994;265:1582.

21. Miyashita T, Reed JC. Tumor suppressor p53 is a direct transcriptional activator of human bax gene. Cell 1995;80:293.

22. Carroll JL, Nielsen LL, Pruett SB, Mathis JM. The role of natural killer cells in adenovirus-mediated p53 gene therapy. Mol Cancer Ther 2001;1:49.

23. Molinier-Frenkel V, Le Boulaire C, Le Gal FA, Gahery-Segard H, Tursz T, Guillet JG, et al. Longitudinal follow-up of cellular and humoral immunity induced by recombinant adenovirus-mediated gene therapy in cancer patients. Human Gene Ther 2000;11:1911.

24. Yen N, Ioannides CG, Xu K, Swisher SG, Lawrence DD, Kemp BL, et al. Cellular and humoral immune responses to adenovirus and p53 protein antigens in patients following intratumor injection of an adenovirus vector expressing wild-type p53 (Ad-p53). Cancer Gene Ther 2000;7:530.

25. Owen-Schaub LB, Zhang W, Cusack JC, Angelo LS, Santee SM, Fujiwara T, et al. Wild-type human p53 and a temperature-sensitive mutant induce Fas/APO-1 expression. Mol Cell Biol 1995;15:3032.

26. Roth JA, Nguyen D, Lawrence DD, Kemp BL, Carrasco CH, Ferson DZ, et al. Retrovirus-mediated wild-type p53 gene transfer to tumors of patients with lung cancer. Nat Med 1996;2:985.

27. Roth JA. Clinical protocol: modification of mutant K-ras gene expression in non-small cell lung cancer (NSCLC). Hum Gene Ther 1996;7:875.

28. Roth JA. Clinical protocol: modification of tumor suppressor gene expression and induction of apoptosis in non-small cell lung cancer (NSCLC) with an adenovirus vector

expressing wildtype p53 and cisplatin. Hum Gene Ther 1996;7:1013.

29. Swisher SG, Roth JA, Nemunaitis J, Lawrence DD, Kemp BL, Carrasco CH, et al. Adenovirus-mediated p53 gene transfer in advanced non-small cell lung cancer. J Natl Cancer Inst 1999;91:763.

30. Yver A, Dreiling LK, Mohanty S, Merritt J, Proksch S, Shu C, et al. Tolerance and safety of RPR/INGN 201, an adeno-viral vector containing a p53 gene, administered intratumorally in 309 patients with advanced cancer enrolled in phase I and II studies world-wide. Proc Am Soc Clin Oncol 1999;19:460a.

31. Ramqvist T, Magnusson KP, Wang Y, Szekeley L, Klein G. Wild-type p53 induces apoptosis in a Burkitt lymphoma (BL) line that carries mutant p53. Oncogene 1993;8:1495.

32. Shaw P, Bovey R, Tardy S, Sahli R, Sordat B, Costa J. Induction of apoptosis by wild-type p53 in a human colon tumor-derived cell line. Proc Natl Acad Sci U S A 1992;89:4495.

33. Yonish-Rouach E, Resnitzky D, Lotem J, Sachs L, Kimchi A, Oren M. Wild-type p53 induces apoptosis of myeloid leukemic cells that is inhibited by interleukin-6. Nature 1991;352:345.

34. Dewey WC, Ling CC, Meyn RE. Radiation induced apoptosis: relevance to radiotherapy. Int J Radiat Oncol Biol Phys 1995;33:781.

35. Fujiwara T, Grimm EA, Mukhopadhyay T, Zhang WW, Owen-Schaub LB, Roth JA. Induction of chemosensitivity in human cancer cells in vivo by adenovirus-mediated transfer of the wild-type p53 gene. Surgical Forum 1994;45:524.

36. Hamada M, Fujiwara T, Hizuta A, Gochi A, Naomoto Y, Takakura N, et al. The p53 gene is a potent determinant of chemosensitivity and radiosensitivity in gastric and colorectal cancers. J Cancer Res Clin Oncol 1996;122:360.

37. Meyn RE, Stephens LC, Hunter NR, Milas L. Apoptosis in murine tumors treated with chemotherapy agents. Anticancer Drugs 1997;6:443.

38. Nguyen DM, Spitz FR, Yen N, Cristiano RJ, Roth JA. Gene therapy for lung cancer: enhancement of tumor suppression by a combination of sequential systemic cisplatin and adenovirus-mediated p53 gene transfer. J Thorac Cardiovasc Surg 1996;112:1372.

39. Roth JA. Clinical protocol for modification of tumor suppressor gene expression and induction of apoptosis in non-small cell lung cancer (NSCLC) with an adenovirus vector expressing wildtype p53 and cisplatin [review]. Hum Gene Ther 1995;6:252.

40. Nguyen D, Spitz F, Kataoka M, Wiehle S, Roth JA, Cristiano R. Enhancement of gene transduction in human carcinoma cells by DNA-damaging agents. Proc Am Assoc Cancer Res 1996;37:347.

41. Akimoto T, Hunter NR, Buchmiller L, Mason K, Ang KK, Milas L. Inverse relationship between epidermal growth factor receptor expression and radiocurability of murine carcinomas. Clin Cancer Res 1999;5:2884.

42. Broaddus WC, Liu Y, Steele LL, Gillies GT, Lin PS, Loudon WG, et al. Enhanced radiosensitivity of malignant glioma cells after adenoviral p53 transduction. J Neurosurg 1999;91:997.

43. Feinmesser M, Halpern M, Fenig E, Tsabari C, Hodak E, Sulkes J, et al. Expression of the apoptosis-related oncogenes bcl-2, bax, and p53 in Merkel cell carcinoma: can they predict treatment response and clinical outcome? Hum Pathol 1994;30:1367.

44. Jasty R, Lu J, Irwin T, Suchard S, Clarke MF, Castle VP. Role of p53 in the regulation of irradiation-induced apoptosis in neuroblastoma cells. Mol Genet Metab 1998;65:155.

45. Sakakura C, Sweeney EA, Shirahama T, Igarashi Y, Hakomori S, Nakatani H, et al. Overexpression of bax sensitizes human breast cancer MCF-7 cells to radiation-induced apoptosis. Int J Cancer 1996;67:101.

46. Brachman DG, Becket M, Graves D, Haraf D, Vokes E, Weichselbaum RR. p53 mutation does not correlate with radiosensitivity in 24 head and neck cancer cells lines. Cancer Res 1993;53:3667.

47. Danielsen T, Smith-Sorensen B, Gronlund HA, Hvidsten M, Borresen-Dale AL, Rofstad EK. No association between radiosensitivity and TP53 status, G(1) arrest or protein levels of p53, myc, ras or raf in human melanoma lines. Int J Radiat Biol 1994;75:1149.

48. Slichenmyer WJ, Nelson WG, Slebos RJ, Kastan MB. Loss of a p53-associated G1 checkpoint does not decrease cell survival following DNA damage. Cancer Res 1993;53:4164.

49. Nemunaitis J, Swisher SG, Timmons T, Connors D, Mack M, Doerksen L, et al. Adenovirus-mediated p53 gene transfer in sequence with cisplatin to tumors of patients with non-small cell lung cancer. J Clin Oncol 2000;18:609.

50. Schuler M, Herrmann R, De Greve JL, Stewart AK, Gatzemeier U, Stewart DJ, et al. Adenovirus-mediated wild-type p53 gene transfer in patients receiving chemotherapy for advanced non-small-cell lung cancer: results of a multi-center phase II study. J Clin Oncol 2001;19:1750.

51. Swisher S, Roth JA, Komaki R, Hicks M, Ro J, Dreiling L, et al. A phase II trial of adenoviral mediated p53 gene transfer (RPR/INGN 201) in conjunction with radiation therapy in patients with localized non-small cell lung cancer (NSCLC). Am Soc Clin Oncol 2000;19:461a.

52. Peng Z, Han D, Zhang S, Pan J, Tang P, Xiao S, et al. Clinical evaluation of safety and efficacy of intratumoral administration of a recombinant adenoviral-p53 anticancer agent (Genkaxin®). Mol Ther 2003;7:422.

53. Ito I, Ji L, Tanaka F, Saito Y, Gopalan B, Branch CD, et al. Liposomal vector mediated delivery of the 3p FUS1 gene demonstrates potent antitumor activity against human lung cancer in vivo. Cancer Gene Ther 2004;11:733.

54. Uno F, Sasaki J, Nishizaki M, Carboni G, Xu K, Atkinson EN, et al. Myristoylation of the FUS1 protein is required for tumor suppression in human lung cancer cells. Cancer Res 2004;64:2969.

Non-Small-Cell Lung Cancer: Clinical Studies in Europe

37

Christian Manegold, Annette Mueller
and Sebastian Belle

Contents

37.1 Introduction

The currently available treatment approaches are still unsatisfactory for most patients with lung cancer, and the chance of cure is limited to a minority, even at an early stage of the disease [1, 2]. For the majority of patients therapy is palliative, aimed at reducing tumor-related symptoms and maintaining or improving quality of life, while offering some prospects for prolongation of life. The mainstays of treatment for lung cancer are surgery, radiotherapy, and systemic chemotherapy. They are used as a standard of care in modern bi- or trimodality strategies for the treatment of early lung cancer. For the treatment of metastatic disease, systemic chemotherapy plays the principal role, despite its limitations regarding efficacy and tolerability. The use of chemotherapy should follow the recommendations of national and international guidelines [3–5]. Especially regarding chemotherapy, there is an urgent need for improvement, and any opportunity should be taken to investigate promising new approaches in clinical studies. Actually, the use of different new drugs as well as innovative therapy strategies offers the hope for substantial progress against the disease in the near future. Most noteworthy is the large number

of targeted antineoplastic agents (i.e., small molecules, monoclonal antibodies) which were developed on the basis of new molecular biologic findings. Further advances in the treatment of patients with localized disease are expected from an improved timing of surgery and/or radiation therapy in relation to chemotherapy. Such approaches are known as inductive (neoadjuvant, preoperative) chemotherapy or chemoradiotherapy, adjuvant (postoperative) chemotherapy, and concurrent or sequential chemoradiotherapy.

Europe has always played a major role in the development of improved therapies for lung cancer, through national or international clinical studies as well as preclinical research. In this review we will give an overview of the current activities of national and international cooperative groups in Europe that deal with clinical trials, and outline the main research topics addressed in these studies. The information presented in this review was collected from different sources including personal communications with experts and cooperative study groups, and through modern communication and information technology (Table 37.1).

37.2 Early-Stage Non-Small-Cell Lung Cancer

37.2.1 Studies of Neoadjuvant (Inductive, Preoperative) Treatment of Non-Small-Cell Lung Cancer

The aim of induction therapy is to improve survival compared with surgery alone by early delivery of systemic therapy and further intensification of local treatment. These approaches are based on the rationale that lung carcinoma, like other solid tumors, tend to disseminate early and are clinically occult, and thus can be considered in most cases systemic diseases from the outset. The administration of full doses of chemotherapy prior to surgery is primarily aimed at the eradication of micrometastases. Another desired effect of preoperative chemotherapy is to shrink potentially resectable primary tumors

Table 37.1. Source data

UICC	International Union Against Cancer	*http://www.uicc.org/* International
IASLC	International Association for the Study of Lung Cancer	*http://www.iaslc.org/* International
ELCWP	European Lung Cancer Working Party	*http://www.elcwp.org/* Europe
CECOG	Central European Cooperative Oncology Group	*http://www.cecog.org/* Vienna, Austria
AKH-Wien	Allgemeines Krankenhaus Universitätskliniken Wien, Klinik für Innere Medizin I	*http://www.akh-wien.ac.at/* Vienna, Austria
EORTC	European Organization for Research and Treatment of Cancer	*http://www.eortc.be* Brussels, Belgium
LLCG	The Leuven Lung Cancer Group	*http://www.LLCG.be/* Leuven, Belgium
IFCT	Intergroupe Francophone de Cancérologie Thoracique	*http://www.ifct.asso.fr/* Paris, France
IGR	Institute Gustave Roussy	*http://www.igr.fr* Villejuif, France
KKS	Arbeitsgemeinschaft der Koordinierungszentren für Klinische Studien	*http://www.kks-info.de/* Germany
CuLCaSG	Associazione Cuneese per lo Studio e la Cura del Cancro del Polmone	*http://www.culcasg.org/links.html* Italy
IST	Istituto nazionale per la ricerca sul cancro	*http://www.istge.it* Italy
INTF-GP	Institutio Nazionale Tumori Fondazione G. Pascale	*http://uosc.fondazione-pascale.it* Italy
IKA	Integraal Kanker-centrum	*http://www.ikca.nl/* Amsterdam, the Netherlands
Oncoline	Oncoline	*http://www.oncoline.nl/* The Netherlands
NVALT	Nederlandse Vereniging van Artsen voor Longziekten en Tuberculose	*http://www.nvalt-oncology.nl/* The Netherlands
SIAK	Schweizerisches Institut für angewandte Krebsforschung	*http://www.siak.ch* Switzerland
NRCT	National Register of Cancer Trials	*http://212.219.75.236/ukcccr/* UK
CR-UK	Cancer Research United Kingdom	*http://science.cancerresearchuk.org* UK
MRC	Medical Research Council	*http://www.ctu.mrc.ac.uk/default.asp* UK
NCRN	National Cancer Research Network	*http://www.ncrn.org.uk/* UK
University of Southampton		*http://www.som.soton.ac.uk* UK

Table 37.1 (continued)

Clinical Trials Gov.	US National Institute of Health	*http://www.clinical-trials.gov/ct* USA
CCT	Current Controlled Trials	*http://www.controlled-trials.com/* USA
NCI	National Cancer Institute	*http://www.cancer.gov* USA
CCT-USA	Cancer Clinical Trials	*http://www.cancerindex.org* USA
Cancer Care Ontario	Cancer Care Ontario	*http://www.cancercare.on.ca/* Ontario, Canada

and involved lymph nodes. Local tumor reduction can be further enhanced by preoperative bimodality strategies, utilizing additional radiation therapy.

Induction chemotherapy or chemoradiotherapy administered prior to definitive surgical resection has been used for more than two decades [6–10] and, in the meantime, has been adopted as the treatment standard for a selected group of patients with resectable non-small-cell lung cancer (NSCLC). This development was fostered by some major European randomized studies, the first results of which were published nearly 10 years ago [9–18]. At present, preoperative therapy is being investigated in at least nine European studies. These trials vary in their design, the treatment strategies and chemotherapy regimens used, the role of radiotherapy, and patient numbers.

While neoadjuvant, unlike adjuvant, therapy is considered being in favor of medical oncology, surgeons tend to prefer the adjuvant approach because most patients with early NSCLC who are admitted to a surgical department or clinic are primarily referred for the purpose of surgical resection. Nevertheless, based on the promising results reported from Europe and North America, several randomized phase II and III trials have been initiated. Some of them are still open for accrual. These studies can be categorized as follows.

Chemotherapy Versus No Chemotherapy

These studies are designed to obtain "proof of principle." Two of these studies are randomized phase III trials with two arms. The LU22/EORTC-08012/NVALT is a cooperative study of the British Medical Research Council (MRC), the EORTC Lung Cancer Group, and Dutch investigators. Patients in the experimental arm receive three preoperative cycles of standard cisplatin-based chemotherapy (gemcitabine/cisplatin, vinorelbine/cisplatin, mitomycin/vinblastine/cisplatin [MVP], mitomycin/ifosfamide/cisplatin [MIC], or taxane/carboplatin). Patients with potentially resectable disease (stage

Table 37.2. NSCLC: operable limited stage, neoadjuvant therapy

Trial	Country	Phase	Stage	Number	Intervention	Primary endpoint	Status
ChEST	Italy	III	IB–IIIA no N2	236	iCT vs none	PFS	Open
MRC-LU22	Europe	III	I–IIIB	450	iCT vs none	OS	Open
NATCH	Spain	III	IB–IIIA	600	iCT vs conCT vs iCT vs none	EFS	Open
IFCT 0002	France	III	IA–IIB	520	iCT + conCT vs iCT	OS	Open
GIP	Belgium	II	IIA N2	46	iCT	OS	Open
SAKK-16/00	Switzerland	III	IIIA,N2	120	iCT + Rad vs iCT	EFS	Open
SAKK-16/01	Switzerland	II	IIIB	46	iCT + Rad	RR	Open
IFTC-0101	France	II	IIIA, N2	150	iCT vs iCT + Rad	Feasibility	Open
EORTC-08013	The Netherlands	II	IIIA, N2	55	iCT	OS	Open

iCT Induction chemotherapy, *conCT* consolidation chemotherapy, *Rad* radiation, *PFS* progression-free survival, *OS* overall survival, *EFS* event-free survival, *RR* remission rate

I–III) are eligible for study entry, and the primary endpoint of the study is overall survival.

The Italian ChEST (Chemotherapy in Early Stages Trial) has an identical design and enrolls patients with potentially resectable stage I–III disease. Chemotherapy in the experimental arm consists of three preoperative cycles of gemcitabine/cisplatin. Resectable stages include T2-3N0, T1-2N1, and T3N1. The primary endpoint of the study is progression-free survival.

The NATCH (Neo-Adjuvant Taxol-Carboplatin-Hope) trial is a randomized, three-arm phase III study from Spain with international participation that compares surgery alone with surgery plus preoperative (neoadjuvant) or postoperative (adjuvant) chemotherapy. Chemotherapy consists of three pre- or postoperative cycles of carboplatin/paclitaxel. Patients with potentially resectable disease including the stages IA (>2 cm), IB, II, or IIIA (T3N1) are eligible for enrollment.

The randomized phase III study IFCT 0002 initiated by the French Thoracic Oncology Intergroup has a complex design with four study arms. It is scheduled to enroll 520 patients with stage I or II disease. Treatment consists of either gemcitabine/cisplatin or paclitaxel/carboplatin for a total of 4 cycles. Chemotherapy is administered either entirely prior to surgery, or 2 cycles are given before and 2 cycles after surgery.

Finally, we became aware of two non-randomized phase II studies investigating the preoperative use of three-drug regimens in patients with stage IIIA, N2 disease. The Leuven Lung Cancer Group (LLCG) is evaluating the chemotherapy triplet gemcitabine, ifosfamide, and cisplatin (GIP), while patients in the EORTC-08013 study are treated with gemcitabine, cisplatin, and gefitinib (Iressa).

Preoperative Chemoradiotherapy

Neoadjuvant chemoradiotherapy is primarily expected to improve long-term survival of patients with stage IIIA and IIIB disease, both through enhanced local tumor control and early inhibition of distant metastasis.

This treatment approach has recently been investigated by two German study groups [8, 19]. A subsequent randomized phase III trial was closed after accrual of more than 500 patients. Results have been published only in abstract form so far. All patients first received 3 cycles of chemotherapy with cisplatin and etoposide. In the control arm, this was immediately followed by surgery and conventionally fractionated postoperative radiotherapy. In the experimental arm, patients were treated after chemotherapy with concurrent chemoradiation including carboplatin/vindesine and hyperfractionated accelerated radiotherapy. There were no differences in progression-free survival, time to progression, response rate, and R0 resection rate [20].

Two Swiss and one French study are still open to accrual. SAKK-16/00 of the Swiss Cooperative Group for Clinical Cancer Research is a randomized phase III study to compare the feasibility and efficacy (event-free survival) of neoadjuvant chemotherapy with or without radiotherapy. The target population are patients with stage IIIA, N2. Sequential chemoradiotherapy begins with 3 cycles of docetaxel/cisplatin. Three weeks after the last chemotherapy administration, patients undergo radiotherapy with once daily fractions, 5 days a week, for 3 weeks and boost-radiotherapy on days 2, 5, 9, 12, 15, 17, and 19 during the same weeks. In contrast SAKK-16/01 is a non-randomized trial evaluating preoperative chemoradiotherapy in patients with stage IIIB (T4N0-3 or T1-4N3) disease. Chemoradiotherapy is also administered sequentially, with three initial cycles of docetaxel and cisplatin. Beginning 3 weeks after the last chemotherapy dose, patients without progressive disease then receive radiotherapy 1–2 times daily on days 1–5, 8–12, and 15–19. In a third treatment step, patients undergo surgery within 3–4 weeks after completion of radiotherapy.

The French IFCT-0101 is a randomized phase II study with three treatment arms, targeting patients with stage IIIA, N2 disease. Chemotherapy consists of three preoperative cycles of gemcitabine/cisplatin (arm A), vinorelbine/cisplatin (arm B), or paclitaxel/carboplatin (arm C). In arms B and C, chemotherapy is given concurrently with radiotherapy from the second cycle. Study endpoints are feasibility and toxicity of the three different approaches which are considered for further study in the group's planned phase III trial.

37.2.2 Studies of Adjuvant (Postoperative) Treatment of Non-Small-Cell Lung Cancer

Adjuvant chemotherapy and/or radiotherapy may be an alternative to induction therapy in the effort to improve outcome after surgical treatment. This attractive treatment approach has proven successful in other solid tumors and has been used for decades in clinical trials for the treatment of lung cancer [21–23]. Only recently, however, it was demonstrated that adjuvant chemotherapy following successful radical resection of NSCLC improved survival to a statistically significant and clinically meaningful extent [24–29]. It was the International Lung Adjuvant Trial (IALT), a study initiated and led by French investigators, whose results ushered in the paradigm shift in postoperative care for patients with NSCLC. IALT is now considered a "proof of principle" trial that has provided strongest evidence for the use of adjuvant treatment in routine practice. However, IALT also revealed substantial deficits in the understanding of the rationale underlying the general recommendation for adjuvant chemotherapy. Therefore, it is another merit of IALT to have rekindled research interest in early NSCLC and to have stimulated the initiation of new clinical studies worldwide.

The current situation of adjuvant chemotherapy for NSCLC is as follows. In the 5 years since 2000, several national and international studies have demonstrated that patients undergoing successful radical surgery benefit from postoperative chemotherapy in terms of a statistically significant and clinically relevant prolongation of survival. Many institutions have considered the available evidence strong enough to recommend and utilize adjuvant chemotherapy as the new treatment standard. Potential treatment candidates are patients with stage IB–IIIA disease, although evidence is most convincing for stage II. Treatment usually consists of 4 cycles of a modern platinum-based doublet with proven efficacy in the advanced or neoadjuvant setting.

European investigators have been continuously involved in the lively debate that was sparked by the relatively slim scientific evidence supporting the general use of adjuvant chemotherapy. Many questions around chemotherapy are still unresolved or need to be discussed and investigated in more detail, including the beginning and duration of treatment, the choice of drugs, and their activity and tolerability. What is also important for a chemotherapy regimen given with curative intent is its feasibility, patient acceptability, and compliance. Another interesting topic is the use of new targeted agents, including small molecules and monoclonal antibodies, with its new possibilities but also incalculable risks. Furthermore, radiotherapy administered after surgery as adjuvant treatment still remains a matter for debate. It is rather clear that the radiation techniques of the past have not been beneficial or have even been detrimental. Modern radiotherapy, however, with its definitely improved technology and accuracy, has claimed a firm place in the current clinical development toward multimodality treatment of NSCLC. Another subject to be addressed in future studies is the proper selection of patients and the definition of risk groups. Modern imaging techniques including positron emission tomography, magnetic resonance imaging, and computerized tomography, as well as new prognostic or predictive molecular markers are expected to provide useful information in this context.

Despite this broad and in-depth discussion reflecting the enormous interest in adjuvant chemotherapy, no large new project has been initiated in Europe or elsewhere recently. This is by no means due to a lack of ideas. As the debate has shown, large two-armed randomized phase III trials are considered the most appropriate research tool. They could be used to determine the relative value of adjuvant and neoadjuvant chemotherapy, of novel drug combinations, and the optimal duration of treatment. However, it is well known that such research is expensive and time-consuming. It requires a large number of patients and is very demanding with regard to logistics and national as well as international cooperation. Therefore, it is very difficult

Table 37.3. NSCLC: operable limited stage, adjuvant therapy

Trial	Country	Phase	Stage	Number	Intervention	Primary endpoint	Status
IALT	France	III	I/II/III	1,867	adCT vs OBS	OS	Closed
ALPI	Italy	III	I/II/III	1,209	adCT vs OBS	OS	Closed
ANITA	Europe	III	I/II/IIIA	840	adCT vs OBS	OS	Closed
BMJ-Meta	UK	Randomized	I/II/III/IV	9,387	Meta-analysis	OS	Closed
IGN 101/2-02	Europe	II/III	II/IIIA	760	Immunotherapy vs OBS	PFS	Open
ZOMETA	Europe	III	III	446	Prevention of BM	TBM	Planned

adCT Adjuvant chemotherapy, *OBS* observation, *BM* bone metastasis, *OS* overall survival, *PFS* progression-free survival, *TBM* time to bone metastases

to put such a project into practice at a time when scientific research is aimed at achieving rapid results. Randomized or non-randomized phase II trials would be more appropriate in this situation. They could be used to investigate important issues of acceptability, feasibility, and tolerability of adjuvant chemotherapy including supplementary high-quality molecular research programs at lower cost compared with phase III studies. We are eagerly awaiting more details of the recently completed studies, and their full publications and planned meta-analyses of pooled study results. These data will, hopefully, encourage investigators to initiate new adjuvant trials.

Of the more recent studies, a multicenter, placebo-controlled phase II/III study investigating the active cancer vaccine IGN 101 (Igeneon, Vienna, Austria) is worthy of note. The vaccine contains edrecolomab, an aluminum-absorbed murine monoclonal antibody against the cell-surface glycoprotein 17-1A that was designed to prevent or delay the formation of metastasis. IGN 101 has been shown to induce an immune response that reduces the number of circulating epithelial cell adhesion molecule (EpCAM)-positive tumor cells in peripheral blood. EpCAM is a cell surface glycoprotein that is expressed, and often overexpressed, on virtually all epithelial cancers but is also present on normal epithelial cells. EpCAM mediates homophilic adhesion of epithelial cells and may also be involved in the mediation of cellular growth or developmental signals. It is planned to recruit a total of 760 patients with stage IB–IIIA NSCLC. Vaccination starts immediately after radical surgery, and the primary endpoint of the study is relapse-free survival.

Another prospective multicenter randomized phase III study is designed to evaluate the efficacy of zoledronic acid (Zometa) to prevent bone metastases in patients with locally advanced stage IIIA and IIIB NSCLC. The primary objective is time to bone metastases. Patients are eligible if they have completed primary treatment of their disease according to local standard practice (surgery, radiotherapy, chemotherapy, or multimodality treatment), with no progression having occurred. Patients will be randomized to receive either Zometa 4 mg every 3–4 weeks or no Zometa. Therapy with Zometa will continue for 24 months. A total of 446 patients will be enrolled in the study.

37.2.3 Studies of Chemoradiotherapy for Unresectable Localized Non-Small-Cell Lung Cancer

Radiotherapy has long been considered the primary local treatment option for patients with unresectable or inoperable stage I–III NSCLC. More recently, however, both radiotherapy alone and surgery alone have been challenged by multimodality treatments, and combined chemoradiotherapy is now recommended as standard of care for patients in appropriate clinical conditions [30–32]. This change reflects a wealth of practical experience and the results of extensive clinical research conducted during recent years, having provided ample evidence for the role of distant metastasis as the major determinant of outcome.

The concept of chemoradiotherapy is the well-timed combination of full-dose radiation therapy and systemic chemotherapy, the latter given with the intent to enhance the effect of radiotherapy in providing local tumor control and at the same time to prevent or delay distant metastasis. In clinical studies of chemoradiotherapy the two modalities were given either concurrently or sequentially, and both approaches were shown to improve survival significantly compared with radiotherapy alone [30–33]. Moreover, in direct comparisons conducted by Japanese and American groups, concurrent chemoradiotherapy was found to be superior to sequential chemoradiotherapy and therefore has been widely accepted as treatment standard [34–38]. Nevertheless, treatment results still remain unsatisfactory and improvements are urgently needed. Innovative approaches including the use of new radiation techniques

Table 37.4. NSCLC: inoperable limited stage

Trial	Country	Phase	Stage	Number	Intervention	Primary endpoint	Status
CHARTWEL	Europe	III	I–III	665	Rad vs CHART	OS	Closed
XRP 6976B/2505	Belgium	II	IIIA multiple N2, IIIB		iCT + cRCT vs cCRT + conCT	n.r.	Open
INRC-ITA	Italy	III	III	300	iCT + cRCT vs cCRT + OBS	OS	Open
GERCOR-B00-1	France	III	II, III	390	cRCT + conCT vs cRCT + OBS	PFS	Open
LU3001	UK	III	I–III	461	CT + Rad vs Rad	OS, QoL	Closed
INCH	UK	II/III	I–III	500	CT + CHART vs CHART	3-y S	Planned
SOCCAR	UK	III	III	508	CT + Rad vs cRCT + conCT	OS	Planned
LU3002	UK	III	I–III	350	CT vs OBS	OS	Closed
GRIN	UK	III	I, IIB no T3	450	CT vs cRCT	PFS	Open

Rad Radiation, *CHART* continuous hyperfractionated accelerated radiotherapy, *iCT* induction chemotherapy, *cRCT* concurrent radiochemotherapy, *cCRT* concurrent chemoradiotherapy, *conCT* consolidation chemotherapy, *OBS* observation, *OS* overall survival, *n.r.* not reported, *PFS* progression-free survival, *QoL* quality of life, *3-y S* 3-year survival

and novel drugs offer hope for progress in the future, and European study groups are actively involved in such research.

CHARTWEL (Continuous Hyperfractionated Accelerated Radiation Therapy–Weekend Less)-Bronchus is a German, Czech, and Polish prospective, randomized, multicenter phase III trial comparing conventionally fractionated radiotherapy (66 Gy given in five daily 2-Gy fractions per week) with the CHARTWEL regimen (60 Gy given in 15 fractions of 1.5 Gy per week, Monday to Friday TID, for 3.5 weeks). The three daily fractions are separated by at least 6 h. In both treatment arms a shrinking field technique is applied (conventional radiotherapy at 50 Gy; CHARTWEL at 39 Gy). The main endpoint of the trial is overall survival. It has been calculated that 665 patients need to be enrolled to detect a 10% improvement in 2-year survival.

XRP 6976B/2505 is a randomized phase II trial comparing induction chemotherapy, consisting of 2 cycles of docetaxel/cisplatin followed by concurrent chemoradiotherapy, with weekly low-dose single-agent docetaxel versus concurrent chemoradiotherapy with weekly low-dose single-agent docetaxel followed by 2 cycles of docetaxel/cisplatin for consolidation. Patients with stage IIIA-multiple cN2 or IIIB are eligible for the trial. Radiotherapy is conventional, with daily fractions of 2 Gy given from Monday to Friday to a total dose of 66 Gy. Primary endpoints of the study are the feasibility and toxicity of treatment. Enrollment of 150 patients is planned.

INRC-ITA is an Italian phase III study of paclitaxel plus carboplatin or cisplatin followed by radiotherapy with or without concurrent paclitaxel. Three hundred patients with unresectable stage III disease will be accrued. After completion of two courses of paclitaxel/carboplatin or paclitaxel/cisplatin they will be randomized to proceed to either concurrent chemoradiotherapy consisting of weekly paclitaxel and conventionally fractionated radiotherapy (five fractions per week from Monday to Friday) for 6 weeks, or the same radiotherapy for 7 weeks without paclitaxel. Trial objectives are overall survival, 1-year survival rate, response rate (local control), and tolerability.

The French GERCOR group has initiated a randomized multicenter phase III study for unresectable stage II or III NSCLC patients. All patients receive initial concurrent chemoradiotherapy consisting of paclitaxel/carboplatin once weekly for up to 6 weeks and radiotherapy 5 days a week for 7–7.5 weeks. Three weeks after completion of chemoradiotherapy, patients with complete response, partial response, or stable disease are randomized to receive either chemotherapy for consolidation or three more cycles of paclitaxel/carboplatin or immediate routine follow-up. A total of 390 patients will be accrued, and the main study objective is progression-free survival.

The British LU3001 trial is a randomized phase III trial comparing sequential chemotherapy and radiotherapy with radiotherapy alone in inoperable patients with localized disease. Patients are randomized to receive 4 cycles of mitomycin, ifosfamide, and cisplatin (MIC) combination chemotherapy, followed by radiotherapy as decided by the radiotherapist (with a total minimum dose not less than 40 Gy in 15 fractions and adequate field size to encompass the known extent of the tumor) or radiotherapy alone as described. Two hundred patients will be included, and the main study endpoint is time to tumor progression.

The MRC-INCH study of the British Medical Research Council is a randomized multicenter two-arm phase II/III trial. Patients receive either continuous hyperfractionated accelerated radiotherapy (CHART) 3 times daily for 12 consecutive days to a total of 54 Gy alone or induction chemotherapy with 3 cycles of vinorelbine/cisplatin followed by CHART. Eligible patients must have inoperable stage I–III localized disease and must be fit enough to receive chemotherapy and CHART radiation. If the chemotherapy is considered feasible and safe in the first 80 patients, the trial will continue to recruit a total of 500 patients. The main study endpoint is survival.

The SOCCAR (sequential or concurrent chemotherapy and radiotherapy) trial is another British randomized two-arm phase III study that is open for patients with stage III disease considered unsuitable for surgery. Eligible patients will receive concurrent chemoradiotherapy consisting of vinorelbine/cisplatin and radical radiotherapy of 55 Gy in 20 fractions over 4 weeks followed 4 weeks later by consolidation chemotherapy with vinorelbine/cisplatin for 2 cycles, or sequential chemoradiotherapy with vinorelbine/cisplatin for 4 cycles followed 4 weeks later by radical radiotherapy (55 Gy in 20 fractions over 4 weeks). Approximately 500 patients will be included, and the primary study endpoint is overall survival.

LU3002 of the British Medical Research Council compares mitomycin, ifosfamide, cisplatin (MIC) chemotherapy with symptomatic treatment only in patients having clinically localized disease deemed not suitable for surgery or radical radiotherapy. Patients will receive 4 cycles of chemotherapy. Radiotherapy is an option for patients with symptoms not responding to systemic therapy (in this case chemotherapy should be stopped), and for patients developing symptoms after completion of chemotherapy. Short and simple radiotherapy schedules of 1–10 fractions, not exceeding a total dose of 30 Gy should be given. The other option for patients is to receive palliative care only, with radiotherapy given where appropriate. The primary study endpoint is survival.

The GRIN (Gemcitabine and Radiotherapy in Non-Small-Cell Lung Cancer) trial initiated by British investigators is a multicenter randomized phase III study designed to determine whether the addition of gemcitabine as a radiosensitizer to radical thoracic radiotherapy improves progression-free survival in patients with T1-2, N0-1 localized disease who have received no prior chemotherapy and are deemed unfit for resection. All patients will receive 55 Gy of radiotherapy administered over 4 weeks in daily fractions of 2.75 Gy, 5 days per week, with randomization to concurrent gemcitabine administered on days 1, 8, 15, and 22 of the radiotherapy course at a dose of 100 mg/m^2 or this radiotherapy regimen given alone, or 60 Gy of radiotherapy over 6 weeks in daily fractions of 2 Gy, 5 days per week, with randomization to concurrent gemcitabine delivered on days 1, 8, 15, 22, 29, and 36 of the radiotherapy course at a dose of 100 mg/m^2 or this radiotherapy regimen given alone. The primary endpoint is progression-free survival at 2 years. Two hundred and thirty patients will have to be randomized to radiotherapy alone and another 230 patients to radiotherapy plus gemcitabine.

37.3 Advanced-Stage Non-Small-Cell Lung Cancer

For NSCLC patients with locally advanced disease or distant metastases ("wet" IIIB, IV) cytotoxic chemotherapy is given solely for palliation. However, chemotherapy may improve survival, reduce tumor-related symptoms, and help to maintain quality of life, as has been demonstrated by a variety of randomized studies and meta-analyses over recent years [1]. The use of modern chemotherapy is nowadays guided by treatment standards. These have been elaborated upon the results of clinical trials, including numerous studies from European investigators, and are summarized in regularly updated national and international consensus papers [3–5]. Considering the modest treatment results, however, chemotherapy standards need to be improved, even though significant clinical advances have recently been achieved with a number of novel agents including gemcitabine or the taxanes, as well as improved supportive care or risk-adapted, individualized chemotherapy. It was due to these research efforts and the high incidence of NSCLC that in the decade since 1995 clinical development programs for new agents and innovative treatment approaches were often initiated in advanced NSCLC as a prototype of malignant disease. Meanwhile, virtually all promising experimental agents for the treatment of solid tumors are being investigated in clinical trials of NSCLC with participation of national as well as cooperative groups from Europe. The increased understanding of molecular biology has given new impetus to the development of innovative drugs and increased the interest in clinical trials. Thus, it has improved the chance to complete randomized trials with large patient numbers within a relatively short time.

The number of clinical trials offered in Europe for patients with advanced (stage IIIB/IV) NSCLC is striking. This is not only due to the discontent with the current standards of systemic therapy and their indisputable limitations, it also reflects the availability of a broad range of potential improvements including the novel agents referred to as "targeted therapies." This applies to first-line therapy as well as the further development of the recently defined standards for second-line therapy [39–41].

37.3.1 Second-line Therapy

Patients who failed prior chemotherapy should be considered for enrolment in one of the numerous ongoing randomized single-agent trials that investigate the therapeutic role of novel drugs that can be easily administered and/or have favorable toxicity profiles. These agents include erlotinib and gefitinib, the angiogenesis inhibitor ZD6474, the glutathione analog prodrug TLK286, vinflunine, a third-generation vinca alkaloid, aplidine, a new anticancer agent of marine origin that inhibits vascular endothelial growth factor, and the multitargeted antifolate pemetrexed. Most of these studies are using single-agent docetaxel as standard. Pemetrexed (Alimta) was not generally available until the middle of 2004.

INTEREST (Iressa NSCLC Trial Evaluating Response and Survival Against Taxotere) is a randomized international phase III trial with European participation. Patients receive gefitinib 250 mg daily or standard docetaxel 75 mg/m^2 every 3 weeks. Target recruitment is 1,440 patients, and the primary endpoint of the study is overall survival. INTEREST has been designed as a non-inferiority study. Its exploratory part aims at investigating the correlation of epidermal growth factor receptor (EGFR) expression and other related biomarkers with the efficacy of gefitinib in patients with available tumor samples, and evaluating pulmonary symptom changes.

IBREESE (Iressa vs. BSC: Randomised Evaluation of Effect on Pulmonary Symptom Endpoint) is a global placebo-controlled randomized trial with European participation. Patients either receive gefitinib (250 mg/day) plus best supportive care (BSC) or placebo plus BSC. The primary endpoint is the pulmonary symptom improvement rate as measured by the four pulmonary questions of the FACT-LCS in symptomatic patients. Target recruitment is 324 patients (2:1 randomization).

Patients are eligible for the ISEL (Iressa Survival Evaluation in Lung Cancer) trial if they have failed one or two prior chemotherapy regimens including platinum and docetaxel. As in the IBREESE trial, patients either receive gefitinib 250 mg daily plus BSC or placebo plus BSC. To reach the aim of including at least 577

Table 37.5. NSCLC: advanced stage, second-line therapy

Trial	Country	Phase	Stage	Number	Intervention	Primary endpoint	Status
INTEREST	International	III	IIIB, IV	1,400	Iressa vs CT	OS	Open
IBREESE	International	II	IIIB, IV	200	Iressa vs OBS	PSI	Closed
ISEL	International	III	IIIB, IV	1,692	Iressa vs OBS	OS	Closed
JMGX	International	III	IIIB, IV	1,000	Pe500 vs Pe900	OS	Open
ASSIST-2	International	III	III, IV	520	TLK286 vs Iressa	OS	Open
JAVALOR	International	III	IIIB, IV	500	Vinflunine vs docetaxel	PFS	Open
ZD6474	Czech Republic	II	IIIB, IV	129	ZD6474/D vs ZD6474	RR	Open
ITA-INTN-DI STAL	Italy	III	IIIB,IV	200	Weekly CT vs q3w	QoL	Open

CT chemotherapy, *OBS* observation, *Pe* pemetrexed, *D* docetaxel, *q3w* every 3 weeks, *OS* overall survival, *PSI* pulmonary symptom improvement, *PFS* progression-free survival, *RR* remission rate, *QoL* quality of life

patients with adenocarcinoma in the gefitinib arm and 398 patients with adenocarcinoma in the placebo arm, it was estimated that a total of 1,600 patients would have to be randomized. The primary endpoint is overall survival. This study is a global study with participation of many countries from Eastern Europe, Asia, and South America.

The ASSIST-2 trial is another global randomized phase III trial with significant North American and European participation. It is to compare gefitinib with TLK286 (Telcyta). TLK286 is a novel glutathione analog prodrug activated by glutathione S transferase P1-1 that induces apoptosis via the stress-response pathway. Patients receive either gefitinib 250 mg daily or TLK286 1,000 mg/m^2 every 3 weeks. The main purpose of this study is to determine if TLK286 is more effective than gefitinib as measured by survival.

Another second-line trial (JAVALOR) compares single-agent vinflunine 320 mg/m^2 every 3 weeks with standard docetaxel. The primary study objective is progression-free survival, and a total of 550 patients will be included. The Italian ITA-INTN-DISTAL study is a randomized phase III trial of two regimens of docetaxel. Patients receive docetaxel either every 3 weeks for a maximum of six courses or weekly for 6 out of 8 weeks for a maximum of two courses. Two hundred patients will be included, and the main study endpoint is survival.

JMGX is a randomized phase III study of two doses of pemetrexed (Alimta). Patients receive standard-dose pemetrexed at 500 mg/m^2 or pemetrexed 900 mg/m^2 every 3 weeks. The main study objective is to determine if higher doses of Alimta will improve treatment outcome with an acceptable toxicity profile. The accrual target is 300 patients.

Investigators from the Czech Republic have initiated a randomized study comparing oral ZD6474, a novel antiangiogenic agent, with docetaxel at different doses and schedules. The trial objectives are safety, tolerability, and efficacy [42].

37.3.2 First-line Therapy

In Europe we have rather well-organized national groups (e.g., in France, Greece, the UK, the Netherlands, Italy, and Spain) as well as international collaborative groups (e.g., EORTC) capable of planning and conducting even large and demanding trials. Often, the treatment concepts followed in these studies are different from and complementary to those used in North America. As seen in the past and, even more impressively at present, this opens the possibility to substantially broaden scientific evidence, an advantage that has been recognized and is currently being exploited by globally operating sponsors for their drug development programs.

Noteworthy are the contributions to platinum-free combination chemotherapy made by Greek groups [43, 44]. Italy is leading in the development of treatment programs for elderly patients [5, 45] and European investigators have made valuable contributions to the role of single-agent chemotherapy for patients with poor performance status (PS 2) [4]. "Customized chemotherapy" was inaugurated by investigators from Spain [46], and groups from the UK added significant work regarding the role of carboplatin in modern combination regimens [47]. Europe was intensively involved in the development of small molecules, such as erlotinib and gefitinib, as first-line treatment [48–52] and thus had also to share the worldwide disappointment of the negative results. The use of gemcitabine has been significantly advanced in Europe, and the use of modern vinca alkaloids and docetaxel in chemotherapy of advanced NSCLC was promoted in France. At present, it appears that stage IIIB/IV disease is still being extensively studied in Europe.

Improving standard combination chemotherapy by classical means is of continued interest. The BTOG-2 trial of the British Thoracic Oncology Group examines the relative role and dosage of different platinum compounds (cisplatin, carboplatin) in modern chemother-

Table 37.6. NSCLC: advanced stage, first-line therapy

Trial	Country	Phase	Stage	Number	Intervention	Primary endpoint	Status
BTOG-2	UK	III	IIIB/IV	1,350	G/P 50 vs G/P 80 vs G/C	OS	Open
JMDB	International	III	IIIB/IB	17,700	G/P vs Pe/P	OS	Open
GILT	Spain	III	IIIB/IB	369	custCT vs CT	RR	Open
NVALT-4	The Netherlands	II/III	IIIB/IB	540	D/C vs D/C + COX-2 Inh	OS	Open
LLCG 14	UK	II/III	IIIB/IB	720	G/C + Thal vs G/C	OS	Open
BO-17704	International	III	IIIB/IB	1,150	P/G + Beva vs P/G	Toxicity	Open
EORTC-080 21	Europe	III	IIIB/IB	736	IR maintenance	OS	Open
CHNT-GEM-HOSP	UK	III	IIIA/IIIB/IV	400	G/P vs G/C	HOSP	Open
INVITE	Italy	II	IIIB/IV	192	IR vs Vin	PFS	Open
GEM-TAX I V	Germany	II/III	IIIB/IV	233	G/C + Cet vs seqG/D + Cet	NI	Planned
TOPICAL	UK	III	IIIB/IB	664	Tar vs OBS	OS	Open

G Gemcitabine, *P* cisplatin, *C* carboplatin, *Pe* pemetrexed, *custCT* customized chemotherapy, *CT* chemotherapy, *D* docetaxel, *COX-2 Inh* cyclooxygenase-2 inhibitor, *Thal* thalidomide, *Beva* bevacizumab, *IR* Iressa, *Vin* vinorelbine, *Cet* cetuximab, *seqG/D* sequential gemcitabine/carboplatin, *Tar* Tarceva, *OBS* observation, *OS* overall survival, *RR* remission rate, *HOSP* hospitalization, *PFS* progression-free survival, *NI* no inferiority

apy doublets (gemcitabine and cisplatin 80 mg/m^2 versus gemcitabine and carboplatin AUC 5).

JMDB is a global registration study with European participation, designed to establish the promising doublet pemetrexed (Alimta) plus cisplatin as a new treatment standard. This randomized two-arm phase III trial therefore compares pemetrexed/cisplatin with gemcitabine/cisplatin.

GILT (Genotypic International Lung Trial) is investigating the rationale underlying modern combination chemotherapy and its individually tailored use based on the platinum resistance marker ERCC1-mRNA. Patients in this two-arm randomized trial are treated with docetaxel/cisplatin in the control arm, while treatment in the experimental arm depends on the ERCC1 expression status of the individual patients, consisting of either a platinum-based (gemcitabine/cisplatin) or platinum-free (gemcitabine/CPT-11) regimen [46].

Despite the negative experience made with targeted therapies, adding these agents to standard platinum-based doublets is still considered an interesting option. The Dutch phase II/III trial NVALT-4 evaluates the addition of the COX-2 inhibitor celecoxib to chemotherapy with docetaxel/carboplatin. The proposed mechanism of action of celecoxib involves inhibition of angiogenesis, induction of apoptosis, and reduced cell proliferation. The British phase II/III trial LLCG-14 is designed to determine if survival is improved by the addition of thalidomide to standard gemcitabine/carboplatin. Thalidomide has antiangiogenic and anticachectic effects which may complement the antitumor effect obtained with chemotherapy.

Particularly noteworthy is the BO-17704 trial (Hoffmann-La Roche), a global randomized phase III study with significant European participation that evaluates the role of the monoclonal antibody bevacizumab (Avastin) in combination with gemcitabine/cisplatin, a regimen that is widely favored as standard chemother-

apy in Europe. This trial is considered pivotal and confirmative to ECOG-4599, a randomized phase II/III trial of paclitaxel/carboplatin with or without bevacizumab. This study has recently demonstrated that in patients with non-squamous histology, bevacizumab given in combination with platinum-based doublets significantly prolongs survival compared with chemotherapy alone [53].

Another randomized phase III trial is planned to evaluate the immunomodulator CPR 7909 (Promune; Coley/Pfizer), a toll-like receptor inhibitor, in combination with gemcitabine/cisplatin (Europe) or paclitaxel/carboplatin (USA). Initiation of this trial was inspired by the results of a randomized phase II study with European participation that combined Promune with platinum-taxane regimens at various doses. Unspecific immune stimulation with Promune resulted in improved response rate, progression-free survival, and overall survival [54].

In contrast, the EORTC-08021 trial is investigating the sequential use of standard chemotherapy and targeted therapies. After completion of 3–4 cycles of platinum-based combination chemotherapy, patients in the experimental arm receive maintenance therapy with gefitinib (Iressa) 250 mg daily aimed at improving overall survival compared with chemotherapy alone.

The GEM Hospitalization Study is a phase III trial examining the combination of gemcitabine with either cisplatin or carboplatin. Study endpoints are feasibility measures such as the rate of overnight stays in the hospital due to toxicity (e.g., blood transfusions, antibiotic use, and to obtain relief from treatment-related symptoms). In addition, this study compares the need for hospitalization for chemotherapy administration in patients treated with these different regimens.

Another important objective of clinical research is to develop appropriate treatments for patients who are, for various reasons, poor candidates for combination chemotherapy. One trial addressing this subject is TOPI-CAL (Tarceva or Placebo in Clinically Advanced Non-Small-Cell Lung Cancer) initiated by the British London Lung Cancer Group (LLCG). The study involves chemo-naive patients considered unsuitable for chemotherapy, having PS 2 or 3, or PS 0–1 with a calculated creatinine clearance of ≤60 ml/min. Patients are randomized to receive erlotinib (Tarceva) or matched oral placebo daily for up to 24 months. The primary study endpoint is survival.

The French IFCT 0301, a three-arm randomized trial, also evaluates first-line therapy in patients with poor performance status (PS 2–3). Patients are treated with either single-agent gefitinib, gemcitabine, or doce-taxel. The main endpoint of the study is time to tumor progression.

The INVITE study (Iressa in NSCLC vs. Vinorelbine Investigation in the Elderly) from Italy is designed to improve single-agent therapy for elderly patients. It is a randomized phase II trial of gefitinib (Iressa) versus vi-norelbine in a population of nearly 200 patients aged >70 years. The primary endpoint is time to progression.

Another randomized phase II/III study is planned in order to optimize the intensity and quality of che-motherapy in patients with stage IIIB/IV disease (GEM-TAX IV). The study compares sequential single-agent therapy consisting of 2 cycles of gemcitabine followed by 2 cycles of docetaxel with 4 cycles of the platinum-based two-drug combination gemcitabine/carboplatin. In addition to their chemotherapy and thereafter as sin-gle agent until tumor progression, all study patients will receive weekly cetuximab (Erbitux). The primary study endpoint is the "clinically relevant toxicity." The study is scheduled as an international cooperative trial (UK, Germany, Spain, Ireland). Its design is a logical conse-quence of the results obtained in our pilot studies of se-quential single-agent chemotherapy using gemcitabine and docetaxel [55, 56].

37.4 Conclusion

Investigators from Europe have always played an active role in the clinical development of new treatment strate-gies and innovative drugs, and they have made valuable contributions to establishing new treatment standards for patients with NSCLC. The most recent results of the IALT study are particularly noteworthy because they mark a first step toward postoperative, adjuvant che-motherapy of NSCLC. Clinical research in Europe pre-pared well for its tasks over the three decades since 1975, giving rise to a large number of national and su-pranational high-quality, high-performance cooperative groups. As a result of their close connections with na-tional tumor centers, and especially their clinical and

diagnostic units, these groups clearly meet the increas-ing requirements of current and future clinical research. A good example is the growing cooperation between the EORTC, the primary European organization for clin-ical cancer research, and highly renowned North Amer-ican study groups as well as national tumor centers. And there is no doubt that the political changes of the last 15 years have expanded Europe's capability to per-form high-quality clinical trials even further, irrespec-tive of the differences in framework conditions for re-search that are still evident between the European re-gions. Rather, border-crossing clinical research in Eu-rope could be seriously threatened by the ever-increas-ing legal and bureaucratic requirements while research budgets are being reduced.

Key Points

- Investigators from Europe have played an active role in the continuous improvement of treatment for lung cancer and have made valuable contribu-tions to establish new effective treatments in clin-ical routine practice.
- Current activities and clinical studies initiated by European cooperative groups cover all clinical as-pects of lung cancer, from early stages up to pal-liation of patients with advanced disease.

References

1. Pfister DG, Johnson DH, Azzoli CG, et al. American So-ciety of Clinical Oncology treatment of unresectable non-small-cell lung cancer guideline: update 2003. J Clin Oncol 2004;22:330.
2. Farray D, Mirkovic N, Albain KS. Multimodality therapy for stage III non-small-cell lung cancer. J Clin Oncol 2005;23:3257.
3. Felip E, Stahel RA, Pavlidis N. ESMO Minimum clinical recommendations for diagnosis, treatment and follow-up of non-small-cell lung cancer (NSCLC). Ann Oncol 2005;16(suppl 1):i28.
4. Gridelli C, Ardizzoni A, Le Chevalier T, et al. Treatment of advanced non-small-cell lung cancer patients with ECOG performance status 2: results of a European experts panel. Ann Oncol 2004;15:419.
5. Gridelli C, Aapro M, Ardizzoni A, et al. Treatment of ad-vanced non-small-cell lung cancer in the elderly: results of an international expert panel. J Clin Oncol 2005;23:3125.
6. Pincus M, Reddy S, Lee MS, et al. Preoperative combined modality therapy for stage III M0 non-small cell lung car-cinoma. Int J Radiat Oncol Biol Phys 1988;15:189.
7. Albain KS, Crowley JJ, Turrisi AT 3rd, et al. Concurrent cisplatin, etoposide, and chest radiotherapy in pathologic stage IIIB non-small-cell lung cancer: a Southwest Oncol-ogy Group phase II study, SWOG 9019. J Clin Oncol 2002;20:3454.

8. Eberhardt W, Wilke H, Stamatis G, et al. Preoperative chemotherapy followed by concurrent chemoradiation therapy based on hyperfractionated accelerated radiotherapy and definitive surgery in locally advanced non-small-cell lung cancer: mature results of a phase II trial. J Clin Oncol 1998;16:622.

9. Rosell R, Gomez-Codina J, Camps C, et al. A randomized trial comparing preoperative chemotherapy plus surgery with surgery alone in patients with non-small-cell lung cancer. N Engl J Med 1994;330:153

10. Rosell R, Gomez-Codina J, Camps C, et al. Preresectional chemotherapy in stage IIIA non-small-cell lung cancer: a 7-year assessment of a randomized controlled trial. Lung Cancer 1999;26:7.

11. Depierre A, Milleron B, Moro-Sibilot D, et al. Preoperative chemotherapy followed by surgery compared with primary surgery in resectable stage I (except T1N0), II, and IIIa non-small-cell lung cancer. J Clin Oncol 2002;20:247.

12. Splinter TA, van Schil PE, Kramer GW, et al. Randomized trial of surgery versus radiotherapy in patients with stage IIIA (N2) non small-cell lung cancer after a response to induction chemotherapy. EORTC 08941. Clin Lung Cancer 2000;2:69:73.

13. De Marinis F, Nelli F, Migliorino MR, et al. Gemcitabine, paclitaxel, and cisplatin as induction chemotherapy for patients with biopsy-proven stage IIIA(N2) non-small cell lung carcinoma: a phase II multicenter study. Cancer 2003;98:1707.

14. Manegold, C, Biesma B, Smit H, et al. Docetaxel and cisplatin as induction chemotherapy in stage IIIA N2 non-small cell lung cancer (NSCLC): an EORTC phase II trial (08984). J Clin Oncol (meeting abstracts) 2004;22(14 suppl):7166.

15. Van Zandwijk N, Smit EF, Kramer GW, et al. Gemcitabine and cisplatin as induction regimen for patients with biopsy-proven stage IIIA N2 non-small-cell lung cancer: a phase II study of the European Organization for Research and Treatment of Cancer Lung Cancer Cooperative Group (EORTC 08955). J Clin Oncol 2000;18:2658.

16. Betticher DC, Hsu Schmitz SF, Totsch M, et al. Mediastinal lymph node clearance after docetaxel-cisplatin neoadjuvant chemotherapy is prognostic of survival in patients with stage IIIA pN2 non-small-cell lung cancer: a multicenter phase II trial. J Clin Oncol 2003;21:1752.

17. Betticher DC, Rosell R. Neoadjuvant treatment of early-stage resectable non-small-cell lung cancer. Lung Cancer 2004;46(suppl 2):S23.

18. O'Brien ME, Smith I, Postmus PE, et al. Taxol and carboplatin induction chemotherapy in stage III non-small cell lung cancer (NSCLC): an EORTC 08958 phase II trial. J Clin Oncol (meeting abstracts) 1999;18:492a.

19. Thomas M, Rube C, Semik M, et al. Impact of preoperative bimodality induction including twice-daily radiation on tumor regression and survival in stage III non-small-cell lung cancer. J Clin Oncol 1999;17:1185.

20. Thomas M, Macha HN, Ukena D, et al. Cisplatin/etoposide (PE) followed by twice-daily chemoradiation (hfRT/CT) versus PE alone before surgery in stage III non-small cell lung cancer (NSCLC): a randomized phase III trial of the German Lung Cancer Cooperative Group (GLCCG). J Clin Oncol (meeting abstracts) 2004;22(14 suppl):7004.

21. Non-small Cell Lung Cancer Collaborative Group. Chemotherapy in non-small cell lung cancer: a meta-analysis using updated data on individual patients from 52 randomised clinical trials. BMJ 1995;311:899.

22. Scagliotti GV, Fossati R, Torri V, et al. Randomized study of adjuvant chemotherapy for completely resected stage I, II, or IIIA non-small-cell lung cancer. J Natl Cancer Inst 2003;95:1453.

23. Waller D, Peake MD, Stephens RJ, et al. Chemotherapy for patients with non-small cell lung cancer: the surgical setting of the Big Lung Trial. Eur J Cardiothorac Surg 2004;26:173.

24. Arriagada R, Bergman B, Dunant A, Le Chevalier T, Pignon JP, Vansteenkiste J. Cisplatin-based adjuvant chemotherapy in patients with completely resected non-small-cell lung cancer. N Engl J Med 2004;350:351.

25. Kato H, Ichinose Y, Ohta M, et al. A randomized trial of adjuvant chemotherapy with uracil-tegafur for adenocarcinoma of the lung. N Engl J Med 2004;350:1713.

26. Winton TL, Livingston R, Johnson D, et al. A prospective randomised trial of adjuvant vinorelbine (VIN) and cisplatin (CIS) in completely resected stage 1B and II non small cell lung cancer (NSCLC) Intergroup JBR.10. J Clin Oncol (meeting abstracts) 2004;22(14 suppl):7018.

27. Winton T, Livingston R, Johnson D, et al. Vinorelbine plus cisplatin vs. observation in resected non-small-cell lung cancer. N Engl J Med 2005;352:2589.

28. Strauss GM, Herndon J, Maddaus MA, et al. Randomized clinical trial of adjuvant chemotherapy with paclitaxel and carboplatin following resection in stage IB non-small cell lung cancer (NSCLC): report of Cancer and Leukemia Group B (CALGB) Protocol 9633. J Clin Oncol (meeting abstracts) 2004;22(14 suppl):7019.

29. Douillard JY, Rosell R, Delena M, Legroumellec A, Torres A, Carpagnano F. ANITA: phase III adjuvant vinorelbine (N) and cisplatin (P) versus observation (OBS) in completely resected (stage I–III) non-small-cell lung cancer (NSCLC) patients (pts): final results after 70-month median follow-up. On behalf of the Adjuvant Navelbine International Trialist Association. J Clin Oncol (meeting abstracts) 2005;23(16 suppl):7013.

30. Dillman RO, Herndon J, Seagren SL, Eaton WL Jr, Green MR. Improved survival in stage III non-small-cell lung cancer: seven-year follow-up of cancer and leukemia group B (CALGB) 8433 trial. J Natl Cancer Inst 1996;88:1210.

31. Schaake-Koning C, van den Bogaert W, Dalesio O, et al. Effects of concomitant cisplatin and radiotherapy on inoperable non-small-cell lung cancer. N Engl J Med 1992;326:524.

32. Sause W, Kolesar P, Taylor SI, et al. Final results of phase III trial in regionally advanced unresectable non-small-cell lung cancer: Radiation Therapy Oncology Group, Eastern Cooperative Oncology Group, and Southwest Oncology Group. Chest 2000;117:358.

33. Le Chevalier T, Arriagada R, Quoix E, et al. Radiotherapy alone versus combined chemotherapy and radiotherapy in unresectable non-small cell lung carcinoma. Lung Cancer 1994;10(suppl 1):S239.

34. Curran WJ, Scott CB, Langer CJ, et al. Long-term benefit is observed in a phase III comparison of sequential vs concurrent chemo-radiation for patients with unresected stage III NSCLC: RTOG 9410 [abstract 2499]. Proc Am Soc Clin Oncol 2003;22:621.

35. Furuse K, Fukuoka M, Kawahara M, et al. Phase III study of concurrent versus sequential thoracic radiotherapy in combination with mitomycin, vindesine, and cisplatin in unresectable stage III non-small-cell lung cancer. J Clin Oncol 1999;17:2692.

36. Pierre F, Maurice P, Gilles R, et al. A randomized phase III trial of sequential chemo-radiotherapy versus concurrent chemo-radiotherapy in locally advanced non small cell lung cancer (NSCLC) (GLOT-GFPC NPC 95-01 study) [abstract]. 2001 ASCO Annual Meeting 2001;20:1246.

37. Gandara DR, Chansky K, Albain KS, et al. Consolidation docetaxel after concurrent chemoradiotherapy in stage IIIB non-small-cell lung cancer: phase II Southwest Oncology Group Study S9504. J Clin Oncol 2003;21:2004.

38. Zatloukal P, Petruzelka L, Zemanova M, et al. Concurrent versus sequential chemoradiotherapy with cisplatin and vinorelbine in locally advanced non-small cell lung cancer: a randomized study. Lung Cancer 2004;46:87.

39. Shepherd FA, Dancey J, Ramlau R, et al. Prospective randomized trial of docetaxel versus best supportive care in patients with non-small-cell lung cancer previously treated with platinum-based chemotherapy. J Clin Oncol 2000;18:2095.

40. Fossella FV, DeVore R, Kerr RN, et al. Randomized phase III trial of docetaxel versus vinorelbine or ifosfamide in patients with advanced non-small-cell lung cancer previously treated with platinum-containing chemotherapy regimens. The TAX 320 Non-small Cell Lung Cancer Study Group. J Clin Oncol 2000;18:2354.

41. Hanna N, Shepherd FA, Fossella FV, et al. Randomized phase III trial of pemetrexed versus docetaxel in patients with non-small-cell lung cancer previously treated with chemotherapy. J Clin Oncol 2004;22:1589.

42. Heymach JV, Dong RP, Dimery I, et al. ZD6474, a novel antiangiogenic agent, in combination with docetaxel in patients with NSCLC: results of the run-in phase of a two-part, randomized phase II study. J Clin Oncol (meeting abstracts) 2004;22(14 suppl):3051.

43. Kosmidis P, Mylonakis N, Nicolaides C, et al. Paclitaxel plus carboplatin versus gemcitabine plus paclitaxel in advanced non-small-cell lung cancer: a phase III randomized trial. J Clin Oncol 2002;20:3578.

44. Georgoulias V, Ardavanis A, Tsiafaki X, et al. Vinorelbine plus cisplatin versus docetaxel plus gemcitabine in advanced non-small-cell lung cancer: a phase III randomized trial. J Clin Oncol 2005;23:293.

45. Gridelli C, Perrone F, Gallo C, et al. Chemotherapy for elderly patients with advanced non-small-cell lung cancer: the Multicenter Italian Lung Cancer in the Elderly Study (MILES) phase III randomized trial. J Natl Cancer Inst 2003;95:362.

46. Rosell R, Cobo M, Isla D, et al. ERCC1 mRNA-based randomized phase III trial of docetaxel (doc) doublets with cisplatin (cis) or gemcitabine (gem) in stage IV non-small-cell lung cancer (NSCLC) patients (p). J Clin Oncol (meeting abstracts) 2005;23(16 suppl):7002.

47. Rudd RM, Gower NH, Spiro SG, et al. Gemcitabine plus carboplatin versus mitomycin, ifosfamide, and cisplatin in patients with stage IIIB or IV non-small-cell lung cancer: a phase III randomized study of the London Lung Cancer Group. J Clin Oncol 2005;23:142.

48. Giaccone G, Herbst RS, Manegold C, et al. Gefitinib in combination with gemcitabine and cisplatin in advanced non-small-cell lung cancer: a phase III trial—INTACT 1. Clin Oncol 2004;22:777.

49. Herbst RS, Giaccone G, Schiller JH, et al. Gefitinib in combination with paclitaxel and carboplatin in advanced non-small-cell lung cancer: a phase III trial—INTACT 2. Clin Oncol 2004;22:785.

50. Herbst RS, Prager D, Hermann R, et al. TRIBUTE: a phase III trial of erlotinib HCl (OSI-774) combined with carboplatin and paclitaxel (CP) chemotherapy in advanced non-small cell lung cancer (NSCLC). J Clin Oncol (meeting abstracts) 2004;22(14 suppl):7011.

51. Gatzemeier U, Pluzanska A, Szczesna A, et al. Results of a phase III trial of erlotinib (OSI-774) combined with cisplatin and gemcitabine (GC) chemotherapy in advanced non-small cell lung cancer (NSCLC). J Clin Oncol (meeting abstracts) 2004;22(14 suppl):7010.

52. Fukuoka M, Yano S, Giaccone G, et al. Multi-institutional randomized phase II trial of gefitinib for previously treated patients with advanced non-small-cell lung cancer (The IDEAL 1 Trial) [corrected]. J Clin Oncol 2003;21:2237.

53. Sandler AB, Gray R, Brahme J, et al. Randomized phase II/III trial of paclitaxel (P) plus carboplatin (C) with or without bevacizumab (NSC # 704865) in patients with advanced non-squamous non-small cell lung cancer (NSCLC): an Eastern Cooperative Oncology Group (ECOG) trial—E4599. Clin Oncol (meeting abstracts) 2005;22(LBA4):1090s.

54. Leichman G, Gravenor D, Woytowitz D, et al. CPG 7909, a TLR9 agonist, added to first line taxane/platinum for advanced non-small cell lung cancer: a randomized, controlled phase II study. J Clin Oncol (meeting abstracts) 2005;23(16 suppl):7039.

55. Mueller A, Thatcher N, Kortsik C, et al. A phase II/III randomized study in advanced non-small cell lung cancer (NSCLC) with first line combination versus sequential gemcitabine and docetaxel: interim study results. J Clin Oncol (meeting abstracts) 2004;22(14 suppl):7095.

56. Manegold C, Thatcher N, Kortsik C, et al. A phase II/III randomized study in advanced non-small cell lung cancer (NSCLC) with first line combination versus sequential gemcitabine (G) and docetaxel (D): update on quality of life (QoL), toxicity, and costs. J Clin Oncol (meeting abstracts) 2005;23(16 suppl):7057.

North American Cooperative Group Research Efforts in Lung Cancer

38

Heather Wakelee and David R. Gandara

Contents

38.1 Introduction

Lung cancer is the leading cause of cancer death in North America and claims more lives than breast, prostate, and colon cancer combined [1]. Since 1985 have witnessed gradual progress in treatment, with most of the pivotal phase III trials in North America conducted within the National Cancer Institute (NCI)-sponsored cooperative group framework. Within the USA, there are four general oncology cooperative groups: the Eastern Cooperative Oncology Group (ECOG), the Southwest Oncology Group (SWOG), the Cancer and Leukemia Group B (CALGB), and the North Central Cancer Treatment Group (NCCTG). ECOG, SWOG, and CALGB include member institutions from throughout the country, while NCCTG is a regional cooperative group centered around the Mayo Clinic. Within Canada, the National Cancer Institute Canada (NCIC) oversees cooperative oncology efforts. Two more focused cooperative oncology groups who play a pivotal role and cross the US/Canadian border are the American College of Surgeons Oncology Group (ACOSOG) and the Radiation Therapy Oncology Group (RTOG). Here we outline the current and planned trials of each of these organizations and give an overview of the vision of each group. Trials which have recently been completed, but have not yet been reported, are also listed.

Recent contributions of the North American cooperative group in advanced non-small cell lung cancer (NSCLC) include the NCIC pivotal trial showing a survival benefit with single-agent erlotinib in second- or third-line treatment of NSCLC [2], and the ECOG trial showing a survival benefit first-line with the addition of bevacizumab to standard chemotherapy [3]. SWOG has continued to investigate treatment options for early-stage NSCLC by comparing preoperative chemotherapy to surgery alone [4] and locally advanced NSCLC with several phase II and III trials of chemoradiotherapy [5, 6]. Many of the most important contributions have been conducted through the Lung Intergroup, where several or all of the North American cooperative groups collaborate together to enhance accrual, such as recent studies on the use of adjuvant chemotherapy for resected early-stage NSCLC [7, 8]. The cooperative groups have performed a service of equal importance by defining which new therapies should not be adopted as standard of care, such as the CALGB-led Intergroup trial in extensive-stage small cell lung cancer (SCLC) showing no differences in survival for cisplatin/etoposide with or without paclitaxel [9].

There are currently seven open phase III trials within the North American cooperative group framework (Table 38.1). Most of these are collaborative efforts between several groups. They will be discussed in detail within the section of the leading cooperative group.

38.2 Eastern Cooperative Oncology Group (ECOG)

ECOG recently reported positive results from a phase III trial of chemotherapy with or without bevacizumab, an antibody against vascular endothelial growth factor (VEGF), for patients with newly diagnosed NSCLC, who met strict eligibility criteria (non-squamous histology,

Table 38.1. Open North American Cooperative Group phase III trials

	Subtype and stage	Treatment	Primary endpoint	Patients	Projected completion
ECOG 3598	Stage III NSCLC	Carboplatin, paclitaxel, radiotherapy, ± thalidomide	Survival and TTP	588	Early 2007
ECOG 5597	Resected stage I NSCLC	Selenium supplementation vs placebo	Second primary NSCLC prevention	1,960	2010
SWOG 0124	E-SCLC, first line	Cisplatin/etoposide vs cisplatin/irinotecan	Survival	620	Late 2006
ACOSOG Z4032	Stage I NSCLC, poor pulmonary function	Sublobar resection ± brachytherapy seeds (^{125}I)	Local recurrence	226	Opened July 2005
RTOG 0412	Stage IIIA (N2) NSCLC	Preoperative chemotherapy vs chemoradio-therapy then surgery + consolidation chemotherapy	Survival	574	2009
RTOG 0214	Locally advanced NSCLC	PCI vs observation	Survival	1,058	?
RTOG 0212	L-SCLC	Standard vs high dose and q.d. vs b.i.d. PCI	Incidence of brain metastases	264	2009

ECOG Eastern Cooperative Oncology Group, *SWOG* Southwest Oncology Group, *ACOSOG* American College of Surgeons Oncology Group, *RTOG* Radiation Therapy Oncology Group, *NSCLC* non-small cell lung cancer, *E-SCLC* extensive-stage small cell lung cancer, *L-SCLC* limited-stage small cell lung cancer, *vs* versus, *PCI* prophylactic cranial irradiation, *q.d.* daily, *b.i.d.* twice daily, *TTP* time to progression

no hemoptysis, no central tumors, no anticoagulation, no brain metastases) [3]. Many ongoing and planned trials will build on this success. ECOG currently has six open NSCLC trials and three SCLC trials, with several others about to open.

Of these trials, two are phase III studies, E3598 and E5597. On E3598, an Intergroup trial, patients receive two cycles of carboplatin and paclitaxel every 3 weeks and, in the absence of progressive disease (PD), are then randomized to receive either carboplatin and paclitaxel weekly with daily thoracic radiotherapy to 60 Gy, or the same regimen with thalidomide given daily. The primary endpoint of the trial is overall survival (OS). Extensive correlative studies are included. E5597 consists of 4 years of selenium supplementation versus placebo in patients with resected NSCLC who have received no other cancer therapy ($n = 1,960$). After a 4-week run-in to assess compliance, patients are randomized to either selenium (200 µg in the form of selenized yeast) or placebo yeast tablet. Stratification is by gender and smoking status. The primary endpoint for this study is the incidence of

second primary lung cancer. Correlative studies looking at oxidative stress are incorporated.

ECOG has three phase II studies open for patients with advanced NSCLC, E3503, E1503, and E2501 (Table 38.2). Patients with newly diagnosed advanced-stage disease on E3503 receive erlotinib, an epidermal growth factor receptor (EGFR) inhibitor, at 150 mg orally daily until PD. Dose escalation by 25 mg/day up to 250 mg/day until a grade 3 acneiform rash or a dose-limiting toxicity (DLT) develops is included in the study. Response rate (RR) will be calculated, as will time to progression (TTP), OS, and disease control rate. ECOG will try to determine if a grade 2 rash is a predictor of response and/or patient survival.

E1503 is open to NSCLC patients who require second-line therapy. Patients on this trial receive triapine and gemcitabine and are evaluated for RR, stable disease (SD) rate, TTP, duration of response, survival, safety, and tolerability of the combination.

E2501 is open to patients who have had at least two prior regimens for advanced NSCLC and employs a ran-

Table 38.2. ECOG phase II trials: advanced NSCLC

	Line of therapy	Treatment	Primary endpoint	Patients	Projected completion
E1503	Second line	Triapine/gemcitabine	RR	48	2006
E2501	Third line +	BAY 43-9006 (sorafenib)	RR/SD	227	2007
E3503	First line	Erlotinib	Identify predictive markers of EGFR response	129	Early 2006

RR Response rate, *SD* stable disease, *EGFR* epidermal growth factor receptor

domized discontinuation design in which all patients are started on sorafenib (raf kinase inhibitor and VEGF receptor [VEGFR] inhibitor) for 8 weeks. At the end of 8 weeks, those with PD are discontinued, those with partial response (PR) or complete response (CR) are continued and those with SD are randomized to continue drug or get placebo for 8 weeks. For those randomized, at the time of disease progression, the drug is unblinded and those on placebo may receive active drug until evidence of progression. The primary endpoint is RR, but median survival time (MST) and progression-free survival (PFS) will also be determined. Molecular markers will be correlated to response.

E4503, a phase II study of 110 patients, enrolls patients with resectable, biopsy proven stage IA–IIIA NSCLC to receive 14 days of preoperative erlotinib (150 mg orally daily). Blood and skin samples are collected prior to treatment, at completion of therapy, and 4–6 weeks postsurgery. The primary response of pMAPk and pAKT to daily erlotinib for 14 days will be assessed, along with the safety and tolerance of the drug. Patterns of gene and protein expression, pretherapy and posttherapy, that are associated with response will also be evaluated.

There are currently three open ECOG trials for patients with extensive-stage SCLC (E-SCLC) (Table 38.3). On E3501, patients with newly diagnosed E-SCLC receive 4 cycles of chemotherapy (cisplatin and etoposide) plus bevacizumab, which continues for 1 year or until disease progression. RR and OS will be evaluated in addition to the primary endpoint of PFS. Pretreatment levels of plasma VEGF and other proteins will be collected to see if they predict for response to the combination regimen and survival.

E5501, also open to patients with newly diagnosed E-SCLC, is a randomized phase II trial of sequence applications of two topoisomerase inhibitors (topotecan and irinotecan). This study will look at toxicity, RR, PFS, and OS. The two arms of the study are arm A: topotecan days 1–3 followed by etoposide and cisplatin days 8–10 or arm B: irinotecan and cisplatin days 1 and 8 plus etoposide days 3 and 10. Both arms are repeated up to 6 times (or more at the discretion of the investigator) with each cycle lasting 3 weeks.

E6501 is open to patients with relapsed SCLC who receive interferon alpha plus 13-cis-retinoic acid plus weekly paclitaxel for 6 weeks with a 2-week rest period. The 13-cis-retinoinc acid is given to modulate bcl-2 and paclitaxel is given to improve interferon alpha drug response. Bcl-2 levels in peripheral blood monocytes, prior to therapy and on day 3 of the first cycle of therapy, will be monitored. Toxicities will be evaluated as well as RR, and OS.

ECOG also has a trial open through the Lung Intergroup, for patients with thymoma or thymic carcinoma, E1C99. The primary objective of this trial is to assess the response rate of carboplatin and paclitaxel in this patient population. A total of 68 patients will be accrued, and it is estimated that the first stage of accrual will be reached in June 2006.

There are multiple trials in development within the ECOG framework, four of which, E1505, E1504, E2504, and E1B03, are discussed below:

1. E1505 – phase III trial of adjuvant therapy for resected stage IB–IIIA NSCLC. Patients with completely resected disease will be randomized to receive 4 cycles of platinum-based chemotherapy, or the same chemotherapy plus bevacizumab. The bevacizumab will be continued for up to 1 year. The primary endpoint will be OS, but disease-free survival (DFS), and toxicity will also be followed. Multiple correlative studies are planned as well.

2. E1504 – phase II study of the anti-EGFR antibody cetuximab (C225) in patients with advanced-stage bronchioloalveolar carcinoma (BAC) or adenocarcinoma with BAC features.

3. E2504 – randomized phase II trial of cetuximab in patients with a poor performance status (PS 2) and advanced NSCLC. Patients will be randomized to either cetuximab followed by paclitaxel and carboplatin for 4 cycles at the time of disease progression, or paclitaxel, carboplatin, and cetuximab initially for 4 cycles (with continuation of the cetuximab until progression).

Table 38.3. ECOG phase II trials: SCLC

	Stage	Treatment	Primary endpoint	Patients	Projected completion
E3501	Extensive; first line	Cisplatin/etoposide/bevacizumab	PFS, toxicity	66	Early 2006
E5501	Extensive; first line	Topotecan d1–3, etoposide + cisplatin d8–10 vs Irinotecan + cisplatin d1, 8 and etoposide d3, 10	RR	60	2007
E6501	Extensive; second line +	Interferon alpha and 13-cis-retinoic acid d1, 2 for 6/8 wks paclitaxel d2 weekly for 6/8 wks	RR	83	2009

d Days, *wks* weeks, *PFS* progression-free survival

4. E1B03 – randomized phase II trial of pemetrexed plus either carboplatin or gemcitabine in newly diagnosed mesothelioma. The trial will evaluate RR (primary objective), relative toxicities, and survival with the two regimens. An additional component of the trial is to explore incidence and prognostic implications of SV40.

38.3   Southwest Oncology Group (SWOG)

Two phase III SWOG trials, S9900 and S0023, were recently closed prematurely due to results from outside trials. Preliminary results of both S9900 and S0023 were presented at the American Society of Clinical Oncology (ASCO) meeting in 2005. Preliminary results from S9900, a randomized trial of neoadjuvant paclitaxel/carboplatin chemotherapy prior to surgical resection of early-stage NSCLC, are inconclusive, but point to the need for randomized studies of neoadjuvant versus adjuvant therapy in this setting [4]. S0023 investigated the role of the EGFR tyrosine kinase inhibitor gefitinib as maintenance therapy following chemoradiotherapy, building on earlier SWOG phase II data in the setting of inoperable stage IIIB NSCLC [5]. Patients received the SWOG regimen of cisplatin/etoposide/concurrent radiation therapy followed by consolidation docetaxel, and were then randomized to receive gefitinib or placebo. The study was closed early based on the negative Iressa Survival Evaluation in Lung Cancer (ISEL) trial of gefitinib versus placebo [10]. Preliminary results of S0023 showed no benefit with the addition of gefitinib [6].

Two recently closed, but not yet reported, SWOG phase II studies explored the use of bortezomib in lung cancer. Sixty patients with previously treated E-SCLC were treated with single-agent bortezomib on S0327. S0339 enrolled 121 patients with chemonaive advanced NSCLC to receive bortezomib with carboplatin and gemcitabine. Ongoing SWOG trials are discussed below. SWOG has also developed a tissue repository trial

(S9925) through its Lung Correlative Science Subcommittee. This study is open to participants of other SWOG lung cancer protocols, in order to investigate potential biomarkers predictive of patient outcomes. Using this resource, S0424 is a recently opened SWOG-led Intergroup study investigating molecular epidemiology of NSCLC in smoking and non-smoking men and women. This study assesses the influence of smoking, hormonal and reproductive factors, and other exposures on gender differences in lung cancer risk.

S0124 is a randomized phase III comparison of the standard cisplatin and etoposide combination to the Japanese regimen of cisplatin and irinotecan for newly diagnosed E-SCLC. The primary endpoint of this trial is OS. Correlative trials will include UGT1A1 (irinotecan metabolism), ERCC-1 (cisplatin metabolism), and XRCC-1 polymorphism analysis.

S0222, a phase II study for limited-stage SCLC (L-SCLC), builds on prior SWOG experience by evaluating the hypoxic cytotoxin tirapazime in combination with concurrent cisplatin-etoposide and thoracic radiation. The primary endpoint of the trial is OS, but TTP, RR, and toxicity will also be evaluated. Exploratory laboratory analyses include PAI-1, VEGF, osteopontin, and other plasma markers. This study is expected to complete accrual by late 2006.

SWOG has four open NSCLC trials, S0341, S0342, S0310, and S0220 (Table 38.4). S0220 is a SWOG-led Intergroup study open for patients will locally advanced, superior sulcus tumors, while the other three studies are for patients with advanced disease.

S0220 is limited to patients with superior sulcus (Pancoast) tumors (T3-4) who do not have mediastinal or supraclavicular nodal involvement (N0-N1). Treatment consists of the standard SWOG regimen of concurrent cisplatin and etoposide with concurrent radiotherapy (61 Gy) followed by surgical resection if feasible, followed by 3 cycles of consolidation docetaxel given every 21 days. In addition to OS, other criteria including RR, resectability rate, and toxicity will be evaluated, as well as several laboratory correlates.

Table 38.4. SWOG phase II trials: NSCLC

	Disease; line of therapy	Treatment	Primary endpoint	Patients	Projected closure
S0220	Pancoast tumors (N0, N1); first line	Cisplatin + etoposide + radiotherapy followed by surgical resection followed by consolidation docetaxel	OS	144	Slow accrual
S0342	Advanced NSCLC; first line	Carboplatin + paclitaxel concurrent with or followed by cetuximab	OS	180	2006
S0341	Advanced NSCLC, PS 2; first line	Erlotinib	OS	65	2006
S0310	Advanced bronchiolo-alveolar carcinoma; any line of therapy	Autologous cancer vaccine	OS	117	September 2005

PS Performance status, *OS* overall survival

S0342 is open to all newly diagnosed, advanced NSCLC patients. In this phase II selection design trial, all patients receive standard carboplatin and paclitaxel followed by maintenance with the EGFR antibody cetuximab. In order to determine whether sequence specificity exists for cetuximab and chemotherapy, half of the patients are randomized to receive the cetuximab starting concurrently with the chemotherapy, and half to start it after completion of all cycles of chemotherapy. Survival will be the primary endpoint, but RR, toxicity, and exploratory molecular correlative studies will also be evaluated. A total of 180 patients will be accrued. This study is designed to select a regimen for comparison with chemotherapy alone in a subsequent phase III trial.

Poor performance status (PS 2) patients with newly diagnosed NSCLC are eligible for S0341, a trial of single-agent erlotinib. This study which will look at OS, RR, functional and symptomatic status, and toxicities. EGFR expression levels and polymorphisms will be correlated with PFS and OS, as will other signaling pathways such as p27. If encouraging, this study will be followed by a subsequent phase III trial in which PS 2 patients with EGFR-positive tumors by fluorescence in situ hybridization (FISH) [11] will be randomized to erlotinib or chemotherapy.

S0310 is limited to patients with advanced bronchioloalveolar carcinoma who have tumor that is accessible for harvest via thoracentesis or surgical procedure. The harvested tumor is processed to make the vaccine (CG8123, formerly GVAX) which is given to the patient. Patients who have and have not been previously treated are eligible. The primary endpoint is survival, but PFS, RR, and toxicity will also be evaluated.

An ancillary trial to S0023, S0229, randomizes patients who had completed the consolidation chemotherapy phase of the protocol (currently receiving either gefitinib or placebo) to 12 weeks of an exercise program versus education about exercise. The study opened in September 2004 and S0023 closed to accrual in March 2005. It is therefore unlikely that the full 164 planned patients will be accrued.

SWOG has multiple trials in development, four of which are discussed below:

1. S0429 – phase II trial of weekly docetaxel and cetuximab with radiation therapy for patients with poor-risk stage III NSCLC.
2. S0436 – phase II combination of pemetrexed and bevacizumab in advanced NSCLC patients who have progressed after first-line therapy.
3. S0435 – phase II trial of sorafenib (BAY 43-9006) for previously treated E-SCLC.
4. S0509 – phase II trial of the oral agent AZD2171 (VEGFR inhibitor) in malignant pleural mesothelioma.

38.4 Cancer and Leukemia Group B (CALGB)

CALGB has led several important NSCLC trials presented recently, including a positive adjuvant therapy trial in resected stage IB disease [8], and a negative trial in locally advanced disease which failed to show a survival benefit with induction chemotherapy prior to concurrent chemoradiotherapy [12]. CALGB currently has three NSCLC trials open and four in SCLC.

C30102, a phase III trial in patients with a malignant pleural effusion from any malignancy, recently closed without meeting its accrual goal. The study was open to any patient with a unilateral pleural effusion requiring sclerosis or drainage and no prior intrapleural therapy. Patients were randomized to either receive a chest tube placement and talc slurry (standard pleurodesis) versus placement of a small catheter (pleurX).

Table 38.5 outlines the currently open phase II NSCLC trials, C39904, C140203, and C30303. C39904, phase I, dose escalates accelerated three-dimensional conformal radiotherapy in patients with stage I NSCLC with pulmonary dysfunction or other co-morbidities which make them inoperable. The primary objective will be determination of the maximum-tolerated dose (MTD), but toxicity, local control, failure-free survival (FFS), and OS will be followed as well. Pulmonary toxicity will also be correlated with the effect of the radiotherapy dose volume and pretreatment pulmonary function.

Table 38.5. CALGB phase II trials: NSCLC

	Stage; line of therapy	Treatment	Primary endpoint	Patients
C39904	Stage I (4 cm), pulmonary dysfunction; phase I	3-D conformal radiotherapy	MTD	8–32
C140203	Stage I; phase II	Sentinel LN mapping	Feasibility and accuracy of mapping	150
C30303	Advanced; first line, randomized phase II	Dose dense cisplatin, docetaxel, with or without dimesna (BNP7787)	RR, toxicity (neuropathy)	142

3-D Three-dimensional, *MTD* maximum-tolerated dose, *LN* lymph node

Sentinel lymph node mapping has been a standard therapy in breast cancer, but is not commonly utilized in lung cancer. C140203, a phase II trial in 150 patients, looks at intraoperative sentinel lymph node mapping using technetium Tc99 sulfur colloid in patients with stage I NSCLC. The primary objective of the study is to determine the feasibility and accuracy of this technique with a focus on the percentage of patients who are found to have positive sentinel lymph nodes, particularly in the absence of other positive lymph nodes. The presence of positive sentinel lymph nodes (especially micrometastases) will be correlated with survival. The presence of skip metastases will also be evaluated.

The primary objective of C30303, a randomized phase II trial in patients with newly diagnosed NSCLC, is to determine if the addition of dimesna (BNP7787) to cisplatin and docetaxel will reduce peripheral neuropathy without altering RR (n=142). OS, FFS, and other toxicity (including nephrotoxicity) will also be assessed. It should be noted that the cisplatin and docetaxel (both at 75 mg/m^2) are given in a "dose-dense" fashion every 2 weeks with growth factor support (pegfilgrastim and darbepoetin alfa) in this trial for a total of 6 cycles.

CALGB has four open phase II SCLC trials: C30206, C30306, C30103, and C30304 (Table 38.6). C30206 includes induction chemotherapy with 2 cycles (6 weeks total) of cisplatin and irinotecan followed by concurrent carboplatin and etoposide (given every 21 days for 3 cycles) with daily radiotherapy over 6–7 weeks (to 70 Gy) for patients with newly diagnosed, untreated, L-SCLC. The percentage of patients alive at 2 years will be the primary endpoint of efficacy of this regimen. RR, OS, FFS, toxicity, and tolerability will be assessed, as will response to the cisplatin/irinotecan induction.

Two CALGB trials in E-SCLC, and one in relapsed SCLC are exploring novel agents: bevacizumab, oblimersen, and depsipeptide (FK228). Patients with previously untreated E-SCLC on C30306 receive cisplatin and irinotecan on days 1 and 8 and bevacizumab day 1 every 21 days for up to 6 cycles. The primary endpoint is percentage of patients alive at 12 months, but toxicity, RR, and VEGF levels will also be assessed. C30103, a randomized phase II trial of carboplatin and etoposide with or without oblimersen (antisense agent to bcl-2) for newly diagnosed, E-SCLC patients, will look at 12-month survival, RR, and toxicity. The majority (41/55)

of patients on this trial will receive oblimersen. C30304 will determine the RR, OS, FFS, and toxicity of weekly depsipeptide (FK228), a histone deacetylase inhibitor, when given to patients with recurrent SCLC. Biologic markers of activity of the agent are included in this trial of 36 patients.

C30307 is exploring sorafenib (BAY 43-9006) in patients with mesothelioma. A total of 44 patients will be enrolled in this phase II single-agent trial in previously untreated (or treated with only one prior regimen) mesothelioma. Sorafenib will be given at 400 mg orally twice daily. RR is the primary endpoint, but OS, FFS, toxicity, and extensive correlative studies are included.

Four planned CALGB future trials are outlined below:
1. C30502 – single-arm pharmacogenetic cohort study of second-line pemetrexed for patients with advanced NSCLC which will explore whether survival is associated with differences in thymidylate synthase (TS) genotype.
2. C30406 – randomized phase II study of erlotinib with or without carboplatin/paclitaxel in patients with adenocarcinoma of the lung who were never or light smokers. PFS is the primary endpoint in this study, which will include extensive correlative studies in all 180 patients.
3. C30402 – randomized phase II study in patients with previously untreated advanced NSCLC who have a poor performance status (PS 2). Patients will receive weekly docetaxel for 4 monthly cycles with either bortezomib or cetuximab (both of which may be continued beyond the 4 cycles).
4. C30407 – randomized phase II study in patients with inoperable stage IIIA/B NSCLC who will receive pemetrexed, carboplatin, and radiation (70 Gy) with or without cetuximab.

38.5   North Central Cancer Treatment Group (NCCTG)

The NCCTG, centered at the Mayo clinic in Minnesota, focuses primarily on phase II studies with novel therapeutics. Additionally, they actively participate in many Intergroup protocols. NCCTG currently has five NSCLC trials and one SCLC trial open.

Table 38.6. CALGB phase II trials: SCLC

	Stage; line of therapy	Treatment	Primary endpoint	Patients
C30206	L-SCLC; first line	Cisplatin + irinotecan followed by carboplatin + etoposide + radiation	2-year survival	75
C30306	E-SCLC; first line	Cisplatin, irinotecan, bevacizumab	1-year survival	72
C30103	E-SCLC; first line	Carboplatin, etoposide with or without oblimersen	1-year survival	55
C30304	Recurrent SCLC	Depsipeptide (FK228)	RR	36

Table 38.7. NCCTG phase II trials: advanced NSCLC

	Line of therapy	Treatment	Primary endpoint	Patients	Projected closure
N0323	First line	CCI-779, mTOR inhibitor	RR, toxicity	55	Late 2005/early 2006
N0326	First line	Sorafenib (BAY 43-9006)	RR, toxicity	42	2006
N0222	Patients at least 65 years old	Gefitinib alone versus weekly carboplatin and paclitaxel followed by gefitinib	Progression at 6 months	107	?

There are three NCCTG advanced NSCLC phase II trials open, N0323, N0326, and N0222 (Table 38.7). N0323 is a phase II study of the mTOR inhibitor CCI-779 given weekly to patients with newly diagnosed advanced NSCLC. The RR and toxicity of this agent will be assessed as well as TTP, and OS. Laboratory correlates are included. N0326 has a very similar design to N0323 and is open to the same patient population. This phase II study of the raf kinase inhibitor sorafenib (BAY 43-9006), which also blocks VEGFR, gives the agent orally twice daily. RR and toxicity will be the primary endpoints, but PFS at 24 weeks, TTP, OS, and laboratory correlates will be included.

N0222 is a randomized phase II trial of single-agent gefitinib versus weekly carboplatin/paclitaxel followed by single-agent gefitinib in elderly patients (at least 65 years old) with advanced NSCLC. The regimen is chosen by the treating oncologist and is not randomized. In addition to progression at 6 months, the RR, quality of life (QoL), impact of social support, rationale for choosing different regimens, and EGFR levels will also be evaluated. Given the recent data with gefitinib, it is unclear if this study will remain open to complete accrual.

Both N0028 and N0321 explore chemoradiotherapy in locally advanced NSCLC (Table 38.8). N0028 is a phase I/II study of concurrent chemotherapy (carboplatin and paclitaxel weekly) and escalating doses of three-dimensional conformal radiotherapy (2.0 Gy daily fractions), followed by 3 cycles of chemotherapy (carboplatin and paclitaxel every 3 weeks) for unresectable NSCLC. The phase I dose escalation portion is completed, and phase II accrual is ongoing. Patients will be followed for 2-year survival, PFS, and QoL.

On trial N0321, the MTD of bortezomib (days 1, 4, 8, and 11 every 3 weeks) with carboplatin, paclitaxel (both on day 2 every 3 weeks), and radiation therapy (2 Gy daily to 60 Gy) will be determined in phase I. Phase II will evaluate 1-year survival, tolerability, RR, PFS, and p27 expression in a population of locally advanced NSCLC patients.

The NCCTG currently has one trial open in SCLC, N9923, for limited-stage disease. The treatment regimen for N9923 consists of 2 cycles of topotecan and paclitaxel followed by high-dose twice-daily thoracic radiation therapy (60 Gy total) with concomitant cisplatin/etoposide orally daily and amifostine subcutaneously daily, followed by consolidation with topotecan and paclitaxel for 2 cycles. The phase I portion of the study was completed with 18 patients, and phase II accrual is ongoing to a total of 70 patients. The primary endpoint is 2-year survival, but OS, PFS (2-year and overall), toxicity, and antitumor activity are also being evaluated. Accrual is expected to be complete in 2008.

The NCCTG has several trials in development including:

1. N0426 – phase II trial of pemetrexed and bevacizumab in second-line therapy for advanced NSCLC.
2. N0425 – randomized phase II trial of PTK 787 (VEGFR inhibitor) versus pemetrexed for second-line therapy of NSCLC.
3. N0423 – phase II trial of pemetrexed and carboplatin in E-SCLC.
4. N0422 – cetuximab and radiotherapy for stage IIIA/B unresectable NSCLC in elderly patients.
5. N0428 – randomized phase II trial of two schedules of carboplatin/paclitaxel in combination with bortezomib as first-line therapy in patients with advanced NSCLC.

Table 38.8. NCCTG trials: locally advanced NSCLC

	Stage	Treatment	Primary endpoint	Patients	Projected closure
N0028; phase I/II	Unresectable stage I–IIIB	Chemotherapy + concurrent radiotherapy (3-D, conformal)	MTD of 3-D conformal radiotherapy + concurrent chemotherapy, phase II – 2-year survival	15 phase I, 48 phase II	Phase I completed; phase II 2007 +
N0321; phase I/II	Unresectable stage III	Bortezomib, carboplatin, paclitaxel, and radiation	MTD phase I/ 1-year survival phase II	66	Opened 2004

38.6   National Cancer Institute Canada (NCIC)

The National Cancer Institute of Canada has recently published two landmark positive trials in NSCLC. BR.10 was one of the recent positive adjuvant NSCLC trials [7], and BR.21 established a role of erlotinib in the second- and third-line treatment of NSCLC [2]. A large adjuvant trial of gefitinib in NSCLC (BR.19) was closed prior to completion of enrollment after the results of two large trials of gefitinib in other settings in NSCLC were negative, ISEL [10] and SWOG 0023 [6]. Over 500 patients were enrolled on the trial, which randomized patients to 2 years of adjuvant gefitinib after complete resection of early-stage NSCLC (with or without adjuvant chemotherapy prior to randomization), or to placebo. The primary endpoint was survival. The study was closed in the spring of 2005, but will not be analyzed for another 3 years. There will be a large tumor bank associated with this trial and correlative studies of EGFR are planned. In addition to Intergroup trials, the NCIC currently has two open lung cancer trials (Table 38.9), and others are in development.

IND.171 is a standard phase I trial to determine the proper phase II dose of the antiangiogenesis agent AZD2171 in combination with front-line carboplatin and paclitaxel for advanced-stage NSCLC. The total enrollment will be determined by the dose at which significant toxicity is seen.

Patients with responsive SCLC, either limited or extensive stage, who have just completed chemotherapy, will be eligible for BR.20 which randomizes patients to the dual anti-EGFR and anti-VEGFR agent, ZD6474, or placebo. In addition to the primary endpoint of PFS, other measures including RR, toxicity, pharmacokinetics and correlative studies to include VEGFR levels, and microvessel density will be measured in this randomized phase II trial. The results of this trial will determine whether a phase III study is justified.

Proposed trials within the NCIC are listed below:

1. BR.24 – phase II–III randomized trial in advanced stage IIIB and IV NSCLC will compare treatment with carboplatin and paclitaxel with the oral VEGFR tyrosine kinase inhibitor, AZD2171, versus the same chemotherapy plus placebo. If sufficient activity is demonstrated in phase II, the study will continue to phase III, where the primary endpoint will be survival. Correlative studies of markers of angiogenesis are planned.
2. BR.(25?) – phase I–II trial will examine the value of hypofractionated radiotherapy in medically inoperable patients with localized NSCLC. Doses of 52–60 Gy administered over 2.5–3 weeks will be assessed.
3. IND.174 – phase II study of BMS-275183, a new oral taxane for the second-line treatment of NSCLC.

Another phase II trial in development will explore the bcl-2 inhibitor GX15-070 for the second-line treatment of SCLC.

38.7   American College of Surgeons Oncology Group (ACOSOG)

ACOSOG, based in North Carolina, includes thoracic surgery participation from across the USA and Canada. ACOSOG has looked into many important surgically focused questions in lung cancer treatment. Most recently, Z0030, a large phase III trial of mediastinal lymph node sampling versus complete lymphadenectomy was completed, and results are awaited. The study was conducted in patients undergoing pulmonary resection who had N0 or N1 (less than hilar) NSCLC. During surgery, patients were randomized to no further lymph node surgery beyond the mediastinal lymph node sampling done prior to randomization, or to complete mediastinal lymph node dissection at the time of pulmonary resection. The primary endpoint is OS and the study was closed with complete accrual of 1,000 patients in 2004. Complications of the complete lymph node dissection are also being followed and tumor specimens were collected for the ACOSOG central specimen bank.

ACOSOG currently has two open NSCLC trials. Z4032 is a randomized phase III trial set to enroll 226 patients, which opened in July 2005. Patients in Z4032 are randomized to receive a sublobar resection with or without the additional placement of brachytherapy seeds (^{125}I) at the operative site. The study is open to patients with stage I NSCLC who are not candidates for lobectomy due to poor lung function. The primary objective will be to determine the effect on local recurrence, but morbidity and mortality will also be evaluated.

Table 38.9. NCIC lung cancer trials

	Disease; line of therapy	Treatment	Primary endpoint	Patients
IND171; phase I	Advanced NSCLC; first line	AZD2171 plus carboplatin and paclitaxel	MTD and recommended phase II dose	Up to 30
BR.20; phase II	E- or L-SCLC, responsive to prior therapy; consolidation	ZD6474 vs placebo	PFS	120

Z4031 is a specimen collection trial of serum from patients who are suspected of having stage I NSCLC. Serum is collected from patients with suspicious lung lesions who then undergo lung resection. The goal is to enroll 1,000 patients (including those on Z4032). The serum will undergo proteomic analysis to correlate the proteomic profile with pathologic nodal status and histopathologic diagnosis. Serum will also be collected postoperatively to correlate changes in the proteomic profile with outcome.

ACOSOG has one trial which is set to open shortly:

1. Z4033 – pilot trial of radiofrequency ablation for NSCLC tumors under 3 cm in size, in patients without lymph node involvement or distant metastases.

38.8 Radiation Therapy Oncology Group (RTOG)

Recently completed RTOG trials for which results are awaited include RTOG 0324, RTOG 0017, and RTOG 0213. RTOG 0324 was a phase II trial which enrolled 84 stage IIIA/B NSCLC patients who received weekly cetuximab plus weekly carboplatin and paclitaxel for 7 weeks concurrently with radiotherapy to 63 Gy (35 daily fractions over 7 weeks). This was followed by consolidation weekly cetuximab plus carboplatin and paclitaxel given every 3 weeks for two cycles. RTOG 0324 closed in June 2005. RTOG 0017 was a phase I trial of gemcitabine plus carboplatin or gemcitabine plus paclitaxel with radiation therapy for inoperable stage III NSCLC which was closed to accrual in April 2005. RTOG 0213 closed in June 2005. This trial enrolled NSCLC patients with stage III disease who were not fit to receive surgery or concurrent chemoradiotherapy, to receive the COX-2 inhibitor celecoxib plus full-course thoracic radiotherapy. RTOG currently has five open NSCLC trials (two are phase III) and three SCLC trials (one phase III).

The three open RTOG phase III trials are outlined in Table 38.1. The recently opened RTOG 0412/SWOG S0332 is a randomized phase III trial designed to determine if radiotherapy is beneficial when added to chemotherapy as preoperative therapy for favorable prognosis stage IIIA (N2) (<3 cm in size) NSCLC. Eligible patients (n=574)

are stratified by number of involved mediastinal nodal stations, whether involvement is clinical or microscopic, and T stage. They are randomized to receive either cisplatin (75 mg/m^2)/docetaxel (75 mg/m^2) both on days 1 and 22, or cisplatin (50 mg/m^2)/docetaxel (20 mg/m^2) both on days 1, 8, 15, and 22 plus thoracic radiotherapy to 50.4 Gy. After re-evaluation, patients undergo surgical resection 4–8 weeks after completion of the induction therapy and then receive 3 cycles of consolidation docetaxel. The primary endpoint is OS. Secondary endpoints include PFS, toxicity, RR, and extensive correlative laboratory work.

RTOG 0214 randomizes patients with stage IIIA or IIIB NSCLC who have completed definitive therapy for their disease (with or without surgery) to either prophylactic cranial irradiation (PCI) (2 Gy per fraction for a total of 15 fractions to a total dose of 30 Gy) or observation. Patients must have at least stable disease after completion of therapy. In addition to the primary endpoint of survival, neuropsychologic impact of PCI, QoL impact of PCI, and impact of PCI on central nervous system metastases will be determined.

RTOG 0212 is open to L-SCLC patients who have had a complete response to definitive therapy. The trial consists of three arms of radiation schedules. Arm 1 will accrue 50% of the patients and consists of 2.5 Gy daily M-F in 10 fractions to a total of 25 Gy. Arm 2 consists of 2.0 Gy given daily M-F in 18 fractions for a total of 36 Gy (25% of patients). Arm 3 will give 1.5 Gy twice daily M-F in 24 fractions for a total dose of 36 Gy (25% of patients). The phase III question of the trial is whether a higher total dose (36 Gy) is superior to the standard 25 Gy dose of PCI. An additional phase II question is the comparison of the daily versus twice daily (b.i.d.) dosing of the higher dose of PCI (36 Gy). The primary endpoint of the trial is to determine the impact of the higher dose of PCI (36 Gy) on the incidence of brain metastases; DFS and OS as well as QoL and late treatment sequelae will also be followed. The impact of PCI dose and schedule on the incidence of chronic neurotoxicity and QoL will be determined in the phase II portion of the trial.

In addition to the phase III studies outline above, RTOG has three open phase II trials in NSCLC (Table 38.10). Patients with locally advanced NSCLC on

Table 38.10. RTOG phase II studies: NSCLC

	Stage	Treatment	Primary objective	Patients
RTOG 0229; phase II	Locally advanced	Chemotherapy plus high-dose radiotherapy followed by resection followed by consolidation chemotherapy	Mediastinal lymph node clearance and rate of pathologic complete response	60
RTOG 0236; phase II	T1-3 (<5 cm) N0M0 medically inoperable	Stereotactic radiotherapy	Local control	52
RTOG 0117; phase I/II	Inoperable stage I–IIIB (if can be encompassed by a radiation field)	3-D conformal radiation therapy + concurrent chemotherapy	Percentage of patients alive at 12 months	46 on phase II

RTOG 0229 receive weekly paclitaxel and carboplatin for 6 weeks with concurrent radiotherapy (1.8 Gy/day to a total of 50.4 Gy in 28 fractions plus a boost of 1.8 Gy/day to a total of 10.8 Gy in 6 fractions), followed by surgical resection (if possible), followed by consolidation chemotherapy (paclitaxel and carboplatin every 21 days for 2 cycles). Eligible patients have stage IIIA (N2) or IIIB (N3, not supraclavicular involvement) NSCLC. In addition to assessment of mediastinal lymph node clearance and rate of pathologic complete response, the feasibility of surgical resection with this regimen, toxicity, DFS, and OS will be evaluated.

RTOG 0236 is a phase II trial of stereotactic body radiation therapy (SBRT) given in three total fractions of 20 Gy each over 1.5–2 weeks (total dose of 60 Gy). Only patients with T1-3 tumors (<5 cm in size), and no lymph node involvement, who are medically not operative candidates, will be eligible. In addition to the primary objective of local control rate, the toxicity and patterns of failure will be watched closely.

RTOG 0117 is now accruing as a phase II trial after completing phase I testing. The treatment consists of paclitaxel 50 mg/m^2 and carboplatin AUC=2 on days 1, 8, 15, 22, 29, 36, and 43 with concurrent radiotherapy (three-dimensional conformal radiation) which is given as 2.0-Gy fractions to a total of 74 Gy in phase II. Now that the MTD has been established, the primary objective in phase II is the percentage of patients alive at 12 months. Toxicity and RR will also be determined.

RTOG is collaborating with the American College of Radiology Imaging Network (ACRIN) on a protocol of FDG-PET scanning for patients with stage II/III NSCLC who are undergoing definitive chemoradiotherapy. On ACRIN 6668/RTOG 0235 all patients receive an FDG-PET scan prior to initiation of therapy and then at 14 weeks after completion of therapy. The maximum standard uptake value (SUV) is measured for both scans and correlated for survival. The trial was opened in the spring of 2005 and plans to enroll 250 patients.

SCLC RTOG trials, RTOG 0241 and RTOG 0239, are outlined in Table 38.11. For the phase I RTOG 0241, patients with L-SCLC are enrolled in dose-escalation cohorts with irinotecan starting at 40 mg/m^2 (up to 60 mg/m^2) days 1 and 8 and cisplatin fixed at 60 mg/m^2 day 1 every 3 weeks, with radiation either given as 1.5 Gy b.i.d. M-F in 30 fractions for 45 Gy total, or 2.0 Gy once daily M-F to a total of 70 Gy. The primary objective is to determine the MTD.

RTOG 0239 consists of large field radiation therapy to 28.8 Gy given as 1.8 Gy fractions daily for patients with L-SCLC. On days 23–26 the therapy is b.i.d. at 1.8 Gy per day b.i.d., then off-cord boost of 1.8 Gy b.i.d. for 5 days to a total of 61.2 Gy. This is given with concurrent cisplatin (60 mg/m^2 day 1)/etoposide (120 mg/m^2 i.v. days 1–3; or oral equivalent) and followed by consolidation cisplatin/etoposide (same doses for 2 cycles). This phase II trial will evaluate RR, PFS, OS, and toxicity with this regimen.

The RTOG has several studies in early development. Along with the other cooperative groups, a proposed trial of bevacizumab in locally advanced disease is under consideration. The use of cetuximab in locally advanced disease with concurrent chemoradiotherapy is also under consideration.

38.9   Conclusions

The cooperative groups of North America have contributed significantly to our understanding of the optimal treatment of lung cancer. Though progress has been slow, the past few years have given us several exciting results, and several new standards of care have evolved from these clinical trials. In particular, the cooperative groups of North America have been pivotal in defining a role for the novel agents erlotinib and bevacizumab in the treatment of advanced NSCLC with NCIC BR.21 [2] and ECOG E4599 [3], as well as contributing greatly to our new knowledge of the benefit of adjuvant therapy for early-stage NSCLC with NCIC BR.10 [7] and CALGB 9633 [8]. With the results of multiple trials, they have also brought us closer to an understanding of how best to treat locally advanced NSCLC. Increasingly, North American cooperative group studies are also defining the underlying biology of lung cancer and identifying associated biomarkers predictive of patient outcomes [11, 13]. This chapter has outlined current trials of the North American cooperative groups, as well as giving a glimpse at some of the studies in development that will continue to lead us forward.

Table 38.11. RTOG studies: SCLC

	Stage; line of therapy	Treatment	Primary objective	Patients
RTOG 0241	L-SCLC; phase I	Irinotecan + cisplatin plus b.i.d. XRT (45 Gy) or daily XRT (70 Gy)	Definition of MTD/tolerability	Max 36 (or to MTD)
RTOG 0239	L-SCLC; phase II	Accelerated high dose thoracic XRT + cisplatin/etoposide	RR, PFS, OS, and toxicity with this regimen	71

XRT Radiation therapy

Acknowledgements

We would like to thank the respective chairs of the thoracic committees of each of the cooperative groups discussed: Dr. Joan Schiller (ECOG), Dr. David Gandara (SWOG), Dr. Everett Vokes (CALGB), Dr. James Jett (NCCTG), Dr. Frances Shepherd (NCIC), Dr. Joe B. Putnam, Jr. (ACOSOG), and Dr. Hak Choy (RTOG) for generously sharing information with us to make this chapter possible.

Key Points

- The cooperative groups of North America have contributed significantly to our understanding of the optimal treatment of lung cancer. Though progress has been slow, the past few years have given us several exciting results, and several new standards of care have evolved from these clinical trials.
- With the results of multiple trials, they have also brought us closer to an understanding of how best to treat locally advanced NSCLC.
- North American cooperative group studies are also defining the underlying biology of lung cancer and identifying associated biomarkers predictive of patient outcomes.

References

1. Jemal A, Murray T, Ward E, Samuels A, Tiwari RC, Ghafoor A, Feuer EJ, Thun MJ. Cancer statistics, CA Cancer J Clin 2005; 55:10.
2. Shepherd FA, Rodrigues Pereira J, et al. Erlotinib in previously treated non-small-cell lung cancer. N Engl J Med 2005; 353:123.
3. Sandler A, Gray R, Brahmer JR, et al. Randomized phase II/III trial of paclitaxel (P) plus carboplatin (C) with or without bevacizumab (NSC #704865) in patients with advanced non-squamous cell lung cancer (NSCLC): an Eastern Cooperative Oncology Group (ECOG) trial – E4599. J Clin Oncol 2005; 23(16S):2s.
4. Pisters K, Vallieres E, Bunn P, et al. S9900: a phase III trial of surgery alone or surgery plus preoperative (preop) paclitaxel/carboplatin (PC) chemotherapy in early stage non-small cell lung cancer (NSCLC). Preliminary results. J Clin Oncol 2005; 23(16S):624s.
5. Gandara DR, Chansky K, Albain KS, et al. Consolidation docetaxel after concurrent chemoradiotherapy in stage IIIB non-small-cell lung cancer: phase II Southwest Oncology Group study S9504. J Clin Oncol 2003; 21:2004.
6. Kelly K, Gaspar LE, Chansky K, et al. Low incidence of pneumonitis on SWOG 0023: a preliminary analysis of an ongoing phase III trial of concurrent chemoradiotherapy followed by consolidation docetaxel and Iressa/placebo maintenance in patients with inoperable stage III non-small cell lung cancer. J Clin Oncol 2005; 23(16S):634s.
7. Winton T, Livingston R, Johnson D, et al. Vinorelbine plus cisplatin vs. observation in resected non-small-cell lung cancer. N Engl J Med 2005; 352:2589.
8. Strauss GM, Herndon J, Maddaus MA, et al. Randomized clinical trial of adjuvant chemotherapy with paclitaxel and carboplatin following resection in stage IB non-small cell lung cancer (NSCLC): report of Cancer and Leukemia Group B (CALGB) protocol 9633. J Clin Oncol 2004; 22(14S):621s.
9. Neill HB, Herndon JE 2nd, Miller AA, et al. Randomized phase III intergroup trial of etoposide and cisplatin with or without paclitaxel and granulocyte colony-stimulating factor in patients with extensive-stage small-cell lung cancer: Cancer and Leukemia Group B trial 9732. J Clin Oncol 2005; 23:3752.
10. Thatcher N, Chang A, Parikh P, et al. A phase III survival study comparing gefitinib (Iressa) plus best supportive care (BSC) with placebo plus BSC, in patients with advanced non-small-cell lung cancer (NSCLC) who had received one or two prior chemotherapy regimens. Lung Cancer 2005; 49:4.
11. Hirsch FR, Varella-Garcia M, McCoy J, et al. Increased epidermal growth factor receptor gene copy number detected by fluorescence in situ hybridization associates with increased sensitivity to gefitinib in patients with bronchioloalveolar carcinoma subtypes: a Southwest Oncology Group study. J Clin Oncol 2005; 23:6838–6845.
12. Vokes EE, Herndon JE 2nd, Kelley MJ, et al. Induction chemotherapy followed by concomitant chemoradiotherapy (CT/XRT) versus CT/XRT alone for regionally advanced unresectable non-small cell lung cancer (NSCLC): initial analysis of a randomized phase III trial. J Clin Oncol 2004; 22(14S):618s.
13. Tsao MS, Sakurada A, Cutz JC, et al. Erlotinib in lung cancer: molecular and clinical predictors of outcome. N Engl J Med 2005; 353:133.

Clinical Trials for Lung Cancer in Progress in Japan

39

Ikuo Sekine, Yuichiro Ohe, Nagahiro Saijo
and Tomohide Tamura

Contents

39.1 Introduction

Lung cancer has been the leading cause of death from cancer in many countries, despite extensive basic research and clinical trials. About 80% of patients with lung cancer have already developed distant metastases, either by the time of the initial diagnosis or by the time recurrence is detected after surgery for local disease. Systemic chemotherapy is the mainstay of lung cancer treatment, although its efficacy is still limited. Therefore, new chemotherapeutic agents continue to be developed against lung cancer [1].

39.2 Drug Approval System in Japan

Since 1955, 23 anticancer drugs have been approved for use against lung cancer in Japan. Of these, 9 were discovered and developed in Japan, including mitomycin, bleomycin, and the topoisomerase I inhibitor irinotecan, and are routinely used all over the world. The Japanese Pharmaceutical Affairs Law (PAL) was enacted in 1948, and was first amended in 1960 to provide for regulations to ensure the maintenance of the quality, efficacy, and safety of drugs and medical devices, and to promote research and development of these medical and pharmaceutical products. Good Clinical Practice was enforced by the Bureau Notification of the Ministry of Health and Welfare of Japan in 1989. In 1996, PAL and its related laws were amended to strengthen Good Clinical Practice, Good Laboratory Practice, Good Post-marketing Surveillance Practice, and standard compliance reviews, conforming to the International Conference on Harmonization of Technical Requirements for Registration of Pharmaceuticals for Human Use [2]. In contrast to the laws prevailing in the US and EU, in Japan, marketing approval for anticancer agents can be granted based on reports of the antitumor effects of the new agents in phase II studies. Two independently conducted comparative phase III trials with survival as the endpoint are required after the approval, with at least one of these conducted as a post-marketing sponsored (PMS) trial in Japan [2].

39.3 Recent Clinical Trials for Non-Small-Cell Lung Cancer

Several randomized phase III trials for previously untreated advanced non-small cell lung cancer (NSCLC) have been conducted by Japanese pharmaceutical companies. A three-arm trial of cisplatin + vindesine versus cisplatin + irinotecan versus irinotecan alone conducted on 398 patients with stage IIIB or IV NSCLC between 1995 and 1998 showed that the overall response rate (31%, 43%, and 21%, respectively, $p < 0.001$), but not the overall survival rate (median survival time [MST], 47, 52, and 47 weeks, respectively, $p = 0.099$), was significantly better in the cisplatin + irinotecan arm than in the other two arms [3]. A second trial conducted on 210 patients with advanced NSCLC, comparing cisplatin + vindesine versus cisplatin + irinotecan, showed no statistically significant difference in the overall response rate (22% versus 29%) or survival rate (MST, 50 versus 45 weeks) between the two arms [4]. A randomized phase III trial of docetaxel + cisplatin versus vindesine + cisplatin was conducted between 1998 and 2000 on 305 patients with stage IV NSCLC. Both the overall response rate and the survival rate were significantly superior in the docetaxel + cisplatin arm as compared to the vindesine + cisplatin arm (response rate, 37% versus 21%, respectively, $p < 0.01$; MST, 11.3 versus 9.6 months, respectively, $p = 0.014$) [5, 6]. After the commercial use of paclitaxel, gemcitabine, and vinorelbine was approved for NSCLC in 1999, a phase III study was conducted to confirm the efficacy and safety of these agents, to fulfill the requirements of PAL. A four-arm randomized phase III study of these agents for NSCLC was conducted in cooperation with three pharmaceutical companies. The four arms consisted of cisplatin (80 mg/m^2 on day 1) + irinotecan (60 mg/m^2 on days 1, 8, and 15) administered every 4 weeks as the reference arm; carboplatin (area under the curve [AUC] 6 on day 1) + paclitaxel (200 mg/m^2 on day 1) administered every 3 weeks; cisplatin (80 mg/m^2 on day 1) + gemcitabine (1,000 mg/m^2 on days 1 and 8) every 3 weeks; and cisplatin (80 mg/m^2 on day 1) + vinorelbine (25 mg/m^2 on days 1 and 8) administered every 3 weeks. Of a total of 602 patients registered from 44 institutes in Japan between 2000 and 2002, 581 were assessable for response, toxicity, and survival. The overall response rates in the four arms were 31%, 32%, 30%, and 33%, respectively, and the MST was 14.2, 12.3, 14.8, and 11.4 months, respectively. Non-inferiority of the three experimental arms as compared to the reference arm was not demonstrated in this study [5, 6].

Docetaxel monotherapy is the standard second-line treatment for NSCLC patients, based upon the demonstration of improved survival and quality of life in phase III studies [7, 8]. The Japan Clinical Oncology Group (JCOG) conducted a phase III trial (JCOG0104) to evaluate the efficacy and toxicity of gemcitabine combined with docetaxel in NSCLC patients with a history of prior platinum-based chemotherapy. The chemotherapeutic regimens compared in this study consisted of docetaxel alone (60 mg/m^2 on day 1) or doce-

taxel (60 mg/m^2 on day 8) + gemcitabine (800 mg/m^2 on days 1 and 8), repeated every 21 days until disease progression, with a planned sample size of 142 patients per arm. Between January 2002 and April 2003, 65 patients were accrued for each arm. However, this trial was terminated early because of the unexpectedly high incidence of interstitial lung disease (ILD) and three treatment-related (all due to ILD) deaths (5%) in the docetaxel + gemcitabine arm. While the incidence of grade 3–4 neutropenia and febrile neutropenia was similar in both the arms, the incidence of dyspnea (23% versus 14%) and ILD (21% versus 2%) was higher in the docetaxel + gemcitabine arm [9]. A randomized, double-blind, parallel-group, international, multicenter trial of gefitinib, an epidermal growth factor receptor (EGFR) tyrosine kinase inhibitor, was conducted in patients with advanced NSCLC with recurrent or refractory disease following therapy with one or two chemotherapeutic regimens, at institutes in Europe, Australia, South Africa, and Japan. Patients were randomized to receive either 250 or 500 mg/day gefitinib using blinded tablets, until disease progression, intolerable toxicity, or withdrawal of consent. Between October 2000 and January 2001, 102 patients were enrolled from 19 institutes in Japan. The objective tumor response rate in the Japanese patients was 28% in both the 250- and the 500-mg/day arms. Thus, there was no difference in the objective response rate depending on the dose of gefitinib, although the incidence of toxicities, including rash, diarrhea, liver damage, and nausea, was relatively lower in the 250-mg/day arm [10]. A randomized, open-labeled phase III trial of second-line chemotherapy with docetaxel versus gefitinib in patients with advanced NSCLC previously treated with platinum-based chemotherapy is in progress in Japan as a PMS trial,

1. Non-small cell lung cancer

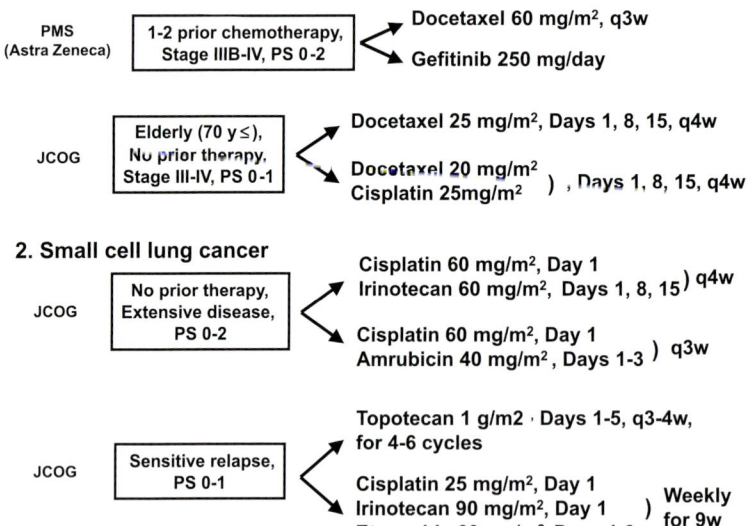

2. Small cell lung cancer

Fig. 39.1. Phase III trials in progress or being planned in Japan. *PMS* Post-marketing sponsored, *JCOG* Japan Clinical Oncology Group

since December 2003. The projected accrual for this study is a total of 484 patients (242 patients per treatment arm) (Fig. 39.1).

Monotherapy with a third-generation cytotoxic agent is widely accepted for the treatment of advanced NSCLC in the elderly, after demonstration of the survival benefit of vinorelbine over standard supportive care alone, without deterioration of the quality of life, in a phase III trial [11]. The West Japan Thoracic Oncology Group (WJTOG) is conducting a phase III trial (WJTOG 9904) of docetaxel (60 mg/m^2 on day 1) versus vinorelbine (25 mg/m^2 on days 1 and 8) administered every 3 weeks for advanced NSCLC in patients aged 70 years or older with no prior history of chemotherapy, a performance status of 0–2, and adequate organ function, as indicated by routine blood counts and blood chemistry, and electrocardiography. The projected sample size for this trial is 90 patients for each arm, and patient accrual for this study has recently been completed.

There are limited data to support the use of platinum-based combination chemotherapeutic regimens in patients over 70 years of age, although platinum doublet is standard treatment for younger patients. A retrospective analysis of 401 patients 65 years of age or older in a large phase III trial of docetaxel + cisplatin versus docetaxel + carboplatin versus vinorelbine + cisplatin revealed no significant differences in the therapeutic outcomes based on the age, although a moderately higher incidence of grade 3–4 asthenia, infection, pulmonary toxicities, diarrhea, and sensory neurotoxicity was noted in the elderly patients [12]. A phase I and a phase II study showed that a combination of cisplatin and docetaxel administered as three consecutive weekly infusions was safe and effective in elderly patients with advanced NSCLC [13, 14]. Based on these data, a JCOG phase III trial of weekly docetaxel versus weekly docetaxel + cisplatin (JCOG0207) is under way (Fig. 39.1). The primary endpoint of this study is the overall survival of the patients treated with these regimens. The secondary endpoints are the response rate, progression-free survival, toxicity, and symptom score. Eligibility includes stage IV or IIIB disease, no history of previous chemotherapy, performance status of 0 or 1, age 70 years or older, and adequate organ functions. The chemotherapeutic regimens consisted of docetaxel (25 mg/m^2) administered on days 1, 8, and 15 every 4 weeks, or docetaxel (20 mg/m^2) + cisplatin (25 mg/m^2) administered on days 1, 8, and 15 every 4 weeks. The projected accrual for this study is a total of 230 patients (115 patients per treatment arm).

39.4 Recent Clinical Trials for Small-Cell Lung Cancer

The JCOG conducted a phase III study of cisplatin (60 mg/m^2 on day 1) + irinotecan (60 mg/m^2 on days 1, 8, and 15) administered every 4 weeks versus cisplatin (80 mg/m^2 on day 1) + etoposide (100 mg/m^2 on days 1, 2, and 3) administered every 3 weeks for untreated extensive small-cell lung cancer (E-SCLC) (JCOG9511). The projected sample size for this study was 230 patients (115 patients per treatment arm), however, enrollment was stopped early because of a statistically significant difference in the survival observed between the two treatment arms on interim analysis. In this interim analysis, 154 patients were randomized to the two treatments, 77 into each arm. The overall response rate and survival were significantly better in the cisplatin + irinotecan group (response rate, 84% versus 68%, respectively, $p = 0.02$; MST, 12.8 versus 9.4 months, respectively, $p = 0.002$) [15]. Based on these observations, the combination of cisplatin + irinotecan is used as the standard chemotherapeutic regimen for E-SCLC in Japan. A three-drug combination of cisplatin, irinotecan, and etoposide was investigated. The maximum tolerated dose of each of the three drugs was determined in phase I studies using two different schedules: a weekly (JCOG9507) and a 4-weekly (JCOG9512) schedule. The antitumor effects of these regimens were evaluated in a randomized phase II study (JCOG9902DI) [16]. The weekly arm consisted of cisplatin (25 mg/m^2 on day 1 at weeks 1–9), irinotecan (90 mg/m^2 on day 1 at weeks 1, 3, 5, 7, and 9), and etoposide (60 mg/m^2 on days 1–3 at weeks 2, 4, 6, and 8), administered with granulocyte colony-stimulating factor (G-CSF) support. The 4-weekly arm consisted of cisplatin (60 mg/m^2 on day 1), irinotecan (60 mg/m^2 on days 1, 8, and 15), and etoposide (50 mg/m^2 on days 1–3) administered with G-CSF support. From August 1999 to October 2000, 30 patients were entered in each of the two treatment arms of this study. Although 70% of all the patients received full cycles of chemotherapy in both arms, treatment delay in the weekly arm and skipping of irinotecan on day 15 in the 4-weekly arm were common because of toxicity. The complete and partial response rates and the MST were 7%, 77%, and 8.9 months, respectively, in the weekly arm, and 17%, 60%, and 12.9 months, respectively, in the 4-weekly arm. Since no overall survival benefit was obtained with the weekly schedule, and the dose of irinotecan on day 15 frequently needed to be skipped in the 4-weekly schedule, a 3-week schedule with irinotecan administered only on days 1 and 8 every 3 weeks might be appropriate for subsequent trials. A randomized phase II trial of cisplatin (60 mg/m^2 on day 1) + irinotecan (60 mg/m^2 on days 1 and 8) versus the same three-drug combination of cisplatin and irinotecan combined with etoposide (50 mg/m^2 on days 1–3) administered every 3 weeks with G-CSF support in patients with previously untreated E-SCLC is in progress.

Amrubicin (SM-5887) is an entirely synthetic anthracycline that has been shown to possess topoisomerase II inhibitory activity. It has been shown to exert more potent antitumor activity than doxorubicin against various experimental tumors and human tumor xenografts in mice, without any cardiotoxicity. A phase II study of single-agent amrubicin using a schedule of 45 mg/m^2 administered on days 1–3 every 3 weeks yielded an overall response rate of 76%, a complete response rate of 9%, and an MST of 11.7 months in 33 previously untreated E-SCLC patients [17]. The recommended dose of amrubicin when combined with cisplatin was determined to be 40 mg/m^2 on days 1–3 every 3 weeks, and the response rate and MST for E-SCLC patients receiving this combination were 88% and 13.6 months, respectively [18]. The next JCOG phase III trial for this patient population should be of a combination of cisplatin + amrubicin versus cisplatin + irinotecan (Fig. 39.1).

Despite a high response rate to chemotherapy, the majority of SCLC patients eventually develop recurrent disease. At the time of recurrence, the tumor is broadly resistant to second-line chemotherapy and death occurs within a few to several months [19]. Thus, there is need for further development of effective salvage chemotherapy. We conducted a phase II study of cisplatin (25 mg/m^2) administered weekly for 9 weeks, etoposide (60 mg/m^2) administered for 3 days on weeks 1, 3, 5, 7, and 9, and irinotecan (90 mg/m^2) administered on weeks 2, 4, 6, and 8, with G-CSF support, in patients with sensitive relapsed SCLC [20]. Since the drug dose and treatment schedule can be easily modified according to the patient condition in the weekly regimen, it is considered that this regimen may be the most suitable for relapsed SCLC patients, who usually present with severe hematological toxicities during salvage chemotherapy because of poor bone marrow reserve. In a total of 40 patients registered, the overall response rate was 78% with 5 complete responses and 26 partial responses, and the MST was 11.8 months. Grade 3–4 neutropenia and thrombocytopenia were observed in 73% and 33% of the patients, respectively, and the non-hematological toxicities were mild and transient in all the patients. The JCOG is planning a phase III study to compare the efficacy of this regimen with that of topotecan monotherapy in sensitive relapsed SCLC patients (Fig. 39.1).

At diagnosis, 25–40% of patients with SCLC are 70 years old or older, and this percentage is expected to increase with the growing population of geriatric patients. Carboplatin is especially useful for the elderly because only minimum hydration of the patients is required, its non-hematological toxicity is mild, and the dose can be adjusted according to the patient's creatinine clearance [21]. The JCOG evaluated the toxicity and efficacy of this drug in a phase II study (JCOG9409), and observed grade 4 neutropenia and

thrombocytopenia in 44% and 12% of the patients, respectively, and complete response and partial response in 6% and 69% of the patients, respectively [22]. We started a large phase III trial in 1998, to compare the clinical efficacy of etoposide (80 mg/m^2 on days 1–3) + carboplatin (AUC = 5) versus etoposide (same dose) + cisplatin (25 mg/m^2 on days 1–3) in elderly patients with SCLC (JCOG9702). The sample size was 220 patients (110 patients for each arm), and registration was completed in February 2004.

39.5 New Agents for the Treatment of Lung Cancer

The development of oral preparations of 5-fluorouracil (5-FU) began in Japan in 1971, based on the finding that 5-FU acts in a time-dependent manner and on the possibility of treating patients on an outpatient basis, without deterioration of the quality of life, when drugs can be administered orally. S-1 (Taiho Pharmaceutical) is a novel oral fluoropyrimidine derivative consisting of tegafur, a prodrug of 5-FU, and two modulators, 5-chloro-2, 4-dihydroxypyridine (CDHP) and potassium oxonate (Oxo), in a molar ratio of 1:0.4:1 [23]. CDHP enhances the serum 5-FU concentrations by competitive inhibition of dihydropyrimidine dehydrogenase, an enzyme responsible for 5-FU catabolism. Oxo reduces 5-FU-induced diarrhea by inhibiting orotate phosphoribosyltransferase, a phosphoenzyme for 5-FU in gastrointestinal tissue. In a phase I trial, the maximum tolerated dose of S-1 was 75–100 mg/body, and the dose-limiting toxicity was myelosuppression. In a phase II trial of S-1 administered orally at approximately 40 mg/m^2 twice a day for 28 days followed by a 2-week rest period in 59 advanced NSCLC patients without prior history of chemotherapy, the response rate was 22% and the MST was 10.2 months, and the incidence of toxicity was relatively low, including grade 3–4 neutropenia in 7%, thrombocytopenia in 2%, diarrhea in 9%, and stomatitis in 2% of the patients [24]. A combination of S-1 and cisplatin was evaluated in a phase II trial for locally advanced and metastatic NSCLC, in which S-1 was administered orally (40 mg/m^2, twice daily) for 21 consecutive days and cisplatin was administered intravenously (60 mg/m^2 on day 8), and this schedule was repeated every 5 weeks. An overall response rate of 47% and MST of 11 months were obtained, with a mild toxicity profile, including grade 3–4 neutropenia in 29%, grade 3 anorexia in 13%, vomiting in 7%, and diarrhea in 7% of the patients [25]. This drug was approved for use in cases of advanced NSCLC by the Ministry of Health, Labor and Welfare of Japan in December 2004, on condition that a phase III trial of S-1 combined with platinum be conducted for advanced NSCLC patients with a reference arm of the standard regimen for this disease.

Several antifolates have been evaluated for the treatment of NSCLC, but none has as yet gained recognition as a useful drug in standard clinical practice. Pemetrexed (LY231514; Eli Lilly Japan) is a novel antifolate with multiple intracellular targets, including thymidylate synthase, dihydrofolate reductase, and glycinamide ribonucleotide formyl transferase, all key folate enzymes involved in the de novo synthesis of purines and pyrimidines [26]. The recommended dose of pemetrexed from early phase I trials is 600 mg/m^2 administered every 3 weeks, and the dose-limiting toxicity was myelosuppression [27]. Phase II studies conducted with this drug at the dose of 500 mg/m^2 yielded response rates of 15–23% in untreated patients and 9% in previously treated patients with advanced NSCLC [28, 29]. A phase III trial of pemetrexed versus docetaxel as a second-line chemotherapy for NSCLC showed that this drug had the same antitumor activity as docetaxel, but with less toxicity [30]. Because folic acid and vitamin B$_{12}$ supplementation was found to decrease the toxicity of this agent [31], a Japanese phase I trial of the drug was conducted with such vitamin supplementation [32]. In a total of 31 patients (19 with NSCLC, 7 with malignant pleural mesothelioma, 2 with thymoma, 1 with rectal cancer, and 2 others), grade 3 neutropenia was observed in 4 patients, elevated liver transaminase levels in 2 patients, and skin rash in 1 patient, and the recommended dose of pemetrexed was determined to be 1,000 mg/m^2 every 3 weeks. The pharmacokinetic profile of pemetrexed with vitamin supplementation in Japanese patients was essentially similar to that in western patients, with or without vitamin supplementation. In a total of 20 patients who were evaluable for antitumor activity, a partial response was observed in 4 of the 13 patients with NSCLC, and 1 of 2 patients with thymoma. A phase II trial of this drug in previously treated cases of NSCLC is under way in Japan.

Erlotinib (Chugai Pharmaceutical) is another selective inhibitor of EGFR tyrosine kinase sharing a common chemical backbone with gefitinib. Erlotinib was consistently twice as potent as gefitinib in preclinical studies, from cell-free systems to in vivo toxicity and efficacy studies [33]. At the dose of 150 mg, the recommended dose for phase II trials, the plasma AUC of erlotinib was higher by one order of magnitude than that of gefitinib administered at the dose of 250 mg/day [33]. The response rate of erlotinib in phase II trials in the USA was 12% in patients with NSCLC and 26% in patients with bronchoalveolar carcinoma. Phase III trials of standard platinum-based doublet with erlotinib versus placebo in patients with stage IIIB or IV NSCLC (TALENT and TRIBUTE) failed to show any survival benefit of erlotinib over placebo in a whole patient population [34]. A Japanese phase I trial of erlotinib was conducted in 11 patients with NSCLC, 3 patients with colon cancer, and 1 patient with head and neck cancer, using a dose in the range 50–150 mg/day [35]. The toxicity profile was mild, with grade 1–2 skin rash in 87%, grade 1 diarrhea in 53%, and grade 1–2 elevation of liver transaminases in 40% of patients, except for 1 patient who developed fatal ILD following treatment with 100 mg/day erlotinib. The C$_{max}$ increased in a dose-related manner, but there was no clear trend in the AUC. A partial response was observed in 4 (36%) of the 11 NSCLC patients. A phase II trial in previously treated patients with NSCLC is in progress.

Vascular endothelial growth factor (VEGF) is a potent and specific mitogen for endothelial cells that activates the angiogenic switch in vivo through binding to two distinct receptors on endothelial cells: Flt-1 (VEGFR-1) and Flk-1/KDR receptor (VEGFR-2). Enhanced expression of VEGF is generally correlated with increased neovascularization within the tumor [36]. ZD6474 (AstraZeneca) is an orally bioavailable, small-molecule VEGFR-2 tyrosine kinase inhibitor that also possesses activity against the EGFR tyrosine kinase [37]. Oral administration of ZD6474 to athymic mice bearing various established human tumor xenografts produced a dose-dependent regression of the tumors in all the cases [37]. In addition, ZD6474 inhibited the growth of tumors resistant to EGFR inhibitors [38]. A phase I trial of ZD6474 in 18 Japanese patients with solid tumors refractory to standard therapy showed that ZD6474 was well tolerated when administered at the dose of 100–300 mg/day, with common toxicity, including skin rash in 14, asymptomatic QTc prolongation in 11, diarrhea in 10, and hypertension in 7 patients [39]. The C$_{max}$ and AUC of ZD6474 increased linearly with the dose, and the terminal half-life was long, ranging from 72 to 167 h (median 96 h). The dose level of 100–300 mg/day yielded trough concentrations of the non-protein-bound drug of 0.08–0.31 μmol/l in 10 patients, which was over the IC$_{50}$ (0.04 μmol/L) of ZD6474 for VEGFR-2. Preliminary suggestion of tumor regression was observed in 4 out of 9 patients with NSCLC. A phase II trial in advanced NSCLC patients with a history of prior chemotherapy is in progress in Japan.

Since 1995, the quality of clinical trials has improved remarkably in Japan, and large-scale phase III trials have been conducted with the support of the JCOG, WJTOG, and Japanese pharmaceutical companies:

1. Molecular-target drugs, including gefitinib, erlotinib, and ZD6474, have been evaluated in phase II–III trials of NSCLC in Japan.
2. Amrubicin, a new anthracycline, is promising for the treatment of SCLC, and phase III trials are being planned.

Acknowledgements

We thank Ms. Yuko Yabe for her assistance in the preparation of this manuscript.

Key Points

- Since 1955, 23 anticancer drugs have been approved for use against lung cancer in Japan; of these, 9 were discovered and developed in Japan, including mitomycin, bleomycin, and the topoisomerase I inhibitor irinotecan, and are routinely used all over the world.
- Since 1995, the quality of clinical trials has improved remarkably in Japan, and large-scale phase III trials have been conducted with the support of the JCOG, WJTOG, and Japanese pharmaceutical companies.

References

1. Sekine I, Saijo N. Novel combination chemotherapy in the treatment of non-small cell lung cancer. Expert Opin Pharmacother 2000; 1:1131.
2. Fujiwara Y, Kobayashi K. Oncology drug clinical development and approval in Japan: the role of the pharmaceuticals and medical devices evaluation center (PMDEC). Crit Rev Oncol Hematol 2002; 42:145.
3. Negoro S, Masuda N, Takada Y, et al. Randomised phase III trial of irinotecan combined with cisplatin for advanced non-small-cell lung cancer. Br J Cancer 2003; 88:335.
4. Niho S, Nagao K, Nishiwaki Y, et al. Randomized multicenter phase III trial of irinotecan (CPT-11) and cisplatin (CDDP) versus CDDP and vindesine (VDS) in patients with advanced non-small cell lung cancer (NSCLC). Proc Am Soc Clin Oncol 1999;18:492a.
5. Kubota K, Nishiwaki Y, Ohashi Y, et al. The Four-Arm Cooperative Study (FACS) for advanced non-small-cell lung cancer (NSCLC). Proc Am Soc Clin Oncol 2004; 23:616.
6. Kubota K, Watanabe K, Kunitoh H, et al. Phase III randomized trial of docetaxel plus cisplatin versus vindesine plus cisplatin in patients with stage IV non-small-cell lung cancer: the Japanese Taxotere Lung Cancer Study Group. J Clin Oncol 2004; 22:254.
7. Dancey J, Shepherd FA, Gralla RJ, Kim YS. Quality of life assessment of second-line docetaxel versus best supportive care in patients with non-small-cell lung cancer previously treated with platinum-based chemotherapy: results of a prospective randomized phase III trial. Lung Cancer 2004; 43:183.
8. Shepherd FA, Dancey J, Ramlau R, et al. Prospective randomized trial of docetaxel versus best supportive care in patients with non-small-cell lung cancer previously treated with platinum-based chemotherapy. J Clin Oncol 2000; 18:2095.
9. Takeda K, Negoro S, Tamura T, et al. Docetaxel (D) versus docetaxel plus gemcitabine (DG) for second-line treatment of non-small cell lung cancer (NSCLC): results of a JCOG randomized trial (JCOG0104). Proc Am Soc Clin Oncol 2004; 23:622.
10. Fukuoka M, Yano S, Giaccone G, et al. Multi-institutional randomized phase II trial of gefitinib for previously treated patients with advanced non-small-cell lung cancer (the IDEAL 1 trial) [corrected]. J Clin Oncol 2003; 21:2237.
11. ELVIS. Effects of vinorelbine on quality of life and survival of elderly patients with advanced non-small-cell lung cancer. The Elderly Lung Cancer Vinorelbine Italian Study Group. J Natl Cancer Inst 1999; 91:66.
12. Fossella F, Belani C. Phase III study (TAX 326) of docetaxel-cisplatin (DC) and docetaxel-carboplatin (DCb) versus vinorelbine-cisplatin (VC) for the first-line treatment of advanced/metastatic non-small-cell lung cancer (NSCLC): analyses in elderly patients. Proc Am Soc Clin Oncol 2003; 22:629.
13. Ohe Y, Niho S, Kakinuma R, et al. Phase I studies of cisplatin and docetaxel administered by three consecutive weekly infusions for advanced non-small cell lung cancer in elderly and non-elderly patients. Jpn J Clin Oncol 2001; 31:100.
14. Ohe Y, Niho S, Kakinuma R, et al. A phase II study of cisplatin and docetaxel administered as three consecutive weekly infusions for advanced non-small-cell lung cancer in elderly patients. Ann Oncol 2004; 15:45.
15. Noda K, Nishiwaki Y, Kawahara M, et al. Irinotecan plus cisplatin compared with etoposide plus cisplatin for extensive small-cell lung cancer. N Engl J Med 2002; 346:85.
16. Sekine I, Nishiwaki Y, Noda K, et al. Randomized phase II study of cisplatin irinotecan and etoposide combinations administered weekly or every 4 weeks for extensive small-cell lung cancer (JCOG9902-DI). Ann Oncol 2003; 14:709.
17. Yana T, Negoro S, Takada Y. Phase II study of amrubicin (SM-5887) a 9-amino-anthracycline in previously untreated patients with extensive stage small-cell lung cancer (ES-SCLC): a West Japan Lung Cancer Group trial. Proc Am Soc Clin Oncol 1998; 18:450a
18. Ohe Y, Negoro S, Matsui K, et al. Phase I–II study of amrubicin and cisplatin in previously untreated patients with extensive-stage small-cell lung cancer. Ann Oncol 2005; 16:430.
19. Glisson BS. Recurrent small cell lung cancer: update. Semin Oncol 2003; 30:72.
20. Goto K, Sekine I, Nishiwaki Y, et al. Multi-institutional phase II trial of irinotecan cisplatin and etoposide for sensitive relapsed small-cell lung cancer. Br J Cancer 2004; 91:659.
21. Sekine I, Yamamoto N, Kunitoh H, et al. Treatment of small cell lung cancer in the elderly based on a critical literature review of clinical trials. Cancer Treat Rev 2004; 30:359.
22. Okamoto H, Watanabe K, Nishiwaki Y, et al. Phase II study of area under the plasma-concentration-versus-time curve-based carboplatin plus standard-dose intravenous etoposide in elderly patients with small-cell lung cancer. J Clin Oncol 1999; 17:3540.
23. Shirasaka T, Nakano K, Takechi T, et al. Antitumor activity of 1 M tegafur-0.4 M 5-chloro-24-dihydroxypyridine-1 M potassium oxonate (S-1) against human colon carcinoma orthotopically implanted into nude rats. Cancer Res 1996; 56:2602.
24. Kawahara M, Furuse K, Segawa Y, et al. Phase II study of S-1 a novel oral fluorouracil in advanced non-small-cell lung cancer. Br J Cancer 2001; 85:939.
25. Ichinose Y, Yoshimori K, Sakai H, et al. S-1 plus cisplatin combination chemotherapy in patients with advanced non-small cell lung cancer: a multi-institutional phase II trial. Clin Cancer Res 2004; 10:7860.
26. Shih C, Chen VJ, Gossett LS, et al. LY231514 a pyrrolo[23-d]pyrimidine-based antifolate that inhibits multiple folate-requiring enzymes. Cancer Res 1997; 57:1116.
27. Rinaldi DA. Overview of phase I trials of multitargeted antifolate (MTA LY231514). Semin Oncol 1999; 26:82.
28. Rusthoven JJ, Eisenhauer E, Butts C, et al. Multitargeted antifolate LY231514 as first-line chemotherapy for patients with advanced non-small-cell lung cancer: a phase II study. National Cancer Institute of Canada Clinical Trials Group. J Clin Oncol 1999; 17:1194.
29. Smit EF, Mattson K, von Pawel J, et al. Alimta (pemetrexed disodium) as second-line treatment of non-small-

cell lung cancer: a phase II study. Ann Oncol 2003; 14:455.

30. Hanna N, Shepherd FA, Fossella FV, et al. Randomized phase III trial of pemetrexed versus docetaxel in patients with non-small-cell lung cancer previously treated with chemotherapy. J Clin Oncol 2004; 22:1589.

31. Scagliotti GV, Shin DM, Kindler HL, et al. Phase II study of pemetrexed with and without folic acid and vitamin B12 as front-line therapy in malignant pleural mesothelioma. J Clin Oncol 2003; 21:1556.

32. Nakagawa K, Kudoh S, Matsui K, et al. A phase I study of pemetrexed supplemented with folic acid (FA) and vitamin B12 (VB12) in Japanese patients with solid tumors. Eur J Cancer 2004; 40(suppl 2):S148.

33. Perez-Soler R. The role of erlotinib (Tarceva OSI 774) in the treatment of non-small cell lung cancer. Clin Cancer Res 2004; 10:4238s.

34. Fuster LM, Sandler AB. Select clinical trials of erlotinib (OSI-774) in non-small-cell lung cancer with emphasis on phase III outcomes. Clin Lung Cancer 2004; 6(suppl 1): S24.

35. Horiike A, Yamada Y, Yamamoto N, Shimoyama T, Murakami H, Fujisake Y, Takayama K, Sakamoto T, Tamura T. A phase I study of erlotinib (TarcevaTM) monotherapy in Japanese patients with non-small cell lung cancer and other solid tumors. Lung Cancer 2003; 41:S251.

36. Ferrara N. The role of vascular endothelial growth factor in pathological angiogenesis. Breast Cancer Res Treat 1995; 36:127.

37. Wedge SR, Ogilvie DJ, Dukes M, et al. ZD6474 inhibits vascular endothelial growth factor signaling angiogenesis and tumor growth following oral administration. Cancer Res 2002; 62:4645.

38. Ciardiello F, Bianco R, Caputo R, et al. Antitumor activity of ZD6474 a vascular endothelial growth factor receptor tyrosine kinase inhibitor in human cancer cells with acquired resistance to antiepidermal growth factor receptor therapy. Clin Cancer Res 2004; 10:784.

39. Minami H, Ebi H, Tahara M, et al. A phase I study of an oral VEGF receptor tyrosine kinase inhibitor ZD6474 in Japanese patients with solid tumors. Proc Am Soc Clin Oncol 2003; 22:194.

Section VIII:
Mesothelioma

Epidemiology and Etiology of Mesothelioma

40

Spyros A. Papiris and Charis Roussos

Contents

40.1 Mesothelioma

Malignant mesothelioma is a highly aggressive and almost invariably fatal tumor arising from the mesothelial cells that form the serosal lining of the pleura, pericardium, peritoneum, and tunica vaginalis. More than 80% of malignant mesotheliomas are pleural in origin. Peritoneal mesothelioma appears to be more common in heavily exposed individuals [1]. Most of malignant mesotheliomas in the western world develop in individuals with higher than background asbestos exposure and it is unlikely that low environmental exposure to asbestos is associated with more than negligible risk of mesothelioma [2]. Indeed, the incidence of mesothelioma appears clearly parallel to the more widespread use of asbestos observed worldwide during the last half century, and it is actually estimated that about 5% of asbestos workers develop this disease. Mesothelioma can develop 20 or more years after the first exposure, while the peak incidence is between 35 and 45 years after exposure. However, the latency period ranges from a minimum of about 5 years [3] to a maximum of 72 years, so that exposed individuals are at risk for all their lives [4]. Non-occupational asbestos exposure has also been associated with an increase incidence of mesothelioma [5, 6]. In the USA, the incidence of mesothelioma, though difficult to be precisely determined, is estimated to be two to three thousand new cases per year [7]. However, it is estimated that the asbestos cancer epidemic may take as many as 10 million lives before asbestos is banned worldwide and exposures are brought to an end [8]. More recently, the oncogenic simian virus (SV) 40, a DNA virus of the family of papovaviridae, has also been implicated as a potential etiologic agent, though some controversy still exists [9]. Rare cases of mesothelioma have been associated with radiation exposure and the intravenous administration of the contrast medium Thorotrast [10]. Finally, in a restricted geographic area of three villages of Cappadocia, a region of central Anatolia in Turkey, more than 50% of all deaths are caused by pleural malignant mesothelioma. These cases are considered to be related to the erionite exposure, another non-asbestos mineral fiber, a type of fibrous zeolite commonly found in the stones of the houses of the villagers. This observation led to the recognition that erionite is one of the most potent chemical human carcinogens [11]. However, it is also known that approximately 20% of mesotheliomas occur in individuals with no history of asbestos exposure and only a small percentage of exposed individuals develop the disease, supporting the concept that genetic factors may play a significant role in its pathogenesis [12]. As appears from the above considerations, mesothelioma seems to have a complex etiology in which environmental carcinogens such as asbestos (by far the most important risk factor) and erionite, ionizing radiation, viruses, and possibly genetic factors act alone or in concomitance to induce malignancy [13]. Whatever the cause and because of its increasing incidence worldwide, the social impact of mesothelioma has become devastating, since no satisfactory treatment exists and survival time after diagnosis is usually less than 18 months.

40.2 Characteristics of Asbestos Fibers

Asbestos is the general name given to certain naturally occurring hydrated magnesium silicate fibrous minerals that form under high pressure in the earth's crust and are commonly found around earthquake faults. Geologists divide asbestos fibers into two groups: (1) serpentines, which include chrysotile (white asbestos), and (2) amphiboles, which include amosite (brown asbestos), crocidolite (blue asbestos), tremolite, anthophyllite, and actinolite. Asbestos fibers have several unique physical properties, such as thermal resistance, tensile strength, acoustic insulation, and resistance to degradation by both acid and alkaline solutions. The aspect ratio (length-to-width ratio) is the distinguishing feature of a particle and classifies it as a fiber when it is 3 or greater. Asbestos degrades by splitting longitudinally into even smaller fibers. This physical characteristic enhances its insulation properties but also increases the fraction of fibers that deposit deeply in the lung when inhaled. Fiber deposition in the lung occurs through five aerodynamic mechanisms: impaction, sedimentation, interception, electrostatic precipitation, and diffusion. Impaction and sedimentation depend on the aerodynamic diameter of the fiber, interception is governed by fiber length, and electrostatic precipitation depends on the electrical charge of the fiber. Processing of asbestos fibers results in aerosols with relatively high levels of electrical charge. Amphibole fibers when inhaled align parallel to the axis of flow and deposit deeply in the lung at the level of the alveolar ducts. Serpentine fibers such as chrysotile when inhaled have a mixed flow pattern and are more frequently deposited at the airway bifurcations. The biologically active or inhalable asbestos particles are those with a diameter of less than 3 µm and a length between 5 and 100 µm. Only 20% of asbestos fibers fall into this category and the most common is crocidolite.

40.3 History of Asbestos Utilization and Exposure

The word asbestos is derived from the Greek «asvestos» which means "inextinguishable or unquenchable" and reflects its resistance to heat and acid as well as its strength, durability, and flexibility. The Romans termed asbestos "amianthus" which means without miasma, undefiled or incorruptible. «Αμίαντος» (amiantos) is also the term actually used by the modern Greeks for asbestos and "amianto" by the Italians. Asbestos has been used by humans since 4,000 years before the Christian Era [14]. One of its first applications was for wicks in lamps and candles. Subsequently, 2–3000 years BCE asbestos was used in clothes to embalm the bodies of the Egyptian pharaohs and in Finland it was used in the same period, 2,500 years

BCE, to strengthen clay pots. Around 1000 years AD Mediterranean people used chrysotile from Cyprus and tremolite from north Italy to make cremation clothes, mats, and wicks for temple lamps. Three to four centuries later Marco Polo visited an asbestos mine in China. In the early 1700s asbestos papers and boards were made in Italy. Subsequent applications were as insulating material in steam engines in the USA (1828), for helmet and jackets by the Parisian Fire Brigade (1853), and for brake linings by Ferodo in England (1896). At the turn of the twentieth century asbestos applications and consequently exposure increased exponentially. One of its last applications was in the insulation of the solid fuel boosters of the space shuttle.

40.4 Epidemiology of Mesothelioma

In the first half of the twentieth century mesotheliomas were so rare that even their existence was debated [15]. In a review of 47 thousand autopsies at the Massachusetts General Hospital from 1896 to 1947 no mesotheliomas were found [16]. However, between 1947 and 1990 about 100 mesotheliomas were observed, and now it is estimated, and probably underestimated, that there are two to three thousand new cases every year in the USA [15]. The modern history of mesothelioma begins with the publication of the article "Diffuse pleural mesothelioma and asbestos exposure in the northwestern Cape province" [17], implicating asbestos exposure in the development of mesothelioma. The authors described a region in South Africa of about 8,000 square miles where crocidolite (locally named "woolstone") was mined. The earliest mining was a "family job" where men quarried the rocks and women and children separated fiber from stone. The increasing demand of asbestos around the years of World War II brought the large companies into the process of mining and processing and resulted in much higher numbers of involved and exposed individuals. Wagner and coworkers identified, in 4 years, 33 cases of mesothelioma almost exclusively in people living around the areas of mine or mill. This pioneering work provided the first and strong evidence of an association between asbestos and mesothelioma. This work also laid the foundation for the definitive investigation of insulation workers in the USA by Irving Selikoff and coworkers [18]. Selikoff's studies demonstrated an enormously increased mortality in these workers and made clear that an epidemic of occupational cancer was under way [18]. In South Africa mining reached its peak in 1977 with more than 380,000 tons being exported and 20,000 miners employed in the industry. South Africa also has large deposits of chrysotile and amosite both of which have been mined extensively. In South Africa the work by Wagner and coworkers was continued, not without difficulties, by Webster (funding was discontinued and the report was denigrated) [14] who reported 232 cases of mesothelioma based on pathology reports sent to the National Centre of Occupational Health [19] and by Zwi and coworkers who reported 1,347 cases diagnosed between 1976 and 1984 [20]. According to these reports, mesothelioma incidence in South Africa is amongst the highest in the world. It is 6 times higher than in England and at least as high as in Western Australia. The male/female ratio is 2.5/1. The incidence in blacks, for obvious reasons, is particularly under reported. Zwi's 9-year study also showed a steady increase in mesothelioma incidence during those years. In South Africa a high proportion of mesotheliomas (26%) is attributed to non-occupational, environmental origin, and among them 93% originate from exposure to crocidolite. Non-occupational exposures to asbestos can be grouped into three main categories: paraoccupational (familial), neighborhood, and true environmental exposures [6]. Among all reported environmental cases more than 70% of women and children are affected. This is presumably related to the asbestos brought home in the hairs and clothes of the miners.

Overall more than 30 million tons of asbestos in its various forms have been mined worldwide in the past century. Actually, the worldwide asbestos production exceeds 2 million tons each year. The greatest asbestos producers are Russia, China, Canada, Brazil, Kazakhstan, and Zimbabwe. Canada is the largest asbestos-exporting country, exporting 300,000 tons of chrysotile annually. All forms of asbestos can cause benign pleural effusions, pleural plaques, round atelectasis, diffuse fibrothorax, asbestosis (interstitial diffuse fibrosing alveolitis), lung cancer, and mesotheliomas. Chrysotile accounts for 90% of the commercially used asbestos worldwide, with the amphiboles constituting the rest. The amphiboles and particularly crocidolite appear to be the most carcinogenic of the fibers [21] though according to Stayner and coworkers it seems prudent "to treat chrysotile with virtually the same level of concern as the amphibole forms of asbestos" [22]. Indeed, on a per fiber basis, the highest risks of lung cancer have been shown for chrysotile [23]. Asbestos exposure affects not only asbestos workers but also their families, users of asbestos products, and the public as asbestos is used in building materials and in heating and ventilating systems [8]. Exposed women develop mesothelioma at rates at least as high as men with the same exposures, though their overall numbers are much lower since fewer women have occupational exposures. Epidemiologic studies attempted to define occupational risks associated with mesothelioma. In a work of the 1980s it was shown that the greater relative risk (RR) was associated with insulation work (RR=46), followed by employment in asbestos manufacture (RR=6.1), heating trades (RR=4.4), shipyards (RR=2.8), and construction (RR=2.0) [24]. Actually, asbestos is present in more than 3,000 manufactured products and justifiably constitutes one of the most pervasive environmental haz-

ards in the world and is a real "health catastrophe". In many developed countries, in specific age groups, mesothelioma may account for 1% of all deaths. In addition to mesotheliomas, 5–7% of all lung cancers can be attributed to asbestos exposure. Peak production and usage of asbestos occurred in many countries during the 1960s, 1970s, and 1980s and, as mesothelioma can develop 20 or more years after the first exposure, with a peak incidence coming 35–40 years after exposure, the incidence of mesothelioma is expected to increase dramatically over the next few years peaking in the developed world in or around the year 2020. In Western Europe it is estimated that deaths from mesothelioma will increase from just over 5,000 per year in 1998 to about 9,000 by the year 2018 [25], a global estimation of a quarter of a million deaths over the next 35 years. Lung cancer deaths caused by asbestos may even be much higher if we accept a ratio 7:1 (lung cancer to mesotheliomas deaths) suggested by some investigators [26]. The International Labor Organization (ILO) estimated that at least 100,000 and maybe as many as 140,000 workers die each year from asbestos exposures resulting in cancer [27]. Current estimations report that the asbestos cancer epidemic may take as many as 10 million lives before asbestos is banned worldwide and exposures are brought to an end [8]. In this conservative estimation, it is assumed that asbestos exposure is going to cease and that the epidemic will run itself out [8]. However, the world's asbestos production seems to have stabilized at around 2 million tons/year (2001–2002 data) and a global ban on asbestos is far from occurring. In future decades, the health problem of asbestos exposure will also occur in developing countries where in recent years most asbestos industries have transferred their economic interests, where protection of workers and communities is scant or non-existent, and where the asbestos cancer epidemic will become even more devastating than in the developed world [8].

40.5 Environmental Asbestos Exposure in the Metsovo Area of North-western Greece

Inhabitants of four villages of the Metsovo area (Metsovo, Milia, Anilio, and Votonosi) in the Epirus region, north-western Greece (population of 4,250 inhabitants on the 1981 census and of 4,494 on the 1991 census) have been exposed, since childhood, to asbestos from a material used for whitewashing. This material locally called "luto" soil contains tremolite and had been used by practically all households until 1950–1960 [28–30]. This tremolite-containing whitewash was taken from outcrops in nearby hills, shaped into balls, and sold. Subsequently, the women of Metsovo crushed the balls into fine powder, boiled it in water, and applied it to the walls once or twice a year. During the extraction process, and particularly while crushing this material, a tremendous amount of fibers was released (>200 fibers per cm^3) and inhaled [31]. Tremolite fibers were indeed identified in the lung parenchyma of the exposed individuals in transbronchial lung biopsy specimens [32]. The exposure of inhabitants of Metsovo to tremolite has resulted in endemic pleural calcifications in at least half of the population [29, 30, 33, 34], a high incidence of malignant pleural mesothelioma [29, 30], sporadic cases of round atelectasis eventually related to the development of a previous benign asbestos pleural effusion [35], and lymphocytic alveolitis especially among inhabitants with pleural calcifications [36], but no diffuse fibrosing interstitial lung pneumonia (asbestosis). The combination of the above findings (and especially the mesothelioma and pleural calcifications) has been named "Metsovo lung" and has been established as an example of non-occupational exposure to tremolite. Metsovo exposure appears to be a unique kind of exposure, differing from the "usual" occupational or non-occupational exposures in the following aspects: (1) it was a "woman's job" and exposure eventually included their small children present during the in-house part of the process (very early in life exposure); (2) the exposure was not continuous; and (3) exposure was very heavy during crushing [37]. The use of "luto" soil gradually diminished during the next three decades and was finally abandoned in the early 1980s. The diminished use of "luto" whitewash was followed by a drop in the incidence of mesotheliomas in the area [37]. Actually it is expected that the "Metsovo mesothelioma epidemic" will fade away by the year 2020–2030, since the material has not been used since 1985 [37]. Environmental asbestos exposure has also been reported in several other geographic areas of Greece "outside Metsovo" [31].

40.6 Malignant Pleural Mesothelioma in Turkey: Geographic Areas with Environmental Asbestos Exposure and Other Geographic Areas with Environmental Exposure to Erionite

Turkey is a country with large natural asbestos deposits and a high prevalence of endemic asbestos-related pulmonary disease [38–41]. Asbestos-contaminated soil mixtures are commonly found in the rural areas around Eskisehir in central Anatolia, where they have been used for many years locally by the rural inhabitants to make a whitewash (in a strikingly similar way to the villagers of Metsovo, Greece) or stucco for the walls, floors, and roofs of the houses and also for baby powder, in pottery, or added to grape juice. These soil mixtures are known in Anatolia as "aktoprak" (white soil)

or "çorak." Mineralogical analysis disclosed that besides tremolite (the most prominent asbestos type found as a contaminant of white stucco in these areas), chrysotile asbestos and, in certain districts (Mihaliççik and Edige), anthophyllite also contaminate white stucco [42]. The above-mentioned environmental exposure to asbestos as a cause of pleural mesothelioma has been documented in many studies [43–46]. Recently it has also been shown that this type of environmental exposure may be responsible for the very high incidence of mesothelioma observed in the villagers exposed, similar to the occupationally exposed asbestos cohorts [40].

In the Nevsehir region of Cappadocia, an informal ancient denomination for parts of central Anatolia, there are three villages, Karain, Tuzköy, and Sarihidir, with a population of around 5,000 people. It has been recently shown that up to 50% of deaths in Karain, between 1970 and 1994, and 36% of deaths in the other two villages, between 1980 and 1994, were due to pleural and, less frequently, peritoneal mesothelioma [11]. Mesothelioma also caused 78% of deaths found in a cohort of 162 Karain villagers who had emigrated to Sweden [46]. These mesotheliomas are attributed to erionite, a fibrous type of zeolite present in stones used to build these villages and mined from nearby caves, and villagers exposed to it have the highest incidence of mesothelioma in the world. Erionite belongs to the mineralogical group of zeolites, a group of hydrated aluminosilicates of alkali and alkaline earths. Zeolites occur in cavities in basic volcanic rocks and in other late-stage hydrothermal environments. Erionite fibers are found in rocks and soils of areas of the above-referred villages, which like many other places in Cappadocia, Turkey, are characterized by ancient rock dwellings and caves dug in soft volcanic tuff. This type of dwelling favors the continuous exposure of inhabitants to erionite fibers. Epidemiologic and experimental data have shown that erionite fibers have the highest carcinogenic potency among any other fibers so far studied [47–50]. Erionite fibers also have a very strong fibrogenic potential. High concentrations of erionite fibers have been found in air samples and in lung tissue and bronchoalveolar lavage fluid of residents from these villages [51]. However, epidemiologic studies in this particular geographic area demonstrated that mesothelioma developed more frequently in certain families and in specific homes, where entire families had died from the disease. Interestingly, in Karlik, a village with a population of about 1,500, 1 km south of Karain, and built with the same stones used to build Karain, no mesothelioma was found except in a woman from Karain who relocated there, suggesting a strong genetic factor contributing to mesothelioma appearance in certain families. To investigate this hypothesis, an analysis of a six-generation extended pedigree of 526 individuals was conducted and it indicated that mesothelioma occurrence, at least in this area, can be explained by genetic susceptibility, which is probably transmitted in an auto-somal dominant way [52]. In these cases erionite might be a cofactor in the cause of mesothelioma, in genetically predisposed individuals.

40.7 Other Geographic Areas with Natural Asbestos Deposits and Environmental Asbestos Exposure

Environmental asbestos exposure is also common in some other rural parts of the world, including other geographic areas of Greece "outside Metsovo" [31], Cyprus, where asbestos deposits contain mostly chrysotile with some tremolite contamination [53], and New Caledonia [54] and Corsica, where both chrysotile and tremolite can be found [55,56]. In all of the above areas an increasing incidence of mesothelioma was described confirming the association between natural asbestos deposits and mesothelioma in non-occupationally exposed populations.

40.8 Etiology of Mesothelioma

After the publication of the "milestone" study by Wagner and coworkers describing mesotheliomas in subjects who lived in the Blue Hills region of Northwest Cape Province of South Africa, and its confirmation by several other studies in the same geographic area and worldwide, asbestos is to be considered the primary etiologic agent of mesothelioma. All asbestos fibers are injurious and carcinogenic for both animals and human, crocidolite (blue asbestos) and amosite (brown asbestos) being the most harmful. In addition several cases of mesothelioma have been associated with erionite fiber exposure, radiation therapy such as in the treatment of Hodgkin's disease [10], chronic inflammation [57], and the Simian virus 40 (SV40), a contaminant of early polio vaccines that were provided to millions of individuals in Europe and in the USA between 1955 and 1963 [58]. Organic chemicals, including polyurethane, polysilicone, ethylene oxide, N-methyl-n nitrosourethane diethylstilbestrol, and mineral oil, have

been shown to cause mesothelioma in rodents [59]. Also other non-asbestos fibers such as fiberglass have been implicated in mesothelioma development in animals [60]. Furthermore, the occurrence of mesothelioma among subjects with blood relations suggests that genetic factors might play a role in determining the susceptibility to asbestos-related cancer [61]. Finally, it is also known that approximately 20% of mesotheliomas occur in individuals with no history of asbestos exposure or to any other putative etiologic factor and that only a small percentage of asbestos-exposed individuals develop the disease, supporting the concept that genetic factors may play some role in mesothelioma development [12] (Table 40.1).

40.9 Simian Virus 40 and Mesothelioma

Simian virus 40 is a small, circular, 5,243-bp, double-stranded DNA polyomavirus of the family of papoviridae of monkey origin. SV40 was found by Sweet and Hilleman to be one of the viruses infecting rhesus and cynomolgus monkey kidney cells used for the preparation of polio and other vaccines [62]. Soon after, it was shown that SV40 had the capacity to infect and transform human cells in vitro [63]. Experimental studies have shown subsequently the potentiality of wild-type SV40 viruses to induce mesotheliomas with at least the same potency as asbestos fibers [64–66]. The primary mechanism of the SV40 oncogenic effect is thought to occur through its linkage with the large T cell antigen Tag and the subsequent inactivation of two tumor suppressor genes, p53 and retinoblastoma protein, Rb, as well as of their products, p107 and p130. The result is a combination of loss of cell cycle regulation associated with genomic instability, cell transformation, immortalization, and tumor development [58]. Hundreds of millions of SV40-contaminated poliovirus vaccine preparations, prepared in Macaca kidney cells, were used between 1955 and 1962 to vaccinate people in USA, Europe, the former USSR, Mexico, Japan, and Central America. Both the inactivated Salk subcutaneous vaccine and the live attenuated Sabin vaccine were contaminated, which were both prepared from macaque rhesus monkey cell cultures. Soon after SV40 was reported to be oncogenic in hamsters, the US government

Table 40.1. Etiologic factors of mesothelioma

Fibers	Radiation	Chemicals	Inflammation	Viruses	Genetic factors
Asbestos (chrysotile, amosite, crocidolite, tremolite, anthophyllite, actinolite) Erionite Fiberglass?	Ionizing radiation Thorotrast	Polyurethane Polysilicone Ethylene oxide N-Methyl-n nitrosourethane diethylstilbestrol Mineral oil	TBC pleuritis?	Simian virus 40?	Autosomal dominant way in Cappadocia

disposed that all newly produced polio vaccine should be free of the contaminant virus but they did not remove the already contaminated ones from the vaccine program. In the following decades SV40 DNA was detected in a variety of human tumors such as mesotheliomas, osteosarcomas, other bone tumors, and brain tumors, and several epidemiologic and experimental studies have suggested a role of SV40 alone or in combination with asbestos fibers [67] in determining an increase of certain human tumors including mesotheliomas. However, the National Institutes of Health and the Food and Drug Administration special joint workshop failed to reach an agreement on the role of SV40 as a potential human carcinogen [68]. Disagreement was based on: (1) the lack of detection of SV40 DNA in human mesothelioma experiments by Shah [69]; (2) the SV40 DNA detection in normal tissue and body fluids; and (3) the inadequacy of epidemiologic data. Furthermore, a recent study has brought more evidence against a role for SV40 infection in human mesotheliomas and the high risk of false-positive PCR results due to the presence of SV40 sequences in common laboratory plasmids [9]. The authors conclude "that clinicians should continue to consider asbestos exposure as the most likely and most thoroughly established etiological factor in individuals with mesothelioma" [9].

40.10 Conclusion

Unequivocally the history of mesothelioma parallels that of asbestos exposure. The estimation that the asbestos cancer epidemic will cause 10 million deaths past and present renders the need to reach urgently a global ban on asbestos an issue of highest priority, so that the asbestos cancer epidemic will not become more devastating and will not continue indefinitely.

Key Points

- Mesothelioma is a highly aggressive and invariably fatal tumor arising from mesothelial cells that form the serosal lining of the pleura, and less frequently of the pericardium, peritoneum, or tunica vaginalis.
- Almost all mesotheliomas develop in individuals with higher than background asbestos exposure. Asbestos is present in more than 3,000 manufactured products and constitutes one of the most pervasive environmental hazards in the world. Asbestos exposure affects not only asbestos workers but also their families, users of asbestos products, and the public as it is exposed to building materials and asbestos in heating and ventilating systems.

References

1. Britton M. The epidemiology of mesothelioma. *Semin Oncol* 2002;29:18.
2. Ware A, Price B. Mesothelioma trends in the United States: an update based on surveillance, epidemiology, and end results program data for 1973 through 2003. Am J Epidemiol 2004;159:107.
3. Booth SJ, Weaver EJM. Malignant pleural mesothelioma five years after domestic exposure to blue asbestos. Lancet 1986;i:435.
4. Bianchi C, Giarelli L, Grandi G, Brollo A, Ramani L, Zuch C. Latency periods in asbestos-related mesothelioma of the pleura. Eur J Cancer Prevent 1997;6:162.
5. Hansen J, de Klerk NH, Musk AW, Hobbs TMS. Environmental exposure to crocidolite and mesothelioma. Exposure-response relationships. Am J Respir Crit Care Med 1998;157:69.
6. Orenstein MR, Schenker MB. Environmental asbestos exposure and mesothelioma. Curr Opin Pulm Med 2000;6:371.
7. Price B. Analysis of current trends in United States mesothelioma incidence. Am J Epidemiol 1997;145:211.
8. LaDou J. The asbestos cancer epidemic. Environ Health Perspect 2004;112:285.
9. López-Rios F, Illei PB, Rusch V, Ladanyi M. Evidence against a role for SV40 infection in human mesotheliomas and high risk of false-positive PCR results owing to presence of SV40 sequences in common laboratory plasmids. Lancet 2004;364:1157.
10. Weissmann LB, Corson JM, Neugut AI, Antman KH. Malignant mesothelioma following treatment for Hodgkin's disease. J Clin Oncol 1996;14:2098.
11. Baris B, Demir AU, Shehu V, Karakoca Y, Kisacik G, Baris YI. Environmental fibrous zeolite (erionite) exposure and malignant tumors other than mesothelioma. J Environ Pathol Toxicol Oncol 1996;15:183.
12. Huncharek M. Genetic factors in the aetiology of malignant mesothelioma. Eur J Cancer 1995;31:1741.
13. Carbone M, Kratzke RA, Testa JR. The pathogenesis of mesothelioma. Semin Oncol 2002;29:2.
14. Abratt RP, Vorobiof DA, White N. Asbestos and mesothelioma in South Africa. Lung Cancer 2004;45S:S3.
15. Hughes RS. Malignant pleura mesothelioma. Am J Med Sci 2005;329:29.
16. Mark EJ, Yokoi T. Absence of evidence for a significant background incidence of diffuse malignant mesothelioma apart from asbestos exposure. Ann N Y Acad Sci 1991;643:196.
17. Wagner J, Sleggs C, Marchand P. Diffuse pleural mesothelioma and asbestos exposure in the northwestern Cape province. Br J Ind Med 1960;17:260.
18. Selikoff IJ, Hammond EC, Churg J, Asbestos exposure and neoplasia. JAMA 1964;188:22.
19. Webster I. Asbestos and malignancy. S Afr Med J 1973;47:165.
20. Zwi AB, Reid G, London SP, Kielkowski D, Sitas F, Becklake MR. Mesothelioma in South Africa 1976–1984: incidence and case characteristics. Int J Epidemiol 1989;18:320.
21. Niklinski J, Niklinska W, Chyczewski E, Laudanski J, Naumnik W, Chyczewski L, Pluygers. The epidemiology of asbestos related diseases. Lung Cancer 2004;45S:S7.
22. Stayner LT, Dankovic DA, Lemen RA. Occupational exposure to chrysotile asbestos and cancer risk: a review of the amphibole hypothesis. Am J Public Health 1996;86:179.
23. Dement JM, Brown DP, Okun A. Follow-up study of crysotile asbestos textile workers: cohort mortality and case-control analysis. Am J Ind Med 1994;26:431.

24. MacDonald AD, MacDonald JC. Malignant mesothelioma in North America. Cancer 1980;46:1650.

25. Peto J, Decarli A, La Vecchia C, Levi F, Negri E. The European mesothelioma epidemic. Br J Cancer 1999;79;566.

26. ILO. Introductory report: decent work-safe work. Geneva: International Labour Organization. 2002.

27. Howie RM. Asbestos and cancer risk. Ann Occup Hyg 2001;45:335.

28. Langer AM, Nolan RP, Constantopoulos SH, Moutsopoulos HM. Association of Metsovo lung and pleural mesothelioma with exposure to tremolite-containing whitewash. Lancet 1987;i:319.

29. Constantopoulos SH, Malamou-Mitsi V, Goudevenos J, Papathanasiou MP, Pavlidis NA, Papadimitriou CS. High incidence of malignant pleura mesothelioma in neighbouring villages of north-west Greece. Respiration 1987;51:266.

30. Constantopoulos SH, Saratzis N, Goudevenos J, Kontogiannis D, Karantanas A, Katsiotis P. Tremolite whitewashing and pleural calcifications. Chest 1987;92:709.

31. Constantopoulos SH, Theodorakopoulos P, Dascalopoulos G, Saratzis NA, Sideris K. Metsovo lung outside Mestovo: endemic pleural calcifications in the ophiolite belts of Greece. Chest 1991;99:1158.

32. Constantopoulos SH, Goudevenos J, Saratzis N, Langer AE, Selikoff IJ, Moutsopoulos HM. Metsovo lung: pleural calcifications and restrictive lung function in north-western Greece; environmental exposure to mineral fiber as etiology. Environ Res 1985;38:391.

33. Bazas T, Bazas B, Kitas D, Gilson JC, McDonald JC. Pleural calcification in northwest Greece [letter]. Lancet 1981;1:254.

34. Bazas T, Oakes D, Gilson JC, Bazas B, McDonald JC. Pleural calcification in north-west Greece. Environ Res 1985;38:239.

35. Papiris SA, Maniati MA, Sakellariou K, Gosios C, Kontogiannis D, Constantopoulos H. Round atelectasis and Metsovo lung. Chest 1993;103:1759.

36. Constantopoulos SH, Dalavanga YA, Sakellariou K, Goudevenos J, Kotoulas OB. Lymphocytic alveolitis and pleural calcifications in nonoccupational asbestos exposure: protection against neoplasia? Am Rev Respir Dis 1992;146:1565.

37. Sakellariou K, Malamou-Mitsi V, Haritou A, Koumpaniou C, Stachouli C, Dimoliatis ID, Constantopoulos SH. Malignant pleura mesothelioma from nonoccupational asbestos exposure in Metsovo (north-west Greece): slow end of an epidemic. Eur Respir J 1996;9:1206.

38. Karakoca Y, Emri S, Cangir AK, Baris YI. Environmental pleural plaques due to asbestos and fibrous zeolite exposure in Turkey. Indoor Built Environ 1997;6:100.

39. Emri S, Demir A, Dogan M, Akay H, Bozkurt B, Carbone M, Baris I. Lung disease due to environmental exposures to erionite and asbestos in Turkey. Toxicol Lett 2002;127:251.

40. Metintas S, Metintas M, Ucgun I, Oner U. Malignant mesothelioma due to environmental exposure to asbestos. Follow-up of a Turkish cohort living in a rural area. Chest 2002;122:2224.

41. Emri S, Demir AU. Malignant pleural mesothelioma in Turkey, 2000–2002. Lung Cancer 2004;45S:S17.

42. Dogan M, Emri S. Environmental health problems related to mineral dusts in Ankara and Eskisehir, Turkey. Yerbilimleri 2000;22:149.

43. Yazicioglu S, Ilcayto R, Balci K, Sayli BS, Yorulmaz B. Pleural calcification, pleural mesotheliomas and bronchial cancers caused by tremolite dust. Thorax 1980;35:564.

44. Hillerdal G, Baris YI. Radiological study of pleural changes in relation to mesothelioma in Turkey. Thorax 1983;38:443.

45. Baris YI. Asbestos and erionite related disease. Ankara, Turkey. Semith Ofset Mat Com 1987;8.

46. Metintas M, Hilllerdal H, Metintas S. Malignant mesothelioma due to environmental exposure to erionite: follow-up of a Turkish cohort. Eur Respir J 1999;13:523.

47. Baris Y, Simonato L, Artvinli M, et al. Epidemiological and environmental evidence of the health effects of exposure to erionite fibers: a 4 year study in the Cappadocian region of Turkey. Int J Cancer 1987;39:10.

48. Maltoni C, Minardi F, Morisi L. Pleural mesotheliomas in Sprague-Dawley rats by erionite: first experimental evidence. Environ Res 1982;29:238.

49. Davis JM, Bolton RE, Miller BG, Niven K. Mesothelioma dose response following intraperitoneal injection of mineral fiber. Int J Exp Pathol 1991;72:263.

50. Wagner JC, Skidmore JW, Hill RJ, Griffiths DM. Erionite exposure and mesotheliomas in rats. Br J Cancer 1985;51:727.

51. Dumortier P, Çoplü L, Broucke I, Emri S, Selcuk T, de Maerelaer V, De Vuyst P, Baris I. Erionite bodies and fibers in bronchoalveolar lavage fluid (BALF) of residents from Tuzköy, Cappadocia, Turkey. Occup Environ Med 2001;58:261.

52. Rousdy-Hamady I, Siegel J, Emri S, Testa JR, Carbone M. Genetic-susceptibility factor and malignant mesothelioma in the Cappadocian region of Turkey. Lancet 2001;357:444.

53. McConnochie K, Simonato L, Mavrides P, Christofides P, Pooley FD, Wagner JC. Mesothelioma in Cyprus: the role of tremolite. Thorax 1987;42:342.

54. Goldberg P, Goldberg M, Marne MJ, Hirsch A, Tredaniel J. Incidence of pleural mesothelioma in New Caledonia: a 10 year survey (1978–1987). Arch Environ Hlth 1991;46:306.

55. Luce D, Brochard P, Quenel P, Salomon-Nekiriai C, Goldberg P, Billon-Galland MA, Goldberg M. Malignant pleural mesothelioma associated with exposure to tremolite. Lancet 1994;344:8939.

56. Rey F, Boutin C, Steinbauer J, Viallat JR, Alessandroni P, Jutisz P, Di Giambattista D, Billon-Galland MA, Hereng P, Dumortier P, et al. Environmental pleural plaques in an asbestos exposed population of northeast Corsica. Eur Resp J 1993;6:978.

57. Roviaro GC, Sartori F, Calabro F, Varoli F. The association of pleural mesothelioma and tuberculosis. Am Rev Respir Dis 1982;126:569.

58. Cerrano PG, Jasani B, Filiberti R, Neri M, Merlo F, De Flora S, Mutti L, Puntoni R. Simian virus 40 and malignant mesothelioma. Int J Oncol 2003;22:187.

59. Bass P, Schouwink H, Zoetmulder FA. Malignant pleural mesothelioma. Ann Oncol 1998;9:139.

60. Stanton MF, Wrench C. Mechanisms of mesothelioma induction with asbestos and fibrous glass. J Natl Cancer Inst 1972;48:797.

61. Bianchi C, Brollo A, Ramani L, Bianchi T, Giarelli L. Familial mesothelioma of the pleura: a report of 40 cases. Ind Health 2004;42:235.

62. Sweet BH, Hilleman MR. The vacualating SV40. Proc Soc Exp Biol Med 1960;105:420.

63. Shein HM, Enders JF. Transformation induced by simian virus 40 in human renal cell cultures. 1. Morphology and growth characteristics. Proc Natl Acad Sci U S A 1962;48:1164.

64. Carbone M, Lewis AM Jr, Matthews BJ, Levine AS, Dixon K. Characterization of hamster tumors induced by simian virus 40 small t deletion mutants as true histiocytic lymphomas. Cancer Res 1989;49:1565.

65. Cicala C, Pompetti F, Carbone M. SV40 induces mesotheliomas in hamsters. Am J Pathol 1993;142:1524.

66. Carbone M, Fisher S, Powers A, Pass HI, Rizzo P. New molecular and epidemiological issues in mesothelioma: role of SV40. J Cell Physiol 1999;180:167.

67. Bocchetta M, Di Resta I, Powers A, Fresco R, Tosolini A, Testa JR, Pass HI, Rizzo P, Carbone M. Human mesothelial cells are unusually susceptible to simian virus 40-mediated transformation and asbestos cocarcinogenicity. Proc Natl Acad Sci U S A 2000;97:10214.

68. Brown F, Lewis AM Jr (eds). Simian virus 40 (SV40): a possible human polyomavirus. Basel: Karger, 1998.

69. Shah KV. Search for SV40 in human mesothelioma. In: Brown F, Lewis AM Jr (eds) Simian Virus 40 (SV40): A Possible Human Polyomavirus. Basel: Karger, 1998:68.

Molecular Epidemiology and Biology of Mesothelioma

41

Riccardo Puntoni and Rosangela Filiberti

Contents

41.1 Etiopathogenesis

Nowadays, molecular events leading to the development of malignant pleural mesothelioma (MPM) have not yet been completely elucidated. The long latent period between the exposure to asbestos, the major determinant of MPM, and clinical diagnosis indicates that multiple genetic alterations are required for malignant transformation of the mesothelium [1–3].

Genomic instability, reduced DNA repair capacity, disruption of programmed cell death, and inherited susceptibility are involved in the etiology of the disease [4].

Asbestos causes structural and numerical chromosome aberrations in cultured mammalian cells. It produces cell transformations, induces genotoxicity characterized by the formation of aneuploid cells, abnormal anaphases, chromosomal aberrations, DNA single strand breaks, and abnormal DNA repair in human mesothelial cells and increases apoptosis [5–9]. An important role played by DNA double strand breaks at the initial stage of asbestos injury has been suggested [10].

Two major mechanisms have been recently proposed for asbestos-induced genotoxicity: one involves the physical effects of fibers on chromosome and spindle apparatus, and the second relies on the assumption that asbestos toxicity and carcinogenicity are mediated by reactive oxygen or nitrogen species (ROS/RNS), such as hydrogen peroxide (H_2O_2), superoxide anion (O_2^-) and the hydroxyl radical ($HO^\bullet$) [11, 12]. Inflammatory cells such as pulmonary alveolar macrophages and neutrophils are able to release ROS and RNS as a result of prolonged phagocytic activity against asbestos fibers [12–14]. The free radicals generated by these processes may cause cellular toxicity and carcinogenicity by damaging DNA, inducing lipid peroxidation, and altering signal transduction pathways. The role of oxidative damage in asbestos-induced mutagenicity has been recently demonstrated in vivo [15, 16]. Oxidative stress and oxidative DNA damage have been observed in workers highly exposed to asbestos fibers in the past [17].

Early studies on SV40 suggested a possible role of this virus in the impairment of DNA repair mechanisms in mesothelial cells, hypothesizing an additive effect with asbestos fibers, recently reported also in humans [18]. In SV40 immortalized cell lines an interference of T antigen with DNA repair has been reported [19]. SV40 transformation was shown to reduce the level of DNA repair, most likely because of the inhibition of normal p53 function by LTAg [20].

It has been supposed that asbestos exposure induces stem cell proliferation and that the carcinogenic process progresses with activation of proto-oncogenes and inactivation of tumor suppressor genes. SV40 increases the risk of MPM inducing DNA alterations and accelerating malignant transformation. Nevertheless, due to the lack of data for early stages of MPM, a temporal sequence of these alterations is not determined [21].

Most human MPM are linked to various non-random chromosomal deletions involving specific regions in chromosome arms 1p, 3p, 4q, 6q, 9p, 13q, 14q, 15q, and 22q. These losses may occur in combination in the same tumor. Less common are chromosomal gains that may be present in chromosome 5p, 5, 7, and 20 [7, 10, 22, 23]. These alterations are caused by asbestos, SV40, and other carcinogens, but likely they also reflect an intrinsic predisposition of the cell to accumulate genetic damage. It is plausible that MPM risk factors act with a stimulatory or an inhibitory effect, triggering off a cascade of molecular events.

The rarity of the disease among exposed subjects and the presence of MPM cases among subjects with very low or unknown levels of asbestos exposure suggest again a complex carcinogenic process with the involvement of susceptibility or other unknown cofactors.

41.2 Molecular Epidemiology

In the 20 years since 1985, the so-called "Traditional Epidemiology", or "Black Box Epidemiology", has been considered inadequate to study the causes of cancer and the mechanistic aspects of the progression of the neoplasias. Therefore, the design of the epidemiological studies has been enriched by introducing biological markers and a "Molecular Epidemiology" approach has been created. This new research, as written by Perera [24], "seeks to combine the precision of laboratory methods to quantify carcinogenic dose or preclinical response in humans, with the relevance and rigor of analytic epidemiology." This new method of study is based on properly designed epidemiological studies that take into account the control of confounding factors, the selection of appropriate control groups, the power of the studies, and the extent to which a biological marker can predict cancer occurrence [25, 26].

Molecular epidemiology has a great potential in the study of MPM, for example, in the detection of early effect markers in people exposed to occupational or environmental carcinogens or in the assessment of susceptibility factors that might predispose to cancer, as well as in the identification of prognostic factors.

Malignant pleural mesothelioma is largely preventable because the causative factors are mostly of environmental origin. Recently, new findings concerning the role of genetic factors have changed the research perspective of MPM prevention. A better understanding of molecular pathogenesis of MPM is a clue factor to organize screening programs for early diagnosis in workers exposed in the past to asbestos fibers and to establish new therapeutic protocols.

In this chapter we have concentrated our discussion in the field of biological markers of susceptibility and of markers of diagnosis and prognosis for pleural malignant mesothelioma. To this aim, we have focused our attention on some phase I and II polymorphic metabolic genes. Then, we have reported some data on the role of oncoproteins as possible markers of risk as well as markers of early disease and as prognostic factors.

41.3 The Micronucleus Test (MNT)

Heritable differences in host resistance to genetic changes may be identified at different phases of the carcinogenic process, such as DNA repair competency and chromosome stability.

Human neoplasms exhibit chromosomal aberrations in tumor tissue samples, as well as in peripheral blood lymphocytes (PBLs). PBLs offer the advantage of non-invasive sample collection and provide a large quantity of cells for analysis. Cytogenetic damage, measured as chromosomal aberrations in PBLs, is a reliable biomarker for human cancer risk independent of the exposure to carcinogens [27].

The MNT in PBLs has been applied as a simple and reliable method for the detection of cytogenetic damage. This assay could be used to assess the chromosomal damage as chromosomal fragments or whole chromosome that is excluded from the nucleus at mitosis. MNT in PBLs seems to be useful for monitoring individuals with genetic instability [28] and as a screening test for carriers of specific mutations in evaluating cancer susceptibility [29, 30].

Elevated levels of micronuclei (MN) in PBLs of cancer patients prior to chemotherapy or radiotherapy have been reported in a number of papers [31–33]. Ad hoc biomonitoring studies dealing with specific types of cancer could help to understand the importance of this biomarker in terms of individual genetic cancer susceptibility and of reduced individual DNA repair capability.

Polyomaviruses such as SV40 and JC virus (JCV) are oncogenic in animal models and transform animal and human cells of different types [34, 35]. Moreover, SV40 and JCV are able to infect human PBLs inducing chromosomal instability [36, 37].

A study to evaluate the MN frequency in PBLs of patients with MPM with respect to lung cancer (LC) and two control groups, as a marker of cancer risk, was carried out [38]. The study included 21 patients with MPM and 37 patients with lung cancer. Sixty-two subjects as healthy controls (HC) and 33 with benign respiratory diseases, as at risk controls (RC), were also studied. Benign diseases were mostly chronic obstructive pulmonary disease (27 patients). The other patients had asbestosis (1), silicosis (3), and emphysema (2). Neoplastic patients were incident consecutive cases with no previous chemotherapeutic and radiotherapy treatment. Blood samples from these patients were collected on average within 20 days of the disease diagnosis. The blood samples of HCs were recruited from a group of blood donors working in the study areas or from patients hospitalized for non-neoplastic, non-respiratory diseases. The epidemiological data were collected through a questionnaire given to all subjects. Information was obtained on demographic data, smoking and

Table 41.1. Micronuclei frequency (MN×1,000 PBL) according to smoking habits and asbestos exposure

	N	Mean	Median	Range
Smoking habits[a]				
Never	26	8.9	6.8	1.0–21.7
Former	67	7.1	6.2	1.1–28.0
Current	59	7.2	6.3	1.2–15.5
Cig. pack/year				
<19.5	26	6.8	6.1	1.1–15.5
19.5–43.6	46	7.8	6.6	1.2–28.0
≥43.7	57	7.1	6.2	1.5–15.8
Asbestos exposure				
No exposure	116	7.0	6.2	1.0–21.7
Exposure	36	8.9	6.4	1.2–28.0

[a] The sum may not add up to the total because of missing values

lifestyle habits, occupational and environmental exposure, tumor familiarity, clinical anamnesis, and medical treatments. Exposure to asbestos for each group was assessed according to the type of activity leading to the exposure and length of exposure. The modified cytokinesis-blocked method of Fenech and Morley [39] was used to determine MN frequency.

Data on MN frequency by type, age, gender, smoking status, and asbestos exposure are reported in Table 41.1. In each group, MN distribution was no different in subjects with a previous asbestos exposure with respect to non-exposed subjects. No relationship was evident between MN and the other explanatory variables such as age, smoking habits, and polyoma virus. A significant increase in micronucleated binucleated (BNMN) lymphocytes was observed in patients with malignant mesothelioma in comparison with all other subjects. A significant higher median frequency was recorded for MPM patients (11.4 BNMN/1,000 BN) with respect to

LC (5.1, $p < 0.0001$), RC (6.1, $p = 0.002$), or HC (6.2, $p < 0.0001$) (Fig. 41.1). The patient with asbestosis in the RC group showed an MN value of 5.7 BNMN/1,000 BN, no different from the non-MPM groups. Two MPM patients (female, aged 63 and 68 years) did not report asbestos exposure. MN frequency in these subjects was 13.6 and 14.5 BNMN/1,000 BN, respectively. Also the third (out of four) woman affected by mesothelioma, despite a low level of asbestos exposure as wife of a dockyard worker, showed a very high frequency of MN (21.4 BNMN/1,000 BN).

Various types of asbestos fibers show their capability to induce MN using the MNT. The loss of whole chromosomes as well as clastogenic events are involved in the induction of MN by asbestos fibers [40, 41].

The evidence of cytogenetic damage revealed as MN frequency in mesothelioma patients could be related to exogenous and endogenous co-factors, besides asbestos exposure.

41.4 Polymorphisms of Metabolic Genes

The study of polymorphisms of metabolic genes may permit to assess differences among individuals or populations that affect the response to the environmental agents. These differences do not depend on the exposure under investigation, but on genetic or other endogenous features influencing the internal dose, the biologically effective dose, and, consequently, the response of the target tissue. These markers can account for interindividual variations in the activities of metabolizing enzymes responsible for activation (phase I reactions) or deactivation (phase II reactions) of carcinogens [42, 43].

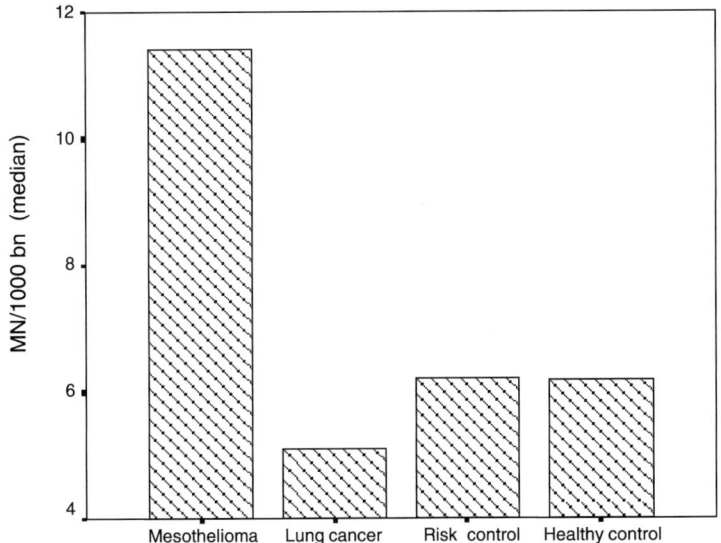

Fig. 41.1. Micronuclei frequency in mesothelioma and lung cancer cases and controls. (*MN* Micronuclei, *BN* binucleated lymphocytes)

A single base change may create a different amino acid sequence with a functional alteration of the gene activity. This genetic profile may be inherited and can lead to conspicuous differences in the individual sensitivity to the effects of chemical exposures. The accumulated evidence supports the hypothesis that cancer susceptibility following exposure to environmental carcinogens depends on the combined effect of exposure and genetic capacity to activate or inactivate carcinogens. For this reason, metabolic genes encoding for enzymes involved in conjugation and detoxification of environmental or endogenous toxicants are considered involved in the carcinogenic pathway of MPM. Recently, some metabolic susceptibility genes have been considered important for human MPM.

1. The genes of the cytochrome P450 (CYP) family, which mediate the phase I reactions of metabolic activation; for example, CYP1A1 may produce epoxide metabolites that are reactive and unstable and may be inactivated by the microsomal epoxide hydrolase (mEH).

2. The phase II genes glutathione S-transferases (GSTs) and N-acetyltransferases (NATs); GSTM.

3. The mEH gene, which plays a dual role in bioactivation and detoxification of procarcinogens. mEH is involved in general oxidative defenses against a number of environmental substances [44, 45]. This enzyme is inducible by oxidative stress, and chrysotile has been shown to decrease its activity in vitro [46–48]. Polymorphisms in the mEH gene have also been associated with respiratory diseases [49].

A study by Smith et al. [50] showed that non-malignant asbestos-related diseases develop more frequently in occupationally asbestos-exposed subjects carrying homozygous deletion (null genotype) of the GSTM1 gene. Hirvonen et al. [51] reported that "individuals with homozygous deletion of the GSTM1 gene and a NAT2 slow-acetylator genotype who are exposed to high levels of asbestos appear to have enhanced susceptibility to asbestos-related pulmonary disorders." In a paper by Stucker et al. [52] results showed that the GSTM1 genotype did not interact with asbestos exposure in the risk of lung cancer.

The first paper on MPM was published in 1995 by Hirvonen et al. [53] and reported that individuals with combined GSTM1 and NAT2 defects had about a 3.6-fold risk of developing MPM compared to those with the GSTM1 gene and NAT2 fast-acetylator genotype. Moreover, the risk among subjects highly exposed to asbestos with the double at-risk genotype was more than 7 times greater compared to those with the more beneficial genotypes of both GSTM1 and NAT2 genes.

In a recent study [54] we have analyzed the distribution of CYP1A1, mEH, GSTM1, GSTT1, and NAT2 polymorphic genotypes in an Italian study group consisting of 80 MPM patients and 255 population controls. MPM patients were classified into two categories according to the estimated intensity of asbestos exposure, i.e., subjects with a high probability of exposure ($n = 57$, mostly shipyard workers) and subjects with low probability of exposure ($n = 23$). A significant association was found between MPM and the NAT2 fast-acetylator genotype (OR 1.74, 95% CI 1.02–2.96). Significantly increased risks of MPM in subjects with low mEH activity (OR 2.51, 95% CI 1.11–5.68) and a double risk in those with the intermediate activity genotype (OR 2.16, 95% CI, 0.96–4.87) were also observed. The test for the linear trend was highly significant (LRT for trend $p < 0.04$). No other polymorphism showed a significant association with MPM, though subjects with GSTM1 null genotype had an increased risk of 48%.

When MPM patients were stratified according to the estimated degree of asbestos exposure, the association of NAT2 fast acetylators with MPM appeared to be confined to the highly exposed cases (OR 2.14, 95% CI 1.15–3.98). An even stronger interaction with asbestos exposure was found for the polymorphisms determining mEH activity, which showed notably high ORs in the group of subjects with low exposure, i.e., 6.63 (95% CI 0.83–52.97) and 7.83 (95% CI 0.98–62.60) for intermediate and low mEH activity, respectively (LRT for trend $p < 0.04$).

When the combined effect of the mEH variants with other genotypes was evaluated, a significant association was observed between MPM and the simultaneous condition of NAT2 fast acetylator and mEH low activity (OR 4.36, 95% CI 1.62–11.79) (Table 41.2). A similar pattern of gene–gene interaction was also observed between GSTM1 and mEH. The highest risks were found in those subjects with GSTM1 null and mEH low activity (OR 3.70, 95% CI 1.37–10.01). A statistically significant association was found also for the combinations of NAT2 fast acetylator with GSTM1 null genotype (LRT $p < 0.049$).

The most remarkable finding of this study was the increased risk of MPM observed in subjects with an mEH low-activity genotype. The evidence that mEH may have a major role in the early stages of asbestos carcinogenesis is strengthened by two findings, the high odds ratios in the subgroup of subjects exposed to low levels of asbestos, and the synergism with the NAT2 fast-acetylator genotype. The almost complete lack of mEH high-activity genotypes among the MPM patients with lower exposure to asbestos (1 subject out of 23) is a surprising finding, and undoubtedly this category deserves to be further explored in future studies with a larger study size. Other examples of a stronger effect of metabolic gene variants in low exposure groups have been published [55, 56].

These results strengthen the hypothesis that metabolic gene polymorphisms involved in oxidation processes have a role in modulating individual susceptibility to MPM in subjects with different degrees of asbestos exposure.

Table 41.2. Association between malignant pleural mesothelioma and selected combinations of genotypes/predicted activities (logistic regression analysis)

	mEH	MPM	Controls	OR (95% CI)
NAT2				
Slow acetylator	High activity	4	31	1.0 (ref)
Slow acetylator	Intermediate activity	14	60	2.16 (0.96–4.87)
Slow acetylator	Low activity	15	51	2.51 (1.11–5.68)
Fast acetylator	High activity	5	27	1.74 (1.02-2.96)
Fast acetylator	Intermediate activity	19	44	3.76 (1.41–10.07)
Fast acetylator	Low activity	17	35	4.36 (1.62–11.79)
	LRT for heterogeneity			$p = 0.023$
GSTM1				
Functional	High activity	3	23	1.0 (ref)
Functional	Intermediate activity	12	54	2.16 (0.96–4.87)
Functional	Low activity	13	37	2.51 (1.11–5.68)
Null	High activity	6	35	1.48 (0.86–2.54)
Null	Intermediate activity	21	50	3.19 (1.16–8.75)
Null	Low activity	19	49	3.70 (1.37–10.01)
	LRT for heterogeneity			$p = 0.061$

NAT N-Acetyltransferase, *mEH* microsomal epoxide hydrolase, *MPM* malignant pleural mesothelioma, *OR* odds ratio, *CI* confidence interval, *LRT* likelihood ratio test

41.5 Gene Alterations in Malignant Pleural Mesothelioma

Chromosomal alterations may lead to gene silencing, amplification, or rearrangement, complete gene loss, and modified expression of their protein products. In this way the DNA damage/repair and apoptotic pathways are inhibited.

Table 41.3. Genes as possible diagnostic or prognostic markers in malignant pleural mesothelioma

Gene	Potential role
CDKN2/p16^{INK4}	Differentiation between benign mesothelial reactive cells and malignant cells Treatment (following inhibition of DNA methylation)
WT1	Differentiation between mesothelioma and adenocarcinoma in tissue from pleural tumors
Ras/p21	Early diagnosis among subjects with asbestos-related diseases Prognosis
PDGF/PDGFR	Marker of progression in benign asbestos-related diseases Use of inhibitors of PDGF receptors as therapeutic agent Prognosis
EGF/EGFR	Use of inhibitors of EGF receptors as therapeutic agent
HGF/SF/c-met	Expression of met supports the diagnosis of malignant mesothelioma Use of inhibitors of c-met as therapeutic agent
VEGF	Differentiation between malignant and benign pleural effusions Prognostic role Therapeutic target
b-FGF	Prognostic role

According to a theory on genesis of malignant mesothelioma, damage induced by asbestos accumulate over years and malignant transformation is more likely if some key regulatory genes are deleted or silenced [21].

The alterations in tumor suppressor genes and dominant oncogenes may be useful markers for the study of the carcinogenic processes in exposed populations. The impairment of the genes might be a marker of exposure and a tool for diagnostic tests, since the expression of certain markers may occur prior to the development of some overt malignancies [57]. They are sometimes associated with tumor aggressiveness and may prove useful as prognostic markers. Moreover, gene therapy-based approaches can be addressed in the treatment of MPM patients (Table 41.3) [58].

The gene products, the oncoproteins, have access to the extracellular environment and are detectable in peripheral fluids such as serum or plasma. Their circulating level provides an opportunity to assess the diagnostic and prognostic value of a marker overexpression in patients with tumors not easily accessible to biopsy [59].

About 300 genes seem to differ between mesothelioma cells and pleural cells, and most of them influence cell growth and invasiveness [58, 60, 61].

41.6 Tumor Suppressor Genes

Loss and/or inactivation of tumor suppressor genes play a substantial role in the development and progression of MPM [62]. In addition, the consequent alterations of the proteins encoded by these genes, carrying a critical cell cycle regulatory role, make them an important candidate for cancer treatment based on gene replacement strategies.

Deletion of the 9p21 region leads to an alteration of the CDKN locus which encodes the tumor suppressor gene products p16^{INK4a} and p14^{ARF}. Loss/inactivation of p16^{INK4a} seems to lead to cell cycle deregulation through the loss of a key inhibitor of G1/S progression. Homozygous loss of p16^{INK4a} and of p14ARF interferes with the p53 and the pRb cellular pathways, contributing to the MPM pathogenesis. p16^{INK4} is being studied as one of the most interesting markers in MPM, as a diagnostic marker to characterize malignant mesothelial cells from benign reactive cells [63] and from a therapeutic point of view [64–66]. Deletion of p16^{INK4} protein expression can also be caused by epigenetic mechanisms, such as an abnormal DNA hypermethylation. The inhibition of methylation is seen as a potential treatment target in some MPM [67, 68].

Deletion of p16^{INK4a} has been reported in 22–70% of MPM [23, 69], and it seems to occur in a relatively susceptible subset of MPM that carry a p16 alteration even in the presence of a low asbestos exposure [70].

Homozygous deletions of p16^{INK4a} can lead to the inactivation of p14^{ARF} and have been reported in 22–70% of MPM [23].

The p53 gene, which is frequently alternated in most human cancers, is rarely mutated in MPM [71–74], but immunoreactivity in tumor tissue was shown for 25–86% of cases [75, 76]. It has been supposed that the lack of mutations is due to an inactivation following the interaction between p53 and the SV40 large T antigen [21]. Very few data exist in the literature on p53-Abs in MPM and results are not encouraging concerning their value as diagnostic or prognostic indicators [77, 78]. We analyzed the anti-p53 autoantibody level in 30 MPM patients, in 48 lung cancer (LC) patients, 55 subjects with benign lung diseases (BLD), and in 51 healthy controls (HC). In our investigation 7.4% of the MPM, 17% of the LC, 3.6% of BLD, and none of the HC had elevated serum levels of the anti-p53 autoantibodies. So, the presence of detectable p53-Abs in serum of patients with MPM does not seem to serve as either a diagnostic or a prognostic indicator. Nevertheless, the presence of two positives among patients at high risk of developing pleuropulmonary malignancies underlines the need for further investigation with prolonged follow-up and an increased number of subjects [79].

Among the genes recognized as hallmarks of MPM, the Wilms' tumor 1 susceptibility (WT1) is selectively expressed in MPM [80, 81]. The detection of WT1 mRNA and of the WT1 protein is particularly useful in the distinction of MPM from adenocarcinoma in tissue sections of pleural tumors.

The deletion of chromosome 22 may lead to frameshift and nonsense mutations and deletions of the neurofibromatosis type 2 tumor suppressor gene NF2 [82, 83]. NF2 codes for merlin, a protein that links the cytoskeleton to the plasma membrane. The loss of stabilizing function from a normal NF2 gene product may favor the mechanism of transformation of mesothelial cells from asbestos [23]. Allelic loss of the NF2 locus has been found in more than 70% of MPM [82].

41.7 Oncogenes and Growth Factors

The role of ras in the development of MPM is uncertain. Results from some studies indicate that neither K-ras or H-ras have a critical role in the induction of MPM mesothelioma by asbestos, either in humans or in rats [84, 85]. p21 was found in 35% of MPM tissues examined by Isik et al. [78]. In this study, a relationship between asbestos exposure and positivity for p21 (35% of MPM examined tissues) was found, since immunopositivity was higher for patients with environmental asbestos exposure and was correlated to exposure times. The role of an early diagnostic marker of p21 has been suggested by a cohort study on serum samples of 46 pneumoconiosis patients. Two patients, both positive for p21, had a diagnosis of MPM 11 and 26 months after the blood test, respectively [86]. Also controversial is the role of p21 as a prognostic marker [78, 87, 88].

Asbestos also seems to influence other types of proto-oncogenes, such as c-fos and c-jun, involved in the activation of some genes responsible for initiation of DNA synthesis [21].

In recent years, attention has been focused on growth factors and/or their receptors, with intrinsic tyrosine kinase activity, as targets for molecularly aimed therapies for MPM.

Platelet-derived growth factor (PDGF) is a mitogenic factor for connective tissue cells present as a dimeric combination of two peptide chains. Many transformed or tumor cells express PDGF and PDGF receptors, suggesting a role of this growth factor in tumor pathogenesis [89]. PDGF is also overexpressed in human MPM cells [90–93], as an autocrine growth factor for mesothelioma. Brandt-Rauf et al. found a higher serum level of PDGF in advanced pneumoconiosis cases than in patients with disease at an earlier stage. Patients with higher PDGF levels had a increased probability to have disease progression, suggesting that serum PDGF levels may be a marker for the development of severe and progressive asbestos-related diseases [86]. We investigated the role of PDGF in serum of 93 MPM patients, 33 primary lung cancers (NSCLC), 51 subjects exposed to asbestos, defined as high-risk controls (RC), and 24 healthy controls (HC) [94]. Positive values in 43% of MPM, in 30% of NSCLC, and in 18% of RC have been found. Higher circulating PDGF levels were associated with a shorter survival, although data did not reach statistical significance. The data, to be confirmed with a larger series, suggest that PDGF could be of clinical usefulness to identify MPM patients with better prognosis and more likely to benefit from available treatments. Some trials are testing a highly selective inhibitor of the PDGF receptor tyrosine kinase as a therapeutic agent [95].

The epidermal growth factor receptor (EGFR) family is a group of four structurally similar tyrosine kinases, comprising the EGFR and HER2/neu protein, encoded by the HER-2/neu gene. The protein has been detected at higher levels in serum of asbestosis patients, who later developed lung cancer [96]. In patients with MPM, tissue immunoreactivity for HER2/neu has been found in 97% of MPM [97]. EGF and its receptor (EGFR) may cooperate in MPM development and progression [98, 99]. Following asbestos exposure, autophosphorylation of the EGFR may occur in mesothelial cells, initiating a cell-signaling cascade influencing carcinogenesis [100]. Studies in vitro or on animal models have shown that an agent that significantly inhibits EGFR may be an effective therapeutic option for patients with MPM and that modification of phosphorylation provides a rationale in preventive and therapeutic approaches to lung cancers and mesothelioma [101, 102].

A diagnostic and therapeutic importance in MPM is also reported for the hepatocyte growth factor/scatter factor (HGF/SF) and its receptor c-Met [97, 103–105]. In our experience, concentration of both HGF and EGF markers, which were significantly correlated, was double in MPM than in healthy subjects (HC). Positivity was found in 60% of MPM and 0% of HC for HGF, and in 50% of MPM and 18% of HC for EGF.

Survival of MPM patients is also negatively associated with two angiogenic factors, namely the vascular endothelial growth factor (VEGF) and basic fibroblast growth factor (b-FGF). The latter marker is more expressed in non-malignant pleural effusions [106, 107], while the former has been found to be more frequent in pleural effusions of MPM patients [106, 107] and plays a crucial role in the tumor progression potential induced by SV40 Tag [108, 109]. As is the case for other growth factors, the VEGF and VEGF-C autocrine loops might constitute a therapeutic target in MPM [110, 111].

41.8 Conclusion

Molecular events leading to the development of malignant mesothelioma (MPM) have not yet been completely elucidated, but it is known that multiple genetic alterations are required for malignant transformation of the mesothelium.

Studies on SV40 suggested a possible role of this virus in the impairment of DNA repair mechanisms in mesothelial cells, hypothesizing an additive effect with asbestos fibers. Most human MPM are linked to various non-random chromosomal deletions involving specific regions in chromosome arms. These alterations may be caused by asbestos, SV40, and other carcinogens, but likely they also reflect an intrinsic predisposition of the cell to accumulate genetic damage.

The rarity of the disease among exposed subjects and the presence of MPM cases among subjects with very low or unknown levels of asbestos exposure, suggests the involvement of individual (susceptibility) cofactors in the etiology of MPM.

Molecular epidemiology has a great potential in the study of MPM, for example, in the detection of early effect markers in people exposed to occupational or environmental carcinogens or in the assessment of susceptibility factors that might predispose to cancer, as well as in the identification of prognostic factors.

Among biomarkers that can be used to measure genetic effects, the micronucleus test in peripheral blood lymphocytes appears to be one of the most suitable. Moreover micronuclei reflect chromosome damage and may be an interesting marker of individual DNA repair capability.

The study of polymorphisms of metabolic genes may permit to evaluate the interindividual variations in the activities of metabolizing enzymes responsible for activation (phase I reactions) or deactivation (phase II reactions) of carcinogens.

So far, the results available indicate that metabolic gene polymorphisms involved in oxidation processes, particularly mEH, GSTM1 null, and NAT2 acetylators have a role in modulating individual susceptibility to MPM in subjects with different degrees of asbestos exposure.

Concerning gene impairment in MPM, the alterations in tumor suppressor genes and dominant oncogenes may be useful markers for the study of the carcinogenic process in exposed populations. The impairment of some genes might be a marker of exposure and a tool for diagnostic tests, since the expression of certain markers may occur prior to the development of some overt malignancies. They are sometimes associated with tumor aggressiveness and may prove useful as prognostic markers, enabling clinicians to identify patients eligible for new therapeutic strategies.

Acknowledgements

We thank the Fondazione Buzzi and the Italian Group of Study and Therapy of Malignant Mesothelioma (G.I.M.E.) for the financial and technical support.

Key Points

- Asbestos exposure causes DNA damage, chromosome aberrations, cell transformations, and increased apoptosis.
- SV40 inhibits the normal p53 function. A role of this virus in the impairment of DNA repair mechanisms in mesothelial cells has been hypothesized with an additive effect with asbestos fibers.
- Among biomarkers that can be used to measure genetic effects, the micronucleus test in peripheral blood lymphocytes and the study of polymorphisms of metabolic genes may permit to evaluate the interindividual variations in the activities of metabolizing enzymes responsible for activation or deactivation of carcinogens.
- Concerning gene impairment in malignant pleural mesothelioma (MPM), the alterations in tumor suppressor genes and dominant oncogenes may be useful markers of exposure and a tool for diagnostic tests. Moreover, gene therapy-based approaches can be addressed in the treatment of MPM patients by the knowledge of the genes involved in the carcinogenic process of each patient.

References

1. Bianchi C, Giarelli L, Grandi G, Brollo A, Ramani L, Zuch C. Latency periods in asbestos-related mesothelioma of the pleura. Eur J Cancer Prev 1997;6:162.
2. Pira E, Pelucchi C, Buffoni L et al. Cancer mortality in a cohort of asbestos textile workers. Br J Cancer 2005;92:580.
3. Puntoni R, Vercelli M, Merlo F, Valerio F, Santi L. Mortality among shipyard workers in Genoa, Italy. Ann N Y Acad Sci 1979;330:353.
4. Huncharek M. Genetic factors in the aetiology of malignant mesothelioma Eur J Cancer 1995;31:1741.
5. Dopp E, Seedler J, Stopper H., Weiss DG, Schiffman D. Mitotic disturbances and micronucleus induction in Syrian hamster embryo fibroblast cells caused by asbestos fibers. Environ Health Perspect 1995;103:268.
6. Kodama Y, Boreiko CJ, Maness SC, Hesterberg TW. Cytotoxic and cytogenetic effects of asbestos on human bronchial epithelial cells in culture. Carcinogenesis 1993;14:691.
7. Liu W, Ernst JD, Courtney Broaddus V. Phagocytosis of crocidolite asbestos induces oxidative stress, DNA damage, and apoptosis in mesothelial cells. Am J Respir Cell Mol Biol 2000;23:371.
8. Ollikainen T, Linnainmaa K, Kinnula VL. DNA single strand breaks induced by asbestos fibers in human pleural mesothelial cells in vitro. Environ Mol Mutagen 1999;33:153.
9. Speit G. Appropriate in vitro test conditions for genotoxicity testing of fibers. Inhalat Toxicol 2002;14:79.
10. Okayasu R, Takahashi S, Yamada S, Hei TK, Ullrich RL. Asbestos and DNA double strand breaks. Cancer Res 1999;59:298.
11. Kamp DW, Weitzman SA. The molecular basis of asbestos induced lung injury. Thorax 1999;54:638.
12. Knaapen AM, Borm PJA, Albrecht C, Schins RPF. Inhaled particles and lung cancer. Part A: mechanisms. Int J Cancer 2004;109:799.
13. Borm PJA, Schins RPF, Albrecht C. Inhaled particles and lung cancer. Part B: paradigms and risk assessment. Int J Cancer 2004;110:3.
14. Schins RPF. Mechanism of genotoxicity of particles and fibers. Inhalat Toxicol 2002;14:57.
15. Schurkes C, Brock W, Abel J, Unfried K. Induction of 8-hydroxydeoxyguanosine by man made vitreous fibres and crocidolite asbestos administered intraperitoneally in rats. Mutat Res 2004;553:59.
16. Topinka J, Loli P, Georgiadis P, et al. Mutagenesis by asbestos in the lung of λ-lacI transgenic mice. Mutat Res 2004;553:67.
17. Marczynski B, Kraus T, Rozynwwk P, Schlosser S, Raithel HJ, Baur X. Changes in low molecular weight DNA fragmentation in white blood cells of workers highly exposed to asbestos. Int Arch Occup Environ Health 2001;74:315.
18. Cristaudo A, Foddis R, Vivaldi A, et al. SV40 enhances the risk of malignant mesothelioma among people exposed to asbestos: a molecular epidemiologic case-control study. Cancer Res 2005;65:3049.
19. Digweed M, Demuth I, Rothe S, et al. SV40 large T-antigen disturbs the formation of nuclear DNA-repair foci containing MRE11. Oncogene 2002;21:4873.
20. Bowman KK, Sicard DM, Ford JM, Hanawalt PC. Reduced global genomic repair of ultraviolet light-induced cyclobutane pyrimidine dimers in simian virus 40-transformed human cells. Mol Carcinog 2000;29:17.
21. Carbone M, Carbone M, Kratzke RA, Testa JR. The pathogenesis of mesothelioma. Semin Oncol 2002;29:2.
22. Berwick M, Vineis P. Markers of DNA repair and susceptibility to cancer in humans: an epidemiologic review. J Natl Cancer Inst 2000;92:874.
23. Lechner JF, Tesfaiqzi J, Gerwin BI. Oncogenes and tumor-suppressor genes in mesothelioma: a synopsis. Environ Health Perspect 1997;105:1061.
24. Perera FP. Molecular cancer epidemiology: a new tool in cancer prevention. J Natl Cancer Inst 1987;78:87.
25. Hulka BS, Wilcosky T. Biological markers in epidemiologic research. Arch Environ Health 1988;43:83.
26. Wogan GN. Molecular epidemiology in cancer risk. Assessment and prevention: recent progress and avenues for future research. Environ Health Perspect 1992;98:167.
27. Bonassi S, Hagmar L, Stromberg U, Heikkila P. Chromosomal aberrations in lymphocytes predict human cancer independently of exposure to carcinogens. European Study Group on Cytogenetic Biomarkers and Health. Cancer Res 2000;15:1619.
28. Maluf SW, Erdtmann B. Genomic instability in Down syndrome and Fanconi anemia assessed by micronucleus analysis in single-cell gel electrophoresis. Cancer Genet Cytogenet 2001;124:71.
29. Rothfub A, Schutz P, Bochum S, et al. Induced micronucleus frequencies in peripheral lymphocytes as a screening test for carriers of a BRCA1 mutation in breast cancer families. Cancer Res 2000;60:390.
30. Trenz K, Rothfuss A, Schutz P, Speit G. Mutagen sensitivity of peripheral blood for women carrying a BRCA1 or BRCA2 mutation. Mutat Res 2002;500:89.
31. Fellay-Reynier I, Orsiere T, Sari-Minodier I, et al. Evaluation of micronucleated lymphocytes, constitutional karyotypes and anti p53 antibodies in 21 children with various malignancies. Mutat Res 2000;467:31.
32. Fenech M, Denham J, Francis W, Morley A. Micronuclei in cytokinesis-blocked lymphocytes of cancer patients fol-

lowing fractionated partial-body radiotherapy. Int J Radiat Biol 1990;57:373.

33. Venkatachalam P, Paul S, Mohankumar M, Prabhu BK, Gajendiran N, Kathiresan A, Jeevanram RK. Higher frequency of dicentrics and micronuclei in peripheral blood lymphocytes of cancer patients. Mutat Res 1999;425:1.

34. Barbanti-Brodano G, Sabbioni S, Martini F, Negrini M, Corallini A, Tognon M. Simian virus 40 infection in humans and association with human diseases: results and hypotheses. Virology 2004;318:1.

35. White MK, Khalili K. Polyomaviruses and human cancer: molecular mechanisms underlying patterns of tumorigenesis. Virology 2004;324:1.

36. Dolcetti R, Martini F, Quaia M, et al. Simian virus 40 sequences in human lymphoblastoid B-cell lines. J Virol 2003;82:1595.

37. Neel JV, Major EO, Awa AA. Hypothesis: "rogue cell"-type chromosomal damage in lymphocytes is associated with infection with the JC human polyoma virus and has implications for oncogenesis. Proc Natl Acad Sci U S A 1996;93:2690.

38. Bolognesi C, Filiberti R, Neri M, et al. High frequency of micronuclei in peripheral blood lymphocytes as index of susceptibility to pleural malignant mesothelioma. Cancer Res 2002;62:5418.

39. Fenech M, Morley AA. Cytokinesis-block micronucleus method in human lymphocytes: effect of in vivo aging and low dose X-irradiation. Mutat Res 1986;161:193.

40. Dopp E, Schuler M, Schiffman D, Eastmond DA. Induction of micronuclei, hyperploidy and chromosomal breakage affecting the centric/pericentric regions of chromosomes 1 and 9 in human amniotic fluid cells after treatment with asbestos and ceramic fibers. Mutat Res 1997;377:77.

41. Lu J, Keane MJ, Ong T, Wallace WE. In vitro genotoxicity studies of chrysotile asbestos fibers dispersed in simulated pulmonary surfactant. Mutat Res 1994;320:253.

42. Bartsch H, Aitio A, Camus AM, Malaveille C, Ohshima H, Pignatelli B, Sabadie N. Carcinogen metabolizing enzymes and susceptibility to chemical carcinogenesis. IARC Sci Publ 1982;39:337.

43. Hanke JZ. Genetic susceptibility to toxic substances and its relationship to carcinogenesis. IARC Sci Publ 1984;59:99.

44. Harrison DJ, Hubbard AL, MacMillan J, Wyllie AH, Smith CA. Microsomal epoxide hydrolase gene polymorphism and susceptibility to colon cancer. Br J Cancer 1999;79:168.

45. Smith CA, Harrison DJ. Association between polymorphism in gene for microsomal epoxide hydrolase and susceptibility to emphysema. Lancet 1997;350:630.

46. Arif JM, Khan SG, Mahmood N, Aslam M, Rahman Q. Effect of coexposure to asbestos and kerosene soot on pulmonary drug-metabolizing enzyme system. Environ Health Perspect 1994;102:181.

47. Fretland AJ, Omiecinski CJ. Epoxide hydrolases: biochemistry and molecular biology. Chem Biol Interact 200;129:41.

48. Kandaswami C, O'Brien PJ. Effect of chrysotile asbestos and silica on the microsomal metabolism of benzo(a)pyrene. Environ Health Perspect 1983;51:311.

49. Gsur A, Zidek T, Schnattinger K, et al. Association of microsomal epoxide hydrolase polymorphisms and lung cancer risk. Br J Cancer 2003;89:702.

50. Smith CM, Kelsey KT, Wiencke JK, Leyden K, Stephen L, Christiani DC. Inherited glutathione S-transferase deficiency is a risk factor for pulmonary asbestosis. Cancer Epidemiol Biomarkers Prev 1994;3:471.

51. Hirvonen A, Saarikoski ST, Linnainmaa K, Koskinen K, Husgafvel-Pursiainen K, Mattson K, Vainio H. Glutathione S-transferase and N-acetyltransferase genotypes and as-
bestos-associated pulmonary disorders. J Natl Cancer Inst 1996;88:1853.

52. Stucker I, Boffetta P, Antilla S, Benhamou S, Hirvonen A, London S, Taioli E. Lack of interaction between asbestos exposure and glutathione S-transferase M1 and T1 genotypes in lung carcinogenesis. Cancer Epidemiol Biomarkers Prev 2001;10:1253.

53. Hirvonen A, Pelin K, Tammilehto L, Karjalainen A, Mattson K, Linnainmaa K. Inherited GSTM1 and NAT2 defects as concurrent risk modifiers in asbestos-related human malignant mesothelioma. Cancer Res 1995;55:2981.

54. Neri M, Filiberti R, Taioli E, et al. Pleural malignant mesothelioma, genetic susceptibility and asbestos exposure. Mutat Res 2005 (in press).

55. Garte SJ, Zocchetti C, Taioli E. Gene-environment interactions in the application of biomarkers of cancer susceptibility in epidemiology. In: Toniolo P, Boffetta P, Shuker DEG, Rothman N, Hulka B, Pearce N (eds) Application of Biomarkers in Cancer Epidemiology. IARC Scientific Publications 142. Oxford: Oxford University Press, 1997:251.

56. Vineis P, Bartsch H, Caporaso N, et al. Genetically based N-acetyltransferase metabolic polymorphism and low level environmental exposure to carcinogens. Nature 1994;369:154.

57. Partanen R, Koskinen H, Oksa P, Hemminki K, Carney W, Smith S, Brandt-Rauf P. Serum oncoproteins in asbestosis patients. Clin Chem 1995;23:1844.

58. Rihn BH, Mohr S, McDowell SA, et al. Differential gene expression in mesothelioma. FEBS Lett 2000;480:95.

59. Brandt-Rauf PW. Biomarkers of gene expression: growth factors and oncoproteins. Environ Health Perspect 1997;105:807.

60. Ascoli A, Aalto Y, Carnovale-Scalzo C, Nardi F, Falzetti D, Mecucci C, Knuutila S. DNA copy number changes in familial malignant mesothelioma. Cancer Genet Cytogenet 2001;127:80.

61. Kettunen E, Nissen AM, Ollikainen T, et al. Gene expression profiling of malignant mesothelioma cell lines: cDNA array study. Int J Cancer 2001;91:492.

62. Lee WC, Testa JR. Somatic genetic alterations in human malignant mesothelioma (review). Int J Oncol 1999;14:181.

63. Illei PB, Ladanyi M, Rusch VW, Zakowski MF. The use of CDKN2A deletion as a diagnostic marker for malignant mesothelioma in body cavity effusions. Cancer 2003;99:51.

64. Frizelle SP, Grim J, Zhou J, Gupta P, Curiel DT, Geradts J, Kratzke RA. Re-expression of p16INK4a in mesothelioma cells results in cell cycle arrest, cell death, tumor suppression and tumor regression. Oncogene 1998;16:3087.

65. Papp T, Schipper H, Pemsel H, et al. Mutational analysis of N-ras, p53, p16INK4a, p14ARF and CDK4 genes in primary human malignant mesotheliomas. Int J Oncol 2001;8:425.

66. Yang CT, You L, Lin YC, Lin CL, McCormick F, Jablons DM. A comparison analysis of anti-tumor efficacy of adenoviral gene replacement therapy (p14ARF and p16INK4A) in human mesothelioma cells. Anticancer Res 2003;23:33.

67. Kratzke RA, Otterson GA, Lincoln CE, Ewing S, Oie H, Geradts J, Kaye FJ. Immunohistochemical analysis of the p16INK4 cyclin-dependent kinase inhibitor in malignant mesothelioma. J Natl Cancer Inst 1995;87:1870.

68. Wong L, Zhou J, Anderson D, Kratzke RA. Inactivation of p16(INK4a) expression in malignant mesothelioma by methylation. Lung Cancer 2002;38:131.

69. Xio S, Li D, Vijg J, Sugarbaker DJ, Corson JM, Fletcher JA. Codeletion of p15 and p16 in primary malignant mesothelioma. Oncogene 1995;11:511.

70. Hirao T, Bueno R, Chen CJ, Gordon GJ, Heilig E, Kelsey KT. Alterations of the p16(INK4) locus in human malignant mesothelial tumors. Carcinogenesis 2002;23:1127.

71. Attanoos RL, Griffin A, Gibbs AR. The use of immunohistochemistry in distinguishing reactive from neoplastic mesothelium. A novel use for desmin and comparative evaluation with epithelial membrane antigen, p53, platelet-derived growth factor-receptor, P-glycoprotein and Bcl-2. Histopathology 2003;43:231.

72. Kitamura F, Araki S, Suzuki Y, Yokoyama K, Tanigawa T, Iwasaki R. Assessment of the mutations of p53 suppressor gene and Ha- and Ki-ras oncogenes in malignant mesothelioma in relation to asbestos exposure: a study of 12 American patients. Ind Health 2002;40:175.

73. Metcalf RA, Welsh JA, Bennett WP, et al. p53 and Kirsten-ras mutations in human mesothelioma cell lines. Cancer Res 1992;52:2610.

74. Mor O, Yaron P, Huszar M, et al. Absence of p53 mutations in malignant mesotheliomas. Am J Respir Cell Mol Biol 1997;16:9.

75. Esposito V, Baldi A, De LA, et al. p53 immunostaining in differential diagnosis of pleural mesothelial proliferations. Anticancer Res 1997;17:733.

76. Ramael M, Lemmens G, Eerdekens C, Buysse C, Deblier I, Jacobs W, van Marck E. Immunoreactivity for p53 protein in malignant mesothelioma and non-neoplastic mesothelium. J Pathol 1992;168:371.

77. Creaney J, McLaren BM, Stevenson S, Musk AW, de Klerk N, Robinson BW, Lake RA. p53 autoantibodies in patients with malignant mesothelioma: stability through disease progression. Br J Cancer 2001;84:52.

78. Isik R, Metintas M, Gibbs AR, et al. p53, p21 and metallothionein immunoreactivities in patients with malignant pleural mesothelioma: correlations with the epidemiological features and prognosis of mesotheliomas with environmental asbestos exposure. Respir Med 2001;95:588.

79. Neri M, Betta P, Marroni P, et al. Serum anti-p53 autoantibodies in pleural malignant mesothelioma, lung cancer and non-neoplastic lung diseases. Lung Cancer 2003;39:165.

80. Amin KM, Litzky LA, Smythe WR, et al. Wilms' tumor 1 susceptibility (WT1) gene products are selectively expressed in malignant mesothelioma. Am J Pathol 1995;146:344.

81. Hecht JL, Lee BH, Pinkus JL, et al. The value of Wilms tumor susceptibility gene 1 in cytologic preparations as a marker for malignant mesothelioma. Cancer 2002;96:105.

82. Bianchi A, Mitsunaga SI, Cheng JQ, et al. High frequency of inactivating mutations in the neurofibromatosis type 2 gene (NF2) in primary malignant mesothelioma. Proc Natl Acad Sci U S A 1995;92:10854.

83. Sekido Y, Pass HI, Bader S, Mew DJ, Christman MF, Gazdar AF, Minna JD. Neurofibromatosis type 2 (NF2) gene is somatically mutated in mesothelioma but not in lung cancer. Cancer Res 1995;55:1227.

84. Cristaudo A, Vivaldi A, Sensales G, Guglielmi G, Ciancia E, Elisei R, Ottenga F. Molecular biology studies on mesothelioma tumor samples: preliminary data on H-ras, p21, and SV40. J Environ Pathol Toxicol Oncol 1995;14:29.

85. Ni Z, Liu Y, Keshava N, et al. Analysis of K-ras and p53 mutations in mesotheliomas from humans and rats exposed to asbestos. Mutat Res 2000;468:7.

86. Brandt-Rauf PW, Smith S, Hemminki K, Koskinen H, Vainio H, Niman H, Ford J. Serum oncoproteins and growth factors in asbestosis and silicosis patients. Int J Cancer 1992;50:881.

87. Baldi A, Groeger AM, Esposito V, et al. Expression of p21 in SV40 large T antigen positive human pleural mesothelioma: relationship with survival. Thorax 2002;57:353.

88. Baldi A, Santini D, Vasaturo F, et al. Prognostic significance of cyclooxygenase-2 (COX-2) and expression of cell cycle inhibitors p21 and p27 in human pleural malignant mesothelioma. Thorax 2004;59:428.

89. Ross R. Platelet-derived growth factor. Lancet 1989;1:1179.

90. Ascoli V, Scalzo CC, Facciolo F, Nardi F. Platelet-derived growth factor receptor immunoreactivity in mesothelioma and nonneoplastic mesothelial cells in serous effusions. Acta Cytol 1995;39:613.

91. Langerak AW, De Laat PA, Van der Linden-Van Beurden CA, et al. Expression of platelet-derived growth factor (PDGF) and PDGF receptors in human malignant mesothelioma in vitro and in vivo. J Pathol 1996;178:151.

92. Metheny-Barlow LJ, Flynn B, van Gijssel HE, Marrogi A, Gerwin BI. Paradoxical effects of platelet-derived growth factor-A overexpression in malignant mesothelioma. Antiproliferative effects in vitro and tumorigenic stimulation in vivo. Am J Respir Cell Mol Biol 2001;24:694.

93. Pogrebniak W, Lubesnsky A, Pass HI. Differential expression of platelet-derived growth factor-beta in malignant mesothelioma: a clue to future therapies? Surg Oncol 1993;2:235.

94. Filiberti R, Marroni P, Neri M, et al. Serum PDGF-AB in pleural mesothelioma. Tumour Biol 2005;26:221.

95. Nowak AK, Lake RA, Kindler HL, Robinson BW. New approaches for mesothelioma: biologics, vaccines, gene therapy, and other novel agents. Semin Oncol 2002;29:82.

96. Brandt-Rauf PW, Luo JC, Carney WP, et al. Detection of increased amounts of the extracellular domain of the c-erbB-2 oncoprotein in serum during pulmonary carcinogenesis in humans. Int J Cancer 1994;56:383.

97. Thirkettle I, Harvey P, Hasleton PS, Ball RY, Warn RM. Immunoreactivity for cadherins, HGF/SF, met, and erbB-2 in pleural malignant mesotheliomas. Histopathology 2000;36:522.

98. Morocz IA, Schmitter D, Lauber B, Stahel RA. Autocrine stimulation of a human lung mesothelioma cell line is mediated through the transforming growth factor alpha/epidermal growth factor receptor mitogenic pathway. Br J Cancer 1994;70:850.

99. Vogelzang NJ. Emerging insights into the biology and therapy of malignant mesothelioma. Semin Oncol 2002;29:35.

100. Pache JC, Janssen YM, Walsh ES, et al. Increased epidermal growth factor-receptor protein in a human mesothelial cell line in response to long asbestos fibers. Am J Pathol 1998;152:333.

101. Manning CB, Cummins AB, Jung MW, et al. A mutant epidermal growth factor receptor targeted to lung epithelium inhibits asbestos-induced proliferation and proto-oncogene expression. Cancer Res 2002;62:4169.

102. Janne PA, Taffaro ML, Salgia R, Johnson BE. Inhibition of epidermal growth factor receptor signaling in malignant pleural mesothelioma. Cancer Res 200;15:5242.

103. Harvey P, Warn A, Newman P, et al. Immunoreactivity for hepatocyte growth factor/scatter factor and its receptor, met, in human lung carcinomas and malignant mesotheliomas. J Pathol 1996;180:389.

104. Maulik G, Shrikhande A, Kijima T, Ma PC, Morrison PT, Salgia R. Role of the hepatocyte growth factor receptor, c-Met, in oncogenesis and potential for therapeutic inhibition. Cytokine Growth Factor Rev 2002;13:41.

105. Tolnay E, Kuhnen C, Wiethege T, Konig JE, Voss B, Muller KM. Hepatocyte growth factor/scatter factor and its receptor c-Met are overexpressed and associated with an increased microvessel density in malignant pleural mesothelioma. J Cancer Res Clin Oncol 1998;124:291.

106. Strizzi L, Catalano A, Vianale G, Procopio A, et al. Vascular endothelial growth factor is an autocrine growth factor in human malignant mesothelioma. J Pathol 2001;193:468.

107. Strizzi L, Vianale G, Catalano A, et al. Basic fibroblast growth factor in mesothelioma pleural effusions: correlation with patient survival and angiogenesis. Int J Oncol 2001;18:1093.

108. Cacciotti P, Strizzi L, Vianale G, et al.. The presence of simian-virus 40 sequences in mesothelioma and mesothelial cells is associated with high levels of vascular endothelial growth factor. Am J Respir Cell Mol Biol 2002;26:189.

109. Catalano A, Romano M, Martinotti S, Procopio A. Enhanced expression of vascular endothelial growth factor (VEGF) plays a critical role in the tumor progression potential induced by simian virus 40 large T antigen. Oncogene 2002;25:2896.

110. Catalano A, Graciotti L, Rinaldi L, et al. Preclinical evaluation of the nonsteroidal anti-inflammatory agent celecoxib on malignant mesothelioma chemoprevention. Int J Cancer 2004;1093:322.

111. Masood R, Kundra A, Zhu S, Xia G, Scalia P, Smith DL, Gill PS. Malignant mesothelioma growth inhibition by agents that target the VEGF and VEGF-C autocrine loops. Int J Cancer 2003;04:603.

Pathology of Malignant Mesothelioma

42

Catherine M. Corbishley

Contents

42.1 Introduction

The diagnosis of malignant mesothelioma has long been a challenge for the pulmonary pathologist but with increasing sophistication of both surgical and laboratory techniques together with advances in imaging it has become relatively easier to give a definitive opinion provided adequate diagnostic material is available. Additional information, such as subtyping, gives valuable information to aid treatment decisions and predict prognosis. Distinction of some complex proliferative lesions from mesothelioma and the characterization of primary and metastatic pleural malignancy have also been aided by new special staining techniques. It is no longer acceptable for pathologists to simply make a diagnosis of pleural malignancy without further comment on tumor type and histogenesis.

There are still many pitfalls in this difficult diagnostic area and the development of multidisciplinary specialist cancer teams who review clinical, pathological, and radiological findings together are proving invaluable in consolidating a secure diagnosis and producing an appropriate treatment plan in consultation with the patient [1].

42.2 Pathological Findings in Malignant Mesothelioma

42.2.1 Macroscopic Appearances

The morphological findings in malignant mesothelioma depend on the stage at diagnosis (Table 42.1) [2]. Initially there may be just pleural nodules on the visceral and/or parietal pleural surfaces which are often associated with pleural effusion (Fig. 42.1). Later on the nodules become confluent and there is often a thick layer of tumor coating the lung, particularly in its lower parts, with extension into fissures (Fig. 42.2). Invasion

Table 42.1. Staging of malignant mesothelioma

TNM staging	Pathological staging
pT1	Tumor involves ipsilateral parietal pleura, with or without focal involvement of visceral pleura
pT1a	No visceral pleura involvement
pT1b	Visceral pleura
pT2	Tumor involves any ipsilateral pleural surfaces with at least one of the following: ipsilateral lung invasion, diaphragm muscle invasion, confluent involvement of visceral pleura including fissure
pT3	Tumor involves any ipsilateral pleural surfaces, with at least one of the following: endothoracic fascia, mediastinal fat, focal chest wall, non-transmural pericardium
pT4	Tumor involves any ipsilateral pleural surfaces, with at least one of the following: contralateral pleura, peritoneum, rib, extensive chest wall or mediastinal invasion, myocardium, brachial plexus, spine, transmural pericardium, malignant pericardial effusion
pN0	No regional node metastasis
pN1	Ipsilateral bronchopulmonary, hilar
pN2	Subcarinal, ipsilateral mediastinal, internal mammary
pN3	Contralateral mediastinal, internal mammary, hilar, ipsi/contralateral supraclavicular, scalene

(Modified by: *TNM Classification of Malignant Tumours*, Sobin LH, Wittekind IN (eds), 2002 [2])

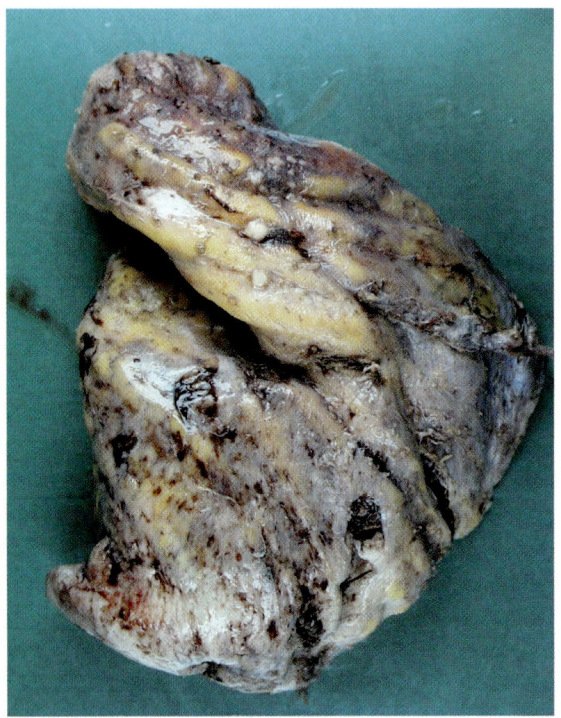

Fig. 42.1. Visceral surface of the lung in diffuse malignant mesothelioma of the pleura showing pleural thickening with nodules

of the mediastinum, pericardium, diaphragm, and chest wall is common as the tumor progresses. The tumor usually appears solid and firm but may show areas of necrosis or more mucoid gelatinous areas depending on tumor type and amount of glycoprotein present in connective tissue. These appearances may be modified by treatment such as pleurodesis, repeated drainage of effusions associated with loculation, or infection. It is therefore vital for the pathologist to be aware of the clinical history and radiological findings when undertaking biopsy diagnosis of pleural disease.

Metastatic mesothelioma involving lung, lymph nodes, and distant sites is also seen in the later stages, particularly in the most aggressive types of tumor such as the sarcomatoid type. The propensity of diffuse malignant mesothelioma to track into biopsy sites and surgical scars is well recorded making post-biopsy radiation of biopsy site advisable [3, 4]. It is, however, unusual for mesothelioma to initially present with metastases. Recurrence in scars is uncommon with most other pleural tumors both primary and metastatic.

The presence of pleural plaques confirms asbestos exposure but they are not precursor lesions for malignancy as they consist only of relatively acellular dense fibrous tissue.

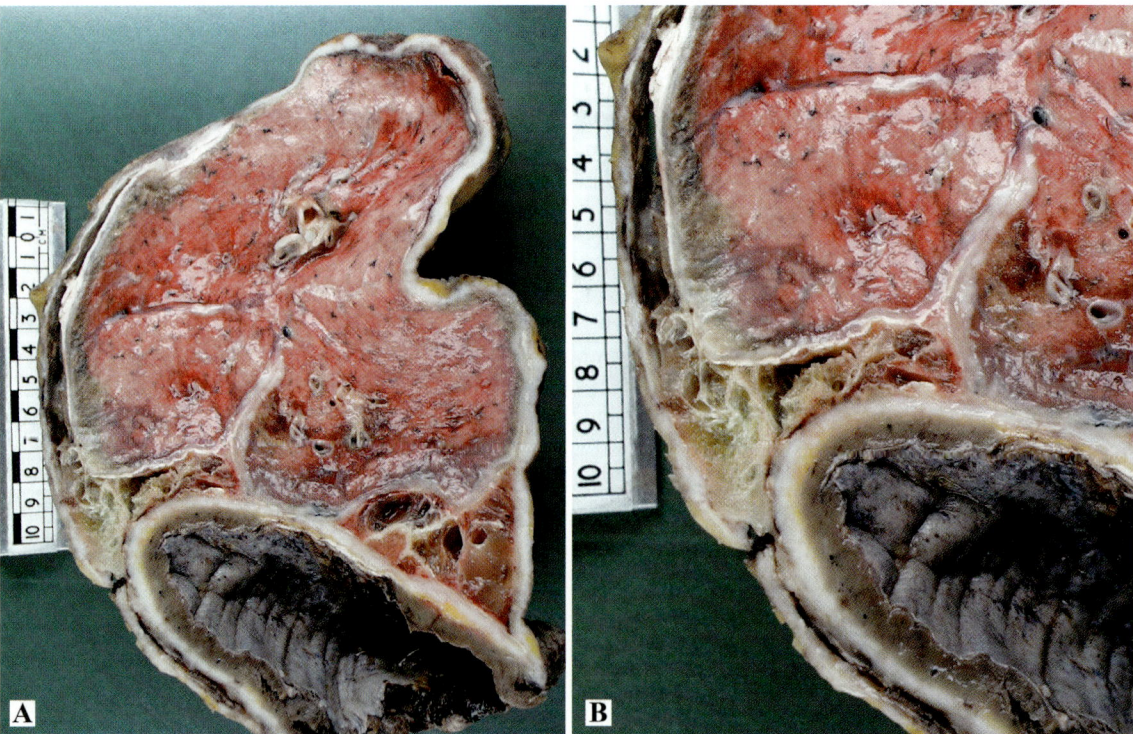

Fig. 42.2. Section of resected lung showing extensive global thickening of the pleura (**A**) which extends into fissures and is associated with a loculated pleural effusion (**B**)

42.2.2 Microscopy

Malignant mesothelioma is subtyped but not graded unlike many other tumors such as carcinomas. Diffuse malignant mesothelioma is divided into three major histological types on the basis of microscopic appearances (Table 42.2) [5]. The commonest is the epithelial (or epithelioid) type where the appearance often resembles that of a glandular or tubulopapillary tumor and/or shows sheets of confluent malignant epithelial-appearing cells. This pattern is seen in up to 80% of tumors (Fig. 42.3 a, b). Other rarer subtypes of the epithelial type occur including small cell, pleomorphic, lymphoplasmacytoid, and clear cell variants [6, 7].

The terms "epithelial" and "epithelioid" are often used interchangeably in pathological literature but the former is preferable to avoid confusion with the morphological changes seen in the epithelioid macrophages in tuberculosis and to reflect the differentiation path of the mesothelial cells and their tumors.

Table 42.2. WHO classification of mesothelial tumors

Mesothelial tumors	Snomed code
Diffuse malignant mesothelioma	9050/3
Epithelioid mesothelioma	9052/3
Sarcomatoid mesothelioma	9051/3
Desmoplastic mesothelioma	9051/3
Biphasic mesothelioma	9053/3
Localized malignant mesothelioma	9050/3
Other tumors of mesothelial origin	
Well-differentiated papillary mesothelioma	9052/1
Adenomatoid tumor	9054/0

Morphology code of the International Classification of Diseases for Oncology (ICD-O) and the Systematized Nomenclature of Medicine. Behavior is coded /0 for benign tumors, /3 for malignant tumors, and /1 for borderline or tumors of uncertain malignant potential
(Modified by: *WHO Classification of Tumours of the Lung, Pleura, Thymus and Heart*, Travis WD, et al. (eds), 2004 [5])

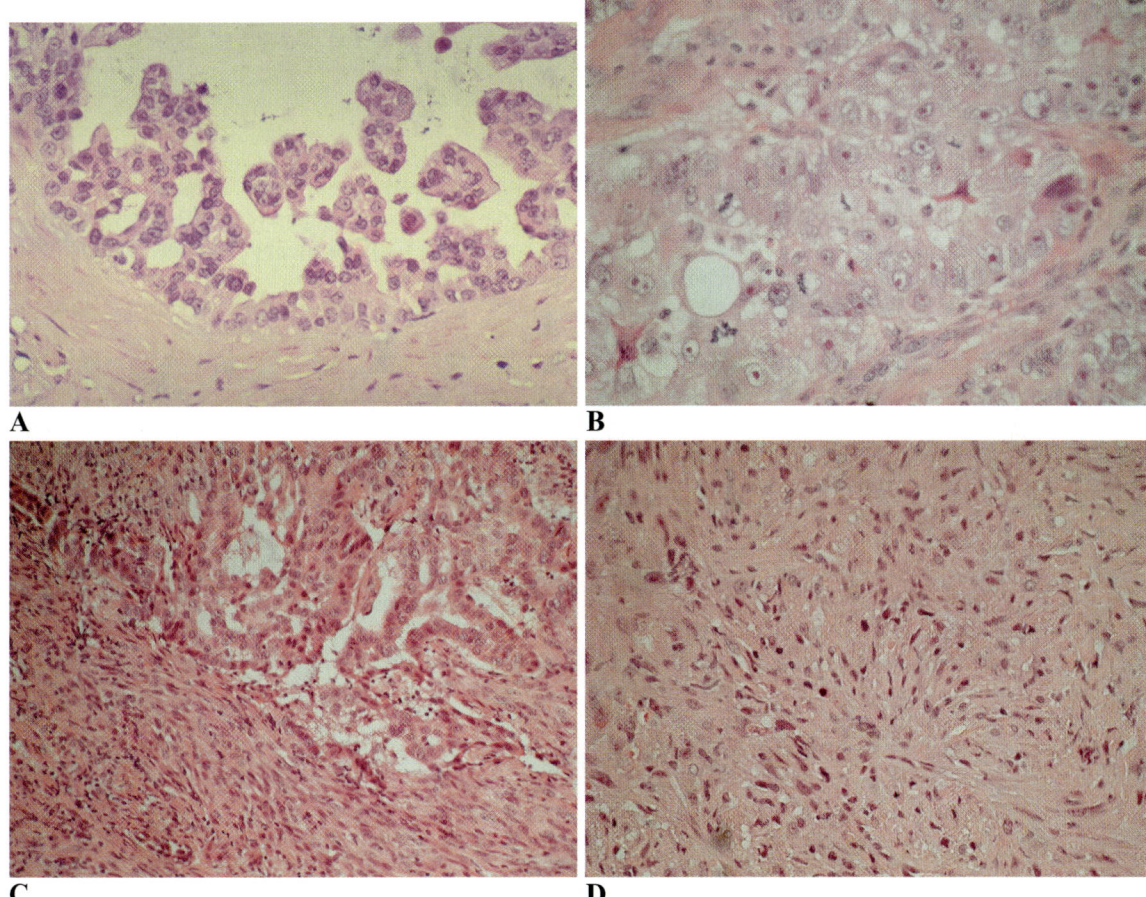

Fig. 42.3. Histological subtypes of malignant mesothelioma (hematoxylin and eosin). **A** Epithelial — tubulopapillary pattern. **B** Epithelial — solid sheets of cells. **C** Biphasic subtype. **D** Sarcomatoid subtype

The most aggressive form of the disease is the sarcomatoid type which is associated with the shortest overall survival and is seen in up to 10% of cases. Mixed/biphasic tumors make up the remainder of the cases (Fig. 42.3 c, d). Tumors may vary greatly from area to area and many tumors diagnosed initially on biopsy as epithelial type may turn out to be biphasic on immunohistochemistry or when more tumor is available for examination following decortication/resection or at postmortem examination [8, 9]. Desmoplastic mesothelioma is a subtype of sarcomatoid mesothelioma associated with marked fibrous reaction where areas of frank malignant tumor may be hard to find making diagnosis on limited amounts of pathological material difficult.

Occasionally malignant mesothelioma may be localized rather than diffuse and reports exist of long survival in these uncommon cases following surgical resection alone [10]. Another rare variant, seen predominantly in women, is the well-differentiated papillary mesothelioma which tends to spread locally but not invade or metastasize [11]. Benign adenomatoid tumors, histologically identical with those seen at other sites such as the testis, also occur rarely in the pleura [12].

Sampling of the underlying lung to look for asbestos bodies does not aid the diagnosis of mesothelioma and is not usually undertaken routinely. It may also increase the risk to the patient of the procedure if the pleural surface of the lung is breached during open biopsy.

42.3 Diagnosis of Malignant Mesothelioma

The two main challenges in the pleural diagnostic process are the distinction between reactive pleural processes and neoplastic ones and the distinction between mesothelioma and other neoplastic processes. A wide variety of specimens may be submitted for pathological examination including pleural fluid for cytology, Abrams needle-type closed pleural biopsy, radiologically directed pleural biopsies, and open pleural procedures. Pleural fluid and closed pleural biopsies are often nondiagnostic but may be able to give limited information on the likelihood that the lesion is a mesothelioma rather than metastatic carcinoma.

With marker studies some metastatic carcinomas may be definitively diagnosed on cytology or small biopsy particularly if the original primary tumor is available for comparison. Radiologically guided core biopsies have the highest yield of the closed biopsies, however the variability of the appearances in mesothelioma often necessitates surgical video-assisted (VATS) or open biopsy to make the diagnosis.

Sometimes the diagnosis in an unfit patient may not be made until after death where in many countries the possibility of the diagnosis of mesothelioma makes referral of the case to the medical examiner/coroner/pro-

curator fiscal mandatory because of the medicolegal implications of industrial disease associated with asbestos exposure. Macroscopic morphological appearances and radiological findings are insufficient in such cases as mesothelioma can mimic both reactive pleural disease and malignancy of all types macroscopically making detailed microscopic examination with special staining essential.

Pleural fluid containing morphologically neoplastic appearing cells which stain for mesothelial markers but not carcinoma markers may be seen in both epithelial and biphasic tumors but the pleural fluid cytology is frequently negative in the sarcomatoid and desmoplastic tumors as the cells are not shed into the fluid. Cytological cell block preparations for immunohistochemistry may be more successful than centrifuged or thin-layer cytological specimens, as antigens within the cell and nuclei may be more readily unmasked.

Radiologically directed core biopsies have a higher diagnostic yield than cytology or closed blind biopsies and give potentially more material for immunohistochemical studies if VATS or open biopsy cannot be performed. Material from VATS biopsies or decortications/resections has the highest diagnostic yield but only if adequately sampled microscopically.

Electron microscopy to look for typical mesothelial microvilli was used extensively in the 1980s to make the diagnosis but has essentially been superseded by immunohistochemistry. It requires special rapid fixation using glutaraldehyde and is relatively more expensive than immunohistochemistry so is now seldom used. Electron microscopy is, however, still used for analysis of lung tissue for numbers and types of asbestos fibers and may be useful in proving high-level exposure in medicolegal cases. However, mesothelioma, unlike asbestosis, may occur in association with a wide range of asbestos body loads and this analysis may not always be required to link causation.

Mucin stains were also used in the past as mesotheliomas usually did not contain the neutral mucins seen in adenocarcinomas and the ground substance of some mesotheliomas contained specific types of acid mucins. These techniques are seldom used now in modern laboratories because of their lack of specificity and the rapid expansion of immunohistochemical markers.

Postmortem histological material is often morphologically suboptimal if there has been an interval of greater than 1–2 days following death, however many of the special immunohistochemical techniques will still work even on autolyzed tissues.

As yet flow cytometry, genetic markers, and the recently reported association with SV40 virus have not made major contributions to routine diagnostic techniques.

A note of caution should be made when evaluating any new technique and/or marker in this field, all of which need to be carefully evaluated and compared to existing markers to look for advantages in specificity and sensitivity.

The literature is full of small studies which show initially enthusiastic results which are not always reproduced in other laboratories and larger studies. Variability in laboratory techniques and different antibody clones may explain some of the variability but observer interpretation still plays a part, particularly where differential staining of membrane/cytoplasm or nucleus is important in determining whether a stain is positive or not. Care must be taken before a new "wonder marker" is introduced into a diagnostic panel.

42.4 Neoplastic Versus Reactive Mesothelial Proliferation

There are no markers that can truly distinguish benign from malignant mesothelial proliferation and the diagnosis of neoplasia must be accompanied by cytological changes in cells that indicate neoplasia, such as cellular pleomorphism, increased mitotic rate, necrosis, and invasion, none of which are usually present in reactive processes.

Normal, reactive, and neoplastic mesothelial cells will stain with low molecular weight cytokeratins such as CAM 5.2 but in histological preparations the growth pattern of the cells, the presence or absence of maturation in proliferating submesothelial cells, and the presence of invasion of lung, fat, or muscle of chest wall are pointers to a neoplastic rather than reactive process. Reactive pleural thickening of submesothelial fibrous tissue usually shows laminar ordered layers of proliferating cells rather than the disordered, focally storiform proliferation seen in sarcomatoid mesothelioma. The

vascular proliferation in granulation tissue may also cause problems particularly if it is mitotically active, however the endothelial cells do not stain with cytokeratins and are CD31/34 positive.

Some pathologists find the presence or absence of epithelial membrane antigen (EMA) staining useful in distinguishing reactive surface mesothelial epithelial proliferation, which is usually EMA negative, from neoplastic proliferation, which is EMA positive. Many carcinomas also express EMA so it is less useful in distinguishing mesothelioma from metastatic tumors. It is not usually expressed in sarcomatoid mesothelioma [13,14]. Desmin is often expressed in reactive mesothelium but is not seen in epithelial mesotheliomas [13]. Sarcomatoid mesotheliomas may express desmin but less frequently than actin expression (Table 42.3).

Florid histiocytic proliferations may be distinguished using macrophage markers such as CD68 but sometimes secondary inflammatory reactive processes may induce a histiocytic reaction particularly following pleurodesis where a foreign body-type giant cell reaction to talc or other substances may be seen. This can cause diagnostic problems if the pathologist is not aware of the history or lacks experience in this area. Pleurodesis also often causes marked pleural thickening. Diagnostic specimens taken after this procedure need to be sampled extensively to make sure that any neoplastic-associated process is not disguised and may be difficult to interpret even with immunohistochemistry. The most often missed type of tumor in this circumstance is the desmoplastic mesothelioma, however it may also lead to overinterpretation of reactive fibrosis associated with epithelial mesothelioma which is subsequently interpreted as biphasic [4].

The presence of invasion of lung, fat, or muscle is almost always indicative of malignancy and may be dem-

Table 42.3. Immunohistochemical staining patterns of reactive and neoplastic mesothelium

Immunohisto-chemical marker	Normal mesothelium	Reactive mesothelium	Reactive fibrosis	Malignant mesothelioma	Comments
Low molecular weight keratins (e.g., CAM 5.2)	+	+	Weakly positive in submesothelial cells but laminar growth pattern and maturation	+ Positive in both epithelioid and sarcomatous areas	Useful in identifying growth pattern and invasion
Epithelial membrane antigen (EMA)	–	–	–	+	Positive in epithelial mesothelioma
Desmin	–	+	–	±	May be positive in sarcomatoid mesothelioma
Macrophage marker (e.g., CD68)	–	–	–	–	Macrophage s positive in inflammatory lesions
Vascular markers (e.g., CD34)	–	– Positive in granulation tissue	± Identifies vascular proliferation	–	Positive in solitary fibrous tumor

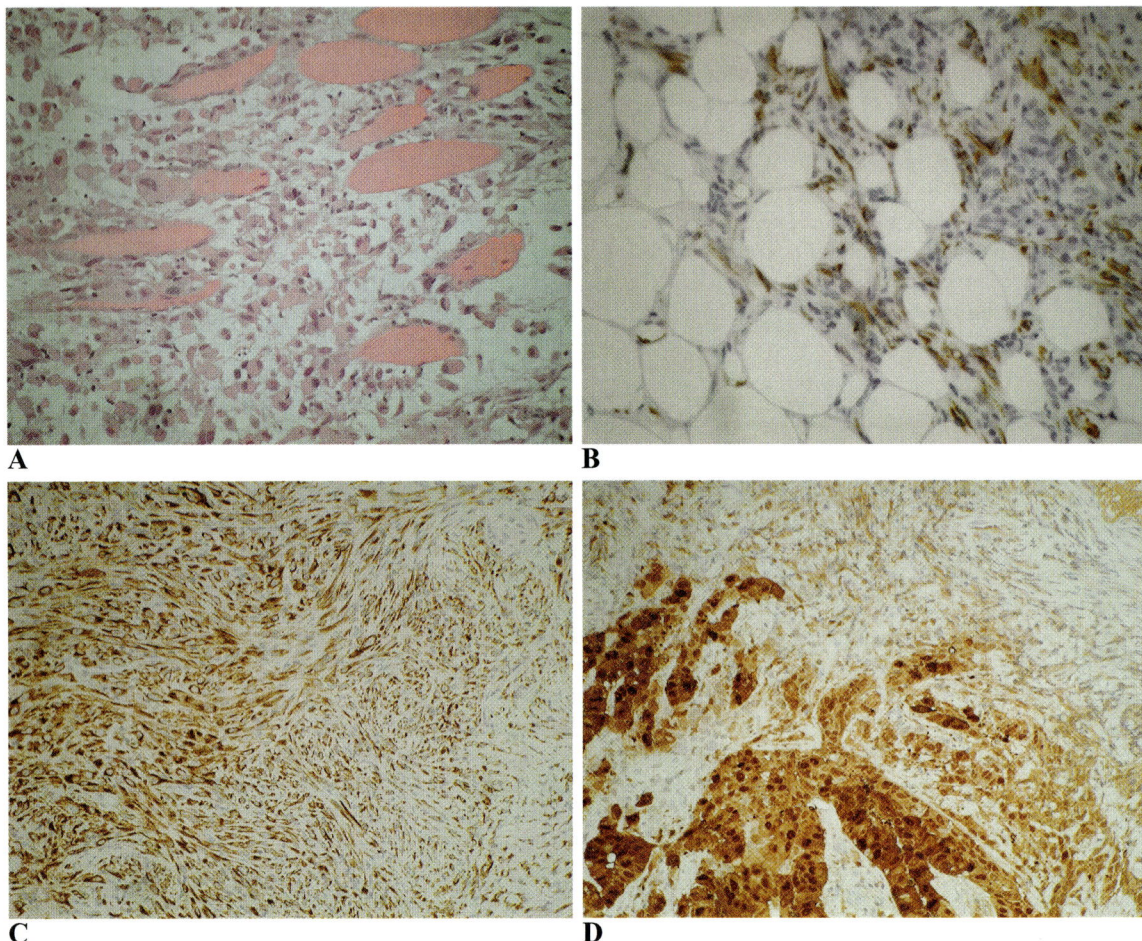

Fig. 42.4. A Invasion of muscle by epithelioid mesothelioma.
B Invasion of fat by sarcomatoid mesothelioma (CAM 5.2
stain). **C** Sarcomatoid mesothelioma showing storiform pattern
highlighted by CAM 5.2 staining. **D** Biphasic mesothelioma
stained with calretinin, the epithelial areas stain more strongly
than the sarcomatoid areas

onstrated with cytokeratins (Fig. 42.4a,b), however
pseudoinvasion of fibrous tissue by bland mesothelial
cells may be seen in reactive processes as may mitotic
activity. In these cases the lack of cytological pleomorphism should suggest a benign diagnosis rather
than a malignant one. Florid surface multilayered mesothelial proliferation may be seen in association with
pneumothorax. True necrosis is rare in reactive mesothelium but must be distinguished from entrapped fi-
brinous exudates.

In those cases where there is felt to be mesothelial
hyperplasia with features suspicious but not diagnostic
of mesothelioma, the designation atypical mesothelial
hyperplasia may be useful to indicate to the clinician
that further investigation and follow-up are required
[6].

42.5 Malignant Mesothelioma Versus Metastatic Tumors and Other Primary Pleural Neoplasms

The many histological types and variable patterns of malignant mesothelioma allow it to mimic numerous other
tumor types. Although special techniques, particularly
immunohistochemistry, have revolutionized the diagnostic process in the last decade or so these adjuncts to diagnosis have to be interpreted with caution as there is much
variation of staining patterns between tumor types [8].
This has led to the development of immunohistochemical
panels which need to be modified according to the histological appearances and clinical background of the patient to make sure that the diagnosis is secure.

The most common differential diagnosis lies between
epithelial malignant mesothelioma of tubulopapillary or
glandular type and adenocarcinoma, particularly of lung
primary origin [15, 16]. However, some of the more solid

and pleomorphic/clear cell variants can mimic tumors such as undifferentiated non-small cell lung cancer, melanoma, renal cell carcinoma, or lymphoma. Whereas melanomas and lymphomas are usually readily distinguished with relevant immunohistochemical markers as they do not routinely express epithelial antigens, metastatic renal cell carcinoma may be difficult to diagnose because of the variability in histological appearances and the marked overlap in immunohistochemical panels [17]. In these cases clinical history and radiological investigation are useful as renal tumors giving rise to metastases are usually readily apparent on CT scan. Panels should therefore include both "positive" mesothelial markers, such as CK5/6, calretinin, thrombomodulin, WT1, and mesothelin, as well as "negative" markers, such as CEA and BerEP4 (Table 42.4) [7, 18–23].

The differential diagnosis of mesothelioma versus adenocarcinoma will also differ in men and women, and breast carcinoma metastatic to pleura may mimic both benign and malignant processes particularly if the cells are small and bland as in lobular carcinoma. Estrogen (ER) and/or progesterone receptor (PR) markers, if positive, may help make the correct diagnosis in these cases.

Some of the tumor markers such as mesothelin and WT1 crossreact with ovarian surface-derived adenocarcinomas [23]. Calretinin, although a very useful mesothelial

Table 42.4. Immunohistochemical staining patterns of mesothelioma and other tumors involving the pleura

Immunohisto-chemical marker	Epithelial mesothelioma	Sarcomatoid mesothelioma	Squamous cell carcinoma (SCC)	Adeno-carcinoma	Comments
Low molecular weight cytokeratin (e.g., CAM 5.2) Cytoplasmic staining	+	+ Useful in identifying storiform growth pattern	–/+ Positive in 30%	+	Useful in identifying mesothelioma type and invasion
Epithelial membrane antigen (EMA) Membrane staining	+	–	+	+	
Cytokeratin CK5/6 Cytoplasmic staining	+	–/+	+	–/+ depending on tumor type	Negative in renal cell carcinoma except papillary type (34%)
Calretinin Cytoplasmic staining	+	+/–	–/+ Positive in 25%	–	May be positive in renal cell carcinoma, papillary type
Thrombomodulin Membrane staining	+	–/+	+	–	Also stains urothelial tumors and endothelial cells
Wilms tumor gene product (WT1) Nuclear staining	+	–/+	Unknown	–	Also stains ovarian serous tumors
Mesothelin Membrane staining	+	+	+/–	–/+ Depends on type of tumor	Also stains ovarian serous tumors and some lung adeno-carcinoma Negative in renal cell carcinoma
BerEP4	–	–	–	+	Focal staining sometimes seen in epithelial mesothelioma
Carcinoembryonic antigen (CEA)	–	–	+ Positive in 50%	+	
MOC 31	–	–	+	+	
P63	–	–	+	–	Useful in distinguishing SCC
Thyroid transcription factor 1 (TTF1) Nuclear staining	–	–	–	Positive in lung and thyroid adeno-carcinomas	Also seen in small cell carcinomas
RCC	–	–	–	Positive in renal cell carcinoma	
Smooth muscle actin	–	+	–	–	Negative in renal cell carcinoma

+ >75% cases positive, +/– 50–75% cases positive, –/+ 25–50% cases positive, – <25% cases positive

marker not seen in many adenocarcinomas [24], stains a significant proportion of squamous carcinomas and papillary renal cell carcinomas as well as other tumors. P63 may be useful in distinguishing squamous carcinomas from mesotheliomas [21], however this is a less common problem than with adenocarcinomas as the morphology and usual presence of keratin lead toward the correct diagnosis, as does careful study of the radiological picture in many cases. Although some studies have found vimentin useful in distinguishing mesothelioma from carcinoma, this author has found it relatively non-specific.

Sarcomatoid and desmoplastic mesotheliomas, although positive with cytokeratins CAM 5.2 (Fig. 42.4 c), do not stain so readily with some mesothelial markers such as calretinin (Fig. 42.4 d) and may stain with muscle markers such as smooth muscle actin and sometimes also desmin [19]. The differential diagnosis of this tumor type may include other primary or metastatic sarcomas with tumors such as sarcomas of muscle or synovial sarcomas producing particular diagnostic dilemmas unless the diagnosis is considered on morphological grounds and appropriate markers performed. Solitary fibrous tumor (previously known as benign mesothelioma) may also lead to confusion if immunohistochemical panels including CD34 and BCL-2 are not used and radiological correlation undertaken, however these tumors are uniformly cytokeratin negative unlike malignant mesothelioma.

The small cell variant of mesothelioma has a significant immunohistochemical overlap with small cell anaplastic tumors of other types so still must be a diagnosis of exclusion [25]. Pulmonary and some extrapulmonary small cell carcinomas have been shown to express TTF1 although as yet little work has been undertaken on primary mesothelial small cell tumors because of their rarity.

In summary a basic reliable panel of markers for mesothelial tumor diagnosis should include a low molecular weight cytokeratin such as CAM 5.2, CK5/6, EMA, calretinin, WT1, CEA, and Ber EP4 in order to show tumor pattern and type and both include positive and negative mesothelial markers (Table 42.4). Other useful markers often included in routine panels include mesothelin, Leu M1 (CD15), and E cadherin. Additional markers may be added as required such as TTF1 for lung and thyroid tumors, ER and PR in breast and endometrial cancers, prostatic-specific antigen (PSA) for prostate cancer, CK7 and 20 to distinguish upper and lower gastrointestinal adenocarcinomas [26], RCC for renal cortical tumors, HMB45 and melan A for metastatic melanoma, P63 for squamous cell carcinoma, etc. according to the morphology of the tumor cells. In sarcomatoid mesothelioma, CAM 5.2 shows infiltrative and storiform morphology which are the most important diagnostic criteria. Other markers which showed initial promise but have been found to be less useful in mesothelioma diagnosis include CD44, HBME1, and human milk fat globule antigen [7, 8].

Thymomas can present particular problems as they may also show a variety of patterns and have marked associated lymphocytic infiltrates. Radiology and relevant immunohistochemical panels will usually lead to the diagnosis but in some cases the distinction from non-small cell carcinoma and mesothelioma may be difficult unless the usually bland cytological appearances are appreciated together with the intimate association with reactive lymphoid cells which is often present.

It cannot be stressed highly enough that detailed knowledge by the pathologist of radiological and clinical findings including previous history of neoplasia are vital in leading to the correct diagnosis in pleural neoplasia. For rare subtypes of pleural neoplasia and atypical proliferations, referral to a specialist team may help secure a diagnosis or help determine a diagnostic strategy.

In all cases good communication between specialist physicians, surgeons, radiologists, and pathologists with multidisciplinary case conferences will improve diagnostic accuracy and inform patient-centered decision-making.

Key Points

- The pathological diagnosis of malignant mesothelioma may be difficult particularly in pleural fluid or small biopsies, however radiologically directed core biopsies and video-assisted biopsies have a higher diagnostic yield.
- A diagnosis of malignant mesothelioma should not be made in the absence of neoplastic cell morphology that is usually associated with invasion.
- There are a multitude of immunohistochemical markers that may assist in the differential diagnosis of both reactive pleural proliferations and pleural tumors.
- Malignant mesothelioma may mimic a number of other tumor types including carcinomas and sarcomas but advances in immunohistochemistry have made major contributions to accurate diagnosis of tumor type.
- Desmoplastic mesothelioma presents a particular diagnostic challenge and requires adequate sampling of a sufficient amount of material usually from an open procedure in order to make the diagnosis with confidence.
- Clinicoradiological correlation and the development of integrated specialist teams containing physicians, surgeons, radiologists, and pathologists are important in improving diagnostic accuracy and in formulating treatment plans.

References

1. Attanoos RL, Gibbs AR. Pathology of malignant mesothelioma. Histopathology 1997; 30:403.

2. Sobin LH, Wittekind IN (eds). Pleural mesothelioma. In: TNM Classification of Malignant Tumours, 6th edn. UICC International Union Against Cancer. New York: Wiley-Liss, 2002:104.

3. Denton KJ, Cotton DWK, Nakielny RA, Goepel JR. Secondary tumour deposits in needle biopsy tracks: an underestimated risk? J Clin Pathol 1990; 43:83.

4. Attanoos RL, Gibbs AR. The pathology associated with therapeutic procedures in malignant mesothelioma. Histopathology 2004; 45:393.

5. Churg A, Roggli V, Galateau-Salle F, et al. Tumours of the pleura. Tumours of the lung, pleura, thymus and heart. In: Travis WD, Brambilla E, Muller-Hermelink HK, Harris CC (eds) Pathology and Genetics of Tumours of the Lung, Pleura, Thymus and Heart. World Health Organisation Classification of Tumours. Lyon, France: IARC Press, 2004:125.

6. Battifora H, McCaughey WTE (eds). Tumours of the serosal membranes. In: Atlas of Tumour Pathology, 3rd series, Fascicle 15 Armed Forces Institute of Pathology. Washington DC: AFIP, 1995.

7. Battifora H. The pleura. In: Mills SE, Carter D, Greenson JK, et al. (eds) Diagnostic Surgical Pathology. Philadelphia: Lippincott Williams and Wilkins, 2004; 1223.

8. Attanoos RL, Webb R, Dojcinov SD, Gibbs AR. Malignant epithelioid mesothelioma: anti-mesothelial marker expression correlates with histological pattern. Histopathology 2001; 39:584.

9. Roberts F, McCall AE, Burnett RA. Malignant mesothelioma: a comparison of biopsy and post-mortem material by light microscopy and immunohistochemistry. J Clin Pathol 2001; 54:766.

10. Allen TC, Cagle PT, Churg AM, Colby TV, Gibbs AR, Hammar SP, Corson JM, Grimes MM, Ordonez NG, Roggli V, Travis WD, Wick MR. Localised malignant mesothelioma. Am J Surg Pathol 2005; 29:866.

11. Galateau-Salle F, Vignaud JM, Burke L, Gibbs A, Brambilla E, Attanoos R, Goldberg M, Launoy G; Mesopath Group. Well differentiated papillary mesothelioma of the pleura: a series of 24 cases. Am J Surg Pathol 2004; 28:534.

12. Kaplan MA, Tazelaar HD, Hayashi T, Schroer KR, Travis WD. Adenomatoid tumours of the pleura. Am J Surg Pathol 1996; 20:1219.

13. Attanoos RL, Griffin A, Gibbs AR. The use of immunohistochemistry in distinguishing reactive from neoplastic mesothelium. A novel use of desmin and comparative evaluation with epithelial membrane antigen, p53, platelet derived growth factor receptor, P-glycoprotein and Bcl-2. Histopathology 2003; 43:231.

14. Mangano WE, Cagle PT, Churg A, Vollmer RT, Roggli VL. The diagnosis of desmoplastic malignant mesothelioma and its distinction from fibrous pleurisy. Am J Clin Pathol 1998; 110:191.

15. Abutaily AS, Addis BJ, Roche WR. Immunohistochemistry in the distinction between malignant mesothelioma and pulmonary adenocarcinoma: a critical evaluation of new antibodies. J Clin Pathol 2002; 55:662.

16. Ordonez NG. The immunohistochemical diagnosis of mesothelioma: a comparative study of epithelioid mesothelioma and lung adenocarcinoma. Am J Surg Pathol 2003; 27:1031.

17. Ordonez NG. The diagnostic utility of immunohistochemistry in distinguishing between mesothelioma and renal cell carcinoma: a comparative study. Hum Pathol 2004; 35:697.

18. Amin KM, Litzky LA, Smythe WR, Mooney AM, Morris JM, Mews DJY, Pass HI, Kari C, Rodeck U, Rauscher FJ III, Kaiser LR, Albeida SM. Wilms' tumour 1 susceptibility (WT1) gene products are selectively expressed in malignant mesothelioma. Am J Pathol 1995; 146:344.

19. Attanoos RL, Dojcinov SD, Webb R, Gibbs AR. Anti-mesothelial markers in sarcomatoid mesothelioma and other spindle cell neoplasms. Histopathology 2000; 37:224.

20. Clover J, Oates J, Edwards C. Anti-cytokeratins 5/6: a positive marker for epithelioid mesothelioma. Histopathology 1997; 31:140.

21. Kaufmann O, Fietze E, Mengs J, Dietel M. Value of P63 and cytokeratin 5/6 as immunohistochemical markers for the differential diagnosis of poorly differentiated and undifferentiated carcinomas. Am J Clin Pathol 2001; 116:823.

22. Kennedy AD, King G, Kerr KM. HMBE and antithrombomodulin in the differential diagnosis of malignant mesothelioma of the pleura. J Clin Pathol 1997; 50:859.

23. Ordonez NG. Application of mesothelin immunostaining in tumour diagnosis. Am J Surg Pathol 2003; 27:1418.

24. Doglioni C, Tos APD, Laurino L, Iuzzolino P, Chiarelli C, Celio MR, Viale G. Calretinin: a novel immunocytochemical marker for mesothelioma. Am J Surg Pathol 1996; 20:1037.

25. Mayall FG, Gibbs AR. The histology and immunohistochemistry of small cell mesothelioma. Histopathology 1992; 20:47.

26. Chu P, Wu E, Wiess LM. Cytokeratin 7 and 20 expression in epithelial neoplasms: a survey of 435 cases. Mod Pathol 2000; 13:962.

Surgical Management of Mesothelioma

43

Michael S. Kent, Sebastien Gilbert
and James D. Luketich

Contents

43.1 Introduction

Despite its rarity, malignant pleural mesothelioma (MPM) has attracted intense interest among epidemiologists, medical oncologists, and surgeons. This is partly due to the rising incidence of the disease, both in the USA and in Europe. Although asbestos has been banned for 30 years in the USA, it was used in Europe well into the 1990s. Mesothelioma will probably continue to be a public health concern for the next several decades given the long latency periods between exposure and disease development. It is predicted that the peak incidence of mesothelioma will occur in the year 2020, and that over the next two decades 200,000 deaths will occur as a result of the disease [1].

Mesothelioma has also attracted interest due to the apparent resistance of the tumor to standard forms of therapy. The disease is often approached with a degree of therapeutic nihilism, given that response rates to either single-agent or combined chemotherapy are in the range of 10–20%, and that survival is rarely prolonged by such therapy. Although mesothelioma cell lines are radiosensitive, the high dose required to achieve palliation of symptoms and the large surface area of the hemithorax that must be treated render radiation unsuitable as primary therapy for the majority of patients.

From the surgeon's perspective, mesothelioma is an equally formidable adversary. The tumor tends to spread diffusely over the parietal pleura. Adjacent structures such as the chest wall and mediastinum may be invaded by tumor which often precludes surgical resection. Also, the surgical procedures available for patients with mesothelioma are technically demanding. The tumor often invades the underlying lung, making a lung-sparing operation such as pleurectomy/decortication difficult. For those that undergo an extrapleural pneumonectomy (EPP), the challenges of achieving a complete resection along with reconstruction of the pericardium and diaphragm can be significant, even in experienced centers. Furthermore, the complication rate associated with this operation remains significant, although the mortality rate has declined in recent surgical series compared to earlier studies.

In this chapter the surgical management of malignant pleural mesothelioma will be reviewed. The selection of patients for operation, and the specific technical issues related to surgery and postoperative care will be discussed. In addition, some of the recent approaches to address the high rate of local recurrence following surgery, such as photodynamic therapy and intrapleural chemoperfusion, will be described.

43.2 Diagnosis of Mesothelioma

Patients with mesothelioma often present with advanced locoregional disease. In part this is due to the insidious nature of the tumor. Symptoms such as shortness of breath may be present for a long time, and patients

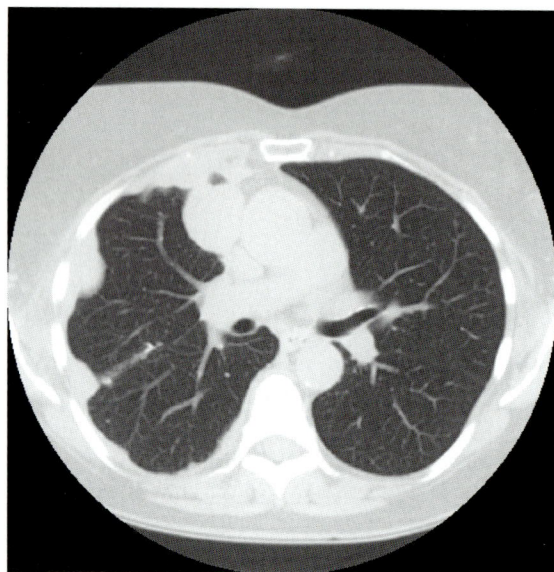

Fig. 43.1. Pleural thickening on computed tomography of a patient with malignant pleural mesothelioma

may not seek attention until symptoms of advanced disease such as chest wall pain and cachexia develop. In addition, mesothelioma is an uncommon disease. Most clinicians will see only a few cases in their lifetime and, as a consequence, the diagnosis is rarely considered when a patient presents with dyspnea, cough, or a pleural effusion. Likewise, the history of asbestos exposure may be remote and not apparent from a routine occupational history.

Ultimately, the diagnosis of mesothelioma usually requires a pleural biopsy, obtained through surgical or percutaneous approaches. However, findings on non-invasive imaging by chest X-ray or computed tomography (CT) can suggest the diagnosis of mesothelioma. The chest X-ray will often show a pleural effusion. In addition, pleural thickening or plaques may be visible. There may also be volume loss of the affected hemithora with a shift of the mediastinum toward the tumor [2]. These findings are better visualized on chest CT (Fig. 43.1). In addition, chest CT may show thickening of the pleura behind an effusion, and in advanced cases extension of the tumor into the lung or chest wall. Once the diagnosis of mesothelioma has been established, both CT and magnetic resonance imaging (MRI) are useful in staging patients and for the selection of therapy [3].

Positron emission tomography (PET) may also be of benefit in evaluating whether a pleural effusion is benign or malignant. For instance, in a series of 28 patients with the suspicion of MPM referred for PET, the uptake of the fluorodeoxyglucose (FDG) tracer was significantly higher in patients with malignant disease [4]. With a cutoff standardized uptake value (SUV) of 2, PET had a sensitivity of 91% and a specificity of 100%

to differentiate malignant from benign disease. In similar studies of 14 [5] and 16 patients [6], PET scanning correctly distinguished benign from malignant pleural disease in all but 1 patient. However, these studies are limited by the small number of patients and the low proportion of patients with benign disease. Furthermore, PET scanning is unable to differentiate MPM from carcinoma metastatic to the pleura, either from a distant site or from the lung. As a consequence, positive findings on PET may raise the suspicion of malignancy but do not obviate the need for a histological diagnosis.

Diagnosis should be confirmed by biopsy of the pleura. Thoracentesis alone is frequently insufficient to provide a diagnosis. Usually, the fluid is hemorrhagic and exudative, with a significant number of reactive mesothelial cells. However, cytology of the fluid has a sensitivity of only 25–30% [7, 8]. Furthermore, it is rare that primary mesothelioma can be differentiated from metastatic adenocarcinoma on the basis of cytology alone. CT-guided biopsy of the pleura has been shown to have a sensitivity of 60%, although this may be increased to 85% with repeat biopsies [9]. As a consequence most patients in whom the diagnosis of MPM is suspected undergo surgical biopsy.

Usually surgical biopsy can be performed thoracoscopically. An effort is made to perform thoracoscopy and biopsy through a single port site remote from obvious pleural involvement on the CT, as implantation of tumor along biopsy tracts is well reported. The port site is placed along the course of a future thoracotomy incision, and is resected should the patient undergo definitive surgery. MPM has a typical appearance when viewed thoracoscopically. It is usually described as a grape-like cluster, which represents confluent, poorly vascularized tumor nodules. The tumor rarely bleeds on biopsy. The sarcomatoid variant of mesothelioma appears as a smooth raised sheet on the parietal pleura that strips easily [10]. On occasion, findings at thoracoscopy, particularly when the disease is suspected at an early stage, are non-specific [7]. For this reason it is important to take several biopsies of the pleura at varying locations. Early-stage disease is often most visible at the diaphragmatic sulcus, and this area must be carefully inspected. In the case of advanced disease, complete fusion of the pleural space may render thoracoscopy technically very difficult. In this circumstance a small cut down to the parietal pleura may be performed, and in some cases a limited rib resection allows access to a generous pleural biopsy. It is rare that a full thoracotomy incision is needed, and thoracoscopy is always preferred when possible as it not only allows ample access to tissue but gives the surgeon information regarding resectability. In a prospective study thoracoscopy was shown to have a sensitivity of 100% in diagnosing MPM [8].

Some research has focused on methods to increase the diagnostic yield of thoracoscopy for early-stage

MPM. One such technique is based on the abnormal fluorescence of reflected laser light from tumor tissue. Small studies have investigated the role of "photodynamic diagnosis" for esophageal [11] and lung cancer [12], and the technique has applicability to MPM as well. With this technique the patient is injected with the compound 5-aminolevulinic acid (5-ALA). This is a naturally occurring precursor to hemoglobin, and may be given orally or intravenously. In normal cells this compound is converted to protoporphyrin IX, and subsequently to hemoglobin. Malignant cells often lack the enzyme necessary to convert protoporphyrin IX to hemoglobin. When exposed to green light, cells with a high concentration of protoporphyrin IX emit red light of a specific wavelength. During thoracoscopy this allows the extent of tumor to be appreciated, and may direct the biopsy of abnormal pleura that appears benign under normal white light. This technique is currently under investigation but holds promise to improve detection of early-stage disease [13]. In our own experience and given the already 100% diagnostic yield of thoracoscopy, this approach will likely only hold promise for investigational protocols for very early stage diagnosis.

43.3 Staging of Mesothelioma

The staging of MPM is complicated by the diffuse nature of the tumor, and its inconstant pattern of nodal metastases. This is in contrast to non-small cell lung cancer, in which patterns of lymph node spread have been well described and an international staging system is accepted and widely used. In the effort to adequately stage patients with MPM, two issues are critical. The first is to determine which patients are technically resectable. Advanced-stage disease frequently invades the chest wall, diaphragm, and mediastinum at multiple sites, precluding complete surgical resection. Accurate staging may help avoid unnecessary thoracotomy in some patients. The clinical importance of this local staging problem is illustrated by the observation that even with extensive preoperative evaluation including CT and MRI, up to 24% of patients with MPM who undergo exploratory thoracotomy are found to be unresectable [14]. The second value of staging lies in its ability to predict survival. It becomes difficult if not impossible to compare different treatment strategies of chemotherapy, radiation, and surgery if an accepted and accurate staging system is not used.

The most utilized staging system used for mesothelioma was proposed by the International Mesothelioma Interest Group (IMIG) in 1995, and is based on the TNM classification system [15]. The T descriptor attempts to quantify the degree of local invasion by the tumor. T1a lesions involve the parietal pleura only, T1b tumors exhibit scattered foci of visceral pleural involvement, and T2 tumors have involvement of both pleura layers. T3 tumors include those which are locally advanced but potentially resectable, such as with invasion of the endothoracic fascia or mediastinal fat, whereas T4 tumors are technically unresectable. This classification is intended to describe the appropriate surgical procedure required for tumor debulking: for T1 tumors a pleurectomy and decortication may be sufficient, however an EPP is often necessary for T2 and T3 tumors. The N and M descriptors are similar to those used for non-small cell lung cancer. N1 disease represents nodal metastases to the hilar nodes, N2 to ipsilateral mediastinal nodes (including internal mammary nodes), and N3 contralateral disease. Any distant metastases (in the case of MPM, transdiaphragmatic invasion and metastases to the peritoneal cavity are particularly important) renders the patient stage IV.

Unfortunately, there is a poor correlation between preoperative and intraoperative staging. This is due to the inability of current imaging, such as CT an MRI, to accurately determine the degree of involvement of the chest wall, visceral pleura, and draining lymph nodes. In a series of 65 patients with MPM who underwent evaluation with CT and MRI followed by surgical exploration, the accuracy of preoperative staging was between 55% and 75% [16]. These modalities were equally poor in all areas except in the determination of diaphragmatic invasion, for which MRI was slightly more accurate.

Non-invasive imaging by CT or MRI is particularly insensitive in defining which patients with MPM have nodal metastases. Up to 50% of patients at the time of thoracotomy were found to have either nodal or hilar metastases, unsuspected by imaging [17]. MPM patients with metastases to either N1 or N2 nodes are considered to have stage III disease, and face a dismal prognosis. The inability of CT or MRI to predict nodal disease has been attributed to the manner in which the tumor may diffusely involve the visceral and mediastinal pleura, obscuring the resolution of adjacent hilar and mediastinal nodal basins.

Recently, the accuracy of PET to stage patients with mesothelioma has been investigated. Results of this technology have been reported in a series of 63 patients treated at the Memorial Sloan-Kettering Cancer Center [18]. In this review, the primary tumor was FDG avid in all but one case of a very early stage (T1a) tumor. However, the sensitivity of PET to detect nodal disease was only 11%. It was found that a high SUV in the primary tumor did correlate with the presence of nodal disease, although this finding remains to be confirmed in other centers. PET scanning did identify 6 patients with distant metastases, however the report did not compare the results of PET with standard imaging such as CT and MRI. The authors concluded that PET was insensitive for determining nodal disease, but may identify unsuspected distant disease in a small number of patients.

The poor results with non-invasive imaging and the high rates of unresectability found at thoracotomy have led to an interest in surgical staging of these patients. This may include laparoscopy to rule out transdiaphragmatic invasion and mediastinoscopy to evaluate nodal metastases. This protocol has been performed at the MD Anderson Cancer Center, and the results in 118 patients were recently presented in abstract form [19]. These patients had already undergone imaging with CT and MRI, and were felt to be technically resectable. Unsuspected transdiaphragmatic invasion was found in 10% of patients. However mediastinoscopy was found to only have a sensitivity of 31% in determining N2/3 disease. The poor sensitivity of mediastinoscopy is attributable to two factors. First, only a minority of patients underwent a complete mediastinoscopy in which both contralateral and ipsilateral nodes were biopsied. This was due to the philosophy of the participating surgeons that ipsilateral mediastinal disease was not a contraindication to surgery. Second, mesothelioma has a propensity to metastasize to internal mammary and diaphragmatic nodes, stations which are inaccessible by mediastinoscopy [14].

Although the IMIG staging system is most frequently used, it must be noted that another staging system has been proposed by the group at the Brigham and Women's Hospital [20]. This staging system is based on this single institution's experience with combined modality treatment for mesothelioma, and has been validated in their series of 328 patients. This system is simpler to use than the IMIG classification, and attempts to account for the completeness of surgical resection. However, it is only applicable for patients who have undergone EPP, and is consequently not relevant for the vast majority of patients diagnosed with mesothelioma.

43.4 Preoperative Evaluation

Both pleurectomy/decortication and EPP can be associated with significant morbidity; although the mortality rate associated with these procedures has been less than 5% in recent series [21]. Furthermore, patients with mesothelioma are often elderly, debilitated, and have significant pulmonary dysfunction due to smoking and asbestos exposure. Because of this, it is important to carefully evaluate a patient's physiological reserve prior to recommending one of these procedures.

Poor performance status is considered by most groups to be a contraindication to EPP, for two reasons. First, it has been shown that poor performance status is an independent predictor of prognosis in patients with mesothelioma, regardless of the method of treatment used [22, 23]. Second, pneumonectomy places considerable physiological and emotional strains on both the patient and caregivers. Those who are unable to ambu-

late or perform their activities of daily living without assistance are felt to have a prohibitive operative risk. In some centers, these patients are considered for pleurectomy/decortication [10]. In other centers, these patients may be referred for chemoradiotherapy, or palliative care alone.

Pulmonary reserve is quantified by pulmonary function testing. Patients who are candidates for EPP should be predicted to have a postoperative FEV1 of at least 800 mL. Patients whose preoperative FEV1 is greater than 2 L physiologically should require no further pulmonary assessment, however in our practice we generally obtain quantitative ventilation-perfusion scanning in any patient considered for EPP. Arterial blood gases are also part of the routine preoperative evaluation. A room air PO_2 less than 65 or PCO_2 greater than 45 raise serious concerns about a patient's ability to tolerate EPP.

A cardiac evaluation is particularly critical for this patient population. As with non-small cell lung cancer, many of these patients have associated coronary disease. In addition, following pneumonectomy the vascular resistance to the right ventricular outflow tract is essentially doubled. Patients with poor ventricular function may develop acute right heart failure in this setting. In addition, the arrhythmias frequently encountered following pneumonectomy are poorly tolerated by these patients. In general, an ejection fraction below 40% or the presence of pulmonary hypertension would raise concerns for a planned EPP. Echocardiography may also detect unsuspected mediastinal invasion, and can provide a baseline measurement of cardiac function that may be impaired by cardiotoxic chemotherapy [10].

Finally, some surgeons consider age to be a relative contraindication to EPP. Although older patients may have adequate cardiopulmonary reserve, many centers have adopted a policy of not recommending EPP to patients older than 70. In our own experience, age greater than 70 is not used as a single criteria to exclude consideration for EPP.

43.5 Extrapleural Pneumonectomy

43.5.1 Surgical Technique

The intent of an EPP is to provide optimal cytoreduction by resecting the involved lung within an envelope of parietal pleura, pericardium, and diaphragm. The technical aspects of the procedure are described below. Anesthetic issues and the management of postoperative complications specific to this procedure are discussed subsequently.

The patient is intubated with a double-lumen endotracheal tube, and is placed in the lateral decubitus position. A full posterolateral thoracotomy incision is made, and any port sites from prior thoracoscopy are excised. This incision is made over the sixth rib, and may extend from the costovertebral to the costochondral junction, although lesser incisions may be adequate in some cases. Rib removal may facilitate exposure and, if so, the periosteum of the rib is stripped and the rib is removed. The posterior periosteum is then excised, and a plane is developed between the parietal pleura and the endothoracic fascia. This plane can usually be developed bluntly, although sharp dissection may be necessary in some cases. Bleeding from this dissection is well-controlled with laparotomy sponges. The plane is first developed toward the apex of the chest and then inferiorly toward the diaphragm. Care is taken to preserve the internal mammary artery and vein, which are easily injured. This plane is continued until the structures of the hilum of the lung are visualized. Absence of mediastinal invasion of the aorta or esophagus is ruled out by careful palpation. A nasogastric tube greatly facilitates identification of the esophagus. Next, if involved, the pericardium is opened to rule out invasion of the heart.

Once the tumor is clearly evaluated and found to be resectable, the diaphragm is resected if removal allows clearance of the costophrenic angles. This is done by incising the diaphragm, taking care to preserve the underling peritoneum if possible. The diaphragm is elevated with clamps and the plane between the diaphragm and the peritoneum is developed with a sponge stick. The attachments of the diaphragm to the chest wall are then divided circumferentially. This can usually be done bluntly. It is important to preserve a 2-cm rim of the crus to allow suturing of the prosthetic patch. This also decreases the incidence of postoperative gastric herniation [24]. Once the incision in the diaphragm is extended medially, the opening in the pericardium is extended to allow the inferior vena cava to be visualized and protected.

After the diaphragm is completely resected, the pericardium is fully opened to expose the intrapericardial pulmonary artery and veins. These structures are then individually divided using a vascular stapler. The pericardium is then divided posterior to the hilum, completing the dissection. The mainstem bronchus is then divided and the specimen removed. Bleeding from the chest wall can be easily controlled with the argon beam laser. The final step before reconstruction is a complete mediastinal lymph node dissection. Areas of residual disease in the mediastinum are marked with clips to facilitate postoperative radiation therapy.

The reconstruction portion of the procedure is perhaps the one which requires the greatest technical experience. First, the bronchial stump should be buttressed to lessen the risk of developing a bronchopleural fistula, a complication associated with a high mortality. This can be done with either pericardial fat or intercos-

tal muscle. Next, the diaphragm and pericardium must be reconstructed. We prefer to reconstruct the diaphragm using a patch of 2-mm Goretex. Two separate 20×30-cm patches may be sewn together to create a larger patch, which is felt to lower the incidence of postoperative patch rupture. This patch is attached to the chest wall using non-absorbable sutures that are secured with a pledget or polypropylene button. The medial edge of the patch is sewn to the pericardium and a rim of diaphragmatic crus which had been preserved. The pericardium is also reconstructed with a Goretex patch, usually of 0.1 mm thickness. It is important that this be done, particularly on the right side. Failure to reconstruct the pericardium may allow the heart to fall out into the empty right chest, obstructing venous return to the heart and leading to immediate hemodynamic collapse. This patch is sewn into place loosely and is fenestrated to prevent excessive buildup of fluid within the pericardium and the development of tamponade. Inferiorly this patch is sewn to the medial leaf of the diaphragmatic patch. The thoracotomy wound is then closed in the usual fashion. In the first 24 h, we prefer to leave a chest tube specifically designed for the pneumonectomy space (Pleur-evac balanced pneumonectomy drainage system; Genzyme, Cambridge, MA) to monitor bleeding and avoid destabilization of the mediastinum. Excessive mediastinal shift may still occur either toward or away from the operated side and lead to significant hemodynamic instability. If no drainage system is used, mediastinal shift can be corrected by either aspirating fluid or withdrawing air from the operated pleural space. The pneumonectomy drainage system maintains a slightly negative pressure within the pneumonectomy space, preventing excessive mediastinal shift.

The technique of a left EPP is generally similar to that of a right-sided resection, although there are some important technical considerations. Isolation of the left lung may be achieved by using either a right-sided double-lumen tube or by a bronchial blocker. Dissection under the aortic arch is performed with care to avoid injury to the recurrent laryngeal nerve. Resection of the diaphragm and division of the pulmonary hilum is performed as for the right side. Unlike right EPP, reconstruction of the pericardium from the left chest is not mandatory if the pericardium is completely resected. However, resection of the pericardium without reconstruction has been reported to lead to the development of a thick pericardial peel, which has led to constrictive pericarditis [25]. This may be prevented by reconstructing the pericardium with a patch.

43.5.2 Anesthetic Considerations

Extrapleural pneumonectomy presents several unique challenges for the anesthesiologist as well as surgeon. The risk of significant blood loss, hypoxemia related to single-lung ventilation, and cardiac instability require the close attention of the entire operating room staff.

Before the induction of anesthesia, arterial and central venous lines are placed. If the potential for injury to the superior vena cava exists, a large-bore venous line is placed in the lower extremity. In general, the interpretation of data from pulmonary artery catheters is difficult during pneumonectomy and they are used rarely [26]. Transesophageal echocardiography is a much more reliable tool to measure right heart function intraoperatively, although it is operator-dependent and not available in all centers.

The choice of anesthetic agents will have a significant impact on the conduct of the operation. Most centers favor insertion of an epidural catheter preoperatively to facilitate early extubation and postoperative pain control. In our center we have found a paravertebral catheter to provide excellent pain control with a superior side effect profile (less sedation, nausea, and hypotension) compared with epidural catheters. The benefits of paravertebral versus epidural catheters for thoracic patients have been shown in a randomized trial [27]. Since early extubation is a priority, short-acting anesthetic agents, whether inhalational or intravenous, are preferred over longer-acting narcotics. It is important to know that inhalational agents are eliminated slowly in patients with significant chronic obstructive pulmonary disease. Also, these agents inhibit pulmonary vasoconstriction in response to hypoxemia. This may lead to significant shunting during single-lung ventilation [28].

Hypoxemia is not uncommon during single-lung ventilation. In part this is due to atelectasis in the dependent, ventilated lung from the weight of the tumor. Other causes, such as endotracheal tube misplacement and inspissated secretions can be ruled out by bronchoscopy. Adding positive end-expiratory pressure to the dependent lung, and continuous positive pressure to the non-dependent lung often solves this problem. A reduction in the use of inhalational agents, for the reasons described above, is also useful. Division of the pulmonary artery prevents shunting of blood to the non-ventilated lung and will significantly improve hypoxemia during single-lung ventilation.

Expeditious diagnosis and management of intraoperative hypotension is also critical to the success of the operation. A common cause of hypotension is compression of the heart leading to an impediment to venous return. Venous return is also impaired by surgical manipulation and positive-pressure ventilation. It is important to not treat hypotension with a significant infusion of crystalloid. Instead, vasopressors and blood transfusion should be used. Often, hemodynamics will improve significantly once the specimen is removed. Less common causes of hypotension to consider during the operation include myocardial ischemia or sympathetic blockade from the epidural catheter.

Hemodynamics may also change rapidly once the chest is closed and the patient is turned supine. This may be due to herniation of the heart into the right chest, and the presentation can be dramatic. The patient must be turned again to the lateral decubitus position, the thoracotomy incision reopened, and the pericardial patch revised. A more common scenario is a subtle degree of hypotension at the end of the operation. Potential causes include mediastinal shift, inadequate volume resuscitation, or tamponade from a constricting pericardial patch. Intraoperative transesophageal echocardiography and a chest X-ray are useful in evaluating these problems.

43.5.3 Postoperative Management

In a review of 328 consecutive patients undergoing EPP at the Brigham and Women's Hospital, the overall complication and mortality rates were 60% and 3.4%, respectively [24]. By far the most common complication was atrial fibrillation, which occurred in 44% of patients. Although a rare cause of mortality, this arrhythmia often prolongs hospital stay and increases utilization of hospital resources. Intravenous calcium channel blockers have shown some efficacy in lowering the incidence of this complication [29]. Other cardiac complications were quite uncommon in this series. Acute myocardial infarction occurred in 1.5% of patients and cardiac arrest in 3% of patients. It is important to note that should a patient develop a sudden cardiac arrest, the treatment should be immediate opening of the thoracotomy and open heart massage. The cause is most often cardiac tamponade or herniation of the heart through a loose pericardial patch. In either case, closed chest compressions and intravenous agents are ineffective.

Significant pulmonary complications are rare after EPP. Prolonged intubation (8%), pneumonia (3%), and the need for tracheostomy (2%) were uncommon in the Brigham series. These complications are closely related to injury of the recurrent laryngeal nerve. Injury to this nerve places the patient at substantial risk for poor clearance of bronchial secretions and the development of aspiration pneumonia. The most feared complication following pneumonectomy is the development of adult respiratory distress syndrome (ARDS) in the remaining lung. This is often attributed to excessive administration of crystalloid in the postoperative period (pulmonary edema is due to fluids, however, ARDS is probably secondary to diffuse alveolar damage occurring during the operation as a result of barotrauma and high FiO_2, among other things). Fluid intake is normally limited to 1 L/day for this reason. However, the majority of research suggests that the cause is more likely due to hyperpermeability within the pulmonary microcirculation [30, 31]. Additional factors that may be contributory are decreased lymphatic drainage after mediastinal lymph node dissection, and excess mediastinal shift and resultant trauma to the remaining lung. Some evidence exists that the use of a balanced postpneumonectomy chest tube may diminish this complication [32]. Finally, it should not be forgotten that esophageal dysmotility is well described after pneumonectomy [33]. Aspiration after pneumonectomy is often a fatal event, and for this reason we leave a nasogastric tube in place for the first postoperative day and advance the patient's oral intake cautiously.

Infection within the pneumonectomy cavity is another rare but potentially catastrophic complication. The management of this is individualized, but greatly depends on whether breakdown of the bronchial stump and a bronchopleural fistula has developed. Details of the management of this complication are beyond the scope of this text. The issue unique to patients who have undergone an EPP relates to the presence of prosthetic material within the infected space. Often, this complication can be managed with thoracoscopic debridement of the chest cavity followed by irrigation with antibiotics through chest tubes, assuming that a bronchopleural fistula is not present [24]. The prosthetic patches can often be saved with this approach. If the patches must be removed, this can be safely done 2 weeks after the pneumonectomy. By this time the mediastinum is sufficiently stabilized by scar that significant shift will not occur.

Complications related to the pericardial patch have already been addressed. The diaphragmatic patch may also rupture, leading to herniation of bowel contents into the chest. The incidence of this complication is thought to be lowered by using a larger patch with less surface tension [24]. The diagnosis is suspected by chest X-ray and confirmed by CT. Immediate reoperation is necessary.

43.6 Pleurectomy and Decortication

Pleurectomy and decortication is used for selected patients with MPM. The benefit of this procedure is that the underlying lung is preserved, and the morbidity following this procedure is generally less than that following EPP. Some centers prefer EPP and reserve pleurectomy and decortication for patients with limited cardiopulmonary reserve and performance status. In other centers a pleurectomy/decortication is performed if all gross disease can be removed by this approach [34]. A pleurectomy/decortication is not possible if there is significant invasion of the underlying lung, and an EPP would be required.

The operation is essentially that of the initial phase of an EPP. A thoracotomy is performed and the extrapleural plane is entered and bluntly dissected to the apex of the chest and the diaphragm. When this dissection is complete the parietal pleura is opened and the visceral pleura and associated tumor is stripped off the lung. This step can be quite difficult in all but the earliest stages of disease. The extensive raw surface of the lung following this dissection may lead to significant bleeding and is the cause for the prolonged air leaks that may follow this type of surgery.

Two other considerations have limited enthusiasm for this procedure. The first is that tumor often remains after pleurectomy/decortication. One study has estimated that this occurs in up to 78% of patients. As a consequence the local recurrence after pleurectomy/decortication is as high as 80% [34]. Secondly, the presence of functional lung limits the amount of adjuvant radiation therapy that may be given to the hemithorax. This is not a concern following EPP where maximal radiation dosage may be given.

Pleurectomy does offer significant palliation of symptoms, however. The operation offers quite durable treatment of pleural effusions. In addition, by removing the parietal pleura involved by tumor the compliance of the chest wall is often improved and symptoms of chest pain, cough, and dyspnea may be diminished [8, 35].

The perception that pleurectomy/decortication is a limited operation with minimal morbidity is not one supported by recent surgical series. Among patients treated at Memorial Sloan-Kettering, the operative mortality was 3.5% for patients treated with pleurectomy/decortication compared with 5.2% for those who underwent EPP. Morbidity can be significant and can include prolonged air leak, empyema, and respiratory failure. The relatively high published morbidity associated with pleurectomy/decortication may reflect a selection bias toward patients who are probably older and more debilitated than EPP candidates.

43.7 Survival Following Surgical Management of Mesothelioma

Surgery as single therapy for patients with mesothelioma is associated with high recurrence rates and a survival that does not differ appreciably from the natural history of the disease [36]. Because of this, recent studies have focused on the role of surgery as a component of multimodality therapy which may include adjuvant radiation therapy or radiation combined with chemotherapy. To the best of our knowledge, no randomized studies have been performed that define the benefit of surgery for patients with mesothelioma. For the time being, the impact of surgery on the outcome of patients with mesothelioma is largely based on the analysis of single institution series and historical controls.

The largest experience with EPP followed by combined chemoradiation therapy was reported by Sugarbaker in 1999 [21]. The protocol of adjuvant therapy was not consistent among the 183 patients, which reflects the long period of time over which these patients were treated (17 years). The majority of patients received a platinum-based regimen with concurrent radiation therapy. The median survival for all patients was 19 months with a 5-year survival of 15% (these figures do not include the 3.8% of patients who died within 30 days of the operation). Survival was then stratified by histology, the presence of extrapleural nodal disease, and the completeness of resection. There were no 5-year survivors of patients who had either mixed cell or sarcomatous subtypes, or patients who had nodal disease in the mediastinum. A positive microscopic margin was associated with a 9% 5-year survival. It was emphasized by the authors that the survival of patients in the most favorable prognostic group (epithelial cell histology, negative margins, and no mediastinal nodal disease) was 46% at 5 years. However, only 31 of 183 patients (17%) were in this favorable prognostic group.

Recurrence among a subset of mesothelioma patients treated by EPP at the Brigham was reported separately [37]. Despite radical surgery and radiation therapy, the rate of local recurrence among 46 patients analyzed was 50%. Compared to historical controls, patients treated with this protocol had an apparent increase in the rate of distant recurrence (41%). This shift from local to distant recurrence may reflect improved local control following trimodality treatment.

Similar results were reported from a large series of patients treated at Memorial Sloan-Kettering Cancer Center. Unlike the Brigham group, a pleurectomy/decortication was selected if all gross disease could be resected with this procedure. An EPP was reserved for those who had extensive involvement of the underlying lung. The majority of patients received some form of adjuvant therapy. Median survival following treatment was 30 months for stage I tumors, 19 months for stage II, 10 months for stage III, and 8 months for stage IV. Of note 170 of the 231 patients in this series were stage III or IV. In a multivariate analysis, stage, histology (epithelial versus non-epithelial), and female gender were independent predictors of improved survival. Patients treated with adjuvant therapy were also noted to have improved survival, although this must be interpreted with caution as only a small number of patients were not given adjuvant therapy and a wide variety of treatment protocols were used. An important finding of this study was that the type of resection did not impact on overall survival. Clearly, this was not a randomized

study and patients only underwent pleurectomy/decortication if no lung invasion was present. However, the results suggest that for the rare patient with early-stage disease, a lung-sparing procedure may be an acceptable alternative to EPP.

43.8 Investigational Strategies to Improve Local Control After Surgery

The behavior of mesothelioma is one of relentless local progression and high rates of local recurrence following radical surgery. This is in contrast to non-small cell lung cancer, in which the majority of patients who die after surgery do so from distant metastases [38]. As a consequence, several centers are investigating additional means of local control that may be utilized after cytoreductive surgery. The aim of these efforts is to address microscopic disease which is invariably present following surgery. Photodynamic therapy and intrapleural chemoperfusion are two forms of adjuvant treatment targeted at residual disease following cytoreduction.

43.8.1 Photodynamic Therapy

Photodynamic therapy (PDT) is a technique in which a sensitizer that is taken up by both normal and tumor cells is injected into a patient. The photosensitizer is activated by visible light and reactive oxygen species are generated that cause cell death. The specificity of this technique lies in the selective application of the light to tumor-bearing tissue. There is evidence that the sensitizer is preferentially absorbed by tumor cells [39], although normal tissue may also be injured if exposed to light of the appropriate wavelength. In addition, the application of PDT is thought to lead to damage of the microvasculature of neoplastic tissue. The occlusion of these vessels after treatment is felt to be an important, secondary mechanism of action of PDT [13].

The most common toxicity seen after PDT is cutaneous photosensitivity due to exposure to sunlight. Generally, this is limited to a mild sunburn, but on occasion, it can include serious third-degree burns. More serious complications, such as esophageal perforation may be seen if PDT is applied to treat disease in the mediastinum [40]. PDT has become an accepted modality for the palliation of esophageal cancer [41] and endobronchial lung cancer [42]. Some centers have also investigated the use of PDT as adjuvant therapy following pleurectomy/decortication or EPP for mesothelioma.

An important consideration in the use of PDT for the treatment of mesothelioma is the lack of a precise method of measuring the amount of light delivered to the chest and mediastinum, to minimize the incidence of complications. Studies have found that a calculation of light doses is often inaccurate, as opposed to direct intraoperative measurement [43]. Consequently, studies of PDT for mesothelioma have used light sensors placed in several locations within the chest (for example, the apex of the chest and adjacent to the bronchial stump). The hemithorax is then filled with a dilute lipid solution which allows the scattering of the laser light. This is meant to prevent the shielding of tissue in the chest from pooled blood. The light source itself is moved around until all light sensors have received the desired dose of light.

The difficulty in obtaining good light exposure to all of the pleural surfaces and the results of a randomized phase III trial have lessened the enthusiasm for this approach in mesothelioma patients [44]. In this study 25 patients underwent cytoreductive surgery (both EPP and pleurectomy/decortication were performed) and intraoperative PDT. This was followed by cisplatin, interferon-alpha, and tamoxifen chemotherapy. The control group of 23 patients underwent the same protocol without PDT. There was no difference in complications between the two groups, but overall survival was also equivalent (14.4 months for PDT versus 14.1 months without). At the present time, therefore, there is no clear benefit for PDT in the treatment of patients with mesothelioma.

43.8.2 Intrapleural Chemoperfusion

The installation of intracavitary chemotherapy has been investigated in a variety of abdominal malignancies [45, 46]. This practice is designed to increase local concentrations of the drug while diminishing systemic absorption and toxicity. However, like PDT, the depth at which chemotherapy remains cytotoxic when delivered in this manner is less than 1 cm. This therapy is unlikely to be effective if gross microscopic disease remains following surgery. In addition, instillation of the drug is ideally performed at the time of surgery, before adhesions form (or, in the case of pneumonectomy a gelatinous effusion that fills the hemithorax) which will limit contact of the drug with the operative bed.

Cisplatin is the agent most commonly used in studies including MPM. Cisplatin has shown some efficacy against mesothelioma when administered systemically [47] Furthermore, in studies of intraperitoneal delivery the local concentration can be 50 times higher than that of intravenous administration [48]. The use of hyperthermia has been shown to increase cell permeability and blood flow to tissues, and several studies have demonstrated a synergistic effect between hyperthermia and chemotherapy [49, 50].

Renal failure is the major toxicity associated with intracavitary cisplatin. Measures taken to diminish this in mesothelioma studies include adequate hydration of the patient and the concurrent administration of sodium thiosulfate, which is believed to bind covalently to cisplatin and lead to an inactive complex [51].

Earlier studies investigating intrapleural chemotherapy did not utilize hyperthermia. For example, Rusch administered cisplatin at a dose of 100 mg/m^2 and mitomycin after pleurectomy/decortication [52]. The agents were instilled through the chest tube in the recovery room following surgery. There was one death and two grade 4 toxicities associated with treatment. Recent studies in which hyperthermia is used in conjunction with chemotherapy utilize a cardiopulmonary bypass circuit adapted for this purpose. The therapy is performed in the operating room after the chest is closed. Large-bore chest tubes are used as the inflow and outflow cannulae. The bypass circuit allows chemotherapy to be administered at a precise temperature and rate.

Complications associated with this regimen have been investigated in two phase I trials from the Brigham and Women's Hospital [53]. These trials were designed as dose-escalation studies, so the maximum tolerated dose could be determined. In the first study, 50 patients underwent EPP followed by hyperthermic chemoperfusion and sodium thiosulfate. The maximum tolerated dose was determined to be 250 mg/m^2, a dose which is significantly higher than that used in earlier studies. There was no additional morbidity of chemoperfusion when compared with matched controls, with the exception of an increased rate of DVT and patch dehiscence. Patch dehiscence occurred in 12% of treated patients, compared with none in the control group. This was thought by the authors to result from high tension on the patch suture line secondary from bowel edema. The incidence of this complication has declined since a larger patch has been used for reconstruction.

The second trial investigated chemoperfusion after pleurectomy/decortication. These patients were older and had a lower performance status than those who underwent EPP. Five deaths occurred among 44 patients. The major dose-limiting toxicity was renal failure, with one patient at the highest dose (250 mg/m^2) requiring dialysis. Subsequent phase II and III trials are planned which may help determine whether hyperthermic chemoperfusion has a survival benefit for patients with mesothelioma.

43.9 Future Directions

Despite significant research efforts to define the etiology and biology of mesothelioma, there is no standard treatment for this disease. Surgery, as part of a combined modality approach, has been associated with prolonged survival in patients with early-stage disease. To date, no randomized study has been performed to evaluate the role of surgery in the treatment of this malignancy. Current therapy for mesothelioma patients is largely based on retrospective case series from single institutions. Although EPP is common in dedicated centers in the United States, this is not the case in Europe. For example, fewer than 50 EPPs are performed in the UK annually [54].

The completion of two randomized trials in Europe may allow for a more evidence-based approach to the treatment of mesothelioma patients [55]. The first trial, known as mesoVATS, seeks to compare the benefit of thoracoscopic pleurectomy to talc pleurodesis alone. The trial is accruing patients, and quality of life as well as survival will be compared between the two treatment arms. The second trial, MARS (Mesothelioma and Radical Surgery) is currently in the planning stage. This trial will be designed to compare treatment arms with and without EPP. The difficulty in designing this study stems from a lack of consensus regarding the "standard therapy" of mesothelioma. Completion of these two trials will hopefully provide useful information in determining the role and benefit of surgical resection for patients diagnosed with mesothelioma.

Key Points

- Malignant pleural mesothelioma (MPM) is a rare and deadly malignancy of the pleura. The tumor spreads in a diffuse manner, and commonly invades the chest wall and mediastinum. The majority of patients present with advanced disease and are not candidates for surgical resection.
- For patients physiologically able to undergo surgery, two procedures have been proposed. The first, extrapleural pneumonectomy, removes the lung, diaphragm, and pericardium within an envelope of pleura. The second, pleurectomy and decortication, removes only the parietal and visceral pleura. Both procedures can be associated with significant morbidity and mortality. The local recurrence rate appears to be lower after pneumonectomy, although it is not clear if this translates into a survival benefit.
- Prolonged survival has been associated with resection of early-stage disease. However survival following resection of locally advanced disease is less than 1 year. To date no randomized study investigating the role of surgery compared to a control group has been performed. Such a study is planned in Europe.

References

1. Peto J, Decarli A, La Vecchia C, Levi F, Tomei F, Negri E. The European mesothelioma epidemic. Br J Cancer 1999; 79:666.
2. Miller WJ, Gefter W, Miller WT. Asbestos-related chest diseases: plain radiographic findings. Semin Roentgenol 1992; 27:102.
3. Yilmaz U, Utkaner G, Yalniz E, Kumcuoglu Z. Computed tomographic findings of environmental asbestos-related malignant pleural mesothelioma. Respirology 1998; 3:33.
4. Benard F, Sterman D, Smith RJ, Kaiser LR, Albelda SM, Alavi A. Metabolic imaging of malignant pleural mesothelioma with fluorodeoxyglucose positron emission tomography. Chest 1998; 114:713.
5. Carretta A, Landoni C, Melloni G, Ceresoli G, Compierchio A, Fazio F, et al. 18-FDG positron emission tomography in the study of malignant pleural diseases: a pilot study. Eur J Cardiothorac Surg 2000; 17:377.
6. Buchmann I, Guhlmann C, Elsner K, Gfrorer W, Schirrmeister H, Kotzerke, et al. F-18 FDG PET for the primary diagnosis of pleural processes. Nuklearmedizin 1999; 38:319.
7. Boutin C, Schlesser M, Frenay C, Astoul P. Malignant pleural mesothelioma. Eur Respir J 1998; 12:972.
8. Grossebner M, Arifi A, Goddard M, Ritchie A. Mesothelioma: VATS biopsy and lung mobilization improves diagnosis and palliation. Eur J Cardiothorac Surg 1999; 16:619.
9. Metintas M, Ozdemir N, Isikoy S, et al. CT-guided pleural needle biopsy in the diagnosis of malignant pleural mesothelioma. J Comput Assist Tomogr 1995; 19:370.
10. Paul S, Neragi-Miandoab S, Jaklitsch M. Preoperative assessment and therapeutic options for patients with malignant pleural mesothelioma. Thorac Surg Clin 2004; 14:505.
11. Mayinger B, Neidhardt S, Reh H, Martus P, Hahn E. Fluorescence induced with 5-aminolevulinic acid for the endoscopic detection and follow-up if esophageal lesions. Gastrointest Endsoc 2001; 54:572.
12. Lam S, MacAulay C, le Rich J, Palcic B. Detection and localization of early lung cancer by fluorescence bronchoscopy. Cancer 2000; 89(suppl):2468.
13. Rodriguez E, Baas P, Friedberg J. Innovative therapies: photodynamic therapy. Thorac Surg Clin 14; 2004:557.
14. Rusch V, Venkratraman E. Important prognostic factors in patients with malignant pleural mesothelioma, managed surgically. Ann Thorac Surg 1999; 68:1799.
15. Rusch V. The International Mesothelioma Interest Group. A proposed new international TNM staging system for malignant pleural mesothelioma. Chest 1995; 108:1122.
16. Heelan R, Rusch V, Begg C, Panicek D, Caravelli J, Eisen C. Staging of malignant pleural mesothelioma: comparison of CT and MR imaging. Am J Roentgenol 1999; 172:1039.
17. Rusch V, Venkratraman E. The importance of surgical staging in the treatment of malignant pleural mesothelioma. J Thorac Cardiovasc Surg 1996; 111:815.
18. Flores R, Akhurst T, Gonen M, Larson S, Rusch V. Positron emission tomography defines metastatic disease but not locoregional disease in patients with malignant pleural mesothelioma. J Thorac Cardiovasc Surg 2003; 126:11.
19. Rice D, Vaporciyan A, Stevens C, et al. Extended surgical staging for potentially resectable mesothelioma. Presented at the Society for Thoracic Surgeons Annual Meeting, 2005.
20. Sugarbaker D, Mentzer S, DeCauld M, Lynch TJ Jr, Strauss G. Extrapleural pneumonectomy or pleurectomy in the

setting of multimodality approach to malignant mesothelioma. Chest 1993; 104:3775.

21. Sugarbaker D, Flores R, Jaklitsch M, et al. Resection margins, extrapleural nodal status and cell type determine postoperative long-term survival in trimodality therapy of malignant pleural mesothelioma: results in 183 patients. J Thorac Cardiovasc Surg 1999; 117:54.

22. Curran D, Sahmoud T, Therasse P, et al. Prognostic factors in patients with pleural mesothelioma: the European Organization for Research and Treatment of Cancer experience. J Clin Oncol 1998; 16:145.

23. Herndon J, Green M, Chahinian A, et al. Factors predictive of survival among 337 patients with mesothelioma treated between 1984 and 1994 by the Cancer and Leukemia Group B. Chest 1998; 113:723.

24. Sugarbaker D, Jaklitsch M, Bueno R, et al. Prevention, early detection and management of complications after 328 consecutive extrapleural pneumonectomies. J Thorac Cardiovasc Surg 2004; 128:138.

25. Byrne J, Karavas A, Colson Y, et al. Cardiac decortication for occult constrictive cardiac physiology and left extrapleural pneumonectomy. Chest 2002; 122:2256.

26. Wittnich C, Trudel J, Zidulka A, Chiu R. Misleading "pulmonary wedge pressure" after pneumonectomy: its importance in post-operative fluid therapy. Ann Thorac Surg 1986; 42:192.

27. Richardson J, Sabanathan S, Jones J, Shah RD, Cheema S, Mearns AJ. A prospective, randomized comparison of preoperative and continuous balanced epidural or paravertebral bupivacaine on post-thoracotomy pain, pulmonary function and stress responses. Br J Anaesth 1999; 83:387.

28. Hartigan P, Ng J. Anesthetic strategies for patients undergoing extrapleural pneumonectomy. Thorac Surg Clinic 2004; 14:575.

29. Amar D, Roistacher N, Rusch V, et al. Effects of diltiazem prophylaxis on the incidence and clinical outcome of atrial arrhythmias after thoracic surgery. J Thorac Cardiovasc Surg 2000; 120:790.

30. Mathru M, Blakeman B, Dries D, Kleinman B, Kumar P. Permeability pulmonary edema following lung resection. Chest 1990; 98:1216.

31. Shapira O, Shahian D. Postpneumonectomy pulmonary edema. Ann Thorac Surg 1993; 56:190.

32. Alvarez J, Panda R, Newman M, Slinger P, Deslauriers J, Ferguson M. Postpneumonectomy pulmonary edema. J Cardiothorac Vasc Anesth 2003; 17:388.

33. Suen H, Hendrix H, Patterson G. Physiologic consequences of pneumonectomy: consequences on the esophageal function. Chest Surg Clin N Am 1999; 9:475.

34. Hilaris B, Nori D, Kwong E, et al. Pleurectomy and intraoperative brachytherapy and postoperative radiation in the treatment of malignant pleural mesothelioma. Int J Radiat Oncol Biol Phys 1984; 10:325.

35. Soysal O, Karaoglanoglu N, Demiracan S, et al. Pleurectomy/decortication for palliation in malignant pleural mesothelioma: results of surgery. Eur J Cardiothorac Surg 1997; 11:210.

36. Van Ruth S, Baas P, Zoetmulder F. Surgical treatment of malignant pleural mesothelioma: a review. Chest 2003; 123:551.

37. Baldini E, Recht A, Strauss G, et al. Patterns of failure after trimodality therapy for malignant pleural mesothelioma. Ann Thorac Surg 1997; 63:334.

38. Mamon H, Yeap B, Janne P, et al. High risk of brain metastases in surgically staged IIIA non-small-cell lung cancer patients treated with surgery, chemotherapy, and radiation. J Clin Oncol 2005; 23:1530.

39. Young S, Woodburn K, Wright M, et al. Lutetium texaphyrin: a near-infrared, water soluble photosensitizer. Photochem Photobiol 1996; 63:892.

40. Luketich JD, Westkaemper J, Sommers KE, et al. Bronchoesophagopleural fistula after photodynamic therapy for malignant mesothelioma. Ann Thorac Surg 1996; 62:283.

41. Litle VR, Luketich JD, Christie NA, et al. Photodynamic therapy as palliation for esophageal cancer: experience in 215 patients. Ann Thorac Surg 2003; 76:1687.

42. Freitag L, Ernst A, Thomas M, Prenzel R, Wahlers B, Macha H. Sequential photodynamic therapy (PDT) and high dose brachytherapy for endobronchial tumour control in patients with limited bronchogenic carcinoma. Thorax 2004; 59:790.

43. Murrer H, Mariginissen H, Star W. Ex vivo light dosimetry and Monte Carlo simulations for endobronchial photodynamic therapy. Phys Med Biol 1995; 40:1807.

44. Pass H, Temecj B, Kranda K, et al. Phase III randomized trial of surgery with or without intraoperative photodynamic therapy, and postoperative immunochemotherapy for malignant pleural mesothelioma. Ann Surg Oncol 1997; 4:628.

45. Alberts D, Liu P, Hannigan E, et al. Intraperitoneal cisplatin plus intravenous cyclophosphamide versus intravenous cisplatin plus intravenous cyclophosphamide for stage III ovarian cancer. N Engl J Med 1996; 335:1950.

46. Sugarbaker P. Treatment of peritoneal carcinomatosis from colon or appendiceal cancer with induction intraperitoneal chemotherapy. Cancer Treat Res 1996; 82:317.

47. Tomek S, Mangold C. Chemotherapy for malignant pleural mesothelioma: past results and recent developments. Lung Cancer 2004; 455:S103.

48. Howell S, Pfeifle C, Wung W, Olshen R. Intraperitoneal cis-diamminedichloroplatinum with systemic thiosulfate protection. Cancer Res 1983; 43:1426.

49. Stehlin JS. Hyperthermic perfusion for melanoma of the extremities: experience with 165 patients, 1967 to 1979. Ann N Y Acad Sci 1980; 335:352.

50. Giovonella B, Lohman W, Heidelberger C. Effects of elevated temperatures and drugs on the viability of L1210 leukemia cells. Cancer Res 1970; 30:1623.

51. Howell S, Taetle R. Effect of sodium thiosulfate on cisdichlorodiammineplatinum (II) toxicity and antitumor activity in L1210 leukemia. Cancer Treat Rep 1980; 64:611.

52. Rusch V, Slatz L, Venkratraman E, et al. A phase II trial of pleurectomy/decortication followed by intrapleural and systemic chemotherapy for malignant pleural mesothelioma. J Clin Oncol 1994; 12:1156.

53. Chang M, Sugarbaker D. Innovative therapies: intraoperative intracavitary chemotherapy. Thorac Surg Clin 2004; 14:549.

54. Kukreja J, Jaklitsch M, Wiener D, et al. Malignant pleural mesothelioma: overview of the North American and European experience. Thorac Surg Clin 2004; 14:435.

55. Treasure T, Sedrakyan A. Pleural mesothelioma: little evidence, still time to do trials. Lancet 2004; 364:1183.

The Role of Chemotherapy in the Management of Mesothelioma

44

Julian R. Molina and Alex A. Adjei

Contents

44.1 Introduction

Many chemotherapy agents have been tested either as single agents or in combination for the therapy of malignant pleural mesothelioma (MPM) [1]. The response rates of these regimens are never more than 20% and comparison across studies is most often meaningless because of the rarity of this tumor: there are only about 2,500 cases a year in the USA. In addition, most studies involve only a few patients, are non-randomized, and there is significant heterogeneity in patient population, staging systems, prognostic factors, and criteria for tumor response [1, 2]. The recently introduced International Mesothelioma Interest Group (IMIG) staging system and the Response Evaluation Criteria In Solid Tumors (RECIST) guidelines should allow for a more uniform evaluation of staging and tumor response in MPM [3, 4].

44.2 Single-agent Chemotherapy

Most available chemotherapy drugs have been tested in MPM as single agents. In general, single-agent response rates are under 20%, and no survival advantage for single-agent chemotherapy has ever been clearly demonstrated. Platinum derivatives, anthracyclines, and the antimetabolites are the most active agents in malignant mesothelioma. Among the antimetabolites, recent evidence suggests that the folic acid antagonists and nucleoside analogs have the most activity. Although older drugs such as doxorubicin, ifosfamide, carboplatin, cisplatin, methotrexate, and mitomycin have some activity, response rates are usually about 15% and never more than 20% (Table 44.1) [5].

44.2.1 Anthracyclines

Doxorubicin was one of the first and certainly most studied single agents tested for MPM. In 1983, the Eastern Cooperative Oncology Group (ECOG) reported the results of a retrospective analysis of single-agent and doxorubicin-containing regimes for MPM. A response rate of 14% in 51 patients, with a median survival of 7.3 months was

Table 44.1. Single-agent chemotherapy response rates in MPM

Agent	Response rate (%)	Reference
Doxorubicin	14	Byrne et al. (1999) [30]
Cisplatin	14.3	Eisen et al. (2000) [73]
Carboplatin	7	Fizazi et al. (2000) [36, 37]
Methotrexate	37	Giaccone et al. (2001) [16]
Edatrexate	25	Govindan et al. (2003) [68]
Vinorelbine	24	Harvey et al. (1984) [19]

taken as encouraging news [6]. Unfortunately, subsequent randomized studies failed to prove any significant beneficial effect. A recent phase III study of doxorubicin compared to ranpirnase, published only in abstract form, demonstrated a disappointing median survival of 8.2 months [7]. Paradoxically, for many practicing oncologists, doxorubicin is still the gold-standard treatment for MPM. Formulations of liposomal doxorubicin, epirubicin, pirarubicin, and mitoxantrone have also been tested yielding response rates no higher than 15% and median survivals of only 4–17 months [8–11].

44.2.2 Platinum Compounds

Since the introduction of cisplatin, platinum analogs have been studied both as single agents and in combination regimens for MPM. Single-agent cisplatin at a dose of 100 mg/m^2 given every 21 days in patients with MPM demonstrated an overall response rate of 14.3% and a median survival of 7.5 months [12]. Higher doses of cisplatin (80 mg/m^2 weekly for 6 weeks) were tested in a phase II trial [13]. Response rates were similar and associated with significant ototoxicity [13]. Carboplatin at a dose of 150 mg/m^2 per day intravenously (IV) for 3 days gave a response rate of 16% in one trial [14] and a 7% response rate in a similar phase II study [15]. Median survival ranged from 5–8 months in both trials [14,15]. Oxaliplatin as a single agent has not been tested in MPM. However, the new generation platinum compound ZD0473 was tested in a phase II study of patients with MPM who had relapsed after previous platinum-based chemotherapy [16]. When administered at a dose of 120 mg/m^2 on day 1 of a 21-day cycle, 50% of patients (5 of 10) had stable disease and 20% experienced tumor shrinkage [16].

44.2.3 Antifolates/Antimetabolites

Antifolates are one of the most active classes of agents in MPM and have shown consistent antitumor activity in multiple trials. A phase II Norwegian trial of 63 patients with MPM treated with four to eight courses of high-dose methotrexate (3 g/m^2) resulted in a response rate of 37%; median survival ranged from 5 months for the sarcomatoid type to 11 months for the epithelioid type [17]. Edatrexate, a methotrexate analog produced by alkylation and substitution of carbon for nitrogen at the 10 position of 4-aminofolate was tested alone and with leucovorin rescue in a phase II multicenter study of the Cancer and Leukemia Group B (CALGB). Fifty-eight patients with MPM were entered into this CALGB Protocol 9131 study. The overall response rate was 25% with a complete response rate of 5% and a median survival of 9.6 months. However, this study was associated with unacceptable

toxicity due to myelosuppression [18]. The leucovorin rescue arm resulted in less toxicity but also decreased efficacy [18]. Pemetrexed and raltitrexed, two new antifolate agents, are the most promising new drugs for the mesothelioma field and will be discussed later.

Other "older" antimetabolites such as 5-fluorouracil (5-FU) have shown minimal activity in this tumor [19]. Likewise, capecitabine, an oral derivative of 5-FU, trimetrexate, and dehydro-5-azacytidine (DHAC) have been tested in studies conducted by the CALGB and shown to have little antitumor activity in MPM [20–22].

44.2.4 Vinorelbine

Vinorelbine, a semisynthetic derivative of vinblastine, is the only vinca alkaloid with proven single-agent activity in MPM. A study by Steele et al. of 29 patients with MPM treated with weekly injections of vinorelbine 30 mg/m^2 for cycles of six weekly injections resulted in seven partial responses (24%), 16 patients had stable disease (55%), and 6 patients had disease progression on therapy (21%). The median survival was 10.6 months and the toxicity associated with this regimen was low. Furthermore, quality-of-life (QOL) analyses demonstrated improvements in psychologic and physical indices for patients receiving treatment with vinorelbine [23]. Other agents such as mitomycin C, cyclophosphamide, and temozolomide, have also been studied as single agents in mesothelioma, with poor results overall [24–26].

44.3 Combination Chemotherapy

44.3.1 Gemcitabine

Although gemcitabine has demonstrated in vitro activity against mesothelioma cell lines, the role of single-agent gemcitabine in patients with mesothelioma is limited (Table 44.2). Three phase II trials treated a total of 60 patients and achieved disappointing response rates of 0%, 7%, and 31% [27–29]. Contrary to this limited activity as a single agent, gemcitabine has shown promising activity in MPM when combined with cisplatin or carboplatin in phase II trials. A phase II study of 21 patients with MPM treated with combined cisplatin 100 mg/m^2, given intravenously on day 1, and gemcitabine 1,000 mg/m^2, given intravenously on days 1, 8, and 15 of a 28-day cycle for 6 cycles, yielded a response rate (complete response + partial response) of 47.6% with a median survival of 9.5 months. Improvement in symptoms was detected in 90% of radiologically responding patients and 33% of unresponsive patients [30]. Unfortunately, these impressive results were not validated by the Rotterdam Oncological Thoracic Study Group

Table 44.2. Combination chemotherapy response rates in MPM

Agent	Response rate (%)	Reference
Gemcitabine/cisplatin	16–47.6	Kindler et al. (2000) [32]; Kindler et al. (1999) [18]
Gemcitabine/epirubicin	9	Kindler et al. (2001) [27]
Irinotecan/docetaxel	15	Langerak et al. (1996) [69]
Cisplatin/irinotecan	41	Lerner et al. (1983) [6]
Methotrexate/interferon	29	Liani et al. (2003) [54]
Oxaliplatin/raltitrexed	26	Mikulski et al. (2002) [67]
Oxaliplatin/gemcitabine	40	Millward et al. (2003) [71]
Raltitrexed/cisplatin	23	Ohta et al. (1999) [72]
Pemetrexed/cisplatin	41.3	Schultz et al. (1999) [50]

(ROTSG). The ROTSG conducted a study of 25 patients with MPM in which gemcitabine 1,250 mg/m^2 was administered on days 1 and 8 and cisplatin 80 mg/m^2 was administered on day 1 in a 3-week cycle with a maximum of 6 cycles. The overall response rate was 16%; time to progression was 6 months (5–7 months) with a median survival from registration of 9.6 months [31]. In a phase II study of the North Central Treatment Group (NCCTG), gemcitabine was given in combination with epirubicin to 41 patients with MPM. This study showed a very limited activity for this regimen with a response rate of only 9% and a time to progression of 4.4 months (S. Okuno, personal communication).

44.3.2 Irinotecan

Irinotecan (CPT-11) is a topoisomerase I inhibitor with very limited activity as a single agent in MPM. A study of 28 patients conducted by the CALGB showed no complete or partial response and a median overall survival of 7.9 months [32]. Few phase II studies have evaluated irinotecan in combination with other agents (Table 44.2). In a study done in Finland of 15 previously untreated patients with MPM, docetaxel 60 mg/m^2 followed by irinotecan 190 mg/m^2 were given on day 1 every 3 weeks. No objective responses (complete or partial) were achieved, but there were two minor responses (overall response rate 15%) each with a duration of 4 months and a median time to progression of 7 months. These results are in sharp contrast with results from two phase II studies done in Japan combining irinotecan with cisplatin or irinotecan, cisplatin, and mitomycin that resulted in response rates of 40% and 41%, respectively, with tolerable toxic effects [33, 34].

44.3.3 Methotrexate

In a study by Halme et al. of 26 patients with MPM treated with either high-dose methotrexate (3 g/m^2) with leucovorin rescue or with methotrexate in combination with interferon, a response rate of 29% and a median survival of 17 months was reported (Table 44.2) [35]. One-year and 2-year survival rates were 62% and 31%, respectively. Median duration of response was 10 months (range 3–24 months). The toxicity of this regimen was acceptable with only one patient stopping treatment due to grade IV neurologic toxicity [35].

44.3.4 Oxaliplatin

Oxaliplatin is a platinum analog that has been studied in several combination regimens for MPM and is currently approved by the Food and Drug Administration (FDA) and European Medicine Evaluation Agency (EMEA) for colon cancer. After very encouraging results from the oxaliplatin–raltitrexed phase I study [36, 37], a phase II study in MPM was done using the same regimen and dosages [38]. Seventy-two patients were included in the study, and 16 of them were previously treated with a cisplatin-based chemotherapy. Data were available for analysis in 58 patients. There were 15 partial responses (26%), 2 in cisplatin-refractory patients. Median time to progression was 4.5 months [38]. When used with vinorelbine in a phase II trial, however, oxaliplatin significantly increased toxicity and did not seem to offer any additional advantage in response rate over vinorelbine alone [10, 11]. A multicenter phase II trial conducted in Germany evaluated the activity of combined gemcitabine and oxaliplatin in MPM. Twenty-five patients received gemcitabine 1,000 mg/m^2 intravenously over 30 min and oxaliplatin 80 mg/m^2 intravenously over 3 h on days 1 and 8 of a 21-day cycle for a maximum of 6 cycles. Partial responses were seen in 10 patients (40%) and stable disease in 6 patients (24%). Median time to disease progression was 7 months, and median survival was 13 months. This study concluded that the combination of gemcitabine and oxaliplatin in MPM was active with tolerable toxicity [39].

44.3.5 Raltitrexed

Raltitrexed (Tomudex) is a quinazoline folate analog that is a specific inhibitor of thymidylate synthase [40]. Raltitrexed is also a substrate for the enzyme folylpolyglutamate synthase, which converts raltitrexed into its polyglutamate forms. The polyglutamate forms are retained for long periods of time within the cell and are 60 times more potent inhibitors than the parent compound [40]. The activity and toxicity of raltitrexed as single-agent treatment in patients with MPM was investigated in a phase II multicenter trial conducted by the European Organization for Research and Treatment of Cancer (EORTC) [41]. Twenty-four chemotherapy-naive patients were given raltitrexed at a dose of 3 mg/m^2 by intravenous bolus every 3 weeks. Five patients (20.8%) had a partial response. Toxicity was mild, with diarrhea, nausea, vomiting, fatigue, and neutropenia as the major side effects, but not exceeding grade 3 toxicity [41]. The combination of raltitrexed and oxaliplatin was evaluated in a French phase II trial. In this study 15 pretreated and 55 chemotherapy-naive patients received raltitrexed 3 mg/m^2 followed by oxaliplatin 130 mg/m^2 every 3 weeks. Fourteen patients (20%) had a partial response, and 32 patients (46%) had stable disease [36,37]. At the 2004 American Society of Clinical Oncology (ASCO) meeting, the results of a phase III trial of raltitrexed plus cisplatin versus cisplatin alone were presented in abstract form. This study was conducted by the EORTC and the National Cancer Institute of Cancer of Canada (NCIC) [42]. Two hundred and fifty patients were randomized to receive cisplatin 80 mg/m^2 or cisplatin 80 mg/m^2 plus raltitrexed 3 mg/m^2. Both regimens were given every 3 weeks. The median overall survival in patients treated with raltitrexed and cisplatin was 11.2 months and was 8.8 months in the cisplatin-only group. The 1-year survival rates were 45% for patients treated with raltitrexed and cisplatin and 40% for patients treated with cisplatin only ($p = 0.06$). The investigators concluded that the combination of cisplatin and raltitrexed was well tolerated and should be considered as an alternative regimen in MPM [42].

44.3.6   Pemetrexed

Pemetrexed (Alimta) is a new multitargeted antifolate that inhibits several enzymes involved in the folate pathway, and has demonstrated clinical activity in MPM as well as in a broad array of other solid tumors including non-small cell lung cancer, breast, colorectal, bladder, cervical, gastric, and pancreatic cancer [43]. Pemetrexed is transported into cells via the reduced folate carrier (RFC), with transport kinetics similar to that of methotrexate, and binds to folate receptor-a (FR-a) with a very high affinity, similar to that of folic acid [44, 45]. Pemetrexed also appears to be a substrate for multidrug resistance protein (MRP) exporters [46]. Once it enters cells, this agent is polyglutamated to the active pentaglutamide. This reaction is catalyzed by folylpolyglutamate synthase (FPGS). Pemetrexed has been shown to be one of the best substrates for FPGS, when compared to other classic antifolates [47]. The pentaglutamate form of pemetrexed is the predominant intracellular form, and is 100 times more potent than the monoglutamate [48]. Polyglutamation traps pemetrexed and enhances its intracellular retention. The parent drug is polyglutamated 90–195 times more efficiently than methotrexate and 6–13 times more efficiently than lometrexol [47]. The increased cellular retention of polyglutamated pemetrexed forms may explain the success of its 3-weekly administration schedule.

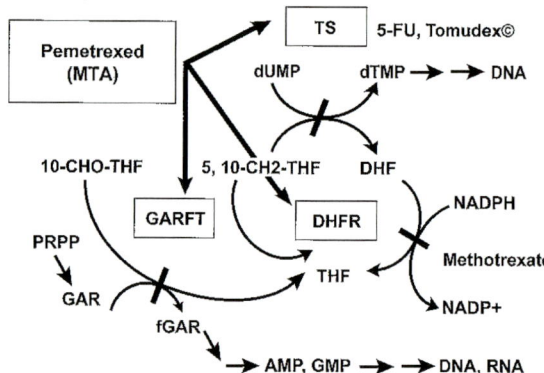

Fig. 44.1. Pemetrexed inhibits multiple folate-dependent enzymes. *TS* Thymidylate synthase, *DHFR* dihydrofolate reductase, *GARFT* glycinamide ribonucleotide formyltransferase, *5-FU* 5-fluorouracil, *dUMP* deoxyuridine monophosphate, *dTMP* deoxythymidine monophosphate, *PRPP* phosphoribosylpyrophosphate, *THF* tetrahydrofuran

Mechanism of Action

One of the primary targets of action is thymidylate synthase (TS) (Fig. 44.1) [49, 50]. TS, a folate-dependent enzyme, catalyzes the transformation of deoxyuridine monophosphate (dUMP) to deoxythymidine monophosphate (dTMP). Inhibition of TS results in decreased thymidine necessary for DNA synthesis [50, 51]. In addition to TS, pemetrexed inhibits dihydrofolate reductase (DHFR), as well as glycinamide ribonucleotide formyltransferase (GARFT); the latter is a folate-dependent enzyme that is involved in purine synthesis [48]. These targets are related to the cytotoxicity of pemetrexed, since both thymidine and hypoxanthine are required to circumvent cellular death caused by pemetrexed at high doses [48]. It should be pointed out that pemetrexed is 30–200 times more potent an inhibitor of TS than of 5-aminoimidazole-4-carboxamide ribonucleotide formyltransferase (AICARFT) or GARFT, suggesting that its cytotoxicity may be mediated predominantly through TS inhibition. However, pemetrexed demonstrates activity against H630 colon cancer cell lines, which are resistant to raltitrexed and 5-fluorouracil because of TS amplification [50]. Thus, inhibition of the other folate enzymes is important for pemetrexed clinical activity.

Mechanisms of Resistance

Different mechanisms of resistance to methotrexate have been described in preclinical systems including: (1) increased overexpression of DHFR, or decreased affinity of methotrexate for DHFR due to single amino acid substitutions in this enzyme; (2) defective membrane transport due to qualitative or quantitative alterations in the RFC; (3) increased ATP-driven antifolate efflux via members of the MRP family including MRP1 and MRP3; and (4) decreased antifolate polyglutamylation due to quantitative or qualitative alterations in

FPGS activity [52]. Because of its inhibition of multiple folate-dependent enzymes, it has been hypothesized that resistance to pemetrexed will be less prevalent than resistance to methotrexate. Other properties of pemetrexed supporting this hypothesis are the efficient transport by the RFC and the high affinity for FPGS.

While this may be true, resistance mechanisms to pemetrexed have been described. First, decreased expression of FPGS has been shown to be a possible resistance mechanism. In a recent study, decreased expression of FPGS was correlated with resistance of L1210 cells to pemetrexed [53]. In addition, Liani et al. [54] used an FPGS mutation screening assay to demonstrate that depressed FPGS activity is the predominant mechanism of high-level resistance to pemetrexed and other polyglutamylation-dependent antifolates upon a clinically relevant exposure schedule in leukemia cells.

Second, pemetrexed polyglutamates have been shown to be excellent substrates for folylpolyglutamate hydrolase, having higher rates of hydrolysis by this enzyme than methotrexate polyglutamates. Thus, the clinical effectiveness of pemetrexed may be inversely related to cellular glutamyl hydrolase activity [55]. Finally, the MRPs, particularly MRP2 and MRP5, have been shown to transport pemetrexed, and may confer resistance to this agent [46].

Toxicity of Pemetrexed is Related to Folate Deficiency

Severe, unpredictable, and occasionally fatal myelosuppression and gastrointestinal toxicities have been associated with antifolate agents. The amelioration of these toxicities by the administration of folic acid is well known [56]. However, it has been extremely difficult to correlate antifolate-induced toxicity with pretreatment folate levels, measured as red blood cell folate or serum folate, in patients. Data accumulated in the past few years suggest that plasma homocysteine is a much more sensitive measure of the functional folate status of patients than red blood cell or serum folate [57]. With this insight into cellular folate metabolism, the role of the folate status of patients in the toxicity of pemetrexed has been delineated.

The major donor of methyl groups for a variety of fundamental processes in mammals is S-adenosylmethionine (SAM). Methionine, which is utilized in the synthesis of SAM, is generated by the transfer of a methyl group from N^5-methyltetrahydrofolate (CH_3FH_4) to homocysteine (Fig. 44.2). Thus, under conditions of folate deprivation, plasma homocysteine levels increase. This is the most sensitive indicator of functional folate status [58]. Vitamin B_{12} (cobalamin) and vitamin B_6 (pyridoxine) deficiencies can also result in high homocysteine levels. However, cystathionine levels are markedly elevated in vitamin B_6 deficiency and are elevated to a lesser extent in folate and vitamin B_{12} deficiency [59]. Thus cystathionine levels can distinguish vitamin B_6 deficiency from folate or vitamin B_{12} deficiency; however it should be noted that isolated vitamin B_6 deficiency is very uncommon.

Amelioration of Pemetrexed Toxicity

Initial phase I and phase II studies of pemetrexed indicated that myelosuppression was the main toxicity. Niyikiza and coworkers [60] used multivariate stepwise regression methods to analyze baseline physiologic and demographic data from individuals enrolled in these early pemetrexed trials. The objective was to identify predictive variables for severe toxicity. Variables analyzed included serum homocysteine, cystathionine, methylmalonic acid, albumin, and other hepatic enzymes. These analyses indicated that an elevated plasma homocysteine concentration was indicative of preclini-

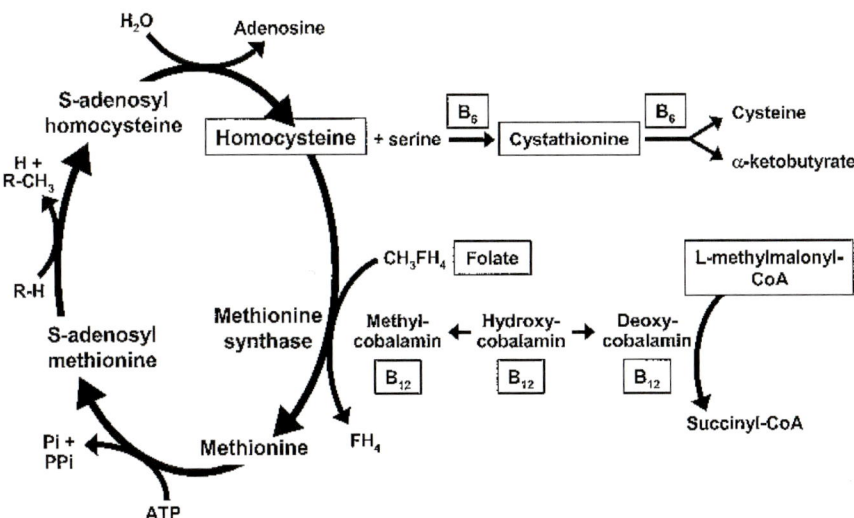

Fig. 44.2. The role of vitamins B_6, B_{12}, and folate in methyl-donor reactions in humans. Deficiencies in any or a combination of these vitamins will lead to elevated serum homocysteine levels. Methylmalonic and cystathionine levels can distinguish between vitamin B_{12} or vitamin B_6 deficiency and folate deficiency, respectively

cal folate deficiency, and resulted in a more severe toxicity profile that typically included thrombocytopenia, neutropenia, and severe diarrhea and mucositis. The threshold baseline homocysteine value of 10 µmol/L appeared to be the cut-off for these toxicities after cycle 1 ($\chi^2 = 6.2$, $p=0.01$), with levels > 10 µmol/L predicting for an increased rate of toxicity. All patients enrolled in pemetrexed clinical trials over the past 2–3 years received folic acid and vitamin B_{12} supplementation, as described below. Current data indicate that this supplemental use of vitamins can ameliorate some of the severe drug-induced toxic effects resulting in an improved safety profile and efficacy for this drug [61, 62].

Administration of Pemetrexed

Currently, pemetrexed is administered as a 10-min infusion every 3 weeks at a dose of 500 mg/m^2. Co-administration with NSAIDS is not allowed, because of the potential for decreased renal clearance and enhanced toxicity.

Patients receive folic acid and vitamin B_{12} supplementation, as follows: oral folic acid tablets 350–1,000 µg starting at least 5 continuous days before pemetrexed administration and continuing throughout the course of therapy. Intramuscular vitamin B_{12} at 1,000 µg is administered with folic acid and repeated every 9 weeks while the patient is on the study.

Clinical Studies of Pemetrexed in Malignant Pleural Mesothelioma

In a phase II study by Scagliotti et al. in 64 patients with chemotherapy-naive and measurable MPM, pemetrexed was administered at a dose of 500 mg/m^2 intravenously every 3 weeks. After a protocol amendment, most patients also received folic acid and vitamin B_{12} supplementation to improve safety [63]. Nine out of 64 patients (14%) experienced a partial response (30.5–50% reduction in measured lesions), with seven out of nine responses (78%) seen in vitamin-supplemented patients. Median survival was 10.7, 13.0, and 8.0 months for all patients, supplemented patients, and non-supplemented patients, respectively. Myelosuppression was the most common toxicity. Grade 3–4 neutropenia occurred in 52% of non-supplemented patients and 9% of supplemented patients. Vitamin-supplemented patients tolerated treatment better and received a median of 6 cycles of treatment, while non-supplemented patients received a median of only 2 cycles [63].

A pivotal phase III randomized study of 456 patients compared pemetrexed 500 mg/m^2 and cisplatin 75 mg/m^2 on day 1, to cisplatin 75 mg/m^2 on day 1. Both regimens were administered intravenously every 21 days. In this study, 226 patients received pemetrexed and cisplatin, 222 received cisplatin alone, and 8 never received

therapy. Median survival time in the pemetrexed/cisplatin arm was 12.1 months versus 9.3 months in the control arm ($p=0.020$). Median time to progression was significantly longer in the pemetrexed/cisplatin arm: 5.7 months versus 3.9 months ($p=0.001$). Response rates were 41.3% in the pemetrexed/cisplatin arm versus 16.7% in the control arm ($p < 0.0001$). After 117 patients had enrolled, folic acid and vitamin B_{12} were added to reduce toxicity, resulting in a significant reduction in toxicities in the pemetrexed/cisplatin arm [62]. Toxicity was more common in the pemetrexed/cisplatin arm, with grade 3/4 neutropenia (28%) and leukopenia (18%) being the most common toxic effects. Pulmonary function tests (PFT) and clinical benefit measures were also collected in this study. Pemetrexed/cisplatin showed improvement in both PFT and major disease-related symptoms such as dyspnea and pain. This study clearly established pemetrexed as the most promising new agent in the treatment of MPM [62], and led to its approval by the FDA and EMEA for the therapy of MPM.

Hughes and colleagues conducted an atypical phase I trial with pemetrexed and carboplatin. All patients enrolled had MPM, and had no prior chemotherapy treatment [64]. Pemetrexed was administered through a 10-min IV infusion followed by 30 min of rest and carboplatin administered over 30 min once every 21 days. No vitamin supplementation was given. Patients were assigned to one of five different dose combinations with pemetrexed given at 400–500 mg/m^2 and carboplatin given at AUC 4–6 (mg/ml×min, calculated from ^{51}Cr-EDTA GFR). Eight out of 25 assessable patients achieved a partial response for a response rate of 32%. Median survival was 14.8 months and median time to progression was 10 months. Seventy percent of patients showed symptom improvement, typically within 2 treatment cycles. Myelosuppression (primarily neutropenia and leukopenia) was the major toxicity. The recommended dose for subsequent studies was pemetrexed 500 mg/m^2 and carboplatin AUC 5 mg/ml×min. This combination, which substitutes carboplatin for cisplatin, is therefore seen as a viable alternative to the approved combination of pemetrexed combined with cisplatin.

44.3.7   Ranpirnase

Based upon the initial work of Shogen and Yoanv it was found that extracts of *Rana pipiens* (leopard frog) early embryos (up to four blastomere stage of development) exert an antiproliferative and cytotoxic activity against numerous cancer cell lines in vitro [65]. Ranpirnase (Onconase) a compound with ribonuclease activity was isolated from these extracts and subsequently tested in preclinical and clinical studies. The phase I study of ranpirnase as a single agent administered intravenously on a weekly schedule showed that the maximum tolerated dose (MTD) was 960 µg/m². The dose-limiting toxicity was renal as manifested by proteinuria with or without azotemia, peripheral edema, and fatigue. Other toxicities included flushing, myalgias, dizziness, and decreased appetite [66]. A single-arm, open-label, multicenter phase II trial of ranpirnase as a single agent was conducted in 105 patients with MPM [59]. Median survival of 6 months for the intent-to-treat population (ITT) and 8.3 months for the treatment target group (TTG) were reported [67]. A phase III study comparing ranpirnase to doxorubicin demonstrated improvement in survival by 2 months in the ranpirnase arm, however with inferior quality of life over doxorubicin [7].

44.4 Novel Cytostatic Agents

44.4.1 Epidermal Growth Factor Receptor Inhibitors

Govindan et al. have demonstrated that the epidermal growth factor receptor (EGFR), a transmembrane glycoprotein, is overexpressed in over 50% of epithelioid and biphasic mesotheliomas [68]. Based on this observation, the CALGB tested gefitinib (Iressa), an EGFR inhibitor, in a phase II trial of 46 previously untreated patients with MPM. Gefitinib showed no significant activity as monotherapy in EGFR-positive chemonaive MPM [68].

44.4.2 Platelet-derived Growth Factor Inhibitors

Platelet-derived growth factor (PDGF) appears to be another autocrine growth factor for mesothelioma [69]. PDGF is a potent mitogen for connective tissue cells; in vitro, mesothelial cells proliferate in a dose-dependent manner when exogenous PDGF is administered [70]. Two PDGF inhibitors are being tested in clinical trials in mesothelioma patients. Gleevec (imatinib mesylate) is an oral, selective inhibitor of the tyrosine kinases activity of the PDGF receptor, c-kit, and Bcr-Abl. Surprisingly, Gleevec was ineffective and not well tolerated as a single agent in patients with MPM [71]. The CALGB is currently evaluating PTK787, an oral inhibitor of the receptor tyrosine kinases of VEGFs (1, 2, 3) and PDGF, in a phase II trial in 40 mesothelioma patients. The primary endpoint will be time to progression. PDGF and VEGF will be correlated with antitumor activity.

44.4.3 Vascular Endothelial Growth Factor Inhibitors

Vascular endothelial growth factor (VEGF) is released by tumor cells that bind to endothelial cell receptors, initiating a signaling cascade that results in new blood vessel formation and appears to play an important role in the progression and prognosis of MPM [72]. Three VEGF inhibitors are currently being evaluated in clinical trials in mesothelioma patients: SU5416, bevacizumab, and thalidomide. SU5416 (semaxanib; Sugen) is a selective inhibitor of the tyrosine kinase activity associated with the VEGF receptor flk-1. A National Cancer Institute (NCI)-sponsored phase II trial at the University of Chicago has assessed single-agent SU5416 in 23 patients. This agent, however, is no longer being developed. Likewise, a randomized, double-blind, placebo-controlled, multicenter phase II trial of bevacizumab/placebo given with gemcitabine/cisplatin chemotherapy is currently accruing. Thalidomide, which is thought to inhibit VEGF, tumor necrosis factor (TNF)-α, and basic fibroblast growth factor (bFGF), is being evaluated in two phase II trials in mesothelioma patients [73].

44.5 Future Directions

SV40 virus has been identified as a possible cause of human cancer, in particular MPM [74]. This fact has been applied to the production of a potential therapeutic vaccine for malignant mesothelioma. A vaccine produced by cloning the modified SV40 T antigen gene was recently tested preclinically in animal models of malignant mesothelioma with positive results [75]. SS1 (dsFv)-PE38 is an immunotoxin produced by the fusion of pseudomonas exotoxin P38 to a high affinity, disulfide-stabilized antibody to mesothelin. Mesothelin, a cell surface glycoprotein overexpressed in ovarian cancer, mesotheliomas, and some squamous cell carcinomas, is an attractive candidate for targeted therapy because it is not shed in significant amounts into the bloodstream and is not present in significant amounts on normal human tissues except for mesothelial cells. The fused protein retains cytotoxic activity and only targets cells expressing mesothelin [76], such as mesothelioma, epithelial carcinomas of ovary and peritoneum, and squamous cancers of cervix and upper aerodigestive tract (i.e., esophagus, head and neck cancers). SS1 (dsFv)-PE38 is currently being studied in phase I/II trials in advanced mesothelin-expressing tumors.

44.6 Conclusions

Several chemotherapy agents have shown minor activity in MPM. Most of the studies supporting their use as single agents or in combination are misleading because of the sample size, lack of uniform measures of response, and lack of reproducibility. However, the combination of cisplatin with pemetrexed has demonstrated improved survival in phase III studies and is now considered standard therapy for mesothelioma.

Key Points

● Many chemotherapy agents have been tested either as single agents or in combination for the therapy of malignant pleural mesothelioma (MPM), with response rates of these regimens being never more than 20%, while comparison across studies is meaningless because of the rarity of this tumor: there are only about 2,500 cases a year in the USA.

● Pemetrexed (Alimta) is a new multitargeted antifolate that inhibits several enzymes involved in the folate pathway, and has demonstrated clinical activity in MPM. In fact it is the most promising new agent in the treatment of MPM.

● The combination of pemetrexed with cisplatin has demonstrated improved survival in phase III studies and is now considered standard therapy for mesothelioma, while substitution of cisplatin by carboplatin is a viable alternative.

References

1. Price B. Analysis of current trends in United States mesothelioma incidence. Am J Epidemiol 1997; 145:211.

2. Herndon JE, Green MR, Chahinian AP, et al. Factors predictive of survival among 337 patients with mesothelioma treated between 1984 and 1994 by the Cancer and Leukemia Group B. Chest 1998; 113:723.

3. International Mesothelioma Interest Group. A proposed new international TNM staging system for malignant pleural mesothelioma. Chest 1995; 108:1122.

4. Therasse P, Arbuck SG, Eisenhauer EA, et al. New guidelines to evaluate the response to treatment in solid tumors. J Natl Cancer Inst 2000; 92:205.

5. Byrne MJ, Nowak AK. Modified RECIST criteria for assessment of response in malignant pleural mesothelioma. Ann Oncol 2004; 15:257.

6. Lerner HJ, Schoenfeld DA, Martin A, et al. Malignant mesothelioma. The Eastern Cooperative Oncology Group (ECOG) experience. Cancer 1983; 52:1981.

7. Vogelzang N, Taub R, Shin D, et al. Phase III randomized trial of onconase (ONC) vs. doxorubicin (DOX) in patients (pts) with unresectable malignant mesothelioma (UMM): analysis of survival (abstract 2274). Proc Am Soc Clin Oncol 2000; 19:557a.

8. Magri MD, Veronesi A, Foladore S, et al. Epirubicin in the treatment of malignant mesothelioma: a phase II cooperative study. Tumori 1991; 77:49.

9. Baas P. Chemotherapy for malignant mesothelioma: from doxorubicin to vinorelbine. Semin Oncol 2002; 29:62.

10. Steele JP, O'Doherty CA, Shamash J, et al. Phase II trial of liposomal daunorubicin in malignant pleural mesothelioma. Ann Oncol 2001; 12:497.

11. Steele JP, Shamash J, Evans MT, et al. Phase II trial of vinorelbine and oxaliplatin (VO) in malignant pleural mesothelioma (MPM) (abstract 1335). Proc Am Soc Clin Oncol 2001; 20:335a.

12. Zidar BL, Green S, Pierce HI, et al. A phase II evaluation of cisplatin in unresectable diffuse malignant mesothelioma: a Southwest Oncology Group study. Invest New Drugs 1988; 6:223.

13. Planting AST, Schellens JHM, Goey SH, et al. Weekly high-dose cisplatin in malignant pleural mesothelioma. Ann Oncol 1994; 5:373.

14. Raghavan D, Gianoutsos P, Bishop J, et al. Phase II trial of carboplatin in the management of malignant mesothelioma. J Clin Oncol 1990; 8:151.

15. Vogelzang NJ, Goutsou M, Corson JM, et al. Carboplatin in malignant mesothelioma: a phase II study of the Cancer and Leukemia Group B. Cancer Chemother Pharmacol 1990; 27:239.

16. Giaccone G, O'Brien M, Byrne MJ, Van Steenkiste J, Cosaert J. Phase II trial of ZD0473 in patients with mesothelioma relapsing after one prior chemotherapy regimen. Proc Ann Meet Am Soc Clin Oncol 2001; 20:257b.

17. Solheim OP, Saeter G, Finnanger AM, Stenwig AE. High-dose methotrexate in the treatment of malignant mesothelioma of the pleura. A phase II study. Br J Cancer 1992; 65:956.

18. Kindler HL, Belani CP, Herndon JE II, et al. Edatrexate (10-ethyl-deaza-aminopterin) (NSC #626715) with or without leucovorin rescue for malignant mesothelioma. Sequential phase II trials by the Cancer and Leukemia Group B. Cancer 1999; 86:1985.

19. Harvey VJ, Slevin ML, Ponder BAJ, et al. Chemotherapy of diffuse malignant mesothelioma. Phase II trials of single-agent 5-fluorouracil and adriamycin. Cancer 1984; 54:961.

20. Otterson GA, Herndon JE 2nd, Watson D, et al. Cancer and Leukemia Group B. Capecitabine in malignant mesothelioma: a phase II trial by the Cancer and Leukemia Group B (39807). Lung Cancer 2004; 44:251.

21. Vogelzang NJ, Weissman LB, Herndon JE 2nd, Antman KH, Cooper MR, Corson JM, Green MR. Trimetrexate in malignant mesothelioma: A Cancer and Leukemia Group B phase II study. J Clin Oncol 1994; 12:1436.

22. Samuels BL, Herndon JE 2nd, Harmon DC, Carey R, Aisner J, Corson JM, Suzuki Y, Green MR, Vogelzang NJ, et al. Dihydro-5-azacytidine and cisplatin in the treatment of malignant mesothelioma: a phase II study by the Cancer and Leukemia Group B. Cancer 1998; 82:1578.

23. Steele JP, Shamash J, Evans MT, et al. Phase II study of vinorelbine in patients with malignant pleural mesothelioma. J Clin Oncol 2000; 18:3912.

24. Bajorin D, Kelsen D, Mintzer DM. Phase II trial of mitomycin in malignant mesothelioma. Cancer Treat Rep 1987; 71:857.

25. Sörensen PG, Bach F, Bork E, Hansen HH. Randomized trial of doxorubicin versus cyclophosphamide in diffuse malignant pleural mesothelioma. Cancer Treat Rep 1985; 69:1431.

26. van Meerbeeck JP, Baas P, Debruyne C, et al. A phase II EORTC study of temozolomide in patients with malignant pleural mesothelioma. Eur J Cancer 2002; 38:779.

27. Kindler HL, Millard F, Herndon JE 2nd, Vogelzang NJ, Suzuki Y, Green MR. Gemcitabine for malignant mesothelioma: a phase II trial by the Cancer and Leukemia Group B. Lung Cancer 2001; 31:311.

28. van Meerbeeck JP, Baas P, Debruyne C, Groen HJ, Manegold C, Ardizzoni A, Gridelli C, van Marck EA, Lentz M, Giaccone G, et al. A phase II study of gemcitabine in patients with malignant pleural mesothelioma. European Organization for Research and Treatment of Cancer Lung Cancer Cooperative Group. Cancer 1999; 85:2577.

29. Kindler HL, van Meerbeeck JP. The role of gemcitabine in the treatment of malignant mesothelioma. Semin Oncol 2002; 29:70.

30. Byrne MJ, Davidson JA, Musk AW, et al. Cisplatin and gemcitabine treatment for malignant pleural mesothelioma: a phase II study. J Clin Oncol 1999; 17:25.

31. Van Haarst JMW, Baas P, Manegold C, et al. Multicentre phase II study of gemcitabine and cisplatin in malignant pleural mesothelioma. Br J Cancer 2002; 86:342.

32. Kindler HL, Herdon J, Vogelzang N, Green M. CPT-11 in malignant mesothelioma: a phase II trial by the Cancer and Leukemia Group B (CALGB 9733). Proc Am Soc Clin Oncol 2000; 19:1978a.

33. Nakano T, Chahinian AP, Shinjo M, et al. Cisplatin in combination with irinotecan in the treatment of patients with malignant pleural mesothelioma: a pilot phase II clinical trial and pharmacokinetic profile. Cancer 1999; 85:2375.

34. Steele JP, Shamash J, Barlow CS, et al. Phase II trial of irinotecan, cisplatin and mitomycin C (IPM) in malignant pleural mesothelioma (MPM). Proc Am Soc Clin Oncol 2002; 21:307a.

35. Halme M, Knuuttila A, Vehmas T, et al. High-dose methotrexate in combination with interferons in the treatment of malignant pleural mesothelioma. Br J Cancer 1999; 80:1781.

36. Fizazi K, Caliandro R, Soulié P, et al. Combination raltitrexed (Tomudex®)–oxaliplatin: a step forward in the struggle against mesothelioma? The Institut Gustave Roussy experience with chemotherapy and chemo-immunotherapy in mesothelioma. Eur J Cancer 2000; 36:1514.

37. Fizazi M, Ducreux P, Ruffié P, et al. Phase I, dose-finding, and pharmacokinetic study of raltitrexed combined with oxaliplatin in patients with advanced cancer. J Clin Oncol 2000; 18:2293.

38. Fizazi K, Doubre H, le Chevalier T, et al. Combination of raltitrexed and oxaliplatin is an active regimen in malignant mesothelioma: results of a phase II study. J Clin Oncol 2003; 21:349.

39. Schutte W, Blankenburg T, Lauerwald K, et al. A multicenter phase II study of gemcitabine and oxaliplatin for malignant pleural mesothelioma. Clin Lung Cancer 2003; 4:294.

40. Van Cutsem E, Cunningham D, Maroun J, et al. Raltitrexed: current clinical status and future directions. Ann Oncol 2002; 13:513.

41. Baas P, Ardizzoni A, Grossi F, et al., EORTC Lung Cancer Group, et al. The activity of raltitrexed (Tomudex) in malignant pleural mesothelioma: an EORTC phase II study (08992). Eur J Cancer 2003; 39:353.

42. van Meerbeeck JP, Manegold C, Gaafar R, et al. A randomized phase III study of cisplatin with or without raltitrexed in patients with malignant pleural mesothelioma (MPM): an intergroup study of the EORTC Lung Cancer Group and NCIC. Proc Am Soc Clin Oncol 2004; 24:7021.

43. Molina JR, Adjei AA. The role of pemetrexed (Alimta, LY231514) in lung cancer therapy. Clin Lung Cancer 2003; 5:21.

44. Zhao R, Babani S, Gao F, Liu L, Goldman ID. The mechanism of transport of the multitargeted antifolate, MTA-LY231514, and its cross-resistance pattern in cells with impaired transport of methotrexate. Clin Cancer Res 2000; 6:3687.

45. Westerhof GR, Schornagel JH, Kathmann I, Jackman AL, Rosowsky A, Forsch RA, Hynes JB, Boyle FT, Peters GJ, Pinedo HM, et al. Carrier- and receptor-mediated transport of folate antagonists targeting folate-dependent enzymes: correlates of molecular-structure and biological activity. Mol Pharmacol 1995; 48:459.

46. Pratt SE, Emerick RM, Horwit L, Gallery M, Lesoon A, Jin S, Chen VJ, Dantzig AH. Multidrug resistance proteins (MRP) 2 and 5 transport and confer resistance to Alimta. Proc Am Assoc Cancer Res 2002; 43:782.

47. Habeck LL, Mendelsohn LG, Shih C, Taylor EC, Colman PD, Gossett LS, Leitner TA, Schultz RM, Andis SL, Moran RG, et al. Substrate specificity of mammalian folylpolyglu-

48. tamate synthetase for 5,10-dideazatetrahydrofolate analogs. Mol Pharmacol 1995; 48:326.

48. Shih C, Chen VJ, Gossett LS, et al. LY231514, a pyrrolo(2,3-d)pyrimidine-based antifolate that inhibits multiple folate-requiring enzymes. Cancer Res 1997; 57:1116.

49. Schilsky RL. Antimetabolites. In: Perry MC (ed) The Chemotherapy Source Book. Baltimore: Williams & Wilkins, 1992:301.

50. Schultz RM, Patel VF, Worzalla JF, et al. Role of thymidylate synthase in the antitumor activity of the multitargeted antifolate, LY231514. Anticancer Res 1999; 19:437.

51. Grem JL. Fluorinated pyrimidines. In: Chabner BA, Collins JM (eds) Cancer Chemotherapy: Principles and Practice. Philadelphia: Lippincott, 1990:180.

52. Hooijberg JH, Broxterman HJ, Kool M, Assaraf YG, Peters GJ, Noordhuis P, Scheper RJ, Borst P, Pinedo HM, Jansen G, et al. Antifolate resistance mediated by the multidrug resistance proteins MRP1 and MRP2. Cancer Res 1999; 59:2532.

53. Wang Y, Zhao R, Goldman D. Decreased expression of the reduced folate carrier and folylpolyglutamate synthetase is the basis for acquired resistance to the pemetrexed antifolate (LY231514) in an L1210 murine leukemia cell line. Biochem Pharmacol 2003; 65:1163.

54. Liani E, Rothe ML, Bunni MA, et al. Loss of folylpoly-glutamate synthetase activity is a dominant mechanism of resistance to polyglutamylation-dependent novel antifolates in multiple human leukemia sublines. Int J Cancer 2003; 33:589.

55. Rhee MS, Ryan TJ, Galivan J. Glutamyl hydrolase and the multitargeted antifolate LY231514. Cancer Chemother Pharmacol 1999; 44:427.

56. Calvert H. An overview of folate metabolism: features relevant to the action and toxicities of antifolate anticancer agents. Semin Oncol 1999; 26(2 Suppl 6):3.

57. Allen RH, Stabler SP, Savage DG, Lindenbaum J. Metabolic abnormalities in cobalamin (vitamin B_{12}) and folate deficiency. FASEB J Rev 1993; 7:1344.

58. Snow CF. Laboratory diagnosis of vitamin B_{12} and folate deficiency: a guide for the primary care physician. Arch Int Med 1999; 159:1289.

59. Arafa AM, Hussein L. The assessment of the vitamin B_6 status among Egyptian school children by measuring the urinary cystathionine excretion. Int J Vitam Nutr Res 1984; 54:321.

60. Niyikiza C, Baker SD, Seitz De, et al. Homocysteine and methylmalonic acid: markers to predict and avoid toxicity from pemetrexed therapy. Mol Cancer Ther 2002; 1:545.

61. Celio L, Bajetta E, Toffolatti L, et al. Phase II trial of pemetrexed disodium administered every 21 days in patients (pts) with gastric cancer: efficacy and toxicity without and with folic acid. Ann Oncol 2000; 11:65.

62. Vogelzang NJ, Rusthoven JJ, Symanowski J, Denham C, Kaukel E, Ruffie P, Gatzemeier U, Boyer M, Emri S, Manegold C, Niyikiza C, Paoletti Pet al. Phase III study of pemetrexed in combination with cisplatin versus cisplatin alone in patients with malignant pleural mesothelioma. J Clin Oncol 2003; 21:2636.

63. Scagliotti GV, Shin DM, Kindler HL, et al. Phase II study of pemetrexed with and without folic acid and vitamin B_{12} as front-line therapy in malignant pleural mesothelioma. J Clin Oncol 2003; 21:1556.

64. Hughes A, Calvert P, Azzabi A, et al. Phase I clinical and pharmacokinetic study of pemetrexed and carboplatin in patients with malignant pleural mesothelioma. J Clin Oncol 2002; 20:3533.

65. Darzynkiewicz Z, Carter SP, Mikulski SM, Ardelt WJ, Shogen K. Cytostatic and cytotoxic effects of Pannon (P-30 protein), a novel anticancer agent. Cell Tissue Kinet 1988; 21:169.

66. Mikulski SM, Grossman AM, Carter PW, et al. Phase I human clinical trial of Onconase (P-30 protein) administered intravenously on a weekly schedule in cancer patients with solid tumors. Int J Oncol 1993; 3:57.

67. Mikulski SM, Costanzi JJ, Vogelzang NJ, et al. Phase II trial of a single weekly intravenous dose of ranpirnase in patients with unresectable malignant mesothelioma. J Clin Oncol 2002; 20:274.

68. Govindan R, Kratzke RA, Herndon JE, et al. Gefitinib in patients with malignant mesothelioma (MM): a phase II study by the Cancer and Leukemia Group B (CALGB 30101). Proc Am Soc Clin Oncol 2003; 22:630.

69. Langerak AW, De Laat PA, Van Der Linden-Van Beurden CA, Delahaye M, Van Der Kwast TH, Hoogsteden HC, et al. Expression of platelet-derived growth factor (PDGF) and PDGF receptors in human malignant mesothelioma in vitro and in vivo. J Pathol 1996; 178:151.

70. Gerwin BI, Lechner JF, Reddel RR, et al. Comparison of production of transforming growth factor-beta and platelet derived growth factor by normal human mesothelial cells and mesothelioma cell lines. Cancer Res 1987; 47:6180.

71. Millward M, Parnis F, Byrne M, et al. Phase II trial of imatinib mesylate in patients with advanced pleural mesothelioma. Proc Am Soc Clin Oncol 2003; 22:228.

72. Ohta Y, Shridhar V, Bright RK, Kalemkerian GP, Du W, Carbone M, et al. VEGF, VEGF type C, and their receptors play an important role in angiogenesis and lymphangiogenesis in human malignant mesothelioma tumors. Br J Cancer 1999; 81:54.

73. Eisen T, Boshoff C, Mak I, Sapunar F, Vaughan MM, Pyle L, et al. Continuous low dose thalidomide: a phase II study in advanced melanoma, renal cell, ovarian, and breast cancer. Br J Cancer 2000; 82:812.

74. Pass HI, Bocchetta M, Carbone M. Evidence of an important role for SV40 in mesothelioma. Thorac Surg Clin 2004; 14:489.

75. Imperiale MJ, Pass HI, Sanda MG. Prospects for an SV40 vaccine. Semin Cancer Biol 2001; 11:81.

76. Hassan R, Lerner MR, Benbrook D, et al. Antitumor activity of SS(dsFv)PE38 and SS1(dsFv)PE38, recombinant antimesothelin immunotoxins against human gynecologic cancers grown in organotypic culture in vitro. Clin Cancer Res 2002; 8:3520.

Rare Tumors of the Chest

45

Ifigenia Tzannou, Christopher Nutting
and Konstantinos N. Syrigos

Contents

45.1 Introduction

The majority of primary lung carcinomas belong to one of the following histological categories which are all of bronchiogenic origin: adenocarcinoma, squamous cell carcinoma, large cell undifferentiated carcinoma, or small cell lung carcinoma (SCLC). However, a variety of non-bronchiogenic malignant tumors may occasionally affect the lung. These neoplasms represent 3–5% of all primary lung tumors, malignant or benign, and have a broad spectrum of causes. The most frequently encountered malignant primary lung carcinomas are malignant lymphoreticular disorders, carcinoid tumors, sarcomas, and malignant melanomas [1–4].

45.2 Lymphoma

The lungs can be involved in lymphomatogenic diseases in three ways. In the majority of cases, the lungs are involved by hematogenous dissemination of non-Hodgkin lymphoma (NHL), or Hodgkin's disease (HD), or by contiguous invasion from an adjacent site such as the mediastinum [5–8].

Primary pulmonary lymphoma (PPL), which includes all other malignant lymphomas of the lung, is an extremely rare case. PPL is currently defined as a monoclonal lymphoid proliferation that affects one or both lungs or bronchi in an individual with no evidence of extrapulmonary disease at the time of diagnosis and for the first 3 months following NHL [9]. PPL represents 3.6% of extranodal NHL, which in turn represents 24–50% of all NHL. Overall, in relation with all other primary malignancies of the lung, lymphomas account for a mere 0.5–1% [5–8, 10–13].

PPL includes a wide spectrum of histological types of lymphoma. The Revised European–American Classification of Lymphoid Neoplasms, developed by the International Lymphoma Study Group in 2000 in a new approach to classification, took into consideration morphology, immunophenotype, and genetic and clinical features. According to this classification, which is the same for all kinds of lymphoma, PPL can be classified into the following types:

1. Low-grade B-cell lymphoma is the most frequent form and accounts for 58–89% of cases. It includes mucosa-associated lymphoid tissue lymphomas (MALT-type), lymphoblastic (non-MALT-type), and diffuse large-cell NHL. A subset of MALT lymphomas is the bronchus-associated lymphoid tissue lymphoma (BALT).
2. High-grade B-cell lymphoma, may be centroblastic, immunoblastic, Burkitt's type, or without further classification. T-cell lymphomas are rarely encountered. Primary pulmonary HD without nodal involvement is also rare, accounting for less than 1% of all HD cases [14–16].

45.2.1 Clinical Features

The majority of patients with PPL lymphoma are asymptomatic, and the disease is usually identified on screening radiological tests. When present, symptoms usually concern the respiratory system and include cough and sputum, dyspnea, chest pain, and, occasionally, hemoptysis. General extrapulmonary symptoms, which include fever, weight loss, and night sweats, are present in less than 25% of patients.

The physical examination does not typically reveal any significant abnormalities. In some cases, however, pulmonary auscultation may reveal crackles usually over the involved site. Decreased breath sounds, while dullness to percussion, may also be encountered.

The clinical manifestations of PPL tend to be more frequent and severe in cases of high-grade lymphoma. Patients with pulmonary HD tend to present with extrapulmonary symptoms rather than local ones. In any case, endobronchial involvement, which may manifest as a central airway obstruction or as a diffuse submucosal infiltration causing peripheral airway narrowing, is a grave complication. Although rare, it can present as wheezing, dyspnea, obstructive pneumonia, abscess formation, bronchiectasis, atelectasis, and even total respiratory distress [6, 13, 15, 17–21].

45.2.2 Imaging and Diagnosis

X-rays and computed tomography (CT) scans are the indicated methods for primary pulmonary lymphoma imaging. Initially detection via these methods leads to further examination. The radiological findings vary but, in most cases, a solid nodule mass or infiltrate is recognized commonly in the lower lobes. Localized opacities are usually 2–8 cm in diameter. Rarely, they can be large enough to involve more than half of the hemithorax. Contours may be either well-defined or blurred. Air bronchograms may be seen in about 50% of cases. Infrequently, cavitary masses can also be observed. Multiple nodules and diffuse alveolar and interstitial infiltrates are each detected in less than 10% of patients. Atelectasis and pleural effusion has also been reported, but intrathoracic lymphadenopathy, as according to the criteria for PPL, is obviously absent.

In the case of HD, the image is quite different. In contrast to NHL, primary pulmonary melanoma (PPM) typically presents with multiple parenchymal nodules, which are usually located in the upper lobes [1, 5, 15, 17, 20–22]. CT is more sensitive than standard X-ray imaging. This technique is indicated in order to precisely determine the morphology, extent, and distribution of the disease. CT scans have demonstrated that PPL lesions are actually bilateral or multiple in about 70% of patients. Air bronchograms can be more easily examined by this method. Moreover, invasion of the chest wall, pericardium, or esophagus can be detected, while mediastinal and hilar lymphadenopathy, which could not otherwise be seen, are easily revealed [5, 15–18, 20–22].

Even though radiological, laboratory, and CT findings provide extensive information about the disease and are suggestive of the diagnosis, the definitive diagnosis of PPL is actually based on pathology findings and immunohistochemistry methods. An adequate biopsy specimen is therefore required. Bronchoscopy is not recommended since it is often non-conclusive. In contrast, bronchoalveolar lavage (BAL) and transbronchial and transthoracic biopsy are considered better techniques for acquiring pathological review material. Surgical specimens may be acquired either by video-assisted thoracoscopy (VATS) or by open thoracotomy. In this case, surgical excision may also have a therapeutic purpose. However, less invasive methods are the preferred approach on the basis that surgery may be avoided altogether [13, 17, 18, 23–26].

45.2.3 Staging

Once the diagnosis has been made, the extent of PPL, as with all lymphomas, is defined according to the Ann Arbor staging classification. According to this staging system, the following features should be taken into account: involvement of one or both sides of the diaphragm, contiguous or disseminated extranodal involvement, and presence of clinical symptoms [27].

Stages

I.   Single lymph node (LN) region (I) or single extra-lymphatic organ (ELO) or site

II. Two or more LN regions on the same side of diaphragm (II) or localized involvement of ELO or site and one or more LN regions on the same side

III. LN regions on both sides (III) which may be accompanied by involvement of the spleen (III S), or localized involvement of one ELO or site (III E), or both (III ES)

IV. Diffuse or disseminated involvement, one or more ELO, or tissues with or without associated LN involvement

Suffix A: Absence of symptoms

Suffix B: Presence of fever, night sweats, and/or weight loss of 10% or more of body weight in 6 months preceding diagnosis [28].

45.2.4 Treatment and Prognosis

The choice of treatment is based on histological type and stage of the disease, as well as on co-morbid medical conditions. Current treatment options are surgical excision, chemotherapy, and radiotherapy, as monotherapies or combined therapies. However, there is still no consensus in treatment strategy due to inadequate data regarding the respective efficacy [5, 6].

In general, low-grade PPL has a favorable outcome regardless of the treatment modalities. Surgery is preferred for localized lesions. In this case, no further therapy, other than observation, is indicated as most localized tumors do not typically recur especially in the first 5 years after excision. Exclusive chemotherapy should be considered in patients with bilateral involvement or with extrapulmonary disease. Combination regimens have not proven to be more effective than single-agent ones.

High-grade lymphomas are significantly more aggressive than low-grade ones. Progression and local or distant relapses occur more frequently and earlier in high-grade lymphomas, while survival is poorer (5-year survival is only 44–60%). The indicated therapy, in this case, is surgery followed by polychemotherapy regimens and/or radiation.

Primary pulmonary lymphoma, as with HD, is treated with multiple chemotherapy regimens, ABVD (doxorubicin, bleomycin, vinblastine, decarbazine) or MCPP (mustine, vincristine, procarbazine, prednisone), with encouraging results as far as remission and disease-free time [5, 6, 13, 16, 17, 29, 30].

45.3 Bronchial-associated Lymphoid Tissue Lymphoma

Mucosa-associated lymphoid tissue (MALT) lymphoma of the lung arises from bronchial-associated lymphoid tissue (BALT) and accounts for 90% of all low-grade NHL of the lung, comprising less than 5% of all lymphomas and 0.3% of all primary lung cancers [5, 24, 30–32].

Mucosa-associated lymphoid tissue is usually absent from the normal human lung, as with most sites where MALT-type lymphomas arise. However, chronic bronchial inflammatory processes may stimulate the onset of pulmonary MALT lymphoma. In contrast to MALT lymphoma of the stomach where *H. pylori* has been identified as the antigen responsible for the onset of this process, no triggering antigens have been found in regard with BALT lymphoma. In this case, chronic antigenic stimulation that happens in certain autoimmune diseases, especially Sjögren's syndrome, may cause follicular bronchiolitis and therefore give rise to patch-like structures with distinctive lymphoepithelial infiltration resembling Peyer's patches (MALT) of the gastrointestinal tract [17, 22, 31, 33].

Bronchial-associated lymphoid tissue lymphoma affects patients between 25 and 85 years of age, even though the mean age of onset lies in the sixth decade of life. There is no significant difference in epidemiology as far as the sexes are concerned, even though some studies have demonstrated a female predominance [1, 6, 17, 18, 24, 34–36].

As mentioned above, immune disorders and chronic inflammatory diseases are highly associated with BALT lymphoma, as is smoking. The most common autoimmune and other immune-related disorders that may be reported in patients with pulmonary MALT lymphomas are Sjögren's syndrome, Hashimoto's thyroiditis, systemic lupus erythematoides, rheumatoid arthritis, multiple sclerosis, atrophic gastritis, pernicious anemia, primary biliary cirrhosis, pulmonary adenocarcinoma, dysgammaglobulinemia, and AIDS [9, 23, 34, 37–39].

Symptoms are those usually found in all subtypes in PPL. Patients may have non-specific chest symptoms (chest pain, cough, dyspnea, hemoptysis) and, less frequently, general signs (malaise, weight loss, fever). However, one third to one half of the patients are asymptomatic, and the disease is therefore discovered incidentally in chest X-rays [1, 9, 24, 30, 34].

Most BALT lymphomas manifest as well-defined solitary nodules or masses that are usually less than 5 cm in diameter and are often associated, in up to 50% of the cases, with an air bronchogram. Less frequently, the lesions are multiple and, rarely, bilateral. Hilar lymphadenopathy and cavitation are infrequent. A CT scan usually reveals more lesions than an X-ray. Multiplicity is prominent, but not always bilateral. Air-space consolidation, air bronchograms, areas with a ground-glass look, and areas of hypoattenuation of lung tissue have also been described [1, 5, 21, 40–42].

45.3.1 Diagnosis

The diagnosis of BALT lymphoma is made by biopsy. Macroscopically, a BALT lymphoma mass is a poorly defined, soft, whitish mass that preserves the pulmonary architecture. Microscopically, the mass consists mainly of small lymphoid cells resembling the marginal zone cells of Peyer's patches (the centrocyte) like lymphocytes and plasmacytoid lymphocytes. Invasion of lymphoid cells from the marginal zone to the bronchial epithelium as well as reactive follicular hyperplasia is present. Rarely, blastic cells (immunoblasts), amyloid, fibrosis, and granulomatous deposits may be seen.

Immunohistochemistry may also be an important diagnostic procedure in excluding the possibility of low-grade lymphoma, since the specific antigens CD 5 and CD 10 are not detected in BALT. Immunohistochemical analysis reveals B-cell phenotype (CD 19, CD 20, and Bcl 2) and infiltration with small reactive T lymphocytes within the tumor at the margin of peribronchial lymphoid nodules and in the alveolar wall [1, 5, 9, 23, 34, 37, 40, 43, 44].

45.3.2 Treatment and Prognosis

Bronchial-associated lymphoid tissue lymphoma lymphomas seem to have an impressively favorable clinical outcome, regardless of the treatment. The 5-year survival rate is over 80% and the median time of survival exceeds 10 years. There have not been any definite prognostic factors described among presentation, bilateral disease, TNM staging, surgery, adjuvant chemotherapy, and histology in MALT lymphoma. Only a few indicators of poor prognosis have been reported: age over 60, elevated b_2 microglobulin, pleural effusions, and intratumoral amyloid deposition [5, 6, 16–18, 30, 34, 45].

There are no clear guidelines as far as treatment is concerned. In the case of asymptomatic BALT lymphoma, initial observation with no treatment whatsoever is possible. Surgical excision, which serves both a diagnostic and a therapeutic purpose, is another option, especially in symptomatic patients, but its role has not yet been clearly defined. Single-agent chemotherapy may also be used instead of surgery or as an adjuvant chemotherapy. Chloraminophene, cyclophosphamide, azathioprine, and steroids are most commonly administered. Exclusive chemotherapy is used in patients with multifocal disease. However, several trials have shown that combination regimens, such as CHOP (cyclophosphamide, adriamycin, Oncovin, prednisolone), have not proven to be more effective than monotherapy with one of the above-mentioned agents. Radiotherapy is rarely used in BALT lymphoma [5, 6, 17, 24, 29, 30, 40, 42].

45.4 Carcinoid

Pulmonary carcinoids are rare low-grade malignant tumors that originate from neuroendocrine or Kulchitsky cells in the tracheobronchial tree. Carcinoid tumors represent 1–2% of all lung neoplasms. The tumor is most commonly seen between the ages of 40 and 60 years even though carcinoids have been reported in patients as young as 10 and as old as 83 years of age. They seem to affect slightly more Caucasians as well as the female gender [2, 46–49].

45.4.1 Symptoms

Approximately half of the patients are asymptomatic and the disease is detected on routine chest radiogra-

phy. Centrally located carcinoid malignancies tend to produce symptoms earlier, sometimes years before the definite diagnosis is made. These symptoms are usually a result of airway obstruction and include cough, dyspnea, fever, wheeze, hemoptysis, and chest pain. Many of the patients are initially diagnosed with asthma, while persistent or recurrent pneumonia, despite antibiotic therapy, is also common.

Paraneoplastic syndromes are not frequently described. Cushing's syndrome, due to ectopic adrenocorticotropic hormone production is the most common. Ectopic secretion of gastrin may result in Zollinger-Ellison syndrome, and ectopic secretion of growth hormone-releasing factor may result in acromegaly. Occasionally, bronchial carcinoids may occur in association with multiple endocrine neoplasias, type 1 (MEN I) syndrome. The carcinoid syndrome can be found in only 2–3% of all cases. It may present as flushing, diarrhea, abdominal cramping, nausea, vomiting, fever, hypotension, wheezing, dyspnea, and carcinoid heart disease. Furthermore, it is usually present, along with hepatic metastases, even though it has been reported mainly as a localized disease [2, 46, 47, 50–53].

45.4.2 Imaging

A chest X-ray may reveal a variety of findings. Findings can range from insignificant as a normal chest X-ray to significantly pathological as a mass or nodule with or without signs of chronic obstruction (i.e., atelectasis, bronchiectasis, lung abscess).

Computed tomography scanning is accurate in demonstrating the exact location and extent of the tumor and its extra- and intrabronchial components. It may also reveal diffuse or punctate calcification and lymph node metastasis [46, 47, 54, 55].

Carcinoid cells have somatostatin receptors with high affinity to somatostatin peptides. Somatostatin-analog scintigraphy with octreotide is therefore helpful in the identification of both primary and metastatic lesions. However, due to its low sensitivity (which in most studies has been reported to be approximately 50%) it cannot be used as the sole imaging technique [56, 57].

45.4.3 Diagnosis

Bronchoscopy with biopsy is successful in setting the diagnosis in 70–75% of cases. Most bronchial carcinoids are visible bronchoscopically and bronchoscopic biopsy specimens may be easily obtained with a rigid bronchoscope with no significant risk of hemorrhage. Brush cytology with a flexible bronchoscope is often not diagnostic. This is due to the fact that the tissue obtained may be the normal mucosa that covers the carcinoid tumors. Transthoracic needle biopsy (TTNB) or video-assisted thoracoscopy (VATS) may be needed in the case of peripheral lesions [46, 53, 58–60].

In terms of pathology, pulmonary carcinoid tumors may be categorized as typical and atypical. A typical carcinoid is comprised of small, cuboidal cells with an abundant, granular, lightly eosinophilic cytoplasm and small nuclei. The cells are arranged in nests, ribbons, or sheets. Neurosecretory granules are abundant. Even though no vascular or local invasion is detected, lymph node metastasis is present in 10% of cases.

Atypical carcinoids are tumors that present with at least one of the following characteristics:
1. Increased mitotic activity
2. Irregularity and pleomorphism of nuclei
3. Areas of increased cellularity and disorganization of the architecture
4. Areas of tumor necrosis

The pathological differentiation between carcinoid tumors and SCLC may be difficult. This differentiation, however, is of great importance since SCLC is highly anaplastic with a very poor prognosis, and requires a different treatment. Elevated levels of 5-hydroxyindole-acetic acid and serotonin in the urine are indicative of a carcinoid tumor especially in the presence of carcinoid syndrome. Chromogranin A hormones are also useful markers in the differential diagnosis between carcinoid tumors and SCLC [46, 53, 61, 62].

45.4.4 Prognosis and Treatment

Prognosis of carcinoid tumors is very encouraging. Typical carcinoids have a far better prognosis with 5- and 10-year survival at 90–100% and 85–100%, respectively. Most deaths are related to causes other than the carcinoid tumor. Prognosis for patients with atypical carcinoids is poorer with 5- and 10-year survival at 40–76% and 18–60%, respectively. Lymph node metastasis has no impact on the survival of patients with typical carcinoid lesions. In contrast, lymph node metastasis in atypical carcinoid neoplasms renders a dismal prognosis with 5- and 10-year survival at 38–74% and 24–76%, respectively. Moreover, some investigators have concluded that a larger tumor size and a peripheral location predispose to a poorer outcome [46, 48, 49, 59, 61–64].

Surgical resection is the treatment of choice for all types of bronchial carcinoids. It has not been clarified whether lobectomy or pneumonectomy with mediastinal lymph node dissection is superior to the more conservative wedge or segmental resection. It has been noted, though, that lymph node resection is an important part of surgical treatment, since 10% of all typical and 30–50% of all atypical carcinoids present with local lymph node metastasis at the time of surgery [2, 46, 65, 66].

In addition to surgery, adjuvant chemotherapy and/or radiotherapy should be implemented in cases of atypical carcinoids. Chemotherapy is also the treatment of choice in the case of metastatic disease at the time of initial diagnosis. Many agents have been used as monotherapy or as combination regimens with no definite effectiveness (octreotide, alfa interferon, etoposide, cisplatin, cyclophosphamide, 5-FU, adriamycin, doxorubicin, dacarbazine) [48, 53, 61].

In the presence of a carcinoid syndrome and an unresectable primary lesion, symptomatic treatment should be followed. Patients should avoid foods and circumstances that might aggravate symptoms. Diarrhea, wheezing, and cardiac failure are treated symptomatically. Interferon-alfa and octreotide have been proven useful in the control of carcinoid symptoms, while contributing to tumor stabilization and even regression. Octreotide can also control carcinoid tumor-induced Cushing's syndrome [67, 68].

45.5 Melanoma

Malignant melanoma is a neoplasm that arises from melanocytes that are situated in the deeper layers of the skin. It is the most fatal kind of skin cancer and usually develops on sun-exposed sites. Nevertheless, malignant melanoma may also originate from mucous membranes. Extracutaneous melanoma accounts for less than 10% of all primary melanoma lesions, and primary pulmonary melanoma (PPM) is an extremely rare entity. No more than 30 cases have been reported in medical literature. PPM comprises 0.01% of all tumors in the lung. The results of three reviews on PPM showed affected ages ranging from the fifth to the eighth decade of life with the median age being around 50 years [69–72].

The diagnostic criteria for PPM are very rigid and include:
1. No prior history of excision of pigmented skin tumor, or preferably no history of excision of any skin lesion
2. No history of other mucous membrane or ocular malignancy
3. Junctional changes such as "dropping of" or nesting of melanoma cells just beneath the bronchial epithelium
4. Invasion of the bronchial epithelium by melanoma cells
5. Malignant melanoma associated with these epithelial changes
6. Solitary lung tumor with morphological features compatible with a primary tumor
7. No demonstrable melanoma elsewhere at the time of diagnosis [71, 73–75]

45.5.1 Symptoms

Just like most rare tumors of the lung, 30% of patients with PPM do not demonstrate any symptoms and the presence of the disease is discovered incidentally by chest radiography. The tumor is often endobronchial. Therefore, it causes symptoms from the respiratory system including (in order of frequency) cough, hemoptysis, chest pain, postobstructive pneumonia, and upper respiratory system infection [69–71].

45.5.2 Imaging and Diagnosis

Radiological findings in X-rays and CT scans are similar to those found in lung cancer, revealing a solitary lesion with often an associated pleural effusion. In most case, the lesion is central [70, 71].

Commonly, PPM is misdiagnosed as bronchiogenic lung cancer. The final diagnosis is actually made according to the above-mentioned criteria after a histopathological examination has been performed. Apart from the pathological findings that concern cell morphology and architecture, melanin can be detected in the neoplastic tissue on hematoxylin and eosin staining. In addition, immunohistochemistry may prove very helpful, through a positive reaction for S-100 protein and HMB-45 antibody, and a negative reaction for cytokeratin, CAM, and chromogranin [69–71].

45.5.3 Treatment and Prognosis

The best course of treatment for PPM seems to be a combination of surgical resection of the primary lesion and the regional lymph nodes with or without adjuvant chemotherapy (usually with interferon-alfa 2b or interleukin-2) or radiotherapy.

Sufficient data are inconclusive to relate with prognostic factors. Generally, prognosis is dismal regardless of any treatment approach. Extensive resection (lobectomy or pneumonectomy) may result in long-term survival. In two cases the 10-year survival was reported, but the majority of patients usually succumb to metastatic disease within 14 months after surgery. However, patients with an initial metastatic disease do not survive longer than 4 months [69, 71, 76–78].

45.6   Sarcoma

Primary pulmonary sarcomas (PPS) are rare. Most of the malignant tumors of the lung with mesenchymal origin are metastatic. PPS accounts for less than 0.3% of all lung cancers. Primary sarcomas of the thorax may originate from the lung parenchyma, the mediastinum, the pleura, or the chest wall. Of all histological subtypes, the most common are leiomyosarcomas, fibrosarcomas, hemangiopericytomas, and rhabdomyosarcomas. Leiomyosarcoma is the most common type of lung sarcoma representing 30% of PPS in adults with the mean age of appearance at 50 years [79–83].

45.6.1 Symptoms

The clinical presentation of mesenchymal lung malignancies may be asymptomatic. More frequently, symptoms are the result of the local mass effect. Chest pain, dyspnea, cough, hemoptysis, superior vena cava syndrome, and sometimes pneumothorax have been reported [82, 84].

45.6.2 Imaging and Diagnosis

The radiological findings are non-specific and differ according to the subset of the mesenchymal tumor and the site of involvement. Generally speaking, the chest radiogram may demonstrate a well-defined opacity. It is usually a large (>5 cm) peripheral mass. Postobstructive infiltrates and atelectasis may also be present. A CT scan provides additional information, in terms of necrosis, cavitation, and calcification that cannot be seen in X-rays, as well as infiltration of the adjacent thoracic structures [79, 81, 82, 85].

Diagnosis is again attained through biopsy. Preoperative diagnosis by histological examination of bronchoscopically obtained specimens is not always possible. Thoracoscopy and/or thoracotomy are the indicated methods in order to obtain a diagnostic tissue specimen. Histological diagnosis is made by combining morphological features and the immunoprofile of the tumor.

Macroscopically, the tumors are variable in size (median size of 6 cm). Necrosis and hemorrhage are usually present. As far as immunohistochemical features of sarcomas are concerned, positive reaction is observed with vimentin and occasionally with HHF 35 (for leiomyosarcoma) [79, 86, 87].

45.6.3 Treatment and Prognosis

The only curative therapy for PPS is radical surgery, regardless of histological tumor type. Radiotherapy may also be delivered, but the role of adjuvant chemotherapy is still under discussion. Chemotherapy is mainly used in the treatment of metastatic disease. Antineoplastic agents are different from those administered for lung cancer. The regimens proposed for PPS are the doxorubicin- and/or ifosfamide-based ones, but even with this therapy response rates remain low (20%) [84, 88, 89].

Due to the aggressive behavior of sarcoma, prognosis is poor. The histological type, location of primary site, and tumor size seem to have a role in defining prognosis. Follow-up results of several trials have reported median survivals around 24 months and a 3-year survival between 17% and 50% [79, 83, 86, 90].

45.7 Conclusion

Non-bronchiogenic lung carcinomas, although rare, are of great importance for the clinician. Most of these tumors are asymptomatic or present with non-specific symptoms. As a result, the indication of disease is set incidentally in routine radiological examination, sometimes a long time after the onset of the disease. The X-ray findings are similar if not identical with those of a bronchiogenic malignancy, thus leading to incorrect diagnoses. Definite diagnosis in all cases is made by histopathological examination with additional information acquired by immunohistochemistry. Treatment strategies, involve surgical excision that may be followed by adjuvant chemotherapy and/or radiotherapy for non-metastatic disease, and chemotherapy (frequently combination regimens) for metastatic disease. Nevertheless, prognosis remains exceedingly dismal with the exceptions of low-grade PPL and carcinoid tumors.

Key Points

- A variety of non-bronchiogenic malignant tumors may occasionally affect the lungs. These neoplasms represent 3–5% of all primary lung tumors, malignant or benign, and have a broad spectrum of causes. The most frequently seen malignant primary lung carcinomas are malignant lymphoreticular disorders, carcinoid tumors, sarcoma, and malignant melanoma.
- The imaging findings are similar if not identical with those of a bronchiogenic malignancy, thus leading to incorrect diagnoses. Definite diagnosis is in all cases made by histopathological examination.
- Treatment strategies involve surgical excision that may be followed by adjuvant chemo- and/or radiotherapy for non-metastatic disease, and chemotherapy – usually combination regimens – for metastatic disease. Nevertheless, the prognosis remains exceedingly dismal with the exceptions of low-grade primary pulmonary lymphoma and carcinoid tumors.

References

1. Giménez A, Franquet T, Prats R, et al. Unusual primary lung tumors: a radiologic-pathologic overview. Radiographics 2002;22:601.
2. Chan A, Shelton D, Yoneda K. Unusual primary lung neoplasms. Curr Opin Pulm Med 2001; 7:234.
3. Burt M, Zakowski M. Rare primary malignant neoplasms. In: Peerson FG, DesLauriers J, Ginsberg RJ (eds) Thoracic Surgery. New York: Churchill Livingstone, 1995:807.
4. Keller SM, Ktariya K. Primary lung tumors other than bronchogenic carcinoma: benign and malignant. In: Fishman AP (ed) Pulmonary Diseases and Disorders, 3rd edn, vol 2. New York: McGraw-Hill, 1998:1833.
5. Cadranel J, Wislez M, Antoine M. Primary pulmonary lymphoma. Eur Respir J 2002; 20:750.
6. L'Hoste RJ Jr, Filippa DA, Lieberman PH, et al. Primary pulmonary lymphomas. A clinicopathologic analysis of 36 cases. Cancer 1984; 54:1397.
7. Newton R, Ferlay J, Beral V, et al. The epidemiology of non-Hodgkin's lymphoma: comparison of nodal and extra-nodal sites. Int J Cancer 1997; 72:923.
8. Isaacson PG, Wright DH. Malignant lymphoma of mucosa-associated lymphoid tissue: a distinctive type of B-cell lymphoma. Cancer 1983; 52:1410.
9. Subramanian D, Albrecht S, Gonzales JM, et al. Primary pulmonary lymphoma: Diagnosis by immunoglobulin gene rearrangement study using a novel polymerase chain reaction technique. Am Rev Respir Dis 1993; 148:222.
10. Chow W, Ducheine Y, Hilfer J, et al. Primary malignant non-Hodgkin's lymphoma of the lung arising in mucosa-associated lymphoid tissue. Chest 1996; 110:838.
11. Filly R, Blank N, Castellino RA. Radiographic distribution of intrathoracic disease in previously untreated patients with Hodgkin's disease and non-Hodgkin's lymphoma. Radiology 1976; 120:277.
12. Freeman C, Berg JW, Cutler SJ. Occurrence and prognosis of extranodal lymphomas. Cancer 1972; 29:252.
13. Ferraro P, Trastek VF, Adlakha H, et al. Primary non-Hodgkin's lymphoma of the lung. Ann Thorac Surg 2000; 69:993.
14. Harris N, Jaffe E, Diebold J, et al. Lymphoma classification – from controversy to consensus: the R.E.A.L. and WHO classification of lymphoid neoplasms. Ann Oncol 2000; 11(suppl I):S3.
15. Habermann T, Ryu J, Inwards D, et al. Primary pulmonary lymphoma. Semin Oncol 1999; 26:307.
16. Cordier JF, Chailleux E, Lauque D, et al. Primary pulmonary lymphomas. A clinical study of 70 cases in nonimmunocompromised patients. Chest 1993; 103:201.
17. Addis BJ, Hyjek E, Isaacson PG. Primary pulmonary lymphoma: a re-appraisal of its histogenesis and its relationship to pseudolymphoma and lymphoid interstitial pneumonia. Histopathology 1988; 13:1.
18. Hebert A, Wright DH, Isaacson PG, et al. Primary malignant lymphoma of the lung: histopathologic and immunologic evaluation of nine cases. Hum Pathol 1984; 15:415.
19. Radin AI. Primary pulmonary Hodgkin's disease. Cancer 1990; 65:550.
20. Lewis ER, Caskey Cl, Fishman EK. Lymphoma of the lung: CT findings in 31 patients. AJR 1991; 156:711.
21. Kyung D, Jung-Gi I, Soo K, et al. B-cell lymphoma of bronchus-associated lymphoid tissue (BALT): CT features in 10 patients [thoracic imaging]. J Comput Assist Tomogr 2000; 24:30.
22. Wislez M, Cadranel J, Antoine M, et al. Lymphoma of pulmonary mucosa-associated lymphoid tissue: CT scan findings and pathological correlations. Eur Respir J 1999; 14:423.

23. Fiche M, Capron F, Berger F, et al. Primary pulmonary non-Hodgkin's lymphomas. Histopathology 1995; 26:529.

24. Koss M. Malignant and benign lymphoid lesions of the lung. Ann Diagn Pathol 2004; 8:167.

25. Ahmed S, Kussick S, Siddiqui A, et al. Bronchial-associated lymphoid tissue lymphoma: a clinical study of rare disease. Eur J Cancer 2004; 40:1320.

26. Morales FM, Matthews JI. Diagnosis of parenchymal Hodgkin's disease using bronchoalveolar lavage. Chest 1987; 91:785.

27. Carbone PP, Kaplan HS, Musshoff K, et al. Report of the Committee on Hodgkin's Disease Staging Classification. Cancer Res 1971; 31:1860.

28. Glick JH, Portlock C. Hodgkin's disease: clinical manifestations, staging and therapy. In: Hoffman R, Benz E, Shattil S, Furie B, Cohen H (eds) Hematology: Basic Principles and Practice, 3rd edn. New York: Churchill Livingston, 2000:921.

29. Kim JH, Lee SH, Park J, et al. Primary pulmonary non-Hodgkin's lymphoma. Jpn J Clin Oncol 2004; 34:510.

30. Li G, Hansmann ML, Zwingers T, et al. Primary lymphomas of the lung: morphological, immunohistochemical and clinical features. Histopathology 1990; 16:519.

31. Raderer M, Vorbeck F, Formanek M, et al. Importance of extensive staging in patients with mucosa-associated lymphoid tissue (MALT)-type lymphoma. Br J Cancer 2000; 83:454.

32. Ahmed S, Siddiqui AK, Rai KR. Low-grade B-cell bronchial associated lymphoid tissue (BALT) lymphoma. Cancer Invest 2002; 20:1059.

33. Zinzani PL, Tani M, Gabriele A, et al. Extranodal marginal zone B-cell lymphoma of MALT-type of lung: single-center experience with 12 patients. Leukemia Lymphoma 2003; 44:821.

34. Kurtin PJ, Myers JL, Adlakha H, et al. Pathology and clinical features of primary pulmonary extranodal marginal zone B-cell lymphoma of MALT type. Am J Surg Pathol 2001; 25:997.

35. L'Hoste RJ Jr, Filippa DA, Licbcrman PH, et al. Primary pulmonary lymphomas. A clinicopathologic analysis of 36 cases. Cancer 1984; 54:1397.

36. Herbert A, Wright DH, Isaacson PG, et al. Primary malignant lymphoma of the lung: histopathologic and immunologic evaluation of nine cases. Hum Pathol 1984; 15:415.

37. Richmond I, Pritchard GE, Ashcroft T, et al. Bronchus associated lymphoid tissue (BALT) in human lung: its distribution in smokers and non-smokers. Thorax 1993; 48:1130.

38. Bégueret H, Vergier B, Parrens M, et al. Primary lung small B-cell lymphoma versus lymphoid hyperplasia. Am J Surg Pathol 2002; 26:76.

39. Nicholson AG, Wotherspoon AC, Jones AL, et al. Pulmonary B-cell non-Hodgkin's lymphoma associated with autoimmune disorders: a clinicopathological review of six cases. Eur Respir J 1996; 9:2022.

40. Bolton-Maggs PHB, Colman A, Dixon GR, et al. Mucosa associated lymphoma of the lung. Thorax 1993; 48:670.

41. Gibson N, Hansell M. Lymphocytic disorders of the chest: pathology and imaging. Clin Radiol 1998; 53:469.

42. Lazar E, Whitman G, Chew F. Lymphoma of bronchus-associated lymphoid tissue. AJR 1996; 167:116.

43. Nathwani B, Hernandez A-M, Deol I, et al. Marginal B-cell lymphomas: an appraisal. Hum Pathol 1997; 28:42.

44. Harris NL, Isaacson PG. What are the criteria for distinguishing MALT from non-MALT lymphoma at extranodal sites? Am J Clin Pathol 1999; 111:S126.

45. Thieblemont C, Berger F, Dumontet C, et al. Mucosa-associated lymphoid tissue lymphoma is a disseminated disease in one third of 158 patients analyzed. Blood 2000; 95:802.

46. Dusmet ME, McKneally MF. Pulmonary and thymic carcinoid tumors. World J Surg 1996; 20:189.

47. Chughtai TS, Morin JE, Sheiner NM, Wilson JA, et al. Bronchial carcinoid: twenty years' experience defines a selective surgical approach. Surgery 1997; 122:801.

48. Harpole DH, Deldman JM, Buchanen S, et al. Bronchial carcinoid tumors: a retrospective analysis of 126 patients. Ann Thorac Surg 1992; 54:50.

49. Vadesz P, Palffy G, Egervary M, et al. Diagnosis and treatment of bronchial carcinoid tumors: clinical and pathological review of 120 operated patients. Eur J Cardiothorac Surg 1993; 7:8.

50. Oliaro A, Filosso PL, Casadio C, et al. Bronchial carcinoid associated with Cushing's syndrome. J Cardiovasc Surg 1995; 36:511.

51. Nakhoul F, Kerner H, Levin M, et al. Carcinoid tumor of the lung and type-1 multiple endocrine neoplasia associated with persistent hypercalcemia: a case report. Miner Electrolyte Metab 1994; 20:107.

52. Doppman JL, Nieman L, Miller DL, et al. Ectopic adrenocorticotropic hormone syndrome: localization studies in 28 patients [published erratum appears in Radiology 1989; 173:226]. Radiology 1989; 172:115.

53. Davila DG, Dunn WF, Tazelaar HD, et al. Bronchial carcinoid tumors. Mayo Clin Proc 1993; 68:795.

54. Kwekkeboom DJ, Krenning EP, Bakker WH, et al. Somatostatin analogue scintigraphy in carcinoid tumors. Eur J Nucl Med 1993; 20:283.

55. Magid D, Siegelman SS, Eggleston JC, et al. Pulmonary carcinoid tumors: CT assessment. J Comput Assist Tomogr 1989; 13:244.

56. Kvolts LK, Brown ML, O'Connor MK, et al. Evaluation of radiolabelled somatostatin analog (I-123 octreotide) in the detection and localization of carcinoid and islet cell tumors. Radiology 1993; 187:129.

57. Meko JB, Doherty GM, Siegel BA, et al. Evaluation of somatostatin-receptor scintigraphy for detecting neuroendocrine tumors. Surgery 1996; 120:975.

58. Collins BT, Cramer HM. Fine needle aspiration cytology of carcinoid tumors. Acta Cytol 1996; 40:695.

59. Martensson H, Bottcher G, Hambraeus G, et al. Bronchial carcinoids: an analysis of 91 cases. World J Surg 1987; 11:356.

60. Rea F, Binda R, Spreafico G, et al. Bronchial carcinoids: a review of 60 patients. Ann Thorac Surg 1989; 47:412.

61. Warren WH, Faber LP, Gould VE. Neuroendocrine neoplasms of the lung: a clinicopathologic update. J Thorac Cardiovasc Surg 1989; 98:321.

62. Walts AE, Said JW, Sintaku IP, Lloyd RV. Chromogranin as a marker of neuroendocrine cells in cytologic material: an immunocytochemical study. Am J Clin Pathol 1985; 84:273.

63. Lequaglie C, Patriarca C, Cataldo I, et al. Prognosis of resected well-differentiated neuroendocrine carcinoma of the lung. Chest 1991; 100:1053.

64. Oliaro A, Filosso PL, Donati G, et al. Atypical bronchial carcinoids: review of 46 patients. J Cardiovasc Surg 2000; 41:131.

65. Ferguson MK, Landreneau RJ, Hazelrigg SR, et al. Long-term outcome after resection for bronchial carcinoid tumors. Eur J Cardiothorac Surg 2000; 18:156.

66. Chughtai TS, Morin JE, Sheiner NM, et al. Bronchial carcinoid: twenty years' experience defines a selective surgical approach. Surgery 1997; 122:801.

67. Gregor M. Therapeutic principles in the management of metastasising carcinoid tumors: drugs for symptomatic treatment. Digestion 1994; 55(suppl. 3):60.

68. Kvols LK. Therapy of the malignant carcinoid syndrome. Endocrinol Metab Clin North Am 1989; 18:557.

69. Dountsis A, Zisis C, Karagianni E, et al. Primary malignant melanoma of the lung: a case report. World J Surg Oncol 2003; 1:26:1.

70. Ost D, Joseph C, Sogoloff H, et al. Primary pulmonary melanoma: case report and literature review. Mayo Clin Proc 1990; 74:62.

71. Wilson RW, Moran CA. Primary melanoma of the lung: a clinicopathologic and immunohistochemical study of eight cases. Am J Surg Pathol 1997; 2:1196.

72. Jennings TA, Axiotis CA, Kress Y, et al. Primary malignant melanoma of the lower respiratory tract. Am J Clin Pathol 1990; 94:649.

73. Özdemir N, Cangir AK, Kutlay H, et al. Primary malignant melanoma of the lung in oculocutaneous albino patient. Case report. Eur J Cardiothoracic Surg 2001; 20:864.

74. Bagwell SP, Flynn SD, Cox PM, et al. Primary malignant melanoma of the lung. Am Rev Respir Dis 1989; 139:1543.

75. Cagle P, Mace ML, Judge DM, et al. Pulmonary melanoma primary vs metastatic. Chest 1984; 85:125.

76. Marchevsky AM. Lung tumors derived from ectopic tissues. Diagn Pathol 1995; 12:172.

77. Lie CH, Chao TY, Chung YH, et al. Primary pulmonary malignant melanoma presenting with haemoptysis. Melanoma Res 2005; 15:219.

78. Reed RJ III, Kent EM. Solitary pulmonary melanomas: two case reports. J Thorac Cardiovasc Surg 1964; 48:226.

79. Janssen JP, Mulder JJS, Wagenaar SS, et al. Primary sarcoma of the lung: a clinical study with long-term follow-up. Ann Thorac Surg 1994; 58:1151.

80. Travis WD, Travis LB, Devesa SS. Lung cancer. Cancer 1995; 75:191.

81. Çakir Ö, Topal U, Bayram S, et al. Sarcomas: rare primary malignant tumors of the thorax. Diagn Interv Radiol 2005; 11:23.

82. Gladish GW, Sabloff BM, Munden RF, et al. Primary thoracic sarcomas. Radiographics 2002; 22:621.

83. Miller DL, Allen MS. Rare pulmonary neoplasms. Mayo Clin Proc 1993; 68:492.

84. Etienne-Mastroianni B, Falchero L, Chalabreysse L, et al. Primary sarcomas of the lung. A clinicopathologic study of 12 cases. Lung Cancer 2002; 38:283.

85. Suster S. Primary sarcoma of the lung. Semin Diagn Pathol 1995; 26:474.

86. Attanoos RL, Appleton MAC, Gibbs AR. Primary sarcoma of the lung: a clinicopathological and immunohistochemical study of 14 cases. Histopathology 1996; 29:29.

87. Kell SB, Bacha E, Mark EJ, et al. Primary pulmonary sarcoma: a clinicopathologic study of 26 cases. Mod Pathol 1999; 12:1124.

88. Bacha EA, Wright CD, Grillo HC, et al. Surgical treatment of primary pulmonary sarcomas. Eur J Cardiothorac Surg 1999; 15:456.

89. Régnard JF, Icard P, Guibert L, et al. Prognostic factors and results after surgical treatment of primary sarcomas of the lung. Ann Thorac Surg 1999; 68:227.

90. Yang JC, Glastein EJ, Rosenberg SA, et al. Sarcomas of soft tissues. In: de Vita VT, Hellman S, Rosenberg SA (eds) Cancer Principles and Practice of Oncology. Philadelphia: Lippincott, 1993:1436.

Section IX:
Palliation of Lung Cancer Patients

Quality of Life after Lung Cancer Surgery

46

Hugo Esteva, Cristina Pecci,
Nora Taubenslag Grigera, Alejandro T. Newton
and Tamara Portas

Contents

46.1   Introduction

Quality of life is a rather subjective concept. In fact, for a given person, it could change daily on the basis of strong personal feelings and/or events. More specifically, health-related quality of life (HRQOL) links quality of life with health status.

Nevertheless, the idea of quality of life is so deeply linked with cultural values that a comparison between different populations becomes difficult. As an example, we have frequently seen that people living in the rural areas of our country divide life into two very distinct periods, before and after a challenging illness, even though they may be cured. In contrast, as a general rule, people living in our large urban centers usually conceive illness as a temporary state to be quickly dealt with, so they are prone to be intolerant of unsatisfactory results.

Efforts have been made to establish standardized methods to measure HRQOL taking cultural differences into account [1]. But the thrust has been mainly put on language, when concepts about life should be the principal issue.

At the same time, it is very difficult to distinguish between the effects of surgery and the impact of cancer diagnosis itself, creating another difference in diverse cultural groups. In fact, our Latin population is less prone to believe in modern science than the Anglo-Saxons, requiring a different approach when coping with oncological decisions.

Conscious about those limitations, we agree that HRQOL measurement should be part of patient follow-up, especially in our surgically treated lung cancer patients. It would not only be a useful tool in comforting the patient but also a test to detect psychological/psychiatric disorders needing treatment, for which mere clinical follow-up is often insufficient.

After having acquired some experience about late effects of resection surgery, every skilled thoracic surgeon knows that performing a pneumonectomy for a central lung cancer changes a mortal illness into a disabling one. In as far as there is no other choice but to perform lung resection surgery, the early impairment of HRQOL [2] sounds superficial. Even more, it could be a cumbersome mistake if this kind of test led to the denial of a potentially curative operation. In fact, the ultimate reason to evaluate HRQOL after lung surgery is to open the possibility of discovering new aspects that could help patients to feel healthier.

In chronic illnesses, the World Health Organization (WHO) suggests that the medical and the supporting staff should not only focus on treatments but also on the management of disabilities, limitations, and restrictions. The aim should be the promotion and maintenance of an adequate quality of life for the sick person, in relation to his/her caregivers and family.

In addition, our care as health providers should be critically assessed. The wise choice of strictly appropriate postoperative tests should be considered paramount. Are we acting in the best interests of the patient when we ask for tests that will not change our therapeutic approach, or are we avoiding our own sense of unease about the difficulty in patient recovery? Will patient confidence be diminished if he/she learns otherwise? Promoting the best possible HRQOL makes clinicians and surgeons fine tune subjective aspects of their judgments of medical care that have not always been fully appreciated.

So, as with any other tool, how and when to use HRQOL tests will determine how they aid our clinical sense [3].

46.2 Definition

Health-related quality of life is a multidimensional concept. The degree of physical comfort, the capacity to cope with everyday life events, the psychological status, and the ability to interact with others are elements composing it [4]. As respiratory limitations are directly related to HRQOL [5], improving both becomes the aim of medical treatment.

Health-related quality of life includes the patient's point of view regarding the impact of therapy on significant aspects of his/her life. It is also sometimes related to his/her feelings of satisfaction [6]. The definition proposed by Shumaker and Naughton, one of those usually quoted in medical literature, implies that HRQOL is the subjective evaluation of health status, healthcare, and health promotion about the capability to carry on the most important daily activities. The main dimensions included are: social, physical, and cognitive functioning; mobility and personal care; and emotional well-being [7].

The WHO defines HRQOL as the individual perception of one's self-position in relation to goals, expectancy, rules, and worries [8]. According to this, treatments should consider every affected dimension. The WHO defines [6] wide areas describing the main aspects of HRQOL: physical, psychological, independence level, social relationships, personal beliefs, and relationship with the environment.

The patient's subjective evaluation of his/her health status can be different from the doctor's evaluation. The HRQOL instruments can give additional information unseen with the usual clinical tests and are useful to detect relevant problems in different dimensions.

The frequent discrepancy between patients' and doctors' or caregivers' evaluations is one of the reasons for using HRQOL testing [9]. In fact, what doctors usually prefer for the sake of their patients might not be what the patient desires; on the contrary, patients might not be worried about the same situations that doctors presume are bad for them [6]. There is frequently a gap between a surgeon's focus on mortality or complications and the patient's fears about a possible permanent disability [2].

In lung cancer patients the HRQOL evaluation has been considered a significant predictor of survival and therefore an important preoperative test before treatment [2]. Nowadays there are studies including HRQOL as a measure of surgical results and as a descriptor of clinical endpoint [9].

Even if rehabilitation programs, nutrition control, and social training may enhance functional performance of cancer patients, progressive lung function impairment cannot be avoided [10] on account of the usual co-morbidity of progressive chronic obstructive pulmonary disease (COPD) in this population. Sometimes lung volume reduction surgery (LVRS) techniques could be combined with cancer excision [11–13] to avoid functional deterioration, but this is a seldom applicable solution. So, as far as surgical resection is the principal curative treatment, it is also important to recognize its effects on functional status and HRQOL in order to compare its potential benefit against any other treatment modalities. That is the reason why evaluation of HRQOL is becoming a standard complementary tool to evaluate symptoms and quality of survival.

Postoperative HRQOL testing should include factors such as complications, additional treatments, and new operations, but also difficulties in reassuming social life, returning to work, and limitations in familial and everyday life activities [6]. This is due to the fact that not only disease-free status but also functional capacity is important from the patient's point of view.

46.3 Health-related Quality of Life Instruments

Since the 1970s and particularly the 1980s, efforts have been made to assess with standardized methods the presence and distribution of different illnesses in the general population and in care-giving institutions under varied sociocultural conditions. This was associated with the need for more precise definitions of the concepts to be evaluated, in order to justify the logical-methodological structure of the different questionnaires employed.

There are two major types of instrument to measure HRQOL: (1) generic, those used for the comparison of different conditions, either in people considered healthy or in people with some impairment and (2) specific, those that have been designed for a certain illness or condition. These questionnaires systematically cover possible areas of dysfunction by means of questions that measure the patients' self-perceived changes longitudinally [14]. They reflect a range of opportunities and possible alternatives for a competent and informed patient who voluntarily takes part in the medical care of his/her health.

Among some well-known scales and questionnaires, internationally acknowledged for their development, application, and psychometric and linguistic validation in varied contexts are:

1. The *Flanagan Quality of Life Scale* (QOLS) [15, 16], a self-administered questionnaire designed for use in patients with chronic illness. It evaluates physical and material well-being; relationships with other people; social, community, and civic activities; per-

sonal development and fulfillment; recreation; and independence.

2. The *Sickness Impact Profile* (SIP) [17], a generic measure used to evaluate the impact of disease on both physical and emotional well-being. Patients are asked to respond to the items as they feel on that day. The measure has also been used in patients with COPD and asthma. It includes two overall domains (physical and psychosocial) with 12 categories (sleep and rest, eating, work, home management, recreation and pastimes, ambulation, mobility, body care and movement, social interaction, alertness behavior, emotional behavior, and communication).

3. The *Nottingham Health Profile* (NHP) [18], another generic HRQOL measure. This instrument is used to evaluate perceived distress across various populations. It includes different dimensions: physical mobility, pain, social isolation, emotional reactions, energy, and sleep.

4. The *Medical Outcomes Study (MOS) 36-item Short Form (SF-36)*, a multipurpose questionnaire based on the recognition of the importance of the patient's point of view in the evaluation of results of medical care. It assesses functional status and well-being. It is not designed for a specific illness, condition, age, or treatment. It may be used in a general population, for monitoring health services, or in clinical research. It is useful for comparing different populations, to estimate the relative burden of different illnesses, to compare benefits obtained through different treatments, or for individual follow-up of patients [19, 20]. In its present version, the SF-36 groups items in eight scales: physical functioning, role-functioning, physical pain, general health, vitality, social functioning, emotional role, and mental health. These scales are summarized in two indices: the physical health component and the mental health component.

5. The *Euroqol (EQ-5D)* [21, 22], which will be described later, is another generic instrument.

6. The *European Organization for Research and Treatment of Cancer Quality of Life Questionnaire (EORTC)* [23], a cancer-specific core questionnaire for use in relation to various cancers. It may be used in conjunction with the lung cancer-specific questionnaires. It includes functional (physical, role, cognitive, emotional, and social), symptoms (fatigue, pain, and nausea and vomiting), global health status, and quality of life scales, and also several single-item symptom measures. In lung cancer patients, the European Organization for Research and Treatment of Cancer Quality of Life Questionnaire Lung Cancer Module (EORTC QLQ-LC13) [24] may be added.

7. The *Functional Assessment of Cancer Therapy*—General, Version 4 (FACT-G v. 4) [25], another instrument for use with a variety of chronic illness conditions. It was originally validated in a general cancer population that included lung cancer patients.

As specific HRQOL instruments we will mention:

8. The *Chronic Respiratory Disease Questionnaire (CRQ)*, an interviewer administered questionnaire measuring both physical and emotional aspects of chronic respiratory disease [26, 27].

9. The *St. George's Respiratory Questionnaire (SGRQ)* [28], a disease-specific instrument designed to measure impact on overall health, daily life, and perceived well-being in patients with fixed and reversible airway obstruction.

46.4 Some Physiopathological Considerations

Lung resections in cancer patients are usually limited by simultaneous smoking-related COPD that leads to poor respiratory condition. Surgery always requires resection of some functioning parenchyma to get adequate oncological margins. The decision making could be crucial in borderline cases. That is the reason for continuous interest in surgical risk assessment [29, 30].

Alternative incisions to posterolateral thoracotomy have been developed to reduce postoperative functional deficit and pain [31]. Video-assisted thoracic surgery could be employed in highly selected poor functional candidates. Nevertheless it is well known that pneumonectomy reduces ventilatory parameters (forced vital capacity [FVC] and forced expiratory volume in the first second [FEV1]) by about 35% 3 months after surgery, when most of the consequences of thoracotomy itself (i.e., pain, movement impairment, and incision swelling) have almost disappeared; after the same postoperative period lobectomy and minor resections reduce FVC and FEV1 by about 25% and 15%, respectively [32]. Even though some recovery could be observed up until 6 months postoperatively [33], there is usually considerable chronic functional reduction that can impact on HRQOL.

Lung volume reduction surgery (LVRS) has been developed to ameliorate functional and/or subjective level of dyspnea in COPD patients. The resection of malfunctioning portions of lung parenchyma could involve simultaneous resection of lung malignant lesions; conversely, a lobectomy of poorly contributing parenchyma in a lung cancer patient could end in a better postoperative function. But those are exceptional situations: the rule is the unavoidable deterioration of respiratory condition as a consequence of cancer resection.

Pneumonectomy, the oncological operation required to excise central tumors developed from segmental to proximal bronchi, poses specific additional chronic problems. Scoliosis causing back pain and/or postpneumonectomy syndrome causing bronchial stenosis of the remaining lung could be collateral damages leading to unavoidable new problems after surgical treatment. In fact, pneumonectomy for cancer could be considered as an illness in itself, a price paid to avoid a certain death.

Pain poses a similar problem. Chronic thoracic pain, though uncommon, may be present and requires specific measures to be controlled [34]. Nevertheless, everyday practice shows that a clear explanation about the nature of postoperative pain and especially the disclosure of its origin as different from the persistence of malignancy can reassure patients and become a principal measure to control it.

The influence of lung resection on circulation has also been recognized. Increased pulmonary artery pressure, increased pulmonary vascular resistance, reduced systolic volume, and reduced oxygen consumption have been demonstrated after lobectomies [35].

All these facts and limitations may have some degree of influence on HRQOL, typical for the cardiorespiratory system and different from any other kind of surgical intervention [36]. But since surgical excision of lung cancer offers the best chance of curative treatment, to exaggerate the focus on "survival and/or symptom relief" [2] is at least ingenuous. So HRQOL evaluation should be a source of new ways of helping patients to cope with the unavoidable side effects of potentially curative surgical interventions instead of raising a wall between surgeons and patients as some of the literature suggests [2, 37].

46.5 Depression in the Postsurgical Patient

A first issue to be discussed is whether a patient who has suffered a curative lung resection should be considered a chronically ill one. Second, as the resection is an oncological treatment, what has been the emotional impact of the knowledge of cancer? Both situations will most probably interact in the patient's perception of his/her health.

As previously stated there is considerable functional reduction when a part or a whole lung is resected. This would cause a "medical illness" which might be perceived by the patient as a functional impairment. The knowledge of an oncological disease brings the fear of recurrence, the dread of surgical treatment, as well as the expectation of potential cure. A good doctor–patient relationship sustains a clear and optimistic vision of the prognosis.

Depressive mood is a normal, usual aspect of a person's mental status when suffering a chronic illness such as a lung resection due to lung cancer would be. This mood may constitute a transient adaptive reaction implying sadness, anxiety, and fear toward a possible loss of independence that may be gradually replaced by an active tackling of the current conditions. This is what may happen when the personality is well structured and the person is capable of using a variety of coping strategies and defense mechanisms combined with an adequate doctor–patient relationship when the patient is well informed regarding diagnosis, treatment, and prognosis. Rather frequently, though, due to failures in the personality structure and/or in the doctor–patient relationship and/or due to concurrent stressful life events, there is a maladaptive reaction, with a depressive disorder interfering during the immediate and subsequent postoperative period, contributing to pain perception, immobility, and functional impairment. This situation acting as co-morbidity amplifies the deterioration of the HRQOL [38].

In addition, from a neurobiological point of view, behaviors in illness, such as appetite reduction, restlessness, fatigue, sleep disorders, anhedonia, and difficulties in concentration, are related to proinflammatory cytokines. These symptoms are usual components of the depressive syndrome [39, 40].

Diverse mechanisms may be considered in the genesis of depression related to somatic illness, including physiological effects of chronic illness on the organism as a totality, the psychological impact of illness, or the maladaptive behavior occurring in preexisting depressive disorders [41].

Factors affecting the individual vulnerability to illness are recent vital events, chronic stress, personality characteristics, and the previous level of psychological well-being. Another important aspect to be considered is the role of "meaning" in the adaptation to illness and loss. Each person has a global meaning composed of beliefs, aims and values, and a sense of one's self that persists throughout life. This personal perception is attacked by chronic illness and the person must face it, giving a new meaning to life. The difficulty in understanding this new meaning may obscure mental disorders, particularly depression, with or without anxiety [42].

In patients with medical illnesses, then, adaptive disorders with depressive mood or with depression and anxiety or major depression may be found.

High co-morbidity indices should be taken into account because:

1. Even though depression is one of the most prevalent disorders (more than hypertension) among medical outpatients, it is usually underdiagnosed (30–50% subdiagnosis according to different papers) [43]. Studies repeatedly demonstrate an underestimation of depression by the healthcare staff in the medically ill. This is important because depression exacerbates morbidity and mortality, decreasing self-care and altering the capacity to cope with the illness [44].
2. Depressive persons are at a greater risk of suffering arterial hypertension, myocardial infarctions, or stroke.
3. It has been demonstrated that depression is related to a worsening of somatic complaints.
4. Compliance to treatments is altered when depression is present.

5. Depression may exacerbate the dysfunction usually related to somatic illness, affecting: (a) social functioning, (b) productivity, (c) physical functioning, and (d) self-care.
6. Depression interacts with physical illness, amplifying the discomfort and disability often associated with it.

Depression is related to a decrease in the HRQOL due to the deterioration of social functioning, physical functioning, the perception of bodily pain, and general health [45]. From a clinical point of view, the high comorbidity rate of depression and medical illnesses marks the need for the non-psychiatric specialist to remain aware of the possible occurrence of depression among the patient population, its diagnosis, and an adequate treatment.

The treatment is specific with a variety of resources depending on the type of depression: pharmacological (selecting drugs in terms of pharmacokinetics and pharmacodynamics, the clinical status, and possible interactions), psychotherapeutic (choosing the appropriate technique in terms of age, clinical situation, and personality), and environmental (in terms of significant others and possible activity level).

Treatment of depression will lead to the improvement of the health status. Therefore, a greater emphasis should be put on it in order to enhance the HRQOL [46]. Depression may increase the risk of medical illness and medical illness may increase the risk of depression [47]. Not only the physical side effects but also the functional, emotional, and psychosocial effects of a treatment must be taken into account [48].

Depression can be usually detected by means of self-administered questionnaires, such as the Beck Depressive Inventory [49] and the Hospital Anxiety and Depression Scale [50]. It may also be assessed through checklist-based interviews such as with the Hamilton Depression Scale [51] and through a clinical evaluation by a psychiatrist usually identifying depressive disorders in terms of DSM IV criteria. Once detected, depression should be confirmed and treated by specialists.

46.6 Study of Health-related Quality of Life with EuroQol and the Hospital Anxiety and Depression Scale in Surgical Patients

In an ongoing study on patients that were resected for lung cancer in our Thoracic Surgery Division at the University Hospital (Hospital de Clínicas) in Buenos Aires, Argentina, the EuroQol (EQ-5D) [52] was applied for the assessment of the health status and HRQOL. The EQ-5D is an internationally employed, standard-

ized, generic, not complex, self-administered questionnaire that may be sent by mail or completed during a personal interview. It provides a descriptive profile and a self-assessment of the health status. The evaluation covers five basic dimensions: mobility, self-care, functioning during daily activities, presence of pain/discomfort, and anxiety/depression. Each dimension includes three severity levels: complete absence of problems, moderate presence of problems, and severe presence of problems, associated with impairment (e.g., being in bed, being unable to wash or dress without any help, being unable to perform everyday tasks, being in much pain, or very anxious/depressed). The questionnaire also includes a visual analog scale in which the patients are asked to rate their perceived health status in a value ranging from 0 to 100 [53], zero rating the worst imaginable status and 100 the best imaginable one.

To assess the probability of anxiety and/or depression, the Hospital Anxiety and Depression Scale (HADS) was employed [50]. It was selected in this medical/surgical context because it is a short, self-administered questionnaire where depression and anxiety are investigated through characteristics that will not tend to overlap with somatic symptoms usually present in medical illnesses. It therefore allows a specific screening for anxiety and depression, avoiding false-positives that would appear due to the presence of similar symptoms derived from other medical/surgical conditions.

A group of 74 patients who were resected for lung cancer between November 1989 and March 2005 were contacted by telephone and invited to voluntarily participate in this evaluation. The average time between surgery and this evaluation has been 45 months (1–183 months). The majority (88%) completed the questionnaires during a personal interview and 12% answered through regular mail. There were 74 patients (52% male) with ages ranging from 25 to 92 years (mean: 63, standard deviation [SD]: 14.3; 57% were 65 years of age or older). Among them 86% were covered by social security services, 68% were married, 20% were widowers, 7% were single, and 81% lived with their families. Sixty-three percent did not work, the majority of which were retired. Twenty-six persons still worked an average of 38 h per week after surgery. Regarding educational level, 40.5% had not completed 12 years of formal education, 32.5% had achieved university studies, and the rest were at an intermediate educational level. Sixty-three percent were patients at the public University Hospital and 38% were private patients from the personal practice of two of the authors (in Argentina this means a significant social and economic difference).There were 83% lobectomies and 15% pneumonectomies. Among them 12% needed hospitalization during the last 12 months due to respiratory problems; 81% had suffered no severe respiratory crises during the last year.

The EQ-5D showed that 70% acknowledged no mobility difficulties for walking; 97% had no difficulty regarding personal care such as dressing or washing; 76% had no difficulties in daily activities; 63.5% acknowledged no pain; and 58% had no anxiety or depression. According to the HADS, 78% of the cases were classified as "no depression" and 82.5% of the cases as "no anxiety". On the visual analog scale, where patients were asked to mark their perceived health status from 0 to 100, the average mark on the scale was 81 points (SD: 15.8).

The analysis of the results of EQ-5D in this study rendered a statistically significant association between acknowledgement of pain/discomfort and less than 6 months from surgery (Fisher exact test: $p<0.01$). There were no significant differences between type of surgery (lobectomy or pneumonectomy) or type of consultation (public or private) and pain/discomfort. Pain did significantly relate to mobility difficulties ($p<0.0002$) and to daily activities ($p<0.0002$). Feelings of anxiety or depression significantly associated with mobility difficulties ($p<0.03$). Age significantly related to mobility problems ($p<0.003$) and to feelings of anxiety/depression ($p<0.0008$); in both cases a significant difference was observed in older patients (>65 years of age), who marked greater mobility problems and feelings of anxiety/depression. No significant difference was observed between pain and anxiety/depression according to EQ-5D. Significant statistical association was found between probable depression according to HADS and mobility problems ($p<0.0001$) and daily life function ($p<0.0004$). Anxiety, according to HADS, and mobility problems did not associate. Anxiety, according to HADS, and daily life functioning showed a greater frequency of association, though not statistically significant. There was no statistically significant association between gender, age, marital status, educational level, life within a family, and labor condition, and the aforementioned EQ-5D variables, or between time since surgery and the development of depression or anxiety. Main statistical relationships are listed in Table 46.1.

Table 46.1. Statistical relationship between different variables characterizing HRQOL

Relationship between:	Statistical significance
Pain/>6 months from surgery	No
Pain/type of surgery	No
Pain/mobility problems	Yes
Pain/daily life functioning	Yes
Pain/age	No
Pain/anxiety–depression	No
Age/anxiety–depression	Yes
Age/mobility problems	Yes
Depression/mobility problems	Yes
Depression/daily life functioning	Yes
Anxiety/mobility problems	No
Anxiety/daily life functioning	No

46.7 Usefulness of Health-related Quality of Life Evaluation

In a usual approach, efficacy of therapeutic results is basically recognized through changes in clinical signs and symptoms. Incorporating HRQOL measures implies that the patient's perspective becomes another source of useful information about the effects of medical treatments. These are evaluated by the patients themselves who will judge, according to their expectations, understanding, values, and beliefs, the relative benefits that have been reached. The adaptation, attitudes, and behaviors of participation and compliance during curative and rehabilitation processes will depend on the subjective aspects to which the medical practice should not be indifferent.

The specialist and his/her team may have in fact already considered this perspective, and that is a frequent attitude. Then the HRQOL vision adds nothing from a conceptual point of view, but does add from a methodological aspect by making this a systematic process through the use of standardized procedures that examine the impact of illness on different aspects of people's lives. The lack of this type of information about the patients' perceptions hinders our understanding of their needs in terms of care which, integrally taken into account, would increase the efficacy and efficiency of the results.

According to its aim, medical care may be considered as: (a) an intervention designed to improve the health status and to reduce the risk of mortality, impairment, or morbidity; (b) rehabilitation, approximating the real physical, psychological, and social functional level to the potential one; (c) palliative, reducing physical pain and psychological malaise; and (d) health promoting and an enhancer of the personal and social resources of people under treatments. The latter may be simultaneously present with any of the other options and all options may combine into a selected strategy.

Once the major (in relative terms) aspects of the impact of illness and treatment have been identified, the task of an interdisciplinary health team will be to apply programs where the principal aim is the improvement or maintenance of the HRQOL from the afflicted person's point of view.

Our experience agrees with this postulate. On the one hand, lung cancer resection is correlated with a good HRQOL (average 81 points in the visual analogue scale); residual pain or surgery-related discomfort is not significant 6 months postoperatively; and morbidity sensation and feelings of anxiety/depression are significantly linked with aging and so, not necessarily with surgery. On the other hand, the HRQOL tests lead us to detect 17.5% of anxiety and 22% of depression symptoms, both unsuspected through the usual clinical follow-up. Those patients were then referred to the specialists.

In an elderly population (57% of the patients were older than 65 years) it is important to point out that 35% (26/74 cases) are working full-time after lung cancer resection. We did not find social, economic, or educational differences in perception of postsurgical clinical or psychological morbidities as suggested by others [54, 55].

In contrast to other published opinions [2,3 7], the addition of HRQOL evaluation encourages surgical treatment of lung cancer and constitutes, at the same time, a useful tool for improving care to the resected patient.

Acknowledgements

The authors acknowledge Professor Nicholas P. Rossi, M.D. (University of Iowa Hospitals and Clinics) for his important help in turning the manuscript into a better English paper.

Key Points

- Health-related quality of life (HRQOL) testing highlights the patients' point of view about the results of lung cancer resection. It should constitute part of regular follow-up.
- The majority of our patients acknowledged a good HRQOL 6 months after lung cancer surgery.
- Self-administered HRQOL questionnaires are useful to detect probable depression/anxiety usually unseen through clinical follow-up. This should be confirmed and treated by specialists.
- The addition of HRQOL evaluation encourages surgical treatment of lung malignancies, providing better care of the resected patient.

References

1. Bullinger M, Alonso J, Apolone G, et al. Translating health status questionnaires and evaluating their quality: the IQUOLA project approach. International quality of life assessment. J Clin Epidemiol 1998; 51:913.
2. Handy JR, Aspa JW, Skokan L, et al. What happens to patients undergoing lung cancer surgery? Chest 2002; 122:21.
3. Esteva H. Surgery in lung cancer patients. Chest 2004; 126:656.
4. Schipper H, et al. Measuring quality of life of cancer patients: the functional living index-cancer: development and validation. J Clin Oncol 1984; 2:472.
5. Leyenson V, Furukawa S, Kuzma AM, et al. Correlation of changes in quality of life after lung volume reduction surgery with changes in lung function, exercise and gas exchange. Chest 2000; 118:728.
6. Yoshimura H. Quality of life (QOL) versus curability for lung cancer surgery. Ann Thorac Cardiovasc Surg 2001; 7:127.
7. Rajmil L, Estrada MD, Herdman M, et al. Calidad de vida relacionada con la salud (CVRS) en la infancia y adolescencia: revisión de la bibliografía y de los instrumentos adaptados en Espaa. Gac Sanit 2001; 15:34.
8. WHOQOL Group. The World Health Organization Quality of Life Assessment (WHOQOL): position paper from the World Health Organization. Soc Sci Med 1995; 41:1403.
9. Johansen J, Overgaard J, Rose C. Cosmetic outcome and breast morbidity in breast counseling treatment. Acta Oncol 2002; 41:369.
10. Casaburi R. Exercise training in chronic obstructive lung disease. In: Casaburi R, Petty TL (eds) Principles and Practice of Pulmonary Rehabilitation. Philadelphia: Saunders, 1993.
11. McKenna RJ, Gelb A, Brenner M. Lung volume reduction surgery for chronic obstructive pulmonary disease: where do we stand. World J Surg 2001; 25:231.
12. Goldstein AS, Todd TRJ, Guyat G, et al. Chronic obstructive pulmonary disease. Influence of lung volume reduction surgery (LVRS) on health related quality of life in patients with chronic obstructive pulmonary disease. Thorax 2003; 58:405.
13. Hamacher J, Buchi S, Georgesan CL, et al. Improved quality of life after lung volume reduction surgery. Eur Respir J 2002; 19:54.
14. Guyatt GH, Bombardier C, Tugwell P. Measuring disease-specific quality of life in clinical trials. Can Med Assoc J 1986; 134:889.
15. Flanagan JC. A research approach to improving our quality of life. Am Psychol 1978; 33:138.
16. Anderson KL. The effect of chronic obstructive pulmonary disease on quality of life. Res Nurs Health 1995; 18:547.
17. Bergner M, Bobbitt RA, Carter WB, et al. The Sickness Impact Profile: development and final revision of a health status measure. Med Care 1981; 19:787.
18. Jenkinson C, Fitspatrick R, Argyle M. The Nottingham Health Profile: an analysis of its sensitivity in differentiating illness groups. Soc Sci Med 1988; 27:1411.
19. Ware JE, Kosinski M, Gandek B. Health Survey, Manual and Interpretation Guide. Lincoln, RI: Quality Metric, 2003:37.
20. Gandek B, Ware JE, Aaronson NK, et al. Test of data quality, scaling assumptions and reliability of the SF-36 in eleven countries: results from the IQOLA project. J Clin Epidemiol 1998; 51:1149.
21. EuroQol Group. EuroQol: a new facility for the measurement of health-related quality of life. Health Policy 1990; 16:199.
22. Stahl E, Jansson SA, et al. Health-related quality of life, utility, and productivity outcomes instruments: ease of completion by subjects with COPD. Health Quality of Life Outcomes 2003; 1:18.
23. Aaronson NK, Ahmedzai S, Bergman B, et al. The European Organization for Research and Treatment of Cancer QLQ-C30: a quality-of-life instrument for use in international clinical trials in oncology. J Natl Cancer Inst 1993; 85:365.
24. Bergman B, Aaronson NK, Ahmedzai S, Kaasa S, Sullivan M. The EORTC QLQ-LC13: a modular supplement to the EORTC Core Quality of Life Questionnaire (QLQ-C30) for use in lung cancer clinical trials. Eur J Cancer 1994; 30A:635.
25. Cella DF, Tulsky DS, Gray G, et al. The Functional Assessment of Cancer Therapy Scale: development and validation of the general measure. J Clin Oncol 1993; 11:570.
26. Guyatt GH, Berman LB, Townsend M, Puglsey SO, Chambers LW. A measure of quality of life for clinical trials in chronic lung disease. Thorax 1987; 42:773.

27. Redelmeier DA, Guyatt GH, Goldstein RS. Assessing the minimal important difference in symptoms: a comparison of two techniques. J Clin Epidemiol 1996; 49:1215.
28. Jones PW, Quirk FH, Baveystock CM. The St. George's Respiratory Questionnaire. Resp Med 1991; 85(suppl):25.
29. Esteva H, Luna CA, Loterzo A, et al. Predictive capacity of risk indices in pulmonary resections. S Am J Thorac Surg 1995; 1:11.
30. Esteva H, Marchevsky A, Núñez T, et al. Neural networks as a prognostic tool of surgical risk in lung resections. Ann Thorac Surg 2002; 73:1576.
31. Esteva H, Mazzei JA, Newton A. Toracotomía y función respiratoria. Rev Argent Cirug 1990; 60:63.
32. Esteva H, Mazzei JA, Salamanco J. Función respiratoria luego de las resecciones pulmonares. La Prensa Médica Arg 1985; 72:11.
33. Hallfeldt KJ, Siebeck M, Thetter O, Schweiberer L. The effect of thoracic surgery on pulmonary function. Am J Crit Care 1995; 4:352.
34. Esteva H, Cervio RC. Complicaciones Quirrgicas. In: Esteva H, (ed) Prevención y manejo de las complicaciones de la Cirugia Torácica. Buenos Aires: EDUCA, 2003:123.
35. Nezu K, Kushibe K, Tojo T, Takahama M, Kitamura S. Recovery and limitation of exercise capacity after lung resection for lung cancer. Chest 1998; 113:1511.
36. Pelletier C, Lapoint L, Le Blanc P. Effects of lung resection on pulmonary function and exercise capacity. Thorax 1990; 45:497.
37. Chen JC, Johnstone SA. Quality of life after lung cancer surgery (Editorial). Chest 2002; 122:4.
38. Barsky A, Goodson J, et al. The amplification of somatic symptoms. Psychosom Med 1988; 50:513.
39. Lekander M, Elofsson S, et al. Self-rated health is related to levels of circulating cytokines. Psychosom Med 2004; 66:559.
40. Kelley K, Bluthe R. Cytokine-induced sickness behavior. Brain Behav Immun 2003; 17:S112.
41. Cella D, Perry S. Depression and physical illness. In: Mann J (ed) Phenomenology of Depressive Illness. New York: Human Science Press, 1988:220.
42. Holland J. Psychological care of patients: psycho-oncology's contribution. J Clin Oncol 2003; 21:S253.
43. Schulberg H, Katon W, Rush A. Treating major depression in primary care practice: an update of the Agency for Health Care Policy and Research practice guidelines. Arch Gen Psychiatry 1998; 55:1121.
44. Silverstone P, Lernay T, et al. The prevalence of major depressive disorder and low self-esteem in medical inpatients. Can J Psychiatry 1996; 41:67.
45. Gaynes B, Burns B, et al. Depression and health related quality of life. J Nerv Ment Dis 2002; 190:799.
46. Ruo B, Whooley M. Depression and health related quality of life. JAMA 2003; 290:2404.
47. Whooley M. Depression and medical illness (Letter). Ann Epidemiol 1999; 9:281.
48. Kremer B. Quality of life scales in allergic rhinitis. Curr Opin Allergy Clin Immunol 2004; 4:171.
49. Beck A, Steer R, Garbin M. Psychometric properties of the Beck Depression Inventory: twenty-five years of evaluation. Clin Psychol Rev 1998; 8:77.
50. Wilkinson M, Barczak P. Hospital Anxiety and Depression Scale. Psychiatric screening in general practice: comparison of the general health questionnaire and the hospital anxiety depression scale. J R Coll Gen Pract 1988; 38:311.
51. Ramos-Brieva JA, Cordero A. Validación de la versión castellana de la escala de Hamilton para la depresión. Actas Luso-Esp Neurol Psiquiatr 1986; 14:324.
52. Brooks R, with the EuroQOL Group. EuroQOL: the current state of play. Health Policy 1996; 37:53.
53. Badia X, Schiaffino A, Alonso J, et al. Using the EQ-5D in the Catalan general population: feasibility and construct validity. Qual Life Res 1998; 7:311.
54. Montazeri A, Hole DJ, Milroy R, et al. Quality of life in lung cancer patients: does socioeconomic status matter? Health and Quality of Life Outcomes 2003; 1:1.
55. Uchitomi Y, Mikami I, Nagai K, et al. Depression and psychological distress in patients during the year alter curative resection of non-small-cell lung cancer. J Clin Oncol 2003; 21:69.

Pain Management in Palliative Care

47

Eleni Plaisia and Konstantinos N. Syrigos

Contents

47.1 Introduction

Pain often accompanies cancer. Some 20–50% of cancer patients suffer pain at the time of diagnosis and approximately 75% in the terminal stage [1, 2]. This means that every day over four million people are afflicted with cancer-related pain, most of whom do not obtain adequate relief [3].

The main reasons for ineffective pain relief are the following [1]:

- The lack of information on the pain relief methods already established
- The lack of systematic teaching of this subject to medical students and other healthcare professionals
- Poor doctor–patient communication
- The patient's lack of communication with his family and others close to him
- The unavailability of the required analgesics
- The fears and prejudices of both healthcare professionals and patients, along with those close to them, as regards the therapeutic use of opioids
- Legal restrictions on prescribing of opioids
- The lack of interest shown by competent authorities

Cancer pain may be due to [4]:

1. *The presence of the disease* (60–70%). Bone metastasis is the most common cause of pain directly related to cancer. Pressure on and infiltration of the nerves or plexuses, infiltration of soft tissues, skin, or mu-

cosa, or infiltration of the viscera are some of the causes of pain due to the disease.

2. *Treatment for the disease* (20%). Surgery, chemotherapy, radiotherapy, and other various procedures for diagnosis and stabilization of the disease cause pain:
   a) Painful neuropathy may develop after any surgical operation, but most frequently following thoracotomy, mastectomy, or lymph node debridement. Amputees may also develop stump pain or "phantom limb pain."
   b) Chemotherapy may cause stomatitis, venous thrombosis, tissue necrosis, and myalgia, or arthralgia (from the discontinuing use of cortisone).
   c) Radiotherapy may cause painful inflammation in any mucosa under treatment, painful neuropathy months or years after radiotherapy, or painful myelopathy following irradiation of the spine.

3. *Causes directly or indirectly related to the disease and its treatment* (>10%). Some patients develop pain due to debilitation and disability caused by the disease or to various side effects of analgesics. Examples of this are:
   a) Myalgia caused by immobility or by unaccustomed activity
   b) Thromboembolic episodes
   c) Stomatitis
   d) Postherpetic neuralgia
   e) Reflux esophagitis
   f) Gastric distension
   g) Constipation
   h) Bladder spasms (from catheterization), etc.

4. *Causes unrelated to the disease and its treatment* (<10%). A small percentage of patients suffer from pain that is unrelated to the disease and is usually due to:
   a) Various forms of arthritis
   b) Ischemic cardiopathy
   c) Peripheral vascular disease

The perception of pain is, however, affected by many other factors: physical, psychological, social, cultural, and intellectual. Cicely Saunders has introduced the concept of "total pain," which is the sum of all these factors, to emphasize the complex nature of pain and the need to view it as being the total of multiple factors. Inversely, if we add pain to all these factors along with their interaction, the concept of "total suffering" is introduced. Thus, effective pain management requires the evaluation of all the other factors as well, and the treatment must be part of a well-coordinated comprehensive care plan. This need has led to the concept of *clinical pain*, which is what the patient describes and what must be treated; represents the interaction between various other causes of the patient's suffering and the perception of pain; and, lastly, stresses the fact that the evaluation of the other factors constitutes a clinical necessity.

Therefore, the basic principle for effective pain relief is that a full evaluation of its cause must be made, always bearing in mind that most people have more than one type of pain and that different types of pain need to be dealt with in different ways. With proper evaluation and a systematic approach to the choice of analgesics, more than 80% of cancer patients can find relief with the use of inexpensive medication and methods.

The therapeutic options could be summed up as follows:

- Treatment of the underlying disease
- The pharmaceutical approach
- Invasive, with anesthesiological and neurosurgical methods
- Non-invasive and non-pharmaceutical approaches, such as TENS, acupuncture, physical therapy, psychotherapy, etc.
- Palliative, with surgery, chemotherapy, and radiation therapy

Different kinds of pain respond differently to various treatments. Thus, in practice, combinations of various treatment plans are often used.

47.2 The Pharmaceutical Approach

Today, managing cancer pain pharmaceutically constitutes the cornerstone of treatment. It is effective, entails relatively little risk, is not costly, and usually works quickly. Various categories of drugs are used: non-opioid analgesics (aspirin, paracetamol, non-steroidal antiinflammatory drugs [NSAIDS]), opioids, and adjuvant drugs (corticoids, antidepressants, anticonvulsants, anxiolytics, NMDA receptor antagonists, etc.).

Drugs are selected based on the WHO analgesic scale (Fig. 47.1). It is suggested that when implementing the scale, drugs should be replaced by those in the same category before moving on to another stage in the scale. But, for effective drug treatment, the following general principles should be taken into account:

1. The dose should be adequate.

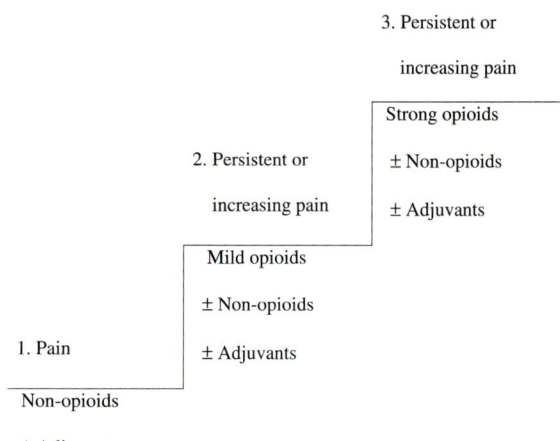

Fig. 47.1. Selection scale of analgesic drugs suggested by the World Health Organization

2. The dosage should be titrated for each patient.
3. Each drug should be administered according to its pharmacological properties.
4. Drugs are administered at regular intervals rather than when pain occurs.
5. Instructions are given for breakthrough pain management.
6. Information is given and medication administered to manage side effects.
7. Written instructions are provided.
8. The simplest methods for administering medication are used when possible.
9. The analgesic regimen is maintained at the simplest level possible.
10. The effectiveness and safety of the treatment are rechecked and reassessed.

47.2.1 Non-opioid Analgesics

The term non-opioid analgesic is used to denote aspirin, paracetamol, and NSAIDS. They are effective in relieving moderate pain and act in synergy with opioids when the latter are administered for moderate to severe pain, which helps to reduce dosages and thus side effects. The non-opioid analgesics all have a ceiling effect for their painkilling action with many similarities in their action mechanism, side effects, and toxicity.

47.2.2 Opioid Analgesics

The main category of analgesics consists of the opioids, which are used to manage moderate to severe pain. They are effective, easily titrated, and have an extremely satisfactory risk–benefit ratio.

In addition to the analgesia they produce, opioids have other effects on the central nervous system as well as on other systems. Most of these effects are undesirable, most notably:

1. *Respiratory depression*, which is rare in patients suffering pain.
2. *Drowsiness*, which is common with opioid use. It may result from the direct action of the drug, but is also due to the pain relief and a reduced perception of external stimuli. In any case, it usually subsides after several days have elapsed.
3. *Confusion and hallucinations.*
4. *Nausea and vomiting*, which, when opioids are systematically administered, are usually short-lived undesirable effects.

Their manifestation and duration depend on the dosage, the routes of administration, and the type of opioid used, but also the patient's receptivity. These effects are dealt with on a case-by-case basis and by changing the opioid used if the effects persist.

When normal therapeutic doses are used, the effects of opioids on the cardiovascular system are minimal. *Constipation constitutes the most common and persistent undesirable effect of opioids.* This should be considered to be a fact and it should be prevented. The administration of mild laxatives before bedtime usually proves to be a sufficient preventive measure. Furthermore, spasms of the expulsive muscle of the bladder along with the external sphincter can result in urgency for micturition and inability to urinate. Urinary retention is more common in men and more frequent after epidural administration.

The undesirable effects that have given rise to the myths and fear of opioid use (opiophobia) are related mainly to three specific phenomena, namely:

1. Tolerance
2. Physical dependence
3. Psychological dependence and addiction

Tolerance to opioids rarely appears in clinical practice. The increase in patients' demands for opioids usually indicates the progress of the disease rather than tolerance. Nor does physical dependence constitute a problem when the dosage is increased or decreased gradually (20–50%) every 2–3 days. Iatrogenically caused addiction is extremely rare and even full discontinuation is possible without side effects [5, 6].

The opioid selected is based on its pharmacodynamics, pharmacokinetics, and half-life, as well as the pathophysiology, intensity, and nature of the pain in question. Steady, constant pain is best managed when the plasma levels of the drug remain stable. Thus it is particularly important to adhere to a schedule in administering opioids. Controlled-release substances present the advantage of maintaining the concentration of the drug without much variation, thus achieving constant action at therapeutic (analgesic) levels. Implementing p.r.n. dosage is very useful in the management of incident and breakthrough pain. Useful substances for this are those with rapid actions such as water soluble morphine and transmucosal system fentanyl.

Finally, a significant factor in drug selection is the patient's previous experience. Effective pain relief does not, however, depend on the type of substance used alone, but also on the route of administration. Today, opioids may be administered by many routes: sublingually, through the oral and nasal mucosa, orally, rectally, intramuscularly, intravenously, subcutaneously, intraspinally, transdermally (TTS fentanyl), and intraventricularly (intracephalically). For terminal stage patients, WHO scale third-stage drugs are used. In our country, slow-release morphine tablets are used to this end as well as the fentanyl transdermal therapeutic system. Transdermal fentanyl presents quite a few advantages compared to slow-release morphine tablets. Nausea and constipation are less frequent, while the 3-day intervals between patch changes release the patient considerably from adhering to a strict daily medication schedule. As shown by many studies, this form of the drug is far more easily accepted by the patient [1]. Finally, the development of PCA techniques has made possible the widespread use of intraspinal, intravenous, and subcutaneous administration of opioids. This notwithstanding, invasive routes should be chosen only after the failure of other methods [7].

47.2.3 Adjuvants to Analgesics

The term "adjuvant" signifies a drug whose primary indication is not pain relief but which acts as an analgesic in certain painful states. It is usually administered along with traditional painkillers and makes it possible to manage pain that fails to respond adequately to traditional analgesics, to reduce the dosage of analgesics and thus their side effects, and to manage symptoms other than pain (Table 47.1).

Table 47.1. Main indications of the most common adjuvant drugs

Drug	Indications
NSAIDS	Bone pain Soft tissue infiltration Hepatomegaly
Corticosteroids	Increased intracranial pressure Soft tissue infiltration Nerve compression
Antidepressants	Nerve compression or infiltration
Anticonvulsants	Paraneoplastic neuropathies
Antiarrhythmics	Intractable neuropathic pain
Bisphosphonates	Bone pain

Adjuvants to analgesics are the antidepressants, anticonvulsives, corticosteroids, β-2 agonists (clonidine), ketamine, calcitonin, neuroleptics, anxiolytics, sedatives, local anesthetics, muscle relaxants, bisphosphonates, antihistamines, hemotherapeutic drugs, radiation, and hormones.

Dexamethasone (4–6 mg) is the corticosteroid of choice, while the preferred antidepressants are the *selective serotonin reuptake inhibitors* (SSRI) and *noradrenaline* (SNRI) because they entail fewer side effects, but they are less effective than the tricyclic antidepressants. Of the anticonvulsives, *gabapentin* is very effective and causes the fewest side effects, while not interacting with other drugs [8]. In addition, the NMDA receptor antagonist *ketamine* may be very useful as, at subclinical dosages, it enhances the analgesic action of opioids, helping to make it possible to decrease the doses of the latter and thus their side effects [9]. The *benzodiazepines* (mainly diazepam, oxazepam, and lorazepam) are often used for advanced cancer patients. They have no analgesic action but their anxiolytic action benefits the patients. Diazepam is particularly useful in patients afflicted with muscular spasms or acute myoskeletal pain. Their most frequent side effects are drowsiness, weakness, and orthostatic hypotension.

Neuroleptic drugs such as chlorpromazine and haloperidol have no analgesic action but can be used to reduce anxiety or to improve nocturnal sleep. Benzodiazepines have the same effect but without the anticholinergic and extrapyramidal side effects of neuroleptics. Their main indication for using them is to manage nausea and vomiting, and even delirium, which cannot be managed otherwise. Moreover, they can be used in cases of intractable neuropathic pain. *Psychostimulant substances* such as amphetamines and methylphenidate may help in decreasing opioid-related depression and in making adequate analgesia possible without intolerable side effects. Tachyphylaxis and tolerance may appear but at larger doses, and elderly patients more commonly show distress.

Palliative radiotherapy is more effective for pain due to local infiltration and should be applied at the lowest possible dosage. *Palliative chemotherapy* may be applied to chemosensitive tumors, provided that the toxicity it triggers is manageable. The same holds for palliative hormone therapy. In general, the use of these palliative relief methods must be weighed against the benefits of the aforementioned relief in relation to their side effects and the patient's overall quality of life [7].

47.3 Invasive Methods

Nerve blockade may be used to block or modify the feeling of pain during the transmission from the pain source to the central nervous system. It is indicated for the treatment of localized pain and is more effective for somatic and visceral pain than for neuropathic pain. *Peripheral blocks* may be diagnostic, prognostic, and therapeutic. Diagnostic nerve blockade is used to ascertain which nerve or nerves are responsible for the pain and to further differentially diagnose somatic from visceral pain. *Prognostic nerve blockade* is not only carried out to evaluate the analgesia that has been produced, but also to permit the patient to experience it temporarily before deciding on having the block on a more permanent basis. *Therapeutic nerve blockade* may be temporary, prophylactic, or permanent. *Temporary blockade* is achieved with the application of a local anesthetic for the relief of acute pain before other treatments are used. *Prophylactic blockade* is used when a local recurrence of the disease is expected to cause severe pain. *Permanent nerve blockade* should be attempted only when preceded by a prognostic block with a local anesthetic. The neurolytic agents used are alcohol (25–50%) or phenol (3–5%). The most frequent point indicated for a permanent blockade is the intercostal nerves, where the loss of other neurological functions is not compromised.

Intraspinal blocks include the infusion of a local anesthetic or neurolytic agents in the epidural or subarachnoid space for the relief of severe pain. The infusion of a local anesthetic in the epidural space produces excellent analgesia. A permanent catheter can be placed at the desired level, fixed subcutaneously, and connected to a reservoir or provided with a continuous infusion pump. Today a combination of various drugs, such as local anesthetics and opioids, offers the best results while avoiding neurolysis. The implantation of catheters with pumps in the epidural or subarachnoid space solves the problems associated with this method. However, their use in patients with malignant disease depends on expected survival time (at least 3 months). The infusion of neurolytic substances such as alcohol or phenol in the epidural or subarachnoid space has virtually been abandoned as a method due to its unacceptable side effects. The administration of a mixture of a local anesthetic and opioids provides a more superior solution for effective analgesia without the associated risks [2].

In *neurostimulatory techniques*, stimulation of the SCS is achieved by the electrical excitation of the posterior bundles of the spinal cord through electrodes placed epidurally. Although this mechanism which produces analgesia remains undetermined, stimulation of the spinal cord brings considerable pain relief in selected patients (e.g. phantom limb pain, pain from peripheral nerve damage, ischemic pain, etc.). Unfortunately, this method has not yet been established for patients suffering from cancer-related pain.

Neuroamputive techniques include:

1. Chordotomy: surgical destruction of the spinothalamic tract
2. Rhizotomy: destruction of the spinal roots

3. Ganglionectomy: excision of the ganglia of the posterior roots

Neurosurgical methods are indicated only when other methods have failed or are not compliant by the patient.

Intraventricular opioid infusion involves the placing of a catheter intracephalically, or intraventricularly, with a subcutaneous reservoir. The advantage of this method is that a much smaller opioid dose (< 5 mg) is given.

Today, neurosurgical techniques have, to a great extent, been replaced by intraspinal opioid infusion techniques, local anesthetics, and a combination of other drugs. Most importantly, the use of invasive techniques is only confined to patients who have not responded well to other techniques and continually exhibit refractory side effects.

47.4 Non-pharmaceutical, Non-invasive Methods

These comprise two large categories: the natural methods and the psychosocial methods.

Natural methods have a place in cancer pain treatment and sometimes it is the patients themselves who request their application. Massage and pressure may help patients by diverting their attention or relaxing them. Massage should not replace exercise in ambulant patients. Exercise strengthens weak muscles, mobilizes ligaments, and enhances the patient's relief. It must be done with great care or be avoided in phases of severe pain. In cases of bone metastasis, careful attention is indicated.

The application of heat with warm compresses, white or infrared light, and hydrotherapy may provide relief from pain due to muscular spasm and/or muscular weakness commonly associated with the disease. It can cause bone damage and should not be applied to areas with ischemia or hypoesthesia, or to inflamed areas, or over malignant processes.

Cryotherapy has the same topical effect and indications as heat, yet its analgesic effects last longer. It is implemented using cold compresses, ice, and freezing sprays (ethyl chloride). It should not be applied in areas where there is vascular disease or on tissues damaged by radiotherapy.

Although its analgesic action may be due in part to the placebo effect, transcutaneous electrical nerve stimulation (TENS) can be tried. Certain patients may benefit from its use.

Acupuncture is also used for pain relief, despite the fact that its role in relieving cancer pain has not been clarified. In any case, it is a relatively cheap and safe method which may lead to a decrease in analgesic needs.

Psychosocial methods constitute an important part of the polyvalent approach to pain management. They help in giving the patient a feeling of control and in developing the capacity to deal with his/her disease. If they are integrated at the onset of the disease, when the patient is still adequately strong and active, they can be highly successful throughout the course of the disease. The most common techniques are *behavioral* therapy and *cognitive* therapy. In behavioral therapy, the objective is to help patients recognize and change aspects of their behavior and disposition which may exacerbate their pain. The aim in cognitive therapy is to change the way pain is experienced, thereby modifying various cognitive variables (such as belief systems, life stances, expectations, etc.).

In conclusion, treating cancer-related pain is never easy. It demands careful attention and understanding, as well as a persistent approach to alleviate its enigma, especially when the pain is intractable. However, it is believed that the relief from pain and its misery can, in fact, be achieved by a great majority of patients.

Key Points

- Some 20–50% of lung cancer patients suffer pain at the time of diagnosis and approximately 75% of them in the terminal stage.
- Cancer pain may be due to the presence of the disease, treatment for the disease, or unrelated causes.
- Different kinds of pain respond differently to various treatments. Thus, in practice, combinations of various treatment plans are often used.
- Treating cancer-related pain demands careful attention and understanding, as well as a persistent approach to alleviate its enigma, especially when the pain is intractable. However, it is believed that the relief from pain and its misery can, in fact, be achieved by a great majority of patients.

References

1. Twycross RG. The fight against pain. *Ann Oncol* 1994; 5:111.
2. Bonica JJ. Cancer pain: current status and future needs. In: Bonica JJ (ed) *The Management of Pain*, 2nd edn. Philadelphia: Lea & Febiger, 1990; 400.
3. World Health Organization Expert Committee Report. *Cancer Pain Relief and Palliative Care. (Technical report series no. 804)*. Geneva: WHO, 1990.
4. World Health Organization. *Cancer Pain Relief*, 2nd edn. Geneva: WHO, 1996.
5. Joranson DE, Ryan KM, Gilson AM, Dahl JL. Trends in medical use and abuse of opioid analgesics. *JAMA* 2000; 283:1710.

6. Zenz M, Willewewbwe Strumpf A. Opiophobia and cancer pain in Europe. *Lancet* 1993; 341:1075.

7. Portenoy RK, Lesage P. Management of cancer pain. *Lancet* 1999; 353:1695.

8. Mao J, Chen L. Gabapentin in pain management. *Anesth Analg* 2000; 91:680.

9. Mercantante S. Ketamine in cancer pain: an update. *Palliat Med* 1996; 10:225.

Pathophysiology and Management of Bone Metastases in Lung Cancer

48

Evangelos Terpos and Konstantinos N. Syrigos

Contents

48.1   Introduction

The most common cause of death worldwide from a malignant disease is due to lung cancer. Lung cancer frequently metastasizes either locally to the lungs or distally to the bone, liver, kidney, or the systemic lymph nodes. More than 90% of deaths from lung cancer can be attributed to metastases [1]. At autopsies, it has been shown that up to 50% of patients with lung cancer have evidence of skeletal metastasis. More than 33% of patients with advanced lung cancer manifest bone metastases. Worldwide, it is estimated that the 5-year prevalence of bony metastatic disease, as a complication of lung cancer, is in the order of 1,394,000 cases, with an estimated incidence of 30–65% [2].

How long the patient lives with the tumor is likely to influence whether bone metastasis will occur. Bone metastases, often arising in load-bearing bones, present as therapeutic challenges, especially when they are present in the neck or shaft of the femur, or in the pelvis [3]. Bone destruction leads to bone pain, hypercalcemia, nerve compression syndromes, and sometimes pathological fractures. It reduces the quality of life and performance status of these patients [4, 5]. These complications frequently require surgery to correct fractures or spinal deformities, as well as radiation to palliate the severe bone pain that is a hallmark of bone metastases [6]. Furthermore, when tumor cells metastasize to bone they are usually incurable. The median survival after the first skeletal-related event (SRE) in lung cancer patients with bone metastases is only 4.1 months [7].

The cost for the management of bone complications in lung cancer is often devastating for many countries. The estimated lifetime SRE-related cost per patient is approximately \$12,000 [7]. Therefore, the prevention and treatment of osteolytic bone metastases in lung cancer are pertinent in the management of the disease.

48.2   Overview of Bone Function and Remodeling

The skeleton provides the mechanical support of the body and a reservoir for normal mineral metabolism. Bone is an active tissue, constantly remodeling and metabolically changing through the balanced activity of osteoclasts and osteoblasts on trabecular surfaces. On a microscopic level, bone metabolism always occurs on the surface of the bone at a particular site called the bone metabolism unit (BMU).

Osteoclasts and osteoblasts are cells that carry out bone metabolism at these specialized BMU sites. Although these cells account for only a small fraction of bone volume, their function is essential [8]. Bone turnover is always initiated by osteoclasts which erode the

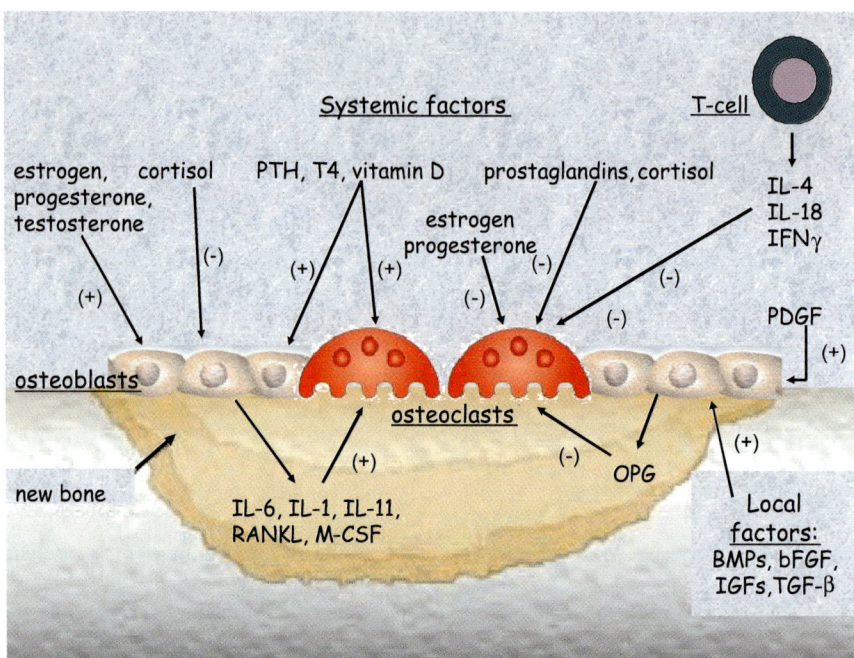

Fig. 48.1. Regulation of bone remodeling. Systemic factors can enhance the proliferation and differentiation of osteoblasts. These include parathyroid hormone, estrogen, progesterone, prostaglandins, and cytokines as well as growth factors produced by circulating lymphocytes, such as platelet-derived growth factor (*PDGF*). Furthermore, locally produced growth factors can also enhance the osteoblast proliferation and function, including bone morphogenetic proteins (*BMPs*), insulin-like growth factors (*IGFs*), fibroblast growth factors (*FGFs*), and transforming growth factor-beta (*TGF-β*). In contrast, corticosteroids can induce apoptosis of osteoblasts and block bone formation. Both systemic factors and locally produced factors also induce the formation and activity of osteoclasts. Osteoclastogenesis requires contact between osteoclast precursors and stromal cells or osteoblasts. Systemic hormones such as

parathyroid hormone (*PTH*), 1,25-dihydroxyvitamin D$_3$, and thyroxine (T$_4$) stimulate the formation of osteoclasts by upregulating the expression of receptor activator of nuclear factor-κB ligand (*RANKL*) on the surface of marrow stromal cells and immature osteoblasts. RANKL then binds its receptor, RANK, on the surface of osteoclast precursors to induce the formation of osteoclasts and promote osteoclast survival. In addition to RANK, a decoy receptor, osteoprotegerin (*OPG*), inhibits RANKL binding to RANK. The ratio of RANKL to OPG determines the level of osteoclastogenesis. Osteoblasts also produce interleukin (*IL*)-6, IL-1, prostaglandins, and macrophage colony-stimulating factor (*M-CSF*), which induce the formation of osteoclasts. Conversely, T cells can produce cytokines, such as IL-4, IL-18, and interferon-γ (*IFN-γ*), that can inhibit the formation of osteoclasts

mineralized surface. After their activation by different factors (mechanical load, growth factors, hormones, and cytokines), osteoclasts are attracted to the new BMU site where they erode the bone matrix, forming a lacuna. Resorption is then halted.

Osteoblasts are then recruited to the outer edge of the erosion cavity where they secrete the organic matrix of the new bone called osteoid. Unmineralized osteoid gradually fills in the cavity. Soon after the lacuna is filled, this newly formed matrix is then mineralized with calcium hydroxyapatite. This gives the BMU its tensile strength [9]. Osteoblasts become trapped as osteocytes in spaces called lacunae in the matrix. Between adjacent lacunae and the central canal are cytoplasmic extensions of the osteocytes. Osteocytes are responsible for the maintenance of the bone matrix. Figure 48.1 depicts the normal bone resorption and formation process.

48.2.1 Osteoclasts

Osteoclasts are multinucleated cells, formed from the fusion of mononuclear progenitors of the monocyte/macrophage family [10]. Osteoclasts resorb bone by secreting proteases that dissolve the organic matrix and by producing organic acids that dissolve bone mineral into the extracellular space under the ruffled border of their plasma membrane [11].

Osteoclastogenesis requires contact between osteoclast precursors and stromal cells or osteoblasts. The adherence of osteoclasts to the bone surface is critical for the bone resorptive process, since agents that interfere with osteoclast attachment, such as cathepsin K, block bone resorption [12]. Osteoblasts produce a few factors that influence osteoclast activity. They are the macrophage colony-stimulating factor (M-CSF), the receptor activator of nuclear factor-κB (RANK) ligand

(RANKL), and osteoprotegerin (OPG). RANKL is a member of the family of tumor necrosis factors [13].

Macrophage colony-stimulating factor is produced by osteoblasts but promotes osteoclast survival and differentiation by binding to a receptor, c-FMS, on early osteoclast precursors. M-CSF expands the pool of osteoclast precursors while RANKL stimulates the osteoclast to commit to a particular phenotype. RANKL is a type II transmembrane glycoprotein expressed on the surface of osteoblast cells. Its soluble form, sRANKL, can be released from its membrane-bound state with the mediation of metalloproteinases [14]. RANKL is a ligand which binds to the RANK receptor on osteoclast precursors and induces a maturation of the osteoclasts by initiating the nuclear factor-κB and Jun N-terminal kinase pathways. These pathways are responsible for the differentiation and activation of the osteoclast into a mature, functional cell.

Stromal cells and osteoblasts are often the target cells of most osteoclastogenic factors that exert their effect by enhancing RANKL expression. Substances, such as parathyroid hormone (PTH), thyroxine, 1,25-dihydroxyvitamin D_3, and cytokines (which use gp130 as part of their receptor, such as interleukin [IL]-6 and oncostatin M), act on these target cells producing osteoclastic activity via RANKL expression [15, 16].

Osteoprotegerin appears to play a role in competing against the RANK receptor for the RANK ligand. It is a member of the tumor necrosis factor receptor family and is secreted by stromal cells as well as osteoblasts. Essentially, it is a decoy receptor for RANKL. OPG blocks the RANKL–RANK interaction by allowing an alternative binding site and thus inhibits osteoclast differentiation and activation [17, 18]. The importance of RANK/RANKL/OPG interactions in the formation of osteoclasts has been demonstrated clearly in mice. Mice that lack either RANKL or RANK, or overexpress OPG develop osteopetrosis due to the decreased osteoclast activity [14, 19]. In addition, mice that lack OPG develop osteoporosis, multiple fractures, a decrease in trabecular bone volume, and an increase in osteoclasts. This proves that OPG plays a role in the regulation of RANK/RANKL, preventing the overactivity of osteoclasts [20].

Therefore, it can be concluded that the intricate balance between the expression of RANKL and OPG is the critical determinant for the degree of bone resorption. The ratio of RANKL to OPG regulates the formation and activity of osteoclasts. The importance of RANKL in bone destruction has led to the development of recombinant OPG as well as antibodies against RANKL as potential treatment options for bone diseases [21, 22].

48.2.2 Osteoblasts

Osteoblasts are the bone-forming cells. Unlike osteoclasts, they arise from mesenchymal stem cells (MSC). The differentiation of osteoblasts is less well understood than the differentiation of osteoclasts [23,24]. Some osteoblastic cells differentiate further and become osteocytes which make up 90% of bone cells in adults.

Bone morphogenetic proteins (BMPs) are critical factors that stimulate the growth and differentiation of osteoblasts [25]. The role of several other factors involved in the activation, proliferation, and control of the mesenchymal stem cells has been partly clarified. Basic fibroblast growth factor (bFGF) increases both osteoblast proliferation and collagen synthesis within bone, but its precise way of action remains unknown [26]. Insulin-like growth factors (IGFs, type I and II) increase the protein content of osteoid by promoting preosteoblastic proliferation, decreasing collagen degradation, and increasing protein synthesis [27]. Transforming growth factors (TGF-β_1 and β_2) and platelet-derived growth factor (PDGF) also stimulate the population of precursor cells committed to becoming osteoblasts [28, 29].

Finally a number of hormones, such as PTH, thyroxine, estrogen, cortisol, insulin, and calcitonin, as well as vitamin D, are involved in the regulation of bone metabolism, effecting osteoblasts, osteoclasts, and their precursors. Systemic hormones such as PTH, 1.25-dihydroxyvitamin D_3, and thyroxine (T_4) stimulate the formation of osteoclasts by inducing the expression of RANKL on marrow stromal cells and osteoblasts. The loss of gonadal hormones increases bone resorption as the normal balance between osteoblasts and osteoclasts is disrupted. Osteoblastic activity is decreased and osteoclastic activity is less suppressed. Calcitonin inhibits bone resorption by blocking osteoclast activity in the presence of high serum calcium. Insulin and IGFs influence osteoblast activity by enhancing their proliferation and differentiation. Cortisol and corticosteroids can induce apoptosis of osteoblasts and block bone formation.

48.3 Biology of Bone Metastases in Lung Cancer

In 1889, Stephen Paget set forth the "seed and soil" hypothesis, which suggests an interplay between the properties of cancer cells and the particular organ microenvironment which determines the selective advantage of cells to grow [30]. More specifically, the ability of cells to survive, clonally expand, and recruit a blood supply is expected to determine successful metastasis.

Bone is a common site of metastasis of lung cancer cells, ranking in frequency only behind that of liver and lung. Several factors account for the increased frequency of bone metastasis in lung cancer. These factors are: (1) the high blood flow in areas of red bone marrow and (2) the presence of tumor cells producing adhesive molecules that bind them to marrow stromal cells [31]. These adhesive interactions lead to increased production of angiogenic factors and bone-resorbing factors that further enhance tumor growth in bone [32]. As mentioned before, bone is a large repository for growth factors, including TGF-β, IGFs, bFGF, PDGF, and BMPs. These growth factors provide suitable conditions for further tumor cell growth [33].

Bone metastasis has been traditionally subdivided into osteolytic or osteoblastic according to different factors. These factors are secreted by either malignant or stromal cells and are responsible for the activation of osteoclasts or osteoblasts. This classification actually represents two extremes of a scale in which dysregulation of the normal bone remodeling process occurs. Patients can have either osteolytic or osteoblastic metastasis or mixed lesions containing both elements. Osseous metastasis from both small cell lung cancer (SCLC) and non-small cell lung cancer (NSCLC) are traditionally considered to be of predominately osteolytic type, resulting in excessive production of bone collagen degradation products, although local bone formation response can also be observed [3, 11].

The mechanisms by which lung cancer cells metastasize to bone are gradually being unraveled. The first step of bone metastasis is the invasion of surrounding tissues by lung cancer cells that produce proteolytic enzymes. These malignant cells traverse the walls of small blood vessels and enter the circulation, traveling to the affected bone. The cancer cells that do survive can enter the wide-channeled sinusoids of the bone marrow cavity [34, 35]. The production of chemokine receptors, cell adhesion molecules, and cell surface receptors by tumor cells enables them to attach to the bone matrix and establish growth in bone.

A specific type of osteolytic metastasis is cortical metastasis, which may also be seen in lung cancer patients and may be particularly relevant for the later stage of disseminated disease. This type of lesion may occur more frequently than previously expected. A cortical metastasis can develop and destroy the cortex without any involvement of the medullary cavity The mechanism of cortical metastasis is not well studied, but an important consideration is the capillary system of the cortex, which likely plays a significant role in the development of cortical metastasis. The cortex receives its vascular supply from anastomotic branches including medullary, periosteal, and nutrient artery vessels. Arterial disseminated metastases can be transported to an intracortical location from any one of the three vessel sources noted above [36].

48.3.1 Increased Osteoclast Activity is Evident in Lung Cancer-induced Bone Disease

Most in vivo studies indicate that osteolysis is not caused by the direct effects of lung cancer cells on bone. The interactions between lung cancer cells and bone microenvironment seem to play an important role on the development of lytic disease, disrupting the balance between osteoclasts and osteoblasts forming a "vicious circle." Lung cancer cells produce osteoclast-activating factors which results in increased osteoclastic activity when they arrive to bone [37]. In turn, bone resorption by osteoclasts releases growth factors from the bone matrix that stimulate tumor growth and bone destruction [38]. This "vicious circle" results in an increase of both bone destruction and the tumor burden (Fig. 48.2).

48.3.2 Parathyroid Hormone-related Peptide

Ectopic paraneoplastic production of parathyroid hormone-related peptide (PTHrP), originally described in breast cancer, is considered to be the main contributing factor of the predominant osteoclastic activity. Most notably in NSCLC, the presence of PTHrP may be the cause of the profound and clinically prevalent hypercalcemia [39, 40]. In SCLC, however, PTHrP production is thought to be less frequent as hypercalcemia is a rarer finding in this subset of lung cancer patients, even in the presence of extensive osseous metastasis [41].

Parathyroid hormone-related peptide was originally discovered in BEN cells, a squamous cell lung carcinoma line [42]. PTHrP is expressed by the majority of lung cancer cells of all histological subtypes [43–45]. Its expression seems to be more common in squamous cell carcinoma and less common in adenocarcinoma than in other lung cancer types, although a large, definitive study has not established this result conclusively.

The expression of PTHrP in eight lung cancer cell lines was directly correlated with the formation of bone metastasis. Malignant cells were injected intravenously into natural killer (NK) cell-depleted SCID mice. The levels of PTHrP and calcium in the mouse serum were increased in a time-dependent manner, suggesting that PTHrP produced by human lung cancer cells plays a crucial role in the formation of bone metastasis and hypercalcemia [46]. Furthermore, repeated intravenous injection with anti-PTHrP antibody inhibited the formation of bone metastasis by SCLL cells in these mice in a dose-dependent way. The same treatment had no significant effect on the metastasis to visceral organs (lung, liver, kidney, and lymph node). In addition, treatment with anti-PTHrP antibody improved the elevated serum calcium level, and inhibited osteolytic bone metastasis

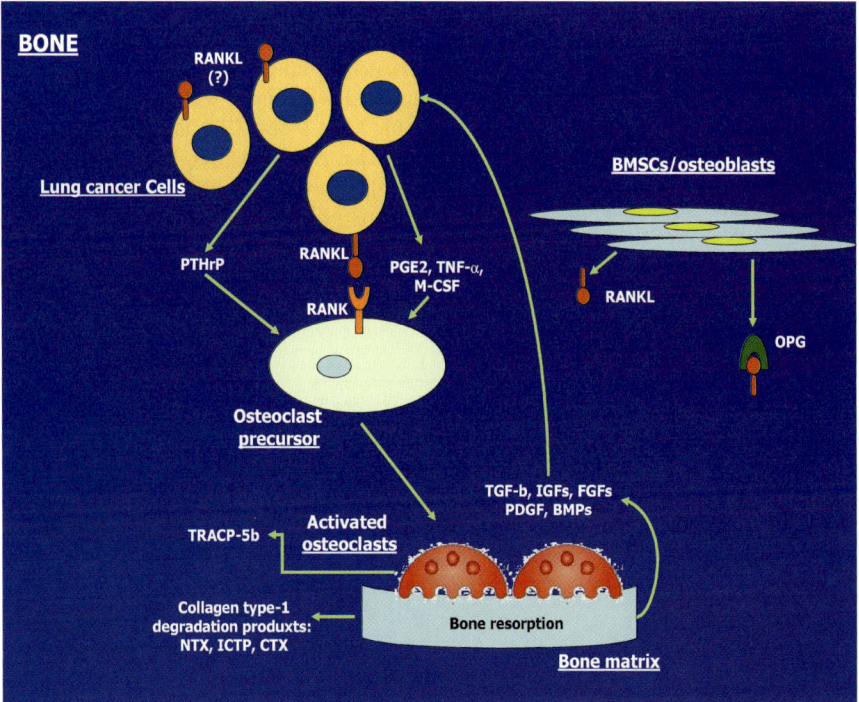

Fig. 48.2. The "vicious circle" hypothesis of osteolytic metastases in lung cancer. Lung cancer cells secrete parathyroid hormone-related peptide (*PTHrP*), which seems to be the primary stimulator of osteoclastogenesis, and possibly other factors with osteoclast activity, such as prostaglandin E_2 (*PGE$_2$*), tumor necrosis factor-α (*TNF-α*), and M-CSF. These factors increase the expression of RANKL by stromal cells, while cancer cells may also produce RANKL. RANKL directly acts on osteoclast precursors leading to osteoclast differentiation, proliferation, and activation, and to increased bone resorption, as is reflected by the increased levels of bone resorption markers, such as TRACP-5b, which are only produced by activated osteoclasts and collagen type I degradation products (NTX, ICTP/CTX). Osteoblasts try to balance this procedure by increasing the production of OPG, which is the decoy receptor of RANKL, but they can not compensate for the increased bone resorption, thus leading to the development of lytic lesions. Furthermore, the process of bone resorption releases factors such as TGF-β, IGFs, FGFs, PDGF, and BMPs, which increase the production of PTHrP by tumor cells as well as growth factors that increase tumor growth. This vicious circle between bone destruction and tumor growth further increases bone destruction and tumor growth

[40]. Serum PTHrP, as determined at the time of onset, appears to be a useful indicator of not only hypercalcemia but also bone metastasis and survival in patients with lung carcinoma [47].

Parathyroid hormone-related peptide is a well-known osteoclast formation factor. It alters the expression of molecules essential for osteoclast activation, such as RANKL [48]. Therefore, PTHrP is considered the most important factor in the pathogenesis of osteolytic bone disease in solid tumors.

48.3.3 RANK/RANKL/OPG Pathway in Osteolytic Lung Cancer Disease

Many researchers have reported that RANKL is mainly expressed by tumor cells when they are found in the bone microenvironment, but it has not yet been sufficiently clarified whether RANKL production by tumor cells is adequate to provoke osteolysis by itself [49]. In contrast, OPG has been shown to prevent bone destruction by blocking the association of RANKL with its receptor. The system RANKL/RANK/OPG seems to play a substantial role in the aforementioned balance of osteoblast and osteoclast activity. It is induced by malignant cells and the result of their interaction seems to determine the direction of bone remodeling. The importance of this system has been initially documented in multiple myeloma, where the ratio of RANKL to OPG has been proposed as an independent prognostic factor for the disease [50]. The substantial role of this system has been expanded in a subset of solid tumors too, including lung cancer [11]. The fact that PTHrP exerts its osteolytic effect by inducing RANKL/RANK/OPG system activation implies that the latter plays a substantial role in bone resorption of lung cancer in studies where PTHrP overproduction is well documented.

48.3.4 Osteopontin

Osteopontin (OPN) is a non-collagenous matrix protein produced by various cells including osteoblasts, osteoclasts, and malignant cells. It is involved in a number of physiological and pathological events including adhesion, angiogenesis, apoptosis, tumor metastasis, and osteoclast function. Osteoclasts bind to OPN deposited in the bone matrix and thus OPN is essential for the migration, attachment, and resorptive activity of osteoclasts [51]. An increase in OPN has been found in the serum of patients with multiple myeloma and correlated with the extent of lytic disease [52].

Osteopontin is among the most abundantly expressed proteins in a range of lung diseases and has been shown to regulate aspects of pulmonary granuloma formation, fibrosis, and malignancy [53]. OPN is also produced by lung cancer cells. Chambers et al. [54] found that OPN RNA levels were elevated in lung cancer patients, and the degree of OPN immunopositivity of the tumor predicted for survival. OPN has also been found to be elevated in the serum of patients with lung cancer [55] and correlated with survival in curatively resected NSCLC patients [56]. These findings suggest that OPN plays a substantial role in both the biology of lung cancer metastases into the bone as well as the lung cancer cell's survival and growth.

48.3.5 Production of Other Cytokines with Osteoclast Activity by Stromal and Lung Cancer Cells

The interactions between lung cancer cells and stromal cells in the bone marrow microenvironment lead to the production of other cytokines with osteoclast activity, such as prostaglandin E_2 (PGE$_2$) [57]. However, no correlation was observed between the formation of bone metastasis and the expression of other osteoclast-related cytokines in SCLL mice models, including IL-1, IL-6, IL-8, IL-10, IL-11, tumor necrosis factor-α (TNF-α), vascular endothelial growth factor (VEGF), and M-CSF [46].

48.3.6 Markers of Bone Resorption are Increased in Lung Cancer with Bone Metastases

Other strong evidence of increased bone destruction and osteoclast activity in patients with lung cancer and bone metastases is provided by the measurement of biochemical markers of bone resorption in such patients. Bone resorption markers include mainly urinary and serum N- or C-terminal crosslinking telopeptide of type I collagen (NTX or ICTP/CTX, respectively), urinary deoxypyridinoline (D-PYD) and pyridinoline

(PYD), and 5b isoenzyme of tartrate-resistant acid phosphatase (TRACP-5b) [58]. Both urinary NTX and D-PYD were elevated in lung cancer patients with bone metastases compared with those without bone involvement [57, 59, 60]. TRACP-5b, ICTP, and PYD were also found elevated in patients with lung cancer and bone metastases [61–63]. These results confirm that increased osteoclast activity is present in these patients. Furthermore, high NTX levels correlate with increased relative risk for skeletal-related events (SREs) and disease progression in NSCLC [64].

48.3.7 Osteoblasts are Functional in Lung Cancer Patients with Bone Metastases

Osteoblasts are also important for the development of bone metastasis in lung cancer patients. In a co-culture system of human osteoblasts with lung cancer cells (Calu-1 lung cancer cell line) the production of local degradation of the collagen matrix was detected. Moreover, in situ hybridization revealed the expression of IGF-1 by osteoblasts [65]. IGFs, and other cytokines produced by stromal cells, including TNF-β (which stimulates PTHrP production in squamous cell carcinoma), FGFs, and BMP-2, are not only able to stimulate the growth of metastatic cancer cells in bone, but also stimulate the production and release of bone-resorbing factors from tumor cells, completing the "vicious circle" of the pathogenic hypothesis of bone metastasis in malignancies (Fig. 48.2) [3, 11, 37].

Osteoblasts try to compensate for the increased bone resorption performed by activated osteoclasts. This is reflected by the increased levels of different molecules that are produced by them, such as bone alkaline phosphatase (bALP), osteocalcin, and OPG [60, 63, 66, 67]. However, osteoblasts do not manage to balance the increased bone destruction thus leading to the development of lytic disease.

48.4 Management of Bone Metastases in Lung Cancer

The goal of therapeutic intervention in the management of bone metastasis includes pain relief combined with restoration of skeletal function and the overall improvement of quality of life and functionality in patients. Traditionally, treatment of bone metastases due to lung cancer consists of radiotherapy, conventional chemotherapy, orthopedic intervention, and analgesics. In addition, the use of osteoclast inhibition substances has become a novel but effective complement to traditional therapies.

48.4.1 Radiotherapy

Radiotherapy (RT) remains the gold standard for palliation of painful bone metastases. The dose fractionation utilized varies widely, from single fractions (in doses usually of 8 Gy) to short fractionation schedules (in doses of 20 Gy for 5 fractions, 30 Gy for 10 fractions) to more radical fractionation schemes (in doses of 50 Gy over 5 weeks). Response rates vary from 65% to 100% [68–70]. However, the response criteria used in studies were variable and included observer interpretations of patients' reports. No concrete definitions of the terms "complete" or "partial relief" of pain existed in the literature for RT and bone metastases. Numerous other methodological differences have lead to contradictory conclusions from reviews of randomized studies [71, 72]. A meta-analysis by the Cochrane Database Systemic Reviews Group [73] reported that palliative external beam RT produced complete pain relief at 1 month after treatment in 25% of patients. Another meta-analysis of single versus fractionated RT schedules for bone metastases demonstrated no difference in pain control between single and multiple fractions [74]. There is a lack of evidence on which treatment is better for the other palliative endpoints, such as prevention of fractures, prevention of neurological deterioration, etc. A published consensus statement offers a uniform set of criteria for the choice and timing of outcome measures in palliative RT trials in bone metastases and will be very useful in future trials [75].

48.4.2 Surgery

Surgery is a mainstay in the treatment of pathological fractures of long bones, hip joints, and/or spinal lesions. Its goal has generally been palliative. Fractures of the femur or humerus require prompt fixation with an intramedullary rod, followed by radiotherapy. Decompression laminectomy is rarely necessary in patients with bone metastasis, although radioresistant disease or retropulsed bone fragments may require surgical intervention [76]. Early diagnosis and early surgical resection can result in improvement in neurological deficits and in the quality of life of patients with an intramedullary spinal cord metastasis [77].

48.4.3 Bisphosphonates

The concept of the "vicious circle," as described before, alters the approach to the treatment of bone metastases. It is theoretically possible that osteoclast inhibitors might also decrease bone tumor burden. Therefore, bisphosphonates that are potent inhibitors of osteoclast function are given to all patients with lung cancer with osteolytic bone disease. There is evidence for an antitumor effect of bisphosphonates in lung cancer which will be discussed in detail.

Bisphosphonates are the most potent treatment for malignant osteolytic bone disease to date. Their core structure is formed by two phosphonate groups attached to a single carbon atom (P-C-P structure), which is similar to endogenous pyrophosphate, but with carbon replacing the central oxygen. This carbon substitution makes bisphosphonates resistant to hydrolysis and allows two additional chains of variable structure. One of these chains includes a hydroxyl moiety, which allows high affinity for calcium crystals and bone mineral. The modification of these side-chains has allowed the biosynthesis of numerous bisphosphonates.

Bisphosphonates have been known for a long time; etidronate was synthesized as early as 1897. They were used for a variety of industrial applications, among them as antiscaling agents [78]. In contrast to pyrophosphates, bisphosphonates are stable in the biological environment. Etidronate and clodronate more closely resemble pyrophosphates, while pamidronate, ibandronate, and zoledronic acid contain nitrogen and other side-chains [79]. First-generation bisphosphonates, such as etidronate and clodronate, are metabolically incorporated into non-hydrolyzable analogs of ATP that may inhibit ATP-dependent intracellular enzymes. Second-generation (amino-) bisphosphonates, including pamidronate, ibandronate, alendronate, and risendronate, inhibit the mevalonate pathway leading to the posttranslational modification of guanidine triphosphatases [80].

All bisphosphonates have a high affinity for bone minerals and are preferentially delivered to sites of increased bone resorption or formation [81]. Bisphosphonates are poorly absorbed when they are taken orally. The bioavailability of clodronate and etidronate is 1–2%, while pamidronate and alendronate have a bioavailability of less than 1% [82, 83]. In addition, there is high individual variability in absorption rate that is decreased by substances such as coffee or orange juice as well as by calcium [84]. Their plasma level drops very rapidly as they bind to bone and they are excreted unchanged in urine. In the bone, they are tightly bound to hydroxyapatite crystals and their release depends on the rate of bone remodeling [85].

Bisphosphonates are potent inhibitors of osteoclastic bone resorption. They do so by inhibiting osteoclastic recruitment and maturation, preventing the development of monocytes into osteoclasts. They also induce osteoclast apoptosis and interrupt their attachment to bone [86]. In view of the accumulation of the bisphosphonates in bone, it is of great clinical interest that the inhibition of bone resorption reaches a certain steady level even when the compounds are given continuously. This suggests that, at the therapeutic dosage, there is no danger of a continuous decrease in bone turnover in the long run, leading to increased bone fragility, as seen in osteopetrosis. The decrease of bone resorption due to bisphosphonates is accompanied by an increase in calcium and mineral content of bone [84].

Although all bisphosphonates have similar physico-chemical properties, their antiresorbing activities differ substantially. Activity is dramatically increased when an amino group is contained in the aliphatic carbon chain. For example, pamidronate and alendronate are approximately 100 and 700 times more potent than etidronate, both in vitro and in vivo, while newer bisphosphonates, such as ibandronate and zoledronic acid show 10,000- to 100,000-fold greater potency than etidronate [85].

In addition to the well-proven antiresorptive efficacy of bisphosphonates, antitumor activity has also been suggested. This has been seen mainly from in vitro studies in different cancer cell lines as well as from preclinical in vivo models, including lung cancer [87–92].

Preclinical Data on Reduction of Bone Metastases and Tumor Burden by Bisphosphonates in Lung Cancer

There is in vivo evidence of inhibition of osteolytic bone metastases in lung cancer. Miki et al. [46] established a model of multiple-organ metastasis with an SCLC cell line, SBC-5, in NK cell-depleted SCID mice. In this model, SBC-5 cells metastasize into multiple organs, such as the lung, liver, kidneys, systemic lymph nodes, and bone, resembling characteristics of SCLC in humans. The same group found that the bisphosphonate minodronate inhibited osteolytic bone metastasis via the inhibition of bone resorption. However, it could not prolong the survival of tumor-bearing mice because of visceral metastasis [93]. The combination of minodronate with etoposide inhibited both bone and visceral metastases in this animal model of SCLC. Together they prolonged survival, suggesting that the combination of bisphosphonates with chemotherapy could prolong survival in humans as well [94].

Furthermore, zoledronic acid, the most potent bisphosphonate to date, induced apoptosis and inhibited the growth of 8/12 SCLC cell lines in vitro. It also significantly inhibited SCLC tumor growth when cancer cells were transplanted subcutaneously into nude mice. In the same study, zoledronic acid augmented the effects of paclitaxel, etoposide, cisplatinum, irinotecan, and imatinib against SCLC cells confirming the previous reported observation that bisphosphonates may enhance the action of chemotherapeutic agents [92]. Zoledronic acid may exert its antitumor effect either directly or indirectly. This can be seen either (1) by the inhibition of both farnesylation and geranylgeranylation of RAS oncoproteins (which are mutated in a variety of human cancers), or (2) by the disruption in interactions between tumor cells and stromal cells, or (3) by the expansion of gamma/delta T cells (which possibly have antitumor activity, including anti-SLCL activity) [95, 96].

Clinical Studies Using Bisphosphonates for Bone Metastases in Lung Cancer

Zoledronic acid has been administered in patients with bone metastases from multiple myeloma and breast cancer. It proved to be as effective and well-tolerated as pamidronate [97, 98]. However, Rosen et al. [99] published long-term follow-up data confirming that zoledronic acid, at a monthly dose of 4 mg, was more effective than pamidronate, at a monthly dose of 90 mg, in significantly reducing the overall risk of skeletal complications. Zoledronic acid is also the first and only bisphosphonate to demonstrate efficacy in both lytic and blastic disease [100].

Zoledronic acid was used in a multicenter, phase III, double-blind, randomized clinical trial for evaluation of its efficacy in patients with solid tumors and bone metastases. This clinical trial included only those with breast cancer or prostate cancer.

A total of 773 patients were enrolled into the three-arm study, one of which was placebo-controlled. Patients with NSCLC comprised the largest subgroup ($n = 378$). All patients were required to have at least one site of bony metastasis and an Eastern Cooperative Group performance status of 2. Patients were excluded if they had liver metastases, a bilirubin level of more than 2.5 g/dl, a creatinine level of more than 3.0 mg/dl, or symptomatic brain metastases. They received zoledronic acid (4 or 8 mg) or a placebo every 3 weeks for a total of 9 months. The study arm with those who took 8 mg zoledronic acid was closed prematurely due to safety concerns with renal toxicity. Approximately 25% of patients completed 9 months of therapy, with a median treatment duration of 4 months.

Zoledronic acid significantly reduced the incidence of SREs including hypercalcemia of malignancy. It also significantly extended the median time for development of SRE by more than 2 months compared with placebo. These results were reconfirmed after 21 months of treatment with zoledronic acid. A subset analysis did not detect a significant difference in NSCLC [101, 102]. Zoledronic acid also reduced skeletal morbidity regardless of SRE history [103]. However, it has to be mentioned that only one fourth of patients in each treatment group completed the study, primarily due to rapid disease progression, making these results more meaningful in view of the advanced nature of the disease in this population. This observation raises the pertinent question of whether earlier intervention prior to development of detectable bone metastasis would be more valuable in a high-risk patient population with advanced NSCLC.

In all rationale, there is a fundamental need to perform further studies to completely investigate preventive measure in patients especially with stage IIIa and IIIb lung cancer (a poor prognosis). The primary objective would be the prevention of bony metastases and its possible survival advantages. Current studies in advanced disease should further elucidate the role of zoledronic acid in the management of lung cancer. Furthermore, ongoing trials should reveal the role of other potent bisphosphonates, such as ibandronate, in the treatment of bone metastasis in lung cancer.

48.4.4 Role of Markers of Bone Turnover in Predicting Bone Metastases and Monitoring Antitumor/Bisphosphonate Treatment

Markers of bone remodeling are useful for the evaluation of bone disease status in patients with lung cancer as mentioned before in the chapter. However, the value of these markers in predicting SREs in lung cancer is still under investigation. A recent study showed that baseline urinary NTX levels could predict bone disease progression and survival in patients with NSCLC. Furthermore, bALP serum levels predicted for survival independently of the time of evaluation (baseline or on-study assessments) in NSCLC [64].

Almost all markers of bone resorption and formation have been used to assess the response to therapy for bone metastases but results have been variable. Urinary NTX and serum CTX appear to be the most useful [104].

48.5 Conclusions and Future Perspectives

Bone metastases are among the most difficult problems to manage in patients with lung cancer. The identification of molecular mechanisms responsible for the tropism of some lung cancer cells to the bones, using gene arrays and proteomics, could help in the earlier detection of bone metastases in these patients. Furthermore, the better understanding of the interactions between lung cancer cells and the bone marrow microenvironment that mediate the process of bone destruction should result in the development of therapeutic agents, such as recombinant human OPG, RANK-Fc, and anti-PTHrP, to treat and possibly prevent this devastating complication of lung cancer.

Key Points

- Bone metastasis is a frequent complication of lung cancer, which leads to impaired quality of life and performance status of the patients and increases the cost of the treatment of patients with lung cancer.
- Bisphosphonates are valuable agents for the management of bone metastases in lung cancer. Zoledronic acid seems to be the more promising, although trials with other bisphosphonates, such as ibandronate, are ongoing.
- The role of bisphosphonates in preventing the metastasis of lung cancer cells into the bone is a matter of investigation.
- Old and novel molecules that are implicated in the pathogenesis of bone metastasis in lung cancer, including PTHrP, RANKL, and OPG, may be targets for the development of novel therapies (RANK-Fc, anti-PTHrP) against bone destruction in lung cancer.

References

1. Quint LE, Francis IR, Wahl RL, Gross BH. Imaging of lung cancer. In: Pass HI, Mitchell JB, Johnson DH, Turrisi AT (eds) Lung Cancer: Principles and Practice. Philadelphia: Lippincott-Raven, 1996:437.
2. Parkin DM, Bray F, Ferlay J, Pisani P. Estimating the world cancer burden: Globocan 2000. Int J Cancer 2001; 94:153.
3. Mundy GR. Metastasis to bone: causes, consequences and therapeutic opportunities. Nat Rev Cancer 2002; 2:584.
4. Coleman R. Skeletal complications of malignancy. Cancer 1997; 80:1588.
5. Bloomfield D. Should bisphosphonates be part of standard therapy of patients with multiple myeloma or bone metastases from other cancers? An evidence-based review. J Clin Oncol 1998; 16:1218.
6. Mercadante S. Malignant bone pain: pathophysiology and treatment. Pain 1997; 69:1.
7. Delea T, Langer C, McKiernan J, et al. The cost of treatment of skeletal-related events in patients with bone metastases from lung cancer. Oncology 2004; 67:390.
8. Mundy GR. Cellular and molecular regulation of bone turnover. Bone 1999; 24(5 suppl):35S.
9. Christenson RH. Biochemical markers of bone metabolism: an overview. Clin Biochem 1997; 30:573.
10. Hodge JM, Kirkland MA, Aitken CJ, et al. Osteoclastic potential of human CFU-GM: biphasic effect of GM-CSF. J Bone Miner Res 2004; 19:190.
11. Roodman GD. Mechanisms of bone metastasis. N Engl J Med 2004; 350:1655.
12. Goldring SR. Inflammatory mediators as essential elements in bone remodelling. Calcif Tissue Int 2003; 73:97.
13. Itoh K, Udagawa N, Matsuzaki K, et al. Importance of membrane- or matrix-associated forms of M-CSF and RANKL/ODF in osteoclastogenesis supported by SaOS-4/3 cells expressing recombinant PTH/PTHrP receptors. J Bone Miner Res 2000; 15:1766.

14. Kong YY, Yoshida H, Sarosi I, et al. OPGL is a key regulator of osteoclastogenesis, lymphocyte development and lymph-node organogenesis. Nature 1999; 397:315.

15. Teitelbaum SL. Bone resorption by osteoclasts. Science 2000; 289:1504.

16. Horowitz MC, Xi Y, Wilson K, Kacena MA. Control of osteoclastogenesis and bone resorption by members of the TNF family of receptors and ligands. Cytokine Growth Factor Rev 2001; 12:9.

17. Simonet WS, Lacey DL, Dunstan CR, et al. Osteoprotegerin: a novel secreted protein involved in the regulation of bone density. Cell 1997; 89:309.

18. Morinaga T, Nakagawa N, Yasuda H, Tsuda E, Higashio K. Cloning and characterization of the gene encoding human osteoprotegerin/osteoclastogenesis-inhibitory factor. Eur J Biochem 1998; 254:685.

19. Kim N, Odgren PR, Kim DK, Marks SC Jr, Choi Y. Diverse roles of the tumor necrosis factor family member TRANCE in skeletal physiology revealed by TRANCE deficiency and partial rescue by a lymphocyte-expressed TRANCE transgene. Proc Natl Acad Sci U S A 2000; 97:10905.

20. Bucay N, Sarosi I, Dunstan CR, et al. Osteoprotegerin-deficient mice develop early onset osteoporosis and arterial calcification. Genes Dev 1998; 12:1260.

21. Body JJ, Greipp P, Coleman RE, et al. A phase I study of AMGN-0007, a recombinant osteoprotegerin construct, in patients with multiple myeloma or breast carcinoma related bone metastases. Cancer 2003; 97(3 suppl):887.

22. Vanderkerken K, Asosingh K, Croucher P, Van Camp B. Multiple myeloma biology: lessons from the 5TMM models. Immunol Rev 2003; 194:196.

23. Stein GS, Lian JB. Molecular mechanisms mediating proliferation/differentiation interrelationships during progressive development of the osteoblast phenotype. Endocr Rev 1993; 14:424.

24. Ahdjoudj S, Fromigue O, Marie PJ. Plasticity and regulation of human bone marrow stromal osteoprogenitor cells: potential implication in the treatment of age-related bone loss. Histol Histopathol 2004; 19:151.

25. Abe E, Yamamoto M, Taguchi Y, et al. Essential requirement of BMPs-2/4 for both osteoblast and osteoclast formation in murine bone marrow cultures from adult mice: antagonism by noggin. J Bone Miner Res 2000; 15:663.

26. Power RA, Iwaniec UT, Magee KA, Mitova-Caneva NG, Wronski TJ. Basic fibroblast growth factor has rapid bone anabolic effects in ovariectomized rats. Osteoporos Int 2004; 15:716.

27. Cornish J, Grey A, Callon KE, et al. Shared pathways of osteoblast mitogenesis induced by amylin, adrenomedullin, and IGF-1. Biochem Biophys Res Commun 2004; 318:240.

28. Ortiz CO, Chen BK, Bale LK, Overgaard MT, Oxvig C, Conover CA. Transforming growth factor-beta regulation of the insulin-like growth factor binding protein-4 protease system in cultured human osteoblasts. J Bone Miner Res 2003; 18:1066.

29. Chaudhary LR, Hofmeister AM, Hruska KA. Differential growth factor control of bone formation through osteoprogenitor differentiation. Bone 2004; 34:402.

30. Paget S. The distribution of secondary growths in cancer of the breast. Lancet 1889; 1:571.

31. Kahn D, Weiner GJ, Ben-Haim S, et al. Positron emission tomographic measurement of bone marrow blood flow to the pelvis and lumbar vertebrae in young normal adults. Blood 1994; 83:958.

32. van der Pluijm G, Sijmons B, Vloedgraven H, Deckers M, Papapoulos S, Lowik C. Monitoring metastatic behavior of human tumor cells in mice with species-specific polymerase chain reaction: elevated expression of angiogenesis and bone resorption stimulators by breast cancer in bone metastases. J Bone Miner Res 2001; 16:1077.

33. Hauschka PV, Mavrakos AE, Iafrati MD, Doleman SE, Klagsbrun M. Growth factors in bone matrix: isolation of multiple types by affinity chromatography on heparin-Sepharose. J Biol Chem 1986; 261:12665.

34. Liotta LA, Kohn E. Cancer invasion and metastases. JAMA 1990; 263:1123.

35. Liotta LA, Kohn EC. The microenvironment of the tumour-host interface. Nature 2001; 411:375.

36. Hendrix RW, Rogers LF, Davis TM Jr. Cortical bone metastases. Radiology 1991; 181:409.

37. Yin JJ, Pollock CB, Kelly K. Mechanisms of cancer metastasis to the bone. Cell Res 2005; 15:57.

38. Chirgwin JM, Guise TA. Molecular mechanisms of tumor-bone interactions in osteolytic metastases. Crit Rev Eukaryot Gene Expr 2000; 10:159.

39. Powell GJ, Southby J, Danks JA, et al. Localization of parathyroid hormone-related protein in breast cancer metastases: increased incidence in bone compared with other sites. Cancer Res 1991; 51:3059.

40. Miki T, Yano S, Hanibuchi M, Kanematsu T, Muguruma H, Sone S. Parathyroid hormone-related protein (PTHrP) is responsible for production of bone metastasis, but not visceral metastasis, by human small cell lung cancer SBC-5 cells in natural killer cell-depleted SCID mice. Int J Cancer 2004; 108:511.

41. Hastings RH. Parathyroid hormone-related protein and lung biology. Respir Physiol Neurobiol 2004; 142:95.

42. Moseley JM, Kubota M, Diefenbach-Jagger H, et al. Parathyroid hormone-related protein purified from a human lung cancer cell line. Proc Natl Acad Sci U S A 1987; 84:5052.

43. Brandt DW, Burton DW, Gazdar AF, Oie HE, Deftos LJ. All major lung cancer cell types produce parathyroid hormone-like protein: heterogeneity assessed by high performance liquid chromatography. Endocrinology 1991; 129:2466.

44. Davidson LA, Black M, Carey FA, Logue F, McNicol AM. Lung tumours immunoreactive for parathyroid hormone-related peptide: analysis of serum calcium levels and tumour type. J Pathol 1996; 178:398.

45. Nishigaki Y, Ohsaki Y, Toyoshima E, Kikuchi K. Increased serum and urinary levels of a parathyroid hormone-related protein COOH terminus in non-small cell lung cancer patients. Clin Cancer Res 1999; 5:1473.

46. Miki T, Yano S, Hanibuchi M, Sone S. Bone metastasis model with multiorgan dissemination of human small-cell lung cancer (SBC-5) cells in natural killer cell-depleted SCID mice. Oncol Res 2000; 12:209.

47. Hiraki A, Ueoka H, Bessho A, et al. Parathyroid hormone-related protein measured at the time of first visit is an indicator of bone metastases and survival in lung carcinoma patients with hypercalcemia. Cancer 2002; 95:1706.

48. Blair HC, Athanasou NA. Recent advances in osteoclast biology and pathological bone resorption. Histol Histopathol 2004; 19:189.

49. Zhang J, Dai J, Qi Y, et al. Osteoprotegerin inhibits prostate cancer-induced osteoclastogenesis and prevents prostate tumor growth in the bone. J Clin Invest 2001; 107:1235.

50. Terpos E, Szydlo R, Apperley JF, et al. Soluble receptor activator of nuclear factor κB ligand (RANKL)/osteoprotegerin (OPG) ratio predicts survival in multiple myeloma. Proposal for a novel prognostic index. Blood 2003; 102:1064.

51. Standal T, Borset M, Sundan A. Role of osteopontin in adhesion, migration, cell survival and bone remodeling. Exp Oncol 2004a;26:179.

52. Standal T, Hjorth-Hansen H, Rasmussen T, et al. Osteopontin is an adhesive factor for myeloma cells and is found in increased levels in plasma from patients with multiple myeloma. Haematologica 2004b;89:174.

53. O'Regan A. The role of osteopontin in lung disease. Cytokine Growth Factor Rev 2003; 14:479.

54. Chambers AF, Wilson SM, Kerkvliet N, O'Malley FP, Harris JF, Casson AG. Osteopontin expression in lung cancer. Lung Cancer 1996; 15:311.

55. Fedarko NS, Jain A, Karadag A, Van Eman MR, Fisher LW. Elevated serum bone sialoprotein and osteopontin in colon, breast, prostate, and lung cancer. Clin Cancer Res 2001; 7:4060.

56. Schneider S, Yochim J, Brabender J, et al. Osteopontin but not osteonectin messenger RNA expression is a prognostic marker in curatively resected non-small cell lung cancer. Clin Cancer Res 2004; 10:1588.

57. Shih LY, Shih HN, Chen TH. Bone resorption activity of osteolytic metastatic lung and breast cancers. J Orthop Res 2004; 22:1161.

58. Terpos E, Politou M, Rahemtulla A. The role of markers of bone remodeling in multiple myeloma. Blood Rev 2005; 19:125.

59. Izumi M, Nakanishi Y, Takayama K, et al. Diagnostic value of bone-turnover metabolites in the diagnosis of bone metastases in patients with lung carcinoma. Cancer 2001; 91:1487.

60. Alatas F, Alatas O, Metintas M, Colak O, Erginel S, Harmanci E. Usefulness of bone markers for detection of bone metastases in lung cancer patients. Clin Biochem 2002; 35:293.

61. Horiguchi T, Tachikawa S, Kondo R, Hirose M, Teruya S, Ishibashi A, Banno K. Usefulness of serum carboxy-terminal telopeptide of type I collagen (ICTP) as a marker of bone metastasis from lung cancer. Jpn J Clin Oncol 2000; 30:174.

62. Koizumi M, Takahashi S, Ogata E. Comparison of serum bone resorption markers in the diagnosis of skeletal metastasis. Anticancer Res 2003; 23:4095.

63. Ebert W, Muley T, Herb KP, Schmidt-Gayk H. Comparison of bone scintigraphy with bone markers in the diagnosis of bone metastasis in lung carcinoma patients. Anticancer Res 2004; 24:3193.

64. Brown JE, Cook RJ, Major P, et al. Bone turnover markers as predictors of skeletal complications in prostate cancer, lung cancer, and other solid tumors. J Natl Cancer Inst 2005; 97:59.

65. Mitsiades C, Sourla A, Doillon C, et al. Three-dimensional type I collagen co-culture systems for the study of cell–cell interactions and treatment response in bone metastases. J Musculoskelet Neuronal Interact 2000; 1:153.

66. Jung K, Lein M, Stephan C, et al. Comparison of 10 serum bone turnover markers in prostate carcinoma patients with bone metastatic spread: diagnostic and prognostic implications. Int J Cancer 2004; 111:783.

67. Naumnik W, Chyczewska E, Izycki T, Ossolinska M. Serum levels of osteoprotegerin (OPG) and progastrin releasing peptide (ProGRP) during chemotherapy of lung cancer. Rocz Akad Med Bialymst 2004; 49(suppl 1):88.

68. Kirkbride P, Mackillop WJ, Priestman TJ, Browman G, Gospodarowicz M, Rousseau P. The role of palliative radiotherapy for bone metastases. Can J Oncol 1996; 6(suppl 1):33.

69. Bezjak A. Palliative therapy for lung cancer. Semin Surg Oncol 2003; 21:138.

70. Ishiyama H, Shibata A, Niino K, Hosoya T. Relationship between morphine and radiotherapy for management of symptomatic bone metastases from lung cancer. Support Care Cancer 2004; 12:743.

71. Ratanatharathorn V, Powers WE, Moss WT, Perez CA. Bone metastasis: review and critical analysis of random allocation trials of local field treatment. Int J Radiat Oncol Biol Phys 1999; 44:1.

72. Wu JS, Bezjak A, Chow E, Kirkbride P. Primary treatment endpoint following palliative radiotherapy for painful bone metastases: need for a consensus definition? Clin Oncol 2002; 14:70.

73. McQuay HJ, Collins SL, Carroll D, Moore RA. Radiotherapy for the palliation of painful bone metastases. Cochrane Database Syst Rev 2000:CD001793.

74. Wu JS, Wong R, Johnston M, Bezjak A, Whelan T. Meta analysis of dose-fractionation radiotherapy trials for the palliation of painful bone metastases. Int J Radiat Oncol Biol Phys 2003; 55:594.

75. Chow E, Wu JS, Hoskin P, Coia LR, Bentzen SM, Blitzer PH. International consensus on palliative radiotherapy endpoints for future clinical trials in bone metastases. Radiother Oncol 2002; 64:275.

76. Wedin R. Surgical treatment for pathologic fracture. Acta Orthop Scand Suppl 2001; 72:1.

77. Kalayci M, Cagavi F, Gul S, Yenidunya S, Acikgoz B. Intramedullary spinal cord metastases: diagnosis and treatment – an illustrated review. Acta Neurochir 2004; 146:1347.

78. Fleisch H. Development of bisphosphonates. Breast Cancer Res 2002; 4:30.

79. Russell RG, Rogers MJ, Frith JC, et al. The pharmacology of bisphosphonates and new insights into their mechanisms of action. J Bone Miner Res 1999; 14(suppl 2):53.

80. Raje N, Anderson KC. The evolving role of bisphosphonate therapy in multiple myeloma. Blood 2000; 96:381.

81. Body JJ. Bisphosphonates. Eur J Cancer 1998; 34:263.

82. Fitton A, McTavish D. Pamidronate. A review of its pharmacological properties and therapeutic efficacy in resorptive bone disease. Drugs 1991; 41:289.

83. Plosker GL, Goa KL. Clodronate. A review of its pharmacological properties and therapeutic efficacy in resorptive bone disease. Drugs 1994; 47:945.

84. Fleisch H. Bisphosphonates: mechanisms of action. Endocr Rev 1998; 19:80.

85. Lin JH. Bisphosphonates: a review of their pharmacokinetic properties. Bone 1996; 18:75.

86. Suda T, Nakamura I, Jimi E, Takahashi N. Regulation of osteoclast function. J Bone Miner Res 1997; 12:869.

87. Fromigue O, Lagneaux L, Body JJ. Bisphosphonates induce breast cancer cell death in vitro. J Bone Miner Res 2000; 15:2211.

88. Coxon JP, Oades GM, Kirby RS, Colston KW. Zoledronic acid induces apoptosis and inhibits adhesion to mineralized matrix in prostate cancer cells via inhibition of protein prenylation. BJU Int 2004; 94:164.

89. Vorotnjak M, Boos J, Lanvers-Kaminsky C. In vitro toxicity of bisphosphonates on human neuroblastoma cell lines. Anticancer Drugs 2004; 15:795.

90. Yang DM, Chi CW, Chang HM, et al. Effects of clodronate on cancer growth and Ca2+ signaling of human thyroid carcinoma cell lines. Anticancer Res 2004; 24:1617.

91. Hashimoto K, Morishige K, Sawada K, et al. Alendronate inhibits intraperitoneal dissemination in in vivo ovarian cancer model. Cancer Res 2005; 65:540.

92. Matsumoto S, Kimura S, Segawa H, et al. Efficacy of the third-generation bisphosphonate, zoledronic acid alone and combined with anti-cancer agents against small cell lung cancer cell lines. Lung Cancer 2005; 47:31.

93. Zhang H, Yano S, Miki T, et al. A novel bisphosphonate minodronate (YM529) specifically inhibits osteolytic bone metastasis produced by human small-cell lung-cancer cells in NK cell-depleted SCID mice. Clin Exp Metastasis 2003; 20:153.

94. Yano S, Zhang H, Hanibuchi M, Miki T, Goto H, Uehara H, Sone S. Combined therapy with a new bisphosphonate, minodronate (YM529), and chemotherapy for multiple organ metastases of small cell lung cancer cells in severe combined immunodeficient mice. Clin Cancer Res 2003; 9:5380.

95. Terpos E, Rahemtulla A. Bisphosphonate treatment for multiple myeloma. Drugs Today 2004; 40:29.

96. Sato K, Kimura S, Segawa H, et al. Cytotoxic effects of gammadelta T cells expanded ex vivo by a third generation bisphosphonate for cancer immunotherapy. Int J Cancer 2005; 116:94.

97. Berenson JR, Rosen LS, Howell A, et al. Zoledronic acid reduces skeletal-related events in patients with osteolytic metastases: a double-blind, randomized dose-response study. Cancer 2001; 91:1191.

98. Rosen LS, Gordon D, Kaminski M, et al. Zoledronic acid versus pamidronate in the treatment of skeletal metastases in patients with breast cancer or osteolytic lesions of multiple myeloma: a phase III, double-blind, comparative trial. Cancer J 2001; 7:377.

99. Rosen LS, Gordon D, Kaminski M, et al. Long-term efficacy of zoledronic acid compared with pamidronate disodium in the treatment of skeletal complications in patients with advanced multiple myeloma or breast carcinoma: a randomized, double-blind, multicenter, comparative trial. Cancer 2003; 98:1735.

100. Lipton A, Small E, Saad F, et al. The new bisphosphonate, Zometa (zoledronic acid), decreases skeletal complications in both lytic and blastic lesions: a comparison to pamidronate. Cancer Invest 2002; 20(suppl 2):45.

101. Rosen LS, Gordon D, Tchekmedyian S, et al. Zoledronic acid versus placebo in the treatment of skeletal metastases in patients with lung cancer and other solid tumors: a phase III, double-blind, randomized trial – the Zoledronic Acid Lung Cancer and Other Solid Tumors Study Group. J Clin Oncol 2003; 21:3150.

102. Rosen LS, Gordon D, Tchekmedyian NS, et al. Long-term efficacy and safety of zoledronic acid in the treatment of skeletal metastases in patients with nonsmall cell lung carcinoma and other solid tumors: a randomized, phase III, double-blind, placebo-controlled trial. Cancer 2004; 100:2613.

103. Hirsh V, Tchekmedyian NS, Rosen LS, Zheng M, Hei YJ. Clinical benefit of zoledronic acid in patients with lung cancer and other solid tumors: analysis based on history of skeletal complications. Clin Lung Cancer 2004; 6:170.

104. Costa L, Demers LM, Gouveia-Oliveira A, Schaller J, Costa EB, de Moura MC, Lipton A. Prospective evaluation of the peptide-bound collagen type I cross-links N-telopeptide and C-telopeptide in predicting bone metastases status. J Clin Oncol 2002; 20:850.

Management of Malignant Pleural Effusions

49

Adrianni Charpidou, Kevin J. Harrington
and Konstantinos N. Syrigos

Contents

49.1   Introduction

Malignant pleural effusion is diagnosed when exfoliated malignant cells are found in pleural fluid or when pleural tissue is invaded by malignant cells. Malignancy is one of the most common causes of exudative pleural effusions. In postmortem examinations of patients who died of cancer, the incidence of malignant effusion was 16% [1]. Carcinoma of any organ can metastasize to the pleura. However, lung cancer is the most common cause of malignant effusions with an incidence of 40%. When first evaluated, approximately 15% of that group of patients exhibited pleural effusion and up to 50% of the patients with an advanced disease may acquire a pleural effusion during the course of their disease [2–4]. Breast cancer is the second cause with an incidence of 25%. Lymphomas account for 10% of all malignant effusions and are the most common cause of chylothorax. Other solid tumors, such as ovarian and gastric cancer, represent the 5% or less of malignant pleural effusions while in 3–10% of patients the effusion is due to malignancy of unknown origin [5]. The incidence of mesothelioma varies according to the geographic location.

49.2   Pathogenesis

The lymphatic drainage from the pleural space occurs through the stomas of the parietal pleura. The liquid travels through lymphatic channels toward the mediastinal lymph nodes. Any interference in its path can result in a pleural effusion. Nevertheless, the latter mechanism cannot solely explain the formation of all malignant effusions. Firstly, these effusions are exudates and the normal pleural fluid has low protein concentration that makes its accumulation a transudate. Secondly, the rate of fluid formation is much higher than normal. The normal rate of pleural fluid formation is 0.01 mL/kg per hour. In many patients with malignant pleural effusions it is common for the fluid egress to exceed the 100 mL/24 h as measured through chest tube drainage. Thirdly, malignant cells are found in more than 90% of these effusions and in addition, many of them are bloody which can be justified only by the invasion of parietal pleura from the tumor as it obstructs the lacunae of the lymphatics.

However, it has been shown that many of these patients have effusions only when their visceral pleura is involved [1, 6]. The visceral involvement represents hematogenous spread of cancer and leads to secondary metastases to the pleural space and parietal side. The presence of pleural metastases may increase the permeability of the capillaries in the visceral and/or parietal pleura. This also explains how malignant effusions are exudates. Furthermore, the existence of mediastinal lymph node involvement decreases the lymphatic drainage and leads to an increase in fluid input in the pleural space by traversing the visceral pleura.

The above suggests that the combination of increased fluid formation and the decreased capacity of the lymphatics are the two mechanisms which can explain the genesis of malignant effusions and the reason why some patients with pleural metastases have effusions while others do not [2, 7]. Postmortem studies indicate that only 55–60% of the patients with proven pleural metastases have developed pleural effusions. Parietal pleural involvement in lung cancer results from either neoplastic spread across the pleural cavity from visceral pleura or by the attachment of exfoliated cells from the visceral pleura. The visceral pleura impairment is due to pulmonary arterial invasion and embolization.

Adenocarcinoma of the lung is the most common histological type associated with malignant pleural infusion; it spreads by contiguity due to its peripheral location and has the propensity to invade the vessels [2]. Some patients with malignancy have cytology-negative pleural effusions and no direct pleural involvement from the tumor. The term "paramalignant effusions" refers to those effusions that are not a direct result of the pleura invasion from the tumor but are still related to the primary malignancy [2, 3]. Not all "paramalignant effusions" exclude operability in lung cancer. Important examples are the parapneumonic effusions due to postobstructive pneumonia and the transudate effusions secondary to postobstructive atelectasis. Other local effects (Table 49.1) of the tumor causing "paramalignant effusions" are: (1) lymphatic obstruction, as mentioned before, (2) obstruction of the thoracic duct with the development of chylothorax, and (3) the trapped lung caused by extensive tumor involvement of visceral pleura. Systemic effects of the tumor can result in effusions with pulmonary embolism, hypoalbuminemia, and cachexia. In addition, adverse events of the therapy can also result in effusions. This category includes radiation therapy and antineoplastic drugs such as bleomycin, methotrexate, cyclophosphamide, and taxanes.

Table 49.1. Causes of "paramalignant" effusions

Local effects of tumor:
  Lymphatic obstruction
  Bronchial obstruction with pneumonia
  Bronchial obstruction with atelectasis
  Trapped lung
  Chylothorax
  Superior vena cava syndrome

Systemic effects of tumor:
  Pulmonary embolism
  Hypoalbuminemia

Complications to therapy:
  Radiation therapy (early or late)
  Chemotherapy

Modified from: Sahn SA. Clin Chest Med 1998; 19:351 [2]

49.3 Clinical Presentation

Dyspnea on exertion and cough are the most common symptoms that patients refer to on admission. The presence and degree of dyspnea depend on the volume of the effusion and the underlying pulmonary function. The mechanism of dyspnea is under scientific research. Decrease of the compliance of the chest wall, contralateral shift of the mediastinum, depression of the ipsilateral diaphragm, decrease in ipsilateral lung volume, and neurogenic reflexes from lung and chest wall may be considered as probable mechanisms. Obstructive pneumonitis, atelectasis, and malignant infiltration of the pulmonary parenchyma may provoke additional causes of dyspnea. Chest pain indicates involvement of parietal pleura and is most common in mesothelioma. It is described as dull and aching rather than sharp and pleuritic. Pleural metastases indicate advanced disease where patients can present with weight loss, anorexia, and malaise. Physical examination can easily detect the presence of fluid of the malignant effusion which commonly exceeds 500 mL.

49.4 Imaging Techniques

Chest radiography shows moderate to large fluid accumulation (500–2,000 mL) in approximately 75% of patients with malignant effusion with 10% having effusions with less than 500 mL and 10% having massive pleural effusions. The term "massive" refers to the occupation of the whole hemithorax with fluid.

Bilateral effusions are common when the primary site of cancer has spread not locally to the lungs but hematogenously. More than 50% of the cases of bilateral effusions with a normal heart size are diagnosed as malignant or paramalignant. Lupus and rheumatoid pleuritis, benign asbestos pleural effusion, hypoalbuminemia, and constrictive pericarditis should also be considered in the differential diagnosis of bilateral effusions.

Usually large effusions push the mediastinum to the contralateral site. Differential diagnosis of mediastinal effusions are: (1) mainstem bronchial obstruction by tumor and atelectasis, (2) trapped lung, (3) fixed mediastinum caused by malignant lymphadenopathy, and (4) extensive infiltration of the ipsilateral lung by tumor radiographically mimicking a large effusion.

Computerized tomography (CT) can provide useful information of lymph node involvement, underlying parenchymal diseases, or co-existing metastases [8, 9]. The role of magnetic resonance imaging (MRI) seems to be limited to malignant pleural effusions but it is considered a useful technique in the assessment of mediastinal and chest wall invasion by virtue of its ability to determine fat-stripe invasion and involvement of the diaphragm [9, 10]. The role of the novel and promising technique of fluorodeoxyglucose positron emission tomography (FDG-PET) is still being evaluated for malignant effusions. Recent studies which compare the efficacy of FDG-PET to CT in differentiating benign pleural effusion from malignant and/or pleural involvement in patients with lung cancer, showed that the new diagnostic method is a highly accurate and reliable non-invasive technique [11, 12].

49.5 Pleural Fluid Characteristics

Diagnostic thoracentesis must be performed in any patient where a pleural effusion of more than 1 cm thick is detected in the lateral decubitus position. Almost all malignant pleural effusions are exudates with a protein concentration of about 4 g/dL. In some cases, such as the pleural fluid accumulation secondary to atelectasis or to lymph node involvement, they can be transudates. The differential cell count is useful to determine the etiology of the fluid. The malignant effusions are characteristically lymphocytic with a range of 50–75% but certainly less than that which can be seen in tuberculous pleurisy (>90%). The reason for this lymphocytosis is unclear. The lymphocytes are predominantly T-type and appear to play a key role in local defense against tumor invasion. Pleural fluid eosinophilia (eosinophils >10%) usually signifies a benign self-limited disease but it cannot exclude malignancy. The frequency of eosinophilia in malignant effusions varies from 10% to 40%. In some populations, eosinophilic effusions are as likely to be malignant as non-eosinophilic ones [2, 13, 14]. Polymorphonuclear leukocytes usually represent less than 25% of the cell population. Although malignancy is the most common cause of bloody effusions, at least half of them are not grossly hemorrhagic (RBC count <;10,000 cells/mL). A bloody malignant pleural effusion can result from either direct invasion of blood vessels, increased capillary permeability caused by vasoactive substances produced from tumor cells, occlusion of venules, or tumor-induced angiogenesis [2]. Although the pleural fluid lactate dehydrogenase (LDH) level is used to distinguish transudative from exudative pleural effusions, it is not useful in the differential diagnosis of malignancy [15]. At the time of the diagnosis, approximately one third of malignant effusions are acidotic with a pH value less than 7. This low pH is associated with low glucose concentrations (<60 mg/dL). The possible mechanism involves the spreading of the tumor within the pleural space. The abnormal thickening of the pleura prevents the glucose transport from blood to pleural fluid. The glucose that does enter the pleura is metabolized by normal and malignant cells to CO_2 and lactate. Additionally, the abnormal pleural barrier impairs the efflux of these end products of glucose metabolism from the pleural space, resulting in the fluid acidosis. Malignant effusions with low pH and glucose concentration are considered to have a higher initial diagnostic yield on cytological examination and a worse survival and response to pleurodesis than those with normal values. Pleural fluid pH correlates with survival [3, 16]. The amylase salivary isoenzyme of the fluid is elevated in 10–14% of malignant effusions. In the absence of esophageal rupture, elevated values of fluid amylase establish the diagnosis of malignancy, especially lung adenocarcinoma.

49.6 Diagnosis

The diagnosis of malignant pleural effusion can be obtained by the demonstration of malignant cells in pleural fluid or in pleural tissue. Cytological examination of pleural fluid is a fast, efficient, non-invasive, and more sensitive technique than the closed pleural biopsy. The percentage of malignant effusions which is diagnosed with cytology varies from 40% to 87% [3, 15]. The frequency of positive cytological results, if the effusion is not "paramalignant", depends on the tumor type. Squamous cell carcinoma, Hodgkin's disease, and sarcomas are less commonly positive. Obviously the frequency also depends on the skills of the cytologist. Overall, if three separate pleural fluid specimens are submitted to an experienced cytologist, the positive diagnosis is about 70–80%. Some clinicians suggest that when the first suspicion is malignancy, several hundred milliliters of fluid should be removed at the initial diagnostic thoracentesis. This procedure, in the case of a negative initial cytological examination, involves the sucking of fluid with fewer degenerative mesothelial cells as well as freshly exfoliated malignant cells in a repeated thoracentesis [2]. In the decade since 1995, the use of other procedures, such as flow cytometry with DNA analysis and immunohistochemical staining with monoclonal antibodies to tumor markers, have been proposed in order to increase the diagnostic accuracy of cytology. Because of their low sensitivity and specificity of these techniques, they can only be used to assist in the diagnosis and not confirm it. Identification of DNA aneuploidy by flow cytometry may add to routine cytology by detecting false-negatives in the initial screening and warrant additional samples for further review. Flow cytometry with immunocytometry can identify the cell lineage (T or B cells) and the clonality of the population of lymphocytes. Therefore, it is useful when lymphoma is suspected. Immunohistochemical staining for tumor markers such as carcinoembryonic antigen (CEA), Leu-M1, mucine, and B72.3 can be used in the differential diagnosis between adenocarcinoma and mesothelioma. If the specimen is positive for at least two of these antibodies, this is a likely indication for adenocarcinoma.

On the contrary, if it is not stained for any of the antibodies and/or it is positively stained for vimentin, the diagnosis is probably mesothelioma [3, 15, 17, 18]. A tumor marker panel, such as CEA, carbohydrate antigen 15-3 (CA 15-3), cytokeratin 19 fragments (CYFRA 21-1), and cancer antigen 125 can reveal the patient that could benefit from a more aggressive and invasive diagnostic procedures when the initial cytological examination is negative [19]. Telomerase activity in recent studies has proven to be a highly diagnostic biomarker for malignancy. Additionally, when it is used as an adjunct to cytology, it significantly increases the diagnostic sensitivity [20].

In malignant effusions, closed pleural biopsies are less sensitive than fluid cytology, with a diagnostic yield of 40–44% [3, 21]. The low sensitivity of this blind biopsy of the parietal pleura is mostly due to the distribution of tumor in unexamined areas and early stage of disease with minimal pleural involvement. Many physicians suggest that if malignancy is suspected and the cytology of thoracentesis is negative, thoracoscopy is then preferred over closed needle pleural biopsy reaching a diagnosis in more than 90% of cases. Medical thoracoscopy compared to surgical thoracoscopy, also known as "video-assisted thoracic surgery" or "VATS," can be performed under local anesthesia or conscious sedation and it is considerably less invasive and less expensive than VATS [22]. Medical thoracoscopy is primarily a diagnostic procedure but it can also be used for staging and in the treatment of malignant effusions. By thoracoscopy, we can achieve direct visualization of the pleural cavity and can obtain biopsies of the chest wall, the parietal or visceral pleura, the lung, the mediastinum, and the diaphragm. Thoracoscopy can also result in the complete evacuation of the pleural fluid, elimination of adhesions hindering lung expandability, and pleurodesis by talc poudrage. The diagnostic sensitivity of medical thoracoscopy is higher than that of both cytology and closed pleural biopsy (96% versus 74%, $p < 0.001$). The combination of all of these methods can result in a 97% diagnosis of malignant pleural effusions. The sensitivity of cytology compared to that of thoracoscopy did not vary among lung carcinomas (67% versus 96%), extrathoracic primary tumors (62% versus 96%), and diffuse malignant mesothelioma (58% versus 92%) [23]. The false-negative thoracoscopic results can be due to a physician's inexperience along with the presence of adhesions that prevent access to the neoplastic tissue. Adhesions can result from multiple attempts of therapeutic thoracentesis. Despite the great usefulness of the procedure, thoracic surgery backup should be available. VATS requires general anesthesia and single-lung ventilation. It usually combines diagnosis and treatment but it is a more extensive procedure than the medical one because several ports have to be used. VATS is not indicated when the patient cannot tolerate single-lung ventilation or if the pleural adhesions prevent the safe insertion of the thoracoscope. In those cases and if diagnosis remains elusive despite a successful exploratory thoracoscopy, thoracotomy is indicated when the patient has a good performance status.

Bronchoscopy has a low diagnostic yield in undiagnosed pleural effusions and it must be performed only if endobronchial lesions are suspected as a result of atelectasis or when the lung fails to expand after therapeutic thoracentesis.

49.7 Prognostic Factors

Many attempts have been made to find prognostic factors in patients with recurrent malignant effusions in order to select the optimum therapeutic strategy. Clinical data and pleural fluid parameters are investigated. Pleural fluid pH and glucose concentration seems to have the best correlation with overall survival [23–25]. Uncertainty remains for the thresholds of their values. A meta-analysis of 400 patients indicated that patients with pH values less than 7.28 had a 3-month survival rate of 38.9% compared to 61.6% for patients with values over this cutoff point. Although pH is a significant predictor of the duration of survival, accuracy is low and only 54.4% of the patients predicted by pH to die within 3 months were classified correctly. Decreasing the cutoff points of pH did not increase accuracy. This study also showed that the primary origin of malignancy influences survival. Patients with neoplasms of the lung, soft tissues, kidney, ovary, gastrointestinal tract, and oropharynx had a worse median survival. It is confirmed that pH correlates with the duration of survival but it cannot be clinically used for the selection of patients who should not undergo pleurodesis based on an estimated survival [26]. In the majority of studies, as well as in the meta-analysis, clinical data such as weight loss and Karnofsky performance status scores (KPS) were not taken into consideration. Performance status measured with Karnofsky's scale has a strong correlation with the survival of patients with lung cancer, other solid tumors, and lymphomas. In recurrent malignant effusions, performance status seems to be a significant predictor of survival. Patients with KPS of more than 70 have a median survival of 395 days, compared with only 34 days for those with KPS less than 30 [27].

49.8 Treatment

The accumulation of pleural fluid in patients with cancer usually signals advanced disease and is associated with a dismal long-term survival rate. Selection of optimal treatment for each individual patient requires a careful assessment of the benefits and the risks of the treatment. Primary treatment targets should involve palliation or elimination of dyspnea, improvement of a patient's overall quality of life in order to restore daily activities, and implementation of oncological therapies. The complexity of confronting malignant effusions is reflected in the official statement of the American Thoracic Society and the European Respiratory Society as it was published in 2000 and 2001, respectively, in their guidelines [3]. The proposed therapeutic options for malignant pleural effusions include repeated thoracentesis, tube thoracostomy or thoracoscopy for the evacuation and pleurodesis, pleuroperitoneal shunts, pleural abrasion, and pleurectomy.

49.8.1 Therapeutic Thoracentesis

Therapeutic thoracentesis must be performed in all symptomatic patients with malignant pleural effusions. This alleviates dyspnea and slows the rate of recurrence. Inability to improve symptoms following therapeutic thoracentesis indicates pathology of the underlying pleura or lung such as trapped lung, atelectasis, lymphangitic carcinomatosis, or tumor embolism. Rapid recurrence of fluid imposes immediate treatment.

Repeated therapeutic thoracentesis, on an outpatient basis, is an acceptable procedure for those with poor performance status, short survival expectancy, and low pH of the pleural fluid. This reduces hospitalization and avoids the more invasive techniques. Periodic thoracentesis in moderate effusions with a combination of systemic chemotherapy can be applied in asymptomatic patients.

The volume of fluid that can be safely removed is unknown. In large effusions with a contralateral mediastinal shift, several liters of drainage are probably safe. In general, when the pleural space pressure is not measured, it is preferred to remove 1–1.5 L as long as the patient does not experience any dyspnea, cough, or chest pain [3]. The main adverse effect in rapidly removing fluid (and air) from the pleural cavity is the on-site re-expanding pulmonary edema. The mechanism of edema progression is not fully clarified, but it is believed that it is mostly related to mechanical forces causing vascular stretching or injury, and increasing capillary permeability rather than the absolute level of negative pleural pressure [28].

The success of pleural fluid drainage can be discriminated on the basis of the relief of dyspnea and by chest X-ray. Determination of pulmonary functions and PaO_2 may be misleading. Pleural effusion tends to increase the volume of the hemithorax rather than decrease the lung volume. Therefore, the improvement of total lung capacity (TLC) after thoracentesis is only one third of the volume of the removed fluid [29]. The effect on PaO_2 varies and it can be increased, remain the same, or temporarily decreased.

49.8.2 Pleurodesis

Pleurodesis is the most suitable palliative treatment in patients with recurrent symptomatic malignant effusions and good performance status. The aim of the procedure is to achieve adhesion of the parietal and visceral pleura by the development of a dense fibrosis in order to prevent accumulation of fluid in the pleural cavity. Lung re-expansion is necessary for a successful pleurodesis. Pleural fluid pH (7.20), glucose levels (60 mg/dL), and pleural space elastance (19 cm H_2O) are used to predict the pleurodesis outcome and/or the absence of trapped lung. The measurement of elastance, defined as the decline in pleural fluid pressure in cm H_2O after the removal of 500 mL of effusion, seems to have a better trend in accuracy than the fluid pH but not significantly. Some suggest that pH levels have more of a discriminative power to predict the outcome of pleurodesis than the trapped lung itself [30, 31].

Pleurodesis is usually performed by installation of a chemical agent through the standard drainage chest tube or small-bore catheter (8–16F). Ideally, the chest tube must be directed posteriorly toward the diaphragm. Confirmation of lung re-expansion with X-ray shortly precedes pleurodesis [3]. A number of antineoplastic and non-antineoplastic agents are used for pleurodesis (Table 49.2). Sterilized asbestos-free talc (3 MgO, 4 SiO_2, and H_2O) consistently produces the highest success rates (>90%) regardless of how it is implemented. It can be insufflated into the pleural space via medical or surgical thoracoscopy or administered in the form of slurry through a chest tube followed by tetracyclines (minocycline and doxycycline) and bleomycin. Minocycline and doxycycline have overall success rates of 73% but the unfortunate requirement of repeated doses and heavy local analgesia is thought to be the main drawback. *Corynebacterium parvum* has limited success while quinacrine can provoke serious toxicity in the central nervous system [2, 3, 32]. Bleomycin is an effective sclerosing agent with similar success rates to tetracycline. With bleomycin, however, there is less chest pain and fever. Generally, talc slurry appears to be more preferred due to its cost. The criticism over the use of bleomycin is that it is relatively more expensive compared with other agents. However, studies of its remarkable success rates have made bleomycin through small-bore chest tubes a more attractive, less invasive option as it reduces hospitalization time [2, 3, 30–33]. Additionally, the use of a standard dose of 60 mg bleomycin mixed with 50–100 cm^3 of sterile saline can be replaced effectively with a lower dose of 30 mg when careful selection is made of patients with no evidence of trapped lung [30].

Table 49.2. Efficacy of the most commonly used sclerosing agents

Agents	Responses (%)	Dose
Bleomycin	64	30–60 mg
Tetracycline[a]	72	500 mg to 20 mg/kg
Doxycycline	73	500 mg (often multiple doses)
Talc	98	2.5–10 g

[a] No longer used.

Modified from: Nguyen DM, Schrump DS. Malignant and pericardial effusions. In: De Vita V, Hellman S, Rosenberg SA (eds) Cancer Principles and Practice of Oncology. Philadelphia: Lippincott, Williams and Wilkins, 2005:2381 [5]

As mentioned above, talc pleurodesis is the most successful therapeutic palliation strategy for malignant effusions. After the pleural cavity has been drained, no more than 5 g talc must be instilled into pleural space as slurry or poudrage. The tube should be closed for 1–2 h after instillation. With slurry, the patient must be repositioned. Slow progressive suction can be applied if trapped lung is suspected. The chest tube can be safely removed when drainage is less than 150 mL/day, usually within 48 h. If after 48 h and up until 72 h the chest tube drainage is still large (>250 mL/day), re-installation of the same dose of talc can be performed [3]. Talc is an inexpensive and highly effective agent. The most common complications seen in talc administration are pain and fever. Pain is ranged from non-existing to severe and can be easily controlled by the administration of local anesthesia and parenteral analgesia before the procedure. Fever is mild, probably related to the inflammatory process, and characteristically occurs 4–12 h after instillation. More serious complications, such as acute respiratory distress syndrome (ARDS), acute pneumonitis, and respiratory failure have been reported. They are mostly related to dose and particle size [3, 34, 35]. Long-term complications, such as an increasing incidence of lung cancer, have not been documented with asbestos-free products [3].

The exact mechanism of pleurodesis has not yet clearly defined. For years, scientists believed that inflammatory cells were responsible for the fibrosis but this hypothesis can not explain the rapidness of the fibrotic procedure. The basic fibroblast growth factor (bFGF) appears to be the cornerstone of the fibrotic cascade. bFGF is a strong mitogen for fibroblasts and, as seen in in vitro studies, pleural mesothelial cells release high levels of biologically active bFGF after talc stimulation. Additionally, it has been proven that normal mesothelial cells synthesize higher amounts of bFGF than malignant ones, indicating that the presence of normal mesothelium is important for the rapid release of bFGF and, also, for a successful pleurodesis. This can support the use of talc pleurodesis by clinicians at an early stage, rather than a later one, and even

for asymptomatic patients, it can be implemented before the pleura is diffusely covered with malignant deposits [32, 36].

49.8.3 Treatment of Pleurodesis Failure

Failure of pleurodesis may be due to either inappropriate patient selection or with its technique. An additional option for these patients is the pleuroperitoneal shunt. This palliation treatment is suitable for patients with trapped lung or malignant chylothorax since chyle is recirculated [3]. Few complications have been associated with shunt placement. The most common is shunt occlusion (12%) and in this case, a replacement is mandatory. The possibility of seeding the peritoneum with malignant cells through the shunt is present, but not clearly documented. For these patients, there is no established alternative treatment [3]. For patients with good performance status, an expected survival of more than 6 months, trapped lung, or pleurodesis failure, pleural abrasion with or without pleurectomy can be a solution. By obliterating the pleural space, pleurodesis can be successful. However, pleurectomy is a major surgical procedure with perioperative mortality of 12% and, thus, the careful selection of patients is important [3].

Lastly, in patients with a short survival expectancy, poor performance status, and symptomatic malignant pleural effusion, implementation of a chronic indwelling catheter can provide an effective, alternative solution.

49.8.4 Systemic Chemotherapy

For patients with chemosensitive tumors, such as small cell lung cancer, lymphomas, and breast cancer, systemic therapy can prove to be equally or more effective than local therapy for relieving malignant effusions. After the initial therapeutic thoracentesis, chemotherapy must be administered and pleurodesis can be delayed until systemic treatment becomes ineffective. However, if a rapid reaccumulation of fluid is present or there is a contraindication to chemotherapy, pleurodesis can be initiated [3]. Malignant effusions due to tumors of the prostate, ovary, or thyroid, or those which have arisen from germ cells, may also respond to chemotherapy.

49.8.5 Intrapleural Therapy

The use of localized intrapleural chemotherapy appears as an attractive therapeutic option to maximize antineoplastic activity and minimize systemic absorption and adverse effects of chemotherapy. Doxorubicin hydrochloride, cisplatin, cytarabine, mitomycin C, and 5-FU are some of the agents used [37–39]. The results from a few studies of small groups of patients were promising. Larger prospective randomized studies are necessary to compare the efficacy of intrapleural therapy with that of pleurodesis. Several studies have investigated the intrapleural use of several active cytokines. Interleukin-2 and interferon-β have been used. Their success varies but, in general, the results were poorer than that of talc [37, 40–42]. It is not yet clear if the responses are due to the immunological effects of cytokines, which increase the natural killer cell population, or if they are due to the sclerosing activity that they possess. Research for new intrapleural therapeutic agents for patients with malignant pleural effusions, a group with dismal prognosis, is needed. Some of the latest studies propose the use of new agents with impressive results. *Staphylococcus aureus* superantigen (SSAg) is one of the newer agents. SSAg has been reported to not only effectively resolve malignant pleural effusion in patients with non-small cell lung cancer and poor performance status (KPS < 50), but also to prolong survival when compared to talc poudrage pleurodesis [43].

49.9 Management of Malignant Effusions in Specific Diseases

49.9.1 Lung Cancer

Although malignant effusion can be due to the invasion of the pleura from malignant cells of any organ, lung cancer is the most common cause. Approximately 15% of these patients are diagnosed with malignant effusion on their first admittance, and 50% of them who have locally advanced or metastatic disease will develop effusion in the course of their sickness. All histological types can metastasize in the pleura but the most frequent is adenocarcinoma, probably because of its peripheral location. For patients with malignant effusion from non-small cell lung cancer, chemotherapy is not the first treatment strategy. Palliative local therapy includes careful drainage of the pleural cavity. If the patient is a candidate for pleurodesis, intrapleural application of a sclerotic agent (talc slurry or poudrage, bleomycin, or doxycycline) is performed. A large phase III study demonstrated that talc insufflation through thoracoscopy has higher success rates (82%) than the use of slurry through thoracostomy in the subgroup of patients with primary lung cancer [44]. In patients with a good performance status (KPS > 70), complementary systemic chemotherapy must be administered. For patients with paramalignant effusions due to postobstructive atelectasis, bronchoscopy is necessary for resolution of obstruction. The prognosis of this group of patients is similar to those at the same stage without effusion [2–4].

Pleural effusion due to small cell lung cancer traditionally stages the disease as extensive. However, if the effusion is the only evidence of metastatic spread, the survival is comparable to those with a limited disease. After the initial thoracentesis, chemotherapy is considered as the first choice of treatment and pleurodesis can be delayed until recurrence [3, 45].

49.9.2 Breast Cancer

Breast cancer is the most common tumor in females and it is the second cause of malignant effusions (25%), following lung cancer [46]. It has been accepted that 46% of patients with disseminating breast cancer will develop pleural metastases. The median time from the initial diagnosis until the development of pleural effusion is 41.5 months with a range of 0 to 246 months [3]. In a retrospective study of 3,856 women with a history of invasive breast carcinoma, Pokieser et al. analyzed the correlation between the site of the primary tumor and the probability to develop a malignant effusion. When the primary tumor was located in the inner quadrants, the probability of malignant pleural or pericardial effusion was 4 times higher [47]. The clinical usefulness of this observation is that a more aggressive adjuvant therapy can be administered to a particular subset of patients with breast cancer. The survival after the onset of effusion is better for breast cancer patients compared to lung cancer ones. It is related to the presence of metastatic sites of the disease in other organs. The median survival is 48 months if pleural effusion is the only evidence of recurrence and 12 months when disseminating disease is present. The diagnosis of malignant effusion due to breast cancer is relatively uncomplicated (by cytological examination of pleural fluid) and more invasive procedures are rarely demanded [48]. The expression of estrogen and progesterone receptors in primary breast tumors is undoubtedly related to the prognosis. The expression of these receptors from metastatic pleural tissue can interfere with the survival of the patient but this hypothesis remains to be confirmed since there is a lack of data [49]. Other prognostic factors such as chromosomal changes, as detected by fluorescence in situ hybridization (FISH), are under investigation but a greater number of prospective studies need to be conducted [50]. The mechanisms of pleural metastases are either through lymphatic spread, which results in an ipsilateral effusion, or through hematogenous spread, which is usually accompanied by hepatic metastases and is associated with bilateral or contralateral effusion. A less common mechanism is the direct invasion through the chest wall. Ipsilateral localization is detected in 50% of patients while contralateral localization is in 40%. Bilateral is seen in 10% of these patients [3, 51]. Systemic chemotherapy and hormone therapy are the recommended first-line therapies for recurrent breast cancer and malignant effusion. If chemotherapy is ineffective or contraindicated, local therapy must be considered. Talc pleurodesis remains the best choice with a tendency to talc insufflation through thoracostomy rather than talc slurry [44]. Distinguishing between pleural effusions due to metastases and those due to post-radiation therapy is important. The latter can occur after adjuvant radiotherapy in patients with breast tumor after segmentectomy. Post-radiation effusions are usually presented within 6 months after radiation and are resolved spontaneously.

49.9.3   Lymphomas and Multiple Myeloma

Lymphomas rank third in frequency (10%) in cancers causing malignant effusions. Effusions occur more often in non-Hodgkin's than in Hodgkin's lymphomas. Fluid characteristics are mostly in accordance with exudate criteria than transudate criteria. Non-Hodgkin's lymphoma is the most common cause of chylothorax [5, 52]. The mechanism of fluid accumulation is blockage of the lymphatic drainage either from mediastinal nodal invasion (Hodgkin's disease) or direct infiltration of the pleura (non-Hodgkin disease). Although the diagnostic usefulness of fluid cytological examinations varies from 30% to 55% (the lowest sensitivity seen in Hodgkin's disease), chromosomal analysis has a higher sensitivity of up to 85%. The application of flow cytometry by using immunocytometry can identify cell lineage (T or B cells) as well as the clonality of the population of lymphocytes [15]. The average overall survival time is usually short and positive fluid cytology is associated with a poor prognosis. Systemic chemotherapy is the recommended treatment for malignant effusions due to lymphomas. Palliative local treatments with sclerosing agents can be provided to achieve relief of symptoms. Mediastinal radiation can help in the resolution of symptomatic pleural effusion when mediastinal node enlargement is the cause of impaired lymphatic drainage. Pleuroperitoneal shunt is a fair approach for patients with chylothorax and chemotherapy failure as chyle is recirculated [3, 53].

Malignant pleural effusion secondary to multiple myeloma is uncommon and occurs in only 6% of patients. The diagnosis can be obtained from the measurement of fluid protein concentration, characteristically from up to 7 g/dL [54]. Electrophoresis and immunoelectrophoresis of the fluid are equally diagnostic. Pleural invasion usually originates from an adjacent lesion (ribs, sternum, and vertebra) or from chest wall plasmatocytoma. Systemic therapy is also recommended.

49.9.4   Malignant Pleural Mesothelioma

Malignant pleural mesothelioma (MPM) has an incidence which varies according to the geographic location. The disease is related to asbestos exposure with predominance in the population of males between 50 and 70 years of age. A long latency period is observed between time of exposure and the development of the disease with a mean time of 40 years (range of 14–72 years). Three histological types of MPM are identified: epithelial, mixed, and sarcomatous. Sarcomatous and mixed types are associated with poor prognosis as well as poor performance status, chest pain, and weight loss. They have a platelet count greater than 400,000/ L, a serum lactate dehydrogenase of more than 500 IU/μL, low hemoglobin levels, high white blood cell count, and are usually greater than 75 years of age [55, 56]. The most recent retrospective studies imply that the simian virus 40 (SV40) correlates with the development of MPM that has a poor prognosis [57]. The importance of molecular biology in cancer research must demonstrate some revolutionary deductions. The analysis of pretherapeutic gene expression in mesothelioma biopsies can predict the clinical outcome of the patient, independently of the histological type [58], and the resistance to treatment [59]. Today, with the use of histochemical and immunohistochemical staining techniques, along with electron microscopic analysis, it is possible to obtain a diagnosis of MPM from pleural effusion in 84% of cases, starkly contrasting the once low diagnostic accuracy of only 33% derived from the cytological examination of pleural fluid associated with mesothelioma. Thoracoscopy (medical or surgical) remains the gold standard for diagnosis and staging. In reviewing the literature, there is no clearly identifiable therapeutic strategy for resectable pleural mesothelioma. Patients who are candidates for surgery are those who theoretically can achieve a complete resection of tumor (stage I–III). The percentage of 2- and 5-year survival time for stage I is 65% and 30%, respectively [60] but a long-term survival for all "resectable" stages is disappointing with a median survival ranging from 9 to 17.3 months [56]. The strategy of a multimodal treatment approach, despite the lack of large phase III trials, appears to be a justifiable choice. Large, but not randomized, reports indicate an improved median survival (13–17 months) for patients with multimodal treatment (surgery, chemotherapy, and/or radiotherapy) compared to the best supportive care (median survival of 7 months) [60, 61]. It is of great importance to notice that these trials were conducted before the arrival of the new antifolates (pemetrexed and raltitrexed) which have changed the course of chemotherapy in MPM. Based on good results of induction/neoadjuvant chemotherapy in non-small cell lung cancer, Weder et al. [62] conducted a neoadjuvant trial for patients with potential operable MPM. They used an acceptable doubled combination of cisplatin and gemcitabine (response rates of 16–48% [63]) for 3 cycles followed by surgery and radiotherapy. Their promising results of median survival of 23 months need further confirmation by larger randomized trials.

The role of radiotherapy as a single-modality therapy is limited. It is most commonly used as a palliative treatment of chest pain and/or as a preventive procedure of scar recurrence when thoracentesis, biopsy, or operation has been obtained. The frequency of malignant seeding after chest wall injury has been reported to have occurred in 20–50% of patients who underwent invasive techniques. Small doses of external beam radiation (21 Gy) to the chest wall, delivered 10–15 days after the invasive procedure, acts as a preventing agent.

Patients who have reached an unresectable stage of the disease are candidates for chemotherapy. Many chemotherapeutic agents have been tested as single agents in MPM with disappointing results. Only vinorelbine given on a weekly schedule has showed any acceptable results with improvement of general physical symptoms and a median survival of 10.6 months [64]. In 2003, the results from a large phase III trial by Vogelzang et al. [65] have changed the role of chemotherapy in MPM. The investigators concluded that the use of a cisplatin plus pemetrexed regimen, compared to a single regimen of cisplatin, improves median survival, pulmonary function tests, and any disease-related symptoms. Another phase III study conducted by the European Organization for Research and Treatment of Cancer (EORTC) that also used a double regimen of a new antifolate raltitrexed and cisplatin, resulted in equally encouraging data with median survival of approximately 12 months. The novel antifolate pemetrexed is a multitargeted inhibitor of dihydrofolate reductase, thymidylate synthase, and glycinamide ribonucleotide formyltransferase. The main toxicities of the double regimen are hematological, with neutropenia grade 3–4 (28%) and leukocytopenia (18%) being the predominant ones. The data of this phase III international study provided level 1 evidence for the treatment of mesothelioma patients with a combination of pemetrexed and cisplatin.

The use of intrapleural cytokine therapy has been investigated in MPM and encouraging results have been reported from small phase II studies. Interleukin-2 has shown the best activity and toxicity profile and a median survival of 18 months [66]. This promising approach remains to be confirmed by larger clinical studies.

49.10 Expectations for the Future

Despite assiduous investigation, in about 3–10% of patients with malignant effusions the primary malignancy is not obvious. Delay of treatment and symptom relief is not justified because the presence of effusion indicates that the tumor is already disseminated. However, it is important to identify tumors that may be sensitive to hormone or chemotherapy, such as breast or ovarian cancer in women or gut and germ cell tumors in both sexes. Imaging examinations such as mammography, abdominal and pelvic ultrasonography, computerized tomography, rectal examination, and use of tumor markers (cancer antigen 125, carcinoembryonic antigen, human chorionic gonadotrophin, and a-fetoprotein) can prove useful in order to localize the primary cause of the effusion.

Malignancy of the pleural space is an area of continuous clinical and biological research. The need for better understanding of the cellular mechanisms of fluid accumulation as well as a better understanding of the administration of more effective and less toxic intrapleural therapy is imperative. The novel technology of gene therapy can be the answer to many malignancies and to malignant effusions, if problems such as therapeutic gene transfer are resolved in the years to come [67, 68].

Key Points

- Malignancy is one of the most common causes of exudative pleural effusions, since in postmortem examinations of patients who died of cancer, the incidence of malignant effusion was 16%.
- Lung cancer is the most common cause of malignant effusions with an incidence of 40%. When first evaluated, approximately 15% of lung cancer patients exhibit pleural effusion and up to 50% of the patients with an advanced disease may acquire a pleural effusion during the course of their disease.
- Adenocarcinoma of the lung is the most common histological type associated with malignant pleural infusion; it spreads by contiguity due to its peripheral location and has the propensity to invade the vessels.
- The term "paramalignant effusions" refers to those effusions that are not a direct result of the pleura invasion from the tumor but are still related to the primary malignancy. Not all "paramalignant effusions" exclude operability in lung cancer. Important examples are the parapneumonic effusions due to postobstructive pneumonia and the transudate effusions secondary to postobstructive atelectasis.
- The accumulation of pleural fluid in patients with cancer usually signals advanced disease and is associated with a dismal long-term survival rate.

References

1. Rodrigues-Panadero F, Borderns Naranjo F, Lopez-Mejias J. Pleural metastatic tumors and effusions. Frequency and pathogenic mechanisms in postmortem series. Eur Respir J 1989; 2:366.
2. Sahn SA. Malignancy metastatic to the pleura. Clin Chest Med 1998; 19:351.
3. Antony VB, Loddenkemper R, Astoul P, et al. Management of malignant pleural effusions. Am J Respir Crit Care Med 2000; 162: 1987.
4. Light RW. Pleural Diseases, 4th edn. Philadelphia: Lippincott, Williams and Wilkins, 2001; 87.
5. Nguyen DM, Schrump DS. Malignant and pericardial effusions. In: De Vita V, Hellman S, Rosenberg SA (eds) Cancer Principles and Practice of Oncology. Philadelphia: Lippincott, Williams and Wilkins, 2005:2381.
6. Canto A, Rivas J, Saumenech J, et al. Points to consider when choosing a biopsy method in cases of pleurisy of unknown origin. Chest 1983; 84:176.
7. Light RW, Hamm H. Malignant pleural effusion: would the real cause please stand up? Eur Respir J 1997; 10:1701.
8. O'Donovan PB, Eng P. Pleural changes in malignant pleural effusions: appearance on computed tomography. Cleve Clin J Med 1994; 61:127.
9. Holling N, Shaw P. Diagnostic imaging of lung cancer. Eur Respir J 2002; 19:722.
10. Bittner RC, Felix R. Magnetic resonance (MR) imaging of the chest: state of the art. Eur Respir J 1998; 11:1392.
11. Empta NG, Rogers JS, Graeber GM, et al. Clinical role of F-18 fluodeoxyglucose positron emission tomography imaging in patients with lung cancer and suspected malignant pleural effusion. Chest 2002; 122:1918.
12. Duysinx B, Nguyen D, Louis R, et al. Evaluation of pleural disease with F-18 fluodeoxyglucose positron emission tomography imaging. Chest 2004; 125:489.
13. Kuhn M, Fitting JW, Lonenberger P. Probability of malignancy in pleural eosinophilia. Chest 1989; 96:992.
14. Rubins JB, Rubins HB. Etiology and prognostic significance of eosinophilic pleural effusion. Chest 1996; 110:12.
15. Light RW. Diagnostic principles in pleural diseases. Eur Respir J 1997; 10:476.
16. Heffner JE, Heffner JN, Brown LK. Multilevel and continuous pleural fluid pH ratios for evaluating malignant pleural effusions. Chest 2003; 123:1887.
17. Wirth PR, Legier J, Wright GL Jr. Immunohistochemical evaluation of seven monoclonal antibodies for differentiation of pleural mesothelioma from lung adenocarcinoma. Cancer 1991; 67:655.
18. Yang PC, Luh KT, Kuo SH, et al. Immunohistochemistry and ELISA quantitation of mucin for diagnosis of malignant pleural effusions. Am Rev Respir Dis 1992; 146:15.
19. Porcel JM, Vives M, Escuerda A, et al. Use of a panel of tumor markers (carcinoembryonic antigen, cancer antigen 125, carbohydrate antigen 15-3 and cytokeratin 19 fragments) in pleural fluid for differential diagnosis of benign and malignant effusions. Chest 2004; 126:1757.
20. Dikmen G, Dikmen E, Kara M, et al. Diagnostic implications of telomerase activity in pleural effusions. Eur Respir J 2003; 22:422.
21. Colt HG. Window to pleural space. Chest 1999; 116:1409.
22. Loddenkemper R. Thoracoscopy: state of the art. Eur Respir J 1998; 11:213.
23. Rondrigues-Panadero F, Lopez-Mejias J. Survival time of patients with pleural metastatic carcinoma predicted by glucose and pH studies. Chest 1989; 95:320.
24. Sahn SA, Good JT. Pleural fluid pH in malignant effusions. Ann Intern Med 1988; 108:3.
25. Rondrigues-Panadero F, Lopez-Mejias J. Low glucose and pH levels in malignant pleural effusions: diagnostic significance and prognostic value in respect to pleurodesis. Am Rev Respir Dis 1989; 139:663.
26. Heffner JE, Nietert P, Barbieri C. Pleural fluid pH as a predictor of survival for patients with malignant pleural effusions. Chest 2000; 117:79.
27. Burrows CM, Mathews WC, Colt HG. Predicting survival in patients with recurrent symptomatic malignant pleural effusions. Chest 2000; 117:73.
28. Sprung CL, Loewenherz JW, Baier H, Hauser JM. Evidence for increased permeability in re-expansion pulmonary edema. Am J Med 1981; 71:497.
29. Light RW, Stansbury DW, Brown SE. The relationship between pleural pressures and changes in pulmonary function after therapeutic thoracentesis. Am Rev Respir Dis 1986; 133:658.
30. Lan RS, Lo SK, Chuang ML, et al. Elastance of pleural space. A predictor for the outcome of pleurodesis in patient with malignant pleural effusion. Ann Intern Med 1997; 126:7.
31. Rondrigues-Panadero F, Sanchez GR, Martin JJ, Castillo Gomez J. Prediction of results of the talc pleurodesis in malignant pleural effusions Am J Respir Crit Care Med 1994; 149:A1103.
32. Rondrigues-Panadero F, Antony VB. Pleurodesis: state of the art. Eur Respir J 1997; 10:1648.
33. Patz EF, McAndams HP, Strange C, Ginsberg RJ, Sahn SA. Sclerotherapy for malignant pleural effusions: a prospective randomized trial of bleomycin vs doxycycline with small bore catheter drainage. Chest 1998; 113:1305.
34. Campos JR, Werebe EC, Vargas FS, et al. Respiratory failure due to insufflated talk. Lancet 1997; 349:251.
35. Rehse DH, Aye RW, Florance MG. Respiratory failure following talk pleurodesis. Am J Surg 1999; 177:437.
36. Antony VB, Nasreen N, Mohammed C, et al. Basic fibroblast growth factor mediates pleural fibrosis. Chest 2004; 126:1522.
37. Kvale PA, Simoff M, Prakash UBS. Palliative care. Chest 2003; 123:284(S).
38. Ike O, ShimizuY, Hitomi S, WadaR, Ikada Y. Treatment of malignant pleural effusions with doxorubicine hydrochloride-containing poly(L-lactic acid) microspheres. Chest 1991; 99:911.
39. Shoji T, Tanaka F, Yanagihara K, et al. Phase II study of repeated intrapleural chemotherapy using implantable access system for management of malignant pleural effusion. Chest 2002; 121:821.
40. Rosso R, Rimoldi R, Salvati F. Intrapleural natural beta interferon in the treatment of malignant pleural effusions. Oncology 1988; 45:253.
41. Astoul PH, Viallat JR, Laurent JC, et al. Intrapleural recombinant IL-2 in passive immunotherapy for malignant pleural effusion. Chest 1993; 103:209.
42. Viallat JR, Boutin C, Rey F, et al. Intrapleural immunotherapy with escalating doses of IL-2 in metastatic pleural effusions. Cancer 1993; 71:4067.
43. Ren S, Terman D, Bohach G, et al. Intrapleural staphylococcal superantigen induces resolution of malignant pleural effusions and survival benefit in non-small cell lung cancer. Chest 2004; 126:15.
44. Dresler CM, Olak J, Herndom JE, Richards WG, Scalzetti E, Fleishman SB, Kernstine KH, et al. Phase III Intergroup study of talc poudrage vs talc slurry sclerosis for malignant pleural effusion. Chest 2005; 127:909.
45. Livingston RB, McCracken JD, Trauth CJ, Chen T. Isolated pleural effusion in small cell lung carcinoma. Chest 1982; 81:208.
46. Wood WC, Muss HB, Solin LJ, Olopade OJ. Cancer of the breast. In: Devita V, Hellman S, Rosenberg SA (eds) Can-

cer Principles and Practice of Oncology. Philadelphia: Lippincott, Williams and Wilkins. 2005:1415.

47. Pokieser W, Cassik P, Fischer G, et al. Malignant pleural and pericardial effusion in invasive breast cancer. Impact of the site of the primary tumor. Breast Cancer Res Treat 2004; 83:134.

48. Dines DE, Pierre RV, Franzen SJ. The value of cells in pleural fluid in the differential diagnosis. Mayo Clin Proc 1975; 50:571.

49. Schwarz C, Lübbert H, Rahn W, et al. Medical thoracoscopy: hormone receptor content in pleural metastases due to breast cancer. Eur Respir J 2004; 24:7.

50. Massoner A, Augustin F, Duba HC, Zojer N, Fielg M. FISH cytogenetics and prognosis in breast and non-small cell lung cancers. Cytometry B Clin Cytom 2004; 62B:52.

51. Feutiman IS, Rubens RD, Hayward JL. Control of pleural effusions in patients with breast cancer. Cancer 1983; 52:737.

52. Weick JK, Kiely JM, Harrison EG, Carr DT, Scanlon PW. Pleural effusion in lymphoma. Cancer 1973; 31:848.

53. Murphy MC, Newman BM, Rodgers BM. Pleuroperitoneal shunts in the management of persistent chylothorax. Ann Thorac Surg 1989; 48:195.

54. Rodrigeuz JN, Pereisa A, Martinez JC, Conde J, Pujol E. Pleural effusion in multiple myeloma. Chest 1991; 105:622.

55. Johansson L, Linden CJ. Aspects of histopathological subtype as a prognostic factor in BS pleural mesotheliomas. Chest 1996; 109:109.

56. Pass HJ, Hahn SM, Vogelzang NJ, Carbone M. Benign and malignant mesothelioma. In: DeVita V, Hellman S, Rosenberg SA (eds) Cancer Principles and Practice of Oncology. Philadelphia: Lippincott, Williams and Wilkins, 2005:1687.

57. Procopio A, Strizzi L, Vianale G, et al. Simian virus 40 sequence is a negative prognostic factor in patients with malignant pleural mesothelioma. Genes Chromosomes Cancer 2000; 29:173.

58. Pass H, Liu Z, Wali AN, Bueno R, Land S, et al. Gene expression profiles predict survival and progression of pleural mesothelioma. Clin Cancer Res 2004; 10:844.

59. Fennell DA, Rudd RM. Defective core-apoptosis signaling in diffuse malignant pleural mesothelioma: opportunities for effective drug development. Lancet Oncol 2004; 5:354.

60. Zellos LS, Sugarbaker DJ. Diffuse malignant mesothelioma of the pleural space and its management. Oncology (Huntingt) 2002; 16:907.

61. Rusch VW, Rosenzweig K, Vankatraman E, et al. A phase II trial of surgical resection and adjuvant high-dose hemithoracic radiation for malignant pleural mesothelioma. Thorac Cardiovasc Surg 2001; 122:788.

62. Weder W, Kestenholz P, Taverna C, Bodis S, Lardinois D, et al. Neoadjuvant chemotherapy followed by extrapleural pneumonectomy in malignant pleural mesothelioma. J Clin Oncol 2004; 22:3451.

63. Steele JPC, Klabasta A. Chemotherapy options and new advances in malignant pleural mesothelioma. Ann Oncol 2005; 16:345.

64. Steele JP, Shamash J, Evans MT, et al. Phase II study of vinorelbine in patients with malignant pleural mesothelioma. J Clin Oncol 2000; 18:39.

65. Vogelzang NS, Rusthoven JL, Symanowki J, et al. Phase III trial of pemetrexed in combination with cisplatin versus cisplatin alone in patients with malignant pleural mesothelioma. J Clin Oncol 2003; 21:2636.

66. Astoul P, Picat-Joosen D, Viallat JR, Boutin C. Intrapleural administration of interleukin-2 for treatment of patients with malignant pleural mesothelioma: a phase II study. Cancer 1999; 83:20.

67. Sterman DH, Treat J, Litzkey LA, et al. Adenovirus-mediated herpes simplex virus thymidine kinase/ganciclovir gene therapy in patients with localized malignancy: results of a phase I clinical trial in malignant mesothelioma. Hum Gene Ther 1998; 9:1083.

68. Bernal RM, Sharma S, Gardner BK, et al. Soluble Coxsackie virus adenovirus receptor is a putative inhibitor of adenoviral gene transfer in the tumour milieu. Clin Cancer Res 2002; 8:19.

Palliation of Dyspnea in the Terminally Ill Patient with Lung Cancer

50

Spyros A. Papiris, Effrosyni D. Manali, and Charis Roussos

Contents

50.1 Definition

Dyspnea is the awareness of uncomfortable breathing, and constitutes one of the most frightening and distressing symptoms for "anyone" including patients with cancer [1]. Like every other symptom it is a subjective experience [2] and has been characterized as a nociceptive phenomenon in response to an aversive stimulus [3]. Dyspnea in patients with cancer is commonly associated with anxiety [4] and can be perceived either as panic, chest congestion, chest tightness, or suffocation [5]. Severity of dyspnea is further aggravated by fatigue or pain, other common symptoms among lung cancer patients [6].

50.2 Epidemiology

Dyspnea constitutes one of the most common symptoms in patients with advanced cancer and may affect as many as 90% of them [7]. Dyspnea is more common when direct (primary or metastatic) pleuropulmonary involvement occurs. However, dyspnea also affects one fourth of patients without evidence of cardiopulmonary involvement [8]. Patients with dyspnea have lower quality of life [7] and a much shorter survival [9].

50.3 Pathophysiology and Etiology of Dyspnea

The pathophysiology of dyspnea is incompletely understood and the cause seems multifactorial. In a prospective analysis of 100 patients with advanced cancer and dyspnea, performed by Dudgeon and Lertzman, it was shown that the average number of potential causes of dyspnea per patient was five. In more detail, the authors found that 65% of patients had pleuropulmonary involvement; 52% had bronchospasm; 49% had lung cancer; 40% had oxygen saturation of less than 90%; 29% had evidence of cardiac disease, ischemia, congestive heart failure, or atrial fibrillation; 20% were anemic; and 12% had hypercapnia ($PaCO_2$ 6.0 kPa) [4]. Pulmonary function tests showed reduced values and 47% presented a mixed obstructive-restrictive pattern, 41% a restrictive pattern, and 5% an obstructive pattern. The measurement of the maximum inspiratory pressure was much lower than predicted indicating severe respiratory muscle weakness.

The etiologic conditions that cause dyspnea in patients with cancer are several and may be: (a) directly related to cancer, (b) indirectly related to cancer, (c) related to cancer therapy, and (d) unrelated to cancer [1]. Causes directly related to cancer include primary or metastatic airway, parenchymal, or pleural involvement, pericardial effusion, superior vena cave syndrome, tumor emboli, phrenic nerve paralysis, chest wall involvement (carcinoma en cuirasse), or pathologic bone fractures. Causes indirectly related to cancer include pneumonia, cachexia, anemia, electrolyte abnormalities, pulmonary embolism, paraneoplastic syndromes, and ascites. Causes related to cancer therapy include surgery (any kind of lung resection), radiation pneumonitis, and chemotherapy-induced lung or heart toxicity. Finally, causes unrelated to cancer include COPD, asthma, congestive heart failure, cardiac ischemia, arrhythmias, pulmonary vascular disease, obesity, neuromuscular disorders, aspiration, anxiety, and any other coexisting lung disease.

The pathologic conditions that produce dyspnea do so by more than one mechanism [2]. To understand better how these pathologic conditions may trigger dyspnea, it is necessary to understand how respiratory sensory information is perceived and processed by the brain and leads to respiratory activity. The pool of neurons that constitute the respiratory center in the medulla and pons coordinates the activity of all the respiratory muscles and ensures ventilation. It receives sensory information from central (medullary) and peripheral (carotid and aortic bodies) chemoreceptors, peripheral mechanoreceptors situated in muscles, tendons, and joints, and pulmonary vagal afferent receptors. The vagal afferents include pulmonary stretch receptors activated by lung inflation, irritant receptors of the airways activated by air flow and smooth muscle tone, and alveolar C fibers sensitive to pulmonary interstitial and capillary pressure. The above afferent information may also directly reach the cerebral cortex and integrate with other cognitive and emotional factors together with the information received from the respiratory center to create the perception of breathing [10, 11]. The anterior insula and the posterior cingulate gyrus have recently been identified by positron emission tomography as the cortical areas involved in the perception and the modulation of dyspnea [12, 13]. The pathophysiology of dyspnea though incompletely understood appears multifactorial and three important components can be independently discerned, the work of breathing, the chemical status (hypercapnia, hypoxemia), and the neuromechanical dissociation (the mismatch between what the brain desires for ventilation and the sensory feedback it receives).

50.4 Diagnosis

The gold standard for the diagnosis of dyspnea is the patient's self-report and no other reliable, objective measure of this condition exists. Pulmonary function tests and arterial blood gases do not measure dyspnea. In the cognitively intact patient scales such as the visual analog scale [14] and the Borg scale [15] may be helpful in the estimation of severity and in the assessment of the response to treatment. Patients history, physical examination as well as further investigation including roentgenograms, complete blood count, oximetry, arterial blood gases, computed tomography, echocardiography, and eventually ventilation–perfusion scans may provide enough evidence to disclose correctable conditions that contribute to dyspnea.

50.5 Specific Treatment

Treatment of dyspnea is based on: (a) management of the underlying cause and/or (b) relief of the symptom. Both etiologic and palliative treatment are deemed to be useful when the benefits are greater than the risks. Specific therapeutic issues should be considered and include the following: (a) palliation of dyspnea caused by pleural effusions, (b) bronchoscopic methods to palliate dyspnea, and (c) pharmacologic measures for reversible superimposed conditions.

50.5.1 Palliation of Dyspnea Caused by Pleural Effusions

The main indication for treating a malignant pleural effusion is to relieve dyspnea. Chest roentgenograms with posteroanterior, lateral, and often decubitus views are necessary to determine if the pleural fluid is free-flowing or loculated. Contralateral shift of the mediastinum with large effusions suggests that fluid removal should provide relief of dyspnea. Trapped lung related to parenchymal or pleural disease is associated with unsuccessful procedures. Pleural fluid removal should not exceed 1–1.5 L per time in order to obviate the formation of re-expansion pulmonary edema. Therapeutic thoracentesis should also be stopped earlier if dyspnea, cough, or pain ensues. In cases of successful initial therapeutic thoracentesis the reaccumulation of pleural fluid can be managed in two basic ways: intermittent therapeutic thoracentesis (to be preferred in the terminally ill patient with poor performance status) or insertion of a chest tube to completely evacuate the pleural fluid, followed by pleurodesis (in the patient with a longer life expectancy) [5]. Chemical pleurodesis via chest tube or medical thoracoscopy is the most common and effective approach. Talc pleurodesis is associated with a 91% complete response rate [16]. Pleural effusions due to small cell lung cancer respond to systemic chemotherapy. Maintenance of symptoms after adequate pleural fluid removal is mainly attributed to other underlying causes of dyspnea.

50.5.2 Bronchoscopic Methods to Palliate Dyspnea

Central airway obstruction (trachea and main bronchi) due either to intraluminal tumor growth or to extraluminal tumor compression is a cause of cough and more importantly that of life-threatening dyspnea. Bronchoscopy provides the visual clues to the nature of the obstructing lesion, the extent of the narrowing, and helps in determining the type of the therapeutic choice. The currently available interventional bronchoscopic therapeutic procedures for the relief of dyspnea include: (a) debulking of intraluminal tumor growth via rigid bronchoscopy, (b) balloon dilatation, (c) laser therapy, (d) electrocautery, (e) cryotherapy, (f) argon plasma coagulation (APC), (g) endobronchial irradiation (brachytherapy), (h) photodynamic therapy, and (i) intraluminal stent placement [17].

Tumor debulking: Intraluminal airway obstruction may be sufficiently relieved by tumor debulking via a rigid bronchoscope. This procedure can easily be followed by stent insertion or Nd:YAG laser resection for better results [18].

Balloon dilatation: This procedure is mostly applied in cases of stenoses that are short in length and proves very helpful in preparing the airway for stent placement [19].

Laser therapy: Laser therapy results in photocoagulation of superficial and deep blood vessels, thermal necrosis, and scatter to adjacent tissues. It may be applied through either a flexible or a rigid bronchoscope. If properly used, immediate relief is achieved in almost 90% of patients [20].

Electrocautery: The effect of electrocautery is determined by coagulation and vaporization of endobronchial lesions through application of alternating electrical current. Immediate alleviation of dyspnea is achieved in 55–75% of patients [21].

Cryotherapy: Cryotherapy acts through the application of repetitive freeze/thaw cycles that cause tissue damage and destruction. Results may be delayed for several days. Repeat bronchoscopy is needed for continued therapy in many patients [22].

Argon plasma coagulation: APC devitalizes tumor gradually by coagulating and desiccating tissue utilizing electrically conductive argon plasma. The procedure can be performed both in an outpatient and an inpatient setting [23].

Endobronchial brachytherapy: This technique allows localized delivery of radiation endobronchially through implantation under direct visual guidance of radioactive seeds. Better results are expected when applied in combination with external radiation or/and laser resection [24].

Photodynamic therapy: Photodynamic therapy causes tissue destruction by applying a selectively retained photosensitizer which, when exposed to the proper amount and wavelength of light, produces an activated oxygen species that oxidizes critical parts of neoplastic cells [25].

Airway stents: Stents are metallic or silicone prostheses used to maintain airway patency in cases of endobronchial obstruction or extraluminal compression. They are mainly used to manage tracheal or main bronchial disease and usually follow bronchoscopic debridement and laser therapy. Immediate relief is expected in more than 80% of patients [26].

All invasive bronchoscopic procedures require special training and expensive equipment. Personnel familiar with the procedures minimize complications, such as severe hemorrhage, pneumothorax, and pneumomediastinum, and maximize patient comfort and safety [27].

50.5.3 Pharmacologic Measures for Reversible Superimposed Conditions

Dyspnea among lung cancer patients is often aggravated by superimposed conditions that could be reversed if appropriately treated, such as infection, anemia, hemoptysis, embolism, and bronchospasm.

In detail, the risk of pulmonary infection increases following intensive chemotherapy and long duration of neutrophilic depletion. *Pseudomonas* represents the most frequent etiology of bacteremic pneumonia, accounting for 43% of cases. Empiric antimicrobial or antifungal treatment should always be provided in a timely manner according to International Guidelines and regional epidemiology data for common pathogens. Sputum and/or bronchoscopic specimen cultures should be obtained where possible [28]. Granulocyte colony-stimulating factor has been shown to shorten the period of neutropenia and could additionally be prescribed [29].

Anemia-related dyspnea could be managed by a combination of red blood cell transfusion and erythropoietin injections [30]. In case of anemia due to severe hemoptysis, further management is required. Airway protection and patient stabilization should be followed either by bronchoscopic therapy (iced saline, topical agents, endobronchial tamponade, laser photoresection), or by bronchial artery embolization and surgical resection, if needed [31].

Another potentially reversible cause of dyspnea in this group of patients is pulmonary embolism. The use of anticoagulants is the treatment of choice.

As far as bronchospasm is concerned, it is attributed either to underlying COPD or cardiac failure. The former is often successfully managed through bronchodilators in combination with corticosteroids. The latter necessitates specific evaluation and is mostly alleviated with the help of diuretics and oxygen therapy.

50.5.4 Symptomatic Relief

For all lung cancer patients with dyspnea, the pharmacologic approaches for its relief may include oxygen, bronchodilators, corticosteroids, anxiolytics, analgesics, and opioids (Table 50.1) [5].

Oxygen: Supplemental oxygen is the most widely used treatment for dyspnea relief in lung cancer patients. Its effectiveness is mostly related to the reverse of hypoxemia but could also be due to a significant placebo effect. Irrespective of the limited number of studies on the issue, it seems that there is a perceived benefit in patients with dyspnea and oxygen therapy should always be considered in this case. Multiple blood gas analyses could be fairly replaced by percutaneous oximetry to assess sufficient oxygenation [9].

Table 50.1. Recommendations for palliation of dyspnea in the terminally ill patient with lung cancer

Evaluation of dyspnea

Mild, moderate, severe, refractory (continuous, intermittent – impact on every day activities)
Presence of reversible superimposed conditions (cardiac failure, arrhythmias, bronchospasm, pulmonary infection, pneumothorax, pericardial or pleural effusion, severe anemia, pulmonary embolism, superior vena cava syndrome, central airway obstruction, ascites)
Coexisting cough, chest pain, bronchial secretions, hemoptysis

Therapeutic measures

Management of reversible superimposed conditions
Cognitive/behavioral interventions for dyspnea
Oxygen therapy ± air blowing on the face for all patients with dyspnea
Bronchodilators
Steroids (carcinomatous lymphangitis, central airway obstruction and stridor [plus evaluation for bronchoscopic management or tracheostomy], superior vena cava syndrome)
Anxiolytic therapy
Opioid therapy
Terminal care (includes, morphine or midazolam, suctioning of secretions, bronchodilators, supplemental oxygen, and psychological support for family carers)

Bronchodilators and corticosteroids: Although it is not proved that lung cancer itself causes bronchospasm, standard bronchodilators such as β_2-agonists and anticholinergics are helpful in alleviating dyspnea in case of underlying COPD or bronchial asthma (2.5–5 mg salbutamol and/or 0.25–0.5 mg ipratropium 4–6 times per day). Corticosteroids could further be used in treating parenchymal toxicity resulting from lung radiation therapy [32] as well as carcinomatous lymphangitis (dexamethasone 4–8 mg or prednisolone 2–50 mg), stridor (dexamethasone 16 mg intravenously), and superior vena cava syndrome (dexamethasone 16 mg/day or prednisolone 60 mg/day) [1].

Anxiolytics: Anxiolytics such as benzodiazepines, buspirone, and chlorpromazine play a limited role in dyspnea management. In patients where anxiety is a major component of dyspnea, anxiolytics in combination with learning breathing control, activity pacing, and relaxation techniques are of great benefit (lorazepam 0.5–1 mg/h orally until settled, then dose routinely every 4–6 h to keep settled; diazepam 5–10 mg/h orally until settled, and then dose routinely every 6–8 h; clonazepam 0.25–2 mg orally every 12 h; midazolam 0.5 mg intravenously per 15 min until settled, then by continuous subcutaneous or intravenous infusion). In all other cases they should either be used in combination or totally be replaced by opioids that have proved very effective in relieving breathlessness and discomfort [1].

Analgesics: Non-narcotic analgesics could be administered for mild pain and discomfort-worsening dyspnea. However, patients with lung cancer mostly suffer from severe pain related to bone metastases and malignant pleural effusions. In this case, response to conventional analgesics is poor and more aggressive pain control is indicated [4].

Opioids: Opioids along with oxygen therapy are the cornerstones of symptomatic relief of dyspnea and at the same time provide adequate control of severe pain and cough. They may be administered both orally and parenterally according to specific guidelines and act mostly through their effect on opioid receptors of the central and peripheral nervous system. After administration of oral morphine (5 mg every 4 h), dyspnea alleviation ensues in 24 h and is maintained with continued therapy. Sedation constitutes opioids major side effect, may lead to ventilatory failure, and should always be taken into consideration in therapeutic and end-of-life management issues [33].

50.6 Conclusions

Dyspnea is the awareness of uncomfortable breathing, and constitutes one of the most frightening and distressing symptoms for patients with cancer. Dyspnea is common in patients with advanced cancer and may affect as many as 90% of them. Both etiologic and palliative treatments are deemed to be useful when the benefits are greater than the risks. Specific therapeutic issues should be considered and include the treatment of pleural effusions, bronchoscopic methods for central airway obstruction, and pharmacologic measures for reversible superimposed conditions. The pharmacologic approaches for its relief may include oxygen, bronchodilators, corticosteroids, anxiolytics, analgesics, and opioids.

Key Points

- Dyspnea is the awareness of uncomfortable breathing, and constitutes one of the most frightening and distressing symptoms for "anyone" including patients with cancer. Like every other symptom it is a subjective experience and has been characterized as a nociceptive phenomenon in response to an aversive stimulus.
- Dyspnea constitutes one of the most common symptoms in patients with advanced cancer and may affect as many as 90% of them. Dyspnea is more common when direct (primary or metastatic) pleuropulmonary involvement occurs. However, dyspnea also affects one fourth of patients without evidence of cardiopulmonary in-

volvement. Patients with dyspnea have lower quality of life and a much shorter survival.

- The pathophysiology of dyspnea, though incompletely understood, appears multifactorial and three important components can be independently discerned: the work of breathing, the chemical status (hypercapnia, hypoxemia), and the neuromechanical dissociation (the mismatch between what the brain desires for ventilation and the sensory feedback it receives).

- Treatment of dyspnea is based on the management of the underlying cause and/or relief of the symptom. Both etiologic and palliative treatments are deemed to be useful when the benefits are greater than the risks. Specific therapeutic issues should be considered and include the treatment of pleural effusions, bronchoscopic methods for central airway obstruction, and pharmacologic measures for reversible superimposed conditions.

- Opioids are the cornerstone of symptomatic relief of dyspnea and at the same time provide adequate control of severe pain and cough. They may be administered both orally and parenterally according to specific guidelines and act mostly through their effect on opioid receptors of the central and peripheral nervous system.

References

1. Thomas JR, Von Gunten CF. Management of dyspnea. Lancet Oncol 2002;3:223.
2. Campbell ML. Terminal dyspnea and respiratory distress. Crit Care Clin 2004;20:403.
3. Steele B, Shaver J. The dyspnea experience: nociceptive properties and a model for research and practice. Adv Nurs Sci 1992;15:64.
4. Dudgeon DJ, Lertzman M. Dyspnea in the advanced cancer patient. J Pain Symptom Manage 1998;16:212.
5. Kvale PA, Simoff M, Prakash UBS. Palliative care. Chest 2003;123:284.
6. Stone P, Richards M, A'Hern R, Hardy J. A study to investigate the prevalence, severity and correlates of fatigue among patients with cancer in comparison with a control group of volunteers without cancer. Ann Oncol 2000;11:561.
7. Smith EL, Hann DM, Ahles TA, et al. Dyspnea, anxiety, body consciousness, and quality of life in patients with lung cancer. J Pain Symptom Manage 2001;21:323.
8. Reuben DB, Mor V. Dyspnea in terminally ill cancer patients. Chest 1986;89:234.
9. Escalante CP, Martin CG, Elting LS, et al. Dyspnea in cancer patients. Etiology, resource utilization, and survival implications in a managed care world. Cancer 1996;78:1314.
10. Manning HL, Schwartzstein RM. Pathophysiology of dyspnea. N Engl J Med 1995;333:1547.
11. American Thoracic Society. Dyspnea: mechanisms, assessment, and management: a consensus statement. Am J Respir Crit Care Med 1999;159:321.
12. Banzett RB, Mulnier HE, Murphy K, Rosen SD, Wise RJ, Adams L. Breathlessness in humans activates insular cortex. Neuroreport 2000;11:2117.
13. Peiffer C, Poline J, Thivard L, Aubier M, Samson Y. Neural substrates for the perception of acutely induced dyspnea. Am J Respir Crit Care Med 2001;163:951.
14. Adams L, Chronos N, Lane R, Guz A. The measurement of breathlessness induced in normal subjects: validity of two scaling techniques. Clin Sci 1985;69:7.
15. Borg G. Psychophysical bases of perceived exertion. Med Sci Sports Exerc 1982;14:377.
16. Walker-Renard PB, Vaughan LM, Sahn SA. Chemical pleurodesis for malignant pleural effusions. Ann Intern Med 1994;120:56.
17. Ernst A, Silvestri GA, Johnstone D, for the ACCP Interventional Chest/Diagnostic Procedures Network Steering Committee. Chest 2003;123:1693.
18. Colt HG, Harrell JH. Therapeutic rigid bronchoscopy allows level of care changes in patients with acute respiratory failure from central airway obstruction. Chest 1997;112:202.
19. Hautmann H, Gamarra F, Pfeifer KJ, Huber RM. Fiberoptic bronchoscopic balloon dilatation in malignant tracheobronchial disease: indications and results. Chest 2001;120:43.
20. Ross DJ, Mohsenifar Z, Koerner SK. Survival characteristics after Nd-YAG laser photoresection in advanced stage lung cancer. Chest 1990;98:581.
21. Sheski FD, Mathur PN. Cryotherapy, electrocautery and brachytherapy. Clin Chest Med 1999;20:123.
22. Mathur PN, Wolf KM, Busk MF, Briete WM, Datzman M. Fiberoptic bronchoscopic cryotherapy in the management of tracheobronchial obstruction. Chest 1996;110:718.
23. Morice RC, Ece T, Ece F, Keus L. Endobronchial argon plasma coagulation for treatment of hemoptysis and neoplastic airway obstruction. Chest 2001;119:781.
24. Anacak Y, Mogulkoc N, Ozkok S, Goksel T, Haydaroglu A, Bayindir U. High dose rate endobronchial brachytherapy in combination with external beam radiotherapy for stage III non small cell lung cancer. Lung Cancer 2001;34:253.
25. McCaughan JS Jr, Williams TE. Photodynamic therapy for endobronchial malignant disease: a prospective fourteen-year study. J Thorac Cardiovasc Surg 1997;114:940.
26. Witt C, Dinges S, Schmidt B, Ewert R, Budach V, Baumann G. Temporary tracheobronchial stenting in malignant stenoses. Eur J Cancer 1997;33:204.
27. Cavaliere S, Venuta F, Foccoli P, Toninelli C, La Face B. Endoscopic treatment of malignant airway obstructions in 2008 patients. Chest 1996;110:1536.
28. Carratala J, Roson B, Fernandez Sevilla A, Alcaide F, Gudiol F. Bacteremic pneumonia in neutropenic patients with cancer: causes, empirical antibiotic therapy, and outcome. Arch Intern Med 1998;158:868.
29. Crawford J, Ozer H, Stoller R, et al. Reduction by granulocyte-stimulating factor of fever and neutropenia induced by chemotherapy in patients with small-cell lung cancer. N Engl J Med 1991;325:164.
30. Mercadante S, Gebbia V, Marrazzo A, Filosto S. Anaemia in cancer: pathophysiology and treatment. Cancer Treat Rev 2000;26:303.
31. Dweik RA, Stoller JK. Role of bronchoscopy in massive hemoptysis. Clin Chest Med 1999;20:89.
32. Muraoka T, Bandoh S, Fujita J, et al. Corticosteroid refractory radiation pneumonitis that remarkably responded to cyclosporine A. Intern Med 2002;41:730.
33. Boyd KJ, Kelly M. Oral morphine as symptomatic treatment of dyspnea in patients with advanced cancer. Palliat Med 1997;11:277.

Endobronchial Treatment of Lung Cancer

51

Michael J. Simoff

Contents

Interventional pulmonary procedures include both therapeutic as well as diagnostic procedures. There is a continual evolution of new diagnostic techniques being developed, with the hope of earlier and more accurate diagnosis of lung cancer. Such techniques include: endobronchial ultrasound, autofluorescence bronchoscopy, and external navigation techniques to name a few. As these technologies continue to expand and evolve, so shall our abilities of identifying, diagnosing, and managing lung cancer patients.

The history of bronchoscopy is actually not that of a diagnostic tool, but rather a therapeutic technique. In 1897, Gustav Killian, a Professor of Oto-Rhino-Laryngology at the University of Freiburg, Germany, successfully removed a bone splinter from the right mainstem bronchus of a farmer using a rigid bronchoscope. His techniques and methods improved with time and expanded to different physicians and countries. In 1904, Chevalier Jackson, of Philadelphia, Pennsylvania, continued to advance the field of therapeutic bronchoscopy by improving upon the equipment first developed by Professor Killian. It was not until the Ninth International Congress of Diseases of the Chest in August 1966 that Professor Dr. Shigeto Ikeda presented his new invention, the broncho-fiberscope [2]. In the early 1970s the fiberoptic bronchoscope went from a novelty to a routine tool in the diagnosis of diseases of the chest. It took about seventy years of use, for the bronchoscope to become a diagnostic tool from its therapeutic roots. As this chapter progresses, we will discuss how the future of this medically historical tool continues to evolve.

51.1 Introduction

Lung cancer is the number one cancer killer in the world. As such, it is important for the treating physicians to understand all of the potential therapeutic modalities available to them for the management of their patients. The growing field of interventional pulmonology is an area that many managing physicians do not recognize as a potential resource for the management of patients with lung cancer. The combined statement of the European Respiratory Society and the American Thoracic Society defines interventional pulmonology as: "… the art and science of medicine as related to the performance of diagnostic and invasive therapeutic procedures that require additional training and expertise beyond that required in a standard pulmonary medicine training program" [1].

51.2 Why Use Endobronchial Techniques?

The traditional thought and role of interventional techniques is that of palliation, which is defined as the relief of symptoms. The symptoms most commonly relieved in the management of lung cancer include: shortness of breath, cough, and hemoptysis. The idea of palliation goes further though, as the term is usually thought to be synonymous with an improved quality of life. This de-

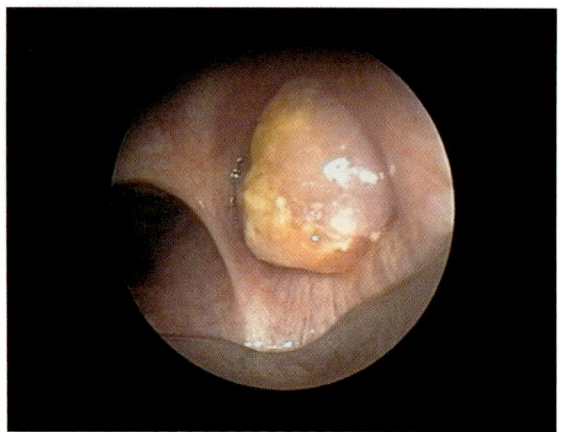

Fig. 51.1. Endobronchial squamous cell carcinoma obstructing the right mainstem bronchus

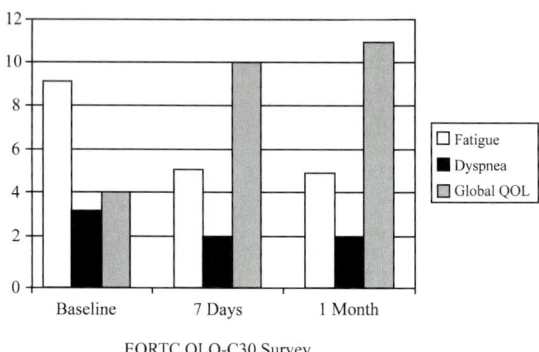

EORTC QLQ-C30 Survey

Fig. 51.3. Patient-assessed QOL scores

finition needs to be further broadened to maximize the potential benefits that the therapeutic techniques of interventional pulmonology can offer patients (Fig. 51.1).

If looking at symptom palliation using laser energy alone in the endobronchial management of lung cancer, the reports of clinical improvement rates are quite high ranging from 84% to 92% following an ablative procedure [3–7]. As an example, Mantovani et al. looked at 89 patients who underwent 133 laser ablative procedures. Both quality of life assessment using the EORTC QLQ-C30 Survey as well as physician-assessed ECOG performance scores were evaluated. In this study, the authors demonstrated a statistically significant decrease in ECOG performance score 3 and 4 patients to ECOG scores of 1 and 2 from baseline to day 7 postprocedure. More significant was the continued statistical improvement of these same scores from day 7 postprocedure to the 1 month follow-up postprocedure (see Fig. 51.2) [8]. The authors also demonstrated statistically significant reductions in fatigue and dyspnea with overall improvements in quality of life (see Fig. 51.3) [8].

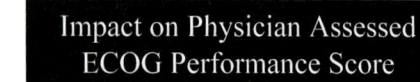

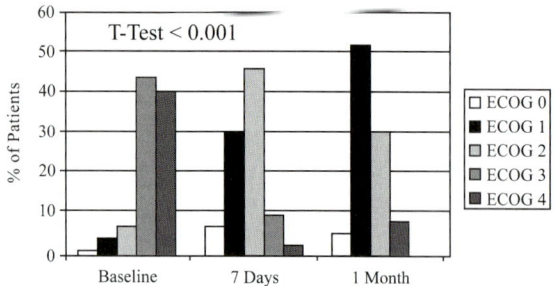

Fig. 51.2. Physician-assessed ECOG performance scores

Further review of the literature identifies studies that demonstrate not only improved quality of life in patients postintervention, but also improved survival in patients treated with laser bronchoscopy [9–12]. Brutinel et al. [9] used 25 historical controls (i.e., patients who would have been candidates for laser management but did not receive it secondary to the unavailability of the procedure at the time of their management) and compared them to 71 patients treated with laser bronchoscopy as part of the treatment program. The authors reported 76% and 100% mortality rates at 4 months and 7 months, respectively, in the control population. In comparison, the group treated with laser bronchoscopy had survival rates of 60% at 7 months and 28% at 1 year. Although no definitive randomized studies are available, review of historical studies would suggest that improved survival in addition to improved quality of life is achievable in lung cancer patients treated with endobronchial techniques.

Not all endobronchial disease causes complete obstruction of the airways. Sometimes patients have partial obstruction, which often has a less severe symptom complex. As these patients enter treatment programs, the endobronchial component of their disease, in response to these treatments, can lead to more complicated concerns. External-beam radiotherapy can induce endobronchial inflammation and swelling, further compromising the airways. Radiation or chemotherapy can lead to necrosis of the endobronchial component of the cancer. The inflammation and necrotic tissue can cause further airway compromise by inducing airway obstruction, lung collapse, and possible postobstructive pneumonia. Therefore, endobronchial techniques should be considered throughout the management of lung cancer patients [13, 14].

Lastly, when all management options have been used, end-stage patients will often develop compromise of their airways as the cancer continues to progress. Endobronchial management options may help to relieve some of their symptoms, allowing them freedom from shortness of breath as they go home in conjunction with hospice or other palliative therapies [13–15].

Most endobronchial techniques are performed on an outpatient basis. Unless a patient presents with respiratory failure, many of the procedures performed provide immediate relief of symptoms. This rapid symptomatic improvement allows patients to return home with an improved quality of life or better prepares them to continue treatment at their local programs. Although interventional procedures are not definitive therapies, they often provide partial to total relief of the strangling sensation produced by complete airway occlusion.

51.3 Ablative Technologies

The ablative techniques are used for the destruction and/or debulking of endobronchial carcinoma that obstructs the airways. There are multiple ways to achieve tissue ablation with opening of the airways. The following sections will describe those most commonly used.

51.3.1 Laser

Laser, an acronym coined from light amplification by stimulated emission of radiation, has many medical uses, including the endobronchial management of lung cancer. Several laser types are currently used within the bronchi: neodymium:yttrium-aluminum-garnet (Nd:YAG), potassium titanyl phosphate (KTP), diode, and carbon dioxide (CO_2). The most common laser used endoscopically is the Nd:YAG, which delivers energy at a wavelength of 1,064 nm. Nd:YAG, KTP, and diode laser energy can be conducted via a quartz monofilament and thus can be easily used with either the rigid or flexible bronchoscope. The CO_2 laser requires direct laryngoscopy and therefore is not commonly used below the proximal several centimeters of the trachea. Normally, the Nd:YAG laser is used at 30–60 W, but it has a wide range of power outputs, up to 100 W. Depending on the energy level used, the laser can affect tissue several millimeters to several centimeters in depth. The KTP and diode lasers both are clinically available with interventionalists who prefer their characteristics, but remain less commonly used.

The predominant tissue effects of Nd:YAG lasers are those of thermal necrosis and photocoagulation. Thermal necrosis uses higher energy levels to destroy tissue, causing the formation of eschar. The problem with this approach is the significant vascularity of most lung cancers. In destroying tissue with laser energy, large blood vessels can also be destroyed. These blood vessels can

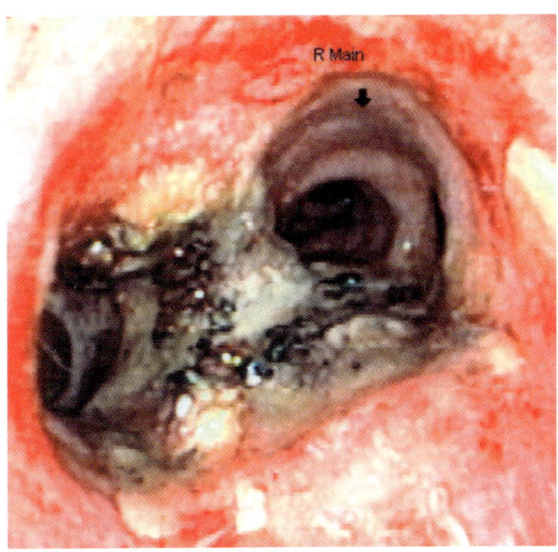

Fig. 51.4. Main carinal squamous cell carcinoma, previously occluding distal trachea and bilateral mainstem bronchi, postlaser ablation

be perforated with the tissue destruction, leading to significant hemorrhage and an increase rather than a decrease in morbidity and mortality with this procedure.

The most commonly used effect of laser energy is photocoagulation. Using lower energy levels, the surface of the tumor is heated, causing shrinkage of the tumor and diminishing the blood flow to that region. By devascularizing the tumor, more rapid mechanical debulking can be performed with improved control of bleeding (Fig. 51.4).

Laser therapy can be performed via either flexible or rigid bronchoscopy. The Nd:YAG laser fibers can be passed through the working channel of most flexible bronchoscopes or via a rigid bronchoscope. The flexible bronchoscope, allows laser energy to be delivered to areas that cannot be reached with the rigid bronchoscope [3, 4, 9–11, 16–25].

As discussed above, using laser energy, there is a high success rate of symptom palliation of 84–92%. The laser is an intricate and important tool in the management of endobronchial lung cancer. As with any modality, lasers have their limitations. A significant one is that they cannot be used in environments with an FiO_2 greater than 40%. Due to their thermal energy, in a high oxygen setting they may cause an endobronchial fire to occur. This can be important as some patients with airway obstruction require high FiO_2s due to their hypoxia, compromising a potential therapeutic technique [3–7]. Further review of the literature identifies studies that demonstrate improved survival in patients treated with laser bronchoscopy [9–12].

Laser is overall very safe when used by an experienced bronchoscopist. Several large studies report complications rates of 0–2.2%. The potential complications

Table 51.1. Dumon's ten commandments of safe laser pulmonary resection

1. Know the anatomic danger zones – aortic arch, pulmonary artery, and esophagus
2. Have a well-trained laser team including an anesthetist specialized in light general anesthesia and two assistants equipped with emergency response procedures
3. Screen patients carefully: any endoluminal growth is amenable to laser resection, but purely external compression is beyond the reach of the technique
4. Use the rigid bronchoscopic technique (custom-made open tube, light general anesthesia, straight telescope, and two suction catheters) for high-grade obstruction, especially if malignancy is involved
5. Monitor blood gases and cardiac performance. At the least sign of hypoxemia, interrupt treatment long enough to oxygenate the patient: if necessary, under closed-circuit conditions
6. Fire laser parallel to the wall of the airway; never aim directly into it
7. Coagulate at will but avoid using the laser at high-power settings; mechanical resection after laser coagulation is preferable to laser resection alone whenever possible
8. Do not neglect hemorrhage: even slow bleeding will lead to hypoxemia if left unattended
9. Terminate each procedure with a thorough laser irradiation of the resected area and a tracheobronchial toilet to remove all secretions or debris
10. Keep the patient under observation in a specially outfitted recovery room for a reasonable period of time

Table 51.2. "Rule of four" for safe and successful endobronchial laser resections

Maximum length of lesion	4 cm
Duration of lung collapse	<4 weeks
Initial power settings	
Power:	
Non-contact	40 W
Contact	4 W
Pulse duration	0.4 s
Distances:	
Endotracheal tube to lesion	>4 cm
Fiber tip to lesion	4 mm
Flexible bronchoscope to tip	4 mm
FiO_2 during procedure	<40%
Number of pulses between cleaning	<40
Total number of repeat laser treatments	<4
Life expectancy	>4 weeks
Laser team individuals	4

of laser resection include: penetration of the airway, hemorrhage, endobronchial fire, pneumomediastinum, and pneumothorax. Another important risk is that of anesthesia, whether it is conscious sedation or general anesthesia (see Tables 51.1, 51.2 regarding safe practice with the use of lasers) [3, 6, 26–28].

51.3.2 Electrocautery

Electrocautery is another form of thermal energy used for endobronchial tumor ablation. Electrical energy, via one of several introducer devices, is delivered to the desired tissues and used to cut and/or destroy tumor cells. There are four probes that are most commonly used: the electrocautery snare (Fig. 51.5), a blunt probe, coagulation forceps, and an electrosurgical scalpel. Each tool has specific characteristics that make it more or less suitable for specific tasks. All of the electrocautery devices are designed to pass through a "grounded" flexible bronchoscope with a 2.8-mm working channel, or a rigid bronchoscope.

The delivery devices of electrocautery are unipolar electrodes, which deliver electric current to the tissue. The delivered energy affects the tissue in three ways: an electrolytic effect (altering chemical bonding of tissue), a capacitance effect (affecting the electrical potential of local structures), and a thermal effect (which is due to the resistance of the tissue to the flow of electrical current). Of these, the thermal effect is clinically that which is most significant.

Endobronchial electrocautery can be used in a similar fashion to Nd:YAG laser ablation in the management of endobronchial lung cancer [29–33]. Two studies, the first by Homasson and the second by Suteja et al., describe relief of dyspnea symptoms in 67% and 70% of their patients treated with electrosurgical procedures [33, 34].

Electrocautery has also been considered an alternative to the management of early-stage endobronchial squamous cell cancer, which was thought to be either carcinoma in situ or superficial. Although only a test study of 13 patients, the long-term response in 10 patients (77%) is encouraging for the management of this disease process [35].

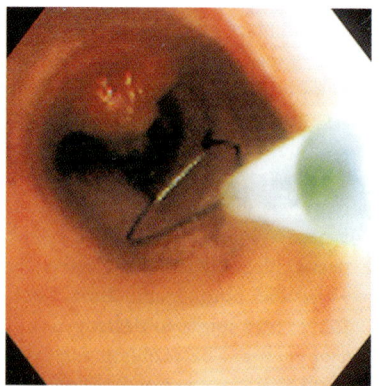

Fig. 51.5. Electrocautery snare being used for endobronchial resection of a small tumor

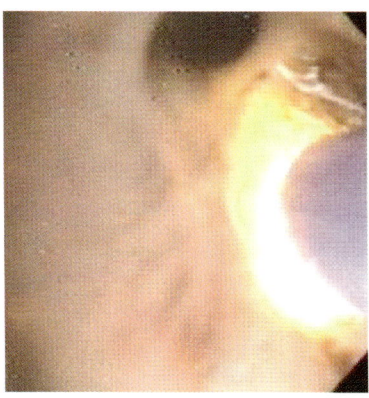

Fig. 51.6. Argon plasma coagulation of superficial metastatic thyroid cancer in right upper lobe

Table 51.3. Cryotherapy

Cryosensitive tissue	Cryoresistant tissue
Skin	Fat
Granulation tissue	Cartilage
Mucus membranes	Connective tissue

51.3.3 Argon Plasma Coagulation

Argon plasma coagulation (APC) is a non-contact form of electrocautery. Instead of using a unipolar contact device to deliver electrical energy, ionized argon gas (argon plasma) is used. The argon plasma in essence, sprays out of the end of the delivery probe. The electrical energy is then transferred to the tissue across the argon plasma. The great advantage of this non-contact mode of delivery, allows "painting" of the surface of a tumor or other area, which might be bleeding (Fig. 51.6) [36, 37].

The disadvantage of APC is that it has a limited depth of penetration and, although an excellent and safe tool, its use in the destruction of endobronchial tumor is more limited than that seen with laser or electrocautery [38].

Crosta et al. described the use of APC for the management of 47 patients with malignant airway obstruction. Of these patients, they were able to achieve immediate airway patency and hemostasis in 91.5% (43/47 patients). Despite the fact that there is little tumor ablation, the authors describe tumor desiccation with some surface shrinkage, which accounted for much of their success [39].

51.3.4 Cryotherapy

Cryotherapy is another modality for the endobronchial destruction of malignant tissue that obstructs the tracheobronchial tree. This technique uses cold instead of the heat used in laser or other thermal-based technologies. A probe is placed onto or into an obstructing tumor mass. Liquid nitrogen (-196 °C) or nitrous oxide (-80 °C) cools the probe tip when performing cryotherapy. This tissue freezing causes eventual destruction of all cells in an area of approximately 1 cm in diameter

from the probe tip. Vascular as well as intracellular crystallization with microthrombosis occurs with the supercooling tissue, initiating tissue necrosis and overall tumor destruction.

Cryoprobes can be used through either a flexible or a rigid bronchoscope. The limiting factor to using cryotherapy is that the tissues destroyed with the freezing procedure take time to die and necrose. This requires performing repeat bronchoscopes to remove the necrosed tissue and, in many cases, repeating the treatments.

Mathur et al. describes a 90% success rate with endobronchial debulking with cryotherapy [40]. Other studies go onto describe up to a 75% subjective improvement in patient's dyspnea [41, 42]. As in electrocautery, small studies have been performed looking at the management of early superficial bronchogenic carcinoma of the airways. Deygas et al. reported a 91% complete response in their study with a 1-year follow-up [43].

An advantage of cryotherapy is the physiologic response of many tissues to cold. Certain tissues are more or less cryosensitive or cryoresistant (see Table 51.3). Due to this, there is a smaller risk of airway injury with the use of cryotherapy. Despite this, there are reports of tissue and cartilage fractures [44] and significant hemorrhage with the use of cryotherapy [45].

Another advantage of cryotherapy is that it can be used at any fraction of inspired oxygen (FiO_2) a patient may require to correct hypoxia. Laser, electrocautery, and argon plasma coagulation all must be used in an environment with an FiO_2 40%. If the FiO_2 is greater than 40%, the risk of an airway fire becomes very high and places the patient at significant risk. Overall, cryotherapy is an excellent modality for the management of endobronchial cancer.

51.3.5 Photodynamic Therapy

Photodynamic therapy (PDT) has received increased attention in recent years. PDT is an important adjunctive modality to the management of endobronchial disease, but it does not replace Nd:YAG lasers, stents, and rigid bronchoscopy. PDT also can be used with bulky disease, but most interventionalists feel that it is of limited benefit in this role [46, 47]. The most suitable lesions for PDT are in situ carcinomas or those early bronchogenic carcinomas limited to 4–5 mm of microinvasion [48].

The procedure of PDT entails injecting a photosensitizing drug intravenously to the patient 48–72 h prior to the time of the procedure. Porfimer sodium (Photofrin) is the most common agent currently used for this. Although studies with other drugs (e.g., mono-L-aspartyl chlorine e6) are being carried out, Photofrin remains the current drug of choice [49]. This photosensitizer penetrates all cells systemically. The drug is not cleared as quickly in cancer cells as in other cells of the airway and is therefore found in higher concentrations in the cancer cells as opposed to the endothelium surrounding the tumor. An argon dye laser or an equivalent wavelength diode laser is then used to provide the 630-nm-wavelength light energy required to activate the intracellular porfimer sodium. The laser energy is transmitted via a flexible quartz fiber, which can be used through either a flexible or a rigid bronchoscope. The fiber tip can be placed in close approximation to the tumor mass, or it can be imbedded into the tumor to provide the energy needed to initiate the intracellular activation of the porfimer sodium. This reaction leads to cellular destruction by a variety of mechanisms. Tissue necrosis is the endpoint of the reaction, causing cellular death of the cancer cells (Fig. 51.7) [48, 50].

As the neoplastic tissue necrotizes, it must be removed by repeated bronchoscopies. Flexible bronchoscopy is commonly performed daily or every other day for up to 1 week after the initial laser treatment to remove the necrotic tissue. The necrosis of bulky tumor can be dangerous to the patient if the necrotic tissue separates from the bronchial wall and occludes the airway. In some programs that use only PDT, patients remain intubated following the procedure for 1–2 days secondary to this concern. If necrotic tissue is removed over the first 24–48 h, a second laser application to the cancer can be performed, thus improving the cancer tissue destruction.

If chosen carefully, the response of superficial bronchogenic carcinomas to PDT can be as significant as 98% [48, 51]. There are further advantages to the use of PDT in patients with multiple synchronous and/or metachronous lesions in the airways, with survival means of up to 52 months reported [52]. PDT has also been used by Kato et al. to reduce the extent of surgical resection required by some patients by eliminating early-stage microinvasive neoplastic processes with PDT from the airways, which if left untreated would have required the inclusion of increased surgical margins [53].

Photodynamic therapy is an excellent therapeutic modality for patients with early-stage cancers. It destroys neoplastic tissue effectively and is an outstanding therapeutic modality in carcinoma in situ and microinvasive cancers. PDT is a necessary tool in our armamentarium of endobronchial treatments, but the time delays and multiple steps of management make it a more cumbersome therapy for the management of late-stage endobronchial lung cancer.

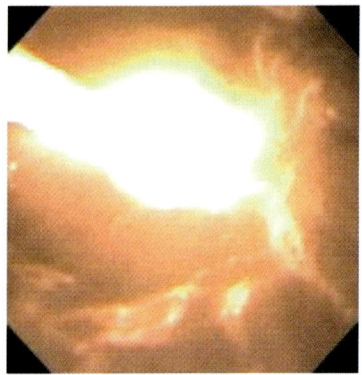

Fig. 51.7. Photodynamic therapy of endobronchial squamous cell carcinoma

51.3.6 Intratumoral Injection

A less commonly discussed endobronchial therapeutic modality is that of intratumoral injection (Fig. 51.8). This type of approach was first reported by Hayata et al. in 1978 [54]. The clinical goal of this approach is to deliver significantly higher drug concentrations to the target tissue by direct injection of a chemotherapeutic or immunotherapeutic agent. Goldberg et al. reported a 6–10 times higher tissue concentration of agent in the injected tissue [55].

Several reports of using intratumoral injection of ethanol describe cell death by lysing cell membranes, denaturing protein, and inducing microthrombosis. Only several small studies discuss the use of ethanol, both describing rapid improvement in obstructed airways in greater than 50% of their patients. Long-term outcomes were unfortunately not available to evaluate for the potential development of bronchial wall erosion or other long-term sequelae of this intervention [56, 57].

Celikoglu and Celikoglu's article describing the use of intratumoral injection with 5-fluorouracil for the adjunctive treatment of bronchogenic carcinoma and the relief of endobronchial obstruction is quite promising. The authors treated 65 patients with at least a 50% obstruction of one of the major bronchi. Fifty-six of the 65 patients treated (86%) were described having a large reduction in the size of their tumors by endoscopic evaluation. Weekly injections were performed with 57 of the 65 patients having symptom relief after 2 weeks. The authors describe no complications and no significant systemic effects of the chemotherapeutic injection [58].

Overall, intratumoral injection appears to demonstrate promise as another endobronchial ablative modality in the management of airway obstruction in lung cancer. Further studies, with an expansion of this practice, may bring the long-term potential benefits of this treatment to more physicians. As advances in immu-

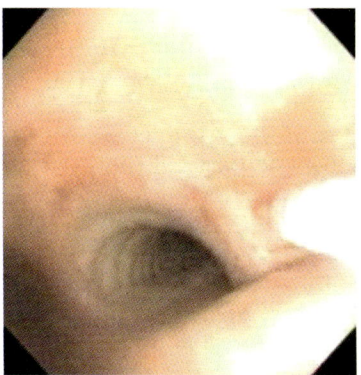

Fig. 51.8. Transbronchial injection

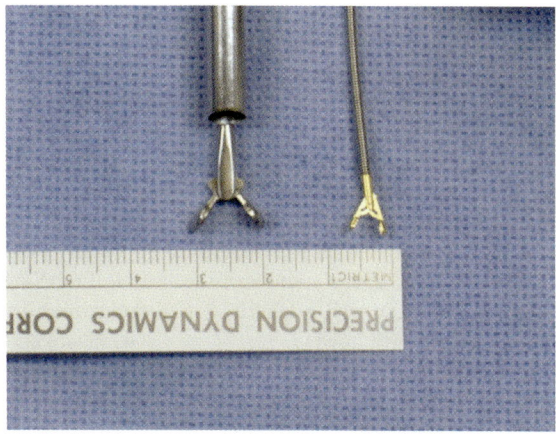

Fig. 51.9. Comparison of rigid bronchoscopy forceps (*left*) with flexible bronchoscopy forceps (*right*)

notherapy progress, variations of this approach may further our progress in treating some advanced cancers.

51.4 Bronchoscopy: Rigid and Flexible

Since the inception of flexible fiberoptic bronchoscopy in the late 1960s in Japan and in 1970 in the USA, the flexible bronchoscope has become the most widespread tool for evaluating and diagnosing diseases of the airways and lungs [2]. The rigid bronchoscope, the flexible bronchoscope's predecessor, was in many regards forgotten as a tool until interventional pulmonology evolved in the 1980s. Interventional pulmonologists reevaluated this tool and found its properties advantageous to the procedures that are currently performed.

51.4.1 Rigid Bronchoscopy

A survey in 1991 by the American College of Chest Physicians reported that only 8% of responding pulmonologists used a rigid bronchoscope [59]. With the growth of interventional techniques the use of rigid bronchoscopy continues to grow in the USA and Europe. The rigid bronchoscope offers many advantages to the interventional pulmonologist, one of which is the superior control of the airway achieved with its use. Ventilation is performed through the scope itself rather than around the flexible bronchoscope. The larger-bore rigid bronchoscopes allow optical systems, large-caliber suction catheters, and the laser to pass through the scope simultaneously with little compromise to the ventilation. Large biopsy forceps are used through the rigid bronchoscope, which can provide more significant tissue biopsies as well as assist in mechanical debulking of lesions (Fig. 51.9).

The rigid bronchoscope itself can be used to debulk tumor from the airway lumen. The distal end of the bronchoscope has a beveled end. This edge can be used to shear large sections of endobronchial tumor away from the airway wall in a technique often referred to as "applecoring." In a report of 56 patients with endobronchial obstruction of the trachea or mainstem bronchi, Mathisen and Grillo reported improvement in 90% of their patients. Only 3 of the 56 patients had more than minor bleeding with this procedure. Applecoring combined with the use of larger biopsy forceps allows tumor to be quickly resected from the obstructed airway [25].

Despite its benefits, the rigid bronchoscope is not the perfect device and has limitations also. The rigid bronchoscope is a more difficult instrument to operate than a flexible bronchoscope. The use of the rigid bronchoscope requires additional training beyond the typical pulmonary fellowship and/or surgical residency. This lack of available training adds to the slow growth of its use. Rigid bronchoscopy is most commonly performed in the operating room with general anesthesia, also limiting its availability to some pulmonary physicians.

51.4.2 Flexible Bronchoscopy

The initial advantage of the rigid bronchoscope was the larger working channel available to perform procedures through. As there continues to be advancements in imaging technologies, flexible bronchoscopes have smaller external diameters with larger working channels. Most diagnostic bronchoscopes have working channels of 2 mm. Most of the endobronchial tools used through a bronchoscope for ablative or advanced diagnostics procedures require a working channel diameter of 2.8 mm. The current therapeutic flexible bronchoscopes available have working channels that are 3.2 mm in diameter.

The "flexibility" of the flexible bronchoscope is another significant advantage to the interventionalists. With a rigid bronchoscope a bronchoscopist can reach surprisingly far into the right lower and middle lobes as well as the left lower lobe, in addition to the main airways. The flexible bronchoscope allows full access to all of the airways within the size and length limitations of the bronchoscope itself. With this maneuverability and the improvement of delivery devices for laser, electrocautery, APC, and cryotherapy, the flexible bronchoscope has become well established as a therapeutic as well as a diagnostic tool.

Overall, the concurrent use of the flexible with the rigid bronchoscope is necessary to provide the fullest extent of treatments to patients with airway obstruction. These two instruments should be thought of as complementary to one another rather than mutually exclusive. It is common to use a flexible bronchoscope through a rigid bronchoscope during a case to provide a finer touch to a procedure. The practice of interventional pulmonology and the management of endobronchial malignancy rely on both.

51.5 Brachytherapy

Brachytherapy is an ablative modality, which uses a radioactive source to treat endobronchial, submucosal, and/or peribronchial bronchogenic carcinoma. The most common source of radiation is iridium 192 (Ir^{192}). Brachytherapy is either provided at a low dose rate (LDR), which is a delivery of 50–100 cGy per hour, or at a high dose rate (HDR), which is usually delivered at 100–500 cGy per hour.

Historically, LDR brachytherapy was the most common approach to this treatment of lung cancer. The disadvantages of LDR brachytherapy is the time required for the intervention, as the radioactive source must stay in for an extended period of time, as well as the increased risk of radiation exposure to medical personnel [60].

The use of HDR brachytherapy together with improved delivery systems has become the most common use of this technique. The technique for brachytherapy requires the placement of a polyethylene catheter into the airway with bronchoscopic guidance. "Dummy" seeds are placed into the catheter. Using fluoroscopy in conjunction with direct visualization, the area to be treated is identified and planning with respect to the area to be treated is completed. The patient is then taken to radiation oncology for afterloading.

Afterloading is accomplished by a remote computerized device. The dummy seeds are removed and the Ir^{192} source is placed into the polyurethane catheter. The radioactive source then moves up the catheter making stops (dwelling) at prescribed locations for calcu-

lated amounts of time to deliver the desired radiation dose to the area being treated. Patients are typically treated with HDR brachytherapy weekly for two or three sessions.

Brachytherapy can be used to relieve airway obstruction, treat early superficial bronchogenic carcinoma, or supplement PDT, external beam radiation, and/or chemotherapy. HDR brachytherapy is the most common technique of brachytherapy currently used in the management of endobronchial carcinoma. Endobronchial response rates of 54–94% have been reported in several outcomes studies [61]. Fifty percent to 100% of patients in these studies experience symptomatic relief of their symptoms of shortness of breath, cough, and/or hemoptysis [62, 63].

Delivering high doses of radiation endobronchially has risks and complications. The most significant of these include hemoptysis (7.4%), radiation bronchitis/airway stenosis (8.7%), esophageal fistula formation, and erosion into the pulmonary artery. Brachytherapy has been used for many years in the management of lung cancer. It continues to be a useful modality independently as well as in conjunction with other treatments for lung cancer.

51.6 Endobronchial Prosthesis

Endobronchial prosthesis involves stenting of the airways, which can be used in several clinical situations: intrinsic, extrinsic, or mixed endobronchial obstruction. Stents work well in conjunction with other modalities such as laser or other ablative techniques and the mechanical debulking of tumors. Vergnon et al. looked at the clinical response of patients with airway obstruction only using endobronchial stenting. They treated 120 patients with 168 tracheal and/or bronchial stents. Twenty-four hours preoperatively and 48 h postoperatively, respiratory function was assessed. Complete data were available for analysis in 24 patients, including 15 further evaluated a mean of 10.1 months later [64].

The authors further divided their grouping to include bronchial, intrathoracic tracheal, and extrathoracic tracheal obstructions. They included both malignant and benign disease in their study. Postprosthesis implantation, airflow parameters demonstrated particular improvement in forced vital capacity in one second or FEV1 (440 ml) and peak expiratory flow rates (0.92 l/s) (see Figs. 51.10–51.12) [64]. Patients had good clinical tolerance to the procedure with uniform improved functionality.

Stents are composed of Silastic rubber, metal alloys, or some combination. No stent is perfect; that design still does not exist. Therefore the choice of which stent to use should be made carefully, weighing the advantages and disadvantages of each, so the proper tool is

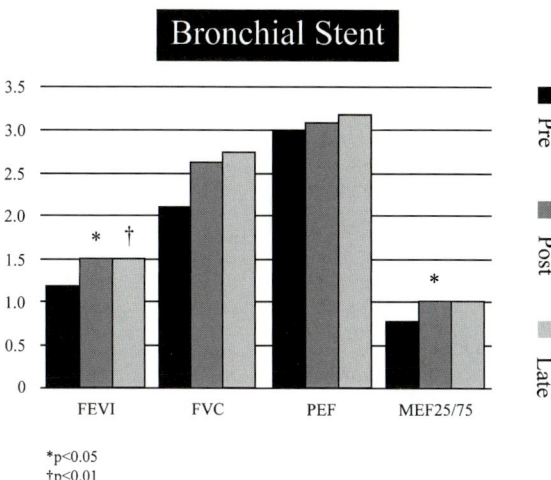

Fig. 51.10. Pulmonary function testing improvements with bronchial stenting

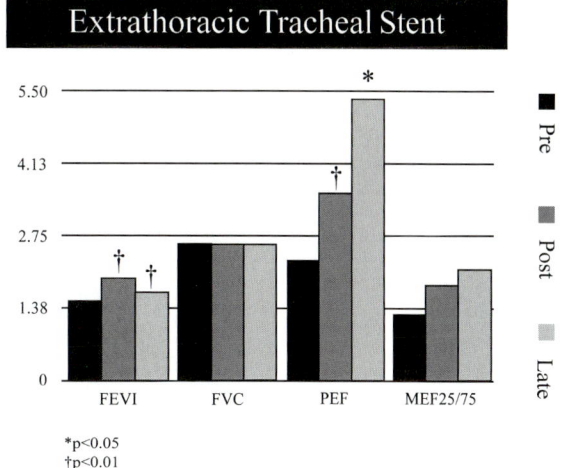

Fig. 51.12. Pulmonary function testing improvements with extrathoracic tracheal stenting

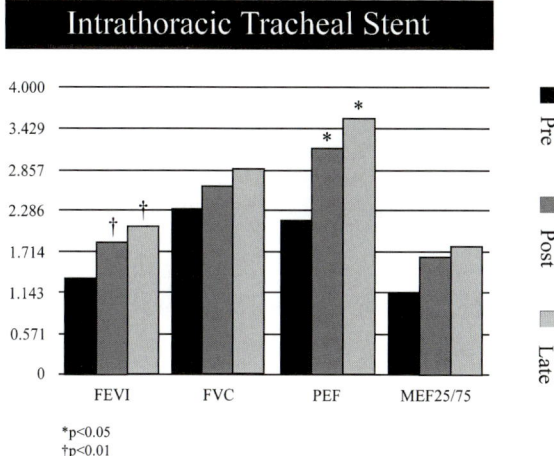

Fig. 51.11. Pulmonary function testing improvements with intrathoracic tracheal stenting

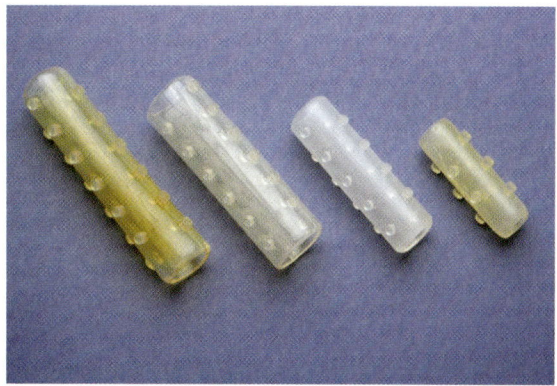

Fig. 51.13. Dumon endobronchial stents

used in each situation. The interventionalist must be knowledgeable of and facile with multiple stent types to match the appropriate stent to the job.

51.6.1 Silastic Stents

Many of the Silastic stents now in use have evolved from the Montgomery T tube, which was first used in the early 1960s. This T-shaped stent supports the entire trachea with an arm that extends through a permanent tracheostomy. Due to the limitation of use with a patent tracheotomy, the use of the Montgomery T tube is limited in the management of endobronchial bronchogenic carcinoma, except in very specific circumstances [65–67].

In 1990, Dumon [68] reported the use of what is now referred to as the Dumon stent (Novatech, Aubagne, France). Developed in 1987, it is a Silastic stent with evenly spaced studs along its outside walls (see Figs. 51.13, 51.14a,b). These studs serve the dual purpose of maintaining stent placement endobronchially and, by keeping the stent from approximating against the airway wall entirely, allowing the clearance of secretions around the outside of the stent. Although the use of expandable wire mesh stents is increasing, the Dumon stent probably remains the most common stent used by interventionalists worldwide.

The Dumon stent is effective in maintaining its structural integrity when placed endobronchially, providing effective support of the compromised airways. Its solid-walled design prevents persistent tumor growth from re-obstructing airways. Another advantage of the Dumon stent is its ease of removal. This can be significant when endobronchial procedures are used early in the management of cancer patients. As part of the en-

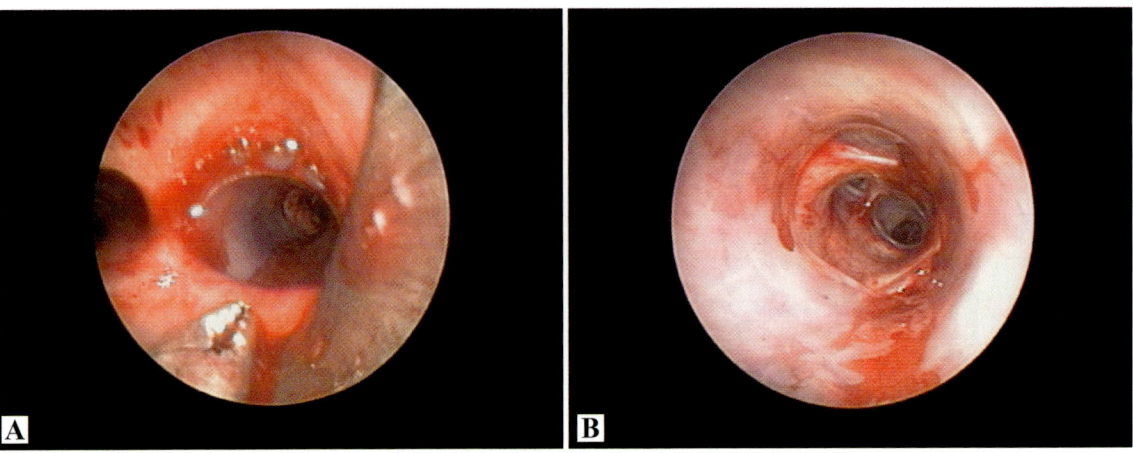

Fig. 51.14. **A** Proximal end of Dumon stent in right mainstem bronchus. **B** Distal end of Dumon stent in right mainstem bronchus

Table 51.4. Advantages and disadvantages of Silastic stents

Advantages	Disadvantages
Removable and replaceable	Potential for migration/dislodgment
No growth through stent	Rigid bronchoscopy needed for placement
Low cost	Possible secretion adherence
Low likelihood of granulation tissue formation	

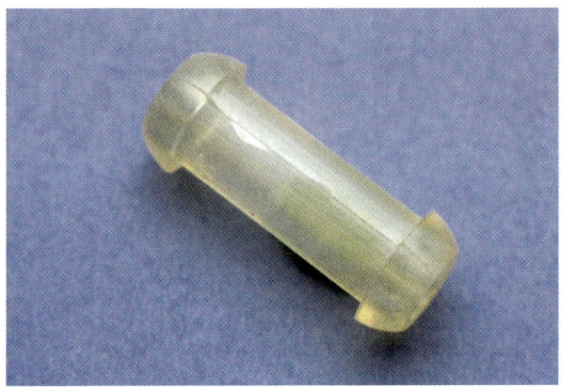

Fig. 51.15. Hood bronchial stent

dobronchial management of tumors, stent placement can be used before the initiation of radiotherapy or chemotherapy to relieve an airway obstruction and the concurrent significant dyspnea. After definitive therapies have been used (radiation, chemotherapy), re-evaluation of the airway can be performed, with the stent being left in place, removed (if deemed of no further clinical advantage), or replaced with a larger stent that would further improve the caliber and stability of the airway [65, 68–73].

Some disadvantages of the Dumon stent include the potential for migration, the difficulty of placement in tortuous or otherwise misshapen airways, as well as an unfavorable wall to inner diameter relationship (Table 51.4). The Dumon stent also requires the need for rigid bronchoscopy for placement. Dumon and Cavaliere reported on the use and complications after 1,574 stents had been placed over 7 years. Six hundred and seventy-seven of these procedures were performed because of malignancy, with 263 for benign tracheal stenosis, and 118 reported as other. The most significant complications were migration, with a rate of 9.5%, recurrent stent obstruction, which occurred in 3.6% of cases, and granulation tissue development in 7.9% [70]. Other studies by Diaz-Jimenez et al. as well as Cavaliere et al. report progressively lower migration rates and granuloma formation, from 13% to 5% and 6% to 1%,

respectively. With regard to migration, experience and studies seem to imply that this becomes a less significant issue with more experience with this stent [23, 71].

Another Silastic stent is the Hood stent (Hood Laboratories, Decatur, GA, USA). The Hood stent is very similar to the Dumon stent in design and use. The Hood stent also requires rigid bronchoscopy for placement and has the same limitations and complications as are found with the Dumon stent. The Hood stent commonly comes in both smooth-walled with capped ends as well as studded versions (see Fig. 51.15) [74].

51.6.2 Metallic Stents

Metal stents, such as the Gianturco (Cook, Bloomington, ID, USA), the Palmaz (Johnson & Johnson Interventional Systems, Warren, NJ, USA), the Wallstent (Schneider, Minneapolis, MN, USA), and the Ultraflex (Boston Scientific, Natick, MA, USA) have been used in the endobronchial management of lung cancer. Due to the limitations and complications seen with the use of

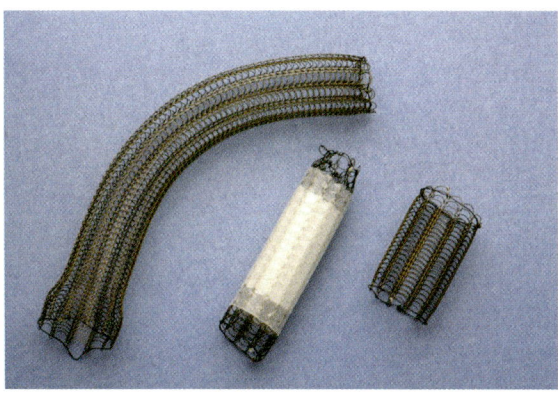

Fig. 51.16. Covered and uncovered Ultraflex stents

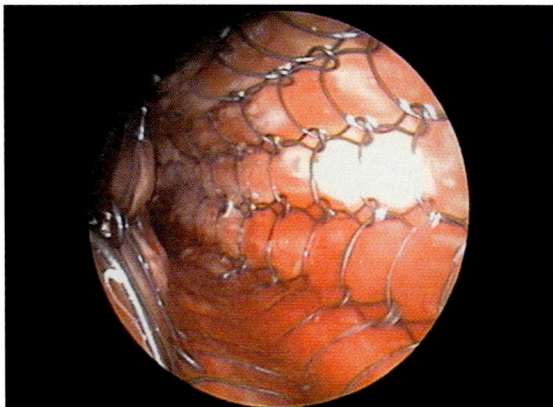

Fig. 51.17. Covered Ultraflex stent in left mainstem bronchus

Table 51.5. Evaluation of dyspnea before and after Ultraflex stent implantation

Dyspnea grade	Before (n=34)	Day 1* (n=33)	Day 30* (n=26)	Day 60* (n=19)
0	0	4	3	1
I	3	14	13	8
II	8	8	6	6
III	8	5	3	2
IV	15	2	1	2

* $p < 0.001$ before versus day 1, 30, and 60

Table 51.6. Pulmonary function tests in patients before and after stent implantation

Variables	Before stent	After stent
VC	1.97 ± 0.54	2.46 ± 0.60*
FEV1	1.40 ± 0.51	1.74 ± 0.52**
PEF	2.9 ± 1.4	3.6 ± 1.2***

  * $p < 0.05$
 ** $p < 0.01$
*** $p < 0.001$

Table 51.7. Advantages and disadvantages of metal stents

Advantages	Disadvantages
Easy to place	Permanent
Good wall/internal diameter relationship	Tumor regrowth (non-covered)
Powerful radial force	Possible migration of covered stents
Excellent conformity for irregular tracheal or bronchial walls	Significant granulation tissue stimulation
Good epithelialization	Epithelialization affecting wall mechanics and secretion clearance
	Radial force causing necrosis of bronchial wall, erosion, fistulas, perforation

the Gianturco, Palmaz, and uncovered Wallstent, they are now rarely used in the management of endobronchial malignancy.

The Ultraflex stent is made of nitinol, a titanium and nickel alloy, which has little bioreactivity. This stent has excellent inner to outer diameter and conforms well to various airway shapes, maintaining an equal pressure along the entire length of the stent. The Ultraflex stent is available in a variety of lengths and diameters. Overall the covered version of this stent is excellent for use in palliation of airway obstruction (see Figs. 51.16, 51.17).

The clinical effectiveness of the Ultraflex stent was evaluated by Miyazawa et al. The investigators evaluated patients at poststent implantation days 1, 30, and 60, for clinical, endoscopic, and pulmonary function response. Most stents placed were performed in conjunction with an ablative procedure. Immediate relief of dyspnea was achieved in 82% of patients with significant improvements in the dyspnea index score (Table 51.5), airways diameter (Fig. 51.18), and pulmonary function testing (Table 51.6) [75].

The Wallstent is composed of woven cobalt-based superalloy monofilaments with exposed proximal and distal ends (Fig. 51.19). These exposed ends imbed in the endobronchial mucosa to fix the stent into place. Due to this, significant stimulation of granulation tissue development at both the proximal and distal ends of the exposed Wallstent is a concern for long-term endobronchial management. Studies using this stent demonstrate excellent initial outcomes, particularly with the release of the covered version [69, 76].

As with all stents, metal stents have limitations (see Table 51.7). The uncovered portions of metal stents epithelialize as they remain in the airways, thereby becoming incorporated into the wall of the bronchus. This epithelization changes the mechanics of the airways

Degree of Airway Obstruction

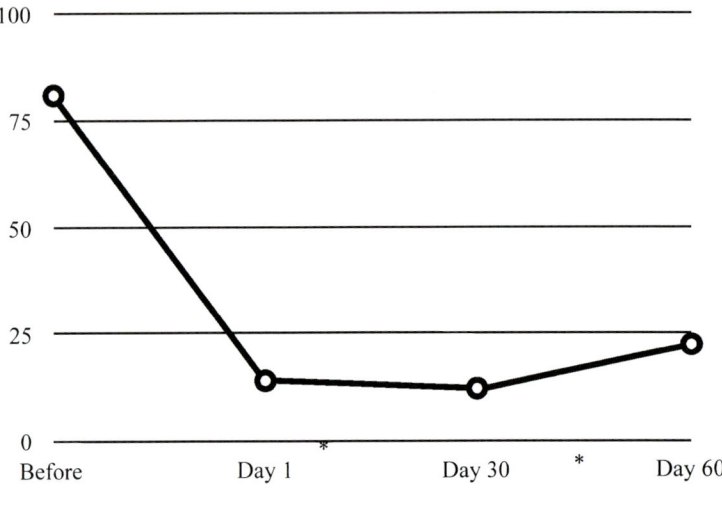

*p<0.001 before vs day 1, 30, 60

Fig. 51.18. Statistically significant improvement from before procedure to 60 days postprocedure

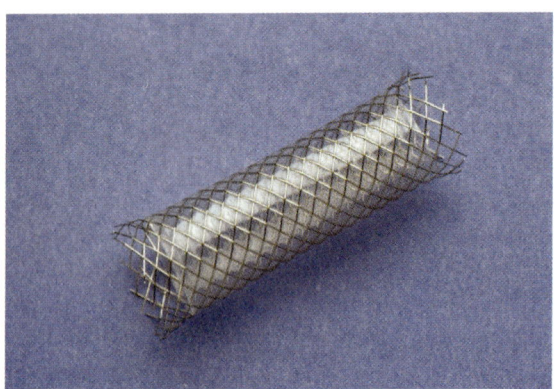

Fig. 51.19. Covered Wallstent

with time by making them stiffer, which may lead to long-term airway complications [77, 78]. Another consideration with the use of metal stents is the fact that once they are endoscopically placed, their removal is difficult and often impossible. Both of these risks are of significant concern with benign disease, but in the management of malignant airway obstruction this process is clinically of less long-term concern. Although uncommon, the risk with the use of metal stents is the erosion that can occur through bronchial/tracheal walls. This can be particularly serious when erosion occurs into blood vessels, leading to massive uncontrollable hemoptysis. Another limitation in the management of malignant airway disease is that the wire mesh design of many of the original metal stents did not prevent the

tumor from growing through the stent over time. The Ultraflex and Wallstent stents are now available in covered versions. A polyurethane wrap is applied to the outside of the wire mesh to prevent tumor invasion through the woven stent walls [65, 69, 78–80].

One of the most significant advantages of metal stents is their relative ease of placement via a flexible bronchoscope with fluoroscopic assistance. This ease of placement allows some bronchoscopists to use these stents as their sole modality in the management of endobronchial disease; however, this practice limits the options to patients that may otherwise be available if all interventional modalities were offered. Patients should always have the option of the technology best suited to their problem, and, therefore, interventionalists should offer more than one option for the management of airway disease [65, 69, 79, 80].

51.6.3 Hybrid Stents

Hybrid stents incorporate multiple materials in their design. The most commonly discussed and used are the Rüsch-Y (Willy Rüsch, Kernan, Germany) and the Polyflex (Boston Scientific, Natkin, MA, USA). The Rüsch-Y stent will be discussed below; the Polyflex stent is a hybrid of polyester and silicone forming a solid-walled stent, with high external radial forces (Fig. 51.20).

The Rüsch-Y stent (Fig. 51.21) is a Silastic stent with stainless steel C rings that artificially represent the cartilage. The posterior wall of the stent is made of a thin-

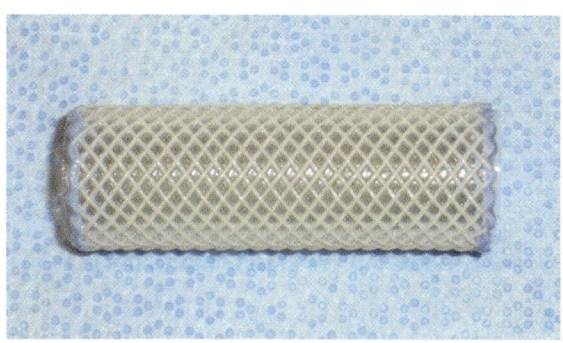

Fig. 51.20. Polyflex stent

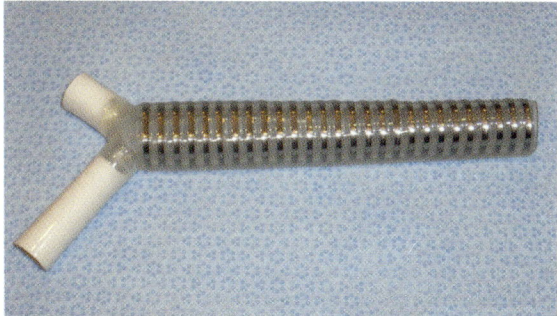

Fig. 51.21. Rüsch-Y stent

ner Silastic plastic to make it more functional, similar to the membranous trachea itself. The three available sizes of this stent are designed to traverse the entire length of the trachea with branches into the right and left mainstem bronchi. The Rüsch-Y stent requires rigid bronchoscopy and is difficult to place.

Freitag et al. describe the use of the Rüsch-Y stent in 94 cases of malignant airway disease of the 135 patients treated in the study. The authors report good results in the control of malignant airway disease, allowing 27 patients to undergo sufficient definitive therapy as to have their stents removed postresponse. The authors also describe good results with the use of this stent in the management of tracheoesophageal fistula formation [81].

51.7 Putting Things Together

The endobronchial management of lung cancer is a vastly expanding field. As is outlined in this chapter there are a significant number of therapeutic modalities, which are available to the physician and the patients they treat. As advanced diagnostics continue to evolve and become more mainstream – endobronchial ultrasound, autofluorescence, and endoscopic coherence tomography to name some – our understanding and diagnosis of endobronchial cancer will improve, giving us

greater opportunities to manage patients as has been suggested in some of our previous references: Furuse et al., Kato et al., Konaka et al., Deygas et al., and Van Boxen et al. All of these novel studies are designed to look at ways of treating cancer endobronchially at earlier stages, allowing complete local therapy [35, 43, 48, 51, 52].

The standard approach to the management of cancer can also be enhanced by the addition of endobronchial techniques. As described in the following references, endobronchial techniques were used to enhance standard therapeutic modalities, allowing patients to feel better and therefore more capable of having the necessary chemotherapy or radiation therapy, or even enhancing the chance of a more conclusive surgical procedure. The knowledge of the entire scope of available endobronchial interventional techniques is not only important to the interventionalist performing these procedures, but also to the physicians seeing the patients who could benefit from them [23, 25, 60, 65, 66, 70, 71, 73–75, 81].

Key Points

- Interventional pulmonary procedures include diagnostic procedures, with the hope of earlier and more accurate diagnosis of lung cancer. Such techniques include: endobronchial ultrasound, autofluorescence bronchoscopy, and external navigation techniques.
- The ablative endobronchial techniques are used for the destruction and/or debulking of endobronchial carcinoma that obstructs the airways.
- Endobronchial prosthesis involves stenting of the airways, which can be used in several clinical situations: intrinsic, extrinsic, or mixed endobronchial obstruction. Stents work well in conjunction with other modalities such as laser or other ablative techniques and the mechanical debulking of tumors.

References

1. Bollinger CT, Mathur PN, Beamis JF, et al. ERS/ATS statement on interventional pulmonology. Eur Respir J 2002;19:356.
2. Ikeda S. Flexible bronchofiberscope. Laryngology 1970; 79:916.
3. Dumon JF, Reboud E, Garbe L, et al. Treatment of tracheobronchial lesions by laser photoresection. Chest 1982; 81:278.
4. Beamis JF Jr, Vergos K, Rebeiz EE, et al. Endoscopic laser therapy for obstructing tracheobronchial lesions. Ann Otol Rhinol Laryngol 1991; 100:413.
5. Cavaliere S, Foccoli P, Farina PL. Nd:YAG laser bronchoscopy. Chest 1988; 94:15.

6. Kvale PA, Eichenhorn MS, Radke JR, et al. YAG laser photoresection of lesions obstructing the central airways. Chest 1985; 87:283.

7. Eichenhorn MS, Kvale PA, Miks VM, et al. Initial combination therapy with YAG laser photoresection and irradiation for inoperable non-small cell carcinoma of the lung: a preliminary report. Chest 1986; 89:782.

8. Mantovani G, Astara G, Manca G, et al. Clin Lung Cancer 2000; 1:277.

9. Brutinel WM, Cortese DA, McDougall JC, et al. A two-year experience with the neodymium-YAG laser in endobronchial obstruction. Chest 1987; 91:159.

10. Desai SJ, Mehta AC, Vanderbug Medendorp S, et al. Survival experience following Nd:YAG laser photoresection for primary bronchogenic carcinoma. Chest 1988; 94:939.

11. Stanopoulos IT, Beamis JF Jr, Martinez FJ, et al. Laser bronchoscopy in respiratory failure from malignant airway obstruction. Crit Care Med 1993; 21:386.

12. Petrovich Z, Stanley K, Cox JD, et al. Radiotherapy in the management of locally advanced lung cancer of all cell types: final report of randomized trial. Cancer 1981; 48:1335.

13. Edell ES, Cortese DA, McDougall JC. Ancillary therapies in the management of lung cancer: photodynamic therapy, laser therapy, and endobronchial prosthetic devices. Mayo Clin Proc 1993; 68:685.

14. Cortese DA, Edell ES. Role of phototherapy, laser therapy, brachytherapy, and prosthetic stents in the management of lung cancer. Clin Chest Med 1993; 14:149.

15. Sutedja G, Schramel F, van Kralingen K, et al. Stent placement is justifiable in end-stage patients with malignant airway tumours. Ann Otol Rhinol Respir 1995; 62:148.

16. Hetzel MR, Millard FJ, Ayesh R, et al. Laser treatment for carcinoma of the bronchus. BMJ 1983; 286:12.

17. Mehta AC, Golish JA, Ahmad M, et al. Palliative treatment of malignant airway obstruction by Nd-YAG laser. Cleve Clin Q 1985; 52:513.

18. McDougall JC, Corese DA. Neodymium-YAG laser therapy of malignant airway obstruction: a preliminary report. Mayo Clin Proc 1983; 58:35.

19. Toty L, Personne C, Colchen A, et al. Bronchoscopic management of tracheal lesions using the neodymium yttrium aluminum garnet laser. Thorax 1981; 36:175.

20. Arabian A, Spagnolo SV. Laser therapy in patients with primary lung cancer. Chest 1984; 86:519.

21. Sonett JR, Keenan RJ, Ferson PF, et al. Endobronchial management of benign, malignant, and lung transplantation airway stenosis. Ann Thorac Surg 1995; 59:1417.

22. Macha HN, Becker KO, Kemmer HP. Pattern of failure and survival in endobronchial laser resection: a matched pair study. Chest 1994; 105:1668.

23. Cavaliere S, Foccoli P, Toninelli C, et al. Nd:YAG laser therapy in lung cancer; an 11-year experience with 2,253 applications in 1,585 patients. J Bronchol 1994; 1:105.

24. Ross DJ, Mohsenifar Z, Koerner SK. Survival characteristics after neodymium:YAG laser photoresection in advanced stage lung cancer. Chest 1990; 98:581.

25. Mathisen DJ, Grillo HC. Endoscopic relief of malignant airway obstruction. A five-year experience with 1,396 applications in 1,000 patients. Ann Thorac Surg 1989; 48:469.

26. Cavaliere S, Foccoli P, Farina PC. Nd:YAG laser treatment of tracheal stenosis. Chest 1983; 84:295.

27. Personne C, Colchen A, Leroy M, et al. Indications and techniques for endoscopic laser resections in bronchology. J Thorac Cardiovasc Surg 1986; 71:710.

28. Lee P, Kupeli E, Mehta A. Therapeutic bronchoscopy in lung cancer. Clin Chest Med 2002; 23:241.

29. Gerasin VA, Shafirowsky BB. Endobronchial electrosurgery. Chest 1988; 93:270.

30. Petrou M, Kaplan D, Goldstraw P. Bronchoscopic diathermy resection and stent insertion: a cost effective treatment for tracheobronchial obstruction. Thorax 1993; 48:1156.

31. Hooper RG, Jackson FW. Endobronchial electrocautery. Chest 1988; 94:595.

32. Suteja TG, van Kralingenk, Schramel F, et al. Fiberoptic bronchoscopic electrosurgery under local anesthesia for rapid palliation in patients with central airways malignancies: a preliminary report. Thorax 1994; 49:1243.

33. Suteja TG, van Boxem TJ, Schramel FM, et al. Endobronchial electrocautery is an excellent alternative for Nd:YAG laser to treat airways tumors. J Bronchol 1997; 4:101.

34. Homasson JP. Endobronchial electrocautery. Semin Respir Crit Care 1997; 18:555.

35. Van Boxen TJ, Venmens BJ, Schramel FM, et al. Radiographically occult lung cancer treated with fiberoptic bronchoscopic electrocautery: a pilot study of a simple and inexpensive technique. Eur Respir J 1998; 11:169.

36. Farin G, Grund KE. Technology of APC, with particular regard to endoscopic application. Endosc Surg 1994; 2:71.

37. Grund KE, Storek D, Farin G. Endoscopic APC: first clinical experiences in flexible endoscopy. Endosc Surg 1994; 2:42.

38. Morice RC, Ece T, Ece F, et al. Endobronchial APC for treatment of hemoptysis and neoplastic airway obstruction. Chest 2001; 119:781.

39. Crosta C, Spaggiari L, De Stefano, et al. Endoscopic APC for palliative treatment of malignant airway obstruction: early results in 47 cases. Lung Cancer 2001; 33:75.

40. Mathur PN, Wolf KM, Busk MF, et al. Fiberoptic bronchoscopic cryotherapy in the management of tracheobronchial obstruction. Chest 1996; 110:718.

41. Maiwand MO, Homasson JP. Cryotherapy for tracheobronchial disorders. Clin Chest Med 1995; 16:427.

42. Walsh DA, Maiwand MD, Nath AR, et al. Bronchoscopic cryotherapy for advanced bronchial carcinoma. Thorax 1990; 45:509.

43. Deygas N, Froudarakis M, Ozenne G, et al. Cryotherapy in early superficial bronchogenic carcinoma. Chest 2001; 120:26.

44. Unger M, Sterman DH. Bronchoscopy, transthoracic needle aspiration and related procedures. In: Fishman AP (ed) Fishman's Pulmonary Diseases and Disorders. New York: McGraw-Hill, 1998:589.

45. Seijo LM, Sterman DH. Interventional pulmonology. N Engl J Med 2001; 344:740.

46. Lam S. Photodynamic therapy of lung cancer. Semin Oncol 1994; 21:15.

47. Sutedja T, Lam S, LeRiche JC, et al. Response and pattern of failure after photodynamic therapy for intraluminal stage I lung cancer. J Bronchol 1994; 1:295.

48. Furuse K, Fukuoka M, Kato H, et al. A prospective phase II study on photodynamic therapy with Photofrin II for centrally located early-stage lung cancer: the Japan Lung Cancer Photodynamic Therapy Study Group. J Clin Oncol 1993; 11:1852.

49. Kato H, Furukawa K, Sato M, Okunaka T, et al. Phase II clinical study of photodynamic therapy using mono-L-aspartyl chlorine e6 and diode laser for early superficial squamous cell carcinoma of the lung. Lung Cancer 2003; 42:103.

50. Hayata Y, Kato H, Konaka C, et al. Photodynamic therapy (PDT) in early stage lung cancer. Lung Cancer 1993; 9:287.

51. Kato H, Okunaka T, Shimatani H. PDT for early stage bronchogenic carcinoma. J Clin Laser Med Surg 1996; 14:235.

52. Konaka C, Okunake T, Furukawa K, et al. Photodynamic therapy for multiple primary lung cancers. Gan T Kagaku Ryoho 1996; 23:31.

53. Kato H, Konaka C, Ono J, et al. Preoperative laser PDT in conjunction with operation in lung cancer. J Thorac Cardiovasc Surg 1985; 90:420.

54. Hayata Y, Ohbo K, Ogawa I, Taira O. Immunotherapy for lung cancer cases using BCG or BCG cell-wall skeleton: intratumoral injections. Gann Monogr Cancer Res 1978; 21:51.

55. Goldberg EP, Hadba AR, Almond BA, Marotta JS. Intratumoral cancer chemotherapy and immunotherapy: opportunities for nonsystemic preoperative drug delivery. J Pharm Pharmacol 2002; 54:159.

56. Fujisawa T, Hongo H, Yamaguchi Y, et al. Intratumoral ethanol injection for malignant tracheobronchial lesions: a new bronchofiberscopic procedure. Endoscopy 1986; 18:188.

57. Sawa T, Ikoma T, Yoshida T, et al. Intratumoral ethanol injection therapy using endoscopic video information system (english abstract). Gan To Kagaku Ryoho 1999; 26:1865.

58. Celikoglu F, Celikoglu S. Intratumoural chemotherapy with 5-fluorouracil for palliation of bronchial cancer in patients with severe airway obstruction. J Pharm Pharmacol 2003; 55:1441.

59. Prakash UB, Stubbs SE. The bronchoscopy survey: some reflections. Chest 1991; 100:1660.

60. Schray MF, McDougall JC, Martinez A, et al. Management of malignant airways compromise with laser and low dose rate brachytherapy. Chest 1988; 93:264.

61. Ofiara L, Roman T, Schwartzman K, et al. Local determinants of response to endobronchial high dose rate brachytherapy in bronchogenic carcinoma. Chest 1997; 112:946.

62. Taulelle M, Chauvet B, Vincent P, et al. High dose rate brachytherapy: results and complications in 185 patients. Eur Resp J 1998; 11:162.

63. Nori D, Allison R, Kaplan B, et al. High dose rate intraluminal irradiation in bronchogenic carcinoma. Technique and results. Chest 1993; 104:1006.

64. Vergnon JM, Costes F, Bayon MC, Emont A. Efficacy of tracheal and bronchial stent placement on respiratory functional tests. Chest 1995; 107:741.

65. Colt HG, Dumon JF. Tracheobronchial stents: indications and applications. Lung Cancer 1993; 9:301.

66. Cooper JD, Pearson FG, Patterson GA, et al. Use of silicone stents in the management of airway problems. Ann Thorac Surg 1989; 47:371.

67. Montgomery WW. T-tube tracheal stent. Arch Otolaryngol 1965; 82:320.

68. Dumon JF. A dedicated tracheobronchial stent. Chest 1990; 97:328.

69. Tojo T, Iioka S, Kitamura S, et al. Management of malignant tracheobronchial stenosis with metal stents and Dumon stents. Ann Thorac Surg 1996; 61:1074.

70. Dumon JF, Cavaliere S, Diaz-Jimenez JP, et al. Seven-year experience with the Dumon prosthesis. J Bronchol 1996; 3:6.

71. Diaz-Jimenez JP, Munoz EF, Ballarin JIM, et al. Silicone stents in the management of obstructive tracheobronchial lesions: 2-year experience. J Bronchol 1994; 1:15.

72. Freitag L, Eicker K, Donovan TJ, et al. Mechanical properties of airway stents. J Bronchol 1995; 2:270.

73. Clarke CP, Ball DL, Sephton R. Follow-up of patients having Nd:YAG laser resection of bronchostenotic lesions. J Bronchol 1994; 1:19.

74. Gaer JA, Tsang V, Khaghani A, et al. Use of endotracheal silicone stents for relief of tracheobronchial obstruction. Ann Thorac Surg 1992; 54:512.

75. Miyazawa T, Yamakido M, Ikeda S, et al. Implantation of Ultraflex nitinol stents in malignant tracheobronchial stenosis. Chest 2000; 118:959.

76. Tsang V, Williams AM, Goldstraw P. Sequential Silastic and expandable metal stenting for tracheobronchial strictures. Ann Thorac Surg 1992; 53:856.

77. Freitag L, Eicker K, Donovan TJ, et al. Mechanical properties of airway stents. J Bronchol 1995; 2:270.

78. Gelb AF, Zamel N, Colchen A, et al. Physiologic studies of tracheobronchial stents in airway obstruction. Am Rev Respir Dis 1992; 146:1088.

79. Colt HG, Dumon J-F. Airway obstruction in cancer: the pros and cons of stents. J Respir Dis 1991; 12:741.

80. Bolliger CT, Probst R, Tschopp K, et al. Silicone stents in the management of inoperable tracheobronchial stenosis: indications and limitations. Chest 1993; 104:1653.

81. Freitag L, Tekolf E, Stamatis G, Greschushna D. Clinical evaluation of a new bifurcated dynamic airways stent: a 5-year experience with 135 patients. Thorac Cardiovasc Surg 1997:45:6.

Delivering Bad News to Patients and Their Families

52

Lidia Schapira

Contents

52.1   Introduction

Preceding chapters have dealt with the specific aspects of diagnosis and treatment of thoracic disease. Now we turn our attention to the therapeutic encounter during which the "bad news" of diagnosis and prognosis is communicated to patients and their families. The past decade has seen a proliferation of articles and courses offering specific methods to effectively deliver bad news. For the most part, recommendations have preceded the evidence and are based, instead, on what is commonly referred to as "best practice." Robert Buckman, an authority on the topic of breaking bad news, has written that there are insufficient research data on the subject to define the best method. And it is difficult to design or even imagine research studies that would settle the issue definitively. The articles and books written in the past twenty years give advice to clinicians based on an individual author's experience. Efforts to improve physicians' communication skills underscore the importance of compassionate and empathic delivery of bad news.

I will avoid a prescriptive approach and instead outline the major themes that physicians need to consider when discussing or sharing serious medical informa-tion. "Bad news" is defined as information pertaining to physical health that will irrevocably damage an individual's concept of self – present and future. For example a diagnosis of diabetes or muscular dystrophy touches the mind, body, and spirit as a person struggles to adapt to the implications of these life-altering diseases. Ptacek and Eberhardt define bad news as information that results in a cognitive, behavioral, or emotional deficit in the person receiving the news that persists for some time [1].

I will begin by addressing the physician's duty to inform, acknowledging the bioethical and legal imperatives for open communication and the emergence of patient autonomy as the single most important ethical value in contemporary medicine. I will then consider from the patient's perspective both the need and the right to know and examine the possibilities for shared decision-making that result from open communication and the uncensored exchange of information. With examples from published memoirs of illness as well as unpublished testimony, I will highlight the importance and the power of the physician's words in shaping an individual's adaptation to chronic illness or transition to end-of-life care.

Generations of physicians before us were guided by the dual obligation of providing information as well as protection to patients. Balancing disclosure with silence in order to maintain hope best sums the oral tradition passed on by many wise physicians throughout the world. The concept of "best practice" has changed dramatically in the past fifty years. Full disclosure of diagnostic and prognostic information, now standard practice in most Western countries, would have shocked many of our mentors and may even today be considered unnecessarily brutal in many societies. Anthropologist Mary-Jo Good argues that in American oncology practice hope is primarily conveyed by providing information in contrast to Europe and Asia, where physicians convey hope primarily by fostering ambiguity [2, 3]. In this arena rich with nuance, the physician's non-verbal communication through gestures, body language, and tone are also likely to impact on patients as they hear information and begin to decipher the medical language.

The following sections will address the patient's and doctor's perspectives, the ethical standards and expectations that frame the doctor–patient encounter, and the societal mores that, although invisible in daily practice, shape personal philosophies of practice and define proper professional behavior.

52.2   The Right and Need to Know

In recent years, lawyers and bioethicists have "excoriated" traditional medical ethics saying it "scants the patient's interest in autonomy." Theorists insist that doctors must inform patients to allow them to decide their own fate. In the USA, the prevailing argument is that a person has the right to decide what is in his or her best interest and requires specific and tailored information in order to make a reasonable medical decision.

Take for example the case of a 65-year-old man just diagnosed with lung cancer who is offered a 4% absolute benefit for adjuvant chemotherapy. He may choose to accept or decline treatment based on his values, perception of benefit, and willingness to experience the burden or discomfort of treatment. The law demands and ethics support the duty to inform patients in order that they may take an active role in deciding whether or not to undergo testing or treatment. The challenge remains in the interpretation of exactly how much information is enough. Patients are often unwilling or unable to share the burden of decision-making – in these circumstances what ethicists wish for them does not match their agenda. Many patients look to their doctors to provide information as well as direction. They may in fact need and want information, but they separate the task of receiving such information from the one of making an active decision regarding treatment.

To complicate matters even more, the emotional impact of hearing life-altering news affects patients' capacity to reason objectively. Suffering may impair a person's ability to imagine goals for the future as well as his or her sense of control and self-efficacy. Yet these are essential for exercising autonomy. Medical decisions often rest on rethinking or regenerating life goals, a process which involves coming to terms with grief as well as clear reasoning. What this tells us is that hearing bad and sad news sets in motion an emotional and cognitive reaction that needs to be acknowledged, addressed, and supported, yet is rarely mentioned in ethical discourse.

Many physicians genuinely strive toward a patient-centered approach, rejecting the older model of paternalistic care in favor of a newer "contractual" one depicting patients and doctors as partners. Yet in practice doctors are constantly sifting through information, picking and choosing just what and how much needs to

be said and how much optimism or pessimism needs to be infused in the telling. Some withholding of information may be considered morally sound and in keeping with the physician's ethical obligation to protect the patient and act on his or her behalf. In the example of disclosure of a terminal illness, the physician may focus entirely on discussion of available treatment and barely touch on the more significant issue of prognosis. Yet most agree that a meaningful discussion of treatment options can be held only when the patient understands the burden of both accepting and refusing treatment as well as the likelihood of treatment-related success [4].

Some are critical of physicians' self-reported constraints on sharing "truthful" information and attribute it to the physician's need to preserve control and power over the patient and the medical encounter [5]. Debate often hinges on definitions of truth ownership. Junior doctors often equate data with truth and inform patients as soon as information is available without attention to language or meaning. This practice is sometimes referred to as "truth dumping." More experienced doctors recognize the need to negotiate and bargain just how much information can be given in order to avoid inflicting unnecessary suffering or harming their patients.

Antonella Surbone describes ways of adapting the need and duty to inform to fit clinical scenarios. By rethinking truth as a relative concept which can be shaped by both patient and doctor, she advocates a respectful bargaining of both quantity and quality of disclosure to fit the needs of the situation as well as the stated goals and boundaries imposed by the patient [6–8]. A patient's information preferences and needs may vary over time and require tactful nurturing by both physician and patient – needs may change reflecting a patient's emotional state, availability of support, or knowledge of inner resources needed to absorb and retain the information. It is also fundamental to recognize the role of the family in both decision-making and caretaking of the cancer patient during the course of the entire illness trajectory. For the individual patient, the tension between wanting to know and needing to know is exemplified in this quote from a patient with advanced disease: "We know I am dying, the doctor knows what therapy I can bear and what is best for me" (personal communication).

Good communication skills help the physician deliver information, but it is ultimately his or her philosophical and ethical view of how much news needs to be given that shapes the clinical encounter. For some, the task of telling a patient of his or her diagnosis is linked to the obligation to forecast or prognosticate. A patient referred to the oncologist following an evaluation for cough and weight loss, found to have stage IV lung cancer, may hear very different things depending on his choice of physician. He may hear not only that he has lung cancer, but also that the disease is not curable. If he then asks for more information he may learn the average life expectancy is typically only a few months.

Nicholas Christakis argues that patient and doctor may negotiate the amount of information that is "allowed" [9]. Some patients with metastatic disease explicitly ask their physicians not to prognosticate. They may find that articulating and repeating estimates of success or measurable life expectancy is simply unhelpful and depressing [9]. They may talk about their need to have their doctor "hope with them" for an improvement, an extension, or symptomatic relief. Often physicians dodge questions by simply offering an empathic response. Practices vary considerably in this regard and reflect an individual physician's personal view of what constitutes "right" or humane practice. On the one hand, if physicians view withholding prognostic information as deceitful they are likely to favor complete disclosure. On the other hand, if they see withholding prognostic information as an important aspect of fostering hope they may steer the conversation away from discussion of timelines and projections of future problems [9]. As with any therapeutic option, the decision of how much to tell depends on the estimates of risk and benefit and ultimately rests with the physician.

52.3 Receiving Bad News

Surprisingly only a very small but informative number of articles have been published in the medical literature addressing the patient's perspective of receiving bad news. Such research is inherently difficult since it involves the subjective and experiential and is hampered by worry that it could add an additional burden to those already maximally stressed. One study conducted by Per Salander in Sweden collected testimonies from 187 patients who had received their cancer diagnosis 2–8 months prior to the outset of the study and were asked to describe the manner in which they learned of their diagnosis in writing [10]. These patients were recruited from a largely rural area and were treated at a tertiary university hospital in Sweden. As stated by the author, the practice in Sweden favors full disclosure although it is uncommon to give prognosis in statistical form, in sharp contrast to the prevailing practice in the USA.

Although the initial letter requested specific information on the doctor–patient encounter, the narratives submitted described a context and a process rather than a single event. Recurrent themes included being unprepared, receiving too much or too little news, wanting to be known as a person, being grateful for a "simple uncomplicated humanity, a hug or a supportive word," and the relief at hearing information related to possible treatment [10]. Salander concludes that the most helpful

strategy from a patient's perspective is one that recognizes the psychological meaning of "togetherness" at diagnosis, of a supportive atmosphere and a personal touch, of being welcomed and acknowledged, and of being spared waiting. This perspective serves to highlight the difference between the patients' experience of receiving bad news and medical theory and concept of best practice. Patients experience the news as a process, while physicians focus on "delivery" of bad news as a single event.

The "bad news" consultation may in some cases confirm a patient's preexisting worries or suspicions. It is delivered through language which has the potential to "unleash a mourning process, a calling into question and readjustment of direction and future plans" [11]. If recognized by the doctor, the patient can be guided to cope and adjust in order to be able to participate in decision-making about treatment. Being summoned to see an oncologist following a chest X-ray or CT scan will likely suggest to the patient that he or she has a serious problem. Patients often comment that the facial expression of a physician lets out the secret of diagnosis long before the word cancer is spoken or dialogue begins.

So in thinking about the physician's delivery of bad news it is crucial to pay attention to each patient's personal relationship with the events and communications that precede the consultation. When a patient presents with a physical symptom such as a cough or a palpable mass, one can imagine that this patient has already entertained the possibility that this is indeed a sign of a serious illness. Although patients are unprepared to estimate the magnitude of risk associated with illness, they have most likely either sketched a likely explanation (stress, a virus, a terminal cancer) for their symptom or formulated a series of questions to ask the expert. Along with a cognitive effort to integrate the new event into the known framework of experience, the patient must make an emotional shift to absorb and prepare for the eventuality of grave danger. In this scenario, there is a period of anticipation that gives the patient some time to adapt to the possibility of life-altering news.

Alternatively, some seem unaware and shocked at hearing the news of a grave diagnosis. A 40-year-old non-smoker with a persistent winter cough who consults with his primary physician and is found to have a thoracic malignancy may be shocked to hear the word cancer. By avoiding assumptions and remaining open and curious to the patient's perspective, clinicians can provide the supportive atmosphere necessary to establish a therapeutic alliance.

Anthropologist and cancer patient Julie Goldman spoke eloquently about the meaning of achieving a "new normal," a process by which an individual learns to incorporate into his or her life the knowledge, tasks, and skills necessary to live in a state of harmony with a catastrophic illness. Goldman describes the painful process through which she came to consider maintenance chemotherapy a normal part of her daily routine. Illness narratives written as text or poems by cancer patients serve to illustrate a few fundamental themes. From the patient's perspective, the primary theme is the need to be known and heard. The physician's empathic response, therapeutic presence, as well as the ability to provide a clear course of action emerge clearly as the most valuable attributes of the "good doctor." As described by lawyer and cancer patient Patricia Barr in her journal, "good doctors know they can't make this go away, they can only hope with me it will continue to move slowly, very slowly" (personal communication). In a classic memoir of life as a cancer patient, literary critic Anatole Broyard wrote: "Now that I know I have cancer of the prostate, the lymph nodes, and part of my skeleton, what *do* I want in a doctor? I would say that I want one who is a close reader of illness and a good critic of medicine ... Someone who can treat body and soul ... " [12].

52.4 How Much Information is Enough?

There are no guidelines addressing just how much information is enough. Individual practices vary as do patients' stated needs for information. Miscalculations and misunderstandings are common. A person may ask for detailed information and then appear overwhelmed when it is given. A physician may consider he or she has adequately informed a patient only to discover the same patient made a comment to another team member indicating a glaring knowledge deficit. Stage and grade are often confused, and goals of treatment and prognostic information frequently misunderstood. The profession as a whole has focused more on how and when to inform, than on how much is retained or understood. Senior physicians often decide how much information to provide based on the patient's educational level. Rather than making assumptions based on education or ethnicity, it is safer to ask the patient. Giving information to patients of limited verbal proficiency with low literacy skills is far more challenging and language barriers add another tier of difficulty.

Several convincing studies from the UK, USA, Australia, and several northern European countries support a preference for complete disclosure. Although estimates vary, we know that approximately 50–97% of patients surveyed wanted to know the truth [12–14]. Elegant studies done by Butow and Tattersall and their colleagues in Australia provide information and insight into the decision-making process as it evolves and proceeds in real time [15, 16]. Based on analysis of audiotapes of consultations and patient interviews, Tatterhall found most patients eagerly elicit and value the recommendation of the doctor [16, 17].

Ideally, consultations involve the exchange of information in an atmosphere of mutual trust followed by deliberation and finally a recommendation from the physician, based on what the patient stated were his or her goals and preferences. Such an approach also promotes good coping. David Spiegel pointed out that gathering and processing information, sorting through different options, and mobilizing inner resources is the key for a successful adaptation to illness [18]. An important and underutilized communication tool involves the discussion of alternatives to the recommended or preferred treatment. Doctors need to help patients think through their options, verbalizing what could happen if the patient chose to forego all treatment or used an "alternative" or "parallel" therapy. In a non-judgmental exchange, the doctor can help patients sort through their options and imagine the consequences of their decision. This "active" approach to decision-making is in sharp contrast to a passive one, where the patient accepts a recommendation for treatment without questions, deliberation, or clear understanding.

Even though studies show the majority of individuals wish to be informed, we cannot lose sight of the fact that a respectable minority has a different view, equally deserving of respect and personalized attention. It is in situations where the need to inform clashes with the individual's legitimate request and right not to receive information that physicians perceive the delivery of bad news as abusive. In real life we face competent, educated individuals who simply do not wish to know the detailed side effects of a chemotherapeutic agent or radiation therapy and prefer instead to skip the explanations and move on to treatment. They prefer to sign the consent authorizing treatment without reading the document or hearing explanations of possible risk. Case by case, physicians need to decide if the patient's unwillingness to listen invalidates or trivializes the process of obtaining consent for treatment.

Since patients are unaccustomed to hearing medical jargon it seems best to keep it at a minimum. Terms routinely employed by physicians may have a completely different meaning for patients and might alarm or falsely reassure a patient. A "negative" biopsy indicates either no tissue or no tumor and thus may have a "positive" implication for the medical team but requires an appropriate explanation for an average patient [19]. A "positive" lymph node confirms spread of tumor and thus negatively impacts on stage and outcome. Sadly, patients and their families learn the language of medicine as they spend more and more time in medical environments and often repeat technical terms even though they may not really comprehend their significance. Doctors can promote understanding and coping by using clear language, avoiding jargon, and asking patients to explain what they know and understand. The use of graphics, audiotapes, and video may facilitate retention of knowledge and help improve communication [20]. Nowadays patients have a responsibility as well as a right to be well informed, and this impacts on relationships with professional caregivers. Both physician and patient need to weigh the benefits and burdens of information and knowledge as they negotiate a mutual level of comfort with disclosure.

52.5 Message, Metaphors, and Meaning

Experienced doctors say they are the first ones to receive bad news such as a laboratory test confirming a recurrence of cancer. When the patient and doctor have an established relationship and the news concerns progression of disease or treatment failure, the doctor may also experience a keen sense of disappointment, sorrow, guilt, and frustration [21]. These feelings need to be acknowledged and processed or they may undermine the physician's therapeutic potential [22]. In an effort to protect the patient, some doctors may use euphemisms to soften the blow which may only add to confusion [23, 24].

In sharp contrast is the situation in which the doctor is the messenger. In this case, the doctor is an agent detached from the news and patient, serving only as conduit for information. No practicing physician can really imagine himself or herself a mere vehicle for transmission of information, yet the concept has persisted among professionals. To complicate matters, many physicians fear that a public accustomed to stories of medical prowess may blame them for the bad news because of a belief that all diseases are either preventable or fixable.

Metaphors illuminate complex issues and help to provide clarity and depth of meaning [25]. There is a long history of using military metaphors in medicine and nursing that has permeated the language of cancer medicine. To understand oncologists' attitudes about disclosing prognostic information to cancer patients with advanced disease, Gordon and Dougherty interviewed 14 oncologists and conducted a focus group of medical fellows. It is perhaps troubling that these physicians used terms such as "hitting over the head," "pounding," "hammering," "bludgeoning," and "dumping" to describe their practice of disclosing sad and bad news [26]. The language clearly conveys the underlying belief that truth is injurious, the physician abusive, and the practice harmful. It also articulates the unspoken distress experienced by many physicians [21, 22]. Many doctors remember past experiences of delivering bad news as harrowing and describe being overcome by painful memories for many years [27, 28].

Metaphors can bridge the gap between the illness experience and the world of technology and treatment. By paying attention to patients' metaphoric speech, physicians may gain insight into the cognitive and affective underpinnings of their illness experience, and this may help make sense of their questions, their demands, their emotional responses, and their treatment decisions [29]. Imagination, curiosity, and sensitivity are important in creating rapport and shaping the language that promotes understanding. Metaphors help bring the patient's subjective view of illness into the forefront of the medical encounter, give meaning to the experience, and allow the doctor and patient to strengthen the therapeutic alliance around a shared vision [25].

Military metaphors are common. Patients speak of waging war and fighting battles and are often praised by family, friends, and physicians for putting up a "good fight." Another recurrent theme is that of a journey with changing landscapes and milestones. Whatever the theme – be it a road race, a journey, a roller coaster, or a battle – metaphors allow clinicians and patients to discuss goals, direction, progress, and possibilities. Together they can agree on what defines success and how best to find it.

52.6 Guidelines for Delivering Bad News to Patients and Families

A well-conceived treatment plan is essential to producing a good outcome. The same concept applies to the delivery of bad and sad news. If the ultimate objective of providing information is to allow the patient and physician to move on with treatment, then it is indispensable to establish a sound working relationship between the doctor, the treatment team, and the patient and family. This positive dynamic is critical if the therapeutic relationship is to prosper [30]. Preparing in advance is a key task for successful communication. The physician needs to be well informed of the medical situation and treatment options, and, if possible, about the patient's own state of knowledge. Allotting the necessary time and safeguarding the encounter to minimize or avoid interruptions is crucial.

Every physician knows there is a well-defined organizational structure shaping the consultative process, a format with a clear beginning, middle, and end. However, most patients are unaware of the rationale for such "structural scaffolding" and may thus wonder why their surgeon and oncologist ask the same questions. To this end, it may be beneficial to explain how the process of information works in clinical medicine and assure the patient that each physician needs to flesh out details directly in his or her own manner. Cancer patients are often relieved to peer behind the curtain to learn why consultations flow the way they do, and why a history and examination must precede discussion of treatment – usually a patient's primary concern [30]. By providing clarity and letting a patient know exactly how much time is available and being flexible enough to negotiate with him or her how it will be spent, the physician can help set the right tone for a respectful partnership and allow the patient to participate without unnecessary stress or anxiety. Giving the patient a ten- or five-minute warning before the end of the meeting allows time to review the strategy and plan. Taking the time to make the process, personnel, and expectations clear helps to set the foundation for a good doctor–patient relationship.

Protocols and guidelines for delivering bad news shed light on both delivery and reception by identifying a series of steps that flow smoothly and cover the important points required for effective communication. By matching process and content [31] and providing a useful framework of linked steps, these guidelines serve to assuage the anxiety of junior doctors and standardize an effective approach to giving bad and sad news. It is important to bear in mind that available guidelines were developed by and for English-speaking physicians and patients in the UK, Canada, USA, and Australia but have been effectively taught and adapted for use in broader multicultural settings.

A very useful six-step protocol was developed by Buckman and Baile and is commonly referred to as the "SPIKES" protocol [32, 33]. The mnemonic helps remember the six steps of the protocol, which are: setting, perception, invitation, knowledge, empathic response, and strategy and summary. It reminds doctors to prepare for the interview and set it up properly by finding a calm and comfortable space, minimizing interruptions, and ensuring the right participants attend the meeting. A simple detail, such as sitting in direct eye contact with the patient helps set the stage for a comfortable interchange. The protocol then shifts to the patient and reminds the physician to check the patient's understanding of the situation. After the patient's knowledge is reviewed and clarified the physician is guided to obtain an invitation to proceed to "tell" the news that needs to be discussed.

At this juncture the clinician needs to ask how much information the patient desires and, if the patient flatly refuses to be informed, to help him or her designate someone who can receive the information and act on his or her behalf. Here too, the clinician needs to ascertain the level of detail the patient wishes to have or is able to comprehend. By taking the time to explore the patient's informational preferences, the physician conveys a keen interest in meeting the patient's needs and shows respect for his or her rights. If the family says clearly "don't tell" then it falls on the physician to take the time to explore the concerns and articulate cultural norms that may underlie the request. These situations add yet another level of complexity and require skillful negotiation of mutual agendas. In the USA it is almost impossible for a cancer patient to undergo treatment without being informed of the diagnosis and thus it is best to encourage families to allow the physician to give

the patient at least a minimum amount of information. Sharing information or imparting the "knowledge" is what physicians commonly refer to as "communicating" with patients.

The SPIKES protocol serves as a useful reminder that information exchange is merely one in a series of important communicative acts and gestures. Guidelines encourage clarity, honesty, avoidance of jargon and ambiguity, and delivering the content in small segments with frequent pauses to check the patient's understanding. There is general agreement that efforts to minimize the impact or soften the blow are best avoided in favor of a steady, supportive, and clear rendering of facts.

The final two steps focus on the patient's reception of the news and end with the medical summary and action plan. The fifth step of SPIKES, the "empathic response" is perhaps the one most frequently neglected in medical and surgical practice and yet is crucial for facilitating coping. Patients and families respond to bad news in a variety of ways. Some respond with emotional outbursts, others express disbelief, fear, and guilt, and some may find the news intolerable and leave the room or pace up and down a hallway. Perhaps the simplest approach is to provide a steady, calm, and accepting presence. At times this may be best accomplished by sharing the silence, other times it may require expressions of sorrow and support or a gentle touch.

Empathic responses refer to the clinical skill of imagining another person's experience, a form of emotional reasoning. Patients may give non-verbal cues that need to be explored with gentle questioning. Asking the patient to share his or her worries, feelings, and concerns encourages disclosure and cements the therapeutic alliance. In so doing the doctor reinforces the clear message that the well-being of the patient is his or her primary concern. Those who are uncomfortable responding to emotion may limit their response to a simple phrase conveying sadness. This validates the patient's suffering even if it fails to address the complex facets of distress. Two important aspects of this protocol deserve to be emphasized: physicians should take care not to block patient's expressions of emotion and avoid reassuring a patient before he or she has had a chance to express his or her feelings and concerns.

While it is both common and desirable for physicians to comfort patients, it bears repeating that premature reassurance in a bad news consultation may in fact be deleterious and is best avoided. Rushing to discuss treatment and practical ways of "fixing" the problem deprives the patient of the opportunity to acknowledge and express his or her feelings and concerns. Just as one cannot assume that an educated person wants to know detailed information, so too it is best to ask the patient what are his or her sources of support. Marriage does not guarantee a supportive spouse and a religious affiliation is no proxy for personal conviction or faith. Asking the patient directly is the only way to obtain accurate information.

To bring the meeting to a close, the physician needs to summarize the facts, and make a recommendation for treatment. This may involve referrals to colleagues, additional testing, and an appointment to initiate chemotherapy or have an operation. Assuming there are options for treatment and a decision needs to be made, the process of information exchange and deliberation needs to begin. A smooth delivery of news with attention to the patient's emotional response forms the foundation for shared decision-making. If a patient is overcome by sadness or anger, he or she will be unable to participate in any meaningful way and treatment-related decisions will need to be postponed. As was discussed in prior sections, the patient is most grateful to the physician who provides clear guidance and expresses concern and a willingness to remain involved.

A single individual rarely delivers all the information. If the patient is hospitalized, he or she will likely hear different iterations of the "bad news" from junior and senior doctors, nurses, and consultants. Sometimes doctors keep giving the bad news over and over because they assume that if the patient seems to have recovered and expresses optimism they may not have fully "understood" the prognosis.

In an outpatient setting most patients are likely to receive care from more than one doctor and nurse and will likely hear the news repeated and re-interpreted. This may serve either to promote retention and understanding or cause confusion. Not infrequently physicians describe the same situation using different expressions or emphasis. Some dwell on treatment options, others insist on discussing both the short- and long-term outcome. Agreement among team members and specialists helps patients and families feel safe and minimizes opportunities for misunderstanding.

52.7 Setting Goals of Care

Despite considerable progress in thoracic oncology and supportive care, the sad fact remains that many patients die as a result of their disease. Delivering bad news is routine practice for busy clinicians in this field. Guidelines such as the ones presented in the prior section help standardize and normalize the process. Physicians who use the SPIKES protocol adapt it to conform to their individual style and typically use a handful of phrases to signal a change from one step to the next. Language varies but consistency helps physicians remain "grounded" during difficult situations and moments of high emotion.

When cure is not an option, decision-making focuses on setting goals of care. Sometimes there is an array of possible interventions ranging from clinical trials of varying levels of aggressiveness and toxicity to standard second-line therapy or palliative care. Other times it may be more appropriate to focus only on comfort measures which can be delivered in the home or hospice setting.

Doctors may experience a personal sense of failure and disappointment at the lack of available options. Patients and their families are likely to feel sad and possibly desperate. Adapting the SPIKES protocol and focusing on setting goals of care allows the physician to take control of the encounter and guide the patient and family as they learn the new language and territory of symptom-focused care. Data show that physicians who avoid discussing prognosis and are uncomfortable talking about end-of-life care are more likely to continue to administer chemotherapy until the last few days or weeks of life.

In keeping with the professional obligation to support and encourage autonomous decision-making, physicians need to let patients know when death is near. Eliciting patients' preferences for treatment and end-of-life care can be accomplished by inviting patients to share their hopes as well as their fears. Some may need to "fight" until the last moment and could not conceive of waiting to die at home. Others may cherish the opportunity to be free from medical centers, procedures, and possibly uncomfortable treatments and choose to focus on quality time with loved ones. When it comes to preferences for end-of-life care it is certainly true that one size does not fit all. Articulating and revisiting goals of care allows both physician and patient to remain grounded in reality and work together even as treatments fail.

52.8 Practical Tips for Delivering Bad News

Consistency of delivery and mastery over the steps required to promote understanding and facilitate coping transform this difficult task into a routine procedure that minimizes the stress experienced by the doctor.

The SPIKES protocol provides a rich platform for reflection on individual styles and a road map for novices. In the final paragraph I offer some word tools and probes that I have found help to keep the conversation going:

Setting: Refers to location, privacy, introductions, and preparation.

Perception: Refers to the patient's understanding of the problem and situation.
Can you tell me what Dr. Z told you about the current problem?
To start us off this morning, I would like to hear from you what you believe is going on?

Invitation: Addresses the patient's need to receive and refuse information and clarifies the level of detail required in the subsequent information exchange.

Are you the kind of person who wants to know every detail?

Is it all right for me to tell you the results of the latest scans or blood test?

Knowledge: Refers to the actual information, i.e., the bad news itself. It is best transmitted in clear language, without jargon, with frequent pauses.

A warning shot: *I'm afraid the news is more serious than we suspected.*

Unfortunately the PET scan showed the cancer has spread to other organs.

Empathic response: Refers to the doctor's acknowledgement of the seriousness and sadness inherent in the situation and the way in which he or she responds to the patient's emotion.

I am sorry ...

This must be very hard to hear ...

What are you most concerned about?

Linked to the empathic response is the doctor' engagement that conveys a promise of non-abandonment.

I want to make it clear that we are here to support you and help.

We have a terrific team and will work together to control your pain.

I will ask the nutritionist to meet with you and go over some sample menus ...

Strategy and summary:

Review of the medical information and concerns expressed.

Let me close by reviewing what we discussed this morning.

We need to bring this meeting to an end. Let me take a moment to go over the main points of our conversation.

Strategy and plans for treatment.

You have an appointment with my colleague in radiation oncology tomorrow at 3 o'clock.

I would like you to call my nurse tomorrow morning to tell her if this medication helped with your pain.

We'll meet again in two weeks and see if you're ready for the next treatment.

Acknowledgements

I am grateful to Dr. Paula Rauch and Rabbi Susan Harris for their helpful comments and review of the manuscript and to Ms Christine Cleary for her editorial assistance.

Key Points

- Giving bad news is a common task for chest physicians and thoracic oncologists. A consistent approach helps ensure a steady delivery. Guidelines provide a road map for physicians and help assuage fears and anxieties. Mastering an approach or routine helps the doctor remain calm and provide useful information as well as support.
- Respect for patients requires that the physician first establish rapport and negotiate the ground rules for information exchange. Only then can the physician provide the knowledge necessary for a person to take an active role in deciding what course of action best meets his or her needs. This task is crucial for procuring meaningful consent for treatment.
- Patients experience receiving bad news as a process that takes place over time instead of a single encounter. It takes time to integrate the information. When news is grim it may be helpful to remember that compassion and engagement are therapeutic tools in their own right.

References

1. Ptacek JT, Eberhardt TL. Breaking bad news, a review of the literature. JAMA 1996; 276:496.
2. Delvecchio Good MJ. The practice of biomedicine and the discourse on hope. Anthropologies of Medicine 1991; 7:121.
3. Delvecchio Good MJ, Good BJ, Schaffer C, Lind S. American oncology and the discourse on hope. Cult Med Psychiatry 1990; 14:59.
4. Fried TR, Bradley EH, Towle VR, et al. Understanding the treatment preferences of seriously ill patients. N Engl J Med 2002; 346:1061.
5. Miyaji, NT. The power of compassion: truth-telling among American doctors in the care of dying patients. Soc Sci Med 1993; 36:249.
6. Surbone A, Zwitter M. Communication with the cancer patient. Information and truth. Ann N Y Acad Sci 1997; 809:421.
7. Surbone A. The quandary of cultural diversity guest editorial. J Palliat Care 2003; 19:3.
8. Surbone A. Persisting differences in truth-telling throughout the world. Supportive Care in Cancer 2004; 12:143.
9. Christakis NA. Death Foretold. Chicago: University of Chicago Press, 1999:87.
10. Salander P. Bad news from the patient's perspective: an analysis of the written narratives of newly diagnosed cancer patients. Soc Sci Med 2002; 55:721.
11. Fraisse P. Breaking bad news by the respiratory physician: a therapeutic process. Rev Mal Respir 2004; 21:75.
12. Broyard A. Intoxicated by My Illness and Other Writings on Life and Death. New York: Fawcett Columbine, 1992:26.

13. Fallowfield L, Ford S, Lewis S. No news is good news: information preferences of patients with cancer. Psychoongcology 1995; 4:197.
14. Butow P, Kazemi J, Beeney L, Friffin A, Dunn S, Tattersall M. When the diagnosis is cancer: patient communication experiences and preferences. Cancer 1996; 77:2630.
15. Butow P, Maclean M, Dunn SM, Tattersall MH, Boyer MJ. The dynamics of change: cancer patients' preferences for information, involvement and support. Ann Oncol 1997; 8:857.
16. Tattersall MH. Consultation audio-tapes: an information aid, and a quality assurance and research tool. Support Care Cancer 2002; 10:217.
17. Gattellari M, Butow PN, Tattershall MH. Sharing decisions in cancer care. Soc Sci Med 2001; 52:1865.
18. Spiegel DA. A 43-year old woman coping with cancer. JAMA 1999; 282:371.
19. Chapman K, Abraham C, Jenkins V, Fallowfield L. Lay understanding of terms used in cancer consultations. Psychooncology 2003; 12:557.
20. Roter DL, Hall JA. Doctors Talking with Patients, Patients Talking with Doctors. Improving Communication in Medical Visits. Westport, CT: Auburn House, 1992.
21. Fallowfield L, Jenkins V. Communicating sad, bad, and difficult news in medicine. Lancet 2004; 363:312.
22. Meier DE, Back AL, Morrison S. The inner life of physicians and care of the seriously ill. JAMA 2001; 286:3007.
23. Fallowfield L, Clark AW. Delivering bad news in gastroenterology. Am J Gastroenterol 1994; 89:473.
24. Dunn SM, Patterson PU, Butow PN, Smartt HH, McCarthy WH, Tattershall MH. Cancer by another name: a randomized trial of the effects of euphemisms and uncertainty in communication with cancer patients. J Clin Oncol 1993; 11:989.
25. Penson RT, Schapira L, Daniels KJ, Chabner BA, Lynch TJ. Cancer as metaphor. Oncologist 2004; 9:708.
26. Gordon E, Daugherty CK. Hitting you over the head: oncologists' disclosure of prognosis to advanced cancer patients. Bioethics 2003; 17:142.
27. Fallowfield L. Giving bad and sad news. Lancet 1993; 341:476.
28. Orlander JD, Fincke BG, Hermanns D, Johnston GA. Medical residents' first clearly remembered experiences of giving bad news. J Gen Intern Med 2002; 17:825.
29. Reisfield G, Wilson G. Use of metaphor in the discourse on cancer. J Clin Oncol 2004; 22:4024.
30. Schapira L. Communication corner: one size doesn't fit all. Research Advocacy Network Update. Breast Cancer 1997; 1:12.
31. Baile WF, Beale EA. Giving bad news to cancer patients: matching process and content. J Clin Oncol 2003; 21(9 suppl):49.
32. Baile WF, Buckman R, Lenzi R, Glober G, Beale EA, Kudelka AP. SPIKES – a six step protocol for delivering bad news: applications to the patient with cancer. Oncologist 2000; 5:302.
33. Baile WF, Lenzi R, Kudelka AP, et al. Improving physician–patient communication in cancer care: outcome of a workshop for oncologists. J Cancer Educ 1997; 12:166.

Section X:
Social Issues in the Management of Lung Cancer

Chemoprevention of Lung Cancer

53

Victor Cohen and Fadlo R. Khuri

Contents

53.1 Introduction

Lung cancer is one of the most common malignancies and is the leading cause of cancer mortality in the Western World. In the USA, the disease has been the leading cause of cancer deaths in men for years, and since 1988 it has also become the number one cause of cancer death in women. It is estimated that in the year 2005, approximately 172,570 people will be diagnosed with lung cancer and 163,510 will die of the disease, surpassing the combined death rates from breast, prostate, and colon cancers [1].

In addition to being the biggest cancer killer, lung cancer is one of the few cancers with a well defined etiology, namely, the inhalation of tobacco smoke. Cigarette smoking is estimated to be responsible for approximately 87% of lung cancer cases, and evidence for this link is indisputable [2]. Estimates of the relative risk of disease in the long-term smoker vary from 10- to 30-fold. The cumulative lung cancer risk among heavy smokers may be as high as 30% compared with a lifetime risk of 1% or less in non-smokers [3, 4]. The

risk of carcinoma increases with the number of cigarettes smoked, years of smoking, earlier age of onset, degree of inhalation, tar and nicotine content, and use of unfiltered cigarettes. Other risk factors for lung cancer include exposure to asbestos, haloethers, polycyclic aromatic hydrocarbons, nickel, arsenic, genetic factors, and the presence of underlying benign forms of parenchymal lung disease, especially pulmonary fibrosis. Recent interest has focused on the potential roles of exposure to environmental tobacco smoke (passive exposure to second-hand smoke) and to radon.

Two major subdivisions are recognized: non-small cell lung cancer (NSCLC) and small cell lung cancer (SCLC). This is due to the major clinical differences in presentation, metastatic spread, and response to therapy. SCLC accounts for 15–25% of all lung cancers and although the disease is sensitive to both chemotherapy and radiotherapy, the duration of response is usually short-lived. The majority of patients of SCLC patients die from progressive disease [5–8].

Non-small cell lung cancer accounts for the remaining cases and composes a heterogeneous aggregate of at least three histological subtypes including adenocarcinoma, squamous cell carcinoma, and large cell carcinoma [9]. About 30% of patients with NSCLC present with stage I and II disease. Surgery is currently the treatment of choice for these patients and represents the best chance of a cure. Despite apparent complete resection, however, patients with pathologic stage Ia disease have an 80% survival rate after resection, whereas 5-year survival rates are 60% in those with stage Ib disease and 40–50% in those with stage IIa/IIb disease [10].

A further 25–30% of patients have locally advanced or stage IIIa and IIIb disease at presentation. While multimodality therapy is routinely recommended for this patient group, its exact nature and sequence remain controversial. In the past, radiation therapy was considered standard of care, however long-term survival with this approach was poor, in the range of 5–10%, with poor local control and early development of distant metastatic disease. Recent studies indicate that the addition of chemotherapy improves survival in these patients, however the magnitude of improvement is small [11–15].

The outcome for patients with stage IV disease is particularly bleak. Systemic chemotherapy has been used in an attempt to prolong symptom-free survival. Treatment with modern cisplatin-containing regimens improves median survival by a modest 6–12 weeks and 1-year survival from 5% to 15% with best supportive care alone to 30–40% in treated patients [16]. Therefore, despite improvements in diagnostic imaging, surgery, radiotherapy, and chemotherapy, the overall survival for NSCLC remains poor with only about 14% of patients surviving 5 years from the date of diagnosis. Furthermore, it appears unlikely that additional marked improvements with these practices alone will occur in the near future. This grim overview argues powerfully for new, emerging approaches such as biologic or molecularly targeted therapy and chemoprevention for controlling lung cancer.

53.2 Chemoprevention

Dr. Michael Sporn is widely credited with launching the modern era of cancer chemoprevention and prevention research. He was the first to put forward the notion that the goals and objectives of clinical efforts in the treatment of some types of cancers should be the process rather than the state of carcinogenesis. He intensely promoted the concept of treatment of precancerous conditions and coined the term *chemoprevention* to describe "the use of specific natural or synthetic chemical agents to reverse, suppress or prevent carcinogenic progression to invasive cancer" [17, 18]. Although at first regarded with skepticism, this approach has led to significant advances in cancer prevention. Clinical validation for the cancer prevention concept was provided by a randomized trial using the selective estrogen receptor modulator tamoxifen in women who are at high risk for breast cancer development based on age, lobar carcinoma in situ, or the Gail model [19]. In women who received tamoxifen, there was a highly statistically significant reduction in the risk of both invasive and non-invasive breast cancers. Studies in colon and head and neck cancers have provided further proof of principle for the concept of chemoprevention as a serious and practical approach to the control of cancer in humans [20–22].

This article will focus on several issues related to lung cancer chemoprevention including current and new chemopreventive agents and endpoint biomarkers. Also, the results of completed clinical chemoprevention trials are reviewed.

53.3 Lung Cancer Biology and Chemopreventive Approaches

Primary carcinoma of the lung appears to develop from a pluripotent stem cell involved in the generation of the bronchial epithelium and capable of differentiation along several pathways [6]. The biology of this process is based on two themes: *field cancerization* and *multistep carcinogenesis* [23–25]. Field carcinogenesis denotes diffuse epithelial injury resulting from carcinogenic (e.g., tobacco smoke) exposure in an entire epithelial field or region, setting off a chronic pattern of tissue damage and wound healing where changes can be detected at the gross, microscopic, and molecular levels [26]. The clinical importance of this phenomenon is best illustrated in aerodigestive cancers for which both synchronous and metachronous second primary tumors are common.

Chronic carcinogenic insults sets off a multistep process characterized by the occurrence of initiation, promotion, and progression events occurring over latent periods of a decade or more. These events produce an accumulation of genetic and epigenetic alterations of at least three groups of genes: proto-oncogenes, tumor suppressor genes, and mutator genes resulting in imbalances between cellular proliferation, apoptosis, and shedding. Imbalance in cellular population kinetics promotes a build-up of cells that, if sufficiently abnormal, have malignant capability. Numerous systems including repair, replacement, recruitment, replication, and redundancy mechanisms become operational to help restore structural and functional integrity. In some instances, however, these mechanisms fail or are overwhelmed and unrepaired injury not only occurs but also is propagated, resulting in the triggering of a transformation from normal to premalignant cells and eventually to invasive carcinoma.

The essence of chemoprevention is intervention within the multistep carcinogenic process and throughout the tobacco/carcinogen-damaged field. Using pharmacologic or natural compounds, chemoprevention is meant to interrupt this clonal propagation of aberrant cells by blocking DNA damage, retarding or reversing malignant phenotype, or inducing apoptosis in the damaged cells of premalignant lesions. Chemopreventive approaches can be considered at three different major levels: primary, secondary, and tertiary (Table 53.1). Primary prevention is defined as an intervention intended to delay the development of cancer or hinder its progression. Normal "healthy" individuals represent the population at which primary prevention is directed. Smoking prevention and cessation treatments or the use of chemoprevention drugs in a group of asymptomatic smokers are good examples of this strategy. Secondary chemoprevention is aimed at persons with evidence of early disease, but without well-established can-

Level	Definition	Example
Primary	Diminish risk for normal healthy individuals	Smoking cessation or prevention Chemoprevention in asymptomatic smokers
Secondary	Decrease progression of preneoplasia	Reversal of preneoplasia or biomarkers of preneoplasia with chemoprevention
Tertiary	Decrease morbidity for patients treated or cured of an initial cancer	Chemoprevention of second primary tumors

cer, and tertiary prevention involves decreasing the morbidity of the established disease. Chemoprevention of second primary tumors in patients treated for or cured of an initial malignancy is a good example of tertiary prevention.

53.4 The ABCs of the Lung Cancer Chemopreventive Strategy: Agents, Biomarkers, and Cohorts

53.4.1 Chemopreventive Agents

An important objective of chemoprevention research is the identification and development of active agents that inhibit the development of cancer. Candidate chemoprevention agents must possess a relevant mechanism of action, optimal pharmacokinetics, preclinical efficacy in in vitro and animal models, a favorable cost-to-benefit ratio, and an acceptable toxicity profile. The last two of these criteria are of critical importance because a large number of patients (the majority of whom are both symptom- and disease-free) would need to be treated for an extended period. With these general principles in mind researchers have investigated a number of potentially active agents. A partial list of these agents appears in Table 53.2.

The best-studied agents in human cancer chemoprevention have been the class of drugs known as retinoids. The term *retinoids* generally refers to the entire set of compounds including both naturally occurring and synthetic vitamin A (retinol) metabolites and analogues [18]. Retinoids are physiologic regulators of a large number of essential biologic processes including embryonic development, vision, reproduction, bone formation, metabolism, hematopoiesis, differentiation, and apoptosis [27–30]. Pharmacologically, they have been recognized as modulators of cell growth, differentiation, and apoptosis.

Support for the role of these compounds in cancer prevention derived from results obtained from experimental animal models, epidemiologic studies, and clinical trials. In 1925 Wolbach and Howe first identified vitamin A-dependent pathways essential for epithelial cell homeostasis [31]. They discovered that vitamin A deficiency in animals caused squamous metaplasia in the trachea as well as other epithelial sites and that repletion of the vitamin reversed these histopathologic changes. These changes were similar to those that arose in smokers implicating a function for vitamin A signaling pathways in suppressing carcinogenesis. Further evidence for a link between vitamin A and cancer came from epidemiologic data establishing an inverse relationship between vitamin A levels and lung cancer incidence [32]. These findings led to the conduct of successful clinical studies treating premalignant lesions that include oral leukoplakia, cervical dysplasia, and xeroderma pigmentosum [32]. Other clinical trials revealed retinoid activity in reducing secondary head and neck, lung, and liver cancers [22, 33–35].

Two main types of natural vitamin A exist: the carotenoids such as beta-carotene and the preformed vitamin A usually in the form of retinol, retinal, and retinyl esters.

Carotenoids

The carotenoids constitute a class of over 600 compounds found predominantly in fruits and vegetables. They have been reported to have a number of biologic actions including important antioxidant activity and enhancement of immune function. The mechanisms for these actions, however, are not well characterized [36, 37]. Many of these compounds can quench singlet oxygen through a physical reaction in which the energy of the excited oxygen is transferred to the carotenoid. In addition to singlet oxygen, these compounds are also thought to quench oxygen-free radicals. A well-reported, strong body of work has linked oxygen free radicals to carcinogenesis, thus there is considerable interest in antioxidant compounds and antioxidant activity as a mechanism for cancer prevention [36–39]. It is unclear whether antioxidant activity is responsible for the chemopreventive effects of carotenoids observed, however. For instance, immune enhancement by the various carotenoids could have an important role in tumor inhibition or killing by increasing natural killer cells and activating immunoregulatory lymphocytes essential in host defense [40, 41]. In addition, various carotenoids have been reported to affect various growth regulatory pathways inducing apoptosis of transformed cells in vitro [42, 43]. These and other potential mechanisms described elsewhere suggest that it is biologically plausible that carotenoids may have chemopreventive activity.

Among the carotenoids, beta-carotene has received considerable clinical investigation and was the darling of the lay press for much of the 1980s and 1990s. Currently, its role in cancer chemoprevention remains controversial showing cancer preventive effects in some situations although pharmacologic doses in large clinical trials have shown neutral or sometimes detrimental effects. For example, in the alpha-tocopherol beta-carotene (ATBC) study and the beta-carotene and retinol efficacy trial (CARET), chemopreventive treatment with beta-carotene for primary lung cancer prevention in high-risk individuals did not result in a reduction of lung cancers and appeared harmful in this setting, especially when subjects continued to smoke or to consume ethanol. These results are discussed in detail in the section on randomized chemoprevention trials. Other carotenoids currently being investigated are alpha-carotene, lutein, zeaxanthin, lycopene, beta-cryptoxanthin, fucoxanthin, astaxanthin, capsanthin, crocetin, and phytoene [44].

Lycopene has recently attracted the most attention. This molecule is a naturally occurring hydrocarbon found primarily in tomatoes and their products. It is the one of the more common dietary carotenoids and the most abundant in human serum. The molecule ranks highest among major natural carotenoids in its capacity for quenching singlet oxygen and scavenging free radicals [45]. In addition to its antioxidant actions, biologic activities include growth control and induction of cell–cell communication. Lycopene at physiologic concentrations can inhibit human cancer cell growth by interfering with growth factor receptor signaling and cell cycle progression without evidence of toxic effects or apoptosis of cells [46, 47]. In human fetal skin fibroblasts, lycopene stimulates gap junctional communication [48]. Gap junctional communication is deficient in many tumor types and its restoration or upregulation is associated with decreased proliferation. Animal trials assessing its chemopreventive effects in a multiorgan carcinogenesis model found pulmonary adenoma and carcinoma formation was reduced with lycopene [44]. Additionally, epidemiologic studies measuring dietary intake (primarily tomato products) or serum concentrations have provided evidence, albeit weak, for a protective association with lung cancer [49]. Collectively these works have offered enough data to warrant the further study of lycopene as a potential chemopreventive agent. Before large intervention trials can be justified, however, small human trials will need to be performed to determine if the agent has biologic activity and toxicity.

Retinoids
Retinoids as mentioned already play an important role in homeostatic maintenance of growth, differentiation, and apoptosis of various epithelial tissues. They also play a regulatory role in the activation of cytokines and the extracellular matrix. Most effects of this class of compounds are mediated by the complex interactions

of their cognate nuclear receptors [50]. These receptors belong to the superfamily of receptors that mediate the effects of many compounds, including steroid and thyroid hormones, vitamin D, prostaglandins, and drugs that activate peroxisomal proliferation [51]. There are two major classes of retinoid receptors: nuclear retinoic acid receptors (RAR) and retinoid receptors or RXR each of which comprise alpha, beta, and gamma subtypes with distinct amino- and carboxy-terminal domains as well as several isoforms generated by alternative splicing or promoter use [50, 52–54]. RAR usually forms a heterodimer with RXR. These heterodimers have two signaling modes: they regulate the transcription of target genes upon binding to retinoic acid response elements or RAREs and they affect the signaling capacity of other pathways (crosstalk) by still indefinable mechanisms. In the absence of ligands, or in the presence of antagonists, target genes that can be accessed by the receptor are repressed; DNA bound RAR-RXR heterodimers form multiprotein complexes with co-repressor and histone deacetylases resulting in deacetylation, chromatin compaction, and silencing of target gene promoter regions [55–58]. Agonist binding generates a conformational transition of the ligand-binding domain [59] which disrupts co-repressor binding and enables the interaction of RAR-RXR with histone acetyl transferase-containing complexes inducing derepression of the chromatin. Subsequently, the association of multiprotein complexes comprising thyroid hormone receptor protein (TRAP), vitamin D_3 receptor-interacting protein (DRIP), and activated recruiter cofactor (ARC) with RAR-RXR enables the recruitment of basal transcription machinery to the promoter and the activation of various genetic programs [57, 58].

In contrast to RAR, RXR are promiscuous in that they can form heterodimers with different partners including thyroid hormone receptors, vitamin D receptors, peroxisomal proliferators-activator receptors, and a number of orphan receptors such as LXR, PXR, and FXR suggesting that RXR ligands (rexinoids) modulate or affect multiple signal transduction pathways [52, 60–63]. One of these ligands, the RXR agonist LGD1069-Bexarotene (Targretin), was shown to effectively prevent the formation and progression of N-nitroso-N-methylurea (NMU)-induced rat mammary carcinomas. These effects were also observed in tamoxifen-refractory breast tumors of the NMU rat model and in mammary carcinogenesis of C3(1)-SV40 Tag transgenic mice [64, 65].

To date, most clinical work has involved the natural retinoids/ligands, i.e., 13-*cis*-retinoic acid (13cRA), all-*trans*-retinoic acid or ATRA, and 9-*cis*-retinoic acid, all having considerable toxicity. These toxicities are similar to that of hypervitaminosis A and include varying severity of anorexia, involuntary weight loss, fever, hepatosplenomegaly, skin and mucous membrane changes, alopecia, cheilitis (cracking and bleeding lips), bone and joint pain, hyperostosis, thrombocytopenia, elevated cerebral fluid pressure, and "night blindness" or impaired visual adaptation to darkness. The latter appears to be asymptomatic in a significant percentage of patients, is often reversible, and can be minimized or averted by allowing drug-free intervals [66, 67]. Some of these toxicities can occasionally be ameliorated by the concomitant use of alpha-tocopherol without any loss of retinoid activity [68, 69] A study by Besa et al. in transfusion-dependent patients with myelodysplastic syndrome reported that alpha-tocopherol significantly reduced the severe skin and constitutional toxicities observed with 13cRA therapy, allowing long-term treatment with the retinoid [69].

Because the natural retinoic acids are pan-agonists or non-selective, there is intense interest in developing synthetic retinoid ligands with greater selectivity than that of the natural ligands. Selective retinoids are designed to increase the therapeutic index by, for example, "dialing out" specific adverse effects. Efforts have concentrated on the development of receptor-selective and function-selective retinoids through molecular targeting strategies and structure–activity relationship studies based upon binding and transactivation assays. Many structurally diverse synthetic ligands have been developed. Selected examples of synthetic ligands in or near clinical testing include AM580, AM80, AGN193836, BMS185411, SR11254, CD666, CD437, SR11237, and LGD100268. Retinoid drug development is proceeding along several other novel avenues. For example, new retinoid-regulated genes (e.g., RARE identified in HoxA-1 and Stat1 promoters) are being identified as potential downstream molecular drug targets [70]. Other avenues include identification of orphan-receptor ligands and functions, elucidation of the mechanism of novel retinoids with potent receptor-independent apoptosis-inducing activity (e.g., 4-HPR or anhydroretinol), synergistic combinations, and novel retinoid delivery systems (liposomal and aerosolized) [71–73].

COX-2 Inhibitors

Cyclooxygenase-2 (COX-2) is the inducible isoform of cyclooxygenase. This enzyme catalyzes the rate-limiting step in prostaglandin synthesis from arachidonic acid. Various prostaglandins are produced in a cell-type-specific manner and they elicit cellular functions via signaling through G protein-coupled membrane receptors and in some cases through the nuclear receptor PPAR. COX-2 utilization of arachidonic acid also alters the level of intracellular free arachidonic acid and subsequently affects cellular functions. Several lines of evidence have provided a rationale for targeting the COX-2 pathway in lung cancer prevention. Preclinical studies indicated that COX-2 overexpression suppressed antitumor immunity, inhibited apoptosis, and increased angiogenesis [74–78]. COX-2 regulated synthesis of pros-

taglandins that promoted tumorigenesis and COX-2 inhibition reduced 4-(methylnitrosamino)-1-(3-pyridyl)-1-butanone (NNK)-mediated lung adenomas in the A/J mouse [79, 80]. Differential overexpression of COX-2 was reported in bronchial premalignancy, lung adenocarcinoma, and squamous carcinoma compared to normal lung tissues and this portended a poorer survival in early-stage disease [81–84]. Epidemiologic evidence also was consistent with a role for COX-2 inhibition in lung cancer therapy or prevention [85, 86].

A number of COX-2 inhibitors are now commercially available and others are currently being researched. One of the first agents to be heavily marketed as a COX-2 selective inhibitor was Celecoxib (Celebrex). A subsequent agent was rofecoxib (Vioxx) produced by Merck Sharp & Dohme. Vioxx was recently withdrawn from the market because of its cardiovascular toxicity and all ongoing and planned studies with this drug have now been cancelled. The "Vioxx story" has now prompted serious efforts to determine whether the cardiovascular and procoagulant effects of Vioxx are a class effect applicable to all COX-2 inhibitors, and, if so, how selective the COX-2 inhibition needs to be to have this adverse effect. Cardiovascular expertise was recently added to the safety monitoring committees for clinical trials including chemoprevention trials testing all COX-2 inhibitors. Data from these trials are being intensely scrutinized for similar problems to assure long-term patient safety. On December 17, 2004, the National Institutes of Health announced that it had suspended the use of Celebrex for all participants in a large colorectal cancer prevention clinical trial conducted by the National Cancer Institute (NCI). The study, called the Adenoma Prevention with Celexocib (APC) trial, was stopped because analysis by an independent Data Safety and Monitoring Board showed a 2.5-fold increased risk of major fatal and non-fatal cardiovascular events for participants taking the drug compared to those on a placebo. In light of these new findings, the NIH has now requested a full review of all NIH-supported studies involving this class of drug.

Epidermal Growth Factor Receptor and Farnesyltransferase Inhibitors

More recently, molecularly targeted agents have been developed as a result of the growing body of knowledge in lung tumor development and biology. Although these agents are currently being tested for their potency in cancer chemotherapy for established malignancies, importantly, they may also be potentially applicable to chemoprevention if their toxicity can be minimized. Examples of such molecules include the farnesyltransferase inhibitors (FTIs) and the epidermal growth factor receptor small molecule tyrosine kinase inhibitors.

The FTIs are among the first wave of signal transduction inhibitors to be tested for antitumor properties.

They were initially designed to attack Ras oncoproteins, the function of which depends upon posttranslational modification by farnesyl isoprenoid [87]. Additional evidence describes the alteration of prenylation and function of additional cellular proteins as a mechanism of action, independently of the presence of the activating Ras oncogene [88]. Extensive preclinical studies have demonstrated that FTIs compromise neoplastic transformation and tumor growth [87]. In preclinical models, FTIs display limited effects on normal cell physiology and in early phase human trials have been largely well-tolerated with very few side effects [87, 89]. Dose-limiting toxicities in these studies included myelosuppression, diarrhea, nausea and vomiting, fatigue, reversible renal dysfunction, and peripheral neuropathy. The scientific reasons for considering FTIs in premalignant lesions was strengthened by work carried out by various investigators demonstrating the existence of K-ras mutations in premalignant lesions of the lung. Perhaps the most compelling descriptions are those of K-ras oncogene activation in atypical alveolar hyperplasia and lung adenocarcinoma [90]. Also, FTIs have been shown to prevent the development of lung tumors in mouse carcinogenesis models. Lantry et al. tested the efficacy of FTI-276 on established lung adenomas, considered to be a premalignant lesion of the lung in A/J mice that were induced by NNK [91]. Analysis of the tumors showed a 60% reduction in tumor multiplicity and a 42% reduction in tumor incidence as well as a significant reduction in tumor volume. Mutational analysis of the lung tumors from both treatment groups revealed that most of the tumors harbored mutations in codon-12 of K-ras and that there were no significant differences in the incidence and types of mutations between tumors from the treated and control animals. This was a demonstration not only of the therapeutic efficacy of an FTI in a primary lung tumor model but also a possible model for the reversal of premalignant disease in this setting.

Epidermal growth factor receptor (EGFR) tyrosine kinase inhibitors are orally active agents that target EFGR, a transmembrane protein involved in the regulation of a complex array of essential biologic events. Overexpression and dysregulation of the EGFR signaling network has been frequently reported in multiple human cancers including NSCLC and has been associated with the processes of tumor development, growth, proliferation, metastasis, and angiogenesis [92, 93]. Importantly, this has been correlated in many cases with a poor prognosis [94–97]. There is also increasing evidence that EGFR is overexpressed in premalignant lesions including early bronchial neoplasia. Kurie et al. showed that increased EGFR expression was widely demonstrable in metaplastic bronchial epithelium in moderate to early premalignant lesions [98]. In active smokers, EGFR expression was higher in metaplastic biopsies than in normal biopsies. Rusch et al. have shown that aberrant expression of EGFR or p53 is frequently present in early bronchial neoplasia and that their co-expression appears to precede and predict squamous cell carcinoma development [99]. These observations argue powerfully for the full development of therapeutics targeting the EGFR as a chemopreventive strategy to reduce the incidence of lung cancer development (Fig. 53.1) [100].

Currently, at least five EGFR tyrosine kinase inhibitors are undergoing various phases of clinical testing; ZD1839-gefitinib (Iressa; AstraZeneca, Wilmington, DE), OSI-774-erlotinib (Tarceva; Genetech, South San Francisco, CA), PD-153053, PD-168393, and CI-1033. Of these gefitinib is the furthest along in clinical development. Preclinically, this agent has shown activity against a wide variety of EGFR-overexpressing human cancer cell lines and xenografts. Subsequent single-agent human studies and trials in combination with chemotherapy have shown tumor growth inhibition in a substantial number of patients with a wide variety of different solid tumors including lung cancer. In May 2003, the US Food and Drug Administration approved gefitinib for the treatment of patients with advanced NSCLC previously treated with chemotherapy. The FDA approval was based upon data from phase II trials showing improved disease-related symptoms and radiographic tumor regressions in patients receiving gefitinib following failure of both platinum-based and docetaxel chemotherapies [101]. When used at a dosage of 250 mg per day, the drug has been shown to be generally well tolerated. Most of its side effects are mild consisting mainly of diarrhea and skin rash and unusual or unexpected adverse events are rare. One such rare event is lung toxicity in the form of interstitial lung disease (ILD). Analysis in over 92,000 patients worldwide who had received gefitinib has shown that the incidence of ILD-type events to be less than 1% [102].

At the time of approval of gefitinib, there was little understanding of the predictive markers of drug activity. Retrospective analyses of patients showed that responses were more frequent among patients who had never smoked, women, and patients with bronchoalveolar carcinoma or adenocarcinoma with bronchoalveolar features. However, there was no correlation between the intensity of the immunohistochemical staining of the tumor for EGFR and the presence and absence of a response, and no obvious candidate biomarker to select patients for treatment with gefitinib. The first reports of a predictive marker for drug sensitivity have recently been published. Two seminal studies by Lynch et al. and Paez et al. have described somatic mutations in the EGFR gene in patients with NSCLC who experienced striking responses to gefitinib [103, 104]. The frequencies of these EGFR mutations as well as their biologic and clinical consequences await clarification. Mutations have also been identified in patients experiencing responses to erlotinib, another targeted small molecule

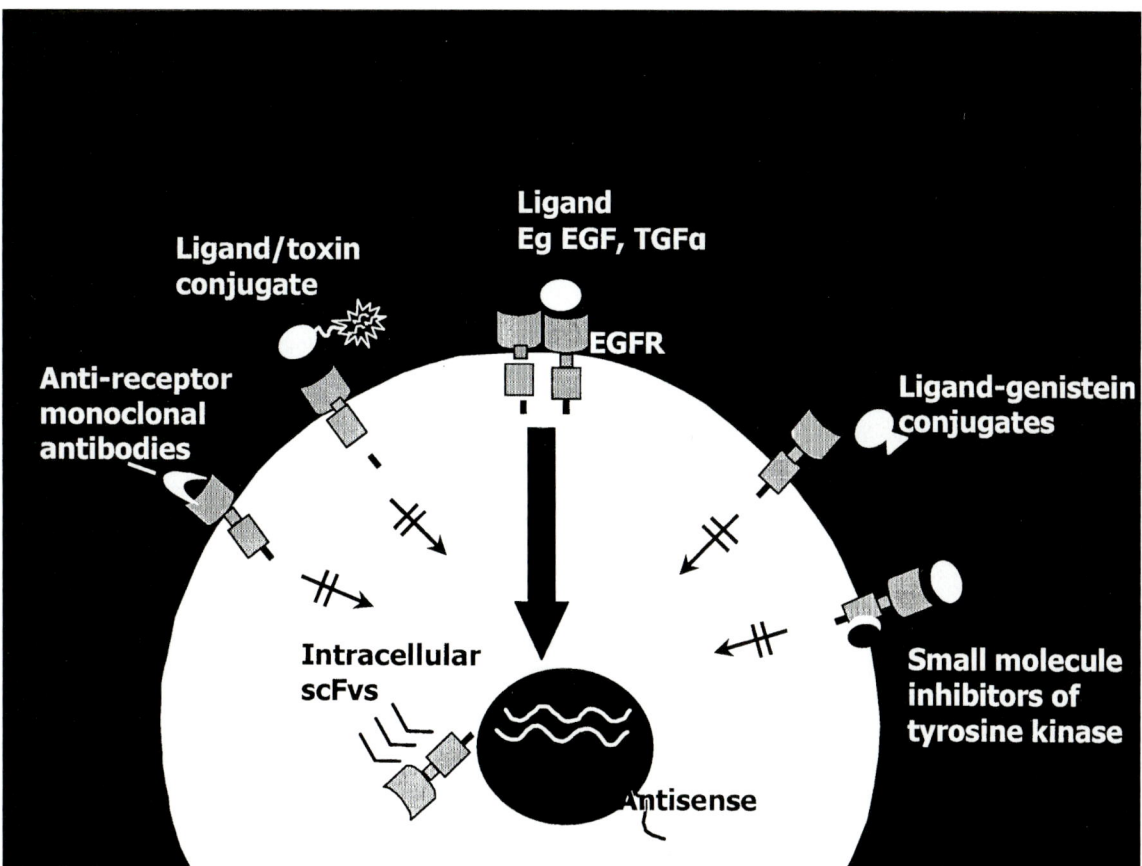

Fig. 53.1. A simplified schematic representation of the EGFR signaling pathway and selected examples of strategies for EGFR inhibition. *EGF* Epidermal growth factor, *EGFR* epidermal growth factor receptor, *scF vs* single-chain antibody

inhibitor of EGFR in late-stage clinical trials recently approved for the treatment of patients with locally advanced or metastatic NSCLC after failure of at least one prior chemotherapy regimen [105].

In the USA, the Lung Cancer Biomarkers Chemoprevention Consortium was, until recently, preparing to conduct two novel projects called *SPORE* (Specialized Programs of Research Excellence) *Trials of Lung Cancer Prevention*, or STOP. The trials were randomized phase IIb studies designed to evaluate the effects of tipifarnib, a farnesyltransferase inhibitor (STOP-FTI) and gefitinib (STOP-TKI) in former and current smokers with a previous specified smoking-related cancer. Patient eligibility requirements and trial conduct were identical in the two studies and borrowing of control groups was to be employed to minimize overall sample size. The major objectives were to evaluate the effectiveness of these compounds in the response of histology and modulation of the Ki-67-labeling index and to assess intermediate serologic and tissue markers as preliminary predictors for efficacy. The FTI study because of safety reasons has been permanently halted. The gefitinib study also for safety reasons has been indefinitely side-lined and very likely will not receive the necessary regulatory approval to proceed.

Peroxisome Proliferator-activator Receptor Agonists

The peroxisome proliferator-activator receptors (PPARs) belong to the nuclear receptor superfamily that includes nuclear hormone receptors and orphan nuclear receptors [106]. Three isoforms have been identified so far; PPAR-α, PPAR-δ/β also known as Nuc 1, and PPAR-γ [107]. PPARs bind to RXR and the resulting dimeric transcription factor binds to peroxisome proliferator response elements (PPREs) in the promoters of PPAR-regulated genes [108]. The resulting PPAR-RXR-PPRE complex elicits expression of targeted genes. Many PPAR-regulated genes are involved in controlling lipid metabolism, insulin signaling, adipocyte differentiation, and apoptosis [109, 110].

Perhaps the most widely studied form of PPAR is PPAR-γ. In humans, PPAR-γ is expressed in multiple tissues including the breast, colon, lung, ovary, and placenta [111–113]. Several ligands have been described for this receptor including the synthetic thiazolidinedione class of agents, such as troglitazone, rosiglitazone, and pioglitazone currently approved for the treatment of hyperglycemia and certain non-steroidal antiinflammatory drugs. Additionally, a number of natural ligands for PPAR-γ have been identified, including the prostanoids, prostaglandin D_2, 15-deoxy-Δ12,14-prostaglandin J_2, and certain polyunsaturated fatty acids [109]. Whether these natural ligands regulate PPAR-γ in vivo is yet to be determined. Few studies have examined the efficacy of these agonists in animal models of tumorigenesis and their mechanisms of action are still not clear. Recent data from Keshamouni et al. demonstrate that activation of PPAR-γ impedes lung tumor progression and suggest that PPAR-γ ligands may serve as potential therapeutic agents in NSCLC [114]. Studies in other tumor types including breast cancer suggest that these ligands may also be useful cancer-preventive agents as well [115].

Cell Cycle Inhibitors

Cell cycle progression leading to cell division and proliferation is strictly controlled by the timed expression of various cyclins that associate with specific cyclin-dependent kinases (CDKs). For example, passage through the G1 phase of the cell cycle is regulated by cyclin D1 and CDK4/6. Inappropriate expression or activity has been found in lung cancer and it has been suggested that the expression of these proteins may be a marker of early carcinogenesis. Immunohistochemical studies have revealed that cyclin deregulation is frequently detected in bronchial preneoplasia. Lonardo et al. studied cyclin expression in a series of bronchial biopsies and found that cyclin D1 was detected in 7% with squamous metaplasia, 15% with atypia, 18% with low-grade dysplasia, and 47% with high-grade dysplasia [116]. These findings indicated that altered cyclin expression could play a critical role in the maintenance or progression of a preneoplastic bronchial lesion. Furthermore, these findings implicated these species as chemopreventive targets. This has been confirmed by analysis of bronchial epithelial cellular models, carcinogen-induced lung tumors in animal models, as well as examination of cyclin D1 expression in tissues harvested during the course of a retinoid clinical trial [117–119]. Selective cyclin D1 inhibitors such as the indolocarbazoles have recently been identified and preclinical studies indicate potent inhibitory properties and antiproliferative activity against several human cancer cell lines [120]. Clinical data about the safety and tolerance of these agents must be available before these drugs can be used in chemoprevention studies.

Demethylating Agents

DNA methylation as an epigenetic abnormality plays an important role in gene expression in many types of cancers [121]. In lung cancer, several genes have been reported to be frequently methylated including the p16 gene and RAR-beta gene located at 3p24. Since epigenetic changes are potentially reversible, demethylating agents have been proposed as potential chemopreventive agents. One such drug is 5-aza-2-deoxycytidine (5-aza-CdR), a potent inhibitor of DNA methylation and an inducer of cellular differentiation. Recent studies have demonstrated that genes that have been silenced by methylation can be re-expressed after treatment with 5-aza-CdR in vitro [122–125]. Although it is too early to make any conclusions about the effect and possible side effects of these drugs in lung cancer patients, this is a very promising concept that needs to be tested in clinical trials with monitoring of methylated markers.

Other Agents

Other candidate agents include soy isoflavones, green tea polyphenols, low-calcemic vitamin D analogues, triterpenoids, alpha-difluoromethylornithine and other inhibitors of polyamine biosynthesis, monoterpenes, lipoxygenase modulators, protein kinase C inhibitors, matrix metalloproteinase inhibitors, histone deacetylase inhibitors, and demethylating agents. Gene-based interventions (p53 adenovirus) are also being explored in the future chemoprevention of lung cancer.

53.4.2 Biomarkers

Surrogate endpoint biomarkers (SEBs) are used as intermediate indicators of cancer incidence reduction in chemoprevention studies. This intermediate biomarker concept is used as well in the management of other diseases. For example, cholesterol quantification is used to indicate the progression of atherosclerosis as a surrogate in determining the risk of myocardial infarction. Although there are currently no validated SEBs for lung cancer, criteria for the discovery and validation of surrogates have been proposed. These are outlined by Kelloff et al. [126–129]: the SEB must be expressed differentially in normal and high-risk tissue; the marker should appear at a well-defined stage of carcinogenesis; the marker and its assay must provide acceptable sensitivity, specificity, and accuracy; the marker should be easily measured; the marker should be modulated by chemopreventive agents; and finally modulation of the SEB should correlate with a decrease in the cancer incidence rate.

Potential markers include morphologic changes of the bronchial epithelium, as well as cytogenetic and molecular changes. Research is focusing on intraepithelial neoplasia (IEN), a premalignant condition exemplified by colorectal adenomas or cervical intraepithelial neoplasia. One specific example is bronchial dysplasia.

Importantly, morphologic criteria for this tissue marker have been defined in the recent World Health Organization classification. This classification of bronchial preneoplastic changes has been found to be highly reproducible by a panel of lung cancer pathologists. However, more data are needed to determine the prognostic implications of the different levels of epithelial changes in the bronchi of high-risk individuals and sparse data are available for the natural course of the different levels of bronchial dysplastic changes.

Biochemical or molecular markers are also being evaluated as SEBs. These include markers such as RAR-beta and other retinoid receptors, proliferating cell nuclear antigen (PCNA), Ki-67, TGF-beta, and EGFR. Genomic instability markers may be the most important biologic markers of all, possibly reflecting the sum of the changes in all other categories. DNA abnormalities (DNA hypomethylation, LOH, point mutations, gene amplification) and chromosome aberrations including chromosomal polysomy and deletions at 3p, 5q, 9p, 11q, 13q, and 17p have been proposed as promising markers for lung cancer trials. Because of the complexity and multifaceted nature of carcinogenesis, it is unlikely that any one of these markers alone will be able to encapsulate all the information necessary to be a viable endpoint. Rather a panel of markers probably will be required to gather sufficient information to assess the effects of preventive agents and perhaps one day to function as a valid endpoint for cancer prevention trials.

Validation of these markers that predict for clinical benefit or risk reduction in randomized controlled trials will be critical to the progress of lung cancer chemoprevention. It is important to recognize though that this may not be readily achievable. The identification and establishment of a biomarker as surrogate for cancer represents a very complex task necessitating multidisciplinary collaboration between epidemiologists, basic scientists, clinicians, and industry. The NCI has recently formed the Early Detection Research Network to facilitate this process and this group has suggested that the process may be divided into five phases analogous to the clinical trial structure used in testing new drugs [130, 131]. Such a structure also helps in the evaluation of published biomarker studies. Detailed discussions of some of these issues together with the statistical considerations involved in the process of marker validation have been published elsewhere [132, 133]. If successful, SEBs will offer several potential benefits in the conduct of lung cancer prevention trials, including shorter latency and hence shorter trials, reductions in size and cost of trials, and the opportunity to study prevention measures where previous studies have been excessively invasive or unethical.

53.4.3 Cohorts

Not all persons who are exposed to cigarette smoke and other potentially carcinogenic environmental influences develop lung cancer. The evaluation of predisposing factors for the disease – mainly by ecologic or case-control studies, prospective population-based research, and familial aggregation studies – has produced little success in identifying the characteristics that single out individuals who possess the highest smoking-related risk. This is regrettable since the ability to identify smokers with the highest risks of developing cancer has substantial implications for the success of chemopreventive interventions. During recent years, intensive research has focused on accurate quantitative risk estimation for lung cancer using multivariable risk models and the molecular epidemiology approach. Multivariate models allow determination of an individual's composite relative risk for lung cancer as well as this person's cumulative lifetime risk adjusted simultaneously for all risk factors and for other causes of mortality. One such model recently proposed by investigators at the Memorial Sloan-Kettering Cancer Center was derived using data from a large, multicenter, randomized, controlled trial of lung cancer prevention in which there was regular ascertainment of lung cancer risk factors, meticulous follow-up, and validation of outcomes [134]. Model inputs included the subject's age, sex, asbestos exposure history, and smoking history. To the extent that this model can differentiate individuals of different risks, it may at some point serve as a useful adjunct to both researchers and patients, paralleling the Gail model, a risk prediction model for breast cancer, and its successful employment in the NASBP-P1 phase III breast cancer chemoprevention trial [19]. Molecular epidemiology integrates advances in molecular biology and cancer genetics to allow among other things the incorporation of genetic susceptibility measures into the quantitative risk assessment process. A major topic of interest in this area has been the study of smoking-related risk factors based on the interactions between tobacco carcinogens, genetic polymorphisms, which are involved in activating and detoxifying these carcinogens, and host-cell efficiency in monitoring and repairing tobacco carcinogen-DNA damage [135, 136].

53.5 Randomized Chemoprevention Trials in Lung Cancer

53.5.1 Primary Chemoprevention

There have been two completed large NCI-sponsored chemoprevention trials with lung cancer as a primary endpoint. The alpha-tocopherol beta-carotene (ATBC) cancer prevention study used a 2×2 factorial design to test alpha-tocopherol and beta-carotene in 29,133 Finnish chronic male smokers aged 50–69 years [137]. Subjects were randomized to one of four groups: alpha-tocopherol 50 mg/day alone, beta-carotene 20 mg/day alone, both alpha-tocopherol and beta-carotene at the above dosages, or placebo, and were followed for 5–8 years. Subjects receiving beta-carotene either alone or in combination with alpha-tocopherol had an 18% increase in the incidence of lung cancer (relative risk [RR] = 1.18; 95% confidence interval [CI] 1.03–1.36; $p = 0.01$) and an 8% increase in total mortality ($p = 0.08$).

The beta-carotene and retinol efficacy trial (CARET) confirmed the results of the Finnish trial [138]. This randomized, double-blinded, placebo-controlled trial tested the combination of 30 mg beta-carotene and 25,000 IU retinyl palmitate against placebo in 18,314 men and women aged 50–69 years at high risk for lung cancer development. Fourteen thousand two hundred and fifty-four individuals had at least a 20-pack-year smoking history and were either current or former smokers. Four thousand and sixty men had extensive occupational exposure to asbestos. This trial was stopped after 21 months because no benefit and possible harm was seen. Lung cancer incidence increased by 28% in the active intervention group (RR = 1.28; 95% CI 1.04–1.57; $p = 0.02$). Overall mortality also increased 17% in this group ($p = 0.02$).

The results of these two trials were in sharp contrast with prior epidemiologic data (showing beta-carotene to be inversely related to the risk of lung cancer) emphasizing the importance of carefully controlled intervention trials to confirm epidemiologic studies and in determining the role of dietary supplements or any intervention agent [139–142]. A recent review by Peter Greenwald of the issues surrounding the ATBC and CARET studies mentions several possible reasons for the discrepancy including concerns over beta-carotene dosing, the possibility that beta-carotene might inhibit the absorption of other nutrients, and queries over the duration of the studies [143]. Dosage of beta-carotene used in the trials was 5–10 times the normal dietary intake resulting in higher serum concentrations than those reported in observational studies. At these higher doses, it was proposed, beta-carotene would inhibit the absorption of other dietary carotenoids or antioxidants with cancer protective properties, although this premise was later questioned. Regarding study duration, active treatment occurred for an average of 6 years in the ATBC study and 4 years in the CARET study. It has been suggested that lag-to-effect and occurrence of events may take considerably longer raising the possibility that the trials underestimated the maximum achievable effects of treatment.

Additionally, since there is now proof that exposure to tobacco has a direct biochemical effect on serum lev-

els of beta-carotene [144] and because as mentioned earlier smoking causes the large majority of lung cancer cases, an explanation has been put forward that the observed association between serum beta-carotene and lung cancer was largely the result of residual confounding with imperfectly reported tobacco exposure – specifically that levels of beta-carotene simply served as a biomarker for true smoking level producing false-positive results [145]. This explanation of course is based on the assumption that a poor correlation existed in the studies between self-reported smoking and biologically relevant tobacco exposure.

The findings of an adverse interaction of cigarette smoke and beta-carotene also raised the suspicion that beta-carotene may even possess co-carcinogenic properties. Recent preclinical studies are beginning to provide biologic plausibility for this theory. Beta-carotene has been found to be an antigenotoxic agent in several in vitro studies [146,147]. Animals given high doses of beta-carotene were found to have significantly increased levels of carcinogen-metabolizing enzymes in their lungs associated with the generation of oxidative stress [148]. The molecule has also been described as an enhancer of cell transferring activity of carcinogens (e.g., benzo(a)pyrene) and cigarette smoke condensate on BALB/c 3T3 cells, inducing p53-dependent enzymes and oxygen-centered radical formation [149]. It has also been shown that beta-carotene oxidation products and oxygen reactive species generated by beta-carotene prooxidant activity can covert benzo(a)pyrene to mutagenic forms [150].

However, it is worth noting that the above findings showing harmful effects of beta-carotene were by no means universal. The Physicians Health Study, a randomized double-blind placebo-controlled trial studied 22,071 healthy male physicians and randomized them to either 15 mg beta-carotene on alternate days versus placebo [151]. Only 11% of participants were current smokers and 39% were former smokers at study entry. The use of supplemental beta-carotene showed no adverse or beneficial effects on cancer incidence or overall mortality during a 12-year follow-up.

53.5.2 Secondary Chemoprevention

Several lung chemoprevention trials used progressive histologic changes in the bronchial epithelium as a study endpoint. A total of five randomized trials have been conducted (Table 53.2). Collectively these results demonstrated that retinoids added no significant benefit to the effects of smoking cessation in the reversal of squamous metaplasia or dysplasia [152–156]. One study showed improvement of sputum atypia in smokers with folate and vitamin B_{12} supplements [156]. This result is questionable, however, because of the small sample size,

Table 53.2. Completed secondary chemoprevention trials in lung cancer

	Intervention	Endpoint	Outcome
Lee et al. [152]	Isotretinoin	Metaplasia	Negative
Kurie et al. [153]	Fenretinide	Metaplasia	Negative
Arnold et al. [154]	Etretinate	Metaplasia	Negative
McLarty et al. [155]	Beta-carotene Retinol	Sputum atypia	Negative
Heimburger et al. [156]	Vitamin B_{12} Folic acid	Sputum atypia	Negative
Kurie et al. [158]	9-cis-Retinoic acid	Retinoic acid receptor-beta	Positive
Lam et al. [160]	Anethole dithiolethione	Dysplasia	Positive

substantial spontaneous and interobserver variability in atypia assessments, and complex and non-standard statistical analytical methods. A reanalysis of these data using standard analytical methods found no significant difference between the two groups [157].

Among recent studies targeting reversal of premalignancy, one trial randomized former smokers to 13-cis-retinoic acid plus alpha-tocopherol versus 9-cis-retinoid acid, a pan-retinoid agonist, versus placebo in an attempt to reverse premalignancy in former smokers with the desired biomarker being the upregulation of RAR-beta (retinoic acid receptor-beta), the loss of which in bronchial epithelium is considered a biomarker of preneoplasia [158]. While 9-cis-retinoic acid was more effective than placebo in upregulating RAR-beta, data implicating maintenance of RAR-beta intratumorally in stage I lung cancers in individuals with a poorer prognosis [159], cast these results in a less than optimal light. A second trial reported by Lam et al. investigated the effects of anethole dithiolethione (ADT) in smokers with bronchial dysplasia [160]. ADT belongs to the dithiolethione class of organosulfur compounds which have antioxidant, chemotherapeutic, radioprotective, and chemopreventive properties. The study concluded that the progression rate of pre-existing dysplastic lesions by two or more grades and/or the appearance of new lesions were statistically significantly lower with treatment. The magnitude of this benefit, while positive, was small.

53.5.3 Tertiary Chemoprevention

Patients diagnosed with a first primary lung cancer have a high incidence of second primary lung tumors (SPT). SPTs must be distinguished from recurrent lesions and are defined as: new cancers separated from the original tumor by 2 cm of normal epithelium, cancers consisting of a different histologic type, or cancers occurring after an interval of more than 5 years from the original tumor. They develop at a rate of 2–5% annually for the first few years following resection of stage I lung cancer. Three definitive phase III studies evaluating retinoids in lung SPT prevention have been completed. The rationale for testing retinoids in this setting came largely from head and neck chemoprevention data showing that these agents significantly reversed oral premalignancy and prevented SPT associated with head and neck cancer [22, 34]. In the first study, the adjuvant effect of high-dose retinyl palmitate (300,000 IU/day) was evaluated in 307 patients with stage I lung cancer, randomly assigned to treatment or placebo after surgery [35]. After median follow-up of 46 months, the number of patients with either recurrence or SPTs was 37% in the treatment arm and 48% in the control arm. Eighteen patients in the treated group developed an SPT and 29 patients in the control group developed 33 SPTs. A statistically significant difference in favor of treatment was observed concerning time to SPT development within the aerodigestive field ($p = 0.045$).

These encouraging results were followed by a European multicenter study, the European Study on Chemoprevention with Vitamin A and N-Acetylcysteine (EUROSCAN) trial, studying the efficacy of chemoprevention following both lung and head and neck cancers [161]. The trial consisted of two parallel trials, one for each organ site and used a 2×2 factorial design to study the efficacy of retinyl palmitate and the antioxidant N-acetylcysteine. There were 2,592 randomized and eligible patients, approximately 1,000 of whom had lung cancer. Results showed no difference between treatment and control arms for SPTs ($p = 0.54$), event-free survival ($p = 0.750$), or long-term survival rates ($p = 0.925$).

The last of these trials carried out through the Oncology Intergroup involving all NCI Cooperative Oncology groups studied the efficacy of isotretinoin in the prevention of SPT following stage I NSCLC [162]. In this randomized, double-blind, placebo-controlled trial more than 1,000 participants received 3 years of intervention and an additional 4 years of follow-up. Time to SPT was the primary endpoint. The results were recently reported showing no statistically significant differences between the two arms with respect to the time to SPTs (RR = 1.08; 95% CI 0.78–1.49), recurrences (RR = 0.99; 95% CI 0.76–1.29), or mortality (RR = 1.07; 95% CI 0.84–1.35). The SPT rate was 3.9% per year and was exceeded by the recurrence rate (6.2%) even in T1N0 patients. Univariate analyses of three stratification factors (tumor stage, histology, and smoking status) on the major endpoints indicated that tumor stage T2 was associated significantly with recurrence (RR of T2 versus T1 = 1.74; 95% CI 1.33–2.27) and mortality (RR of T2 versus T1 = 1.42; 95% CI 1.12–1.80) and that histology (RR of squamous versus non-squamous = 1.42; 95% CI 1.12–1.80) and smoking status (RRs of current and former smokers versus non-smokers = 2.44 [95% CI

1.32–4.53] and 1.94 [95% CI 1.05–3.58], respectively) correlated with mortality. The significant correlations between tumor stage and histology carried on into the multivariate analyses but smoking was no longer associated with mortality. This led to a *post hoc* analysis of a possible treatment intervention–smoking interaction which found that isotretinoin was harmful in current smokers and beneficial in never smokers. Mortality and recurrence were increased in current smokers but were decreased in never smokers in the isotretinoin arm versus in the placebo arm. Possible reasons for this finding include potential adverse interactions of retinoic acid with tobacco smoke. For example, tobacco carcinogens can suppress RAR-beta expression and can induce retinoic acid metabolism and DNA methylation leading to augmentation of mitogenic activities (e.g., increased activity of the transcription factor AP-1, a complex of the proto-oncogenes c-*fos* and c-*jun*) [122]. Retinoic acid and smoking can increase gastrin-releasing peptide (GRP) expression which can promote lung tumorigenesis in model systems and smoking can increase GRP receptor expression [163, 164]. Finally, the tobacco carcinogen benzo(a)pyrene and retinoic acid can induce activation of nuclear factor kappaB, a transcription factor for a number of genes involved in tumor progression and a major regulator of the apoptotic pathway [165, 166]. It is important to recognize that although this finding of a differential retinoid-smoking interaction appears to be important, it must be viewed as exploratory at best given the problematic nature of *post hoc* secondary analyses and the high likelihood of type I and II error rates.

More recently, Mayne et al. reported the results of a randomized trial evaluating the efficacy of supplemental beta-carotene on reducing failure attributable to second primary tumors (head and neck, esophagus, and lung) and local recurrences in individuals curatively treated for early-stage cancers of the head and neck [167]. Patients were randomly assigned to receive 50 mg beta-carotene per day or placebo and were followed for up to 7.5 years. The trial was stopped early after the results of the ATBC and CARET studies were available. After a median follow-up of just over 4 years, there was no difference between the two groups in the time to failure (RR = 0.90; 95% CI 0.56–1.45). In site-specific analyses none of the effects were statistically significant (RR = 0.69; 95% CI 0.39–1.25 for second head and neck cancer and RR = 1.44; 95% CI 0.62–3.39 for lung cancer). However the point estimates suggest a possible decrease in second head and neck cancer risk but a likely increase in lung cancer risk. These results, if reproduced in already completed or future studies, could serve as an important starting point for mechanistic studies addressing differential responses of chemopreventive interventions in one epithelial site versus another.

Subsequent results in this area with retinoids have also been disappointing. In 1991, investigators at the

MD Anderson Cancer Center launched a large Intergroup trial of low-dose, long-term isotretinoin in stage I and II head and neck squamous cell carcinoma patients definitively treated with radiation therapy or surgery. Results of this trial were presented at the 2003 American Society of Clinical Oncology meeting [168]. One thousand three hundred and eighty-four patients were registered and 1,190 were eligible and randomized to receive either isotretinoin or placebo for 3 years with a subsequent 4 years of follow-up. No significant difference was found between the two groups with respect to overall survival, SPT-free survival, or recurrence-free survival ($p = 0.79$, 0.99, and 0.18, respectively). The annual SPT rate was 4.7% for both arms. The most common secondary tumor site in both groups was lung followed by the oral cavity, larynx, and pharynx. These negative results may be explained by the fact that the dose chosen may have been too low. A higher dose, however, although potentially more effective, would have likely resulted in increased toxicity (toxicity that would be unacceptable for a population of patients with early-stage disease and good prognosis). A way forward may be the study of retinoid combinations, such as a retinoid and an interferon, which currently are being tested in ongoing clinical and mechanistic studies.

In addition to the completed SPT trials, there is an ongoing Intergroup trial of selenium for reducing the incidence of lung cancer-associated SPT. The basis for this study includes observational studies showing lower serum levels of selenium in lung cancer patients compared with control subjects and encouraging secondary lung cancer findings of two NCI phase III trials involving selenium. In a study by Clark et al. designed to determine selenium effects on the incidence of skin basal cell or squamous cell carcinomas, nutritional supplementation with this agent showed no consequences on skin cancer incidence, however secondary analyses revealed that it was associated with significantly fewer lung cancers [169]. Another large-scale trial produced similar encouraging findings showing a 0.55 relative risk of death from lung cancer associated with the combination of alpha-tocopherol, selenium, and beta-carotene [170].

53.6 Conclusion and Future Directions

In conclusion, all the prospective randomized controlled trials in lung cancer chemoprevention have so far produced either neutral or harmful primary end point results whether in the primary, secondary, or tertiary setting. The data suggest that lung cancer was not prevented by beta-carotene, alpha-tocopherol, retinal, retinyl palmitate, N-acetylcysteine, or isotretinoin in smokers. On the basis of these findings, at present no agent either alone or in combination should be used for lung cancer prevention outside of a clinical trial. The results from the recently completed Canadian study of ADT in smokers with bronchial dysplasia, secondary analyses of the phase III trials involving selenium and vitamin E as well as data from the US Intergroup NCI-91-0001 supporting the treatment with isotretinoin in never and former smokers are all hopeful and present a promising direction for future clinical study.

There are several other areas of promise for future lung cancer chemoprevention study. A major area involves the characterization of molecular targets for new drug development and molecular and genomic biomarkers that can be used to identify and quantify risk in prospective cohorts as well as finding use as surrogate endpoints in clinical studies. Promising molecular/targets currently drawing attention include retinoic acid receptors, ornithine decarboxylase, PPAR, p53, and molecules implicated in the apoptotic pathways such as the caspases and polyadenosine phosphate ribose polymerase-3, vascular endothelial growth factor, telomerase, Ras association domain family 1, LOH, fragile histidine triad or FHIT, COX-2, lipooxygenases, and certain transcription factors such as AP-1 [171].

Another area of study will be leads to new animal models of carcinogenesis. These afford a strategic framework for evaluating agents according to defined criteria and not only provide evidence of efficacy, but also serve to generate important dose-response, toxicity, and pharmacokinetic data required prior to early-phase clinical testing in humans. Currently, potential inhibitors of lung carcinogenesis are evaluated using models developed in both hamster and mouse species. Of the hamster lung cancer models, one model utilizes the direct-acting carcinogen methylnitrosurea and the other utilizes diethylnitrosamine [172]. Tumors appear within 6 months and both models are responsive to modulation by several classes of potential chemopreventive drugs. Another practical and useful model for the study of lung cancer prevention is the A/J mouse model that reliably produces lung tumors with an oncogenic K-ras mutation when induced by 4-(methylnitrosoamino)-1-(3-pyridyl)-1-butanone, a tobacco-related carcinogen [91]. Cutting-edge methods in genetic engineering in the mouse have recently produced far more superior and sophisticated models. One type involving K-ras uses a new gene targeting procedure to create mouse strains carrying oncogenic alleles of K-ras that can be activated only on a spontaneous recombination event in the whole animal [173, 174]. This approach of course has one large advantage over traditional strategies including transgenic strategies in that it more closely recapitulates spontaneous oncogene activation as seen in human cancers. Another example of one of these newly generated models representing a true breakthrough in the study of lung cancer is the Meuwissen et al. model, a rationally designed, conditional p53 and Rb allele-based and lung-targeted mouse model of human SCLC

[175]. While much work remains in the validation and application of these models, they are likely to improve our understanding of disease development and provide a crucial means to test potential prevention strategies.

Novel treatment regimens to improve the therapeutic ratio of chemopreventives will also be important. At least three strategies may be employed to achieve this goal: improved mechanistic specificity, local drug delivery to cancer targets, and combination therapy. The series of preclinical and clinical studies that led to the approval of celecoxib for the treatment of adenomas in persons with FAP show the merits of applying the second strategy in order to move a promising agent from theory to practice. An example of local agent delivery in lung is the use of topical administration of agent by aerosol delivery which minimizes systemic toxicity and circumvents bioavailability problems. Aerosol formulations of the antiasthmatic glucocorticoid budesonide and the phase 2 metabolic enzyme modulators oltipraz and phenethyl isothiocyanate were found to prevent lung cancers in the A/J model [176, 177]. Budesonide was the most effective of the three agents and showed a dose response related inhibition of tumor multiplicity up to 90%. Combination chemoprevention therapy involves the concomitant use of multiple agents with different mechanisms of action. Targeting different chemopreventive pathways allows for agents to be administered at doses lower than when these agents are used alone potentially reducing the clinical toxicity of each drug. The combination of a promoter of differentiation, an antiproliferative agent, and an inducer of apoptosis would be particularly appropriate for the treatment of malignant lesions. An example of combination chemopreventive regimens to consider would involve the use of a rexinoid with an EGFR inhibitor. Alternatively, a retinoid might be used together with a compound that would modify chromatin structure such as a histone deacetylase inhibitor. Other potential combination regimens exist.

A last and equally important priority will be education and specialized training for physicians. Most physician investigators presently carrying out clinical prevention activities entered the field through other more traditional or established areas such as community or public health and cancer therapy clinical trials. As interest in cancer prevention as an important complement to other cancer control approaches increases, scientific schooling will need to concentrate on the recruitment and development of future researchers for this type of work. Possibly even more essential will be the need to implement structured curricula in medical schools and postgraduate programs to help bridge the gap between research and general application of new knowledge by teaching future primary care physicians, lung-oriented specialists, and healthcare professionals how to appropriately make use of the results of prevention trials for the benefit of the public. In order for the findings of cancer prevention trials to have their intended influence, they must be employed broadly. Embedding the important principles of cancer prevention in physicians early on in their careers should help accomplish that objective.

Key Points

- Lung cancer is the commonest cause of cancer death in developed countries and throughout the world
- Chemoprevention shows promise as a new approach to this disease
- Chemoprevention builds on the concepts of multistep carcinogenesis and field carcinogenesis and can be defined as the use of natural or chemical compounds to prevent, inhibit, or reverse the process of carcinogenesis
- Chemoprevention trials in lung cancer have so far produced either neutral or harmful primary end point results whether in the primary, secondary, or tertiary setting. The data suggest that lung cancer was not prevented by beta-carotene, alpha-tocopherol, retinal, retinyl palmitate, N-acetylcysteine, or isotretinoin in smokers.
- No drug or drug combination should be used for lung cancer prevention outside of a clinical study.

References

1. Jemal A, Tiwari RC, Murray T, et al. Cancer statistics, 2005. CA Cancer J Clin 2005; 55:10.
2. Wingo PA, Reis LA, Giovino GA, et al. Annual report to the nation on the status of cancer, 1973–1996, with a special section on lung cancer and tobacco smoking. J Natl Cancer Inst 1999; 91:675.
3. Samet JM. Health benefits of smoking cessation. Clin Chest Med 1991; 12:669.
4. Samet JM, Wiggins CL, Humble CG, et al. Cigarette smoking and lung cancer in New Mexico. Am Rev Respir Dis 1988; 137:1110.
5. Chute JP, Chen T, Feigal E, et al. Twenty years of phase III trials for patients with extensive-stage small cell lung cancer: perceptible progress. J Clin Oncol 1999; 17:1794.
6. Simon GR, Wagner H. Small cell lung cancer. Chest 2003; 123:259S.
7. Albain KS, Crowley JJ, LeBlanc M, et al. Survival determinants in extensive-stage non-small cell lung cancer: the Southwest Oncology Group experience. J Clin Oncol 1991; 9:1618.
8. Sandler AB. Chemotherapy for small cell lung cancer. Semin Oncol 2003; 30:9.
9. Sekido Y, Fong K, Minna J. Cancer of the luna. In: DeVita VT Jr, Hellman S, Rosenberg SA (eds) Cancer: Principles and Practice of Oncology, 6th edn. Philadelphia: Lippincott-Raven, 2001; 917.
10. Mountain C. Revisions in the international system for staging lung cancer. Chest 1997; 17:1.
11. Dillman RO, Hemdon J, Seagren SL, et al. Improved survival in stage III non-small-cell lung cancer: seven-year follow-up of Cancer and Leukemia Group B (CALGB) 8433 trial. J Natl Cancer Inst 1996; 88:1210.
12. Sause W, Kolesar P, Taylor S IV, et al. Final results of phase III trial in regionally advanced unresectable non-small cell lung cancer. Radiation Therapy Oncology Group, Eastern Cooperative Oncology Group, and Southwest Oncology Group. Chest 2000; 117:358.
13. Curran WJ Jr, Scott C, Langer C, et al. Phase III comparison of sequential vs concurrent chemoradiation for patients with unresected stage III non-small cell lung cancer: initial report of Radiation Therapy Oncology Group (RTOG) 9410. Proc Am Soc Clin Oncol 2000; 19:484a.
14. Furuse K, Kubota K, Kawahara M, et al. Phase II study of concurrent radiotherapy and chemotherapy for unresectable stage III non-small-cell lung cancer. Southern Osaka Lung Cancer Study Group. J Clin Oncol 1995; 13:869.
15. Furuse K, Fukuoka M, Kawahara M, et al. Phase III study of concurrent versus sequential thoracic radiotherapy in combination with mitomycin, vindesine, and cisplatin in unresectable stage III non-small-cell lung cancer. J Clin Oncol 1999; 17:2692.
16. Non-small Cell Lung Cancer Collaborative Group. Chemotherapy in non-small cell lung cancer: a meta-analysis using updated data on individual patients from 52 randomised clinical trials. BMJ 1995; 311:899.
17. Sporn MB. Approaches to prevention of epithelial cancer during the preneoplastic period. Cancer Res 1976; 36:2699.
18. Sporn MB, Dunlop NM, Newton DL, et al. Prevention of chemical carcinogenesis by vitamin A and its synthetic analogues (retinoids). Fed Proc 1976; 35:1332.
19. Fisher B, Constantino JP, Wickerham DL, et al. Tamoxifen for prevention of breast cancer: report of the National Surgical Adjuvant Breast and Bowel Project P-1 study. J Natl Cancer Inst 1998; 90:1371.
20. Steinbach G, Lynch PM, Phillips RK, et al. The effects of celecoxib, a cyclo-oxygenase inhibitor, in familial adenomatous polyposis. N Eng J Med 2000; 342:1946.
21. Hong WK, Endicott J, Itri LM, et al. 13-cis-Retinoic acid in the treatment of oral leukoplakia. N Engl J Med 1986; 315:1501.
22. Hong WK, Lippman SM, Itri LM, et al. Prevention of second primary tumors with isotretinoin in squamous cell carcinoma of the head and neck. N Engl J Med 1990; 323:795.
23. Auerbach O, Gere JB, Forman JB, et al. Changes in the bronchial epithelium in relation to smoking and cancer of the lung. N Engl J Med 1957; 256:98.
24. Auerbach O, Hammond EC, Garfinkel L. Changes in bronchial epithelium in relation to cigarette smoking, 1955–1960 vs. 1970–1977. N Eng J Med 1979; 300:381.
25. Auerbach O, Stout AP, Hammond EC, et al. Changes in bronchial epithelium in relation to cigarette smoking and in relation to lung cancer. N Engl J Med 1961; 265:253.
26. Slaughter DP, Southwick HW, Smejkal W. Field cancerization in oral stratified squamous epithelium: clinical implications of multicentric origin. Cancer 1953; 6:963.
27. Gudas LJ, Sporn MB, Roberts AB. Cellular biology and biochemistry of the retinoids. In: Sporn MB, Roberts AB, Goodman DS (eds) The Retinoids: Biology, Chemistry and Medicine, 2nd edn. New York: Raven, 1994:443.
28. Deluca LM. Retinoids and their receptors in differentiation, embryogenesis and neoplasia. FASEB J 1991; 5:2923.
29. Lotan R. Retinoids and apoptosis: implication for cancer chemoprevention and therapy. J Natl Cancer Inst 1995; 87:1655.

30. Nagy L, Thomazy VA, Heyman RA, et al. Retinoid-induced apoptosis in normal and neoplastic tissues. Cell Death Differ 1998; 5:11.

31. Wolbach SB, Howe PR. Tissue changes following deprivation of fat-soluble vitamin A. J Exp Med 1925; 42:597.

32. Kitareewan S, Pitha-Rowe I, Ma Y, et al. The retinoids and cancer prevention mechanisms. In: Kelloff GJ, Hawk ET, Sigman CC (eds) Cancer Chemoprevention, vol I. Promising Cancer Chemopreventive Agents. Totowa, NJ: Humana (in press)

33. Muto Y, Moriwaki H, Ninomiya M, et al. Prevention of second primary tumors by an acyclic retinoid, polyprenoic acid, in patients with hepatocellular carcinoma. N Engl J Med 1996; 334:1561.

34. Benner SE, Pajak TF, Lippman SM, et al. Prevention of second primary tumors with isotretinoin in patients with squamous cell carcinoma of the head and neck: Long-term follow-up. J Natl Cancer Inst 1994; 86:140.

35. Pastorino U, Infante M, Maioli M, et al. Adjuvant treatment of stage I lung cancer with high-dose vitamin A. J Clin Oncol 1993; 11:1216.

36. Mavne ST, Lippman SM. Retinoids, carotenoids and micronutrients. In: Devita VT, Hellman S, Rosenberg SA (eds) Cancer: Principles and Practice of Oncology, 6th. ed. Philadelphia: Lippincott-Raven, 1997:575.

37. Krinsky NI. Actions of carotenoids in biologic systems. Annu Rev Nutr 1993; 13:561.

38. Peto R, Doll R, Buckley JD, et al. Can dietary β-carotene materially reduce human cancer rates? Nature 1981; 290:201.

39. Floyd RA. Role of free radicals in carcinogenesis and brain ischemia. FASEB J 1990; 4:2587.

40. Chew BP, Wong TS, Shultz TD, et al. Effects of conjugated dienoic derivatives of linoleic acid and beta-carotene in modulating lymphocyte and macrophage function. Anticancer Res 1997; 17:1099.

41. Murata T, Tamai H, Morinobu T, et al. Effect of long-term administration of beta-carotene on lymphocyte subsets in humans. Am J Clin Nutr 1994; 60:597.

42. Toba T, Shidoji Y, Fujii J, et al. Growth suppression and induction of heat-shock protein-70 by 9-cis beta-carotene in cervical dysplasia-derived cells. Life Sci 1997; 61:839.

43. Muto Y, Fujii J, Shidoji Y, et al. Growth retardation in human cervical dysplasia-derived cell lines by beta-carotene through down-regulation of epidermal growth factor receptor. Am J Clin Nutr 1995; 62(6 suppl):1535S.

44. Nishino H, Murakoshi M, Ii T, et al. Carotenoids in cancer chemoprevention. Cancer Metastasis Rev 2002; 21:257.

45. Sies H, Stahl W. Lycopene: antioxidant and biological effects and its bioavailability in the human. Proc Soc Exp Biol Med 1998; 218:121.

46. Amir H, Karas M, Giat J, et al. Lycopene and 1,25-dihydroxyvitamin D_3 cooperate in the inhibition of cell cycle progression and induction of differentiation in HL-60 leukemic cells. Nutr Cancer 1999; 33:105.

47. Karas M, Amir H, Fishman D, et al. Lycopene interferes with cell cycle progression and insulin-like growth factor I signaling in mammary cancer cells. Nutr Cancer 2000; 36:101.

48. Stahl W, von Laar J, Martin HD, et al. Stimulation of gap junctional communication: comparison of acyclo-retinoic acid and lycopene. Arch Biochem Biophys 2000; 373:271.

49. Heber D. Colorful cancer prevention: a-carotene, lycopene and lung cancer. Am J Clin Nutr 2000; 72:901.

50. Mangelsdorf DJ, Umesono K, Evans RM. The retinoid receptors. In: Sporn MB, Roberts AB, Goodman DS (eds) The Retinoids: Biology, Chemistry and Medicine, 2nd edn. New York: Raven, 1994:319.

51. Mangelsdorf DJ, Thummel C, Beato M, et al. The nuclear receptor superfamily: the second decade. Cell 1995; 83:835.

52. Chambon P. A decade of molecular biology of retinoic acid receptors. FASEB J 1996; 10:940.

53. Zelent A, Mendelson C, Kastner P, et al. Differentially expressed isoforms of the mouse retinoic acid receptor beta are generated by usage of two promoters and alternative splicing. EMBO J 1991; 10:71.

54. Napgal S, Zelent A, Chambon P. RAR-beta-4, a retinoic acid receptor isoform is generated from RAR-beta-2 by alternative splicing and usage of a CUG initiator codon. Proc Natl Acad Sci U S A 1992; 89:2718.

55. Hu X, Lazar MA. Transcriptional repression by nuclear receptors. Trends Endocrinol Metab 2000; 11:6.

56. Germain P, Iyer J, Zechel C, et al. Co-regulator recruitment and the mechanism of retinoic acid synergy. Nature 2002; 415:187.

57. Rachez C, Freedman LP. Mediator complexes and transcription. Curr Opin Cell Biol 2001; 13:274.

58. Altucci L, Gronemeyer H. The promise of retinoids to fight against cancer. Nat Rev Cancer 2001; 1:181.

59. Renaud JP, Rochel N, Ruff M, et al. Crystal structure of the RAR-gamma ligand-binding domain bound to all-trans-retinoic acid. Nature 1995; 378:681.

60. Davies P, Lippman SM. Biologic basis of retinoid pharmacology: implications for cancer prevention and therapy. Adv Oncol 1996; 12:2.

61. Lala DS, Mukherjee R, Schulman IG, et al. Activation of specific RXR heterodimers by an antagonist of RXR homodimers. Nature 1996; 383:450.

62. Mukherjee R, Davies PJ, Crombie DL, et al. Sensitization of diabetic and obese mice to insulin by retinoid X receptor agonists. Nature 1997; 386:407.

63. Perlman T, Evans RM. Nuclear receptors in Sicily: all in the family. Cell 1997; 90:391.

64. Bischoff ED, Gottardis MM, Moon TE, et al. Beyond tamoxifen: the retinoid X receptor-selective ligand LGD1069 (Targretin) causes complete regression of mammary carcinoma. Cancer Res 1998; 58:479.

65. Gottardis MM, Bischoff ED, Shirley MA, et al. Chemoprevention of mammary carcinoma by LGD1069 (Targretin): an RXR-selective ligand. Cancer Res 1996; 56:5566.

66. Mariani L, Formelli F, De Palo G, et al. Chemoprevention of breast cancer with fenretinide (4-HPR): study of long-term visual and ophthalmologic tolerability. Tumori 1996; 82:444.

67. Costa A, Formelli F, Chiesa F, et al. Prospects of chemoprevention of human cancers with the synthetic retinoid fenretinide. Cancer Res 1994; 54:2032S.

68. Dimery IW, Hong WK, Lee JJ, et al. Phase I trial of alpha-tocopherol effects on 13-cis-retinoic acid toxicity. Ann Oncol 1997; 8:85.

69. Besa EC, Abrahm JL, Bartholomew MJ, et al. Treatment with 13-cis-retinoic acid in transfusion-dependent patients with myelodysplastic syndrome and decreased toxicity with addition of alpha-tocopherol. Am J Med 1990; 89:739.

70. Langston AW, Thompson JR, Gudas LJ. Retinoic acid-responsive enhancers located 3 of the Hox A and Hox B homeobox gene clusters. Functional analysis. J Biol Chem 1997; 272:2167.

71. Clifford JL, Menter DG, Wang M, et al. Retinoid receptor-dependent and -independent effects of N-(4-hydroxyphenyl) retinamide in F9 embryonal carcinoma cells. Cancer Res 1999; 59:14.

72. Oridate N, Suzuki S, Higuchi M, et al. Involvement of reactive oxygen species in N-(4-hydroxyphenyl) retinamide-induced apoptosis in cervical carcinoma cells. J Natl Cancer Inst 1997; 89:1191.

73. Mulshine JL, De Luca LM, Dedrick RL. Regional delivery of retinoids: a new approach to early lung cancer intervention. Clin Biol Basis Lung Cancer Prev 1998; 24:273.

74. Cao Y, Pearman AT, Zimmerman GA, et al. Intracellular unesterified arachidonic acid signals apoptosis. Proc Natl Acad Sci USA 2000; 97:11280.

75. Chan TA, Morin PJ, Vogelstein B, et al. Mechanisms underlying nonsteroidal anti-inflammatory drug-mediated apoptosis. Proc Natl Acad Sci USA 1998; 95:681.

76. Tsuji M, DuBois RN. Alterations in cellular adhesion and apoptosis in epithelial cells overexpressing prostaglandin endoperoxide synthase 2. Cell 1995; 83:493.

77. Majima M, Isono M, Ikeda Y, et al. Significant roles of inducible cyclooxygenase (COX-2) in angiogenesis in rat. Jpn J Pharmacol 1997; 75:105.

78. Sharma S, Stolina M, Yang SC, et al. Tumor cyclooxygenase 2-dependent suppression of dendritic cell function. Clin Cancer Res 2003; 9:961.

79. Cao Y, Prescott SM. Many actions of cyclooxygenase-2 in cellular dynamics and in cancer. J Cell Physiol 2002; 190:279.

80. Castonguay A, Rioux N, Duperron C, et al. Inhibition of lung tumorigenesis by NSAIDS: a working hypothesis. Exp Lung Res 1998; 24:605.

81. Wolff H, Saukkonen K, Anttila S, et al. Expression of cyclooxygenase-2 in human lung carcinoma. Cancer Res 1998; 58:4997.

82. Hida T, Yatabe Y, Achiwa H, et al. Increased expression of cyclooxygenase 2 occurs frequently in human lung cancers, specifically adenocarcinomas. Cancer Res 1998; 58:3761.

83. Hosomi Y, Yokose T, Hirose Y, et al. Increased cyclooxygenase 2 (COX-2) expression occurs frequently in precursor lesions of human adenocarcinomas of the lung. Lung Cancer 2000; 30:73.

84. Khuri FR, Wu H, Lee JJ, et al. Cyclooxygenase-2 overexpression is a marker of poor prognosis in stage I non-small cell lung cancer. Clin Cancer Res 2001; 7:861.

85. Harris RE, Beebe-Donk J, Schuller HM. Chemoprevention of lung cancer by non-steroidal anti-inflammatory drugs among cigarette smokers. Oncol Rep 2002; 9:693.

86. Akhmedkhanov A, Toniolo P, Zeleniuch-Jacquotte A, et al. Aspirin and lung cancer in women. Br J Cancer 2002; 87:49.

87. Sebti SM, Hamilton AD. Farnesyltransferase and geranylgeranyltransferase I inhibitors and cancer therapy: lessons from mechanism and bench-to-bedside translational studies. Oncogene 2000; 19:6584.

88. Hill BT, Perrin D, Kruczynski A. Inhibition of RAS-targeted prenylation: protein farnesyl transferase inhibitors revisited. Crit Rev Oncol Hematol 2000; 33:7.

89. Zujewski J, Horak ID, Bol CJ, et al. Phase I and pharmacokinetic study of farnesyl protein transferase inhibitor R115777 in advanced cancer. J Clin Oncol 2000; 18:927.

90. Westra WH, Baas IO, Hruban RH, et al. K-ras oncogene activation in atypical alveolar hyperplasias of the human lung. Cancer Res 1996; 56:2224.

91. Lantry LE, Zhang Z, Yao R, et al. Effect of farnesyltransferase inhibitor FTI-276 on established lung adenomas from A/J mice induced by 4-(methylnitrosamino)-1-(3-pyridyl)-1-butanone. Carcinogenesis 2000; 21:113.

92. Salomon DS, Brandt R, Ciardiello F, et al. Epidermal growth factor-related peptides and their receptors in human malignancies. Crit Rev Oncol Hematol 1995; 19:183.

93. Richardson CM, Sharma RA, Cox KJ, et al. Epidermal growth factor receptors and cyclooxygenase-2 in the pathogenesis of non-small cell lung cancer: potential targets for chemoprevention and systemic therapy. Lung Cancer 2003; 39:1.

94. Fontanini G, Vignati S, Bigini D, et al. Epidermal growth factor receptor (EGFr) expression in non-small cell lung cancer carcinomas correlates with metastatic involvement of hilar and mediastinal lymph nodes in the squamous subtype. Eur J Cancer 1995; 31:178.

95. Mukaida H, Toi M, Hirai T, et al. Clinical significance of the expression of epidermal growth factor and its receptor in esophageal cancer. Cancer 1991; 68:142.

96. Neal DE, Mellon K. Epidermal growth factor receptor and bladder cancer: a review. Urol Int 1992; 48:365.

97. Sainsbury JR, Farndon JR, Needham GK, et al. Epidermal-growth factor receptor status as predictor of early recurrence of and death from breast cancer. Lancet 1987; 1:1398.

98. Kurie JM, Shin HJC, Lee JS, et al. Increased epidermal growth factor receptor expression in metaplastic bronchial epithelium. Clin Cancer Res 1996; 2:1787.

99. Rusch V, Klimstra D, Linkov I, et al. Aberrant expression of p53 or the epidermal growth factor receptor is frequent in early bronchial neoplasia, and coexpression precedes squamous cell carcinoma development. Cancer Res 1995; 55:1365.

100. Lonardo F, Dragnev KH, Freemantle SJ, et al. Evidence for the epidermal growth factor receptor as a target for lung cancer prevention. Clin Cancer Res 2002; 8:54.

101. Kris MG, Natale RB, Herbst RS, et al. Efficacy of gefitinib, an inhibitor of the epidermal growth factor receptor tyrosine kinase, in symptomatic patients with non-small cell lung cancer: a randomized trial. JAMA 2003; 290:2149.

102. Forsythe B, Faulkner K. Overview of the tolerability of gefitinib (Iressa) monotherapy: clinical experience in non-small cell lung cancer. Drug Saf 2004; 27:1081.

103. Lynch TJ, Bell DW, Sordella R, et al. Activating mutations in the epidermal growth factor receptor underlying responsiveness of non-small cell lung cancer to gefitinib. N Engl J Med 2004; 350:2129.

104. Paez JG, Janne PA, Lee JC, et al. EGFR mutations in lung cancer: correlation with clinical response to gefitinib therapy. Science 2004; 304:1497.

105. Pao W, Miller V, Zakowski M, et al. EGF receptor gene mutations are common in lung cancer from "never smokers" and are associated with sensitivity of tumors to gefitinib and erlotinib. Proc Natl Aca Sci U S A 2004; 101:13306.

106. Evans RM. The steroid and thyroid hormone receptor superfamily. Science 1988; 240:889.

107. Schoonjans K, Martin G, Staels B, et al. Peroxisome proliferator-activated receptors, orphans with ligands and functions. Curr Opin Lipidol 1997; 8:159.

108. Schoonjans K, Staels B, Auwerx J. The peroxisome proliferator activated receptors (PPARs) and their effects on lipid metabolism and adipocyte differentiation. Biochim Biophys Acta 1996; 1302:93.

109. Berger J, Moller DE. The mechanisms of action of PPARs. Annu Rev Med 2002; 53:409.

110. Auwerx J. PPARgamma, the ultimate thrifty gene. Diabetologia 1999; 42:1033.

111. Theocharis S, Kanelli H, Politi A, et al. Expression of peroxisome proliferator activated receptor-gamma in non-small cell lung carcinoma: correlation with histologic type and grade. Lung Cancer 2002; 36:249.

112. Segawa Y, Yoshimura T, Hase T, et al. Expression of peroxisome proliferator-activated receptor (PPAR) in human prostate cancer. Prostate 2002; 51:108.

113. Mueller E, Sarraf P, Tontonoz P, et al. Terminal differentiation of human breast cancer through PPAR gamma. Mol Cell 1998; 1:465.

114. Keshamouni VG, Reddy RC, Arenberg DA, et al. Peroxisome proliferator-activated receptor-γ activation inhibits

tumor progression in non-small-cell lung cancer. Oncogene 2004; 23:100.

115. Shen Q, Brown PH. Novel agents for the prevention of breast cancer: targeting transcription factors and signal transduction pathways. J Mammary Gland Biol Neoplasia 2003; 8:45.

116. Lonardo F, Rusch V, Langenfield J, et al. Overexpression of cyclins D1 and E is frequent in bronchial neoplasia and precedes squamous cell carcinoma development. Cancer Res 1999; 59:2470.

117. Boyle JO, Langenfeld J, Lonardo F, et al. Cyclin D1 proteolysis: a retinoid chemoprevention signal in normal, immortalized and transformed human bronchial epithelial cells. J Natl Cancer Inst 1999; 91:373.

118. Witschi H, Espiritu I, Suffia M, et al. Expression of cyclin D1/2 in the lungs of strain A/J mice fed chemopreventive agents. Carcinogenesis 2002; 23:289.

119. Papadimitrakopoulou VA, Izzo J, Mao L, et al. Cyclin D1 and p16 alterations in advanced premalignant lesions of the upper aerodigestive tract: role in response to chemoprevention and cancer development. Clin Cancer Res 2001; 7:3127.

120. Engler TA, Furness K, Malhotra S, et al. Novel, potent and selective cyclin D1/CDK4 inhibitors: indolo(6,7-a)pyrrolo(3,4-c)carbazoles. Bioorg Med Chem Lett 2003; 13:2261.

121. Zochbauer-Muller S, Minna JD, Gazdar AF. Aberrant DNA methylation in lung cancer: biological and clinical implications. Oncologist 2002; 7:451.

122. Virmani AK, Rathi A, Zochbauer-Muller S, et al. Promoter methylation and silencing of the retinoic acid receptor-beta gene in lung carcinomas. J Natl Cancer Inst 2000; 92:1303.

123. Burbee DG, Forgacs E, Zochbauer-Muller S, et al. Epigenetic inactivation of RASSF1A in lung and breast cancers and malignant phenotype suppression. J Natl Cancer Inst 2001; 93:691.

124. Zochbauer-Muller S, Fong KM, Maitra A, et al. 5 CpG island methylation of the FHIT gene is correlated with loss of gene expression in lung and breast cancer. Cancer Res 2001; 61:3581.

125. Toyooka KO, Toyooka S, Virmani AK, et al. Loss of expression and aberrant methylation of the CDH13 (H-cadherin) gene in breast and lung carcinomas. Cancer Res 2001; 61:4556.

126. Kelloff GJ, Boon CW, Crowell JA, et al. Risk biomarkers and current strategies for cancer prevention. J Cell Biochem Suppl 1996; 25:1.

127. Lippman SM, Benner SE, Hong WK. Cancer chemoprevention. J Clin Oncol 1994; 12:851.

128. Workshop report. Biomarkers in cancer chemoprevention. In: Miller AB, Bartsch H, Boffeta P, Dragsted L, Vainio H (eds) Biomarkers in Cancer Chemoprevention, no. 154. Lyon, France: IARC Scientific, 2001:1.

129. Lippman SM, Lee JS, Lotan R, et al. Biomarkers as intermediate endpoints in chemoprevention trials. J Natl Cancer Inst 1990; 82:555.

130. Srivastava S, Rossi SC. Early detection research program at the NCI. Int J Cancer 1996; 69:35.

131. Sullivan Pepe M, Etzioni R, Feng Z, et al. Phases of biomarker development for early detection of cancer. J Natl Cancer Inst 2001; 93:1054.

132. Prentice RL. Surrogate endpoints in clinical trials: definition and operational criteria. Stat Med 1989; 8:431.

133. Buyse M, Molenberghs G. Criteria for the validation of surrogate endpoints in randomized experiments. Biometrics 1998; 54:1014.

134. Bach PB, Kattan MW, Thornquist MD, et al. Variations in lung cancer risk among smokers. J Natl Cancer Inst 2003; 95:470.

135. Shields PG. Molecular epidemiology of smoking and lung cancer. Oncogene 2002; 21:6870.

136. Wu X, Zhao H, Suk R, et al. Genetic susceptibility to tobacco-related cancer. Oncogene 2004; 23:6500.

137. Alpha-tocopherol, Beta Carotene Cancer Prevention Study Group. The effect of vitamin E and beta-carotene on the incidence of lung cancer and other cancers in male smokers. New Engl J Med 1994; 330:1029.

138. Omenn GS, Goodman GE, Thornquist MD, et al. Effects of a combination of beta-carotene and vitamin A on lung cancer and cardiovascular disease. N Engl J Med 1996; 334:1150.

139. Block G, Patterson B, Subar A. Fruit, vegetables and cancer prevention: a review of the epidemiological evidence. Nutr Cancer 1992; 18:1.

140. van Poppel G, Goldbohm RA. Epidemiologic evidence for beta-carotene and cancer prevention. Am J Clin Nutr 1995; 62:1393S.

141. Menkes MS, Comstock GW, Vuilleumier JP, et al. Serum beta-carotene, vitamins A and E, selenium and the risk of lung cancer. N Engl J Med 1986; 315:1250.

142. Stryker WS, Kaplan LA, Stein EA, et al. The relation of diet, cigarette smoking, and alcohol consumption to plasma beta-carotene and alpha-tocopherol levels. Am J Epidemiol 1988; 127:283.

143. Greenwald P. Beta-carotene and lung cancer: a lesson for future chemoprevention investigations? J Natl Cancer Inst 2003 Jan 1; 95:E1.

144. Handelman GJ, Packer L, Cross CE. Destruction of tocopherols, carotenoids, and retinol in human plasma by cigarette smoke. Am J Clin Nutr 1996; 63:559.

145. Stram DO, Wu AH. Re: Beta-carotene and lung cancer: a lesson for future chemoprevention investigations? J Natl Cancer Inst 2003 May21; 95:E4.

146. Omaye ST, Krinsky NI, Kagan VE, et al. Beta-carotene: friend or foe? Fundam Appl Toxicol 1997; 40:163.

147. Buiatti E. An overview of recent results of chemoprevention trials. In: Maltoni C, Soffritti M, Davis W (eds) The Scientific Basis of Cancer Chemoprevention. Amsterdam: Elsevier, 1996:257.

148. Paolini M, Cantelli-Forti G, Perocco P, et al. Co-carcinogenic effect of beta-carotene. Nature 1999; 398:760.

149. Perocco P, Paolini M, Mazzullo M, et al. Beta-carotene as enhancer of cell transforming activity of powerful carcinogens and cigarette-smoke condensate on BALB/c 3T3 cells in vitro. Mutat Res 1999; 440:83.

150. Salgo MG, Cueto R, Winston GW, et al. Beta-carotene and its oxidation products have different effects on microsome mediated binding of benzo(a)pyrene to DNA. Free Radic Biol Med 1999; 26:162.

151. Hennekens CH, Buring JE, Manson JE, et al. Lack of effect of long-term supplementation with beta-carotene on the incidence of malignant neoplasms and cardiovascular disease. N Engl J Med 1996; 334:1145.

152. Lee JS, Lippman SM, Benner SE, et al. Randomized placebo-controlled trial of isotretinoin in chemoprevention of bronchial squamous metaplasia. J Clin Oncol 1994; 12:937.

153. Kurie JM, Lee JS, Khuri FR, et al. N-(4-hydroxyphenyl)-retinamide in the chemoprevention of squamous metaplasia and dysplasia of the bronchial epithelium. Clin Cancer Res 2000; 6:2973.

154. Arnold AM, Browman GP, Levine MN, et al. The effect of the synthetic retinoid etredinate on sputum cytology: results from a randomized trial. Br J Cancer 1992; 65:737.

155. McLarty JW, Holiday DB, Girard WM, et al. Beta-carotene, vitamin A, and lung cancer chemoprevention: results of an intermediate endpoint study. Am J Clin Nutr 1995; 62:1431S.

156. Heimbuger DC, Alexander CB, Birch, et al. Improvement in bronchial squamous metaplasia in smokers treated with folate and vitamin B_{12}. Report of a preliminary randomized double-blind intervention trial. JAMA 1988; 259:1525.

157. Lippman SM, Benner SE, Hong WK. Cancer chemoprevention. J Clin Oncol 1994; 12:851.

158. Kurie JM, Lotan R, Lee JS, et al. Treatment of former smokers with 9-cis-retinoic acid reverses loss of retinoic acid receptor-beta expression in the bronchial epithelium: results from a randomized placebo-controlled trial. J Natl Cancer Inst 2003; 95:206.

159. Khuri FR, Lotan R, Kemp B, et al. Retinoic acid receptor-beta as a prognostic indicator in stage I non-small-cell lung cancer. J Clin Oncol 2000; 18:2798.

160. Lam S, MacAulay C, Le Riche JC, et al. A randomized phase II b trial of anethole dithiolethione in smokers with bronchial dysplasia. J Natl Cancer Inst 2002; 94:1001.

161. van Zandwijk N, Dalesio O, Pastorino U, et al. EURO-SCAN, a randomized trial of vitamin A and N-acetylcysteine in patients with head and neck cancer or lung cancer. For the European Organization for Research and Treatment of Cancer Head and Neck and Lung Cancer Cooperative Groups. J Natl Cancer Inst 2000; 92:977.

162. Lippman SM, Lee JJ, Karp DD, et al. Randomized phase III intergroup trial of isotretinoin to prevent second primary tumors in stage I non-small-cell lung cancer. J Natl Cancer Inst 2001; 93:605.

163. Ravi RK, Scott FM, Cuttitta F, et al. Induction of gastrin-releasing peptide by all-trans retinoic acid in small-cell lung cancer cells. Oncol Rep 1998; 5:497.

164. Siegfried JM, DeMichele MA, Hunt JD, et al. Expression of mRNA for gastrin-releasing peptide receptor by human bronchial epithelial cells: association with prolonged tobacco exposure and responsiveness to bombesin-like peptides. Am J Respir Crit Care Med 1997; 156:358.

165. Manna SK, Aggarwal BB. All-trans-retinoic acid upregulates TNF receptors and potentiates TNF-induced activation of nuclear factors-kappaB, activated protein-1 and apoptosis in human lung cancer cells. Oncogene 2000; 19:2110.

166. Pei XH, Nakanishi Y, Takayama K, et al. Benzo(a)pyrene activates the human p53 gene through induction of nuclear factor kappaB activity. J Biol Chem 1999; 274:35240.

167. Mayne ST, Cartmel B, Baum M, et al. Randomized trial of supplemental beta-carotene to prevent second head and neck cancer. Cancer Res 2001; 61:1457.

168. Khuri FR, Lee JJ, Lippman SM, et al. Isotretinoin effects on head and neck cancer recurrence and second primary tumors (abstract 359). Proc Am Soc Clin Oncol 2003; 22:90.

169. Clark LC, Combs GF Jr, Turnbull BW, et al. Effects of selenium supplementation for cancer prevention in patients with carcinoma of the skin. JAMA 1996; 276:1957.

170. Blot WJ, Li JY, Taylor RR, et al. Linxian nutrition intervention trials: supplementation with specific vitamin/mineral combinations, cancer incidence, and disease-specific mortality in the general population. J Natl Cancer Inst 1993; 85:1483.

171. Cohen V, Khuri FR. Chemoprevention of lung cancer: current status and future prospects. Cancer Metastasis Rev 2002; 21:349.

172. Moon RC, Rao KV, Detrisac CJ, et al. Animal models for chemoprevention of respiratory cancer. J Natl Cancer Inst Monogr 1992; 13:45.

173. Johnson L, Mercer K, Greenbaum D, et al. Somatic activation of the K-ras oncogene causes early onset lung cancer in mice. Nature 2001; 410:1111.

174. Meuwissen R, Linn SC, van der Valk M, et al. Mouse model for lung tumorigenesis through Cre/lox controlled sporadic activation of the K-ras oncogene. Oncogene 2001; 20:6551.

175. Meuwissen R, Linn SC, Linnoila I, et al. Induction of small cell lung cancer by somatic inactivation of both Trp53 and Rb1 in a conditional mouse model. Cancer Cell 2003; 4:181.

176. Wattenberg LW, Wiedman TS, Estensen RD, et al. Chemoprevention of pulmonary carcinogenesis by brief exposures to aerosolized budesonide or beclomethasone diproprionate and the combination of aerosolized budesonide and dietary myo-inositol. Carcinogenesis 2000; 21:179.

177. Wattenberg LW, Wiedman TS, Estensen RD, et al. Chemoprevention of pulmonary carcinogenesis by aerosolized budesonide in female A/J mice. Cancer Res 1997; 57:5489.

Smoking Prevention and Cessation Policies

54

Christina Gratziou and Charis Roussos

Contents

54.1 Introduction

In 2002, the Euro barometer survey series estimated that nearly 39.4% of Europeans smoke. The UK (45.2%) and France (44.1%) are the two countries characterized by the highest percentage of smokers, followed by Denmark (42.6%) and Greece (42.0%), while Luxembourg (33.8%), Sweden (33.0%), and Portugal (29.3%) have the lowest percentages (Tables 54.1, 54.2) [1]. Tobacco smoking has a great impact on morbidity and mortality. Tobacco use is a major contributor to the incidence of chronic respiratory disease (80–90%) and myocardial infarction (23–40%) and is the most important etiological factor in the development of lung cancer [2]. Smoking accounts for approximately 80–85% of lung cancer cases and has also been strongly correlated with other types of cancer (e.g., oral, laryngeal, and bladder cancers) [3].

Tobacco use causes 656,000 deaths each year in the European region of the World Health Organization (WHO) (15% of all deaths). Smokers who die in middle age as a result of their smoking lose an average of 22 years of life. On average smokers die 14 years earlier than never smokers [4]. The leading causes of death from tobacco smoking were cardiovascular diseases, chronic obstructive pulmonary disease (COPD), and lung cancer. Lung cancer is the disease with the highest fraction attributable to tobacco smoking, which accounted for 71% of all lung cancer. When the analyses were restricted to industrialized countries only, the fractions of lung cancer attributable to smoking were 91% in men and 71% in women [5]. At present, lung cancer is the biggest "cancer killer" in Europe, accounting for about 20% of all cancer deaths [4]. It has been estimated that about 100 million people worldwide were killed by tobacco in the twentieth century and that the number will increase to one billion in the twenty-first century if this smoking behavior trend continues (Table 54.3). According to recently collected data [4], unless more is done to help the 200 million European adult smokers to stop, the result will be 2,000,000 European deaths a year by 2020.

The WHO has established goals to reduce tobacco related morbidity and mortality [6]. Fighting tobacco use has also been a public health priority for the European Community since 1985 when the Europe Against Cancer program was launched [7]. Since then tobacco control has developed into areas such as legislation and mobilizing of European and International actions. On an international stage the European Community has been instrumental in designing and achieving consensus on the WHO's Framework Convention on Tobacco Control (FCTC), the world's first global health treaty. More recently a very important report *Tobacco or*

Table 54.1. Estimated smoking prevalence by gender and number of smokers in population aged 15 years or more, by World Bank region, 1995. [Adapted from 2]

	Smoking prevalence (%)			Total	
	Men	Women	Overall	Millions	Percent
World Bank region					
East Asia and Pacific	59	4	32	401	35
Eastern Europe and Central Asia	59	26	41	148	13
Latin America and Caribbean	40	21	30	95	8
Middle East and North Africa	44	5	25	40	3
South Asia	20	1	11	86	8
Sub-Saharan Africa	33	10	21	67	6
Smokers					
Low/middle income	49	9	29	933	82
High income	39	22	30	209	18
World	47	12	29	1,142	100

Source: Authors' calculations based on World Health Organization (1997) *Tobacco or Health: A Global Status Report.* Geneva, Switzerland

Table 54.2. Prevalence of smokers and smoking-related deaths among men and women aged >25 years in the European Union, 1999. [Adapted from 1]

Country	Smoking prevalence (%)		Number of smoking-related deaths	
	Men	Women	Men	Women
Austria	47	29	10,897	2,267
Belgium	45	26	16,227	2,668
Denmark	35	43	8,236	3,905
Finland	41	20	5,293	1,351
France	40	30	63,153	13,531
Germany	40	25	112,274	22,212
Greece	61	30	22,131	2,497
Ireland	40	29	4,462	964
Italy	35	19	76,234	14,853
Luxembourg	38	25	475	119
The Netherlands	37	26	17,435	4,703
Portugal	47	15	11,082	1,422
Spain	47	25	53,681	5,858
Sweden	19	25	7,396	2,486
UK	36	31	76,771	26,225
Total	**40**	**26**	**485,657**	**105,061**

Table 54.3. Leading causes of death from respiratory diseases worldwide in 1990 with the prediction for 2020. [Modified from 4]

	Number of deaths (in millions)	
	1990	2020
Respiratory diseases	9.4	11.9
Lung cancer	0.95	2.3
Chronic obstructive pulmonary disease	2.2	4.7
Pneumonia	4.3	2.5
Tuberculosis	2.0	2.4

Health in the European Union: the ASPECT Consortium (analysis of the science and policy for European control of tobacco) was published, with a set of recommendations for tobacco control policy [8].

Three major target areas are important for a tobacco control policy:

1. *Smoking prevention* includes activities to discourage initiation of tobacco use, particularly among young people. This will reduce morbidity and mortality rates; however, changes will not been seen until the year 2015 because lung cancer usually takes 20–30 years to develop.
2. *Smoking cessation programs* to inform, to motivate, and to help smokers to make attempts to quit. They are to be developed worldwide, and ensuring adequate cessation resources exist is critical. Detailed recommendations will be analyzed in this chapter.
3. *Reduction of exposure to passive smoking*, as avoiding involuntary exposure to environmental tobacco smoke protects the health and rights of children and adults.

54.2 Public Health Policy and Regulations for Tobacco Control

Policies to tax tobacco products, restrictions on their use and advertising, regulation of their contents and labeling, and public information and education are some of the common prevention strategies that are proposed by the WHO and recommended by the European Commission (EC) for smoking prevention and cessation [6–8].

Education remains crucially important in informing the general population, both children and adults, as well as smokers in particular about the dangers of smoking and motivating smokers to stop. In many countries health education campaigns are conducted by the healthcare system.

Preventing young people and others from starting to smoke is a very important element in the struggle against tobacco use. Ninety-two percent of adult smokers in the USA tried their first cigarette and 77% became daily smokers before the age of 21 [9]. Preventive approaches with young people, if effective, prevent disease 30–50 years in the future, whereas smoking cessation in current adult smokers brings population health gain more quickly, over 20–30 years.

Some of the important elements in a national strategy to prevent and reduce smoking are presented in Table 54.4, based on elements discussed at an International Association for the Study of Lung Cancer (IASLC) workshop combined with relevant elements from other reports [6, 9, 10].

The EC policies on tobacco control [7, 8] mainly include the following recommendations:

- Taxation is very important because increases in cigarette prices decrease the number of young people who start smoking and also encourage some individuals to quit.
- Legislation aimed at eliminating tobacco advertising is another important tool, in conjunction with regulations to reduce access to cigarettes for minors and policies to prohibit smoking in public places and in workplaces.

- Prohibition of internet sales of tobacco products as well as of sales of tobacco products in vending machines may prevent young people from starting smoking.
- A regulatory framework on comprehensive disclosure of the physical, chemical, and design characteristics of all tobacco products should be required and made public with a common harmonized system for information on ingredients and emissions from tobacco.
- Common policies for cigarette labeling and packaging are recommended. Health warnings should be made mandatory on tobacco packs in order to have a platform for mandatory health promotion messages to help smoking prevention and cessation policies. Requirements for tobacco manufacturers to print tar, nicotine, and CO yields on packs should be enforced.
- Legislation for smoke-free work and public places is very important to reduce exposure to environmental tobacco smoke and avoid the health consequences of passive smoking.
- Development and support of smoking cessation and treatment strategies is essential to be organized at national level. These should include the training of health professionals, the development of a national network for smoking cessation treatment services, and an increase in the accessibility of pharmaceutical therapies.

Table 54.4. National tobacco public health policy programs on tobacco control

1. Stimulate, support, and coordinate national tobacco control activities by maintenance of a national focal point
2. Establishment of a national coordinating organization on tobacco and health aspects
3. Tobacco taxes that increase faster than the growth in prices and incomes. (In EU, harmonize taxes on tobacco at the highest EU taxation rate)
4. Governments should reduce support for tobacco farming and develop strategies to provide economic alternatives to tobacco agricultural workers. (The EC subsidization plan should be rapidly phased out)
5. A portion of tobacco taxes should be used to finance control measures and research into smoking-related diseases and smoking prevention
6. Banning all forms of tobacco advertising, promotion, and sponsorship (eliminating sports sponsorships, free gifts of coupons and merchandise, and banning tobacco billboards and other visible emblems during electronic media programming)
7. A legal requirement for strong, varied warnings on packets of cigarettes. Making health warning labels visible, using a multiple warning rotation system
8. Restriction of access to tobacco products including a prohibition on sale of tobacco products to young people (<18 years), banning vending machine sales of cigarettes, banning tax-free sale of tobacco in airports, etc.
9. Limitations on the level of tar and nicotine permitted in manufactured tobacco products (e.g., a nicotine delivery of <0.5 mg)
10. Mandatory reporting of the levels of toxic constituents in the smoke of manufactured tobacco products
11. Eliminate passive smoke in workplaces, public transport, public buildings, schools, and kindergartens
12. Monitoring of trends in smoking and other forms of tobacco use, tobacco-related diseases, and effectiveness of national control actions
13. Healthcare providers and institutions should set a good example by not smoking themselves, by making institutions smoke-free, and by providing smoking cessation treatment
14. Effective programs of education and promotion aimed at smoking prevention and cessation
15. Voluntary organizations should be involved in smoking prevention and cessation. Ex-smokers might be very useful in these programs
16. Effective and widely available support for cessation of smoking, focusing on self-help programs. Initiate cessation programs in the electronic media. Reimburse behavioral and pharmacological treatment for smoking cessation

Changes in public policy and regulations are required worldwide, although tobacco issues are highly politicized as the tobacco industry has a very powerful lobby that opposes restrictive regulation; additionally, many national governments raise substantial revenues from tobacco monopolies or sales taxes on cigarettes.

Lobbying by antismoking activists in the political arm of professional organizations at national and international levels is crucial. Globally, it is also important to regulate international sales of tobacco products in developing countries which have no policies for protections related to the use of tobacco (e.g., advertising restrictions, smoking cessation programs, etc.).

54.3   Smoking Cessation Strategies

Smoking cessation strategies have tremendous potential to improve public health. The relative risk of developing other conditions, such as chronic obstructive pulmonary disease, lung cancer, and stroke, also decreases with smoking cessation [11–14]. Doll et al. found that ex-smokers had a shorter life expectation than never smokers, but larger than current smokers [12]. The risk of coronary heart disease has been estimated to decrease by 50% 12 months after smoking cessation [12]. Stopping smoking reduces the accelerated decline in pulmonary function and improves long-term prognosis [13].

54.3.1   The Problem of Nicotine Addiction

Quitting smoking requires far more than willpower. There are approximately 1.1 billion people worldwide who use tobacco products, and most of these want to stop [15]. Approximately 70% of smokers report that they want to quit, one third of them try to stop smoking each year, but only 20% of them seek help [15–17]. Most quit attempts are unassisted (willpower alone) and are associated with low success rates (3–5%) [18]. In addition the majority of people who do successfully stop smoking will relapse. Smokers have a higher rate of success when they seek help with quitting. Even then, giving up permanently is difficult and several attempts are often required before long-term abstinence is achieved [15–18]. Cigarette smoking is governed by social, psychological, habitual, and behavioral factors as well as by nicotine addiction.

Nicotine addiction is a chronic relapsing condition that can be difficult to treat. Withdrawal symptoms of nicotine abstinence begin hours after quitting, peak at approximately 7 days, and then gradually decrease over 4–12 weeks. The nicotine withdrawal syndrome may include the following: dysphonic or depressed mood; in-

Table 54.5. The Fagerström test for nicotine dependence

		Points
1. How soon after you wake up do you smoke your first cigarette?	Within 5 min	3
	6–30 min	2
	31–60 min	1
	After 60 min	0
2. Do you find it difficult to refrain from smoking in places where it is forbidden?	Yes	1
	No	0
3. Which cigarette would you most hate to give up?	The first one in the morning	1
	Any other	0
4. How many cigarettes per day do you smoke?	≤10	0
	11–20	1
	21–30	2
	≥31	3
5. Do you smoke more frequently during the first hours after waking than during the rest of the day?	Yes	1
	No	0
6. Do you smoke if you are so ill that you are in bed most of the day?	Yes	1
	No	0

somnia; irritability; frustration or anger; anxiety; difficulty in concentrating; restlessness; decreased heart rate; and increased appetite and weight gain. Nicotine dependence should be assessed and recorded for every smoker using the Fagerström Tolerance Questionnaire (FTQ) or the modified Fagerström Test for Nicotine Dependence (FTND) (Table 54.5) [19].

54.3.2   Smoking Cessation and the Role of Healthcare Providers

Healthcare providers, particularly physicians, dentists, and nurses, have a professional as well as an ethical obligation to discourage tobacco use by their patients. Many professional organizations have stressed the importance of reducing smoking to reduce premature death worldwide. The American College of Chest Physicians, the American Thoracic Society, the Asia Pacific Society of Respirology, the Canadian Thoracic Society, the European Respiratory Society, and the International Union Against Tuberculosis and Lung Diseases have started in an official report that the physician has a responsibility to play a strong and active role in seeking to reduce smoking [20]. Providers can demonstrate their responsibility in their own behavior as well, by: (1) striving for a smoke-free profession; (2) never using tobacco in the presence of their patients; (3) making professional meetings smoke-free; (4) enforcing smoke-free regulations in their hospitals and practices; and (5) using their professional organizations to develop a strong antismoking policy and advocacy position.

The involvement of physicians in smoking prevention and cessation has grown slowly over time and varies substantially between specialties, as well as between nations. While physicians receive training in the adverse pathophysiological consequences of tobacco use, most are not adequately trained in providing smoking cessation counseling [21]. In addition, physicians often believe that cessation counseling takes too much time, and they become discouraged if their patients fail to quit smoking. Physicians may help more actively now as effective treatment resources are available. Engaging other healthcare providers (e.g., nurses or psychologists) to promote smoking cessation is important. Incorporating information about smoking cessation in medical school curricula and in continuing medical education is essential.

54.3.3 Clinical Guidelines for Smoking Cessation

Healthcare providers should deliver state-of-the-art assistance to help their smoking patients to quit. Given that the health benefits of stopping smoking are enormous, and that significant morbidity, mortality, and economic effects are attributed to smoking, a number of smoking cessation guidelines have been published in recent years that provide recommendations for interventions and strategies to promote the treatment of tobacco dependence.

These recommendations reflect a global movement toward evidence-based medicine, and reflect the fact that an increasing number of countries are adopting evidence-based guidelines for the treatment of tobacco dependence. A number of authoritative reviews and guidelines have recently been published [22–27]. These reviews and guidelines draw on hundreds of well-controlled trials, and emphasize not only that treatment for tobacco dependence is effective, but also that it is extremely cost effective.

These guidelines contain patient-oriented material, advice guidelines for primary care providers, and detailed information for smoking cessation specialists. In

Table 54.6. Recommendations for brief interventions. As part of their normal clinical work, health professionals should provide brief interventions including the following essential features

Ask	Ask about and record smoking status; keep record up to date
Advise	Advise smokers of the benefit of stopping in a personalized and appropriate manner (this may include linking the advice to their clinical condition)
Assess	Assess their motivation to stop
Assist	Assist smokers in their attempt to stop, if possible; this might include the offer of support, recommendation to use NRT or bupropion and accurate information and advice about them, or referral to a specialist cessation service if necessary
Arrange	Arrange a follow-up, if possible

NRT nicotine replacement therapy

all of these guidelines there is general agreement about what constitutes effective treatment.

According to these guidelines physicians should routinely assess and record patients' smoking status; advise smokers to quit; assess their readiness to do so; and assist smokers by offering support themselves through counseling, pharmacotherapy, and follow-up or refer them to more intensive specialist support (Tables 54.6, 54.7; Fig. 54.1) [28].

54.3.4 Smoking Cessation Clinics

The healthcare system should offer treatment as back up to brief opportunistic interventions for those smokers who need more intensive support. This support can be offered individually or in groups, and should include coping skills training and social support. A well-tested group format includes around five sessions of about one hour over about one month with follow-up. Intensive support should include the offer of or encouragement to use pharmacotherapy (as appropriate) and clear advice and instruction on how to use them.

Table 54.7. Key points for health professionals and advice to smokers

Health professionals	Advice to smokers
Set a stop day and stop completely on that day	Completely quit at target quit day
Review past experience and learn from it (what helped? what hindered?)	Prevent smoking even a single cigarette during the first 2 weeks
Make a personalized action plan	Withdrawal symptoms last 2–3 min with intervals without symptoms of 20–30 min. Do something physical to distract thoughts from withdrawal symptoms
Identify likely problems and plan how to cope with them	Use adequate NRT or bupropion SR (Zyban)
Ask family and friends for support	Rewarding: self-reward and support from others
	Follow-up should be arranged (general practitioner, smoking cessation clinic)

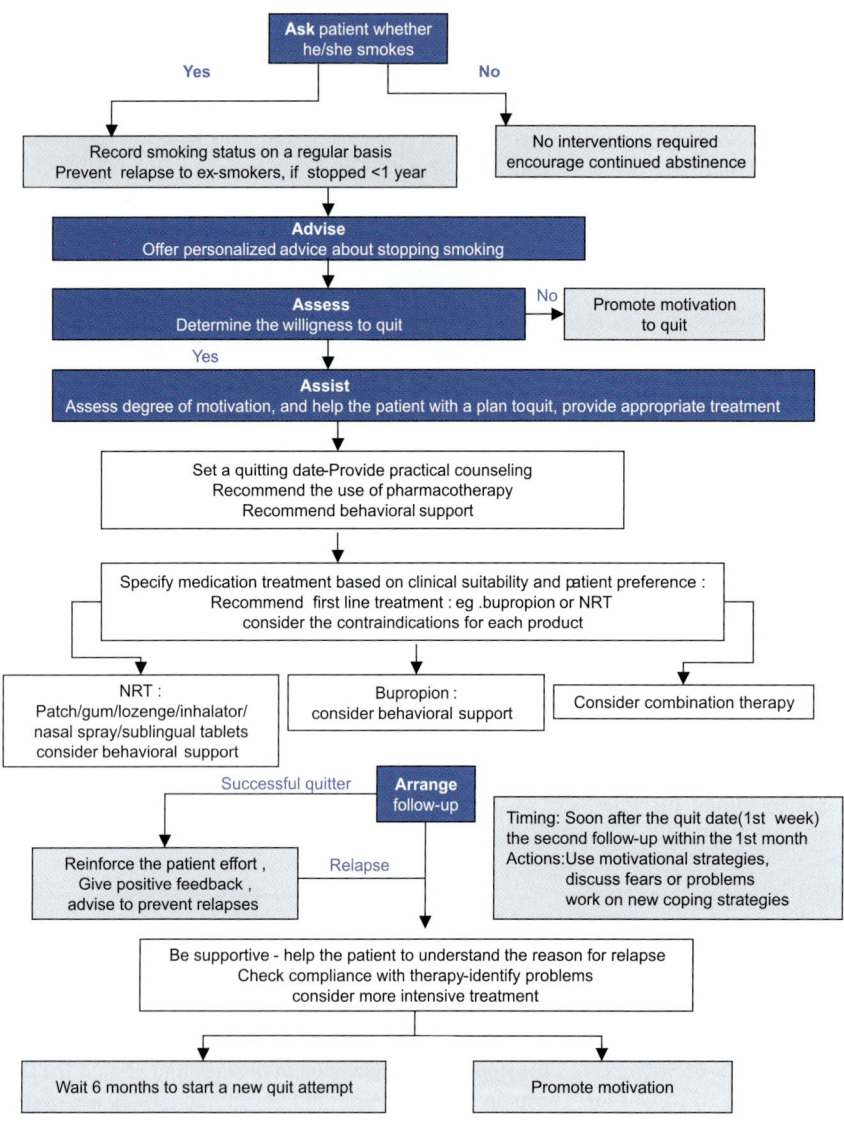

Fig. 54.1. Recommended smoking cessation steps and approved first-line interventions. *NRT* Nicotine replacement therapy

Treatment research has tended to focus on health professionals such as doctors (especially in primary care), nurses, midwives, pharmacists, and smoking cessation specialists. However advising and supporting smokers in stopping is an activity for the whole health-care system and should, eventually, be integrated into as many settings as possible throughout the system. This includes hospital and community settings. However in many countries there is still high smoking prevalence among health professionals, so in addition to the education and training recommended below, health professionals should, where appropriate, be targeted for help in stopping smoking. Hospital staff should ask about patients' smoking status prior to or on admission, and offer brief advice and assistance to those interested in stopping. Patients should be advised of the hospital's smoke-free status before admission. Hospital patients who need it should also be offered medication treatment.

There are three types of intervention:
1. Brief opportunistic interventions delivered by health professionals in the course of their routine work
2. More intensive support delivered by treatment specialists, often in what have been called "smokers clinics"
3. Pharmacological aids, which approximately double cessation in minimal or more intensive settings.

Pharmacotherapy and counseling are effective, but the two in combination achieve the highest rates of smoking cessation. The efficacy of a treatment correlates with its intensity, but even brief interventions by physicians during an office visit promote smoking cessation (Table 54.6). Providing a brief period of counseling (3 min or less) is more effective than simply advising the patient to quit and doubles the cessation rate, as compared with no intervention [23].

An individual approach to smokers by the health professionals with discussion of personal problems following a specific design of a cessation program will enable most smokers to overcome their addiction with success. An intensive program with weekly visits, personal consultation by the respiratory physician, and use of pharmacotherapy can increase the cessation rate of the motivated smokers who try to quit [28, 29].

Telephone help lines can be effective and are very popular with smokers. Although more research is needed on their effectiveness, they seem likely to provide a valuable service to smokers and should be made available where possible.

54.3.5 Pharmacological Treatment

First-line Treatment

Numerous effective pharmacotherapies for smoking cessation now exist. Nicotine replacement therapy (NRT) or sustained-released bupropion (bupropion SR) in conjunction with behavioral intervention for the management of smoking cessation are recommended as the first-line smoking cessation interventions [22–27]. Ex-

cept in the presence of contraindications, these should be used with all patients attempting to quit smoking. Smokers of ten or more cigarettes a day who are ready to stop should be encouraged to use NRT or bupropion as a cessation aid. Health professionals who deliver smoking cessation interventions should give smokers accurate information and advice on these products.

Nicotine Replacement Therapy

Nicotine dependence is a significant element of tobacco addiction and so a standard approach to pharmacological-based smoking cessation has been the use of NRT. NRT aims to replace the nicotine obtained from cigarettes, thus reducing withdrawal symptoms when stopping smoking. Various forms of NRT, such as gum, patches, inhalers, nasal spray, sublingual tablets, and lozenges, have been found to be efficacious and well tolerated (Tables 54.8, 54.9) [30, 31].

Dosages used in NRT may depend on the number of cigarettes smoked per day. Use should normally be restricted to the licensed duration of the form of NRT used. However, use may continue for up to 3 months in cases of continuing nicotine dependency (in the case of nicotine patches, use should be reduced after 3 months). NRT should be discontinued if the user restarts smoking [29, 30].

Table 54.8. Formulations of nicotine replacement therapies

Formulation	Trade name	Supplier
Nicotine transdermal patches:		
5, 10, 15 mg	Nicorette	Pharmacia
7, 14, 21 mg per 24 h	Nicotinell TTS 10, TTS 20, and TTS 30	Novartis Consumer Health
7, 14, 21 mg	NiQuitin CQ	GlaxoSmithKline
Nicotine chewing gum 2, 4 mg	Nicorette	Pharmacia
	Nicotinell	Novartis Consumer Health
Nicotine 2-mg sublingual tablet	Nicorette Microtab	Pharmacia
Nicotine 1-mg lozenge	Nicotinell	Novartis Consumer Health
Nicotine 10-mg inhalation cartridge plus mouthpiece	Nicorette Inhalator	Pharmacia
Nicotine 0.5 mg per puff metered nasal spray	Nicorette	Pharmacia
Nicotine 2- and 4-mg lozenge	NiQuitin CQ	GlaxoSmithKline

Table 54.9. Nicotine replacement formulations and dosages suggested for smoking cessation

NCD	FTND	NNS	Nicotine replacement therapy		
			Nicotine gum	24-h nicotine patch	16-h nicotine patch
10–19	≤3		2 mg/90 min for 6–8 weeks	21 mg/day for 4 weeks 14 mg/day for 2 weeks 7 mg/day for 1 week	15 mg/day for 4 weeks 10 mg/day for 2 weeks
20–30	4–6		4 mg/90 min for 12 weeks	21 mg/day for 6 weeks 14 mg/day for 4 weeks 7 mg/day for 2 weeks	25 mg/day for 6 weeks 15 mg/day for 4 weeks 10 mg/day for 2 weeks
More than 30	≥7	2–3 mg/h for 3–6 months	4 mg/60 min for 3–6 months		

NCD number of cigarettes smoked daily, *FTND* smoking dependence Fagerström scale (0–10 points), *NNS* nicotine nasal spray

Smokers with certain conditions (cardiovascular disease, hyperthyroidism, diabetes mellitus, severe renal or hepatic impairment, and peptic ulcer) are advised to use an NRT only after careful consideration of risks and benefits and after discussion with a healthcare professional. Similar advice applies to women who are pregnant or breastfeeding. Healthcare professionals should take into account the significant harm associated with continuing to smoke and that it can be expected that NRT will deliver less nicotine (and none of the other potentially disease-causing agents) than would be obtained from cigarettes.

Nicotine replacement therapies are generally very well tolerated. Actually this might be underscored by the fact that all six formulations are available from pharmacies without prescription in most countries. The most common adverse effects are localized reactions, particularly skin irritation with patches and nasal irritation with sprays, and do not generally require discontinuation of treatment. Sleep disturbances, which are a feature of withdrawal from tobacco, are also reported with nicotine patches.

The use of NRT increases the long-term rates of smoking cessation and relieves cravings for nicotine and the symptoms of nicotine withdrawal. The Cochrane review of over 90 trials found that nicotine replacement helps people to stop smoking [29]. A total of 96 placebo-controlled randomized trials of the use of NRTs has found them to increase a smoker's chances of stopping smoking for at least 6 months by 7 percentage points. With the addition of behavioral support the cessation rates are increased to 15 percentage points. Early relapse is common in studies of NRT and is predictive of an unsuccessful cessation attempt.

Individual NRT formulations have proven efficacy in smokers motivated to make a quit attempt, and there is little direct evidence that one nicotine product is more effective than another. Thus the decision about which product to use should be guided by individual preferences. In some smokers who are heavily dependent it may be beneficial to combine NRT products. In Europe NRT can be found on prescription, over-the-counter, and on general sale.

Bupropion Hydrochloride SR

Bupropion SR is the first non-nicotine-containing pharmacological agent that has been approved for use in smoking cessation and it received regulatory approval in both the USA and the European Union in 1997 [23–27]. Bupropion SR has proven efficacy in people who smoke more than 10–15 cigarettes per day who are motivated to stop.

Bupropion SR is considered as a useful option for smokers attempting to stop smoking for the first time, and in those who either cannot tolerate NRTs, those who prefer non-nicotine treatment, or those in whom

Table 54.10. Treatment with bupropion SR: advantages, disadvantages, and dosages suggested for smoking cessation

Advantages
It is active via oral route
It is easy to use
Odds ratio for success is 2.10 (95% CI, 1.62–2.73)
While used, it can control weight gain
Disadvantages
It can produce drug interactions
Insomnia and dry mouth are the most common side effects
Dosage
150 mg/day during the first 7–15 days, then dosage should be increased to a maximum daily dose of 300 mg (administered as 150 mg twice daily)
The duration of treatment is 7–12 weeks; in some cases 6–12 months
Bupropion should be initiated 1–2 weeks before the target quit date

NRT has failed [23–27, 32–35]. Recommended dosages are shown in the Table 54.10. A reduced dosage – that is, one tablet daily – is recommended in elderly people and those with liver or renal impairment. The recommended duration of treatment with bupropion SR for smoking cessation is 7–12 treatment weeks. Unlike NRT, bupropion SR therapy is initiated approximately 1 week prior to a cessation attempt. Treatment with bupropion SR should be accompanied by a motivational support program highlighting additional information on quitting and relapse prevention. Bupropion SR is a prescription only medicine.

Studies comparing bupropion to NRT are very limited and there is insufficient evidence at this time to recommend one over the other. Choice based on patient preference and consideration of adverse effects and comorbidity is reasonable given the lack of evidence. More research is also needed on combined treatment with bupropion and NRT. In addition, further research is required comparing the effectiveness of different antidepressants (e.g., nortriptyline) as a smoking cessation treatment.

Mechanism of Action of Bupropion SR

The postulated mechanism of action of bupropion SR differs from that of nicotine replacement therapy, which replaces the nicotine in cigarette smoke with nicotine delivered by an alternative route. Bupropion SR is a non-nicotine treatment acting on neurological pathways involved in nicotine dependence [36]. Bupropion is a selective inhibitor of the neuronal reuptake of catecholamines (noradrenaline and dopamine) with minimal effect on the re-uptake of serotonin and no inhibitory effect on monoamine oxidase. Nicotine is known to produce activation of the mesolimbic system, resulting in dopamine release in the nucleus accumbens. This is the pathway thought to be responsible for reward and cravings, while withdrawal is thought to be related to altered noradrenergic activity in the locus coeruleus. Bupropion has been shown to reduce the activity of these dopamine-releasing neurons and thereby may deactivate the reward circuit and reduce craving. Bupropion has been shown to reduce the activity of norepinephrine-releasing neurons in animals. Moreover, at clinically relevant doses in man, bupropion reduced whole-body turnover of norepinephrine without altering plasma norepinephrine levels. These noradrenergic effects may contribute to the ability of bupropion to mitigate symptoms of withdrawal. Besides inhibiting norepinephrine and dopamine reuptake, recent in vitro data indicate that bupropion SR may be a non-competitive, functional inhibitor of nicotinic acetylcholine receptors [37]. This antinicotinic activity of bupropion SR may also contribute to its efficacy in the treatment of nicotine dependence.

Contraindications and Precautions for Treatment with Bupropion SR

Bupropion SR is contraindicated in patients with current or past epilepsy. It should also be used with extreme caution in patients with conditions predisposing to a low threshold for seizure – history of head trauma, alcohol misuse, diabetes treated with hypoglycemic agents or insulin – and in patients taking drugs that lower the seizure threshold (for example, theophylline, antipsychotics, antidepressants, and systemic corticosteroids). Bupropion is also contraindicated in patients with a history of anorexia nervosa and bulimia, severe hepatic necrosis, or bipolar disorder. Bupropion should not be used with a monoamine oxidase inhibitor, and at least 14 days should elapse between stopping such treatment and starting bupropion. Bupropion interacts with a number of commonly used drugs, including some antidepressants, type 1c antiarrhythmics, and antipsychotics [23–27, 36, 37].

Second-line Smoking Cessation Treatments

Nortriptyline, a tricyclic antidepressant, is the only other antidepressant demonstrating evidence of efficacy. Nortriptyline is related to an increased rate of serious cardiac events among those with ischemic heart disease [38].

Clonidine, an imidazoline used in the management of hypertension, has been reported to have limited efficacy as a smoking cessation therapy [39]. It has been recommended as a second-line therapy in US smoking cessation guidelines [23]. However, adverse effects associated with clonidine, such as drowsiness, fatigue, and dry mouth, may limit its use, and the drug is likely to play only a second-tier role in smoking cessation [39].

54.3.6 Other Alternative Therapies

Acupuncture

The Cochrane review of 20 trials found no benefit of acupuncture compared with sham acupuncture. Acupuncture may be better than doing nothing, but this is likely to be a placebo effect [40].

Hypnotherapy

The Cochrane review of nine small trials of hypnotherapy found it no more effective than other behavioral interventions [41]. Hypnotherapy is difficult to evaluate in the absence of a sham procedure to control for non–specific effects.

54.4   General Recommendations for Smoking Cessation

54.4.1   Addressing Barriers to Smoking Cessation

According to the guidelines [23–27] there are some basic principles relating to successful smoking cessation that are important for the physician to consider:
- Patients must stop smoking completely at quit day. Even 1 or 2 cigarettes per day during the first 2 weeks of cessation are usually followed by relapse.
- Use of nicotine replacement therapy lessens withdrawal symptoms and improves cessation outcomes.
- Use of bupropion can start 1–2 weeks before the quit date with instructions for a progressive reduction in number of cigarettes up to the quitting day.
- Follow-up should be arranged to prevent relapse (which is highest during the first 3–6 weeks and then gradually declines, similar to other addictions).
- If the patient relapses, encourage him or her to make another quit attempt (the average 12-month success rate reported in most studies is 15–25%).

54.4.2   Addressing High-risk Populations

As smoking is a complex, multifactor addiction, the presence of various social and clinical factors can make it harder for some smokers to quit than others. Individuals at highest risk for smoking-related tumors should be targeted for the most intensive interventions. Vulnerable populations include patients with smoking-related prior cancers; other smoking-related diseases (e.g., coronary heart disease, chronic obstructive pulmonary disease, and vascular diseases); chronic heavy smokers; survivors of any cancer site who continue to smoke; and genetically susceptible individuals (once reliable and valid biomarkers are established). Furthermore, intensive smoking cessation treatment (combining behavioral and pharmacotherapy), delivered by clinical specialists, could be integrated into chemoprevention trials which recruit former, but not current smokers. One design suggestion would be to provide such treatment during the run-in period and to incorporate smoking cessation as an eligibility criterion for randomization in such clinical trials. Booster treatments to maintain abstinence could be made readily available. Research might also examine the relationship of nicotine dependence, smoking cessation, and chemoprevention efficacy, involving genetic, behavioral, and biological variables as predictors and endpoints. Another interesting area for research is to clarify what benefits a person can gain in reducing smoking but not quitting and how successful it is in assisting those unwilling or unable to quit to reduce their cigarette intake [42].

54.5 Protection from Environmental Tobacco Smoke

The increasing awareness that passive smoking or environmental tobacco smoke (ETS) is harmful to health has led many governments to provide legislation to protect the general public from passive (involuntary) smoking. The recent declaration (2002) by the WHO's International Agency for Research on Cancer that exposure to ETS is carcinogenic to humans reflects the position of the scientific community as a whole. The focus of occupational legislation is to provide safe work environments. Recent court cases have demonstrated that the protection of workers from ETS at their place of work is becoming an important occupational health issue.

Epidemiological studies have shown that passive smoking has serious health effects (Table 54.11) similar to those seen from active smoking albeit at lower levels [6, 42], namely:

- An increased risk of lung cancer (possibly increased by 20–30%)

- An increased risk of heart disease (estimated at 25–30%)
- An increased risk of stroke (possibly as high as 82%)
- A reduction in birth weight of infants born to mothers exposed to ETS
- An increased frequency of chronic respiratory symptoms such as cough, phlegm production, shortness of breath, and chest colds.

Legislation prohibiting smoking in all public places and workplaces would have most impact in protecting people from second-hand smoke as this has been classified as an occupational carcinogen by the Environmental Protection Agency IARC. The legislation developed in Ireland and Norway should serve as a model for a common European directive. This action is considered very important in the EC recommendation ASPECT consortium [6].

54.6 Cost of Tobacco Control

54.6.1 Cost of Smoking-related Diseases

While both epidemiological and clinical data concerning smoking-related diseases is widely available, less is known regarding the costs of smoking-related diseases borne by the healthcare sector, patients and their families, and society as a whole.

A US study reports the difference in medical expenditure for people with smoking-related diseases, compared to those without, to be 6 billion US dollars [43]. A cost of illness study carried out in Germany estimated the total smoking-related healthcare costs (attributable fraction due to smoking) for chronic obstructive pulmonary disease to be 5.471 billion euros (73%), for lung cancer 2.593 billion euros (89%), for cancer of the mouth and larynx 0.996 billion euros (65%), for stroke 1.774 billion euros (28%), for coronary artery disease 4.963 billion euros (35%), and for atherosclerotic occlu-

Table 54.11. Health effects of second-hand smoke

Adults	Children	Other proven health effects of passive smoking
Lung cancer	Cot death (sudden infant death syndrome)	Shortness of breath
Coronary heart disease	Middle-ear disease (ear infections)	Nausea
Onset of symptoms of heart disease	Respiratory infections	Airway irritation
Asthma attacks in those already affected	Development of asthma in those previously unaffected	Headache
Worsening of symptoms of bronchitis	Asthma attacks in those already affected	Coughing
Stroke		Eye irritation
Reduced fetal growth (low-birth-weight baby)		
Premature birth		

sive disease 0.761 billion euros (28%). The economic burden of smoking-related health care for Germany is 16.6 billion euros, with smoking being responsible for 47% of the total costs of these diseases, that is 35.2 billion euros [44].

The annual costs to the UK National Health Service (NHS) of adult smoking-related diseases approach 2.3 billion euros [45, 46]. In the UK, costs related to premature deaths due to smoking are estimated to be 130 billion euros; lung cancer is associated with 5.7% of all smoking-related NHS costs. Of the healthcare costs, 90% of lung cancer costs are from hospital rather than primary care. The global burden of the healthcare-related cost of smoking for Italy was estimated to be 4,312.71 million euros (cardiovascular disease: 2,464.19; chronic obstructive pulmonary disease: 451.53; small cell lung cancer: 58.06; non-small cell lung cancer: 232.25; stroke: 1,106.67); all amounts are expressed in 1998 million euros [47].

The Health and Economic Consequences of Smoking (HECOS) model estimates the health and economic burden of smoking-related diseases across all the EU countries and Australia, Canada, China, Czech Republic, Hungary, Mexico, New Zealand, Norway, Poland, and the Ukraine. The first version of the model was presented in May 1999, on World No-Tobacco day. The model is in the public domain and can be accessed via a dedicated European WHO website [48].

54.6.2 Cost Effectiveness of Smoking Cessation Interventions

As far as the economics of smoking cessation are concerned, all programs aimed at stopping smoking are highly cost effective when compared to other healthcare programs.

When expressed in 1997 prices, smoking cessation interventions are more cost effective (US$ 2,700 per year of life saved) than other healthcare programs targeted to different diseases, such as mammography screening (US$ 50,000 per year of life saved) and treatment of high cholesterol levels (US$ 100,000 per year of life saved) [23, 47]. According to one of the most important contributions on the cost effectiveness of smoking cessation interventions carried out in UK the cost per year of life saved ranged from 354 euros (GP's brief advice to stop smoking) to 1,458 euros (GP's advice + self-help + advice to purchase NRT with specialist services) when inflated to 1998 prices. All these figures included healthcare and non-healthcare resource use related cost [45, 46].

54.7 Recommendations for Healthcare Purchasers and Systems

Because tobacco-dependence treatment is so cost effective, it should be provided by public and private health care systems.

The general recommendations include as follows [23–27].

54.7.1 Healthcare System

- Healthcare delivery systems (including hospitals) are directed to identify patients' smoking status, offer smoking cessation services, and document these actions.
- Access to both behavioral and pharmaceutical treatments should be as wide as possible with due regard to local regulatory frameworks and other circumstances.
- The Public Health Service guidelines urge health insurers to cover all recommended treatments, including counseling and pharmacotherapy.
- Mechanisms should be found to increase the availability of treatment to low-income smokers, including at a reduced cost or free of charge.

54.7.2 Education of Health Professionals

- Health professionals should be trained to advise and help smokers stop smoking, and healthcare purchasers should ensure the provision of adequate training, budgets, and training programs.
- Education and training for the different types of interventions should be provided not only at the postgraduate and clinical level, but should start at undergraduate and basic level, in medical and nursing schools and other relevant training institutions.

A smoking cessation specialist is someone trained and paid to deliver skilled support to smokers who need help in stopping, over and above brief opportunistic advice. They need not be medically trained but should not be offering this support unpaid and squeezed into their normal work, as the evidence suggests this is not effective.

54.7.3 Other Suggestions

- Healthcare premises and their immediate surroundings should be smoke-free.

● A system for healthcare education, smoking cessation clinics, and protection of workers from exposure to passive smoking can be promoted through smoke-free hospitals.

54.8   Conclusion

Cigarette smoking is one of the leading causes of preventable death and disability in the world as nearly 4 million people globally each year are estimated to die as a result of smoking. Reducing the number of current smokers should substantially lower future smoking-related morbidity and mortality. Health professionals play a vital role in promoting smoking cessation and in discouraging initiation of tobacco use. Physicians have to realize that nicotine addiction is a chronic condition that needs long-term management with interventions that are extremely cost effective but underused. Tobacco users must not be left to stop smoking on their own and most healthcare professionals should help people who are willing to stop smoking. An extra urgency is required in promoting smoking cessation worldwide.

Brief counseling advice and specific pharmacological treatment may be implemented effectively in routine medical care. Special care and more intensive interventions may increase the success rates of smoking cessation among older smokers and patients with chronic diseases.

Assessing smoking status should become as routine as assessing vital signs. Intervention with all smoking patients is critical if reductions in morbidity and mortality are to be achieved. While pharmacotherapy greatly enhances cessation outcomes, cessation counseling and behavioral strategies are important adjuncts for maintaining long-term smoking cessation. Healthcare providers should take advantage of the excellent resources now available which provide effective smoking cessation models that can be easily incorporated into clinical practice. However, support and treatment to help smokers stop is not yet widely available. It is not generally integrated into European healthcare systems, although some countries are now making a start. Paradoxically, in contrast to the restricted availability of help for smokers in stopping (including pharmaceutical products designed to alleviate tobacco withdrawal), the tobacco products whose use causes the enormous burden of death and disease described above are extremely widely available. Governmental contribution to support tobacco-dependence treatment may help more smokers to quit and thus offer more opportunities in overcoming tobacco dependence not only in individuals but also in the population as a whole.

Key Points

● Tobacco dependence is now a well-defined medical condition that is the major cause of avoidable morbidity and early mortality.
● Social attitudes, legislation, and public health measures influence changes in tobacco use.
● The healthcare system has to realise the cost benefit of tobacco use based on the world mortality due to smoking-related diseases.
● Programs for smoking prevention, education, and smoking cessation are essential to control tobacco use.
● An extra urgency is required in promoting smoking cessation worldwide.
● Physicians have to realise that nicotine addiction is a chronic condition that needs long-term management with interventions that are extremely cost effective but underused.
● Recent increases in the number of approved drugs for smoking cessation have given healthcare providers a broad range of treatment approaches.
● Support and treatment to help smokers stop is one of the major approaches to tobacco control. It is an issue not just for individual health professionals in their work with smokers, but for the entire healthcare system.

References

1. European Commission. European Opinion Research Group. Smoking and the environment: actions and attitudes. Special Euro barometer 183/Wave 58.2, 2003; 1. http://europa.eu.int./comm/public_pinion/
2. World Bank. Curbing the epidemic: governments and the economics of tobacco control. Washington DC, 1999. www1.WorldBank.org/tobacco/chapter1.asp
3. Peto R, Lopez AD, Boreham J, Thun M, Heath C Jr, Doll R. Mortality from smoking worldwide. Br Med Bull 1996; 52:12.
4. European Respiratory Society (ERS). The burden of lung disease. In: Loddenkemper R, Gibson GJ, Sibille Y (eds) European Lung White Book: The First Comprehensive Survey on Respiratory Health in Europe. Sheffield, UK: ERSJ, 2003:7.
5. European Respiratory Society (ERS). Lung cancer. In: Loddenkemper R, Gibson GJ, Sibille Y (eds) European Lung White Book: The First Comprehensive Survey on Respiratory Health in Europe. Sheffield, UK: ERSJ, 2003:44.
6. World Health Organization (WHO). Guidelines for Controlling and Monitoring the Tobacco Epidemic. Prepublication draft. Geneva: WHO, 1995.
7. Europe against cancer programme. Official Journal 26/2/1987; C:50:58.
8. European Commission. Tobacco or health in the European Union: the ASPECT Consortium. October 2004 http://europa.eu.int
9. CDC. Reasons for tobacco use and symptoms of nicotine withdrawal among adolescent and young adult tobacco

users. Morbidity and Mortality Weekly Report 1994; 43:745.

10. IASLC Workshop. Prevention and early detection of lung cancer. Clinical aspects proceedings. Elsinore, Denmark, 1996.

11. Lightwood JM, Glantz SA. Short term economic and health benefits of smoking cessation. Circulation 1997; 96:1089.

12. Doll R, Peto R, Boreham J, et al. Mortality in relation to smoking: 50 years observation on male British doctors. BMJ 2004; 328:1519.

13. Scanlon PD, Connett JE, Waller LA, et al. Smoking cessation and lung function in mild to moderate chronic obstructive pulmonary disease: the Lung Health Study. Am J Res Crit Care Med 2000; 161:381.

14. Peto R, Darby S, Deo H, et al. Smoking, smoking cessation, and lung cancer in the UK since 1950: combination of national statistics with two case-control studies. BMJ 2000; 321:323.

15. World Health Organization (WHO). Tobacco or health: a global status report. Geneva: WHO, 1997.

16. Zhu SH, Melcer T, Sun J, et al. Smoking cessation with and without assistance: a population-based analysis. Am J Prev Med 2000; 18:305.

17. Royal College of Physicians. Nicotine addiction in Britain. London: Royal College of Physicians, 2000.

18. Hughes JR, Gulliver SB, Fenwick JW, et al. Smoking cessation among self-quitters. Health Psychol 1992; 11:331.

19. Fagerström K-O, Schneider N. Measuring nicotine dependence: a review of the Fagerström tolerance questionnaire. J Behav Med 1989; 12:159.

20. American College of Chest Physicians, American Thoracic Society, Asia Pacific Society of Respiratory, Canadian Thoracic Society, European Respiratory Society, International Union Against Tuberculosis and Lung Diseases Smoking and Health. A physician's responsibility: a statement of the joint committee on smoking and health. Eur Respir J 1995; 8:1808.

21. USDHHS Tobacco and the Clinician Interventions for Medical and Dental Practice, NCL 94-3693. US Department of Health and Human Services, Public Health Service, National Institutes of Health, 1994.

22. Fiore MC, Bailey WC, Cohen SJ, et al. Smoking cessation. Clinical practice guideline no. 18, AHCPR 96-0692. US Department of Health and Human Services, Public Health Service, Agency for Health Service, Agency for Health Care Policy and Research. The smoking cessation clinical practice guideline. Panel and staff. The Agency for Health Care Policy and Research. JAMA 1996; 275:1270.

23. Fiore MC, Bailey WC, Cohen SJ, et al. Treating tobacco use and dependence: quick reference guide for clinicians. Rockville, MD: US Department of Health and Human Services. Public Health Service, 2000.

24. West R, McNeill A, Ras M. Smoking cessation guidelines for health professionals: an update. Thorax 2000; 55:987.

25. World Health Organization (WHO). European partnership to reduce tobacco dependence: WHO evidence-based recommendations on the treatment of tobacco dependence. Geneva: WHO, 2001.

26. National Institute for Clinical Excellence (NICE). Guidance on the use of nicotine replacement therapy (NRT) and bupropion for smoking cessation. National Institute for Clinical Excellence Technology Appraisal Guidance 2002; 39. www.nice.org.uk

27. Andersson JE, Joremby DE, Scott WJ, Fiore MC. Treating tobacco use and dependence. Chest 2002; 121:932.

28. Gratziou CH. The process of stopping smoking. European Respiratory Seminar on Smoking Cessation. European Respiratory Society School. Budapest Dec 2004. www.ersnet.org/edu

29. Tonnesen P. Essential communication skills in individual smoking cessation. Review series: patient education. Chronic Respir Dis 2004; 1:221.

30. Fiore MC, Smith SS, Jorenby DE, et al. The effectiveness of the nicotine patch for smoking cessation: a meta-analysis. JAMA 1994; 271:1940.

31. Tonnessen P, Paoletti P, Gustavsson G, et al. Higher dosage nicotine patches increase one-year smoking cessation rates: results from the European CEASE-trial. Eur Respir J 1999; 13:238.

32. West R. Bupropion SR for smoking cessation: expert opinion. Drug Evaluation 2003; 533.

33. Coleman T, West R. Newly available treatments for nicotine addiction: smokers wanting help to stop smoking now have effective treatment options. BMJ 2001; 322:1076.

34. Holm KJ, Spencer CM. Bupropion: a review of its use in the management of smoking cessation. Drugs 2000; 59:1007.

35. Gratziou C, Francis K, Maragianni A, et al. Bupropion treatment and cognitive behavioral therapy in smoking cessation program. Eur Respir J 2001; 12

36. Balfour DJK. The pharmacology underlying pharmacotherapy for tobacco dependence: a focus on bupropion. Int J Clin Pract 2001; 55:53.

37. Slemmer JE, Martin BR, Damaj MI. Bupropion is a nicotinic antagonist. J Pharmacol Exp Ther 2000; 295:321.

38. Hall S, Humeet G, Reus V, et al. Psychological intervention and antidepressant treatment in smoking cessation. Arch Gen Psychiatry 2002; 59:930.

39. Benowitz NL, Wilson Peng M. Non-nicotine pharmacotherapy for smoking cessation. Mechanisms and prospects. CNS Drugs 2000; 13:265.

40. White A, Resch K, Ernst E. A metaanalysis of acupuncture techniques for smoking cessation. Tob Control 1999; 8:393.

41. Lancaster T, Stead LF. Individual behavioral counselling for smoking cessation. Cochrane Database Syst Rev 2000; 2:CD001292.

42. British Medical Association. Towards smoke-free public places. London: BMA, 2002.

43. Johnson E, Dominici F, Griswold M, et al. Disease cases and their medical costs attributable to smoking: an analysis of the national medical expenditure survey. J Econometrics 2003; 112:135.

44. Ruff LK, Volmer T, Nowak D, et al. The economic impact of smoking in Germany. Eur Respir J 2000; 16:385.

45. Parrott S, Godfrey C, Raw M, et al. Guidance for commissioners on the cost effectiveness of smoking cessation interventions. Thorax 1998; 53:S1.

46. Godfrey C. The economic and social costs of lung cancer and the economics of smoking prevention. Monaldi Arch Chest Dis 2001; 56:458.

47. WHO – World Health Organization. Economic consequences of smoking (ECOS) model. WHO European Partnership Project to Reduce Tobacco Dependence. Copenhagen-Geneva: WHO, 1999. http://www.who.dk/adt/ecos/whoweb.asp

48. Cromwell J, Bartosch WJ, Fiore MC, et al. Cost-effectiveness of the clinical practice recommendations in the AHCPR guideline for smoking cessation. Agency for Health Care Policy and Research. JAMA 1997; 278:1759.##

Cost Effectiveness of Smoking Cessation Interventions

55

Christine Godfrey and Steve Parrott

Contents

55.1 Introduction

Active and passive smoking cause a range of health and social problems that have associated economic costs. These costs are borne by a range of individuals and institutions in any society. The smoker bears the costs of ill-health and reduced length of life. Smoking-related illnesses may also have an impact on earnings. Families also bear a number of costs including the impact of secondhand smoke in the home on partners and particularly children and the unborn. The costs of care for smoking-related illness including lung cancer may fall partly on the families, other tax payers, or employers depending on the financing of the healthcare system. There are also considerable other costs associated with smoking in the workplace, including reduced productivity, smoking-related fires, and cleaning costs.

Reducing population rates of smoking primarily brings a very large health benefit both immediately and for the future by reducing future smoking-related illness and deaths. However, these reductions in smoking also reduce other costs, which have additional benefits for the smoker, the families, workmates, employers, and the rest of society.

Economic evaluation techniques combine the costs of different prevention or healthcare interventions with gains in health outcomes and reduction in other resource use. The aim is to compare interventions on their value for money per health outcome produced. This comparison can be between smoking and other healthcare interventions or across different types of actions available to reduce smoking. Given the potential benefits from reduced smoking, most available literature on the cost effectiveness of smoking suggest this is a very efficient use of government or healthcare provider's funds. Such interventions yield health gains in terms of increased quality and quantity of life at a much lower cost (or indeed in some cases saving resources) than most other healthcare interventions. However, many healthcare systems have failed to encourage smoking cessation activities. Even where the healthcare system does reward healthcare professionals to undertake such interventions and may also help smokers pay for pharmacotherapies, actual interventional use may be lower than expected.

The purpose of this chapter is to explore the evidence for cost-effective strategies to reduce smoking and, in particular, the role physicians and other healthcare professionals may play. In the second section of this chapter, the identification, measurement, and valuation of the costs and consequences of different smoking cessation interventions are explored. The existing economic evidence base is reviewed in the following two sectors. A range of different prevention strategies is briefly reviewed in the third section. The fourth section contains a more extensive discussion of economic evaluation of health professional-led interventions directed at aiding existing smokers to quit.

55.2 Economic Evaluations of Smoking Cessation: Identifying, Measuring, and Assessing the Costs and Consequences

Economic evaluations involve comparing the costs and consequences of alternative interventions. Such evaluations are directed at providing decision-makers with information about the most efficient use of scarce resources. The task for the evaluator is therefore to identify, measure, and value the different resource use, which would occur in implementing the different interventions being compared.

The evaluation of smoking cessation interventions presents a number of challenges. First is the nature of the main outcome of interest. To compare across smoking cessation interventions, it may be considered adequate to have some sort of validated measure of the change in smoking prevalence. However, expressing results in terms of the net costs per quitter does not allow the results to be put in the context of wider healthcare resource decision-making. For healthcare evaluations, a number of academic experts and policy makers have advocated the use of health utility measures so that the results can be expressed in terms of the net cost per quality adjusted life years (QALYs) saved, for example in the USA [1] and the UK [2]. Using a common outcome measure across healthcare interventions and common rules on methodology as these guidelines suggest allows the compilation of results. It is interesting to note that in such compilations, smoking cessation interventions are among the most cost effective [3].

However, most evaluations of smoking cessation interventions will have at most 12-month outcomes. While quitting can bring some immediate health benefits in terms of reduced morbidity and therefore increased quality of life, gains in mortality would be seen in the medium to longer term. It is therefore necessary to model the potential health gains. This requires a number of assumptions and steps. Fortunately there are now considerable data on gains in life expectancy from quitting smoking, even extending over 50 years of follow-up of the original UK doctors' study [4]. There are however fewer data on the quality of life changes. Tengs and Wallace suggest that there are gains in QALYs for all age bands and for men and women comparing smokers and those that have quit for more than 15 years [5]. These gains increase with age and are slightly higher for men than women.

Gains in mortality arise mainly from permanent quitting. As well as different ways of measuring quitting in interventions, for example biochemically validated or self-reported, there are different lengths of follow-up. Different interventions or different population groups may also be subject to different longer-term relapse rates.

Reduced smoking should also yield benefits in terms of reduced healthcare spending on smoking-related diseases. Who actually gains from such a reduction in expenditure will depend on the healthcare system, from tax payers, private insurers, employers, or the smokers themselves. A number of models have been built to forecast the changes in healthcare expenditure from changes in smoking prevalence [6]. Ironically many of the new detection and treatment possibilities for smoking-related diseases such as lung cancer may increase smoking-related treatment costs and therefore suggest that prevention activities may indeed be more cost effective. In a recent report, for example, the National Institute of Health and Clinical Excellence (NICE) in England estimated that it would cost £ 23 million (US$ 42 million) revenue costs to implement their current evidence-based guidance on lung cancer treatment and an additional £ 62 million (US$ 113 million) in capital costs [7].

More controversial is whether account should be taken of other healthcare expenditure over the projected lifetime. Living longer than the alternative of staying a smoker may over a lifetime result in an overall increase in total healthcare expenditure. Partly this resolves around the relative costs of smoking-related illnesses and chronic diseases more prevalent among older populations. Evidence from population-based studies has been mixed [8] although the majority of studies suggested that there are net overall costs of smoking. Guidance on economic evaluation techniques also reveals some controversy in the question as to whether to include unrelated healthcare costs. Clearly expanding the boundaries of economic evaluations outside the disease or risk factor in question would suggest that the other beneficial consequences of living longer should be included. In general, current economic evaluation guidelines suggest that to aid comparison between evaluations only related healthcare costs should be included.

There are a number of other consequences that arise from reduced levels of smoking. Smoking is related to lower productivity both from smoking-related sickness absences and smoking breaks at work. There are also risks from fires and additional cleaning costs. Environmental tobacco smoke however causes more harm than additional cleaning costs. Recent estimates put the number of deaths attributable to environmental tobacco smoke at 12,200 in the UK [9], compared to 114,000 from active smoking [10].

A more indirect impact occurs through reductions in overall population levels of smoking on the uptake of smoking by young people and quitting attempts by older smokers. These wider consequences are however generally very difficult to attribute to specific interventions and suggest many existing estimates of the cost effectiveness of smoking prevention interventions may be underestimating their value for money.

Finally to calculate the cost-effectiveness ratios of the interventions being considered data are required on the full costs of the interventions. It is perhaps surprising for such an important health intervention that there are few studies that have measured the costs of such interventions alongside primary intervention studies. While there is a rich body of evidence on effectiveness as can be accessed in the Cochrane Library, the economic evidence base is relatively small and the cost data within existing studies are relatively poor in quality. Interventions vary in the type of resource used. Most healthcare interventions involve the use of healthcare professional time and smoking cessation aids whether in terms of educational materials or drug therapies such as nicotine replacement therapies and bupropion. There are a number of different arrangements for the availability of such products, which impacts not only on the direct costs but also the time and search costs smokers may have obtaining such products. Other non-healthcare-based interventions such as changes in regulation or tax levels do not necessarily have the same type of costs but also require resources to enact and enforce. More reliable data are needed on the costs of different policies to correctly resolve the debate on whether resources should be devoted to smoking cessation activities or a mixture of interventions.

55.3 Cost Effectiveness of Tobacco Control Policies

Healthcare professionals have many important roles to play in reducing levels of smoking in the population. Undertaking active interventions with individual smokers to help them quit may be seen as their most obvious role, and the cost effectiveness of these activities is reviewed in the next section. Health professionals have led advocacy efforts to publicize the harms of both active and passive smoking as well as effective policies to reduce these harms. Wider tobacco control policies such as tax changes, advertising bans, and public place restrictions have the potential to have a major impact on population smoking prevalence. The economic aspects of a broad spectrum of policies were recently reviewed by the World Bank and the World Health Organization [11]. The reviews undertaken for this project provide an excellent evidence base for tobacco control policies.

The relationship between the prices of cigarettes and consumption has long been established in developed countries. The estimated price elasticities for such countries center around –0.4 which suggests that a 10% increase in prices would reduce cigarette consumption by 4% [12]. More recently additional studies have been undertaken in a broader range of countries and Chaloupka et al. [12] concluded that price effects in the lower or middle income countries are almost double those in the higher income countries. The impact on overall sales of tobacco include impacts on the fre-

quency and quantity of products consumed by smokers but also help initiate cessation and reduce initiation among young people. The overall costs of taxation and the costs of changing levels of taxation are relatively low and taxation is one of the most cost effective overall tobacco control policies.

Some policies may even be cost saving. Extending restrictions on smoking in the workplace have the ability to increase productivity in the workplace, save fire and cleaning costs as well as achieving health gains. Such bans, as well as saving lives through reducing environmental tobacco smoke, also have an impact on active smokers by encouraging them to quit and with the young by preventing them to start smoking. Recent estimates for the UK suggest that such a comprehensive ban may save over 150,000 lives in the longer term as a result of 300,000 stopping smoking [9].

In contrast, direct school prevention activities have only been found to have limited effectiveness, at most slightly delaying the onset of smoking, and are costly. More success has been gained from peer-led approaches. Tobacco policy advocates have noted that the tobacco industry has been supportive of the type of didactic prevention even though they are of limited effectiveness. However, young people while having knowledge about the health effects of smoking, and may even overestimate the risks of some smoking-related disease, are less knowledgeable about the risk of addiction [13] and some of the shorter-term health impacts [14]. This suggests there is a wider task for information-based approaches both in preventing misinformation from the tobacco industry's advertising and marketing activities and counter-advertising.

The evidence for partial bans on advertising suggests limited effectiveness but there is evidence that comprehensive bans are effective. The costs of imposing such a ban can be significant as considerably lobbying and preparatory work may be necessary to ensure such regulations pass legislative bodies and counter industry lobbying.

Finally there are community level interventions that are directed at increasing quit attempts. These can take the form of mass media campaigns, or supported competitions or events such as "quit and win". Parrott et al. [15] simulated the potential cost effectiveness of such interventions in England and Wales. Three types of policies were considered: a Quit and Win competition; a broader community-wide campaign; and a specific day and associated activities namely National No Smoking Day. Only the costs of the interventions and the health gains in terms of life years gained were considered. No attempt was made to estimate future healthcare cost savings, other consequences of these interventions, or the gains to quality of life of individual smokers and therefore these estimates are likely to overestimate the cost per life year gained. These estimates updated to 2003/04 prices are shown in Table 55.1. Similar low cost

Table 55.1. Cost effectiveness of community smoking cessation interventions, UK, 2003/04

Intervention	Cost per community (500,000 population)	Cost per life year saved[a]
Quit and win (low resource)	£ 19,499	£ 1,020
Quit and win (medium resource)	£ 116,994	£ 982
Quit and win (high intensity)	£ 490,261	£ 1,334
Broader community interventions	£ 35,052	£ 294
National No Smoking Day	£ 6,368	£ 40

[a] Effectiveness estimates discounted at 1.5% per annum
Source: Parrott et al. (1998) [15]. Cost figures uprated by Retail Price Index from 1997 to 2003/04 prices

per life year gained estimates have been found in studies from both the Netherlands [16] and the USA [17]. All estimates suggest these interventions are good value for money.

A recently published study applied modeling and survey methods to examine the impact of introducing comprehensive control measures in a specific location, New York City [18]. This program had four active components: increased taxes; a comprehensive ban on smoking in all workplaces including bars and restaurants; increased smoking cessation activities; and an education program. Over two years there was an 11% drop in adult smoking prevalence from 21.6% to 19.2%. It may postulated from the modeling exercises that approximately 45,000 of the smokers quitting could be attributed to tax increases, 18,000 to the ban on smoking in the workplace, and 11,000 to the free nicotine patch initiative. The survey evidence suggested that smokers

attributed slightly larger impacts to the tax increases and the smoke-free legislation. Also such comprehensive policies have synergistic effects. While not examining the different costs of the components of this initiative, it can be seen that these results are in line with previous research review evidence.

The review work undertaken for the World Bank has been extended and updated as part of the WHO-CHOICE program [19]. They provide estimates of the broad costs of policies and the projected health gains in terms of the net cost per disability adjusted life years (DALYs) for different regions of the world divided by geographical area, development status, and income level. The interventions include several different tax increase strategies, clean indoor air laws in public places through legislation and enforcement, a comprehensive ban on advertising of tobacco products, information dissemination through health warning labels, counter-advertising and various consumer information packages, nicotine replacement therapy, and various combinations of these policies. Each policy or combination was evaluated against the current policy in the region.

The latest results for a selection of these regions are shown in Table 55.2. Across all regions, including those not included in the table, all strategies are very cost effective compared to most healthcare interventions. The intervention to increase nicotine replacement therapy is one of the most costly strategies in every region but this is not surprising given the resource required. Other interventions, such as clean air laws, clearly vary with regional characteristics. Tax is one of the most cost-effective strategies in all regions.

There are some differences in the cost effectiveness of different components of tobacco control measures. Some elements seem cost ineffective especially some education programs. The other broad ranges of policies

Table 55.2. WHO-CHOICE cost-effectiveness estimates of different tobacco control strategies

Intervention	Average cost per disability adjusted life year (I$, 2000[a])					
	Euro A[b]	Euro C[c]	AMRO A[d]	WPR B[e]	SEARO B[f]	AFRO D[g]
Doubling region's maximum tax rate	13	18	18	15	5	58
Clean indoor air law and enforcement	358	201	725	795	513	4,077
Comprehensive advertising ban	189	129	313	268	103	931
Information dissemination	337	243	536	486	202	1,512
Nicotine replacement therapy	2,164	3,689	3,027	3,980	3,167	8,603
Combination of all five policies	274	488	371	429	300	849

[a] Results expressed in international dollars of 2000. Costs in local currency are converted to international dollars using purchasing power parity exchange rates. This and other details of the WHO-CHOICE methodology are set out on the website
[b] Euro A. Higher income Western European countries including UK
[c] Euro C. Central and Eastern European countries including Belarus, Estonia, Hungary, Moldova, and Ukraine
[d] AMRO A. American region including Canada, Cuba, and USA
[e] WPR B. Western Pacific Region including China, Fiji, and Malaysia
[f] SEARO B. South East Asia Region including Indonesia, North Korea, and Thailand
[g] AFRO D. African countries including Angola, Gambia, Madagascar, Nigeria, and Senegal
Source: WHO-CHOICE. Cost-effectiveness analyses. http://www3.who.int/whosis/cea (accessed 12 June 2005)

are very cost effective compared to many other health-care interventions as illustrated by the WHO-CHOICE analyses and other research. Specific thresholds below which health regulatory authorities would definitely recommend the adoption of interventions are difficult to definitely determine but are in the region of US$ 50,000 per QALY (or DALY). In the UK, the NICE [2] suggests that any intervention which yields a QALY at a net cost of less than £ 20,000 (US$ 36,450) would be adopted on economic criteria alone. This suggests all those policies in Table 55.2 would be recommended for adoption on cost-effectiveness criteria. It is important for such information to be widely disseminated and concerned health professionals have an important role to play in pressuring authorities to adopt evidence-based cost-effective tobacco control policies.

55.4 Cost Effectiveness of Health Professional-led Interventions

For most health professionals however their main role will be in identifying smokers and delivering smoking cessation advice, interventions, and referrals to help quit attempts. Considerable evidence exists which is based on the effectiveness of different types and intensities of interventions, delivered by various health professionals and to different types of smokers. Economic evaluations of these interventions are more limited and surprisingly few economic evaluations have been undertaken alongside randomized clinical trials.

In examining health professional-led interventions it may be useful to divide intervention types into those interventions which are focused on motivating smokers to make a quit attempt from those interventions which are designed to help motivated smokers to stop smoking. Levels of intensity and whether or not pharmacotherapies are used can further divide those interventions directed at motivated smokers.

55.4.1 Cost Effectiveness of Brief Interventions

In many countries smokers have quit through a variety of different methods. Some have quit without obvious health professional advice or aids of any kind. However, many smokers will make many quit attempts before they become permanent ex-smokers. Action taken by health professionals action to identify those smokers and then attempt to motivate them to quit is an important part of a tobacco control strategy. However, as may be expected the effectiveness of such interventions alone in increasing the quit rates among smokers may be only marginally increased on the background quit rate in the population.

There are a variety of methods which could be adopted to encourage quit attempts. Some are simple such as computerized systems for generating letters promoting quit attempts. Scott Lennox et al. [20] evaluated such a scheme in Scotland and generated an extra quitter at a cost of £ 89, and a cost-effectiveness ratio of between £ 50 and £ 122 per life year gained. In other cases brief interventions are encouraged by advertised telephone quit lines which may or may not be staffed by health professionals. An economic evaluation of one such telephone quit line in the USA suggests a cost of US$ 1,300 for each 12-month quitter [21]. Expressed in future life years saved the ratio would be lower.

In assessing the cost effectiveness of interventions there is a need to consider the screening and identification costs for smokers as well as the cost of any brief intervention delivered including the training of the health professionals. Sometimes the screening and identification costs could be considerable. Cromwell et al. [22], for example, estimated that in the USA a cost of US$ 14.51 for every smoker for a minimal screening and intervention in 1995 prices. This yielded a cost per QALY of US$ 4,015, which was much higher than the estimated cost effectiveness of more intensive and more effective strategies. In some healthcare systems, however, such monitoring and brief advice can be delivered opportunistically rather than requiring a separate and expensive visit to the healthcare provider and therefore may be delivered at a lower cost and greater cost effectiveness, see for example Parrott et al. [15] for a review of such studies from the UK and Comas-Fuentes et al. [23] for figures for Spain.

There is also potential for brief interventions to be delivered in a range of health settings, such as pharmacies, dentists, specialized healthcare clinics, etc. While there is a body of evidence about the effectiveness of such interventions in increasing quit attempts there are far fewer cost-effectiveness studies. In general all effective brief interventions have been shown to be cost effective despite their low overall effectiveness. This low overall rate of success is difficult for health professionals and perhaps such interventions have not been properly "marketed." The constant monitoring and screening of smokers in a variety of settings are likely to generate far more quit attempts and help smokers in a process of becoming smoke-free than the 12-month direct outcomes may suggest. Such schemes also allow health professionals to give advice on other smoking cessation methods and to refer motivated smokers who have found it hard to quit without further support to specialist and more intensive services.

55.4.2 Cost Effectiveness of Nicotine Replacement Therapies and Other Pharmacotherapies

There has been extensive research on the effectiveness of nicotine replacement therapy (NRT) in addition to other smoking cessation interventions whether brief or more intensive. It has been found that NRT doubles the rate of effectiveness of interventions [24]. However, the costs of such therapy are also considerable and so the relative cost effectiveness is more difficult to predict.

Stapleton et al. [25] demonstrated that contingent prescribing could increase the cost effectiveness of NRT in primary care. Their estimates suggested that such prescribing yields additional life years at a cost of between £ 398 (US$ 724) and £ 758 (US$ 1,380) in 1998 UK pounds compared to brief counseling alone. Similar estimates were found using US data with Wasley et al. [26]. Other studies have also demonstrated the potential cost effectiveness of NRT both in primary care and more specialist smoking cessation services [15, 22].

However, some NRT products are available over the counter. Some researchers have suggested that policies to increase the availability of NRT products are not as cost effective as other tobacco control policies. Ong and Glantz [27], for example, suggest that in Minnesota a free NRT program would generate 18,500 quitters at a cost of US$ 4,440 per QALY compared to a smoke-free workplace policy which would general 10,400 quitters at US$ 506 per QALY. However, the effectiveness of NRT varies with the intensity of the additional counseling as outlined in the next subsection. Making products available without the necessary additional support from health professionals may not be sufficient to impact on population quit rates. It is clear that the price of such products does impact on their use [28]. Also the coverage of smoking cessation interventions through healthcare plans or offering free NRT products or other pharmacotherapies increases their use but this coverage needs to be of sufficient time to be effective [29].

More recently a new therapy, bupropion, has become available and a number of other products are being developed. A few studies have examined the cost effectiveness of bupropion [30–33]. In some of these studies bupropion has been directly compared to NRT and found to be more cost effective but the evidence base for this difference is limited. Also Gilbert et al. [34] demonstrated that both NRT and bupropion are highly cost effective healthcare strategies in low mortality, middle income countries such as the Seychelles as well as the high income countries.

55.4.3 Cost Effectiveness of More Intensive Interventions Delivered to Motivated Smokers

Warner [35], in an early review, suggested that brief interventions may be more cost effective than more intensive therapies. However, these modeling studies did not take into account the potential coverage of different interventions and how they may vary with motivation.

Buck et al. [36] is one of the only economic evaluation studies based on cost data from a trial rather than modeling. This study looked at the cost effectiveness of a general physician-led intervention delivered to motivated smokers. Those smokers assessed by the specially trained physicians as being prepared to quit received a special booklet and a program of three visits and advice on using nicotine chewing tablets. Some modeling was required on the outcomes of the non-motivated smokers but even the most pessimistic assumptions yielded estimates of costs per quitter of US$ 984 in 1995 prices.

Cromwell et al. [22] was another modeling study but did take into account the costs of recruiting non-motivated smokers and the potential choices smokers may make in taking up interventions of different intensities. In this study the more intensive interventions were found to be comparatively more cost effective than the briefer interventions but the take-up was lower.

Feenstra et al. [37] by contrast simulated five face-to-face strategies compared to current practice for the Netherlands. Their model predicted QALY gains over 75 years and savings in future healthcare costs. All five strategies were cost effective compared to current practice but the minimal general practitioner counseling was actually cost saving. For the other strategies incremental cost per QALY gained ranged from € 1,100 for telephone counseling to € 4,900 for intensive counseling with nicotine patches or gum.

Woolacott et al. [32] found both NRT and bupropion SR to be effective interventions to assist smoking cessation. Based on a review of articles from 26 electronic databases, results showed the incremental cost per life year saved to be about £ 1,000–2,400 (US$ 1,820–4,370) for NRT, £ 640–1,500 (US$ 1,165–2,730) for bupropion SR, and £ 900–2,000 (US$ 1,640–3,640) for NRT plus bupropion SR. The estimated cost per life year saved about £ 750 (US$ 1,365). The authors concluded that NRT and/or bupropion SR are cost effective when compared with many accepted healthcare interventions.

Godfrey et al. [38] undertook a specific evaluation of the specialist smoking cessation services that were set up in the UK. These services were aimed at providing more intensive help to motivated smokers and deliver a range of individual and group counseling sessions combined with pharmacotherapies. All these services are free to smokers, apart from the standard prescription charges which patients, apart from the poor, would be required to pay. Data from the services themselves were used to model both costs and effectiveness. This analysis therefore reflects the performance of services in practice rather than the results of research studies often conducted in "ideal" settings. The services were delivering a range of individual and group interventions with and without pharmacotherapies. In this study, which did take future healthcare savings into account, an average cost effectiveness of £ 438 per life year gained (in 2000/01 prices) was found compared to the alternative of no specialized services being available. Even under the most conservative sensitivity analysis the mean cost-effectiveness ratios never exceeded £ 4,500 per life year gained. The figures from this study were very comparable to the results of Cromwell et al. [22], Orme et al. [6], and Woolacott et al. [32].

The main conclusion from the existing economic evaluations is that specialized treatment for smoking cessation compared to the alternative of no specialized treatment being available is a very cost effective healthcare intervention. It is possible to get these results in practice, and the results for face-to-face interventions seem to hold across a range of communities and countries. However, there is less evidence on the most cost effective mix of face-to-face interventions. Also further research is required on determining the incentives required for smokers and for health professionals to ensure the most cost effective coverage of these types of interventions.

55.5 Conclusions

Face-to-face smoking cessation interventions have an important role to play in any smoking cessation strategy. However, on their own such smoking cessation efforts will not have a large impact on overall population smoking prevalence rates. Parrott et al. [15], for example, suggested that in the UK even if 50% of current smokers were identified each year by their family physician and provided with a package of self-help, NRT, and referral a more specialist service the overall result would be a population quit rate of 1.12%. Wider tobacco control policies which have also been shown to be cost effective need to be implemented alongside these treatments for smokers in order to make a sizeable difference to population smoking rates. Health professionals have an important role to play in advocating such strategies.

Cost-effectiveness analysis relies upon complex epidemiological models to translate the impact of changes in smoking behavior into health outcomes such as life years gained, based upon changes in risks for a range of smoking-related diseases. There is also a need for more research to keep updating available models so that health professionals can demonstrate cost effectiveness

of different strategies using data from local populations. A more extensive database on estimating the resources required for different types of interventions as well as effectiveness rates would also be helpful for such modeling.

Current research does show that in terms of cost effectiveness, a number of tobacco control interventions do overwhelmingly provide excellent value for money compared to many other areas of healthcare competing for funds. For example, in the UK, the cost per life year estimated falls well below accepted benchmarks representing good value for money, as set down by commissioning organizations. These findings tend to be robust and hold true in different populations of smokers in different countries. This suggests that investment in tobacco control programs can generate considerable health gains from limited resources, and therefore represent an efficient use of healthcare budgets.

Key Points

- Active and passive smoking cause a range of health and social problems that have associated economic costs. Reducing population rates of smoking primarily brings a very large health benefit both immediately and for the future by reducing future smoking-related illness and deaths. However, these reductions in smoking also reduce other costs, which have additional benefits for the smoker, the families, workmates, employers, and the rest of society.
- Face-to-face smoking cessation interventions have an important role to play in any smoking cessation strategy, but they have a limited impact on overall population smoking prevalence rates.
- Wider tobacco control policies are also cost effective by they need to be implemented alongside the treatments for smokers in order to make a sizeable difference to population smoking rates.
- Investment in tobacco control programs can generate considerable health gains from limited resources, and therefore represent an efficient use of healthcare budgets.
- Health professionals have an important role to play in advocating such strategies.

References

1. Gold MR, Siegel JE, Russell LB, Weinstein MC (eds). *Cost-effectiveness in Health and Medicine*. New York: Oxford University Press, 1996.
2. National Institute for Health and Clinical Excellence (NICE). *Guide to the Methods of Technology Appraisal*. London: National Institute for Health and Clinical Excellence, 2004. http://www.nice.org.uk/pdf/TAP_Methods.pdf (accessed 23 August 2005).
3. Harvard School of Public Health. *The Cost Effectiveness Analysis (CEA) Registry*, 2005. http://www.hsph.harvard.edu/cearegistry/data/1976-2001_CEratios_comprehensive_4-7-2004. pdf (accessed 24 August 2005).
4. Doll R, Peto R, Boreham J, Sutherland I. Mortality in relation to smoking: 50 years' observations on male British doctors. *BMJ* 2004; 328:1519.
5. Tengs T, Wallace A. One thousand health-related quality-of-life estimates. *Med Care* 2000; 38:583.
6. Orme M, Hogue SL, Kennedy LM, et al. Development of the health and economic consequences of smoking (HE-COS) interactive model. *Tob Control* 2001; 10:55.
7. National Institute for Health and Clinical Excellence (NICE). *Lung Cancer: The Diagnosis and Treatment of Lung Cancer. National Cost-impact Report*. London: National Institute for Health and Clinical Excellence, 2005. http://www.nice.org.uk/pdf/cg024 fullguideline.pdf (accessed 23 August 2005).
8. Lightwood J, Collins D, Lapsley H, Novotny T. Estimating the costs of tobacco use. In: Jha P, Chaloupka F (eds) *Tobacco Control in Developing Countries*. Oxford: Oxford Medical Publications, 2000.
9. Royal College of Physicians. *Going Smoke-free: The Medical Case for Clean Air in the Home, at Work and in Public Places*. London: Royal College of Physicians, 2005.
10. Twigg L, Moon G, Walker S. *The Smoking Epidemic in England*. London: Health Development Agency, 2004.
11. Jha P, Chaloupka F (eds). *Tobacco Control in Developing Countries*. Oxford: Oxford Medical Publications, 2000.
12. Chaloupka F, Hu T-W, Warner K, et al. The taxation of tobacco products. In: Jha P, Chaloupka F (eds) *Tobacco Control in Developing Countries*. Oxford: Oxford Medical Publications, 2000.
13. Lundberg P. *Risky Health Behaviour among Adolescents. Lund Economic Studies 100*. Lund, Sweden: Department of Economics, Lund University, 2003.
14. Kenkel D, Chen L. Consumer information and tobacco use. In: Jha P, Chaloupka F (eds) *Tobacco Control in Developing Countries*. Oxford: Oxford Medical Publications, 2000.
15. Parrott S, Godfrey C, Raw M, et al. Guidance for commissioners on the cost effectiveness of smoking cessation interventions. *Thorax* 1998; 53(suppl 5):S1.
16. Mudde A, de Vries H. The reach and effectiveness of a national media-led smoking cessation campaign in the Netherlands. *Am J Public Health* 1999; 89:346.
17. Secker-Walker R, Worden J, Holland R, Flynn B, Detsky A. A mass media programme to prevent smoking among adolescents: costs and cost effectiveness. *Tob Control* 1997; 6:207.
18. Frieden T, Mostashari F, Kerker B, Miller N, Hajat A, Frankel M. Adult tobacco use levels after intensive tobacco control measures: New York City, 2002–2003. *Am J Public Health* 2005; 95:1016.
19. World Health Organization (WHO-CHOICE). Cost-effectiveness analyses. Web site: http://www3.who.int/whosis/cea (accessed 12 June 2005).
20. Scott Lennox A, Osman L, Reiter E, et al. Cost effectiveness of computer-tailored and non-tailored smoking cessation letters in general practice: randomised controlled trial. *BMJ* 2001; 322:1396.
21. McAlister A, Rabius V, Geiger A, et al. Telephone assistance for smoking cessation: one year cost effectiveness estimations. *Tob Control* 2004; 13:85.
22. Cromwell J, Bartosch WJ, Fiore MC, et al. Cost-effectiveness of the clinical practice recommendations in the AHCPR guideline for smoking cessation. *JAMA* 1997; 278:1759.
23. Comas-Fuentes A, Suarez-Gutierrez R, Lopez-Gonzalez M, Cuero Espinar A. Cost-effectiveness of anti-smoking health counseling in primary health care. *Gac Sanit* 1998; 12:126.
24. West R, McNeill A, Raw M. National smoking cessation guidelines for health professionals: an update. *Thorax* 2000; 55:989.
25. Stapleton J, Lowin A, Russell M. Prescription of transdermal nicotine patches for smoking cessation in general practice: evaluation of cost-effectiveness. *Lancet* 1999; 354:210.
26. Walsey M, McNagny S, Phillips V, Ahluwalia J. The cost-effectiveness of the nicotine transdermal patch for smoking cessation. *Prev Med* 1997; 26:264.
27. Ong M, Glantz S. Free nicotine replacement therapy programs vs implementing smoke-free workplaces: a cost-effectiveness comparison. *Am J Public Health* 2005; 95:969.
28. Tauras J, Chaloupka F, Emery S. The impact of advertising on nicotine replacement therapy demand. *Soc Sci Med* 2005; 60:2351.
29. Alberg A, Margalit R, Burke A, et al. The influence of offering free transdermal nicotine patches on quit rates in a local health department's smoking cessation program. *Addict Behav* 2004; 29:1763.
30. Halpern M, Khan Z, Young T, et al. Economic model of sustained-release bupropion hydrochloride in health plan and work site smoking-cessation programmes. *Am J Health Syst Pharm* 2000; 57:1421.
31. Nielson K, Fiore M. Cost-benefit analysis of sustained-release bupropion, nicotine patch, or both for smoking cessation. *Prev Med* 2000; 30:209.
32. Woolacott NF, Jones L, Forbes CA, et al. The clinical effectiveness and cost effectiveness of bupropion and nicotine replacement therapy for smoking cessation: a systematic review and economic evaluation. *Health Tech Assess* 2002; 6:1.
33. Javitz H, Swan G, Zbikowski S, et al. Cost-effectiveness of different combinations of bupropion SR dose and behavioural treatment for smoking cessation: a societal perspective. *Am J Managed Care* 2004; 10:217.
34. Gilbert A, Pinget C, Bovet P, et al. The cost effectiveness of pharmacological smoking cessation therapies in developing countries: a case study in the Seychelles. *Tob Control* 2004; 13:190.
35. Warner K. Cost effectiveness of smoking-cessation therapies. *Pharmacoeconomics* 1997; 11:538.
36. Buck D, Richmond R, Mendelsohn C. Cost-effectiveness of a family physician delivered smoking cessation program. *Prev Med* 2000; 31:641.
37. Feenstra T, Hamberg-van Reenen H, Hoogenveen R, Rutten-van Mölken M. Cost-effectiveness of face-to-face smoking cessation interventions: a dynamic modeling study. *Value in Health* 2005; 8:178.
38. Godfrey C, Parrott S, Coleman T, Pound E. Cost effectiveness of English smoking cessation services: evidence from practice. *Addict* 2005; 100(suppl 2):70.

Financial Aspects of Lung Cancer

56

J. Russell Hoverman

Contents

56.1   Introduction

The economic costs of lung cancer are inextricably associated with tobacco use and have implications for all levels of care, from personal to global. This chapter examines the current state of the financial impact of lung cancer and the prospects for the future. The issues involved with measuring quality and value and associated economic measures, such as cost/effectiveness are discussed. Specific areas of service with their contribution to total costs as well as potential for cost savings are examined.

56.2   National and Global Perspectives

There are simple measures of the impact of a disease, such as deaths. There are more complex measurements that account for the loss to family and society by a death due to a specified disease. An example of this latter is the disability adjusted life year (DALY). A DALY is a year of income-producing life lost to either disability related to treatment or complications of the disease,

or to premature death. As an example, a man who dies at age 50 of lung cancer who lives in a country with working life that on average extends to age 65 has lost 15 DALYs. The actual calculation of a DALY is a complicated event [1] and must include adjustments for degrees of disability, regional differences in longevity, and cultural and age-related differences in work habits. For the purposes of this discussion a DALY is used as a surrogate for the economic value of an income-producing member of society. No monetary value is ascribed to a DALY, as this will vary considerably from region to region, and is subject to interpretation as to how to measure the worth, both present and future, of a productive individual. The proportion of DALYs to deaths is a reflection of the prematurity of the deaths related to the specified disease.

The most accessible cost of lung cancer is the cost of medical care. This is measured by either private or government payers and can account for the complete episode of care from diagnosis to death. Yet these sources may not account for all medical costs, as the payer database may be fragmented, staging and clinical data inaccessible, and information systems cumbersome. The indirect costs, such as time and income lost from work, the costs to families without a primary source of income, and the costs of uncompensated care from friends and family members are all difficult to calculate and are not included in standard cost analyses. Even costs confined to the episode of care will be difficult to compare across borders and across regions. Many studies measure only one aspect of care, such as chemotherapy. For other studies, there are regional or national differences in the locus of care, such that the costs of a predominantly hospital-based system of care will differ from a system with a predominantly outpatient system of care. The costs of chemotherapy drugs will not be the same for all countries. Financial pressures, especially in nationalized healthcare systems will limit treatment choices and supportive drugs.

That said, the global impact of tobacco-related disease including cancers of the lung, bronchus, and trachea is considerable. Currently, lung cancer is a disease of developed countries, principally the USA, Canada,

Western Europe, the Soviet Union, and Eastern Europe. For these countries tobacco-related deaths were about 15% of all deaths and 12% of DALYs [2]. This contrasts with a global burden of 2–3% of DALYs worldwide. However, as developing countries become industrialized the proportion of deaths due to communicable diseases and perinatal illnesses drops and the number of deaths due to smoking and lung cancer increases. Murray and Lopez estimate that worldwide DALYs related to tobacco use will rise from 40 million in 1990 to 120 million by 2020 [2]. Lung cancer will move from the tenth most common cause of death worldwide to fifth [3]. The specter of the future pattern of disease is reflected in the current prevalence of tobacco use in those countries developing market economies. The percentage of men who smoke in the Soviet Union, China, and many Eastern European countries is over 60% [4]. In Korea two thirds of males over 20 are smokers and another 20% are ex-smokers [5]. In Eastern Europe the rates of deaths from lung cancer have doubled or tripled over the last 30 years. Some former Soviet bloc countries have recognized this as an epidemic and have taken a national approach to curb tobacco use. In the 1980s over 60% of Polish males were smokers. By 2002, this percentage had dropped to 40%. With this the incidence of lung cancer has begun to drop, whereas in countries without this approach, such as Hungary, the incidence has continued to climb [6]. The net result of these changes is that the global economic burden of tobacco-related diseases will rise from $ 500 billion (USD) in 2010 to over $ 1 trillion in 2030 [4].

The responsibility for responding to this global burden will fall on healthcare systems. A system may be active on multiple levels, but the usual economic unit falls within national borders. Within a system, there may be allocation of responsibility with governments, national, regional, and local, employers, and individuals. The costs for lung cancer will be part of the economic picture for that system. Reports on a national level will measure either total costs, which include lost income based on lost years of productive life, or direct costs, which measure only the costs of care given. For the USA, the direct costs of lung cancer range from $ 4.68 billion (1995 USD) [7] to $ 8 billion [8]. Cancer care in the USA represents slightly less that 5% of overall direct healthcare costs, of which lung cancer is approximately 12%. [9]. For South Korea total costs for tobacco-related illness may be as high as $ 4.5 billion (1998 USD) at 1.19% GDP [5]. For the UK the proportion of all direct disease costs attributed to cancer has increased from 7.8% to 10.6% from 1990–1 to 2000–1 [9]. For Australia in 1993–1994, lung cancer accounted for 5.6% of health system costs at $ 107 million [10]. The cost for Canada for stage IV lung cancer alone in 1995 Canadian dollars was $ 132 million [11]. For General Motors, one of the largest non-government employers in the world, the years of life lost to disease for the years 1994–1998 were 42,322 with 5,764 deaths. Lung cancer represented 8.64% of all DALYs for the company. The cost per case of lung cancer will vary according to stage, tissue type, and initial health of the patient. Costs may range from as low as $ 10,000 to over $ 100,000. The mean for an insured population in the USA was just over $ 47,000 (USD 1997) [12]. US Medicare payments for lung cancer averaged $ 29,000 from diagnosis to death (USD 1990) in 1990 [13]. For France, the estimated costs ranged from $ 20,000 to $ 32,000 (USD 1998) [14]. These costs per case represent financial hardships to patients responsible for all or part of the costs. The Study to Understand Prognoses and Preferences for Outcomes and Risks of Treatments (SUPPORT) found that for the surrogates of patients dying with lung and colon cancer, over 40% reported that a family member had to quit work to provide care. Nearly one third lost a major source of income. For 25% the illness consumed most or all of their financial resources [15]. Although lung cancer was not specifically mentioned, Himmelstein et al. [16] reported that in 2001 approximately 2 million US citizens experienced a bankruptcy of which medical costs were a significant contributor. The highest cost diagnosis was for cancer at $ 35,878 (USD 2001). For a US cohort of women with breast cancer, monthly out-of-pocket expenses and lost income costs were $ 1,455 (USD 2004) with 98% of the income of low wage earners consumed by the costs of cancer care [17].

An unmeasured cost is that of lost opportunity. Opportunity costs are those spent for little apparent long-term good that could have been spent elsewhere. From the national to the personal, the use of tobacco products diverts money from productive investments to expenditures for the care of preventable diseases. From a shrinking labor pool in Japan, to the loss of infrastructure investment in Poland, to the expenditure of one and a half hours of labor in Kenya, or to forgoing the purchase of a dozen eggs in Panama to buy a single pack of cigarettes, the opportunity costs are substantial [4].

56.3 Assessing Value and Quality

For any level of healthcare delivery there must be a method for comparing needs so as to direct funds to address those needs. In its simplest form, a value (V) is anything that in and of itself is desirable. In medicine, as elsewhere, a value is related directly to an outcome (O), such as pain control or longer survival. However, no value stands alone. Any value must compete with other values for scare resources. Therefore, we have relative values (RV) as any value is associated with a cost (C). This leads to the equation:

RV (relative value) = O (outcome) / C (cost)

Relative values, then, are directly proportional to the outcomes and inversely proportional to the costs.

In this schema, quality is anything that enhances value. This can occur by either improving the outcome or decreasing costs. In more formal terms, quality is equal to the efficient attainment of a defined outcome, where that outcome is as good as or better than that generally obtainable.

Although simple conceptually, determining RVs is not a simple task. There is no shortage of metrics used in RV calculations, such as survival, cure rate, response rate, and time to progression, all measured in expenditures to achieve these outcomes. The difficulty is in measuring these outcomes with a sense of assurance. The vehicle for measuring outcomes has become the randomized clinical trial (RCT). The RCT has a simple logical structure that leads nicely to RV measurements:

$$a(1) + a(2) + a(3) + \dots + a(n) + b = O(1)$$
$$a(1) + a(2) + a(3) + \dots + a(n) = O(2)$$
$$V(b) = O(1) - O(2)$$
$$RV(b) = O(1) - O(2)/C(1) - C(2)$$

In this case, the two arms of the study are identical except for the experimental intervention of b. Any difference in outcome is attributable only to b and the value $V(b)$ is determined by the difference between the two arms. RV may be determined by calculating the incremental cost or savings of adding b to the regimen.

The RCT is the only structure in which O can be tied to a single variable, in this case b. For example, a clinical trial that compares an outcome with historical controls has a different logical structure:

$$a(1) + a(2) + a(3) + \dots + a(n) + b = O(1)$$
$$a(1) + a(2) + a(3) + \dots + a(n+x) = O(2)$$

The general argument is that no additional variables exist between current studies and previous studies. However, this is clearly not true as the simple passage of time is associated with at least new imaging and treatment technologies. Stage migration is a frequent result of these new technologies. The simple fact is that x is unknown and may be a confounding variable. From the structure of the formulas alone, it appears that RV can be assigned. However, this is risky as there is no certainty that the outcome is associated with the intervention.

A process improvement project is, in fact, a trial with historical controls. Its logical structure is as follows:

$$a(1) + a(2) + a(3) + \dots + a(n) + b + c + d = O(1)$$
$$a(1) + a(2) + a(3) + \dots + a(n + x) = O(2)$$

The difference between a typical clinical trial and a process improvement project is that for the latter we are not necessarily looking for an improvement in outcome.

We may be looking for decreased costs. If we do demonstrate decreased costs, we do not know to what exactly that decrease should be attributed, whether new known variables or unknown variables associated with historical controls, but the process may have uncovered important information by improving efficiency. We cannot ascribe relative value to the new variables, but only to the process as a whole.

For a meta-analysis, multiple RCTs with low statistical validity are combined to increase the statistical power and support conclusions. The logical structure is as follows:

$$a(1) + a(2) + a(3) + \dots + a(n) = O(1)$$
$$a(1) + a(2) + a(3) + \dots + a(n + x) = O(2)$$
$$a(1) + a(2) + a(3) + \dots + a(n + y) = O(3)$$
$$a(1) + a(2) + a(3) + \dots + a(n + z) = O(4)$$

The argument is that statistical rules can be applied to the sum of these studies. This form of meta-analyses is based on abstracted data. However, as can be seen from the logical structure, confounding variables have not been ruled out and statistical arguments may be invalid. Other meta-analyses are based on individual patient data, where each patient record is abstracted. Even individual patient data meta-analyses, such as that by the Early Breast Cancer Trialists [18, 19], face difficulties as not all data may be available; they are time consuming and expensive [20]. Any meta-analysis, especially those based on previously abstracted data, runs the risk of being trumped by a large RCT [21–23].

Even recognizing the validity of the RCT, we are left far short of having the information we need for clinical decision-making. RCTs often apply to only a very select population and are not reflective of the bulk of oncology practice. The strengths of RCTs may vary [24]. For lung cancer, we have too little information about the elderly, or poor performance status patients, or women, or costs, for example. The response to this uncertainty has been an attempt to systematize the information we do have into levels of evidence [25]. In this way we at least recognize what we know and do not know. With this, there has been a continued emphasis on clinical trials, but there has also been a recognition that consensus is an important source of decision-making. The resurgence of the systematic review is an example of this [26, 27]. The systematic review recognizes the shortcomings of the meta-analysis and instead looks to build a consensus from a thorough review of current evidence. Cancer-related specialty groups have responded to this uncertainty by establishing levels of evidence. The hierarchy used by the American Society of Clinical Oncology (ASCO) is outlined in Tables 56.1 and 56.2 [28] and that of the National Cancer Center Network (NCCN) in Table 56.3 [29]. This evidence is then synthesized into guidelines outlining current standards of care. The Program in Evidence-based Care, de-

Table 56.1. Levels of evidence

Level	Type of evidence
I	Evidence obtained from meta-analyses of multiple, well-designed, controlled studies. Randomized trials with low false-positive and low false-negative errors (high-power)
II	Evidence obtained from at least one well-designed experimental study. Randomized trials with high false-positive and/or false-negative errors (low power)
III	Evidence obtained from well-designed, quasi-experimental studies such as non-randomized, controlled, single-group, pre-post, cohort, time, or matched case-control series
IV	Evidence from well-designed, non-experimental studies such as comparative and correlational descriptive and case studies
V	Evidence from case reports and clinical examples

Table 56.2. Grades of recommendation

Grade	Grade of recommendation
A	There is evidence of type I or consistent findings from multiple studies of type II, III, or IV
B	There is evidence of type II, III, or IV and findings are generally consistent
C	There is evidence of type II, III, or IV but findings are inconsistent
D	There is little or no systematic empirical evidence

Table 56.3. Categories of consensus

Category	Recommendation
1	The recommendation is based on high-level evidence (i.e., high-powered randomized clinical trials or meta-analyses), and the panel has reached uniform consensus that the recommendation is indicated
2A	The recommendation is based on lower-level evidence, but despite the absence of higher-level studies, there is unknown consensus that the recommendation is appropriate
2B	The recommendation is based on lower-level evidence, and there is non-uniform consensus that the recommendation should be made
3	The recommendation has engendered a major disagreement among the panel members

veloped by Cancer Care Ontario is an example. Draft guidelines are developed by specialty committees based on high-level evidence, predominantly RCTs. The draft guidelines are then sent to practicing physicians for comments. In this way both evidence and consensus are addressed.

With appropriate evidence base for outcomes, the costs and RV of the delivery of care can be addressed. They are four generally accepted mechanisms for as-

sessing cost in cancer care. The first is cost-effectiveness analysis (CEA) where the outcome is measured in natural units, such as disease-free or overall survival. The incremental costs to achieve this additional benefit are then calculated. A shortcoming of this method is that only one outcome can be measured. The gain may be associated with unacceptable toxicity or quality of life [30, 31]. The most used unit of a CEA is the cost per year of life gained. A cost-utility analysis (CUA) uses the same format as a CEA but standardizes the unit of outcome. A CUA uses quality adjusted life years (QALYs). This measures not only the years of life gained, but also adjusts this absolute measurement with an assessment of the quality of those years. Both of these methods have created controversy when used to make coverage decisions in real life. These measurements do not include justice concerns, such as equity, the number of lives benefited, and community compassion [32]. Also, the CUA must make some value decisions regarding the constituents of a quality year of life.

The third mechanism is a cost-benefit analysis (CBA). In this exercise cost units are given to the benefit as well as the costs. The simplicity of a CBA is attractive in that the result is a single number – if the benefits outweigh the costs, the number is <1.0, if the costs predominate it is >1.0. The difficulty is that a value in monetary terms must be placed on the benefit. Again, the process depends on judgments of value that have proven difficult.

The fourth method, and the one used in the economic assessments in the remainder of this chapter, is the cost-minimization study. In this process, two or more clinical interventions with equal outcomes are assessed for cost and compared. The exercise has the limitation of depending on clinical trials directly comparing differing treatments. Again, the RCT is preferred, but some comparisons can be made across trials, albeit with some risks. A selection and substitution of one of a number of equivalent treatments may be called "therapeutic interchange." The second, and possibly more important method of cost minimization is to eliminate aspects of care that prove to be costly, but of no benefit. Again, clinical trials are the most important source of these kinds of data. The assessment of variability is an important indication to ensure that what is being done in the delivery of care is not excessive or necessary. Wennberg [33, 34] has shown wide variability in the costs of specified common procedures throughout the USA. His group has recently shown that this variability may not be associated with quality, in that high costs do not necessarily lead to better outcomes. Others [35] have shown that survival in non-small cell lung cancer (NSCLC) is no better with high-cost physicians than with low-cost physicians. Exploration of the sources of variability is an important avenue to investigate cost minimization. The difficulty is associating the differences in costs with outcomes.

In the following sections, the results of CEAs or CUAs will be mentioned where available. However, recommendations on the basis of a CEA or CUA will be made only if within generally accepted levels as the RV of that intervention will have to be made on a macroeconomic level, such as a health plan or government agency [36]. Cost minimization will be used, either addressing therapeutic interchange or the addition of care that enhances value or omission of care that detracts from value.

56.4 Prevention, Cessation, and Screening

There has been no question that the rise in lung cancer mortality has been associated with the prevalence of tobacco use. Where tobacco use has fallen, there has been an accompanying drop in lung cancer mortality. However, it has been difficult to measure the cost benefit of either prevention or cessation programs in terms of mortality or medical costs. Some have argued that since patients with lung cancer die sooner, their lifetime costs for medical services are actually less than never smokers. However, these arguments do not measure benefits in terms of QALYs, or costs per year of life gained. Nor do they measure indirect costs, such as lost productivity [8]. A recent article helps to quantify this. The Lung Health Study (LHS) results, after 14.5 years of monitoring, reported that smoking cessation had a significant benefit in terms of reduced mortality. The striking finding of this study was that the differences in mortality applied to the intervention group as a whole, even though only 21.7% of the intervention group was sustained quitters (versus 5.4% in the usual care group). For this comparison, the death rate in the intervention group was 8.83 per 1,000 person years versus 10.38 in the usual care group. When death rates were looked at specifically in those who were sustained non-smokers, the mortality was 6.04 per 1,000 person years versus 7.77 in intermittent quitters and 11.09 in continuing smokers. That is, the death rate was cut nearly in half by sustained non-smoking. An important finding of this study was that the greatest effect was in the youngest group of patients [37]. The estimated cost per participant was approximately $ 2,000 (2004 USD). The participants in this study had an average pack year of smoking of 40. This puts in perspective the potential benefit of smoking cessation for younger smokers, or smoking prevention campaigns.

The subjects of smoking prevention (primary smoking prevention) and cessation (secondary smoking prevention) have been extensively reviewed [38, 39]. The findings with consistent high levels of evidence of effective smoking cessation or prevention are: (1) mass media campaigns, (2) tobacco excise taxes, (3) direct workplace restrictions, (4) clinician-based approaches, (5) physician advice, especially if given on four or more occasions, (6) group or individual counseling formats, (7) pharmacotherapy, and (8) reminder systems plus education. Additional counseling support, reminder systems, and telephone support enhanced most of these efforts. An assessment of the incremental costs per year of life saved of cessation programs with pharmacotherapy compared to counseling alone indicate a range of $ 920 (USD 2003) for counseling plus bupropion to $ 3,455 for brief physician advice plus nicotine replacement [40]. Karnath [41] looked at the costs of pharmacotherapy alone and found a fivefold increase in the cost of nicotine inhaler compared to gum or a patch per successful quitter. Bupropion was as cost effective as the best nicotine replacement.

Currently, there is no generally recommended screening program outside of Japan [42, 43]. Clinical trials testing frequent chest X-rays or sputum cytology have not found a reduction on lung cancer-specific mortality [44]. Recent attention has been focused on the use of low-radiation dose spiral computed tomography (LDCT). Results from the Lung Screening Study (LSS) showed a fourfold discovery of early lung cancer (30/1,660 versus 7/1,658) of individuals screened with CT versus yearly chest X-ray [45]. Others have demonstrated similar findings [46]. The LSS findings have led to a large national randomized trial (National Lung Screening Trial) with randomization complete by 2004 and final analysis in 2009. The end point will be lung cancer mortality. The costs per year of life gained range from $ 48,000 (USD 2002) [47] to well over $ 100,000 (USD 2002) [44]. The difference depends on the assumptions of age screened, inclusion of former smokers as well as current smokers, cure rate of surgery, the costs for screening, the duration of repeat screening, and the rate of unnecessary surgery. As seen in the smoking cessation study with a follow-up of over 14 years, the answer to this issue may not be apparent in 2009. In that study, there was no difference in mortality 5 years after the intervention. There are no data as yet on which to base a meaningful cost-effectiveness assessment.

56.5 Imaging, Staging, and Surveillance

Non-small cell lung cancer has been notoriously difficult to stage accurately. A retrospective study by Herder et al. [48] reported that 23% of clinically staged patients who went to thoracotomy had unresectable lesions. Another 13% of patients had benign findings. An additional 15% had local recurrence or metastases within the first 12 months. The net result was that for this cohort of patients staged in the 2-year interval 1993–1994, over half had a thoracotomy that did not change the outcome. A number of studies indicate that staging efficiency has been improved by the introduction of positron emission tomography (PET) using F18-fluorodeoxyglucose. This applies to evaluating solitary pulmonary nodules (SPNs) for malignancy [49, 50] and staging potentially resectable early lung cancer [51, 52]. PET has also been valuable in the evaluation of patients being considered for combined chemoradiation therapy for stage IIIA–B disease. In this situation as many as 30% may be upstaged, and 20% may have previously undetected distant metastases [53, 54]. There is good evidence that in the evaluation of the SPN and in stage III disease for which surgery or chemotherapy, radiation therapy, or combined therapy is considered, PET is cost effective and may be cost saving by avoiding unnecessary treatment.

The cost effectiveness of PET in NSCLC staged as I or II by CT is less certain. One prospective study indicated an 18% occurrence of distant metastases in clinically stage II patients [55]. Another study indicated that the rate of thoracotomy may not be affected by PET in stage I and II [56]. Other models suggest that PET is not needed for tumors with a negative mediastinum by CT scan [57]. All agree that a PET with a positive mediastinum requires mediastinoscopy to exclude non-malignant positives. In some situations, especially peripheral clinical stage 1 tumors and those with mediastinal lymph nodes less than 1 cm by CT, the addition of PET to a standard use of mediastinoscopy may not be cost effective [58–60].

The routine use of other imaging in addition to PET and chest CT scan is not recommended in the absence of organ-specific symptoms. PET is more sensitive than radionuclide bone scanning in detecting bone metastases. The negative predictive value of the physical examination in NSCLC in evaluation for brain metastases is 0.94, for adrenal or liver metastases is 0.95, and for bone metastases is 0.90. In the absence of history, physical examination, or laboratory findings indicating organ-specific disease, routine imaging of the brain, liver, adrenals, or bone is not indicated [61].

Positron emission tomography has also been used to determine prognosis and tumor response to treatment. However, there is no study indicating that PET findings in these circumstances either change treatment or improve survival. There is a potential for cost savings using PET if a cohort of patients can be identified in which the costs of treatment can be lessened by eliminating ineffective chemotherapy or radiation therapy. PET for assessing prognosis or response to treatment cannot be recommended [62].

The results of routine surveillance following surgery with curative intent are conflicting. Current guidelines [63] recommend a physician evaluation with imaging (either chest X-ray or chest CT scan) every 6 months for 2 years and then annually. A recent Swiss study indicates that the cost per year of life saved over 10 years for this strategy was 90,000 Swiss francs [64]. The evidence suggests that a benefit, if any, will come at a high price. This speaks for the potential benefit of LDCT screening as well. Other studies such as undirected organ imaging (e.g., abdominal CT scans, bone scans, or PET) are not indicated. Blood tests, sputum cytology, and tumor markers similarly are not recommended for routine surveillance. The cost savings of strictly following surveillance protocols with these recommendations are unknown.

56.6 Chemotherapy and Supportive Medications

In a study of lung cancer costs in Canada for 1988, the costs of chemotherapy for NSCLC were omitted due to low utilization. Approximately 29% of costs for limited-stage small cell lung cancer (SCLC) were for chemotherapy, and 20% for extensive stage. Hospital costs were 29 and 57%, respectively [65]. In another study looking at patterns in 1989–1991 for a commercial payer in the US State of Virginia, 18.2% of patients with distant disease received chemotherapy either alone or with radiation therapy. This was 11.1% of all patients. The mean overall cost from diagnosis to death for lung cancer was $ 47,941 (USD 1992) [12]. Hospital days accounted for 48% of the costs. Ramsey et al. [66] recently reported an average use of chemotherapy of 30% for Medicare patients with stage III or IV lung cancer diagnosed between 1994 and 1999. However, between those dates the proportion of chemotherapy use rose from 21% to 43%. Patients who had chemotherapy only had a mean cost of $ 57,532, and if combined with radiation therapy $ 75,074 (USD 1994–1999). In the economic analysis of the Southwest Oncology Group (SWOG) trial S9509 comparing vinorelbine/cisplatin (V/C) to paclitaxel/carboplatin (P/C) in advanced NSCLC the mean total cost (excluding initial staging, biopsy, and surgery) for the V/C arm was $ 40,292 (USD 1998) of which 13% or $ 5,231 was drug. The cost for the P/C arm averaged $ 48,940 of which drugs were $ 17,094 or 35% [67]. The implications are clear that chemotherapy costs have become a significant part of the total expense of lung cancer treatment and that the choice of drug can be important.

This change in the utilization of chemotherapy for lung cancer is driven by clinical trial evidence of efficacy [68–70]. Associated with these data are calculations that the costs per QALY fall within generally accepted limits [71–73]. The recent trials indicating a benefit to adjuvant chemotherapy for early-stage disease will only increase this utilization. However, within this context there are ample opportunities for cost minimization. There are at least four combinations used for NSCLC that have shown clinical equivalence [74]. Costs may vary by country but a critical analysis will show differences in costs among these regimens. For conservative estimates Berthelot et al. [72] have shown that V/P is the preferred regimen. For a Spanish group [75] the combination of docetaxel/cisplatin was preferred to paclitaxel combinations. The change of paclitaxel from proprietary to generic may change many of these initial calculations.

The mode of delivery of chemotherapy as well as the total number of cycles both impact overall costs. Weekly chemotherapy for drugs such as docetaxel and paclitaxel instead of q3 weekly will lead to higher overall chemotherapy drug costs, higher supportive drug costs, and more infusion costs. A number of studies for both NSCLC and SCLC have shown that either continuing care beyond 4 cycles of primary chemotherapy or following primary chemotherapy with maintenance chemotherapy has no effect on survival [76–81]. There is now clinical trial evidence for both NSCLC and SCLC that second-line chemotherapy offers a survival benefit [82–85]. The cost effectiveness of docetaxel in a second-line setting for NSCLC was estimated at £ 13,863 (UK pounds 2004) [86]. There is no proven cost effectiveness for third-line therapy or beyond for either NSCLC or SCLS [87]. There is no proven benefit to adding a third drug to any of these two-drug combinations for NSCLC [88]. The recent approval of pemetrexed for second-line NSCLC is another opportunity for cost comparison. Docetaxel is less expensive on a unit dose, but pemetrexed reportedly has less toxicity requiring hospitalization [89]. Overlooked in both this comparison and the V/P–P/C comparison of the SWOG S9509 trial is the importance of effective or threshold dose levels [90]. The dose level of cisplatin in the V/P arm was 100 mg/m^2 whereas a lower dose may have been just as effective with less toxicity [91]. Similarly, in regards to second-line therapy in NSCLC, a lower dose of docetaxel may be as effective with less toxicity [92]. For the SWOG trial a systematic approach to cost minimization would have included a follow-up trial testing lower doses of V/P. The Canadian Health System adopted a lower dose regimen but this has not been rigorously tested elsewhere.

In some unmanaged environments, the use of recombinant erythropoietin or epoetin alone can constitute as much as 45% of all drug costs [93]. In a retrospective study by Hoverman and Robertson [35], a principal driver of costs for NSCLC was growth factors, including epoetin. The role of epoetin in lung cancer treatment remains controversial. There is general agreement that epoetins decrease the use of transfusions when started in patients with moderate anemia (hemoglobin < 10 g/dl) [94, 95]. The difficulty is in justifying treatment for fatigue when the correlation of fatigue to overall quality of life (QOL) is uncertain [96, 97]. In no case is the contribution of expense to overall QOL calculated. The current average selling price (ASP) for Medicare in the USA for epoetin alfa is $ 407 (USD). The monthly cost

not including administration is then $ 1,628. The number of patients needed to treat with epoetin to prevent a transfusion as defined in the highest quality trials is 5.2 [94]. Therefore the rough cost of epoetin use per transfusion avoided is $ 8,465.60. The cost for transfusion of 2 units of packed red blood cells will vary but will be less than 25% of this cost. Looked at in another way, in the study by Witzig et al. [97], 16 weeks of epoetin therapy prevented the transfusion of one unit of blood. This is spending $ 6,400 (USD 2004) to avoid the cost of $ 1,000. Increasing the dose of epoetin in unresponsive patients makes these comparisons even less attractive. These costs must be weighed against the costs, both direct and indirect, of transfusions, as avoiding unnecessary transfusions is a personal and societal value. There does not appear to be a benefit in terms of transfusion avoidance to beginning epoetin at higher levels of hemoglobin [94]. Initiation of guidelines with a treatment threshold of 10.0 g/dl hemoglobin can lower costs for lung cancer patients in unmanaged environments. Scrutiny of the cost effectiveness of escalating doses is warranted.

A second large expense for supportive care is that of white blood cell growth factors, or granulocyte colony-stimulating factors (GCSFs). These are primarily pegfilgrastim, filgrastim, and sargramostim. The routine use of prophylactic pegfilgrastim can double the drug expense for most commonly used NSCLC and SCLC chemotherapy regimens. There are no studies that indicate an improvement in survival for the use of GCSFs to maintain dose intensity in NSCLC. The same holds for SCLC [98]. There is evidence that the use of GCSFs in combined modality therapy for SCLC may be detrimental [99]. There are RCT data indicating that GCSF at the time of afebrile neutropenia is of no benefit [100]. As with epoetins, careful adherence to guidelines using dose reduction rather than growth factors has the potential to substantially reduce costs without compromising benefits.

56.7 Radiation Therapy and Surgery

Between 55% and 75% of patients with lung cancer will receive radiation therapy during the course of their illness [101, 102]. There is good evidence that radiation therapy as part of the initial management of the disease is cost effective [103] but there is little cost information on other aspects of care using this modality. There is evidence of wide variability in effective treatment choices for metastatic bone disease [104]. With PET as an example, there is evidence of rapid adoption of new technology. Intensity-modulated radiotherapy (IMRT) will add to the accuracy with which we can treat tumor volumes [105, 106]. In chest disease as well as brain metastases, there is the potential for stereotactic radiosurgery. However, there is no assessment of the incremental value of these modalities.

The efficiency of surgery for lung cancer has benefited from better staging [107]. As with radiation therapy there are new technologies. Less invasive therapies such as video-assisted thoracic surgery (VATS) or bronchoscopic treatment may be used instead of thoracotomy. The cost effectiveness of these modalities appears promising but await formal value testing [108, 109].

56.8 End-of-life and Palliative Care

In a sense, all care for lung cancer patients with metastatic disease is end-of-life care. However, for cost measurement, most studies measure this as the 6 months before death. A study by Hillner et al. [12] reported that 45% of costs for NSCLC were incurred in the last 6 months of life. Riley et al. [13] showed that two thirds of Medicare payments for all elderly patients dying of cancer occurred in the last 6 months. In France 51% of direct treatment costs for NSCLC corresponded to "terminal care" [110]. In France nearly all patients receive terminal care in the hospital. For the US Medicare populations, lung cancer patients were more likely to enroll in a hospice than those with non-cancer diagnoses, and those who enrolled incurred less cost than those who did not [111]. Although attractive in concept a statistical association of a treatment with less cost does not mean that those cost savings can be achieved in practice. SUPPORT has shown this to be so. In this case, a vigorous attempt to educate both patients and physicians about the disease prognosis did not alter resource utilization [112]. However, more recent studies done as part of the Promoting Excellence Project have shown at least cost neutrality and possibly cost savings by introducing the hospice concept and hospice and palliative care personnel at the time of diagnosis of metastatic NSCLC [113]. These investigators had the luxury of having both aggressive and palliative care paid for by the program.

The cost effectiveness of end-of-life care can be enhanced on both macroeconomic levels and the personal care level. Payment systems may not encourage an integrated approach to end-of-life care, allowing both aggressive palliative chemotherapy and/or radiation therapy, and encouraging the tenets of hospice care, that is, living the remainder of one's life in the best way possible. There are simple things as well, as simple as being comfortable prescribing the lowest cost medications for pain control [114]. Table 56.4 outlines the retail costs for commonly used narcotic analgesics. The cost savings of using methadone compared to other long-acting analgesics is apparent.

56.9 Conclusion

In 2000 Earle and colleagues [115] published an overview of cost-utility assessments in oncology. There were three studies related to lung cancer. Since then concern regarding costs has heightened, as has the need. There is ample evidence of inefficiency in the delivery of lung cancer care.

Key Points

- Lung cancer is a global disease. The expense of treating lung cancer will create a drag on the emergence of developing countries into market economies.
- The most cost effective methods of controlling lung cancer costs are prevention and cessation. This cost effectiveness will only increase with the rising technological costs of treatment.
- Cost analyses cannot be done with assurance except in the context of the randomized clinical trial.
- There are many opportunities in care delivery to address costs. Variability in staging algorithms including PET scans, in chemotherapy, and in supportive drug use may be modified by guidelines and pathways.
- The integration of aggressive treatment with a hospice philosophy of end-of-life care holds promise for improving quality and reducing costs.

Table 56.4. Comparison costs of long-acting narcotic analgesics

Narcotic	Cost ($)
Methadone 10 mg b.i.d., #60	32.00
Morphine sulfate ER 30 mg t.i.d., #90	158.25
MS Contin 30 mg t.i.d., #90	176.00
OxyContin 20 mg t.i.d., #90	286.50
Duragesic 50 mg q3d, #10	287.25

References

1. Murray CJL. Rethinking DALYs. In: Murray CJL, Lopez AD (eds) *Global Burden of Disease Study 1996*. Boston: Harvard School Public Health, 1996:1.
2. Murray CJL, Lopez AD. Global mortality, disability and the contribution of risk factors. Global Burden of Disease Study. *Lancet* 1997; 349:1436.
3. Murray CJL, Lopez AD. Alternative visions of the future: projecting mortality and disability, 1990–2020. In: Murray CJL, Lopez AD (eds) *Global Burden of Disease Study 1996*. Boston: Harvard School Public Health, 1996:361.

4. Mackay J, Eriksen M. *The Tobacco Atlas*. Brighton, UK: Myriad Edition, 2002.

5. Kang HY, Kim HJ, Park TK, Jee SH, Nam CM, Park HW. Economic burden of smoking in Korea. *Tob Control* 2003; 12:37.

6. Sansom C. Provisions of cancer care in Eastern Europe. *Lancet Oncol* 2002; 3:203.

7. Brown ML, Lipscomb J, Snyder C. The burden of illness of cancer: economic cost and quality of life. *Annu Rev Public Health* 2001; 22:91.

8. Goodwin PJ, Shepherd FA. Economic issues in lung cancer: a review. *J Clin Oncol* 1998; 16:3900.

9. Bosanquet N, Sikora K. The economics of cancer in the UK. *Lancet Oncol* 2004; 5:568.

10. NHMRC. National Health and Medical Research Council Clinical Practice Guidelines for the prevention, diagnosis and management of lung cancer. http://www.nhmrc.gov.au/publications/_files/cp97.pdf. (Accessed 9/3/05)

11. Earle CC, Evans WK. Management issues for stage IV non-small-cell lung cancer. *Cancer Control* 1997; 4:307.

12. Hillner BE, McDonald MK, Desch CE, et al. Costs of care associated with non-small cell lung cancer in a commercially insured cohort. *J Clin Oncol* 1998; 16:1420.

13. Riley GF, Potosky AL, Lubitz JD, Kessler LG. Medicare payments from diagnosis to death for elderly cancer patients by stage at diagnosis. *Med Care* 1995; 33:828.

14. Chouaid C, Molinier L, Combescure C, et al. Economics of the clinical management of lung cancer in France: an analysis using a Markov model. *Br J Cancer* 2004; 90:397.

15. McCarthy EP, Phillips RS, Zhong Z, et al. Dying with cancer: patients function, symptoms and case references as death approaches. *J Am Geriatr Soc* 2000; 48:S110.

16. Himmelstein DU, Warren E, Thorne D, Woolhandler S. Market watch: illness and injury as contributors to bankruptcy. http://www.healthaffairs.org/cgi/content/full/hlthaff.w5.63/DCI. (Accessed 9/3/05).

17. Arozullah AM, Calhoun EA, Wolf M, et al. The financial burden of cancer: estimates from a study of insured women with breast cancer. *J Support Oncol* 2004; 2:271.

18. Early Breast Cancer Trialists Collaborative Group. Effects of adjuvant tamoxifen and of cytotoxic therapy on mortality in early breast cancer. An overview of 61 randomized trials among 28,896 women. *N Engl J Med* 1988; 319:1681.

19. Peto R, Collins R, Gray R. Large-scale randomized evidence: large simple trials and overviews of trials. *J Clin Epidemiol* 1995; 48:23.

20. Piedbois P, Buyse M. Meta-analyses based on abstracted data: a step in the right direction, but only a first step. *J Clin Oncol* 2004; 22:3839.

21. LeLorier J, Gregoire G, Benhaddad A, et al. Discrepancies between meta-analyses and subsequent large, randomized, controlled trials. *N Engl J Med* 1997; 337:536.

22. Ioannidis JP, Cappelleri JC, Lau J. Issues in comparisons between meta-analyses and large trials. *JAMA* 1998; 279:1089.

23. DerSimonian R, Levine R. Resolving discrepancies between a meta-analyses and a subsequent large controlled trial. *JAMA* 1999; 282:664.

24. Altman DG, Schulz KF, Moher D, et al. The revised CONSORT statement for reporting randomized trials: explanation and elaboration. *Ann Intern Med* 2001; 134:663.

25. Evidence-Based Medicine Working Group. Evidence-based medicine. *JAMA* 1992; 2668:2420.

26. Slavin RE. Best evidence synthesis: an intelligent alternative to meta-analyses. *J Clin Epidemiol* 1995; 48:9.

27. Jadad AR, Cook DJ, Jones A, et al. Methodology and reports of systematic review and meta-analyses. *JAMA* 1998; 280:278.

28. American Society of Clinical Oncology. American Society of Clinical Oncology recommendations for the use of he-

29. matopoietic colony-stimulating factors: evidence-based clinical practice guidelines. *J Clin Oncol* 1994; 12:2471.

29. Winn R, McClure J. The NCCN clinical practice guidelines in oncology: a primer for users. *J Natl Cancer Center Network* 2003; 1:5.

30. Hayman JA, Weeks JC. Techniques used in the assessment of cost-effectiveness. *Dis Breast Updates* 1999; 3:1.

31. Earle CC, Coyle D, Evans WK. Cost-effective analysis in oncology. *Ann Oncol* 1998; 9:475.

32. Russell LB, Gold MR, Siegel JE, Daniels N, Weinstein MC. Panel on cost-effectiveness analysis in health and medicine. *JAMA* 1996; 276:1172.

33. Fisher ES, Wennberg DE, Stukel TA, et al. The implications of regional variations in Medicare spending. Part 1: the content, quality and accessibility of care. *Ann Intern Med* 2003; 138:279.

34. Wennberg JE. Unwarranted variations in healthcare delivery: implications for academic medical centers. *BMJ* 2002; 325:961.

35. Hoverman JR, Robertson SM. Lung cancer: a cost and outcomes study based on physician practice patterns. *Disease Management* 2004; 7:112.

36. Gelijns AL, Brown LD, Magnell C, et al. Evidence, politics and technological change. *Health Affairs* 2005; 24:29.

37. Anthonisen NR, Skeans MA, Wise RA, et al. The Lun Health Study Research Group. The effects of a smoking cessation intervention on 14.5-year mortality. *Ann Intern Med* 2005; 142:233.

38. Kelley MJ, McCrory DC. Prevention of lung cancer: summary of published evidence. *Chest* 2003; 123:50S.

39. Hopkins DP, Briss PA, Ricard CJ. Reviews of evidence regarding interventions to reduce tobacco use and exposure to environmental tobacco smoke. *Am J Prev Med* 2001; 20:16.

40. Munafo M. Pharmacological therapy is relatively cost-effective when added to counseling. *Evidence-based Healthcare* 2003; 7:44.

41. Karnath B. Smoking cessation. *Am J Med* 2002; 112:399.

42. Koike T, Terashima M, Takizawa T, et al. The influence of lung cancer mass screening on surgical results. *Lung Cancer* 1999; 24:74.

43. Humphrey LL, Teutsch S, Johnson M. Lung cancer screening with sputum cytologic examination, chest radiography and computed tomography: An update for the US Preventative Services Task Force. *Ann Intern Med* 2004; 140:740.

44. Mahadevia PJ, Fleisher LA, Frick KD, et al. Lung cancer screening with helical computed tomography in older adult smokers: a decision and cost-effectiveness analysis. *JAMA* 2003; 289:313.

45. Gohagan J, Marcus P, Fagerstrom R, et al. Baseline findings of a randomized feasibility trial of lung cancer screening with spiral CT scan vs chest radiograph: The Lung Screening Study of the National Cancer Institute. *Chest* 2004; 126:114.

46. Pastorino U, Bellomi M, Landoni C, et al. Early lung-cancer detection with spiral CT and positron emission tomography in heavy smokers: 2-year results. *Lancet* 2003; 362:593.

47. Chirikos TN, Hazelton T, Tockman M, Clark R. Screening for lung cancer with CT: a preliminary cost-effectiveness analysis. *Chest* 2002; 121; 1507.

48. Herder GJM, Verboom P, Smit EF, et al. Practice, efficacy and cost of staging suspected non-small cell lung cancer: a retrospective study in two Dutch hospitals. *Thorax* 2002; 57:11.

49. Gambhir SS, Shepherd JE, Shah BD, et al. Analytical decision model for the cost-effective management of solitary pulmonary nodules. *J Clin Oncol* 1998; 16:2113.

50. Dietlein M, Weber K, Gandjour A, et al. Cost-effectiveness of FDG-PET for the management of solitary pulmonary

nodules: a decision analysis based on cost reimbursement in Germany. *Eur J Nucl Med* 2000; 27:1441.

51. Sloka JS, Hollett JD, Mathews M. Cost-effectiveness of positron emission tomography for non-small lung carcinoma in Canada. *Med Sci Monit* 2004; 10:MT73.

52. Kalff V, Hicks RI, MacManus MP, et al. The clinical impact of F-18 FDG positron emission tomography (PET) in patients with non-small cell lung cancer: a prospective study. *J Clin Oncol* 2001; 19:111.

53. MacManus MP, Wong K, Hicks RJ, et al. Early mortality after radical radiotherapy for non-small cell lung cancer: comparison of PET-staged and conventionally staged cohorts treated at a large tertiary referral center. *Int J Radiat Oncol Biol Phys* 2002; 52:351.

54. Hoekstra CH, Stroobants SG, Hoekstra OS, et al. The value of (18F) fluoro-2-deoxy-D-glucose positron emission tomography in the selection of patients with IIIA-N2 non-small cell lung cancer for combined modality treatment. *Lung Cancer* 2003; 39:151.

55. MacManus MP, Hicks RJ, Ball DL, et al. F-18 fluorodeoxyglucose positron emission tomography staging in radical radiotherapy candidates with non-small cell lung carcinoma: powerful correlation with survival and high impact on treatment. *Cancer* 2001; 92; 886.

56. Viney RC, Boyer MJ, King MT, et al. Randomized controlled trial of the role of positron emission tomography in the management of stage I and II non-small cell lung cancer. *J Clin Oncol* 2004; 22:2357.

57. Esnaola NF, Lazarides SN, Mentzer SJ, Kuntz KM. Outcomes and cost-effectiveness of alternative staging strategies for non-small-cell lung cancer. *J Clin Oncol* 2001; 20:263.

58. Kelly RF, Tran T, Holmstrom A, Murar J, Segurola RJ. Accuracy and cost-effectiveness of [18F]-2-fluoro-deoxy-D-glucose-positron emission tomography scan in potentially resectable non-small cell lung cancer. *Chest* 2004; 125:1413.

59. Harewood GC, Wiersema MJ, Edell EX, Liebow M. Cost-minimization analysis of alternative diagnostic approaches in a modeled patient with non-small cell lung cancer and subcarinal lymphadenopathy. *Mayo Clin Proc* 2002; 77:155.

60. Detterbeck FC, Falen S, Rivera MP, Halle JS, Socinski MA. Seeking a home for a PET, part 2: defining the appropriate place for positron emission tomography imaging in the staging of patients with suspected lung cancer. *Chest* 2004; 125:2300.

61. Toloza EM, Harpole L, McCrory DC. Noninvasive staging of non-small lung cancer: a review of the current evidence. *Chest* 2002; 123:137S.

62. Vansteenkiste J, Fischer BW, Dooms C, Mortensen J. Positron-emission tomography in prognostic and therapeutic assessment of lung cancer: systematic review. *Lancet Oncol* 2004; 5:531.

63. Colice GL, Rubins J, Unger M, American College of Chest Physicians. Follow-up and surveillance of the lung cancer patient following curative-intent therapy. *Chest* 2003; 123:272S.

64. Egermann U, Jaeggi K, Habicht JM, Perruchoud AP, Dalquen P, Soler M. Regular follow-up after curative resection of non-small cell lung cancer: a real benefit for patients? *Eur Respir J* 2002; 19:464.

65. Evans WK, Will BP, Berthelot JM, Wolfson MC. Estimating the cost of lung cancer diagnosis and treatment in Canada: the POHEM model. *Can J Oncol* 1995; 4:408.

66. Ramsey SD, Howlader N, Etzioni RD, Donato B. Chemotherapy use, outcomes, and costs for older persons with advanced non-small-lung cancer: evidence from surveillance, epidemiology and end results-Medicare. *J Clin Oncol* 2004; 22:4971.

67. Ramsey SD, Moinpour CM, Lovato LC, et al. Economic analysis of vinorelbine plus cisplatin versus paclitaxel plus carboplatin for advanced non-small-cell lung cancer. *J Natl Cancer Inst* 2002; 94:291.

68. ELVIS Group. Effects of vinorelbine on quality of life and survival of elderly patients with advanced non-small lung cancer. *J Natl Cancer Inst* 1999; 91:66.

69. Rapp E, Pater VL, Willan A, et al. Chemotherapy can prolong survival in patients with advanced non-small cell lung cancer: report of a Canadian multicenter randomized trial. *J Clin Oncol* 1998; 16:633.

70. Non Small Cell lung Cancer Collaborative Group. Chemotherapy in non-small cell lung cancer: a meta-analysis using updated data on individual patients from 52 randomized clinical trials. *BMJ* 1995; 311:899.

71. Dest CE, Hillner BE, Smith TJ. Economic considerations in the care of lung cancer patients. *Curr Opin Oncol* 1996; 8:126.

72. Berthelot JM, Will BP, Evans WK, Coyle D, Earle CC, Bordeleau L. Decision framework for chemotherapy interventions for metastatic non-small-cell lung cancer. *J Natl Cancer Inst* 2000; 92:1321.

73. Evans WK, Will BP, Bertholet J, Earle CC. Cost of combined modality interventions for stage III non-small-cell lung cancer. *J Clin Oncol* 1997; 15:3030.

74. Schiller JH, Harrington D, Sandler A, et al. A randomized phase III trial of four chemotherapy regimens in advanced non-small cell lung cancer (NSCLC). *Proc Am Soc Clin Oncol* 2000; 19:1a.

75. Rubio-Terres C, Tisaire JL, Kobina S, Moyano A. Cost-minimization analysis of three regimens of chemotherapy (docetaxel-cisplatin, paclitaxel-cisplatin, paclitaxel-carboplatin) for advanced non-small-cell lung cancer. *Lung Cancer* 2002; 35:81.

76. Johnson DH, Adak S, Cella DF, et al. Topotecan vs observation following cisplatin plus etoposide in extensive stage small cell lung cancer (E7593): a phase III trial of the Eastern Cooperative Group. *Proc Am Soc Clin Oncol* 2000; 19:482a.

77. Bleehan NM, Girling DJ, Mackin D, et al. A randomized trial of three vs six courses of etoposide, cyclophosphamide, methotrexate and vincristine or 6 courses of etoposide and ifosfamide in small cell lung cancer (SCLC). I. Survival and prognostic factors. Medical Research Council Lung Cancer Working Party. *Br J Cancer* 1993; 8:1150.

78. Beith JM, Clarke SJ, Woods RL, et al. Long-term follow-up of a randomized trial of combined chemoradiotherapy induction treatment, with and without maintenance chemotherapy in patients with small cell carcinoma of the lung. *Eur J Cancer* 1996; 32a:438.

79. Buccheri GF, Ferrigno D, Curcio A, et al. Continuation of chemotherapy versus supportive care alone in patients with inoperable non-small cell lung cancer and stable disease after two or three cycles of MACC. *Cancer* 1989; 63:428.

80. Smith IE, O'Brien MER, Talbot DC, et al. Duration of chemotherapy for advanced non-small cell lung cancer (NSCLC): a phase III randomized trial of three vs six courses of mitomycin C, vinblastine, cisplatin (MVP). *J Clin Oncol* 2001; 19:1336.

81. Socinski MA, Schell MJ, Peterman A, et al. A phase III trial comparing a defined duration of therapy vs continuous therapy followed by second-line therapy in advanced stage IIIB/IV non-small cell lung cancer. *J Clin Oncol* 2002; 20:1335

82. Sheperd FA, Dancey J, Ramlau R, et al. Prospective randomized trial of docetaxel vs best supportive care in patients with non-small-cell lung cancer previously treated with platinum-based chemotherapy. *J Clin Oncol* 2000; 18:2095.

83. Foscell FV, DeVore R, Kerr RN, et al. Randomized phase III trial of docetaxel versus vinorelbine or ifosfamide in patients with advanced non-small-cell lung cancer previously treated with platinum containing chemotherapy regimens. *J Clin Oncol* 2000; 18:2354.

84. von Pawel J, Schiller JH, Sheperd FA, et al. Topotecan vs cyclophosphamide, doxorubicin and vincristine for the treatment of recurrent small-cell lung cancer. *J Clin Oncol* 1999; 17:658.

85. Huisman C, Smit EF, Postmus PE. Second-line chemotherapy in relapsing or refractory non-small-cell lung cancer: a review. *J Clin Oncol* 2000; 18:3722.

86. Holmes J, Dunlop D, Hemmett L, Sharplin P, Bose U. A cost-effectiveness analysis of docetaxel in the second-line treatment of non-small cell lung cancer. *Pharmacoeconomics* 2004; 22:581.

87. Massarelli E, Andre F, Liu DD, et al. A retrospective analysis of the outcome of patients who have received two prior chemotherapy regimens including a platin and docetaxel for recurrent non-small-cell lung cancer (abstract 1323). *Proc Am Soc Clin Oncol* 2002; 21:331a.

88. Delbaldo C, Michiels S, Syz N, et al. Benefits of adding a drug to a single-agent or a 2-agent chemotherapy regimen in advanced non-small-cell lung cancer: a meta-analysis. *JAMA* 2004; 292:470.

89. Hanna N, Shepherd FA, Fossella FV, et al. Randomized phase III trial of pemetrexed vs docetaxel in patients with non-small-cell lung cancer previously treated with chemotherapy. *J Clin Oncol* 2004; 22:1589.

90. Kelly K, Crowley J, Bunn PA, et al. Randomized phase III trial of paclitaxel plus carboplatin versus vinorelbine plus cisplatin in the treatment of patients with advanced non-small-cell lung cancer: A Southwest Oncology Group trial. *J Clin Oncol* 2001; 19:3210.

91. Gandara DR, Crowley J, Livingston RB, et al. Evaluation of cisplatin intensity in metastatic non-small cell lung cancer: a phase III study of the Southwest Oncology group. *J Clin Oncol* 1993; 11:873.

92. Cole JT, Gralla RJ, Rittenberg CN, et al. Defining the dose of docetaxel in combination chemotherapy of non-small cell lung cancer: preserving efficacy with lower dose regimens (abstract 1671). *Proc Am Soc Clin Oncol* 1997; 16:465a.

93. Costich TD, Lee FC. Improving cancer care in a Kentucky managed care plan: a case study of cancer disease management. *Disease Management* 2003; 6:9.

94. Seidenfeld J, Piper M, Flamm C, et al. Epoetin treatment of anemia associated with cancer therapy: a systematic review and meta-analysis of controlled clinical trials. *J Natl Cancer Inst* 2001; 93:1204.

95. Rizzo DH, Lichtin AE, Woolf SH, et al. Use of epoetin in patients with cancer: evidence-based clinical practice guidelines of the American Society of Clinical Oncology and the American Society of Hematology. *J Clin Oncol* 2002; 19:4083.

96. Browman GP. Standards of proof, standards of practice, and proof of standards: a tale of two trials. *J Clin Oncol* 2005; 23:2583.

97. Witzig TE, Silberstein TP, Loprinzi CL, et al. Phase III, randomized, double-blind study of epoetin alfa vs placebo in anemic patients with cancer undergoing chemotherapy. *J Clin Oncol* 2004; 23; 2606.

98. Adams JR, Lyman GH, Djubegovic B, Feinglass J, Bennett CL. G-CSF as prophylaxis of febrile neutropenia in SCLC. *Expert Opin Pharmacother* 2002; 3:1273.

99. Bunn PA Jr, Crowley J, Kelly K, et al. Chemotherapy with or without granulocyte-macrophage colony stimulating factors in the treatment of limited-stage small-cell lung cancer: a prospective phase III randomized study of the Southwest Oncology Group. *J Clin Oncol* 1995; 13:1632.

100. Hartmann LC, Tschetter LK, Habermann TM, et al. Granulocyte colony stimulating factors in severe chemotherapy-induced afebrile neutropenia. *N Engl J Med* 1997; 336:1776.

101. Delaney G, Barton M, Jacob S, Jalaludin B. A model for decision making for the use of radiotherapy in lung cancer. *Lancet Oncol* 2003; 4:120.

102. Tyldesley S, Boyd C, Schulze K, et al. Estimating the need for radiotherapy for lung cancer: an evidence-based epidemiologic approach. *Int J Radiat Oncol Biol Phys* 2001; 49:973.

103. Barbera L, Walker H, Foroudi F, et al. Estimating the benefit and cost of radiotherapy for lung cancer. *Int J Technol Assess Health Care* 2004; 20:545.

104. McQuay HJ, Carroll D, Moore RA. Radiotherapy for painful bone metastases: a systematic review. *Clin Oncol* 1997; 9:150.

105. Moran JM, Elshaikh MA, Lawrence TS. Radiotherapy: what can be achieved by technical improvements in dose delivery? *Lancet Oncol* 2005; 6:51.

106. Martel MK. Advanced radiation treatment planning and delivery approaches for treatment of lung cancer. *Hematol Oncol Clin North Am* 2004; 18:231.

107. van Tinteren H, Hoekstra OS, Smit EF, et al. Effectiveness of positron emission tomography in the preoperative assessment of patients with suspected non-small-cell lung cancer: the PLUS multicentre randomized trial. *Lancet* 2002; 359:1388.

108. Pasic A, Brokx HA, Noordegraaf AV, Paul RM, Postmus PE, Sutedja TG. Cost-effectiveness of early intervention: comparison between intraluminal bronchoscopic treatment and surgical resection for T1N0 lung cancer patients. *Respiration* 2004; 71:391.

109. Van Schil P. Cost analysis of video-assisted thoracic surgery vs thoracotomy: critical review. *Eur Respir J* 2003; 22:735.

110. Braud A, Levy-Piedbois C, Piedbois P, et al. Direct treatment costs for patients with lung cancer from first recurrence to death in France. *Pharmacoeconomics* 2003; 21:671.

111. Campbell DE, Lynn J, Louis TA, Shugarman LR. Medicare program expenditures associated with hospice use. *Ann Intern Med* 2004; 140:269.

112. SUPPORT Principal Investigators. A controlled trial to improve care for seriously ill hospitalized patients. *JAMA* 1995; 274:1591.

113. Beresford L, Byock I, Twohig J. Promoting excellence: financial implications of promoting excellence in end-of-life care. http://www.promotingexcellence.org/finance/ (Accessed 3/1/2005).

114. Ripamonti C, Bianchi M. The use of methadone for cancer pain. *Hematol Oncol Clin North Am* 2002; 16:543.

115. Earle CC, Chapman, RH, Baker CS, et al. Systematic overview of cost-utility assessments in oncology. *J Clin Oncol* 2000; 18:3302.

Decision-Making in Lung Cancer

57

Geoff P. Delaney and Bruce G. French

Contents

57.1 Introduction

Decision-making for many clinical conditions is complex. This is particularly the case for lung cancer as the illness has a high mortality rate and the treatment options usually have moderate to significant morbidities. In addition, the patients may have complicated medical, psychological, and social issues that may impact upon their fitness for appropriate treatment.

The maze that patients have to negotiate before making a treatment decision is frequently convoluted. Many medical disciplines may be required to assist decision-making. These disciplines include primary healthcare, pathology, diagnostic radiology, respiratory physicians, cardiothoracic surgeons, radiation oncologists, clinical oncologists, medical oncologists, palliative care teams, community healthcare, physiotherapists, social workers, occupational therapists, psychologists, respiratory laboratory technicians, and speech therapists.

The information being provided to patients is often difficult for them to understand and requires the ability to problem-solve when under the emotional strain of receiving information on a new diagnosis that may have lethal consequences. The patient may also have preconceived ideas about the illness and treatment, which may sometimes be incorrect. Therefore, it is imperative that instruments are developed that improve the clinician's ability to choose the appropriate treatment for the patient and can improve the patient's understanding and retention of information so that they are able to make an informed decision.

This chapter will examine some of the issues involved in decision-making, focusing on some of the specific decisions that patients and clinicians need to make, the complexities behind problem-solving in lung cancer, and on tools that have been developed to improve decision-making.

57.2 Factors Involved in Making Decisions

The complexity of the decision-making process results not only from the milieu of evidence for and against treatment but also because the individuals involved in decision-making all may view and value states of health, toxicity, and outcome differently [1]. There are a large number of factors that impact upon decision-making in lung cancer. Some of these factors have been well studied whereas others have had little formal research. Table 57.1 lists some of the factors that contribute to the complexity of decision-making in lung cancer.

57.3 Variations in Decision-Making in Lung Cancer

Population-based patterns of care studies provide useful data to assess the level of care and the proportions of patients that undergo particular treatments and to make comparisons between different areas. Some of the varia-

Table 57.1. Factors that impact upon decision-making in lung cancer

Clinician-related factors	Patient-related factors
Type of clinician (primary health, specialist, etc.)	Age
Level of experience	Performance status
Past experiences with similar patients	Co-morbid conditions
Past training	Race/culture
Degree of nihilism	Geographical location
Referral patterns	Distance from a treating center
Clinical biases	Economic considerations
Understanding and interpretation of literature	Perception of life expectancy
Access to literature and/or evidence-based treatment guidelines	Degree of nihilism
Conference attendance	Perception of illness
Extent of disease	Perception of treatment factors
Histology	Level of understanding of clinical information
Availability of staging investigations	Past experiences
Perception of patient's fitness for treatment	Psychological state
Cultural issues	Ability to make decision under pressure
	Intellect
	Level of support from family and friends
	Rate at which decision needs to be made
	Current symptoms
	Fitness for treatment
	Whether the patient is risk-averse or risk-accepting

tions in treatment relate to variations in decision-making in different regions. Understanding differences in patterns of care helps to formulate strategies to improve decision-making and treatment in areas where these differences in treatment are considered inappropriate.

Table 57.2 summarizes population-based patterns of care data for lung cancer from different geographical regions published in the past 12 years [2–8]. These studies indicate that there are widely disparate patterns of care between regions and there are relatively low rates of specialist referral of lung cancer patients in some regions. Although some differences might be due to variations in socioeconomic, disease-related, and general health demographics, such as stage of disease at presentation or age and fitness level of particular populations, it is known that differences in the patterns of care of lung cancer are not solely based upon cancer-specific factors. This therefore suggests that decision-making factors play a significant role in some areas and may reflect differences in clinician's views about treatment and differences in access to multidisciplinary care.

Variations in patterns of practice have been shown to relate to the type of clinician specialty and training [9–13], the lung cancer patient caseload volume seen by the initial clinician [12, 14], the duration of experience of the clinician [12], patient socioeconomic factors [15, 16], and the overall process of care [4]. The relatively high rates of non-referral for specialist care and the high proportions of patients where a tissue diagnosis is not made when compared with other cancers in some of these studies suggests that "some clinicians had been applying a different set of standards to the management of lung cancer compared with what they might do, for example, in dealing with a cancer of the breast or oro-

pharynx" [17]. In at least one study, even patients with good performance status were not receiving the level of care that would be considered optimal [6]. This relates to the nihilism that some clinicians have about the outcome of lung cancer patients. Surveys of clinicians' attitudes to the management and outcome of lung cancer show variability in attitudes on the worthiness of treatment for specific treatment groups, especially patients with more advanced stages of lung cancer [18, 19]. It is known that patients' attitudes to their illness will be profoundly affected and manipulated by the information provided at the early consultations.

Decision-making requires access to advice about treatment, and patterns of care studies suggest that patients can miss out on this advice. The further one lives from a major city, the less likely one is to receive radiotherapy or chemotherapy [8, 10, 20–23]. Another study showed that establishing a cardiothoracic clinic increased the lung cancer resection rates [24]. The new rates of resection correlated with the resection rates in well-established cardiothoracic practices implying that patients diagnosed with lung cancer prior to the implementation of such a clinic were being denied access to potentially curable treatment by omission of referral. Similarly, non-medical factors, such as access to a medical oncologist rather than tumor- or patient-related prognostic factors, played a major role in determining referral for a chemotherapy opinion thus potentially denying appropriate patients an appropriate intervention [10, 22].

Even within oncology specialties there can be quite disparate interpretations of the evidence and hence the proportion of patients treated with radical or palliative intent. For example, several studies have indicated very

Table 57.2. Population-based patterns of care studies in lung cancer

Area	Victoria, Australia	Glasgow, Scotland	Scotland	US National Cancer Data Base	Southwestern Sydney, Australia	Republic of Ireland	Northern Sydney, Australia	Hunter region, Newcastle, Australia
Reference	Richardson et al. (2000) [2]	Kesson et al. (1998) [3]	Gregor et al. (2001) [4]	Fry et al. (1999) [5]	Vinod et al. (2003) [6]	Mahmud et al. (2003) [7]	Vinod et al. (2004) [8]	Vinod et al. (2004) [8]
Study years	1993	1991–1992	1995	1995	1993 and 1996	1994–1998	1996	1996
Median age (years)	69	NR	NR	NR NR	68	70	73	70
Pathology								
NSCLC (%)	73	54	56		75	62	74	68
SCLC (%)	14	15	18		16	14	16	12
No histology (%)	12	31	26		9	24	10	20
Percent receiving conservative care	25	38	43	19	28	50	22	45
Percent receiving surgery[a]	23	5	12	27	19	12	26	17
Percent receiving radiotherapy[a]	44	20	36	56	56	22	54	39
Percent receiving chemotherapy[a]	18	10	16	30	21	9	34	12
Percent where treatment was unknown	2	20.5	0	0	0	0	0	0
Median survival (months)	NR	NR	3.6	NR	6.7	NR	7.4	6.4
3-Year survival (%)	NR	9	7	NR	11	NR	15	8
5-Year survival (%)	11	NR	NR	NR	8	NR	10	7

NR not reported, *NSCLC* non-small cell lung cancer, *SCLC* small cell lung cancer

[a] Percent receiving treatment adds up to >100% as some patients had more than one treatment modality except for the study by Mahmud et al. where the percent treatment rates are for single modality only. A further 8% had a combination of treatments which were not specified

different proportions of patients treated with radical radiotherapy versus palliative radiotherapy across hospitals and countries [11, 14, 18, 25–27]. These differences are not due to differences in patient population alone and are likely to be related to differing views about the benefits of radical treatment or due to differences in access to particular health services. For example, one study identified that a reduction in radical radiotherapy across a Canadian province correlated with increasing workload of radiotherapy departments, suggesting that decisions were being made based on availability of resources as opposed to clinical factors [11]. Similarly, studies have identified significant variations in chemotherapy regimen used for metastatic non-small cell lung cancer [28] and small cell lung cancer [29].

The patterns of care data are used to improve the standard of care in areas where deficiencies are identified and then re-study the study population to assess the impact that introduction of a new practice has had on patterns of care, survival, and quality of life. A recent large health services research consortium has been established in the USA to determine what characteristics of patients and their providers influence treatment decisions and to evaluate the effects that specific thera-

pies have on survival, quality of life, and satisfaction with care [30]. The results of such a study will be important in our understanding of what factors most impact on decision-making variations.

57.4 Decision-Making from the Clinician's Perspective

The clinician is responsible for considering all of the prognostic factors available and all of the evidence that is known about the particular stage of disease for each individual patient. Before discussing treatment options with the patient, the clinician needs to consider what the treatment alternatives are and whether any treatment options are inappropriate for that patient. This is usually done by assessing all the clinical data and then applying the evidence to best fit that patient's case. Therefore, the clinical factors that go into decision-making are important. This usually involves an assessment of the extent of the disease, the presence of comorbid medical conditions that may complicate or preclude therapy and the overall performance status and life expectancy of the patient. Sometimes the evidence is highly complex and perhaps controversial where conflicting clinical data exist. There are many controversies in the management of lung cancer. The relevant choices available and treatment controversies for each stage of disease are discussed in previous chapters of this textbook. This section mainly discusses the decision-making process that goes into assessing the appropriateness of treatment.

57.4.1 Patient Fitness for Treatment

One of the major factors in deciding on possible therapy options relies on an assessment of the patient's fitness for particular treatment by the clinician. Many of these assessments of fitness for therapy are subjective rather than objective in nature and often rely on the experience of the clinician, which may lead to variations in practice and perhaps the inappropriate treatment or omission of treatment for some patients. There are some tools available that provide a guide as to the fitness required for the various treatment options although further research and the development of more objective measures are required.

57.4.2 Surgery

There are four main considerations when deciding which patients are suitable for surgical resection in lung cancer:
1. Is the pulmonary lesion anatomically able to be excised?
2. Establishing the diagnosis.
3. Performance of the extent of disease workup.
4. Assessment of a patient's fitness for the required surgical resection.

Is the Pulmonary Lesion Anatomically Able to be Excised?

Most patients with resectable lung cancer have a localized pulmonary lesion apparent on a chest computed tomography (CT) scan. From the chest CT scan the clinician can identify the radiological margins of the pulmonary lesion and thus decide whether the lesion is likely to be resectable by lobectomy, bilobectomy or by pneumonectomy.

The chest CT scan may also indicate the possibility of locally advanced but potentially resectable disease, such as chest wall invasion/attachment or hilar nodal enlargement. Thus the clinician can assess whether the lesion might require a contiguous chest wall resection or whether an otherwise more extensive pulmonary resection (such as a pneumonectomy) might be necessary to encompass hilar lymph nodes.

The chest CT scan may also demonstrate local or regional abnormalities indicating inoperability. Direct invasion of the mediastinum or central tumors involving the proximal pulmonary artery or main bronchus origin indicate inoperability. Macroscopic involvement of the ipsilateral superior mediastinal lymph nodes or the subcarinal lymph nodes also indicates inoperability. In some instances these situations may be rendered resectable by induction chemotherapy.

Establishing the Diagnosis

It is a sensible plan to obtain a tissue diagnosis of lung cancer prior to planning any definitive treatment. Rarely small cell lung cancer may be diagnosed and this is not a disease treated by surgical excision. In a few special situations surgical resection may proceed without a definitive cancer diagnosis preoperatively but where the diagnosis of non-small cell lung cancer is likely.

Centrally placed tumors and tumors associated with airway symptoms are likely to yield a diagnosis through diagnostic bronchoscopy, or occasionally from sputum cytology. Peripherally placed tumors are more likely to yield a diagnosis through CT-guided transcutaneous fine-needle aspirate cytology.

Some situations may require bronchoscopic fine-needle (Wang) cytology [31]. Transcervical paratracheal mediastinoscopy enables the biopsy of paratracheal and subcarinal lymph nodes. Lesions in the aortopulmonary window are best biopsied using a transpleural approach either by left anterior incision or by video-assisted thoracoscopic surgery.

In rare situations preoperative diagnostic measures may fail to demonstrate malignancy. If there remains sufficient doubt as to whether the patient may have a potentially resectable malignant lesion then the clinician needs to make a decision about whether to proceed to a surgical resection without a preoperative cancer diagnosis or to further attempts to establish a preoperative diagnosis. Provided the patient is fully informed it is reasonable to perform a thoracotomy and surgical resection. In some situations (small peripheral tumors less than 2 cm in diameter) a limited resection and frozen section may be useful with the plan to proceed to a lobectomy if the diagnosis is malignant.

Performance of Extent of Disease Workup

It is important prior to any resection with curative intent that an appropriate extent of disease workup is performed as metastatic non-small cell lung cancer is incurable.

The vast majority of non-small cell lung cancers are highly glucose avid and can be accurately located by positron emission tomography (PET). For clinicians with access to PET scanning this investigation is probably the only investigation required [32–35].

Clinicians without access to PET scanning should consider including the liver and adrenal glands in the chest CT scan. A bone scan should be considered for patients with bone symptoms or in higher-stage patients. There is no need to perform a bone scan in patients who have had a PET scan, as PET is more accurate in assessing metastatic bone disease [35]. CT imaging of the brain should be considered if symptoms dictate it and in higher-stage patients.

Whether patients with clinical stage I benefit from PET scanning is unclear as the prevalence of occult distant or regional nodal metastases is extremely low in this group.

Assessment of the Patient's Fitness for the Required Surgical Resection

Pulmonary Reserve

The simplest clinical assessment of pulmonary reserve is exercise tolerance. In its basic form this means taking the patient for a walk and assessing their performance in terms of breathlessness and distance traveled. There has been some standardization of the exercise test in the form of the 6- and 12-min walk tests [36, 37].

The forced expiratory volume in one second (FEV1) accurately predicts tolerance to lung resection, particularly when expressed as a percentage of the predicted FEV1. Increased morbidity and mortality begins to occur when the postresection FEV1 falls below 40% of the predicted value [38]. There is also evidence that a reduction of the diffusing capacity of the lung for carbon monoxide (DLCO) to less than 40% predicted is associated with a poor outcome [39].

In cases where the pulmonary tumor is large the lobe/lung is underventilated but very likely perfused. Thus resection has the potential to remove lung without very significantly affecting the FEV1 and improving ventilation perfusion matching. This may be able to be objectively measured using preoperative differential pulmonary ventilation and perfusion scanning [38, 40–42].

In borderline pulmonary reserve cases full ventilatory function tests, room air arterial blood gases, and consideration for exercise oxygen consumption studies should be performed [43–45]. Normal DLCO and normal blood gases would add weight to the decision to proceed in a borderline resection case. A multidisciplinary approach to the assessment of pulmonary fitness is always a good policy in the borderline case.

Cardiac Fitness

Patients with lung cancer have an increased risk of ischemic heart disease mostly due to common risk factors. The increased risk is not however so significant to jus-

tify detailed cardiac investigations in all patients being worked up for lung resection. Symptomatic ischemic heart disease (angina) is the most common symptom requiring investigation. In some situations coronary artery bypass surgery may be required prior to curative lung cancer surgery. Patients with left ventricular dysfunction are particularly at risk of adverse cardiac events complicating lung cancer surgery. Such patients will mostly likely be symptomatic, particularly during the walk test, or have ECG abnormalities. These patients should be assessed by a cardiologist before lung resection.

Other Medical Conditions

Many other medical conditions may affect a patient's fitness for pulmonary resection. These conditions sporadically occur and should be dealt with appropriately on their merits. Their discussion is beyond the scope of this review.

57.4.3 Radiotherapy and Chemotherapy

There are many possible clinical scenarios that could occur in patients referred for consideration of lung cancer radiotherapy and/or chemotherapy. For patients with localized disease, the main aim of the clinician is to assess the appropriateness of radical treatment and the potential risk of giving treatment. For radiotherapy, the assessment will mainly concentrate on the stage of disease, the cell type, the size of the primary tumor, whether the mediastinum requires treatment, and the overall extent of the radiotherapy treatment fields.

In terms of appropriateness of treatment, determining the risk of radiation pneumonitis and radiation fibrosis will be based on the volume of lung to be irradiated, the total dose received, and the lung capacity of the patient. The greater the volume of lung receiving a high dose, the greater the risk is of long-term respiratory sequelae. Nomograms which graph the volume of lung against radiation dose are predictive of pneumonitis risk and are a valuable objective tool for the radiation oncologist to assess potential morbidity and mortality risk [46–49].

For chemotherapy, there are chemotherapeutic agents that have organ-specific toxicity and specific guidelines are available for each drug as to the dose reductions required when organs have impaired function. For the decision regarding whether patients are fit for chemotherapy, there are several physiological parameters that are easily measured to predict organ tolerance such as renal and liver function tests.

However, there are patients with relatively normal renal and hepatic function who are still considered unfit for treatment because they are more likely to suffer toxicity that outweighs benefit. But how should this be measured and how reliable is individual clinician assessment in predicting this? There have been very few studies examining this in detail and no studies that provided clinicians with an objective measure for choosing the patients that are most appropriately treated with chemotherapy. In addition, effective chemotherapy agents with less toxicity have been recently trialed [50]. This suggests that the area requires critical examination in the future.

While these tests and nomograms predict organ-specific toxicity, the difficulty in decision-making is to recognize the point at which the patient's general fitness becomes so poor that treatment would be inadvisable. In terms of using radical radiotherapy, the main determinant of prognosis for patients undergoing radical therapy is the performance status of the patient [51]. Although there are several prognostic performance status measures used in the literature, most studies quote results based on the Karnofsky performance status (KPS). A recursive partitioning analysis of data from 1,592 patients enrolled into Radiation Therapy Oncology Group (RTOG) trials found that KPS was the strongest predictor of outcome. This suggests that using a measure such as KPS can be useful in evaluating patients for the appropriateness of radical radiotherapy [51] with patients over a KPS of 70 being recommended to have radical therapy provided that organ-specific measures and tumor stage are compatible with a radical approach.

Wigren et al. [52, 53] have devised a clinical decision support tool for lung cancer that calculates a prognostic index based upon scores for disease extent, a clinical symptom score, the performance status of the patient, the tumor size, and baseline hemoglobin level, all of which were observed to be of equal significance when predicting survival. This guides the decision-making by differentiating cases into radical or palliative treatment. This measure was found to correlate with actual decision-making in one retrospective study and also identified those patients more likely to have longer survival suggesting that widespread use of this system may reduce some of the differences in treatments identified by patterns of care studies [54]. Prospective assessment of this tool is required before widespread use.

57.4.4 Age and the Management of Lung Cancer

Patient age is a factor that frequently complicates decisions about the aggressiveness of therapy. Lung cancer is a relatively common cancer in the elderly and therefore assessments that consider age are important. Most studies of lung cancer treatment outcomes have been randomized trials or single-arm retrospective or prospective studies from specialist lung cancer clinics. The studies in lung cancer have therefore involved specific patient populations with the elderly underrepresented, with perhaps only the fit elderly patient included. In many randomized trials, eligibility criteria commonly exclude elderly patients and yet extrapolation from these studies to apply therapy to the elderly frequently occurs in clinical practice.

Although it is recognized that fitness for radical treatment diminishes with age, as does desire for treatment particularly when the gains might be modest and the risk of toxicity high, studies have shown that good outcomes can be achieved in carefully selected patients [55–58] and that treatment tailored to a patient's age is well-tolerated [50, 59–62].

Despite this evidence, population-based studies indicate that the elderly are less often referred and receive less treatment for lung cancer [6, 63, 64]. Referral to a lung specialist declines as age increases above 65 years and some studies have identified a dramatic drop-off with age for the use of radiotherapy, surgery, and chemotherapy once patients reached 65 years of age [6, 15, 22, 63–66]. What is most alarming about this is that a significant proportion of people that are over 65 are stated to be in good health and have possible life-spans of 20–30 years.

The best evidence available would suggest that age alone should not be used as a criterion of appropriateness of treatment and that factors relating to the biological or physiological state of the patient would be more appropriate.

57.4.5 Tools that Can Assist a Clinician's Decision-Making

Evidence-based Treatment Guidelines

Published clinical data are applied differently by different clinicians [9, 14, 18, 28, 67]. The choice of treatment will often depend upon the type of specialty in which the clinician was trained, their exposure to new evidence, and their personal interpretation of these data. Another difficulty facing clinicians is an ever-increasing amount of literature to read to maintain knowledge across all aspects of treatment. Lung cancer literature is spread across oncology, respiratory, cardiothoracic, and general medical texts and journals. Many clinicians also have other diseases for which they need to maintain knowledge as well as lung cancer.

One of the ways that treatment can become more standardized is to describe what is considered appropriate treatment by a panel of representative lead clinicians based on their interpretation of the evidence. This is usually by way of evidence-based treatment guidelines or consensus guidelines. These are usually derived by large clinical groups that use a systematic method of grading the evidence and using the best available evi-

Table 57.3. A list of lung cancer guidelines available

Guideline group	Scope	Publication date/last modified date	Reference
Scottish Intercollegiate Guidelines Network	Management of lung cancer	1998	*www.sign.ac.uk*
Royal College of Radiologists' Clinical Oncology Information Network	Non-surgical management of lung cancer	1999	*www.rcr.ac.uk/lung.pdf*
Australian National Health and Medical Research Council	Prevention, diagnosis and management of lung cancer	2004	*http://www7.health.gov.au/n hmrc/ publications/synopses/ cp97syn.htm*
National Cancer Institute (US). PDQ Cancer Information Summaries	NSCLC SCLC	2004 2004	*www.cancer.gov*
British Columbia Cancer Agency, Canada	NSCLC SCLC	2002 Revision date N/A	*www.bccancer.bc.ca*
Cancer Care Ontario, Canada	Approximately 15 specific guidelines on the use of various treatments for specific clinical stages of NSCLC and SCLC	N/A	*www.cancercare.on.ca*
American Society of Clinical Oncology	Unresectable NSCLC	2003	*www.asco.org*
National Comprehensive Cancer Network	Small cell and neuroendocrine lung cancer	2005	*www.nccn.org*
American College of Chest Physicians	Prevention, screening, diagnosis, staging and management of lung cancer	2005	*Chest* 2003; 123 (suppl 1)
National Institute for Clinical Excellence (UK)	Use of chemotherapy for NSCLC	2001	*www.nice.org.uk*
American Association for Thoracic Surgery, Society of Thoracic Surgeons, Southern Thoracic Surgical Association, et al., USA	Surgical management of lung cancer	1993	*Ann Thorac Surg* 1993; 56:1203
American Cancer Society	Early detection of lung cancer	2001	*CA Cancer J Clin* 2001; 51:38
British Thoracic Society	Malignant mesothelioma	2001	*Thorax* 2001; 56:250 *www.brit-thoracic.org.uk/d ocs*
British Thoracic Society and Society of Cardiothoracic Surgeons of Great Britain and Ireland	Selection of lung cancer patients for surgery	2001	*Thorax* 2001; 56:89 *www.brit-thoracic.org.uk/d ocs*
National Health Service, UK	Planning and development of lung cancer services	1998	*www.dh.gov.uk*
British Thoracic Society	Organizing the care of lung cancer patients	1998	*Thorax* 1998; 53(suppl 1):S1 *www.brit-thoracic.org.uk/d ocs*
The Cochrane library	Twenty-three reviews of various aspects of screening, diagnosis, and management of lung cancer	Various	*http://www3.interscience.wi ley.- com/cgi-bin/mrwhome/1 06568753/ HOME*
European Society of Medical Oncology	SCLC NSCLC	2003 2003	*www.esmo.org*
American College of Radiology	Various guidelines on the diagnosis and management of lung cancer	Various	*www.acr.org*
Palliative Radiotherapy Workshop	Palliative radiotherapy	2001	*Clin Oncol* 2001; 13:86

SCLC small cell lung cancer, *NSCLC* non-small cell lung cancer

dence to formulate policy. There are a large number of lung cancer treatment guidelines available with the more common ones being listed in Table 57.3.

However, there are some limitations of treatment guidelines that must be considered by the clinician before they are used:

1. *Some guidelines are not truly evidence-based.*

Harpole et al. [68] reviewed lung cancer guidelines between 1989 and 2001 and found that only one third of guideline groups had used well-described and rigorous scientific methodology when developing the guidelines. A thorough analysis of the more recently published lung cancer guidelines has not been undertaken but one must be aware when using guidelines that the scientific rigor of the guideline process may vary.

2. *The guidelines are only as good as the evidence.*

There are many aspects of lung cancer care where there is insufficient evidence to formulate a decision as there are insufficient studies of adequate quality available. As the quality of the evidence decreases, it becomes increasingly difficult to formulate a meaningful treatment guideline [69]. In addition, very few studies include quality of life as an endpoint even though the majority of lung cancer patients have incurable disease.

3. *The evidence being used to formulate the guidelines is frequently old.*

Due to the long lead time of publication of evidence in peer-reviewed journals and the lack of new studies in some areas, treatment guidelines may rely on old data that may no longer be relevant to the current clinical situation. An example of this is the role of postoperative radiotherapy for N2 non-small cell lung cancer. This area is controversial due to the conflicting interpretations of the current evidence. What complicates this further is that the randomized data are from old clinical trials using relatively primitive treatment. For instance, since execution of these studies, surgical mortality rates have fallen due to better supportive care and surgical techniques, newer chemotherapy drugs are available with better support of hematological toxicity, and radiotherapy techniques used in the past were often without CT planning and conformal radiotherapy — technologies that have widespread use today. In addition, these trials were done prior to the introduction of PET staging. Evidence suggests that at least 20% of patients that would have met the eligibility criteria for the N2 treatment studies would have been upstaged to M1 disease if PET staging were available [70]. This therefore suggests that at least 20% of patients enrolled in these studies were never going to benefit from locoregional treatment as they already had occult metastatic disease that is now detectable using PET. Therefore the original studies are potentially underpowered, as the number of truly eligible patients has been diluted by patients that were never going to derive a benefit and would be detected by PET if treated today. This means that the management of N2 disease in the PET era has very little evidence by which a decision can be appropriately made. Further studies will need to be done with PET staging as routine. In the meantime, the guideline recommendations are unreliable where the data are old.

4. *The guidelines themselves may be old.*

Treatment guideline development involves significant time and resources. It has been estimated that it takes the Cancer Care Ontario Program in Evidence-Based Care approximately 18 months to produce a scientifically rigorous clinical practice guideline even though they have made explicit decisions about streamlining the process, which they acknowledge may impact on the validity of the guideline [71]. Significant resources are required to maintain the guidelines when new evidence is published.

5. *The guidelines do not cover all clinical scenarios.*

The majority of the evidence comes from randomized trials in which eligibility criteria are limited. The atypical nature of the sample population in randomized trials may have an impact on the potential extrapolation of the results to non-trial populations. For example, patients of lower socioeconomic status are less frequently enrolled in randomized clinical trials when compared with a population-based sample of lung cancer patients [72].

It is also not possible to formulate guidelines that lead to total uniformity of care, nor is it appropriate to attempt to do this. Local circumstances, professional judgment, patient choice, co-morbid conditions, and inefficiencies of healthcare facilities all confound attempts to get uniform care [73–75]. In addition, moving all decisions toward a consensus does not always lead to the best care for each individual [73, 76] and some variability in compliance with guidelines may be based on appropriate individual patient variations or clinician judgment rather than clinician refusal [69, 75].

6. *The guidelines may conflict.*

It has been identified that there may be some conflict in treatment recommendations between guidelines for a particular stage of disease even when the guideline committees are using the same evidence [68, 77–79]. These differences often reflect conflicting or relatively poor quality evidence or evidence of a small benefit and additional toxicity where the trade-off between the advantages and disadvantages of treatment may be controversial, for example, the role of postoperative radiotherapy for N2 non-small cell lung cancer.

7. *The guidelines might not have adequate representation from specialty areas.*

Some guidelines list their committee members and their relevant specialties. Other guidelines have lists of names without identifying the specialty or no list of contributors at all. Unless aware of who the contributors are then there is no way of telling whether all relevant specialties have been represented. Palliative care clinicians and nurses seem to be poorly represented in a number of different guideline committees. Type of specialty and training influences decision-making and therefore the constituency of the guideline panel may influence the recommendations [68].

8. *Guidelines do not necessarily alter local practice.*

Guideline publication does not necessarily alter clinical practice. Surveys of clinicians' attitudes to the introduction of lung cancer guidelines found that clinicians were suspicious of guidelines as they felt that they had been introduced to cut treatment costs and up to 20% felt guidelines to be too rigid to be applied to clinical practice [69, 80].

9. *There is disagreement as to what constitutes success of guideline implementation.*

There is conflict between studies as to whether implementation of the majority of clinical guidelines has been successful [81–83] or unsuccessful [74, 75]. This disparity of opinion is largely due to different opinions on the best measure of guideline implementation success. Guideline implementation studies have identified that resultant changes in practice have led to improvements in efficiency, improvements in cost effectiveness, improvements in reduced complication rates, or merely improvement in consistency of treatment. However, these objectives may not be of sufficient benefit to justify the time, effort, and cost involved in setting them up and keeping them up to date. One of the only guideline implementation studies that have found a possible improvement in survival was a breast cancer study that showed that incremental improvements in survival over time corresponded with greater compliance to the clinical guidelines and that the magnitude of the improvements in survival corresponded with the results from randomized trials suggesting that the increase in guideline compliance resulted in a survival benefit as more patients were being treated with optimal therapy [84].

10. *Guidelines are subject to publication bias.*

The majority of guidelines rank published data highest when it comes to assessing the quality of evidence. This potentially introduces publication bias as there may be a large number of trials with negative outcomes which are unpublished. It is imperative that all studies are registered so that the guideline recommendations are not skewed inappropriately toward the publication bias that occurs [71].

While the limitations suggested above limit the usefulness of guidelines, they remain an improvement compared with the relatively haphazard way that lung cancer care has been delivered in the pre-guideline era. Several reviews have shown that the introduction of evidence-based treatment guidelines does lead to a change in practice in the majority of cases [81, 83]. Studies have identified that the best way to implement guidelines and change practice is to ensure wide dissemination of the guidelines and provide feedback to the clinicians about their performance in comparison to the entire treating clinician group [81]. One method for improving the uptake of guidelines is through the use of sophisticated software linked to the clinician's electronic patient database that will alert the clinician when a patient's characteristics match those for which a treatment

recommendation is available [71]. This technology remains the subject of research.

Evidence-based Decision Trees

One further step in using evidence-based treatment guidelines to aid decision-making is to use these treatment guidelines to formulate evidence-based decision trees. For example, the US National Cancer Control Network publish their guideline recommendations in the form of decision trees thus representing the pathway of care in a diagrammatic fashion (www.nccn.org).

Decision trees may also be used to predict the proportions of patients with a particular stage of cancer that should receive treatment. The process was first described to examine the optimal rate of radiotherapy delivery in lung cancer [85]. A radiotherapy decision tree for lung cancer was derived by using evidence-based treatment guidelines. The tree was constructed with branch-points corresponding to patient-, tumor-, or treatment-related attributes that impact on the decision to treat or not to treat with radiotherapy. Epidemiological data on the proportions of the identified attributes were then used to calculate the overall proportion of all lung patients that should receive treatment. The study predicted that 61% of patients should receive at least one course of radiotherapy at some point during their illness; this was substantially higher than occurred in actual practice. A similar study estimated that 76% of patients should receive at least one course of radiotherapy at some time during their illness [65]. The differences in result compared with the original study were a result of differing interpretations of the guidelines and the use of Australian epidemiological data. The small cell lung cancer decision tree for radiotherapy is reproduced in Fig. 57.1 as an example of an evidence-based decision tree.

Despite the difference in results of these two studies, they highlighted that optimal rates of radiotherapy exceed the actual rates of radiotherapy delivery by more than 15%. The strength of the research was that the estimates are actually based on the evidence-based treatment guidelines rather than individual opinions or actual practice and therefore provides an evidence-based benchmark that can then be assessed against actual practice, thus identifying the shortfalls between actual and optimal radiotherapy for subpopulations of patients. To be most useful, the data on actual and optimal rates of radiotherapy could then be presented to the treating group in a format to provide feedback about deficiencies in practice and identify areas of potential improvement. A pilot study at the Johns Hopkins Cancer Center using protocols to formulate treatment policies, provide feedback on performance, and analyze the reasons why some patients were not treated according to protocol identified the potential for such a process [86]. A system such as that described could be set

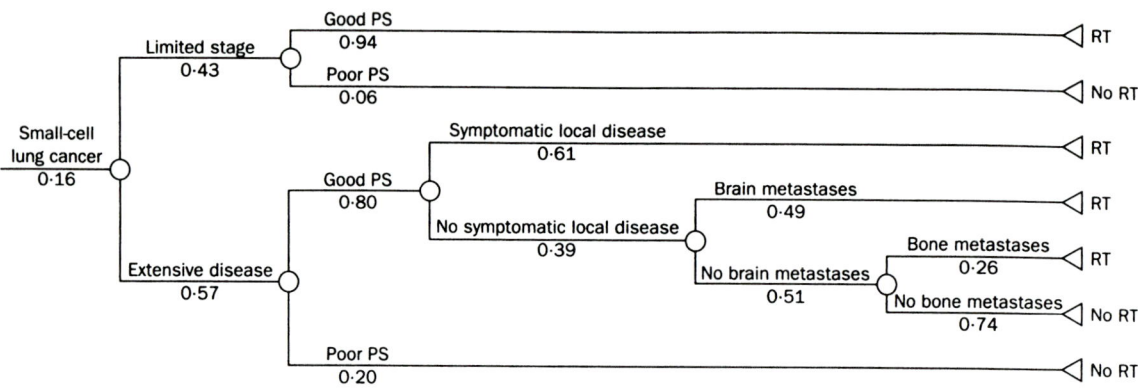

Fig. 57.1. An evidence-based radiotherapy decision tree for small cell lung cancer. *PS* Performance status, *RT* radiotherapy. (Reproduced with permission by Delaney et al. *Lancet Oncol* 2003; 4:120.)

up to evaluate the evidence-based decision trees reported in the last few years.

At the present time, these evidence-based decision trees remain an excellent option for estimating ideal rates of treatment and also to provide clinicians with a decision framework for the management of lung cancer. They can be adapted over time as stage distributions and histology distributions vary. The only lung cancer decision trees reported in the literature to date relate to the use of radiotherapy although treatment decision trees for the use of surgery, chemotherapy, and palliative care based upon evidence-based treatment guidelines would be possible using the same methodology.

57.4.6 Multidisciplinary Management

Is the primary health clinician in the best position to assess the pros and cons of therapy for the patient?

No doubt there are going to be very clear cases of patients not being appropriate for active cancer therapy (e.g., the very elderly or patients of very poor performance status). However, the patterns of care studies of different regions show little similarity in the proportions of patients not receiving any treatment suggesting that some decisions to forego therapy are made in circumstances that might be considered inappropriate. A study of practice patterns in one region of Australia identified that 31% of patients with non-small cell lung cancer who did not receive therapy did not see a specialist [6].

The lack of knowledge about all aspects of lung cancer care for the average primary care physician and the relative biases that specialist clinicians might have about lung cancer treatment might be reduced when there is the opportunity to discuss individual cases openly in a multidisciplinary forum. Studies have identified that patients not discussed in a multidisciplinary setting may be denied access to effective treatment options and ac-

cess to possible clinical trials of new therapies [2]. Some studies have identified that multidisciplinary clinics increase the timeliness of appropriate consultation, timeliness of surgery, and a shorter time from diagnosis to treatment [82, 87, 88]. Research on the benefits of breast cancer multidisciplinary clinics revealed a higher level of patient satisfaction with their choice of treatment when their case was discussed in a multidisciplinary meeting when compared with patients not discussed [82]. However, research evidence is sparse regarding the survival or quality of life impact that managing patients specifically in multidisciplinary clinics provide compared with referral to at least an experienced clinician. Nor is there research into the various different models of multidisciplinary care to recommend one style of clinic over another.

Multidisciplinary clinics have increased in their use despite the lack of evidence of improvements in survival. They do provide the opportunity for clinicians from various different specialties to come together and discuss the various options and provide a reference group for referring doctors to discuss problematic clinical problems particularly when multimodality therapy is appropriate. It is likely that any inherent biases that any one individual might have can be overcome by other members of the group so that more balanced views can be put to the patient. It is for these reasons as well as the likelihood of benefit for the patient in being discussed in a multidisciplinary forum that the development of regional multidisciplinary clinics has been advocated [89].

57.5 Decision-Making from the Patient's Perspective

Consultations with patients with lung cancer are particularly complex. The patient has just been told the diagnosis of a condition with a high mortality rate, they have perhaps been offered treatment of possible benefit but also possible risk, their prognosis has perhaps been discussed with them, and the doctor may then attempt to ask the patient to make a decision about treatment. The consultation is likely to be stressful for the patient, their relatives, and the clinician. This high level of anxiety may impact on the amount of information that the patient might understand, remember, and process. Even without an emotionally charged encounter, patients vary in the amounts of information they can absorb, vary in their capacity to understand and retain information, and doctors vary in their ability to communicate and explain the information. Patients also vary in the amount of information and the amount of decision-making they desire [90]. Differences also exist between patients and clinicians about the type of information considered important when deciding on an intervention [91].

Studies have attempted to examine the factors that might predict for the amount of information required by a patient. Possible factors include age, sex, educational attainment of the patient, type of cancer, stage of disease, type of treatment, and time since diagnosis [90]. A multicenter study examining the information needs of cancer patients found that although the vast majority of patients wanted a lot of detail regarding their diagnosis, prognosis, and treatment options, patients varied in the amount and type of information that they required, and basing a prediction of the amount of information required by an individual on their demographic data was impossible [92]. Although older patients tended to want less information than younger patients, there was sufficient variation across the study group that one cannot make a dogmatic statement about the information needs of a generic cancer patient. To overcome this, the clinician must enquire of the patient the specific type of information that they are seeking and tailor the explanation to the individual patient's requirement.

Not all patients want to make their own decisions about therapy. In one study conducted on breast cancer patients, only 22% wanted complete autonomy of treatment selection, 44% wanted a consultative decision between doctor and patient, and 34% were happier if the treatment selection was delegated to the clinician [93]. The feelings of the patient about their treatment and their level of risk acceptance play a large role in the management decision. This is particularly true in the lung cancer setting as it is such a lethal disease and the treatments have the potential of moderate to severe morbidity. Even when two patients are presented with the same information, their view on whether to proceed with treatment largely relates to their attitude about risk and benefit. Some patients prefer a risk of a very bad outcome if it provides hope for long-term cure whereas others might prefer not to proceed with high-risk treatment provided their intermediate term quality of life is maintained.

57.5.1 Improving Patient Understanding

It is highly important that patients have an accurate understanding of their prognosis when communicating treatment options to them. Patients who overestimate their likelihood of deriving benefit from a treatment were more likely to proceed with treatment compared with patients who do not overestimate their prognosis. The greater the overestimate of prognosis, the greater the aggressiveness of treatment and the higher the risk the patient is willing to take for small benefits. To make an informed decision the discussion around prognosis needs to be understood and accurate [94].

Clinicians have often found it difficult to provide patients with an accurate understanding of prognosis, particularly when the prognosis is poor. It is always easier to give good news or a hope that therapy might work rather than bad news, although doing this will not benefit the patient in the long term [95]. Patients' preferences are also vulnerable to bias and manipulation [96]. This is of particular concern because it has been found that prediction of prognosis in non-small cell lung cancer is highly variable amongst referring doctors [12] and is often intentionally overly optimistic due to the difficulty of discussing bad news [97]. Studies have shown that patients with poorer prognosis have less information discussed with them when compared with patients with a better prognosis, particularly information about prognosis and non-cancer treatment such as supportive care. This suggests that clinicians are more reluctant to provide bad news compared with good news [98–100]. One study identified that although hospitalized patients with cancer had similar survival irrespective of age, the younger patients were less frequently spoken to about issues to do with palliative care, hospice care, or resuscitation, suggesting that doctors were more reluctant to discuss bad news openly with younger patients and that it was easier to have these discussions with patients who were older, frailer, and more accepting about their situation [64]. Furthermore, this study found that younger patients were more aggressively treated with antineoplastic therapy.

The timing of the provision of information, particularly bad news, is important. A survey of patients with incurable malignancy revealed that most patients want information about survival times and likelihood of 5-year survival discussed with them [101]. Their preference was to receive this information in words rather than charts or graphs. However, only 59% of patients wanted to discuss expected survival when first diagnosed with incurable malignancy and most patients wanted to negotiate the amount of information they receive about dying suggesting that clinicians need to attempt to tailor the amount of information to each patient in a consultative way and that multiple consultations are usually required so that the information can be given at a time that best suits each individual patient. The main limitation of this study was selection bias, with non-participants more likely to be unaccepting of the information provided and therefore the data may not reflect the feelings of patients who felt less informed, patients who were poorly informed, and patients who are in denial of their prognosis.

It is also important that clinicians be aware that not all patients understand the information with which they are presented. A group of 287 women of varying education levels were presented with a number of numeracy tasks to assess their ability to understand percentages when discussing the potential benefits of screening mammography [102]. Slightly more than a third of test subjects had a college education. Of three questions presented to the patients, 16% answered all questions correctly, 26% got two correct, 28% one correct, and 30% got no question correct. Although the likelihood of getting the questions correct correlated with education level, the majority of the high education level group were unable to portray the risk accurately enough to suggest that they understood the information being presented to them. Another study showed that patient's recall of risk varied with time with an increasing tendency over time to overestimate the risk of mortality [103].

These studies do not suggest that because of these limitations the patients should be omitted from the role of decision-maker – far from it. However, when a clinician is speaking to a patient, the clinician must understand that there are differences between patients and provide decision-making tools to assist this process. This might be by providing information in different terms apart from percentages and by providing information to the patient in the written as well as the oral form.

57.5.2 Improving Patient Retention of Information

Not all patients accurately recall all of the information provided to them [104]. It is therefore essential that the clinician be aware of this and provide information in several different ways to maximize the chances of the patient retaining the information.

The use of tape-recordings or videotapes of consultations improves patients' recall of the important information given to them to assist with decision-making [104, 105]. Fiset et al. [106] developed a decision aid for metastatic lung cancer patients that included an audiotape and workbook for the patients to take home. Patient knowledge about outcomes was found to be better than pre-intervention suggesting benefit. Further evaluations of these types of aids are warranted.

Websites may also be valuable sources of written information about the management of cancer. The Inter-national Union Against Cancer (UICC) website provides a list of suitable web-based resources for patients. This includes websites with general information for patients. Some oncology groups such as the National Cancer Institute of the United States, the National Comprehensive Cancer Network of the United States, Cancer BACUP, and the National Breast Cancer Centre of Australia have produced consumer versions of the evidence-based treatment guidelines by simplifying the language and removing medical jargon so that patients are able to determine what these groups recognize as appropriate therapy.

There are several limitations to patients using websites. First, with the rapid expansion of the web and lack of editorial control on the information provided on the internet it is difficult for patients to differentiate evidence-based information from non-evidence-based information. Second, trying to make a decision about their specific case can be difficult when the information provided on the internet is usually non-specific. The clinician therefore can play an important role in helping patients find relevant websites and guiding them through the information that they find, making sure the patients understand where the information is relevant and where it is not.

The clinician can also provide in-house information brochures for patients that detail the specifics of treatment. They have the advantage of being able to be more specific than the generic information provided by websites. There are several resources that are available to clinicians to review the quality and completeness of information provided to patients. These include the National Health and Medical Research Council in Australia (www.nhmrc.org.au), the Centre for Health Information Quality in the UK (www.hfht.org/chic/), and the DISCERN questionnaire (www.discern.org.uk) [107].

Another way that clinicians can ensure that patients feel that a shared decision has been made is to encourage their patients to ask questions. In this way, patients can control the amount of information with which they are provided. This may be particularly advantageous as clinicians find it difficult to assess the amount of information each individual feels is optimal. The use of prompt sheets of suggested questions has been evaluated and shown to increase the amount of information patients received, particularly about prognosis [108].

57.5.3 What is the Role of the Family?

Patients have varying decision-making support from family members and therefore the influence that family members might have on a decision will vary between patients. Very few studies have examined the influence that family members have on the decisions made by patients. Zhang and Siminoff [109] identified that up to

65% of families disagreed with the management choice made by patients with locally advanced lung cancer. This had not been previously identified and suggests that significant disagreements between families and the patients need to be identified, explored, and understood by the clinician during the decision-making process. It is particularly important to involve the patient's family in decision-making but by the same token ensure that overbearing family members do not have exaggerated effects on the patient's final decisions and that the patient is comfortable with the decision rather than being cajoled into a treatment decision that they are not comfortable with.

57.5.4 Decision Aids to Assist Patients Analyze the Treatment Options

Decision aids are tools that help patients weigh up the advantages and disadvantages of different treatment options offered when more than one is available. A decision aid is defined as a tool in which the discussion of the pros and cons of treatment are provided in a structured way relevant to the health status of the individual. As stated previously, patients have a need for an accurate understanding of their prognosis and the relative benefits of any treatments being offered in order to make a treatment decision. Therefore, developing decision aids that incorporate clear prognostic information based upon well-researched prognostic factors, rather than providing patients with personal views of evidence and educated prognostic guesses by the referring clinician, is an important issue that requires further research.

There have been more than 50 studies of the use of different decision aids in oncology, with most studies focusing on the decision for adjuvant therapy for breast cancer or the primary treatment of prostate cancer [110]. Most of the studies to date have been small developmental studies. Three randomized studies of the use of a decision aid were performed on breast cancer patients making decisions about treatment for breast cancer [111–113]. Both studies found that the use of a decision aid improved patient knowledge and patient satisfaction regarding their treatment decision-making.

Computerized prognostic index scores based on large databases of patient data have been compiled for breast cancer [113, 114]. They provide nomograms from which individual patient prognostic information can be used to calculate treatment benefits thus providing patients with accurate information. Such a prognostic tool for decision-making in lung cancer has not been developed and the decision analysis tools that have been shown to have some success in the adjuvant breast cancer setting do not necessarily guarantee success in using similar technology in lung cancer as the decisions

are likely to be more complex than deciding on small survival gains in the adjuvant setting. Quality of life, symptom control, and toxicity issues are likely to be of greater importance but as yet no decision analysis tool addressing these issues has been evaluated by randomized trial in the advanced cancer setting [110]. Further research is required.

Several attempts at building decision-making models that include considerations of the pros and cons of therapy have been reported for lung cancer. These include health utility scores which attempt to apply numerical values between 0 and 1 to reflect the quality of life score that the patient attributes to various states of health and includes data within the model of the expected outcome for various treatment options [115–117]. The main limitation of each of these techniques is that although useful as research tools to evaluate decision-making of individuals there has been little research to date on whether using these methods improves the quality of clinical decision-making for the patient compared with standard medical consultation alone [116]. In addition, there is often conflict as to the correct data that should be entered into a model to represent outcomes such as survival, local control, and toxicity and whether these should be generalized results or local figures based upon individual clinician's data and whether clinician biases on the types of data selected make a difference to the utility analysis [117–119].

Another decision aid described for lung cancer decision making is the treatment trade-off technique [120, 121]. This provides patients with a structured description of the treatment options including the possible risks of toxicity and potential gains from additional treatment and involves the clinical picture being discussed as a trade-off. In their small pilot study, Brundage et al. [120] found that patients liked this tool as it strengthened their feelings that they had made the correct decision. It appeared to improve their understanding of the percentage benefits that different treatments conferred. However, the authors did also find that some patients continued to overestimate the benefits of more radical treatment compared to the decision aid and suggested that this warranted further examination.

57.6 End-of-life Care

The vast majority of lung cancer patients will ultimately succumb to their disease. Therefore, a lot of decision-making occurs when discussing end-of-life care. Perhaps surprisingly, treatment guidelines for end-of-life care [122] have only recently been getting the attention warranted with most treatment guidelines previously focusing on active therapy. Studies have shown that a significant proportion of terminal patients do not feel that they have been adequately informed about end-of-life information and feel that the psychosocial aspects of their situation have not been sufficiently discussed [97, 123–126].

One of the most important aspects of decision-making in end-of-life care is communication and the importance of breaking bad news in such a way that patients and relatives can absorb the information, ask questions, and speak openly about their emotions. It is normal for clinicians to feel awkward about communicating information that is likely to be received poorly by the patient. Consensus guidelines have been published on techniques that are useful in achieving these aims in ways that the patient can feel satisfied [127].

Another important aspect of end-of-life care is involving the patients' families and friends. Although many health professionals dislike discussing bad news with patients, studies have revealed that most clinicians have more trouble talking to the relatives of patients than the patients themselves [128]. Relatives reported "feeling in the way" which is of particular concern as family involvement is highly desirable in most clinical situations.

These factors influencing the communication of end-of-life issues between the clinician, the patient, and the patient's support people are profoundly important if the patient is to participate fully in the end-of-life decision-making required. Examples of issues that may need to be discussed are do not resuscitate (DNR) orders, withdrawal of active treatment, and symptom control measures. It is also important that these issues are discussed with the patient before any serious deterioration in the patient's medical condition that may limit the patient's ability to make an informed decision.

When making a decision about the form that end-of-life care will take, it is important to consider the different factors that might impact on their decision. These factors include the medical facts about the patient (i.e., stage of disease, previous treatment, current symptoms), what life factors are important to the patient (their cultural and religious beliefs, quality versus quantity of life, upcoming major life events), what support the patient has, and what the overall wishes of the patient has for their death. When discussing the issues about end-of-life care it is important to define the goals of any therapy, to prevent surprises as much as possible by keeping the patient informed about their illness's progress and setting realistic goals that the patient can understand, and to respond empathically to the patient's response to this news [122, 129].

Key Points

- Decision-making in lung cancer is highly complex and involves a large number of factors.
- Patterns of care studies suggest that variations in practice are not entirely explained by medical factors. This suggests that medical decision-making differs across different patient populations.
- To assist clinicians provide consistent advice to patients, evidence-based treatment guidelines and evidence-based decision trees have been produced and multidisciplinary clinics established.
- To assist the patient understand and retain information, decision aids such as consumer information packs and information websites, treatment trade-off interview techniques, guidelines to clinicians addressing how to better communicate with patients, and taped consultations have been developed and evaluated.
- Breaking bad news to patients should be done in a fashion whereby the patient develops a true understanding of their prognosis but at the same time feels that the person breaking the news has been empathic to their situation.

References

1. Kravitz RL, Melnikow J. Engaging patients in the medical decision making. The end is worthwhile but the means need to be more practical. *BMJ* 2001; 323:584.
2. Richardson GE, Thursfield VJ, Giles GG for the Anti-Cancer Council of Victoria Lung Cancer Study Group. Reported management of lung cancer in Victoria in 1993: comparison with best practice. *Med J Aust* 2000; 172:321.
3. Kesson E, Bucknall CE, McAlpine LG, et al. Lung cancer: management and outcome in Glasgow, 1991–1992. *Br J Cancer* 1998; 78:1391.
4. Gregor A, Thomson CS, Brewster DH, Stroner PL, Davidson J, Fergusson RJ, Milroy R on behalf of the Scottish Cancer Trials Lung Group and the Scottish Cancer Therapy Network. Management and survival of patients with lung cancer in Scotland diagnosed in 1995: results of a national population based study. *Thorax* 2001; 56:212.
5. Fry WA, Phillips JL, Menck HR. Ten-year survey of lung cancer treatment and survival in hospitals in the United States. *Cancer* 1999; 86:1867.
6. Vinod SK, Delaney GP, Bauman AE, Barton MB. Lung cancer patterns of care in south western Sydney, Australia. *Thorax* 2003; 58:690.
7. Mahmud SM, Reilly M, Comber H. Patterns of initial management of lung cancer in the Republic of Ireland: a population-based observational study. *Lung Cancer* 2003; 41:57.
8. Vinod SK, Hui AC, Esmaili N, Hensley MJ, Barton MB. Comparison of patterns of care in lung cancer in three area health services in New South Wales, Australia. *Intern Med J* 2004; 34:677.
9. Raby B, Pater J, Mackillop W. Does knowledge guide practice? Another look at the management of non-small cell lung cancer. *J Clin Oncol* 1995; 13:1904.

10. Earle CC, Neumann PJ, Gelber RD, Weinstein MC, Weeks JC. Impact of referral patterns on the use of chemotherapy for lung cancer. *J Clin Oncol* 2002; 20:1786.

11. Mackillop WJ, Dixon P, Zhou Y, et al. Variations in the management of non-small cell lung cancer in Ontario. *Radiother Oncol* 1994; 32:106.

12. Schroen AT, Detterbeck FC, Crawford R, Rivera P, Socinski MA. Beliefs among pulmonologists and thoracic surgeons in the therapeutic approach to non-small cell lung cancer. *Chest* 2000; 118:129.

13. Jennens RB, de Boer R, Irving L, DL Ball, Rosenthal MA. Differences of opinion: a survey of knowledge and bias among clinicians regarding the role of chemotherapy in metastatic non-small cell lung cancer. *Chest* 2004; 126:1985.

14. Palmer MJ, O'Sullivan B, Steele R, Mackillop WJ. Controversies in the management of non-small cell lung cancer: the results of an expert surrogate study. *Radiother Oncol* 1990; 19:17.

15. Greenberg ER, Chute CG, Stukel T, Baron JA, Freeman DH, Yates J, Korson R. Social and economic factors in the choice of lung cancer treatment. A population-based study in two rural states. *New Engl J Med* 1988; 318:612.

16. Potosky AL, Saxman S, Wallace RB, Lynch CF. Population variations in the initial treatment of non-small-cell lung cancer. *J Clin Oncol* 2004; 22:3261.

17. Ball DL, Irving LB. Are patients with lung cancer the poor relations in oncology? We must abandon the nihilistic attitude to management of lung cancer. *Med J Aust* 2000; 172:310.

18. Perez EA. Perceptions of prognosis, treatment and treatment impact on prognosis in non-small cell lung cancer. *Chest* 1998; 114:593.

19. Yung RC, Orens JB. Radicalism in therapy of lung cancer. *Lancet* 2001; 357:1306.

20. Grosclaude P, Galat JP, Mace-Lesech J, Roumagnac-Macheleard M, Mercier M, Robillard J. Differences in treatment and survival rates of non-small cell lung cancer in three regions of France. *Br J Cancer* 1995; 72:1278.

21. Janssen-Heijnen MLG, Gatta G, Forman D, Capocaccia R, Coeburgh JWW and the EUROCARE Working Group. Variation in survival of patients with lung cancer in Europe 1985–1989. *Eur J Cancer* 1998; 34:2191.

22. Earle CC, Venditti LN, Neumann PJ, Gelber RD, Weinstein MC, Potosky AL, Weeks JC. Who gets chemotherapy for metastatic lung cancer? *Chest* 2000; 117:1239.

23. Jong KE, Smith DP, Yu XQ, et al. Remoteness of residence and survival from cancer in New South Wales. *Med J Aust* 2004; 180:618.

24. Laroche C, Wells F, Coulden R, et al. Improving surgical resection rates in lung cancer. *Thorax* 1998; 53:445.

25. Priestman TJ, Bullimore JA, Godden TP, Deutsch GP. The Royal College of Radiologists' fractionation survey. *Clin Oncol* 1989; 1:39.

26. Maher EJ. The influence of national attitudes on the use of radiotherapy in advanced and metastatic cancer, with particular reference to differences between the United Kingdom and the United States of America: implications for future studies. *Int J Radiat Oncol Biol Phys* 1990; 20:1369.

27. Timothy AR, Girling DJ, Saunders MI, Macbeth F, Hoskin PJ on behalf of the participants of the second Workshop on Palliative Radiotherapy and Symptom Control. Consensus statement. Radiotherapy for inoperable lung cancer. *Clin Oncol* 2001; 13:86.

28. Choy H, Shyr Y, Cmelak AJ, Mohr PJ, Johnson DH. Patterns of practice survey for nonsmall cell lung carcinoma in the U.S. *Cancer* 2000; 88:1336.

29. Sambrook RJ, Girling DJ. A national survey of the chemotherapy regimens used to treat small cell lung cancer (SCLC) in the United Kingdom. *Br J Cancer* 2001; 84:1447.

30. Ayanian JZ, Chrischilles EA, Fletcher RH, et al. Understanding cancer treatment and outcomes: the Cancer Care Outcomes Research and Surveillance Consortium. *J Clin Oncol* 2004; 22:2992.

31. Wang KP, Haponik EF, Britt EJ, Khouri N, Erozan Y. Transbronchial needle aspiration of peripheral pulmonary nodules. *Chest* 1984; 86:819.

32. Gould M, Maclean C, Kuschner W, Rydzak C, Owens D. Accuracy of positron emission tomography for diagnosis of pulmonary nodules and mass lesions: a meta-analysis. *JAMA* 2001; 285:914.

33. Pieterman RM, von Putten JWG, Meuzelaar JJ, et al. Preoperative staging of non-small cell lung cancer with positron-emission tomography. *N Engl J Med* 2000; 343:254.

34. van Tinteren H, Hoekstra OS, Smit EF, et al. Effectiveness of positron emission tomography in the preoperative assessment of patients with suspected non-small-cell lung cancer: the PLUS multicentre randomised trial. *Lancet* 2002; 359:1388.

35. Cheran SK, Herndon JE II, Patz EF Jr. Comparison of whole-body FDG-PET to bone scan for detection of bone metastases in patients with a new diagnosis of lung cancer. *Lung Cancer* 2004; 44:317.

36. Butland RJ, Pang J, Gross ER, Woodcock AA, Geddes DM. Two, six and twelve minute walking tests in respiratory disease. *BMJ* 1982; 284:1607.

37. Bagg LR. The 12 minute walking distance: its use in the preoperative assessment of patients with bronchial carcinoma before lung resection. *Respiration* 1984; 46:342.

38. Markos J, Mullan BP, Hillman DR, et al. Preoperative assessment as a predictor of mortality and morbidity after lung resection. *Am Rev Respir Dis* 1989; 139:902.

39. Ferguson MK, Little L, Rizzo L, et al. Diffusing capacity predicts mortality after pulmonary resection. *J Thorac Cardiovasc Surg* 1988; 86:894.

40. Larsen KR, Lund JO, Svendsen UG, Milman N, Petersen BN. Prediction of post-operative cardiopulmonary function using perfusion scintigraphy in patients with bronchogenic carcinoma. *Clin Physiol* 1997; 17:257.

41. Cordiner A, De Carlo F, De Gennaro R, Pau F, Flore F. Prediction of postoperative pulmonary function following thoracic surgery for bronchial carcinoma. *Angiology* 1991; 42:985.

42. Wernly JA, DeMeester TR, Kirchner PT, Myerowitz PD, Oxford DE, Golomb HM. Clinical value of quantitative ventilation-perfusion lung scans in the surgical management of bronchogenic carcinoma. *J Thorac Cardiovasc Surg* 1980; 80:535.

43. Walsh GL, Morice RC, Putnam JB, et al. Resection of lung cancer is justified in high-risk patients selected by exercise oxygen consumption. *Ann Thorac Surg* 1994; 58:704.

44. Ribas J, Diaz O, Barbera JA, et al. Invasive exercise testing in the evaluation of patients at high risk for lung resection. *Eur Respir J* 1998; 12:1429.

45. Villani F, De Maria P, Busia A. Exercise testing as a predictor of surgical risk after pneumonectomy for bronchogenic carcinoma. *Respir Med* 2003; 97:1296.

46. Graham MV, Purdy JA, Emami B, Harms W, Bosch W, Lockett MA, Perez CA. Clinical dose-volume histogram analysis for pneumonitis after 3D treatment for non-small cell lung cancer (NSCLC). *Int J Radiat Oncol Biol Phys* 1999; 45:323.

47. Kwa SLS, Lebesque JV, Theuws JCM, et al. Radiation pneumonitis as a function of mean lung dose: an analysis of pooled data of 540 patients. *Int J Radiat Oncol Biol Phys* 1998; 42:1.

48. Hernando ML, Marks LB, Bentel GC, et al. Radiation-induced pulmonary toxicity: a dose-volume histogram analysis in 201 patients with lung cancer. *Int J Radiat Oncol Biol Phys* 2001; 51:650.

49. Tsujino K, Hirota S, Endo M, et al. Predictive value of dose-volume histogram parameters for predicting radiation pneumonitis after concurrent chemoradiation for lung cancer. *Int J Radiat Onol Biol Phys* 2003; 55:110.

50. Gridelli C, Perrone F, Gallo C, et al. Chemotherapy for elderly patients with advanced non-small-cell lung cancer: the Multicenter Italian Lung Cancer in the Elderly Study (MILES) phase II randomized trial. *J Natl Canc Inst* 2003; 95:362.

51. Scott C, Sause WT, Byhardt R, Marcial V, Pajak TF, Herskovic A, Cox JD. Recursive partitioning of 1,592 patients on four Radiation Therapy Oncology Group studies in inoperable non-small cell lung cancer. *Lung Cancer* 1997; 17(suppl 1):S59.

52. Wigren T, Kolari. A practical prognostic index for inoperable non-small cell lung cancer. *Methods Inf Med* 1994; 33:397.

53. Wigren T. Confirmation of a prognostic index for inoperable non-small cell lung cancer. *Radiother Oncol* 1997; 44:9.

54. Erkurt E, Tunali C, Erkisi. Primary therapeutic decision making in inoperable non-small cell lung cancer. *Int J Radiat Onc Biol Phys* 2000; 46:439.

55. Damhuis RAM, Schutte PR. Resection rates and postoperative mortality in 7,899 patients with lung cancer. *Eur Respir J* 1996; 9:7.

56. Ishida T, Yokoyama H, Kaneko S, Sugio K, Sugimachi K. Long-term results of operation for non-small cell lung cancer in the elderly. *Ann Thorac Surg* 1990; 50:919.

57. Sherman S, Duidot CE. The feasibility of thoracotomy for lung cancer in the elderly. *JAMA* 1987; 258:30.

58. Earle CC, Tsai JS, Gelber RD, Weinstein MC, Neumann PJ, Weeks JC. Effectiveness of chemotherapy for advanced lung cancer in the elderly: instrumental variable and propensity analysis. *J Clin Oncol* 2001; 19:1064.

59. Gridelli C, Ardizzoni A, Le Chavalier T, et al. Treatment of advanced non-small-cell lung cancer patients with ECOG performance status 2: results of a European Experts Panel. *Ann Oncol* 2004; 15:419.

60. Begg CB, Cohen JL, Ellerton J. Are the elderly predisposed to toxicity from cancer chemotherapy? An investigation using data from the Eastern Cooperative Oncology Group. *Cancer Clin Trials* 1980; 3:369.

61. Chen H, Cantor A, Meyer J, et al. Can older patients tolerate chemotherapy? A prospective pilot study. *Cancer* 2003; 97:1107.

62. Shepherd FA, Amdemichael E, Evans WK, Chalvardjian P, Hogg-Johnson S, Coates R, Paul K. Treatment of small cell lung cancer in the elderly. *J Am Geriatr Soc* 1994; 42:64.

63. Brown JS, Eraut D, Trask C, Davison AG, Age and the treatment of lung cancer. *Thorax* 1996; 51:564.

64. Rose JH, O'Toole EE, Dawson NV, et al. Age differences in care practices and outcomes for hospitalized patients with cancer. *J Am Geriatr Soc* 2000; 48:S25.

65. Delaney G, Barton M, Jacob S, Jalaludin B. A model for decision making for the use of radiotherapy in lung cancer. *Lancet Oncol* 2003; 4:120.

66. Tyldesley S, Zhang-Salomans J, Groome P. Association between age and the utilization of radiotherapy in Ontario. *Int J Radiat Biol Phys* 2000; 47:469.

67. Mackillop WJ, O'Sullivan B, Ward GK. Non-small lung cancer: how oncologists want to be treated. *Int J Radiat Oncol Biol Phys* 1987; 13:929.

68. Harpole LH, Kelley MJ, Schreiber G, Toloza EM, Kolimaga J, McCrory DC. Assessment of the scope and quality of clinical practice guidelines in lung cancer. *Chest* 2003; 123:7S.

69. Evans WK, Newman T, Graham I, Rusthoven JJ, Logan D, Shepherd FA, Chamberlain D. Lung cancer practice guidelines: lessons learned and issues addressed by the Ontario Lung Cancer Disease Site Group. *J Clin Oncol* 1997; 15:3049.

70. MacManus MP, Hicks RJ, Matthews JP, et al. High rate of detection of unsuspected distant metastases by PET in apparent stage III non-small-cell lung cancer: implications for radical radiation therapy. *Int J Radiat Oncol Biol Phys* 2001; 50:287.

71. Browman GP. Improving clinical practice guidelines for the 21st century. Attitudinal barriers and not technology are the main challenges. *Int J Techniques Assess Health Care.* 2000; 16:959.

72. McCusker J, Wax A, Bennett JM. Cancer patients accessions into clinical trials. A pilot investigation into some patient and physician determinants of entry. *Am J Clin Oncol* 1982; 5:227.

73. Lescoe-Long M, Long MT. Defining the utility of clinically acceptable variations in evidence-based practice guidelines for evaluation of quality improvement activities. *Evaluation Health Professions* 1999; 22:298.

74. Gunderson L. The effect of clinical practice guidelines on variations in care. *Ann Intern Med* 2000; 133:317.

75. Ellrodt AG, Connor L, Riedinger M, Weingarten S. Measuring and improving physician compliance with clinical practice guidelines. A controlled intervention trial. *Ann Intern Med* 1995; 122:277.

76. Long MJ. Clinical practice guidelines: when the tool becomes the rule. *J Evaluation Clin Pract* 2001; 7:191.

77. Macbeth F. All evidence was considered when COIN guidelines were drawn up. *BMJ* 2000; 320:1604.

78. O'Brien M, Cullen M. Guidelines must help bring us in line with European standards. *BMJ* 2000; 320:1604.

79. Ardizzoni A, Grossi F, Salvati F, Silvano G, Santi L. Common international guidelines must be developed. *BMJ* 2000; 320:379.

80. Graham ID, Evans WK, Logan D, et al. Canadian oncologists and clinical practice guidelines: a national survey of attitudes and reported use. *Oncology* 2000; 59:283.

81. Smith TJ, Hillner BE. Ensuring quality cancer care by the use of clinical practice guidelines and critical pathways. *J Clin Oncol* 2001; 19:2886.

82. Gabel M, Hilton NE, Nathanson SD. Multidisciplinary breast cancer clinics: do they work? *Cancer* 1997; 79:2380.

83. Grimshaw JM, Russell IT. Effect of clinical guidelines on medical practice: a systematic review of vigorous evaluations. *Lancet* 1993; 342:1317.

84. Olivotto IA, Bajdik CD, Plenderleith IH, et al. Adjuvant systemic therapy and survival after breast cancer. *N Engl J Med* 1994; 330:805.

85. Tyldesley S, Boyd C, Schulze K, Walker H, Mackillop WJ. Estimating the need for radiotherapy for lung cancer: an evidence-based epidemiologic approach. *Int J Radiat Oncol Biol Phys* 2001; 49:973.

86. Lenhard RE Jr, Waalkes TP, Herring D. Evaluation of the clinical management of cancer patients. A pilot study. *JAMA* 1983; 250:3310.

87. Fergusson RJ, Gregor A, Dodds R, Kerr G. Management of ling cancer in South East Scotland. *Thorax* 1996; 51:569.

88. Billing JS, Wells FC. Delays in the diagnosis and surgical treatment of lung cancer. *Thorax* 1996; 51:903.

89. Alberts M, Bepler G, Hazelton T, Ruckdeschel JC, Williams JH Jr. Practice organization. *Chest* 2003; 123:332S.

90. Jefford M, Tattersall MHN. Informing and involving cancer patients in their own care. *Lancet Oncol* 2002; 3:629.

91. Mazur DJ, Hickam DH. Patients' and physicians' interpretations of graphic data displays. *Med Decis Making* 1993; 13:59.

92. Jenkins V, Fallowfield L, Saul J. Information needs of patients with cancer: results from a large study in UK cancer centres. *Br J Cancer* 2001; 84:48.

93. Degner LF, Kristjanson LJ, Bowman D, et al. Information needs and decisional preferences in women with breast cancer. *JAMA* 1997; 277:1485.

94. Weeks JC, Cook EF, O'Day SJ, et al. Relationship between cancer patients' predictions of prognosis and their treatment preferences. *JAMA* 1998; 279:1709.

95. Smith TJ, Swisher K. Telling the truth about terminal cancer. *JAMA* 1998; 279:1746.

96. Cassell EJ. The nature of suffering and the goals of medicine. *N Engl J Med* 1982; 27(suppl 3):S110.

97. Lamont E, Christakis N. Prognostic disclosure to patients with cancer near the end of life. *Ann Intern Med* 2001; 134:1196.

98. GIVIO (Interdisciplinary Group for Cancer Care Evaluation) Italy. What doctors tell patients with breast cancer about diagnosis and treatment: findings from a study in general hospitals. *Br J Cancer* 1986; 54:319.

99. Gattellari M, Voigt KJ, Butow PN, Tattersall MH. When the treatment goal is not cure: are cancer patients equipped to make informed decisions? *J Clin Oncol* 2002; 20:503.

100. Tattersall MH, Gatellari M, Voigt K, Butow PN. When the treatment goal is not cure: are patients informed adequately? *Support Care Cancer* 2002; 10:314.

101. Hagerty RG, Butow PN, Ellis PA, et al. Cancer patient preferences for communication of prognosis in the metastatic setting. *J Clin Oncol* 2004; 22:1721.

102. Schwartz I, Woloshin S, Black W, Welch H. The role of numeracy in understanding the benefit of screening mammography. *Ann Intern Med* 1997; 127:966.

103. Lloyd A, Hayes P, Bell P, Naylor A. The role of risk and benefit perception in informed consent for surgery. *Med Decis Making* 2001; 21:141.

104. Tattersall MH, Butow PN. Consultation audio tapes: an underused cancer patient information aid and clinical research tool. *Lancet Oncol* 2002; 3:431.

105. Thomas R, Daly M, Perryman B, Stockton D. Forewarned is forearmed: benefits of preparatory information on video cassette for patients receiving chemotherapy or radiotherapy: a randomised trial. *Eur J Cancer* 2000; 36:1536.

106. Fiset V, O'Connor AM, Evans W, et al. Development and evaluation of a decision aid for patients with stage IV non-small cell lung cancer. *Health Expect* 2000; 3:125.

107. Charnock D, Shepperd S, Needham G, Gann R. DISCERN: an instrument for judging the quality of written consumer health information on treatment choices. *J Epidemiol Community Health* 1999; 53:105.

108. Brown RF, Butow PN, Boyer MJ, Tattersall MH. Promoting patient participation in the cancer consultation: evaluation of a prompt sheet and coaching in question-asking. *Br J Cancer* 1999; 80:242.

109. Zhang AY, Siminoff LA. The role of the family in treatment decision making by patients with cancer. *Oncol Nurs Forum* 2003; 30:1022.

110. Leighl NB, Butow PN, Tattersall MHN. Treatment decision aids in advanced cancer: when the goal is not cure and the answer is not clear. *J Clin Oncol* 2004; 22:1759.

111. Whelan T, Sawka C, Levine M, Gafni A, Reyno L, Willan A, Julian J, Dent S, Abu-Zahra H, Chouinard E, Tozer R, Pritchard K, Bodendorfer I. Helping patients make informed choices: a randomized trial of a decision aid for adjuvant chemotherapy in lymph-node negative breast cancer. *J Natl Cancer Inst* 2003; 95:581.

112. Whelan T, Levine M, Willan A, Gafni A, Sanders K, Mirsky D, Chambers S, O'Brien MA, Reid S, Dubois S. Effect of a decision aid on knowledge and treatment decision making for breast cancer surgery: a randomised trial. *JAMA* 2004; 292:435.

113. Ravdin PM, Siminoff L, Hewlett J, et al. Evaluation of impact of communication tool generated by the computer program Adjuvant! on patients with early breast cancer and their doctors (abstract 119). *Proc Am Soc Clin Oncol* 2001; 20:31a.

114. De Laurentiis M, De Placido S, Bianco AP, Clark GM, Ravdin PM. A prognostic model that makes quantitative estimates of probability of relapse for breast cancer patients. *Clin Cancer Res* 1999; 5:4133.

115. Torrance G, Thomas W, Sacket D. A utility maximization model for the evaluation of health programs. *Health Serv Res* 1972; 7:118.

116. Elwyn G, Edwards A, Eccles M, Rovner D. Decision analysis in patient care. *Lancet* 2001; 358:571.

117. Dowie J, Wildman M. Choosing the surgical mortality threshold for high risk patients with stage Ia non-small cell lung cancer: insight from decision analysis. *Thorax* 2002; 57:7.

118. Macbeth F. Decision analysis in NSCLC. *Thorax* 2002; 57:919.

119. Treasure T. Whose lung is it anyway? *Thorax* 2002; 57:3.

120. Brundage MD, Feldman-Stewart D, Cosby R, Gregg R, Dixon P, Youssef Y, Davies D, Mackillop WJ. Phase I study of a decision aid for patients with locally advanced non-small-cell lung cancer. *J Clin Oncol* 2001; 19:1326.

121. Brundage MD, Davidson JR, Mackillop WJ, Feldman-Stewart D, Groome P. Using a treatment trade-off method to elicit preferences for the treatment of locally advanced non-small-cell lung cancer. *Med Decis Making* 1998; 18:256.

122. Griffin JP, Nelson JE, Koch KA, Niell HB, Ackerman TF, Thompson M, Cole FH Jr. End-of-life care in patients with lung cancer. *Chest* 2003; 123:312S.

123. Silveira MJ, DiPiero A, Gerrity MS, Feudtner C. Patients' knowledge of options at the end of life: ignorance in the face of death. *JAMA* 2000; 132:825.

124. Maguire P. Improving communication with cancer patients. *Eur J Cancer* 1999; 35:1415.

125. Curtis JR, Wenrich MD, Carline JD, Shannon SE, Ambrozy DM, Ramsey PG. Patients' perspectives on physician skill in end-of-life care. Differences between patients with COPD, cancer and AIDS. *Chest* 2002; 122:356.

126. Gore JM, Brophy CJ, Greenstone MA. How well do we care for patients with endstage chronic obstructive pulmonary disease (COPD)? A comparison of palliative care and quality of life in COPD and lung cancer. *Thorax* 2000; 55:1000.

127. Girgis A, Sanson-Fisher RW. Breaking bad news: consensus guidelines for medical practitioners. *J Clin Oncol* 1995; 13:2499.

128. Speice J, Harkness J, Laneri R, et al. Involving family members in cancer care: focus group considerations of patients and oncological providers. *Psychooncology* 2000; 9:101.

129. von Roenn JH, von Gunten CF. Setting goals to maintain hope. *J Clin Oncol* 2003; 21:570.

Subject Index